Handbook of Pain and Palliative Care

Rhonda J. Moore

Editor

Handbook of Pain and Palliative Care

Biobehavioral Approaches for the Life Course

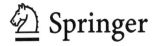 Springer

Editor
Rhonda J. Moore
Department of Health and Human Services
Rockville, MD, USA
moorer2001uk@yahoo.co.uk

ISBN 978-1-4419-1650-1   e-ISBN 978-1-4419-1651-8
DOI 10.1007/978-1-4419-1651-8
Springer New York Dordrecht Heidelberg London

Library of Congress Control Number: 2011943748

Printed on acid-free paper

Springer is part of Springer Science+Business Media (www.springer.com)

*This book is dedicated first and foremost
to the glory of God, the most high for his love, guidance,
refuge, faithfulness, strength, and many blessings.*

*Through him all things are possible. He is eternal and just.
May he continue to bless us and supply all our needs.*

Foreword

"It is easier to find men who will volunteer to die than to find those who are willing to endure pain with patience." *Julius Caesar 75 BCE*

"Pain is inevitable. Suffering is optional." *Unknown*

In his Foreword to the first edition of *Pain and the Neurosurgeon* in 1955, Sir Geoffrey Jefferson noted: "This book is concerned with pain, not as a warning, but as an enemy to be defeated." Wilder Penfield addressed this further in his Foreword to the 1969 edition of this classic: "The problem is vastly complicated by the fact that the enemy presents himself with devilish guile behind so many masks." He was referring to the multiplicity of human afflictions that result in pain and suffering; concepts that can be agonizingly vague and subjectively defined. Penfield describes the physician's dilemma as "running through quicksand" in determining whether the patient's pain complaints are organic, functional, or a subtle combination of both.

A short list of acute and intractable chronic pain patterns includes phantom limb pain, arthritis, angina, cancer pain, the many types of neuralgia, fibromyalgia, multiple classifications of headache, and posttraumatic and postoperative pain. Renewed interest in the heterogeneity, neuroplasticity, and neurocognitive complexity of the human brain promises rewards that can lead to new horizons for understanding these human sensations beyond our ability to conceptualize at the present time. A new lexicon, reflected in such terms as neuroanthropology, cognitive neurobiology, and culture-gene-evolutionary theory, is rapidly developing.

This publication encompasses every aspect of these areas of interest at the highest levels of expertise and promises to be a basic source of information for years to come. Otfrid Foerster, Penfield, Jefferson, Leriche, Sweet, and an esteemed list of others devoted their professional lives attempting to decipher the elusive features of pain sensory mechanisms in humans and to confront the difficulties inherent in devising methods of treatment. Also, for centuries, suffering and pain have been masterfully portrayed in music, literature, and art. Throughout history, scientists and creative artists alike, devoted to the further elucidation of these universal human sensations and emotions, are entranced and probably incredulous of the introduction of the disciplines of neuroanthropology and neuropsychology as enhancements to the neurosciences. With this added perspective to neuroanatomy, neuroendocrinology, physiology, psychiatry, and neuropathology we may be able to further explore the physical and even the transcendental essence of pain in many of its ramifications in the 21st century and beyond. An entire new world of neuroscience, interpersonal neurobiology, is also emerging to further unravel the Gordian knot of our limited understanding of "feelings, pain, and suffering" along with humanity's varying and unpredictable responses thereof. We are witnessing a healthy skepticism of the so-called established markers and evidence-based facts and standards in all of these matters. Questioning "whose evidence and on what basis were their conclusions drawn?" is a welcomed pervading theme throughout.

Any review of the completeness of the gamut of topics in the chapter headings in this volume, along with the stature of their authors and editors reflects a profound new evolutionary approach for the evaluation of pain in its innumerable forms and in a vast new multicentric universe of modalities for palliation.

Richard M. Hirshberg, M.D., FACS

White, J.C., Sweet, W.H., Pain and the Neurosurgeon: A Forty Year Experience, 1969, 2nd Edition, Charles C. Thomas.

Preface

Chronic pain is a major cause of distress, disability, loss of work, and quality of life. A World Health Organization (WHO) cross-continental survey, conducted in 26,000 primary care patients in fifteen centers in Asia, Africa, Europe, and the Americas, indicated that one in five adults suffers from chronic pain (range, 6–33%) (Verhaak et al. 1998; Smith et al. 2011; Power et al. 2007). More than 116 million Americans struggle with chronic pain each year, and associated medical charges and lost productivity cost the nation as much as $635 billion annually (Relieving Pain in 43 America: A Blueprint for Transforming Prevention, Care, Education, and Research. IOM Report. The National Academies Press 2011). About 15–20% of children experience at least one episode of chronic pain. Moreover, despite major advances many chronic pain patients still needlessly suffer due to inadequate assessment, management, and treatment.

New paradigms for chronic pain management and symptom control have recently emerged. These studies have begun to take a life course approach to understand the risks, onset and progression of health and disease based on biological, behavioral, psychosocial, spiritual/existential, and environmental processes that can affect the course and development of illness and disease (Power et al. 2007; Kuh and Ben-Shlomo 1997). The study of life course influences on chronic pain states is still in its infancy (Pang et al. 2010). Nevertheless, this new paradigm emphasizes enhanced biobehavioral pain and symptom assessment and management, improved communication among clinicians, patients, and caregivers, an holistic approach to care including the "context" of care, the integration of psychosocial, narrative, anthropological, and spiritual approaches to pain management and symptom control, and increased insight into the underlying biobehavioral mechanisms of pain.

This book is designed as the beginning of a journey and a conversation about life course perspectives on chronic pain that will be refined over time, and expanded as this wonderful field evolves. It is our belief that this changing paradigm can lead to a broader *and* better understanding of chronic pain conditions, interventions, and treatments that will result in improved pain control and palliative care.

The broad aim of this edited volume is to take a multidisciplinary, biobehavioral, and life course (where applicable) approach to understanding chronic pain. By way of introduction, the contributing authors review biopsychosocial approaches to understanding chronic pain and disability. The second set of chapters describe issues related to communication and pain. The next set of chapters discuss pain and palliative care assessment. The fourth set of chapters highlight biobehavioral approaches to understanding common pain conditions, including pain in pediatric patients, pain in the older person, pain after traumatic brain injury (TBI), pain in the battlefield injured, pain in whiplash associated disorder (WAD), chronic low back pain, and adult cancer-related pain. The subsequent set describe biobehavioral mechanisms associated with chronic pain. These include stress and chronic pain, the biobehavior of hope, temporomandibular disorder and its relationship to fibromyalgia, and pain imaging. The sixth set review interventions for chronic pain including evidence-based pharmaco-therapy's for chronic pain, chronic pain and opioids, nerve block, trigger points and intrathecal therapies for chronic pain, neurosurgical interventions, and rehabilitation treatments for chronic musculoskeletal pain. The next set address broader issues in chronic pain management. These include psychosocial issues associated with chronic pain, spiritual dimensions of chronic pain and suffering, contributions from the humanities and social sciences in terms of understanding the chronic pain experience. The eighth set highlight ethical issues in pain and palliative care. These include disparities in pain management and palliative care, the delineation and explication of pallia-tive options of a last resort, and recognition and resolution of ethical barriers to palliative care. The final chapter provides one endpoint and a framework for how healthcare reform can improve access to quality pain and palliative care services.

The collaborators for this project are from diverse cultural and biomedical settings, including the UK, USA, Italy, England, Singapore, Canada, Australia, and Norway. The expertise in this volume spans the fields of clinical medicine, neuroscience, neurosurgery, literature, anthropology, art, neuro-anatomy, pediatrics, gerontology, pain imaging, health disparities, transportation, rehabilitation, palliative medicine, philanthropy, the medical humanities, oncology, physiology, anesthesiology, pharmacology, genetics, stress management, psychology, dentistry, complementary and alternative medicine, spiritual care, nursing, pain policy, and clinical ethics. While highly multidisciplinary, our collaborators have explored the evidence base for chronic pain and palliative care in their individual professional areas and each has provided valuable insights which we, and they, hope will result in improved pain control and palliative care (Blank et al. 2007).

Rockville, MD, USA   Rhonda J. Moore

References

Blank, A. E., O'Mahony, S., & Selwyn, A. (2007). *Choices in palliative care: Issues in health care delivery.* New York: Springer.

Kuh, D., & Ben-Shlomo, Y. (1997). *A life course approach to chronic disease epidemiology.* Oxford: Oxford University Press.

Pang, D., Jones, G. T., Power, C., & MacFarlane, G. J. (2010). Influence of childhood behaviour on the reporting of chronic widespread pain in adulthood: Results from the 1958 British Birth Cohort Study. *Rheumatology, 49,* 1882–1888.

Power, C., Atherton, K., Strachan, D. P., Shepherd, P., Davis, E. A. et al. (2007). Life-course influences on health in British adults: Effects of socio-economic position in childhood and adulthood. *International Journal of Epidemiology, 36,* 532–539.

Relieving Pain in America: A Blueprint for Transforming Prevention, Care, Education, and Research. IOM Report. The National Academies Press, 2011.

Smith BH, Elliott AM, Chambers WA, Smith WC, Hannaford PC, Penny K. (2011). The impact of chronic pain in the community. *Fam. Pract. 18,* 292–299.

Verhaak PF, Kerssens JJ, Dekker J, Sorbi MJ, Bensing JM. (1998). Prevalence of chronic benign pain disorder among adults: a review of the literature. *Pain. 37,* 215–222.

Acknowledgements

At times our own light goes out and is rekindled by a spark from another person. Each of us has cause to think with deep gratitude of those who have lighted the flame within us.

Albert Schweitzer (14 January 1875 – 4 September 1965)

A thankful heart is not only the greatest virtue, but the parent of all the other virtues. [Lat., Gratus animus est una virtus non solum maxima, sed etiam mater virtutum onmium reliquarum.]

Cicero, Roman orator and philosopher (106–43 bc)

The beginning and completion of any edited volume is never an individual task. Others always help along the way. At this time I thank those individuals who were supportive of this edited volume. I begin by thanking my collaborators for their enthusiasm, commitment, and support of this project. This volume could not have been completed without your insight, intelligence, generosity, and the wisdom of your words. I thank Janice Stern, Bill Tucker, Kathryn Hiler, and Lesley Poliner of the editorial offices of the Springer Publishing House in New York. I also thank Greetal Carolyn Jayananda and Bactavatchalane Gokulnathan of SPi Content Solutions - SPi Global (India) for their insight, assistance, and support of this edited volume. Their encouragement, support, and patience helped to make this dream a reality.

I am trained as a cultural and medical anthropologist and the works of David Spiegel, MD (Stanford Medical School), Bernard Siegel, PhD (Stanford University, deceased), Renato Rosaldo, PhD (New York University), Howard Spiro, MD (Yale University School of Medicine), Arthur Kleinman, MD (Harvard Medical School), Vicktor Emil Frankel, MD, PhD (University of Vienna, Austria, deceased), and David Morris (University of Virginia) have all served as inspiration for my ideas and clarified my thinking on this subject matter, even as I take full responsibility for what has been written.

I am also indebted to the encouraging words and unfailing loving kindness of my colleagues, friends, and family. I thank Richard Hirshberg, MD (Houston, TX) for his unfailing kindness, care, support, friendship, and intellectually inspiring conversations. I thank my mum, Juanita Moore, for her great sense of humor, perseverance, and encouragement. I thank the following individuals for their friendship and kind support of this intellectual endeavor: Dorota Doherty, PhD (Perth, Australia); Gloria Valentine (San Francisco, California); Pat Norfleet (Houston, TX); Karen Walters, DDS (Houston, TX); Mary Carter (Houston, TX); Alan Block (Bethesda, MD); Fran Kleinhenz (Kensington, MD); C. Mike Kerwin, PhD (Midlothian, VA); Judi Ziegler (Silver Spring, MD), Ralph Zinner, MD (The University of Texas MD Anderson Cancer Center); James Alexander (Bowie,

MD); Captain Philip Budashewitz (USPHS, DHHS, HRSA); Captain Betty Chern-Hughes, MS, CNM (USPHS, DHHS, Dallas, Texas); Robert Scholle, MA (Fairfax, Virginia); Vanessa White, MPH (Washington, DC); Jim Hallenbeck, MD (Stanford Medical School); Dr. Marco Montoya (Austin, TX); Captain Leslie Cooper PhD, MPH (USPHS, NCRR-NIH); Cathy X. Ge, OMD (Rockville, MD); James Yates (Washington, DC), Sister Veronica Kerwin (Garrett Park, MD); and Reverend Monsignor Robert Cary Hill (Garrett Park, MD). I thank my dear and wonderful friends Jean Wong, RN (Bethesda, MD) and Lee O. Carter Jr. (Houston, TX) for their unfailing support, love, and care all these years. Finally, I thank my husband, Christopher Schoppet, for his love, faith, prayers, and generosity. Please know that I am grateful to each of you for your friendship, kindness, prayers, and care at this time, and through the years.

Rockville, MD, USA   Rhonda J. Moore

Contents

1 **Biopsychosocial Approaches to Understanding Chronic
Pain and Disability** 1
Robert J. Gatchel, Robbie Haggard, Christina Thomas,
and Krista J. Howard

Part I Communication and Pain

2 **Pain and Intercultural Communication** 19
James Hallenbeck

3 **Truth Telling and Palliative Care** 35
Lidia Schapira and David P. Steensma

4 **Communication and Palliative Care: E-Health Interventions
and Pain Management** 43
Gary L. Kreps

5 **Educating Patients and Caregivers About Pain Management:
What Clinicians Need to Know** 53
Micke Brown, Amanda Crowe, and Stefanie Cousins

Part II Assessment

6 **Pain Assessment Tools in Palliative Cancer Care** 71
Marianne Jensen Hjermstad, Dagny Faxvaag Haugen, Michael I. Bennett,
and Stein Kaasa

7 **Quality Indicators for Pain in Palliative Care** 95
Sydney Dy and Hsien Seow

8 **Palliative Care Clinical Trials: Generalizability and Applicability
in Hospice and Palliative Care Practice** 109
David C. Currow and Amy P. Abernethy

9   **Dynamic Pain Assessment: An Application of Clinical Infometrics
    to Personalized Pain Treatment and Management** 121
    Chih-Hung Chang

10 **Assessing Pain and Unmet Need in Patients with Advanced Dementia:
    The Role of the Serial Trial Intervention (STI)** 131
    Christine R. Kovach

Part III   Common Pain Conditions

11 **Pediatric Chronic Pain** 147
    Thomas R. Vetter

12 **Pain in the Older Person** 169
    Bill H. McCarberg and B. Eliot Cole

13 **Pain After Traumatic Brain Injury** 177
    Jason K. Ough and Devi E. Nampiaparampil

14 **Pain in the Battlefield Injured** 195
    Anthony Dragovich and Steven P. Cohen

15 **Pain, Whiplash Disorder and Traffic Safety** 213
    Michele Sterling

16 **Chronic Low Back Pain** 231
    Stephen May

17 **Adult Cancer-Related Pain** 247
    Sean Ransom, Timothy P. Pearman, Errol Philip, and Dominique Anwar

Part IV   Mechanisms

18 **Neuroanatomy of Pain and Pain Pathways** 273
    Elie D. Al-Chaer

19 **Acute to Chronic Pain: Transition in the Post-Surgical Patient** 295
    Roland T. Short III and Thomas R. Vetter

20 **Pain and the Placebo/Nocebo Effect** 331
    Antonella Pollo and Fabrizio Benedetti

21 **Sex Differences in Pain Across the Life Course** 347
    Edmund Keogh

22 **Stress and Pain** 367
    Catherine M. Stoney

23 **Hope in the Context of Pain and Palliative Care** 383
    Richard T. Penson, Lynette Su-Mien Ngo, and Gillianne Lai

24 **Temporomandibular Disorders and its Relationship with Fibromyalgia** 399
    Ana Mirian Velly, Hong Chen, João R. Ferreira, and James R. Fricton

25 **Phantom Limb Pain** 417
    Jens Foell and Herta Flor

26 **Pharmacogenetics of Pain: The Future of Personalized Medicine**.............................. 431
Lynn R. Webster

27 **Pain Imaging**.. 439
Magdalena R. Naylor, David A. Seminowicz, Tamara J. Somers,
and Francis J. Keefe

Part V   Interventions

28 **Evidence-Based Pharmacotherapy of Chronic Pain**... 471
Howard S. Smith, Sukdeb Datta, and Laxmaiah Manchikanti

29 **Chronic Pain and Opioids**... 497
Regina P. Szucs-Reed and Rollin M. Gallagher

30 **Nerve Blocks, Trigger Points, and Intrathecal Therapy for Chronic Pain**.............. 525
Zirong Zhao and Doris K. Cope

31 **Neurosurgical Interventions for the Control of Chronic Pain Conditions**................. 565
Brittany L. Adler, Mark Yarchoan, and John R. Adler Jr.

32 **Rehabilitation Treatments for Chronic Musculoskeletal Pain**...................... 583
Nalini Sehgal, Frank Falco, Akil Benjamin, Jimmy Henry,
Youssef Josephson, and Laxmaiah Manchikanti

**Part VI   Psychosocial, Complementary and Alternative (CAM) and Spiritual
Approaches for the Control of Symptoms**

33 **Pain, Depression, and Anxiety in Cancer**... 615
Kristine A. Donovan, Lora M.A. Thompson, and Paul B. Jacobsen

34 **Support Groups for Chronic Pain**... 639
Penney Cowan

35 **CAM in Chronic Pain and Palliative Care**.. 649
Jean S. Kutner and Marlaine C. Smith

36 **Spiritual Dimensions of Pain and Suffering**.. 697
Amy Wachholtz and Suzana Makowski

Part VII   Perspectives on Pain from the Humanities and Social Sciences

37 **Suffering, Hope, and Healing**.. 717
Jack Coulehan

38 **Narrative and Pain: Towards an Integrative Model**...................................... 733
David B. Morris

39 **Representations of the Body in Pain: Anthropological Approaches**.......................... 753
Nora L. Jones

40 **The Art of Pain: The Patient's Perspective of Chronic Pain**....................... 763
Yvonne Palermo

Part VIII   Ethical Issues and Future Directions

41   Disparities in Pain Management and Palliative Care... 795
Carmen R. Green

42   The Delineation and Explication of Palliative Options of Last Resort 809
Ben A. Rich

43   Recognition and Resolution of Ethical Barriers to Palliative Care Research 825
Perry G. Fine

**44   How Health Care Reform Can Improve Access to Quality Pain
and Palliative Care Services**... 839
Amber B. Jones and Diane E. Meier

Index... 849

Contributors

Amy P. Abernethy, MD is an Associate Professor in the Division of Medical Oncology at Duke University School of Medicine and School of Nursing, Director of the Duke Cancer Care Research Program, and Medical Director of Oncology Quality, Outcomes, and Patient-centered Care in Duke University Health System. Dr. Abernethy founded and directs Duke Cancer Care Research Program (DCCRP), which conducts a diverse portfolio of studies focused on improving the symptoms and quality of life of cancer patients at all stages of disease and survivorship.

Brittany B. Adler, MD is a medical student at the Case Western Reserve University School of Medicine.

John R. Adler Jr., MD is a neurosurgeon, the Dorothy and Thye King Chan Endowed Professor of Neurosurgery at the Stanford University School of Medicine and Vice Chair for Innovation and Technology in the Department of Neurosurgery at the Stanford University School of Medicine. Clinically, Dr. Adler specializes in the treatment of brain tumors, spinal tumors, and trigeminal neuralgia. Dr. Adler's primary area of academic interest is the development of noninvasive computer controlled tools for neurosurgery. Dr. Adler is a pioneer in the field of radiosurgery and the inventor of the CyberKnife Radiosurgical System. By virtue of such he is widely acknowledged as the father of the rapidly emerging field of image-guided irradiation. In the fields of surgery, medical imaging, and therapeutic radiation, Dr. Adler holds nine United States patents and has authored more than 180 peer-reviewed publications and book chapters.

Elie Al-Chaer, JD, PhD is a Professor of Pediatrics, Internal Medicine – Gastroenterology, Neurobiology and Developmental Sciences, and the Director of the Center for Pain Research at the University of Arkansas for Medical Sciences in the USA. He is also a lawyer and member of the bar in Texas and the District of Columbia. His translational scientific research is centered on the sex differences, hormonal regulation, and neural processing of pain. His research also examines the mechanisms involved in controlling and downregulating chronic pain symptoms in adults, associated with long-term neuroplastic, endocrine, and immunal changes. He is well-published and regularly invited to speak at international symposia on the mechanisms of pain and functional disorders.

Dominque Anwar, MD is an Associate Professor of Medicine and Senior Director of the Palliative Care Program, Section of Internal Medicine and Geriatrics at the Tulane University School of Medicine.

Fabrizio Benedetti, MD is a Professor of Clinical and Applied Physiology at the University of Turin Medical School, Consultant for the Placebo Project at the National Institute of Health in Bethesda (USA), and Member of the Mind-Brain-Behavior Initiative at Harvard University in

Cambridge (USA). His current scientific interests are the placebo effect across diseases, pain in dementia, and intraoperative neurophysiology for mapping the human brain.

Akil Benjamin, DO is a Pain Medicine Fellow, at the Temple University Hospital, Philadelphia, PA.

Michael I. Bennett, MD, FRCP is a Professor at the International Observatory on end-of-life care, School of Health and Medicine, Lancaster, UK.

Micke Brown, BSN, RN is the Director of Communications at the American Pain Foundation. She also served as Past President of the American Society for Pain Management Nursing.

Chih-Hung Chang, PhD is an Associate Professor of Medicine, and Director, Methodology and Infometrics Section, Buehler Center on Aging, Health & Society at the Feinberg School of Medicine, Northwestern University. He also serves as an adjunct Professor, Graduate Institute of Biostatistics, China Medical University, Taiwan.

Hong Chen, DDS, MS is a clinical Assistant Professor at the University of North Carolina School of Dentistry Center for Neurosensory Disorders. She is a Fellow of the American Academy of Orofacial Pain. Her research focuses on pathophysiology, diagnosis, and management of complex persistent orofacial pain conditions. Dr. Chen received her advanced training in Temporomandibular Disorders and Orofacial Pain at the University of Minnesota, MN, USA.

Steven P. Cohen, MD is a Professor at the Uniformed Services University of the Health Sciences and an Associate Professor at Johns Hopkins School of Medicine. Dr. Cohen is a Colonel in the Army Reserve, and serves as Chief, Anesthesia and Operative Services, at the 48th Combat Support Hospital at Fort Meade, and the Director of Chronic Pain Research at Walter Reed Army Medical Center. His major contributions include pioneering the development of lateral branch radiofrequency denervation for treating sacroiliac joint pain, inventing the intravenous ketamine test, and performing the first studies evaluating the local administration of tumor necrosis factor inhibitors. His recent work has focused on improving pain care in wounded soldiers. These include outcome data from the first pain clinic ever established in a combat zone, and conducting epidemiological studies evaluating a wide range of pain conditions, some of which have received international acclaim.

B. Eliot Cole, MD, MPA, FAPA, CPE is a Medical Director for the Shoals Hospital Senior Care Center in Muscle Shoals, AL.

Doris K. Cope, MD is the Professor and Vice Chairman of Pain Medicine, Department of Anesthesiology, University of Pittsburgh School of Medicine and Director, Interprofessional Program on Pain Research, Education and Health Care at the University of Pittsburgh Schools of Health Sciences. Dr. Cope is a Board examiner in Anesthesiology and Pain Medicine. Dr. Cope has published numerous scientific and historical articles, and is the editor-in-chief of the *Bulletin of Anesthesia History* and Assistant Editor of the *American Society of Anesthesiologists Newsletter.*

Jack Coulehan, MD, MPH is an Emeritus Professor of Preventive Medicine and Senior Fellow of the Center for Medical Humanities, Compassionate Care, and Bioethics at Stony Brook University. He has written or edited numerous books, including *Medicine Stone, Chekhov's Doctors, The Medical Interview: Mastering Skills for Clinical Practice*, and *Primary Care: More Poems of Physicians.*

Stefanie Cousins, MPH has more than 15 years of demonstrated success in broadcast media and communications, including more than 5 years of experience in health marketing and communications. She also has 10 years of experience as an award-winning news and documentary producer for ABC News, PBS, and *The New York Times*. Ms. Cousins' projects focus on HIV/AIDS, harm reduction, chronic disease prevention, pain and pain management, and reproductive health.

Penney Cowan is founder and executive director of the American Chronic Pain Association (ACPA). She herself is a person with chronic pain and established the ACPA in 1980 to help others living with the condition. The ACPA provides peer support and education in pain management skills to people with pain and their families. The ACPA also works to build awareness about chronic pain among professionals, decision makers, and the public. Over the past 30 years, Cowan has been an advocate and consumer representative for pain issues. She was awarded the Jefferson Medal for Outstanding Citizen by the Institute for Public Service, Washington, and is listed in Who's Who in America, 24th edition. She is the author of Patient or Person, Living With Chronic Pain, published by Gardner Press. In addition, she has written all manuals and materials used by the ACPA. Cowan began the Partners for Understanding Pain campaign in 2002 in an attempt to raise awareness about the need to better understand, asses, and treat pain. There are more than 80 partner organizations. The campaign, under the direction of the ACPA, successfully established September as Pain Awareness Month.

Amanda Crowe, MA, MPH is a contributing writer or editor for a number of online health toolkits, newsletters, and print publications. She has nearly 15 years practical expertise in strategic health communications, material and program development, media advocacy, healthcare alliance and coalition building, health messaging, and market research. Ms. Crowe's interests are in pain and pain management, infectious diseases, oncology, cardiovascular diseases, diabetes, access to care, and preventive medicine.

David C. Currow, MD is a Professor, Discipline of Palliative and Supportive Services, Flinders University, Flinders Centre for Clinical Change, Flinders University, Adelaide, Australia.

Sukdeb Datta, MD is a Diplomat, American Board of Anesthesiology and Diplomat, American Board of Pain Medicine. He has additionally acquired the Subspecialty Certification in Pain Management awarded by the joint Boards of the American Board of Anesthesiology, American Board of Physical Medicine and Rehabilitation and the American Board of Psychiatry and Neurology. He is also certified as FIPP (Fellow of Interventional Pain Practice) and the American Board of Interventional Pain Physicians as a DABIPP (Diplomat, American Board of Interventional Pain Practice). He has served as the Director, Interventional Pain Management Program, Vanderbilt University, Nashville, and Associate Professor, Department of Anesthesiology, Vanderbilt University Medical School, Nashville, TN, USA. He also served as the Division Chief, Pain Medicine Division within the Department of Anesthesiology and the Program Director of the Multidisciplinary Pain Medicine Fellowship at Vanderbilt University. He has an active interest in translational pain research and his past funded research grant looked at new treatments based on potential mechanisms of neuropathic pain. His research focused on detailed anatomic studies of different markers of neuropathic pain in the SDH like morphine, cholecystokinin, neurokinin, and neuropeptide Y in both normal and neuropathic rats and complex modeling of clinical human neuropathic pain.

Kristine A. Donovan, PhD, MBA is Assistant Member in the Health Outcomes and Behavior and Psychosocial and Palliative Care Programs at the Moffitt Cancer Center and the Department of Oncologic Sciences at the University of South Florida College of Medicine. Dr. Donovan received her PhD in Medical (Clinical) Psychology from the University of Alabama at Birmingham and completed a postdoctoral fellowship in Behavioral Oncology at Moffitt where she was subsequently appointed to the faculty. Her research focuses on the etiology and management of side effects of cancer treatment and the identification of appropriate interventions to alleviate these symptoms and improve quality of life in cancer survivorship. Her research has been funded by the American Cancer Society and National Cancer Institute.

Anthony Dragovich, MD is the Chief of Pain Medicine at Womack Army Medical Center, Ft. Bragg North Carolina. He is an Assistant Professor of Anesthesiology at the Uniformed Services

University of the Health Sciences. His primary interest is the treatment of combat related pain conditions, specifically the transition between acute and chronic pain. His research is focused on clinical protocols and interventions to inhibit the development of chronic pain states.

Sydney Dy, MD, MSc is an Associate Professor, Health Policy and Management, Oncology, and Medicine, at Johns Hopkins, and a hospice and palliative care physician with the Harry J. Duffey Family Palliative Care and Pain Program at the Hopkins Kimmel Cancer Center. She is also researcher and educator in healthcare quality and safety, focusing on evidence-based reviews and development and evaluation of quality indicators, particularly in palliative care.

Frank Falco, MD is an Adjunct Associate Professor, Temple University Medical School, Philadelphia, Pennsylvania; Director, Pain Medicine Fellowship Program, Temple University Hospital, Philadelphia, PA; and Medical Director, Mid Atlantic Spine and Pain Physicians, Newark, Delaware and Elkton, MD.

João R. Ferreira, DDS, MS is an Temporomandibular Disorders (TMD) and Orofacial Pain Senior Fellow at the University of Minnesota, MN, USA.

Perry G. Fine, MD is a Professor of Anesthesiology at the University of Utah. He currently serves as President of the American Academy of Pain Medicine, and he is on the Board of Directors of the American Pain Foundation and on the Steering Committee of the Pain Care Coalition, Washington, DC. Dr. Fine serves as the External Strategic Advisor for Capital Hospice, Washington, DC developing sustainable models of advanced illness coordinated care in community settings, as an integrative component of comprehensive chronic care. Dr. Fine is widely published in the fields of pain management and end-of-life care. He serves on several scientific advisory boards and the editorial boards of several peer-reviewed medical journals. He is the recipient of the 2007 American Academy of Hospice and Palliative Medicine Distinguished Hospice Physician Award, and the 2008 American Pain Society John and Emma Bonica Public Service Award. In addition, in 2008, an endowed lectureship has been created in his name at West Virginia University School of Medicine (Perry G. Fine, MD Annual Lectureship in Pain and Palliative Medicine). He is the recipient of the American Academy of Pain Management's 2010 "Head and Heart" award.

Herta Flor, PhD is Full Professor at the Ruprecht-Karls-University Heidelberg and Scientific Director of the Department of Cognitive and Clinical Neuroscience at the Central Institute of Mental Health, Mannheim, Germany. Her research focuses on the role of neuronal plasticity and learning and memory in chronic pain, anxiety and mood disorders, substance abuse, and neuropsychological rehabilitation. She has received more than 48 research grants and numerous prestigious awards and has more than 480 publications.

Jens Foell, Dipl. Psych is a PhD student working in the Department of Cognitive and Clinical Neuroscience at the Central Institute of Mental Health in Mannheim, Germany. His research focuses on neuronal and behavioral correlates of body perception in chronic phantom limb pain patients and healthy controls.

James R. Fricton, DDS, MS is a Professor in the Department of Diagnostic and Surgical Sciences and Physical Medicine and Rehabilitation at the University of Minnesota. He is also a Senior Research Investigator at HealthPartners Research Foundation. He has over thirty years of experience in clinical care, research, and teaching in the field of chronic pain, orofacial pain, temporomandibular muscle and joint disorders, muscle pain, and, more recently, health informatics.

Rollin M. Gallagher, MD, MPH is the Deputy National Program Director for Pain Management, VA Central Office; Director for Pain Policy Research and Primary Care, Penn Pain Medicine; and Clinical Professor of Psychiatry and Anesthesiology, University of Pennsylvania. He is also editor-in-chief of Pain Medicine, *Official Journal of the American Academy of Pain Medicine*; Faculty of

Pain Medicine of the Australia and New Zealand College of Anesthetists, and the International Spine Intervention Society. Dr. Gallagher's research and writing has covered topics ranging from opioid use in primary care and workers' disability to depression and chronic pain, as well as early interventions to prevent the development of chronic pain. He lectures nationally and internationally and has received the American Academy of Pain Medicine's Founders and Distinguished Service awards.

Robert J. Gatchel, PhD, ABPP is Nancy P. and John G. Penson Endowed Professor of Clinical Health Psychology and Professor and Chairman of the Department of Psychology, College of Science at The University of Texas at Arlington.

Gillianne Lai Geet Yi is a final year medical student at the National University of Singapore, and served an elective clerkship at Massachusetts General Hospital in 2011. Gillianne has done research in B cell lymphoma and intends to pursue a residency in internal medicine with a view to specialize in Medical Oncology.

Carmen R. Green, MD is Professor of Anesthesiology,   Obstetrics and Gynecology, and Health Management and Policy at the University of Michigan Medical School in Ann Arbor, MI.

Robbie Haggard, MS, CRC, LCP is a Certified Rehabilitation Counselor and Licensed Professional Counselor working for the Department of Psychology at the University of Texas at Arlington, where he is the Program Coordinator for the Acute Temporomandibular Jaw Pain Program. His research interests and experience include biobehavioral treatment and interdisciplinary care with acute and chronic pain populations and other chronic illnesses.

James Hallenbeck, MD is an Associate Professor of medicine in the Division of General Medical Disciplines, Department of Medicine, at the Stanford University School of Medicine. He is also an Associate Chief of Staff for Extended Care at VA Palo Alto Health Care Services in Palo Alto, California. Dr. Hallenbeck specializes in palliative medicine. His research interests include cross-cultural communication and clinician education in palliative care.

Dagny Faxvaag Haugen, MD, PhD is a consultant in Oncology and Palliative Medicine, Head of the Regional Centre of Excellence for Palliative Care, Western Norway in Bergen, and Assistant Professor, European Palliative Care Research Centre, Norwegian University of Science and Technology in Trondheim, Norway. His main interests in palliative care are symptom assessment, education, and organization of services.

Jimmy Henry, MD is a Pain Medicine Fellow, at the Temple University Hospital, Philadelphia, PA.

Richard M. Hirshberg, MD, FACS is the Emeritus Chairman of Neurosurgery, St. Joseph Hospital Houston, Texas. His professional career included all modalities and procedures concerned with the Neurosurgical treatment of pain. He introduced groundbreaking clinical findings that led to the identification of a pathway in the dorsal funiculus of the dorsal column that signals visceral pain.

Marianne Jensen Hjermstad, PhD is a senior researcher at the Regional Center for Excellence in Palliative Care in the Department of Oncology at the Oslo University Hospital, Oslo Norway.

Krista J. Howard, PhD is an Assistant Professor of Psychology at the Texas State University.

Paul B. Jacobsen, PhD Dr. Jacobsen received his bachelor's degree from Wesleyan University and his doctoral degree in Clinical Psychology from Michigan State University. Upon completing post-doctoral training in psychosocial oncology at Memorial Sloan-Kettering Cancer Center, he was appointed to the center's professional staff. In 1994, he was recruited by the Moffitt Cancer Center to direct the clinical and research programs in psychosocial oncology. He currently chairs the Department of Health Outcomes and Behavior at Moffitt and is a Professor of Psychology at the

University of South Florida. For the past 25 years, his work has focused on using knowledge from the behavioral and social sciences to promote reductions in cancer risk, earlier of cancer, and improvements in quality of life following cancer diagnosis. Dr. Jacobsen is the author of more than 150 journal articles and the recipient of numerous research grants from the American Cancer Society and the National Cancer Institute. A past president of the American Psychosocial Oncology Society, Dr. Jacobsen is closely involved in the society's efforts to develop and promote quality standards for psychosocial care of cancer patients. He was awarded the society's Holland Distinguished Leadership Award for this and related work in 2010.

Amber Jones is a heathcare consultant who received her undergraduate degree in psychology and her graduate education in psychology and business administration. Since 2001, she has served as a consultant for the Center to Advance Palliative Care (CAPC) and for hospitals, health systems, hospices and State Hospice and Palliative Care Associations. Ms. Jones serves on the Board of Directors of the Visiting Nurse Service of New York Hospice Program, of the Hospice and Palliative Care Association of New York State and on the Executive Committee of the National Hospice Work Group. She is the immediate past President of the Hospice and Palliative Care Association of New York. In addition to the positions outlined above, Ms. Jones has worked as a clinician, a hospital department director, a program manager at the national association for medical education and as the vice president of an academic medical center.

Nora L. Jones, PhD is the Associate Director of Graduate Studies and Senior Fellow at the Center for Bioethics at the University of Pennsylvania School of Medicine.

Youssef Josephson, DO is a Pain Medicine Fellow, at the Temple University Hospital, Philadelphia, PA.

Stein Kaasa, MD, PhD is a Professor in the Department of Oncology, St. Olav's University Hospital, Trondheim, Norway.

Francis J. Keefe, PhD is a Professor of Psychology and Neuroscience at the Duke University. His clinical interests include psychosocial treatment of persistent pain syndromes (low back pain, arthritic pain, and temporomandibular joint pain). Treatment approaches include: biofeedback, cognitive-behavioral group therapy, individual therapy, and spouse training; psychological assessment of patients who are candidates for advanced neurosurgical treatments for pain (e.g., implanted neural stimulators, morphine pumps); the use of early psychosocial intervention to prevent persistent pain; and behavioral approaches to treating anxiety disorders particularly agoraphobia, social phobias, and generalized anxiety.

Edmund Keogh, PhD is a senior lecturer in psychology based at the Department of Psychology. His main area of research is the psychology of pain. He has a specific interest in sex differences in pain, with a focus on identification of potential mechanisms, especially psychological (e.g., emotions, coping), which may help to explain the variability between and within men and women. A second interest is in the role that cognitions and emotions, especially those related to anxiety, play in the experience of pain and pain-related behaviors. He has interests in anxiety sensitivity, which is associated with the fear of bodily sensations, as well as the role attentional processes play in pain. His focus is predominately on the use of experimental methods, although he also has interests in chronic pain management.

Christine R. Kovach, PhD, RN, FAAN is a Professor in the College of Nursing at the University of Wisconsin Milwaukee and directs the research methods core for the Self-Management Science Center. She has done extensive clinical work and research with people who have Alzheimer's disease and other dementias. Her research focuses on developing interventions to assess and treat pain, agitation, comorbid conditions, and activity–rest disturbances of people with advanced dementia in nursing homes.

Gary L. Kreps, PhD is a University Distinguished Professor and Chair of the Department of Communication at George Mason University (GMU) in Fairfax, VA. He also holds a joint faculty appointment with the National Center for Biodefense at GMU. Prior to his appointment at GMU, he served for five years as the founding Chief of the Health Communication and Informatics Research Branch at the National Cancer Institute (NCI) at the National Institutes of Health. At NCI, he planned, developed, and coordinated major new national research and outreach initiatives concerning risk communication, health promotion, behavior change, technology development, and information dissemination to promote effective cancer prevention, screening, control, care, and survivorship.

Jean S. Kutner, MD, MSPH is Gordon Meiklejohn Endowed Professor of Medicine, in the Divisions of General Internal Medicine (GIM), Geriatrics, and Health Care Policy and Research, University of Colorado School of Medicine (UCSOM), and is Division Head for GIM. Dr. Kutner's research involves measurement of complex outcomes, such as symptom distress and quality of life, in a frail population, using both qualitative and quantitative methods. She has significant experience and expertise in measurement issues in the advanced illness population. In addition to building her successful extramurally funded research program, she mentors trainees and junior faculty from multiple disciplines, building investigator capacity in palliative care research.

Suzana Makowski, MD, MMM, FACP is a palliative care physician at the University of Massachusetts Medical School in Worcester, MA. She is also founder and of the Lois Green Learning Community.

Laxmaiah Manchikanti, MD is the Medical Director of the Pain Management Center of Paducah and Ambulatory Surgery Center in Paducah, Kentucky, encompassing a multidisciplinary pain program. He is also an Associate Clinical Professor of Anesthesiology and Perioperative Medicine of the University of Louisville in Louisville, KY. Dr. Manchikanti is certified by the American Board of Anesthesiology along with subspecialty certification in Pain Medicine, the American Board of Interventional Pain Physicians (ABIPP), American Board of Pain Medicine, and is a Fellow in Interventional Pain Practice (FIPP). Dr. Manchikanti is the founder, Chief Executive Officer, and Chairman of the Board of the American Society of Interventional Pain Physicians, the Society of Interventional Pain Management Surgery Centers, and many State Societies of Interventional Pain Physicians. He is also the founder of the Pain Physician Journal, ABIPP, and the ASIPP Foundation. Dr. Manchikanti has multiple academic interests; initially in anesthesiology, followed by Interventional Pain Management, not only the scientific aspects, but also in aspects of practice management.

Stephen May, MA, FCSP, Dip MDT, MSc, PhD is a Senior Lecturer in Physiotherapy at Sheffield Hallam University, Sheffield, UK. He is the coauthor, with Robin McKenzie, of *The human extremities: mechanical diagnosis and therapy* (2000), *The lumbar spine: mechanical diagnosis and therapy* (2nd edn., 2003), and *The cervical and thoracic spine: mechanical diagnosis and therapy* (2nd edn., 2006), several chapters in books, and over 30 publications in peer-reviewed journals. He was awarded a Fellowship from the Chartered Society of Physiotherapists (UK) in 2006 for his contribution to the profession. He has been a subeditor of the *Journal of Manual and Manipulative Therapy* since 2009.

Bill H. McCarberg, MD is the Founder of the Chronic Pain Management Program for Kaiser Permanente in San Diego, CA. He is on the board of directors of the American Academy of Pain Medicine and the National Pain Foundation. He is the President of the Western Pain Society and Adjunct Assistant Clinical Professor at the University of California at San Diego School Medicine. He is board certified by the American College of Pain Medicine, the American Board of Family Practice and additionally certified in Geriatrics.

Diane E. Meier, MD is the Director of the Center to Advance Palliative Care (CAPC), a national organization devoted to increasing the number and quality of palliative care programs in the United States. Under her leadership, the number of palliative care programs in US hospitals has doubled in the last 5 years. She is also the Director of the Lilian and Benjamin Hertzberg Palliative Care Institute; Professor of Geriatrics and Palliative Medicine; and Catherine Gaisman Professor of Medical Ethics at Mount Sinai School of Medicine in New York City. Dr. Meier was named one of 20 People Who Make Healthcare Better in the US by HealthLeaders Media 2010. She received a MacArthur Foundation Fellowship in September of 2008 and an Honorary Doctorate of Science from Oberlin College in 2010. Dr. Meier has published extensively in all major peer-reviewed medical journals, including *The New England Journal of Medicine* and *The Journal of the American Medical Association.*

Rhonda J. Moore, PhD is health scientist with the US Department of Health and Human Services in. Rockville, MD. She is trained as a cultural and medical anthropologist. Her research focus is pain management, complementary and alternative medicine, narrative and empathy in medicine, clinical ethics, and palliative care.

David B. Morris, PhD is recently retired as University Professor at the University of Virginia, where he held an appointment split between English and Medicine. He has written two prize-winning books on British literature – including *Alexander Pope: The genius of sense* (1984), which won the annual award for best book by the American Society of Eighteenth-Century Studies – while *The culture of pain* (1991) won a PEN prize. During twenty years as a self-employed writer, he subsequently lectured and published widely in the field of pain medicine – including recent chapters in *Evidence-based chronic pain management* (2010) and in the fourth edition (2010) of *Bonica's management of pain.* His work in pain has expanded to include a broader interest in so-called *biocultural studies*, which he explores further in three texts: *Illness and culture in the postmodern age* (1998); *Narrative, pain, and suffering* (2005), coedited with pain specialists Daniel Carr and John Loeser; and in "Unforgetting Asclepius: An Erotics of Illness," in *New literary history* (2007).

Devi E. Nampiaparampil, MD is an Assistant Professor of Physical Medicine and Rehabilitation (PM&R) and of Anesthesiology at NYU School of Medicine. She is Chief of Interventional Pain Management at the VA New York Harbor Healthcare System, where she performs procedures to treat spinal disorders, sports injuries, and cancer-related pain. She is board certified in PM&R, Pain Medicine, and Hospice and Palliative Medicine.

Magdalena R. Naylor, MD, PhD is a Professor of Psychiatry at the University of Vermont and Director of the MindBody Medicine Clinic at the University Health Center in Burlington, VT. Dr. Naylor's research has focused on the development of novel modes of treatment and relapse prevention for chronic pain. She has demonstrated that telephone-based therapy through interactive voice response technologies (TIVR) dramatically improve the long-term outcomes for patients participating in cognitive-behavioral therapy. She has also expanded this research and therapeutic approach to obesity and alcohol dependence. She has also studied the effects of coping in chronic pain utilizing functional magnetic resonance imaging (fMRI). In addition, her research has focused on the neuroendocrinology of mood disorders, with special emphasis on depression and cognition in menopausal women. At the CNRU her current research includes studies on the interaction of estrogen and central cholinergic systems in menopausal and elderly women. She is coauthor of the book, "The Search for Meaning."

Jason K. Ough, MD is completing a fellowship in Pain Medicine through New York University (NYU) School of Medicine. He graduated from the University of Wisconsin School of Medicine and Public Health and moved to New York to do a medicine internship at the Montefiore Medical Center in the Bronx. Dr. Ough completed his residency training in Anesthesiology at NYU where he also served as Chief Resident. After completing his subspecialty training, he will be joining a practice based in Brooklyn and Queens, where he will practice both Anesthesiology and Interventional Pain Management.

Yvonne Palermo (Seattle, WA) is a Professional artist, an Advocate through art, and a constant warrior. As a terminal chronic pain patient, she found herself learning that her accomplishments were trivial to the basic need to just get up in the morning. Bringing awareness is a necessity as patients with pain are often neglected and misunderstood. All people need to know that they are one incident away from walking in her shoes, so be aware that the simple things in life should be enjoyed just as much as the bigger ideals in life. She will continue to paint, create her life through visual means to enforce that we exist, all those individuals who live with chronic pain. www.yvonnepalermo.com.

Timothy P. Pearman, PhD is the Director of Supportive Oncology at the Robert H. Lurie Comprehensive Cancer Center of Northwestern University and an Associate Professor in the Departments of Medical Social Sciences and Psychiatry and Behavioral Sciences at the Northwestern University Feinberg School of Medicine. From 2000 to 2008, Dr. Pearman was the Director of Tulane's Psychosocial Oncology Program. He is a member of NCI Subcommittee G (Education), has served on various ACS advisory committees and has lectured nationally and internationally on topics including palliative care, bioethics, and quality of life in oncology.

Richard T. Penson, MD, MRCP is an Assistant Professor, Department of Medicine, Harvard Medical School and Clinical Director Medical Gyneologic Oncology, Medicine, Massachusetts General Hospital. He sits on the national Gynecologic Oncology Group (GOG) committees for ovarian cancer, rare tumors, and quality of life research. Dr. Penson serves as the chairman for two of the Institutional Review Board panels of Dana-Farber/Partners CancerCare, and is very actively involved in the investigation of novel agents and treatment strategies in ovarian cancer, and psychosocial issues related to gynecologic cancer care and general oncology.

Errol Philip, PhD is with the Department of Psychiatry and Behavioral Sciences, Memorial Sloan-Kettering Cancer Center. His research focuses on cancer outcomes and the development of comprehensive care models to promote health across diagnosis, treatment, and long-term survivorship. His current work examines the role of demographic and psychological variables in predicting care outcomes across the illness trajectory. He is also interested in patients' response to cancer and the ability to promote lifestyle change within structured follow-up care, as well as the utility of technology and modern psychometrics in improving survivorship care and support services for patients.

Antonella Pollo, MD is an Assistant Professor of Physiology at the Faculty of Pharmacy of the University of Torino, Italy. She is conducting research studies on the placebo and nocebo effects. Her main areas of interest include placebo analgesia, nocebo hyperalgesia, and placebo responses in motor performance in healthy individuals and in pathological conditions, such as Parkinson's disease. Other lines of research focus on pain in healthy elders and demented patients.

Sean Ransom, PhD is the Director of the Friedler Center for Psychosocial Oncology, Tulane Cancer Center. He is also a Clinical Assistant Professor of Psychiatry and Behavioral Sciences at the Tulane University School of Medicine.

Ben A. Rich, JD, PhD is a Professor and School of Medicine Alumni Association Endowed Chair of Bioethics at the University of California Davis. Professor Rich received his law degree from Washington University in St. Louis in 1973. He did postgraduate work as a Research Associate in Environmental Law at the University of Illinois College of Law (1973–1974) and served as the Antitrust Coordinator for the National Association of Attorneys General (1974–1976) before joining a Raleigh, NC law firm as a litigation specialist (1976–1980). He served as the Deputy Commissioner of the North Carolina Industrial Commission from 1980 to 1982, when he began his involvement in healthcare law as legal counsel to the University of North Carolina Hospitals and Clinics (1982–1984) and as Senior Resident Counsel at the University of Colorado Health Sciences Center (1984–1986). From 1986 to 1989 he served as University Counsel (General Counsel) for the University of Colorado system.

Lidia Schapira, MD is an Assistant Professor, Department of Medicine, Harvard Medical School and Assistant Professor, Medicine, Massachusetts General Hospital. Her research focus is on treatment trials for patients with breast cancer, psychosocial aspects of cancer care, and community attitudes toward cancer clinical trials.

Nalini Sehgal, MD is an Associate Professor at the University of Wisconsin School of Medicine and Public Health and Director of the Pain Medicine Fellowship Program, the Interventional Pain Medicine Program in the Department of Orthopedics and Rehabilitation at the University of Wisconsin School of Medicine and Public Health Madison, WI.

David A. Seminowicz, PhD is an Assistant Professor, Department of Neural and Pain Sciences at the University of Maryland Dental School in Baltimore, MD. His research goals are to understand the brain mechanisms supporting pain and pain relief, with the long-term goal of identifying brain targets for treating chronic pain conditions. He has also examined the effects that treatment for chronic pain conditions has on abnormal functional and anatomical MRI measures.

Hsien Seow, PhD is the Cancer Care Ontario Research Chair in Health Services Research at McMaster University in the Department of Oncology. His PhD is from Johns Hopkins School of Public Health, Department of Health Policy and Management, with a concentration in health services research and a certificate in gerontology. His research interests involve examining ways to better coordinate, organize, and deliver palliative care.

Roland T. Short III, MD is an Assistant Professor in the Division of Anesthesiology and Pain Medicine at the University of Alabama at Birmingham.

Howard S. Smith, MD, FACP, FAAPM, FACNP is an Associate Professor in the Departments of Anesthesiology, Medicine, and Physical Medicine and Rehabilitation and Academic Director of Pain Management in the Department of Anesthesiology at the Albany Medical College in Albany, NY. Dr. Smith is board certified in Pain Medicine, Addiction Medicine, Palliative Medicine, Anesthesiology, Nuclear Medicine, and Internal Medicine. He is a Fellow of the American College of Physicians, American Academy of Pain Medicine, and the American College of Nuclear Physicians, and member of many other professional organizations, including the American Society of Anesthesiology, International Association for the Study of Pain, and the New York State Society of Anesthesiologists.

Marlaine C. Smith, RN, PhD, FAAN is the Dean of the Christine E. Lynn College of Nursing at the Florida Atlantic University. Dr. Smith's main areas of interest are developing knowledge related to processes and outcomes of healing, and analyzing, extending and applying caring-based nursing theories. Dr. Smith is a fellow in the American Academy of Nursing.

Tamara J. Somers, PhD is an Assistant Professor in the Psychiatry and Behavioral Sciences Department at Duke University Medical Center in Durham, NC. Her research focuses on identifying coping variables that either enhance adjustment to pain or predispose patients toward increased pain and disability. She is particularly interested in studying the relationships between pain, pain coping, and weight related factors (eating, activity) in overweight and obese patients with persistent pain (e.g., arthritis, cancer).

David P. Steensma, MD is an Associate Professor, Department of Medicine at the Harvard Medical School. He is also Attending Physician in Hematologic Oncology at the Dana-Farber Cancer Institute and Attending Physician, in the Department of Medicine at the Brigham and Women's Hospital. His primary area of clinical activity and research focus is the myelodysplastic syndromes (MDS) and related conditions. This research activity includes development of new therapies, as well as discovery of new somatic genetic mutations important in the pathobiology of this difficult and poorly understood group of smoldering myeloid neoplasms.

Michele Sterling, BPhty, MPhty, Grad Dip Manip Physio, PhD is Associate Director, Centre of National Research on Disability and Rehabilitation Medicine (CONROD), The University of Qld and the Director of the Rehabilitation (Medical and Allied Health) Research Program (CONROD). Dr. Sterling's main areas of research are: the physical and psychological factors underlying whiplash associated disorders; the prediction of outcome following whiplash injury, improving the timing and nature of interventions for whiplash and neck pain, and the clinical translation of research findings to clinical practice.

Catherine Stoney, PhD is health pychologist/psychophysiologist with specialization in behavioral cardiology and endocrinology. Dr. Stoney has wide-ranging expertise in the areas of clinical trial design, sleep, and stress and disease, with a special emphasis on understanding the behavioral, physiological, social, and psychological mechanisms and pathways by which psychosocial stress and cardiovascular diseases are linked. She is currently the Program Director for Clinical Applications and Population Science in the Division of Population and Prevention Sciences at the National Heart, Lung, and Blood Institute, a component of the National Institutes of Health (NIH). Immediately prior to joining NIH, Dr. Stoney was the Professor of Psychology at the Ohio State University, where she conducted laboratory and clinical investigations of the health impact of psychosocial stress and lifestyle factors, as well as environmental, social and individual difference factors that mediate and moderate these relationships.

Lynette Su-Mien Ngo, MBBS, MRCP is a consultant in the Department of Medical Oncology, National Cancer Centre (NCC), Singapore and a visiting Consultant at KK Women's and Children's Hospital and Khoo Teck Puat Hospital. In addition, she spent 5 years caring for patients in hospice home care and in-patient hospice services in the community. Her areas of interest are in gynecologic cancers and psychosocial oncology. She has contributed to numerous publications in local and international peer-reviewed journals.

Regina P. Szucs-Reed, MD, PhD is currently an addiction psychiatry fellow at the Penn Presbyterian Medical center, University of Pennsylvania. Dr. Szucs-Reed is also participating in a postdoctoral fellowship at the Mental Illness Research, Education, and Clinical Center at Philadelphia Veterans Affairs Medical Center, where her research interests include neuroimaging in substance use disorders, including prescription opioid dependence.

Christina Thomas, LMSW is a Social Worker employed by the Department of Psychology at the University of Texas at Arlington. She is a biobehavioral clinician for the Acute Temporomandibular Jaw Pain Program. Her experience also includes Cognitive-Behavioral Therapy and biofeedback with an acute jaw pain population.

Lora M.A. Thompson, PhD is an Assistant Member in the Health Outcomes and Behavior and the Psychosocial and Palliative Care Programs at the Moffitt Cancer Center and in the Department of Oncologic Sciences at the University of South Florida College of Medicine. Dr. Thompson received her PhD in Clinical Psychology from the University of South Florida and completed a postdoctoral fellowship in Behavioral Oncology at Moffitt Cancer Center where she was subsequently appointed to the faculty. Her primary role is to provide assessment and psychotherapy services to patients experiencing distress or difficulty coping with cancer diagnosis, treatment, and survivorship.

Ana M. Velly, DDS, PhD is an Assistant Professor at Faculty of Dentistry at McGill University, Canada and a Research Associate at the School of Dentistry, University of Minnesota, USA. She is also an investigator on the Centre for Clinical Epidemiology and Community Studies, and Department of Dentistry of the Jewish General Hospital, Montreal, Canada. She is also the Director of the Registry for the National Institute of Health/NIDCR's TMJ Implant Registry and Repository.

Thomas R. Vetter, MD, MPH is the Maurice S. Albin Professor of Anesthesiology at the University of Alabama at Birmingham. He is clinically involved in acute and chronic pain management in children and adults, as well as the preoperative evaluation and treatment of complex surgical patients. He has developed and directed three pediatric chronic pain medicine programs in his career, most recently at the Children's Hospital of Alabama. Dr. Vetter's interests include outcomes research, comparative effectiveness research, performance improvement, patient-reported health measures, healthcare economics, clinical epidemiology, and healthcare disparities, with an emphasis on population-level implementation studies, especially in the area of chronic pain prevention in children.

Amy B. Wachholtz, PhD, MDIV is an Assistant Professor of Psychiatry at the University of Massachusetts Medical School. Her clinical interests include Anxiety/depression, biofeedback, health/medical psychology, religion/spiritual issues, sleep, and stress management.

Lynn R. Webster, MD, FACPM, FASAM is the Cofounder and Chief Medical Officer of Lifetree Clinical Research® and Director-At-Large for the American Academy of Pain Medicine. Dr. Webster is a leading researcher in exploring the relationship of medications and sleep, with particular interest in analgesic-induced sleep-disordered breathing, and is actively working within the industry to develop safer and more effective therapies for chronic pain and addiction.

Mark Yarchoan, MD is a medical student at the University of Pennsylvania School of Medicine.

Zirong Zhao, MD, PhD is a staff physician at the Veterans Affairs Medical Center in Washington, DC. She is also an Associate Professor at the George Washington University Medical Center. Dr. Zhao is Board certified in Internal Medicine and Pain Medicine and is a fellow of the American College of Physicians.

Chapter 1
Biopsychosocial Approaches to Understanding Chronic Pain and Disability

Robert J. Gatchel, Robbie Haggard, Christina Thomas, and Krista J. Howard

Early Theories of Pain

Two definitions are of primary importance in order to comprehend some of the prior theories of pain. While *pain* is a subjective experience, resulting from the transduction, transmission, and modulation of sensory information, *nociception* is a more objective phenomenon resulting from the stimulation of nerves that convey information about potential tissue damage to the brain. The traditional bio-medical model of nociceptive processing dominated the medical views of the nineteenth and twentieth centuries, and considered pain processes within a model of disease processes. These early models were informed by Cartesian views of an isomorphic relationship between reported pain and visible or measurable tissue injury. These early models consist primarily of two schools of thought. The first of these, termed the *specificity theory* required unique receptors and specific pathways in order to transmit painful information from the periphery to the spinal cord and, finally, to the brain. This particular point of view may date back as far as the ancient Greeks, who understood pain transmission as part of a direct transmission line. The work of von Frey (an early modern *specificity* theorist) involved identification and description of mechanical and thermal receptive fields on the skin (Gatchel et al. 2007).

An early twentieth-century theory termed the "pattern response" described nociceptive information as resulting from the particular pattern of responses in afferent systems, instead of activation of specific receptors and pathways, as in specificity theory (Gatchel et al. 2007). According to this theory, the response to pain resulted from stimulus intensity and the processing of the pattern of responses, which in turn determined the perceptual response to the nociceptive trigger. While these preceding theories successfully explained much of the phenomena reported in the literature and prompted a wealth of further scientific publication, they had some serious limitations, lacking specifically in explanations for the relationship between pain and the concept of suffering. A third perspective, popular through the early twentieth century, actually has its origins in concepts associated with the Greek philosopher Aristotle. Instead of a purely sensory model, as with the preceding theories, Aristotle viewed pain as an emotional concept, termed "quality of the soul." Drawing from these ideas, Livingston was one of the first to argue for pain as a subjective experience, resulting from activation of aversive networks in the brain. In exposing the weaknesses of specificity theory, Livingston described certain "appetites," which included pleasure and pain as motivating factors

R.J. Gatchel, PhD, ABPP (✉) • R. Haggard, MS, CRC, LPC • C. Thomas, LMSW • K.J. Howard, PhD
Department of Psychology, College of Science at The University
of Texas at Arlington, Arlington, TX, USA

R.J. Moore (ed.), *Handbook of Pain and Palliative Care: Biobehavioral Approaches for the Life Course*,
DOI 10.1007/978-1-4419-1651-8_1, © Springer Science+Business Media, LLC 2012

(Gatchel et al. 2007). These earlier models fell short, in that observations derived in clinical and experimental settings could not be fully explained by purely sensory and affective models (Beecher 1956). A more complex set of integrative models was eventually proposed in response to the largely ineffective treatments that had been constructed around these earlier theories. These more encompassing models are discussed in the next section, with a specific focus on the *gate control theory of pain* (Melzack and Wall 1965; Melzack and Casey 1968).

The Gate-Control Theory of Pain

The *gate control theory of pain* introduced by Melzack and Wall (1965) emphasized the close interaction between psychosocial and physiological processes affecting the perception of pain. The primary contribution of *gate control theory* to the scientific community was the idea that the central nervous system interacts with various psychosocial factors in the pain perception process. Psychosocial factors in the perception of pain thus took on a more important meaning in the assessment, treatment, and understanding of pain (Melzack 1993). Because scientific understanding is itself a self-correcting process, other researchers contributed to our understanding by pointing out the flaws and unexplained phenomena still to be answered by this model (Schmidt 1972; Nathan 1976). These contributions further strengthened the model by responding to these criticisms with revisions and reformulations of *gate control theory* (Wall 1989). But due to its versatility and simplicity, the gate control model of pain has withstood the rigor of changing scientific data and theoretical challenges, and continues to provide a heuristic conceptualization for a wide array of pain symptomatology encountered in clinical and experimental settings. Still, our understanding of pain phenomena becomes more refined over time by scientific contributions, particularly due to technological advances that allow us to better assess underlying pain neurophysiology, neurotransmission, and opioid receptor processes.

This more complex view was followed up during the next decade by Engel (1977), who first introduced the concept of the biopsychosocial (BPS) approach to medicine. Prior to this development, the term *psychogenic pain* was used to suggest that pain that could not at the time be physiologically measured was a result of underlying psychological etiology. It was often implied, and even outright stated in many cases, that this was not "authentic" pain because it could not be objectively measured. The ideology resulting from this model effectively stunted the development of treatment modalities necessary to address comorbid psychiatric and pain conditions. Fortunately, *psychogenic* pain is no longer classified as a diagnostic disorder in modern psychiatry thanks to the work of the researchers like Melzack, Engel, and others (*DSM–IV*; American Psychiatric Association 1994). However, this does not preclude the dynamic relationship that psychosocial factors and pain can play for any particular patient. *Pain disorder* is instead used to more accurately define and describe various subtypes of conditions, as well as the degree of relationship between physiological and psychosocial factors. More detail pertaining to the BPS perspective is discussed in an upcoming section but, before this, another contributing model of pain based upon neurological factors is described in detail – the *neuromatrix model of pain*.

The Neuromatrix Model of Pain

Melzack (1999, 2005), in building on his prior work with the gate-control theory of pain, has proposed a *neuromatrix model of pain* which integrates models of stress along with a great deal of physiological and psychological factors associated with pain. Specifically, this theory proposes that pain is an elaborate process resulting from the distinctive neurosignature of a widely disbursed neural network in the brain, which Melzack labeled the *body – self neuromatrix* (Melzack 1999). The body – self neuromatrix is responsible for the integration of cognitive – evaluative, sensory – discriminative, and motivational – affective functions originally proposed by Melzack and Casey (1968). According to this model, the output patterns of the neuromatrix are what activate specific perceptual, behavioral, and homeostatic systems in response to injury and chronic stress. Of particular importance in distinguishing *neuromatrix theory* from other pain models is the identification of pain as subsequent to neural network output, as opposed to pain being thought of as a direct antecedent to injury or inflammation (Melzack 2005).

Chronic Pain and Stress

While it is proposed that this neuromatrix is to some degree genetically derived, sensory experience and learning also affect it (Gatchel et al. 2007). Therefore, according to this model, when a person is injured, homeostatic regulation is disrupted or altered. A complex hypothalamic–pituitary–adrenal (HPA) axis response is initiated due to this disruption, in order to restore homeostasis. The effect on this system due to chronic stress can result in a suppressed or compromised immune response and the limbic system. The limbic system is a keystone element in this dynamic interaction because it is responsible for much of human emotion, motivation, and cognitive processes (Gatchel et al. 2007).

As a result of all the aforementioned complex interactions, the neuromatrix is shaped by learning history, cognitive interpretation, and individual physio-behavioral response patterns. This interactive process, in which predisposed factors interact with an acute stressor, is referred to as a *diathesis-stress* model. Pain is a discrete stressor in this process as the body attempts to achieve homeostasis. Chronic pain is therefore an ongoing stressor that continually makes demands on the body's defense systems. A combined threat of fear, anxiety, and cognitive interpretation of the pain then contributes to the ongoing stress, thereby producing a feedback loop of sorts which, without intervention, is likely to maintain an ongoing pain-stress process (Gatchel et al. 2007).

The basis of the neuromatrix model comes from research with patients who have spinal cord injuries and in patients who experience phantom limb syndrome and phantom limb pain (see also Foell and Flor 2011). Findings have demonstrated that a significant number of people who have lost a limb or sensation in another body region, also continue to experience the sensation of the limb or other area. While it is thought that phantom limb phenomena might occur in some cases due to altered peripheral nerve activity in the region of the stump (Gatchel et al. 2007), the available evidence does not fully account for all of the observed phenomena (Katz and Melzack 1990). While traditional sensory-based theories of pain cannot adequately address these phenomena, the neuromatrix theory may be able to, as no actual sensory input is required to produce sensation experiences.

The Biopsychosocial Perspective of Pain

The BPS model of pain, introduced earlier in this chapter, is widely recognized in modern clinical and research settings as the most heuristic approach for conceptualizing and treating pain disorders. Physical disorders (such as pain) often are likely the result of dynamic interactions between physiological and psychosocial factors. As with the neuromatrix model, these interactions perpetuate and contribute to the overall pain experience. While each person experiences pain uniquely, a range of psychosocial and socioeconomic factors also interact with physical symptoms to create the clinical presentation. In a very brief period of time, the BPS perspective has produced a large evidence-based repository of information that has contributed to improved patient care, pain prevention, and clinical understanding of persons with pain conditions (Gatchel and Maddrey 2004).

Turk and Monarch (2002) discussed, in a review of literature regarding the BPS perspective on chronic pain, how individuals differ significantly in the frequency with which physical symptoms are reported, in their likelihood to visit physician, and treatment response. It was observed that, often, treatment response is not directly related to objective physical symptoms. Observations like this have been reported for some time, as with findings by White et al. (1961) that less than one-third of all persons with clinically significant symptoms ever actually consulted a physician. Conversely, Dworkin and Massoth (1994) reported that approximately 30–50% of patients who seek treatment in primary care do not have specific diagnosable disorders. For emphasis, this means that many people with identifiable symptoms do not seek treatment, while many patients who do seek treatment and report pain do not have clinically identifiable or diagnosable ailments.

The terms *disease* and *illness* are further distinguished in the pain literature (Turk and Monarch 2002). Disease typically refers to a process that interferes with the functions of an organ or organ system, resulting from infection, injury, genetics, or other precursors. Illness, however, primarily refers to an individual's experience of that disease, resulting in a range of physical, behavioral, and psychosocial stressors. Similar differences are noted in nociceptive versus pain processes. Two individuals may have similar injuries that, in turn, transmit information regarding nerve and tissue damage to the brain, as an example of nociception. Subjectively, though, they may experience entirely different pain processes. Pain, similar to illness, refers to how physical and psychosocial experiences are subjectively interpreted through the transduction, transmission, and modulation of sensory input. Pain can therefore only be evaluated and fully described from the perspective of the person who has endured the nociceptive process. Illness is the primary focus of assessment and treatment within the BPS model. While patterns and similarities between experiences emerge from this perspective, the biological, psychological, and social factors interact in such a complex manner that no two people are likely to bring the same pain experience to the fore. This diversity of pain experiences requires an empathic clinical understanding of pain, along with the patient's perception and response to that process. It has been demonstrated repeatedly throughout clinical and research literature that any assessment and treatment approach with neglect in these constructs is incomplete. To further emphasize this point, the success of the BPS treatment modality has been consistently demonstrated (Turk and Monarch 2002).

Comorbidity of Chronic Pain and Mental Health Disorders

Identifying comorbid mental health disorders is a vital component in treating pain from the BPS perspective, because subjective experiences of pain may be intensified by comorbid psychopathology, thus perpetuating any associated disability (Dersh et al. 2002; See also Donovan et al. 2011). Patients experiencing chronic pain are at increased risk for depression, suicide, and sleep disorders, and these factors become more significant in the maintenance of dysfunction and suffering as pain becomes more chronic in nature (Gatchel 1996). The three major psychiatric concomitants of chronic pain are mood disorders, anxiety disorders, and substance abuse disorders (Dersh et al. 2002).

Several relationships have been demonstrated between mental health disorders and pain. As evaluated through the multiaxial classification system of the DSM-IV-TR (American Psychiatric Association 2000), mental health disorders are defined and categorized as part of a five axis domain that encompasses more transient states, consistent traits, medical conditions, social factors, and global functioning. The more acute clinical disorders that are often focused on clinically are coded on Axis I, while the more persistent trait disorders (personality disorders (PDs) and mental retardation (MR)) are reported on Axis II. Major depressive disorder (MDD), an Axis I disorder, has a particularly high prevalence among patients being treated for chronic pain symptoms (Kinney et al. 1993; Polatin et al. 1993). Also within the Axis I diagnostic categories, Anxiety disorders (Burton et al. 1997; Fishbain et al. 1986; Polatin et al. 1993) and substance use disorders (Fishbain et al. 1986; Katon et al. 1985; Polatin et al. 1993; Reich et al. 1983) have high prevalence rates among persons being treated for pain symptoms.

In the literature, depression has been defined as a mood, symptom, or syndrome, and assessed by multiple methods that make it difficult to compare results across study designs, further complicating accurate diagnosis and treatment for pain and depression in clinical settings (Dersh et al. 2002). Several researchers (Kinney et al. 1993) have identified high rates of MDD in patients with chronic pain. Prevalence rates for MDD from these studies were reported as current rates of about 45% and lifetime rates of approximately 65%. In a comprehensive meta-analysis of 14 studies that identified MDD in patients with chronic pain, nine studies reported current prevalence of MDD between 30 and 54% (Banks and Kerns 1996). During this time period, estimates of MDD in the US population were reported as 5% for current major depression and 17% for lifetime major depression (Blazer et al. 1994). It is most likely that the high prevalence rate of MDD in patients with chronic pain accounts for much of the research investigating the association between the two.

As mentioned earlier, high prevalence rates of anxiety disorders have also been documented among patients with chronic pain (Fishbain et al. 1986; Polatin et al. 1993; Burton et al. 1997). Within the larger domain of anxiety disorders, panic disorder and generalized anxiety disorder tend to be the most commonly diagnosed of the specific anxiety disorders. These also include agoraphobia, specific phobia, social phobia, posttraumatic stress disorder (PTSD), and obsessive compulsive disorder (OCD) (Dersh et al. 2002). In contrast to findings with MDD, in studies that relied upon DSM diagnostic criteria, the overall prevalence for anxiety disorders was similar to those estimated in the general population. Follow-up findings suggest, however, that anxiety disorders are more often associated with chronic pain than has been previously reported (Dersh et al. 2002). Researchers have reported lifetime prevalence rates similar to the general population, while current prevalence rates of other mental health disorders in patients with chronic pain are significantly higher (Polatin et al. 1993; Burton et al. 1997).

While anxiety disorders have been frequently identified in both acute and chronic pain populations, higher prevalence rates of other mental health disorders have also been indicated in patients with chronic pain (Kinney et al. 1993; Gatchel et al. 1996). It might simply be that, while anxiety is a common reaction to acute pain, other conditions such as MDD develops over time along with chronic pain. This would seem to support a model of progression from acute pain to chronic pain disability (Gatchel 1991a, b). Some patients may have genetic markers that would predispose them to a mental health disorder that, in turn, is then activated by the stress of a chronic pain experience. Following this logic, chronic pain might be exacerbated by physiological mechanisms that "follow on the heels" of an anxiety response. Avoidance of activities that might actually help to reduce pain symptoms, in turn, contributes to the maintenance of pain by avoidance of activities like exercise, primarily due to fear of re-injury. In addition to this, some patients with pain disorders might have unwanted responsibilities and social obligations that they may avoid which, in turn, leads to lowered self-esteem and reinforces their belief that exertion might increase pain. Such a cognitive-behavioral mediation cycle may actually occur with patients who are anxiety-sensitive, and who catastrophically misinterpret physical sensations of arousal as pain related.

Brown et al. (1996) found rates of current substance use disorders ranging from 15 to 28%, while lifetime substance use disorders ranged from 23 to 41%, among patients with chronic pain disorders. It should also be noted that these rates were higher among male patients than female patients in the chronic pain population, similar to findings within the general population. In contrast to the general population, however, the prevalence rates of both lifetime and current substance use disorders were significantly higher for male and female patient in the chronic pain population (Dersh et al. 2002). While chronic pain may not induce substance use disorders as once believed, it was demonstrated by one study that 94% of chronic pain patients have experienced lifetime substance use disorders prior to the onset of a chronic pain disorder (Polatin et al. 1993). While these statistics can be intimidating from a treatment perspective, Brown et al. (1996) found that patients with chronic pain were no more likely than other patients in a medical setting to have current substance use disorders. So, while there is not a unique risk for substance abuse within the chronic pain population, these patients do seem to be at an increased risk for new substance use disorders during the 5 years following the onset of chronic pain (Brown et al. 1996). It may even be that iatrogenic factors (conditions induced inadvertently by a physician or as a result of medical treatment) are at least partly responsible for this increased risk.

One measure to prevent or reduce this risk is for the treatment provider to conduct a comprehensive history and physical during their initial intake with a pain patient. During this exam and interview process, specific issues should be addressed, including opiate use patterns, the pain condition itself, previous treatments utilized and their outcomes, how the patient obtains and utilizes his or her opiate medications, evidence of drug-seeking behaviors or loss of control, and the current level of relief (Bernstein et al. 2007). One important note of caution is that patients habituated to chronic pain are more likely to underestimate medication use and in some circumstances may attempt to hide illicit drug use. For this reason, a comprehensive screening for these issues must include a combination of experienced clinical observation confirmed by physiological testing such as urinalysis. While pain medications can be effective and safe, treatment providers must also balance the risk of prescription drug abuse with the needs of patients in need of effective relief (Bernstein et al. 2007).

A Conceptual Model of How Acute Pain Develops into Chronic Pain

All chronic pain conditions arise from acute occurrences, yet not all acute injuries result in chronic pain situations. Understanding the factors that contribute to the development of chronic pain conditions has been a primary goal in pain research. It is understood that individuals experience acute pain in reaction to noxious stimuli often associated with physical injury (Basbaum and Jessell 2000). In most cases, as the disease state heals, the perception of pain, at this acute level, fades. Most individuals who have sustained injuries report some level of anxiety; yet, this psychosocial response is viewed as an adaptive emotion in that it promotes behaviors associated with healing, such as focusing on the injury and seeking appropriate medical care. Individuals for whom the pain state does not cease with the healing of the injury have been seen to enter an intermediate phase that can last several months following the injury. This secondary phase is marked with prolonged psychosocial distress, which can include emotions such as increased anxiety, fear, or anger, and can lead to behaviors involving learned helplessness. Furthermore, during this phase, secondary symptoms not associated with the original injury are often reported. The increased levels of stress can be associated with other physiological disturbances, such as in the respiratory and digestive systems, that qualify as somatization disorders (Gatchel 2001).

Within 6 months following an injury, the natural healing process should have restored the body back to the original condition. However, some individuals continue to experience pain following the sufficient period of biological repair (Gatchel 1991a, b) (see also Short and Vetter 2011). In fact, long-term pain conditions are repeatedly found to occur in conjunction with psychosocial issues, primarily depression (Gatchel and Maddrey 2004). Physical deconditioning often occurs with chronic pain conditions, in that exercise neglect results in the deterioration of the muscles and skeletal regions associated with the injured site (Mayer and Gatchel 1988). Oftentimes, chronic pain patients also exhibit "deconditioning" of their psychosocial state, such that daily activities are often abandoned and personal relationships can collapse (McMahon et al. 1997). Motivation can become a major factor for the chronic pain patient. Many times, individuals with chronic pain lose interest in normal responsibilities which can have direct negative effects on their family and with their work. In fact, if this lack of motivation becomes problematic with their work, patients with chronic pain can incur financial difficulties that can also contribute to their psychosocial distress. Once the individual has developed a chronic pain condition, it is essential to attend to the patient from a holistic, or BPS approach, to accommodate the biological, psychological, and social needs. Moreover, because each patient's circumstances are unique, it is vital to mold the treatment to match the needs of each individual (Gatchel and Maddrey 2004).

The Biopsychosocial Approach to Pain Assessment and Management

Chronic Pain Assessment

The concept of pain cannot be separated into discrete physical or psychosocial elements (Gatchel and Maddrey 2004). The BPS approach to understanding pain has been identified as the most successful model to date, in that the interactions among the biological, psychological, and social components unique to each individual are taken into account. The complexity of pain manifests not only within the range of psychological, social, and physical attributes, but also with respect to chronicity, such that these intertwined components are seen to modulate the patient's perception of pain and disability. The BPS model, therefore, uses physical, psychological, social, cognitive, affective, and behavioral measures, along with their interactions, to best assess the individual's unique pain condition (Gatchel and Maddrey 2004).

A recent expansion of this model shows a better understanding of how the neuroendocrine system affects the chronic pain condition (Gatchel 2004, 2005). In addition to the impact of general emotional distress, elevations of stress hormones produced by the hypothalamic-pituitary-adrenocortical (HPA) system, such as cortisol, have been shown to exacerbate pain conditions. McEwen (1998) had highlighted the importance of evaluating cortisol dysregulation under condition of allostatic load increases due to stress. Underlying mechanisms related to the HPS axis may therefore help to explain individual differences in stress and pain. Cogntive-behavioral therapy may be helpful in preventing and reducing the physiological and behavioral toll of this stress module (Turner et al. 2006; Gatchel and Rollings 2008).

Furthermore, growing technologies have allowed for a better understanding of the pain experience through various modalities, such as functional magnetic resonance imaging (fMRI) and positron emission tomography (PET) (see also Naylor et al. 2011). These types of imaging techniques focus on the displacement of blood flow within specified regions of the brain. Although there is some controversy regarding the implications derived from imaging procedures, these noninvasive technologies have provided knowledge about the anatomy and pathways related to the central nervous system (Gatchel et al. 2007). In addition to the brain imaging techniques, other developments in pain research have been found in areas of genetics, electrophysiology, molecular biology, and pharmacology (Gatchel et al. 2007). The unification of disciplines focused on pain provides the most effective methods to understanding pain because it gives a comprehensive and holistic view of how the nervous system perceives, interprets, and responds to pain (Gatchel 1999, 2007).

When attempting to assess an individual's pain condition, there are two essential "traps" to avoid. First, although there are numerous pain assessments available, the practitioner cannot assume that any one assessment will have more validity or reliability than another measure in a given pain patient. Secondly, while physical measures of pain are more objective than self-report instruments, both must be taken into consideration in the evaluation of the pain condition. Regardless of the level of accuracy in the objective analysis of pain, the interpretation on the part of the health care professional must be considered for an adequate diagnosis to be made. Furthermore, the individual's psychosocial state can influence the performance on a physical assessment, such that fear of re-injury and lack of motivation may adversely affect the outcome measures (Gatchel 2001).

When considering the types of assessments to use, the measure is only valid if it is aligned with the purpose at hand. Assessments used in chronic pain populations that focus solely on biological and physiological aspects may not be valid in predicting impairment or disability (Gatchel and Maddrey 2004). Not only is it important to consider how each measure will be used but, moreover, it is essential to be able to identify how the various tools assimilate into a complete portrait and analysis of the individual's pain condition (see also Hjermstad et al. 2011; See also Dy and Seow (2011); see also Palermo 2011). A step-wise approach to assessment has been advocated, beginning with a general evaluation of the factors under consideration, leading up to a more definitive diagnosis (Gatchel 2000). By taking this multidimensional view, the BPS approach to assessment will lead not only to a better understanding of the patient's pain condition, but ultimately will lead to a comprehensive treatment protocol customized to the individual's unique situation.

Chronic Pain Management

Similar to other chronic illnesses, such as diabetes or asthma, a chronic pain condition cannot be cured, but it can be managed. Due to the heterogeneity with respect to the biological and psychosocial elements within a chronic pain population, not only is greater diversification of treatment options necessary, it is essential to properly match the treatment to the patient. Because two patients with the same diagnosis differ in physical, social, and psychological compositions, grouping these patients into the same treatment program will not likely produce the best outcomes compared to a tailored treatment regimen (Gatchel 2005).

The overall outcome goal when treating patients which chronic pain conditions is improving functional capacity, which correlates with better physical strength, disability, and mobility, along with an improved affective state and self-esteem. Depending on the circumstances and duration of the injury, there are different levels of care, specifically primary, secondary, and tertiary care, for patients experiencing pain. The focus of *primary care* is to relieve the symptoms associated with the acute pain condition while increasing movement and functionality in the affected area (Mayer et al. 2006). In general, the psychosocial factors addressed in primary care settings correspond to alleviating any anxiety or fear associated with the occurrence of pain. At this phase, it is important to educate the patient about medication compliance and following the prescribed exercise protocol in order to expedite the healing process.

The majority of patients who incur an injury recover well following the *primary care* treatment. When psychological factors and social issues merge with the physiological impairment, though, a more integrated rehabilitation process is necessary to help the patient avoid entering into a full chronic pain condition. Commonly, a subset of the injured population finds recuperation to be difficult at the level of primary care, and will therefore require an expanded treatment program for their injury, which is called *secondary care*. At this level, an interdisciplinary team works together to help the patient to prevent physical deconditioning and to reduce psychosocial barriers that interfere with recovery. Most patients for whom primary care is not sufficient experience positive outcomes following secondary care (Karjalainen et al. 2004).

Some patients do not respond well to either primary or secondary care for reasons relating to poor physical and psychological recovery, or other factors such as legal and work-related issues that may contribute to more pronounced emotional distress. Functional restoration, which is a form of *tertiary care*, has been developed for this chronic pain population. The focus of functional restoration is to avert permanent disability by utilizing a BPS approach. Within the scope of this treatment, the patient receives assistance from an interdisciplinary team of health care professionals, often including, but not limited to, a primary care physician, a psychiatrist or psychologist, a physical therapist, an occupational therapist, and a disability case manager. Together, this team develops a comprehensive plan to help the patient not only regain mobility and function, but also to teach the patient stress management techniques and coping skills necessary for dealing with any lifestyle or work issues that develop as a result of the pain and impairment (Mayer et al. 1985). Oftentimes, chronic pain patients admitted to a tertiary care program are found to be reliant on, or have developed tolerance to their pain medications. Tolerance itself can lead to patients feeling or being stigmatized by their treatment provider. Tolerance is a decreased pharmacological effect that results in administration of higher doses to achieve the same effect (Bernstein et al. 2007; see also Palermo 2011). Although relief from pain symptoms is an appropriate course of action in the primary and secondary care programs, substance use, specifically opioid dependency, is far too common (Dersh et al. 2002). In most functional restoration programs, detoxification is found to be an essential part of treatment which is found to produce positive lifetime outcomes.

Following sufficient assessment measures and the resultant tailored treatment regimen, it is necessary to routinely evaluate the progress of the patient and amend or modify the program when deemed appropriate. The interdisciplinary team should meet on a regular basis to discuss each patient's progress. It is through effective communication, not only within the medical team, but also with the patient, that the BPS approach to pain management is successful (Gatchel and Maddrey 2004).

Functional restoration programs have repeatedly been shown to produce positive outcomes within the chronic pain population. It is through this BPS approach to pain management that patients experiencing chronic pain are able to regain mobility and function, to improve psychosocial conditions such as depression and anxiety, and to allow the patient to return to normal life activities. Besides decreasing self-reported pain and disability, as well as increasing physical functioning, this functional restoration approach (first developed by Mayer and Gatchel 1988) has also produced substantive improvement in various important socioeconomic outcome measures (e.g., return to work and resolution of outstanding medical issues). For example, in patients who were chronically disabled with spinal disorders, Mayer et al. (1987) found that 87% of the functional restoration group was actively working 2 years after treatment, as compared with only 41% of a nontreatment comparison group. Moreover, about twice as many of the comparison group patients had both additional spine surgery and unsettled workers' compensation legal cases, relative to the treatment group. The comparison group continued with an approximately five times higher rate of patient visits to health care professionals and higher rates of recurrence or re-injury. Thus, these results displayed the striking impact that a functional restoration program can have on these important measures in a chronic pain group consisting primarily of workers' compensation patients (traditionally the most difficult cases to treat successfully).

This functional restoration approach has also been found to be effective in the treatment of patients with chronic upper extremity disorders (Mayer et al. 1999). In addition, this type of approach has been found to be an effective early intervention treatment for preventing chronic disability. For example, in a randomized controlled study, acute low-back-pain patients who were identified as "high risk" for developing chronic back pain disability were randomly assigned to an early functional restoration group or a treatment-as-usual group (Gatchel et al. 2003). The functional restoration group displayed significantly fewer indexes of chronic pain disability at 1-year follow-up on a wide range of work, healthcare utilization, medication use, and self-reported pain variables. For example, the functional restoration group was less likely to be taking narcotic analgesics (odds ratio = 0.44), and also less likely to be taking psychotropic medications (odds ratio = 0.24). Moreover, the treatment-as-usual group was less likely to have returned to work (odds ratio = 0.55). The cost-comparison savings data from this study were also quite impressive: the treatment-as-usual group cost *twice* as much as the functional restoration group over a 1-year period.

Besides functional restoration, there have been a host of other studies demonstrating the treatment effectiveness of interdisciplinary pain-management programs (based on the BPS model) in successfully treating various other prevalent chronic pain syndromes. In fact, Gatchel and Okifuji (2006) comprehensively reviewed the literature in demonstrating the therapeutic- and cost-effectiveness of such comprehensive programs, relative to simple, single-modality approaches such as pharmacotherapy, surgery, injections, etc., on a number of measures, as well as on the important variable of return to work. In addition to these, cognitive-behavioral therapy that incorporates biofeedback and coping skills training has been demonstrated to be helpful in reducing the psychosocial stress of chronic and acute pain conditions (Turner et al. 2006; Gatchel and Rollings 2008).

Chronic Pain and Disability

As the role of psychosocial stressors become increasingly recognized in pain management, evidence-based practice that targets these factors is increasingly in demand. Psychosocial stressors that can exacerbate and prolong a patient's pain can include mental health (particularly in regards to coping skills, thinking patterns, and emotionality), dynamics of their family system, employment and socioeconomic environment, access to health care, and one's place in society as a pain patient. Currently, the most validated and practiced methods for treating psychosocial stressors in pain are cognitive behavioral therapy (CBT), relaxation, and biofeedback (see also Kutner and Smith 2011). As noted previously, many chronic pain patients are afflicted with comorbidities of depressive or anxious pathology, or simply dealing with the adjustment of living with pain. Social dislocation refers to the process of pain patients struggling to come to terms with what has been lost in their social life, work life, and interpersonal life in addition to the struggle one faces to refine their role and identity (Roy 2008). Such a process can change a patient's thought process, as well as how they react emotionally and behaviorally to daily life.

Psychosocial stressors trigger the coping skills which play a significant role in the BPS model of pain (e.g., Jensen and Karoly 1991; Gatchel and Maddrey 2004; Samwel et al. 2006; Hanley et al. 2008), with factors and associated variables of coping covering a broad range of psychosocial and behavioral mechanisms. These factors include emotional states, psychopathology, activity adjustment, and pain-related beliefs (e.g., Jensen and Karoly 1991; Samwel et al. 2006; Hanley et al. 2008). Insight into the dynamic role of these variables in relation to chronic pain has been adapted in research from theoretical models such as locus of control (Seligman 1975), the cognitive distortion model (Beck 1967, 1976), and the fear-avoidance model (Lethem et al. 1983). Multiple types of coping have been identified through research as having either an adaptive or maladaptive effect in a chronic pain patient's experience with pain severity, disability, and general interference with functioning and quality of life. In general, one's beliefs and emotions regarding pain are expressed in their behaviors toward their pain, generally resulting in either active or passive coping strategies.

Two basic perspectives exist on the causal relationship of negative emotional states and the onset and etiology of chronic pain. Specifically, whether pain and disability are influenced by negative emotional states and pain-related beliefs, or the noxious experience of pain itself, triggers the onset of negative emotional states and disability (e.g., Banks and Kerns 1996; Gatchel 2006). Regardless of the direction, negative emotional and mood states such as fear, anger, depression, and anxiety have been related to disability and pain intensity in chronic pain (Baker et al. 2008; Tan et al. 2008). Stress and anger are problematic emotions in the development and maintenance of chronic pain. Anger can influence stress and pain level, as well as activity, particularly when internalized (Kerns et al. 1994; Burns 1997). However, an interesting review conducted by Burns et al. (2008) led the authors to conclude that anger inhibition is not necessarily the contributor to pain, but is simply reflective of a patient's emotionally oriented coping response of hyper-vigilance towards any perceived stressors.

Depression has been shown to play a major role in exacerbating pain and hindering one's ability to actively cope (Banks and Kerns 1996; Baker et al. 2008). There is evidence that depression may be the source from which other negative emotional states evolve in chronic pain (Tan et al. 2008). The *Fear-Avoidance Model* is used to explain the etiology of disability and depression in chronic pain patients, wherein patients avoid any activity expected to increase pain and distress due to fear of pain. This avoidance can continue, resulting in increased pain avoiding behaviors in any type of activity including pleasurable and work-related, thereby increasing physical disability due to lack of movement, as well as psychosocial distress due to a lack of exposure to positive reinforcements (Samwel et al. 2006). Emotional affect itself can be a predictor for treatment gain in pain. Although depression is more often researched in chronic pain, anxious affect has also been shown to be related to a higher number of localized pain sites reported as well as a direct affect on disability (Tan et al. 2008).

Activity adjustment is an important factor in predicting disability in chronic pain (Samwel et al. 2006; McCracken et al. 2007). An example of this can be seen in a study conducted by Parrish et al. (2008) which found that increases in positive events for women with fibromyalgia and rheumatoid arthritis predicted less fatigue, whereas increases in negative events produced more fatigue. Level of fatigue had a positive relationship with physical disability.

Passive coping can include resting, help-seeking, and any avoidance of all activities anticipated to cause discomfort (see previous section on the *Fear Avoidance Model*). Active coping, including engaging in activities, distraction, and using self-statements, has been related to better psychosocial and physical functioning, emotional functioning, and pain levels and disability (Jensen and Karoly 1991; Keogh and Eccleston 2006). One's emotional state and pain-related beliefs are antecedents for a patient's pain-related behaviors. For example, in chronic pain patients, the pain-related belief of worrying (rumination over aversive pain experiences and consequences) has a cycle similar to the negative reinforcement paradigm mentioned previously in the Fear Avoidance Model. The passive coping of worrying can lead to a reduction in physical and psychosocial functioning, such as depression, leading to increased disability of the musculoskeletal and cardiovascular system (Samwel et al. 2006). Hence, when examining the coping cycle of pain-related beliefs in chronic pain patients, disability generates further disability both physically and psychologically. Types of psychopathology shown to be significantly higher in pain populations include anxiety disorders, obsessive compulsive personality disorder, avoidant and histrionic personality disorder, PTSD, and alexithymia (Fifield et al. 1998; Edwards et al. 2006; Tennen et al. 2006).

Pain-related beliefs are coping mechanisms that refer to an individual's thinking patterns about their pain, including anticipation of future pain experiences, interpretation of pain signals, and beliefs about the role of one's self and others in effective (or ineffective) treatment (Hanley et al. 2008) (see also Velly et al. 2011). Models, such as *Locus of Control* and the *Cognitive Distortion Model,* provide theoretical insight into the important role that one's pain-related beliefs have in chronic pain. Pain-related beliefs have been shown to predict disability, pain level, psychosocial functioning, and activity in multiple pain populations, including temporomandibular joint disorder, spinal cord injuries, and fibromyalgia (Jensen and Karoly 1991; Glaros and Lumley 2005; Samwel et al. 2006; Hanley et al. 2008). Helplessness in chronic pain refers to how an individual's attitude towards his/her ability to cope with pain is learned from past experiences with pain episodes. With negative experiences over time, an individual develops an attributional style of explaining aversive experiences as being out of their control (Jensen and Karoly 1991; Samwel et al. 2006). In fact, after completing a multiple regression analysis, Samwel et al. (2006) showed that helplessness was the only significant predictor of pain levels after controlling for multiple variables, including fear of pain and passive pain-coping strategies. Locus of control has also been adapted in chronic pain to examine how individuals' perception of control over pain relates to their pain and functioning. Increased perceptions of control have been shown to predict positive adjustment to pain including well-being, activity level, and pain experience (McCrea et al. 2000; Cousson-Gélie et al. 2005; Hanley et al. 2008).

When passive pain-related cognitions such as fear of pain, worrying, and catastrophizing are used by patients to cope, they often have maladaptive consequences of increasing physical and psychological disability (Keogh and Eccleston 2006). Although there are some conflicting results (Samwel et al. 2006; Hirsh et al. 2008), pain-related cognitions, particularly catastrophizing, have been shown to predict depression, disability, and pain intensity (Turner et al. 2000; Severeijns et al. 2001). Models such as the cognitive distortion model (Beck 1967, 1976) also provide additional insight into how cognitions, emotions, and behaviors can perpetuate and exacerbate an individual's pain.

The cognitive distortion model, which explains the etiology of psychopathology through negative schemas, has been adapted to explain the vulnerability of a chronic pain patient's psychopathology as well (Banks and Kerns 1996). This concept can be seen in the cognitive distortion of catastrophizing among chronic pain patients. A study conducted by Severeijns et al. (2001) found that, among chronic pain patients catastrophizing independently predicted pain intensity, disability, and psychosocial distress. Catastrophizing could play a causal role in pain interference and psychosocial functioning (Hanley et al. 2008). Turner et al. showed that after analyzing the roles of pain, beliefs, coping, and physical disability in depression levels, catastrophizing was the only variable independently associated with depression (Turner et al. 2000). In fact, age, sex, and pain intensity only explained 9% of the variance in depression. In contrast, beliefs, coping, and catastrophizing predicted 47%. Another study of patients with temporomandibular disorder showed that catastrophizing accounted for 33% of the variance in depression, 14% of activity interference, and 18% of jaw disability (Turner et al. 2001).

Put differently, chronic pain is often maintained and influenced by one's coping skills emotionally, behaviorally, and cognitively, and such factors need to be a primary concern when implementing treatment in pain patients. Passive and maladaptive coping beliefs are a contributing mechanism to the common relationship between pain and psychopathology across pain populations. Although the direction of the relationship of such factors and chronic pain remains unclear, psychosocial distress can exacerbate pain (Edwards et al. 2006) and the ability to cope adaptively.

Psychological Therapies for the Treatment of Pain and Disability

All of the aforementioned coping factors can grow and become more complex as a patient moves from being acute to chronic. Therefore, interventions that deal with the emotional, psychosocial, existential, and not just the physical, consequences of pain can enable the patient to be treated with multimodal interventions rather than in a direct linear biomedical model that often does not alleviate all the distress and pain-related suffering. Deficits in coping skills are primarily treated in pain management through the use of validated methods such as CBT. CBT has been validated for multiple mental illnesses, including depression and anxiety, and has been more recently validated as a treatment for chronic pain (e.g., Roy 2008). When looking at a dynamic approach to pain management, CBT treats psychosocial stressors that can factor into an individual's pain cycle described earlier. Furthermore, it has been shown to be effective in the treatment of chronic pain (e.g., Roy 2008).

The cognitive behavioral model is the most common and dynamic model used for explaining both acute and chronic pain. According to Okifuji et al. (1999), there are certain assumptions in applying CBT to pain that are summarized and discussed below:

- Individuals perceive the pain experience differently because it is filtered through their own schemas or ways of perceiving the world. When a practitioner takes the individual beliefs and attitudes, and fears towards pain of each patient into account, the diverse array of complaints and treatment responses to seemingly linear medical problems makes more sense.
- Thoughts (adaptive and maladaptive) can affect physiological arousal through emotionality, and thus affect behavior. Furthermore, this relationship is reciprocal; hence, emotions, physiology,

and behavior can affect one's thinking patterns. This can play a major role in factors that lead an acute patient to a chronic one, particularly in terms of treatment adherence to things such as physical therapy as the patients' actual and perceived experiences play a role in their willingness to work on rehabilitation and rebuilding their social and work behaviors and networks.

- If something is learned, then it can be unlearned. Therefore, patients who have developed maladaptive ways of thinking, feeling, and responding can benefit from interventions that focus on targeting maladaptive coping in the form of thoughts, feelings, and behaviors and work to learn more alternative adaptive coping skills.
- A patient's work is instrumental and primary in effecting treatment change. This refers to change of the administration of treatment in the health care system, from a traditionally passive recipient patient role to an active patient role. A patient's work is instrumental and primary in effecting treatment change. Therefore, the clinician and patient must be willing to collaborate wherein the overall goal is to increase the patients' sense of control and efficacy over their pain condition as they learn and implement their new skills.

Conclusion

The development of chronic pain conditions generally occurs in conjunction with other factors, including environmental, psychological, and social factors. Successful treatment of chronic pain conditions involves more than just focusing on the source of pain; it requires adequately assessing and treating the patient from a holistic perspective. The implementation of the BPS approach towards the assessment and treatment of chronic pain conditions has been viewed as the most heuristic approach. Rehabilitation, a treatment option that focuses not only on reducing the severity of the pain systems, but also on increased function, is often seen to enhance quality of life. However, in order to comprehensively and successfully manage all aspects of pain, treatment must be focused on environmental factors such as stress, as well as psychosocial factors such as depressive symptomatology, anxiety and fear-avoidance, catastrophizing, and maladaptive coping skills. Following treatment of these comorbid psychosocial disorders, patients with chronic pain conditions do generally report reductions in pain symptoms. However, one must note that chronic pain conditions are rarely cured. Therefore, the focus of treatment should be on decreasing pain and comorbid symptoms while enhancing the patient's return to function and improving his or her quality of life. Through the combination of BPS approach and palliative care options, patients with chronic pain conditions are able to improve psychosocial factors that lead to a decrease in pain symptoms and an increase in quality of life. Future endeavors in pain management should include objective forms of data collection alongside interdisciplinary treatment in order to determine what works best within the scope of their own practice, based on financial needs, patient characteristics, and the ability to incorporate interdisciplinary modalities into clinical practice. The treatment modalities discussed within this chapter were primarily observed within the scope of clinical research programs, and while they demonstrated much efficacy for interdisciplinary treatment, many factors may not be applicable to all sectors of the population.

References

American Psychiatric Association. (1994). *Diagnostic and statistical manual of mental disorders*. Washington, DC: APA.

American Psychiatric Association. (2000). *Diagnostic and statistical manual of mental disorders (Text Revision)* (4th ed.). Washington, DC: APA.

Baker, T. A., Buchanan, N. T., et al. (2008). Factors influencing chronic pain intensity in older black women: Examining depression, locus of control, and physical health. *Journal of Women's Health, 17*(5), 869–878.

Banks, S. M., & Kerns, R. D. (1996). Explaining the high rates of depression in chronic pain: A diathesis-stress framework. *Psychological Bulletin, 119*(1), 95–110.

Basbaum, A. I., & Jessell, T. M. (2000). The perception of pain. In E. R. Kandel, J. H. Schwartz, & T. M. Jessell (Eds.), *Principles of neural science* (pp. 472–491). New York: McGraw Hill.

Beck, A. (1967). *Beck depression inventory.* New York: Harper & Row.

Beck, A. T. (1976). *Cognitive therapy and the emotional disorders.* New York: International Universities Press.

Beecher, H. K. (1956). Relationship of significance of wound to the pain experienced. *Journal of the American Medical Association, 161,* 1609–1613.

Bernstein, D., Stowell, A. W., et al. (2007). Complex interplay of participants in opioid therapy. *Practical Pain Management, 7,* 10–36.

Blazer, D. G., Kessler, R. C., et al. (1994). The prevalence and distribution of major depression in a national community sample: The national comorbidity survey. *The American Journal of Psychiatry, 151,* 979–986.

Brown, R. L., Patterson, J. J., et al. (1996). Substance abuse among patients with chronic back pain. *Journal of Family Practice, 43*(2), 152–160.

Burns, J. (1997). Anger management style and hostility: Predicting symptom-specific physiological reactivity among chronic low back pain patients. *Journal of Behavioral Medicine, 20*(6), 505–522.

Burns, J., Quartana, P., et al. (2008). Anger inhibition and pain: Conceptualizations, evidence and new directions. *Journal of Behavioral Medicine, 31*(3), 259–279.

Burton, K., Polatin, P. B., et al. (1997). Psychosocial factors and the rehabilitation of patients with chronic work-related upper extremity disorders. *Journal of Occupational Rehabilitation, 7,* 139–153.

Cousson-Gélie, F., Irachabal, S., et al. (2005). Dimensions of cancer locus of control scale as predictors of psychological adjustment and survival in breast cancer patients. *Psychological Reports, 97*(3), 699–711.

Dersh, J., Polatin, P., et al. (2002). Chronic pain and psychopathology: Research findings and theoretical considerations. *Psychosomatic Medicine, 64,* 773–786.

Donovan, K. A., Thompson, L. M. A., & Jacobsen, P. B. (2011). Pain, depression and anxiety in cancer. In R. J. Moore (Ed.), *Handbook of pain and palliative care.* New York: Springer.

Dworkin, S. F., & Massoth, D. L. (1994). Temporomandibular disorders and chronic pain: Disease or illness? *Journal of Prosthetic Dentistry, 72*(1), 29–38.

Dy, S., & Seow, H. (2011). Quality indicators for pain in palliative care. In R. J. Moore (Ed.), *Handbook of pain and palliative care.* New York: Springer.

Edwards, D. M., Gatchel, R. J., et al. (2006). Emotional distress and medication use in two acute pain populations: Jaw and low back. *Pain Practice, 6*(4), 242–253.

Engel, G. L. (1977). The need for a new medical model: A challenge for biomedicine. *Science, 196*(4286), 129–136.

Fifield, J., Tennen, H., et al. (1998). Depression and the long-term risk of pain, fatigue, and disability in patients with rheumatoid arthritis. *Arthritis and Rheumatism, 41*(10), 1851–1857.

Fishbain, D. A., Goldberg, M., et al. (1986). Male and female chronic pain patients categorized by DSM-III psychiatric diagnostic criteria. *Pain, 26,* 181–197.

Foell, J., & Flor, H. (2011). Phantom limb pain. In R. J. Moore (Ed.), *Handbook of pain and palliative care.* New York: Springer.

Gatchel, R. J. (1991a). Early development of physical and mental deconditioning in painful spinal disorders. In T. G. Mayer, V. Mooney, & R. J. Gatchel (Eds.), *Contemporary conservative care for painful spinal disorders* (pp. 278–289). Philadelphia: Lea & Febiger.

Gatchel, R. J. (1991b). Psychosocial assessment and disability management in the rehabilitation of painful spinal disorders. In T. Mayer, V. Mooney, & R. Gatchel (Eds.), *Contemporary conservative care for painful spinal disorders.* Philadelphia: Lea & Febiger.

Gatchel, R. J. (1996). Psychological disorders and chronic pain: Cause and effect relationships. In R. J. Gatchel & D. C. Turk (Eds.), *Psychological approaches to pain management: A practitioner's handbook* (pp. 33–52). New York: Guilford.

Gatchel, R. J. (1999). Perspectives on pain: A historical overview. In R. J. Gatchel & D. C. Turk (Eds.), *Psychosocial factors in pain: Critical perspectives* (pp. 3–17). New York: Guilford.

Gatchel, R. J. (2000). *How practitioners should evaluate personality to help manage chronic pain patients.* Washington, DC, American Psychological Association: Personality Characteristics of Patients with Pain. R. J. Gatchel and J. N. Weisberg.

Gatchel, R. J. (2001). A biopsychosocial overview of pre-treatment screening of patients with pain. *The Clinical Journal of Pain, 17,* 192–199.

Gatchel, R. J. (2004). Comorbidity of chronic mental and physical health disorders: The biopsychosocial perspective. *The American Psychologist, 59,* 792–805.

Gatchel, R. J. (2005). *Clinical essentials of pain management.* Washington, DC: American Psychological Association.

Gatchel, R. J. (2006). The influence of personality characteristics on pain patients: Implications for causality in pain. In G. Young, A. Kane, & K. Nicholson (Eds.), *Causality: Psychological knowledge and evidence in court: PTSD, pain and TBI.* New York: Springer.

Gatchel, R. J., Garofalo, J. P., et al. (1996). Major psychological disorders in acute and chronic TMD: An initial examination of the "chicken or egg" question. *Journal of the American Dental Association, 127*, 1365–1374.

Gatchel, R. J., & Maddrey, A. M. (2004). The biopsychosocial perspective of pain. In J. Raczynski & L. Leviton (Eds.), *Healthcare psychology handbook*. Washington, DC: American Psychological Association Press.

Gatchel, R. J., & Mayer, T. G. (2000). Occupational musculoskeletal disorders: Introduction and overview of the problem. In T. G. Mayer, R. J. Gatchel, & P. B. Polatin (Eds.), *Occupational musculoskeletal disorders: Function, outcomes, and evidence* (pp. 3–8). Philadelphia: Lippincott Williams & Wilkins.

Gatchel, R. J., & Okifuji, A. (2006). Evidence-based scientific data documenting the treatment- and cost-effectiveness of comprehensive pain programs for chronic nonmalignant pain. *The Journal of Pain, 7*(11), 779–793.

Gatchel, R. J., Peng, Y., et al. (2007). The biopsychosocial approach to chronic pain: Scientific advances and future directions. *Psychological Bulletin, 133*, 581–624.

Gatchel, R. J., Polatin, P. B., et al. (2003). Treatment- and cost-effectiveness of early intervention for acute low back pain patients: A one-year prospective study. *Journal of Occupational Rehabilitation, 13*, 1–9.

Gatchel, R. J., & Rollings, K. H. (2008). Evidence-based review of the efficacy of cognitive-behavioral therapy for the treatment of chronic low back pain. *The Spine Journal, 8*, 40–44.

Glaros, A. G., & Lumley, M. A. (2005). Alexithymia and pain in temporomandibular disorder. *Journal of Psychosomatic Research, 59*(2), 85–88.

Hanley, M. A., Raichle, K., et al. (2008). Pain catastrophizing and beliefs predict changes in pain interference and psychological functioning in persons with spinal cord injury. *The Journal of Pain, 9*(9), 863–871.

Hirsh, A. T., George, S. Z., et al. (2008). Fear of pain, pain catastrophizing, and acute pain perception: Relative prediction and timing of assessment. *The Journal of Pain, 9*(9), 806–812.

Hjermstad, M., Haugen, D. F., Bennett, M. I., & Kaasa, S. (2011). Pain assessment tools in palliative care and cancer. In R. J. Moore (Ed.), *Handbook of pain and palliative care*. New York: Springer.

Jensen, M. P., & Karoly, P. (1991). Control beliefs, coping efforts, and adjustment to chronic pain. *Journal of Consulting and Clinical Psychology, 59*(3), 431–438.

Karjalainen, K., Malmivaara, A., et al. (2004). Min-intervention for subacute low back pain: Two-year follow-up and modifiers of effectiveness. *Spine, 10*, 1069–1076.

Katon, W., Egan, K., et al. (1985). Chronic pain: Lifetime psychiatric diagnoses and family history. *The American Journal of Psychiatry, 142*, 1156–1160.

Katz, J. N., & Melzack, R. (1990). Pain "memories" in phantom limbs: Review and clinical observations. *Pain, 43*, 319–336.

Keogh, E., & Eccleston, C. (2006). Sex differences in adolescent chronic pain and pain-related coping. *Pain, 123*(3), 275–284.

Kerns, R. D., Rosenberg, R., et al. (1994). Anger expression and chronic pain. *Journal of Behavioral Medicine, 17*(1), 57–67.

Kinney, R. K., Gatchel, R. J., et al. (1993). Prevalence of psychopathology in acute and chronic low back pain patients. *Journal of Occupational Rehabilitation, 3*(2), 95–103.

Kutner, J. S., & Smith, M. S. (2011). CAM in chronic pain and palliative care. In R. J. Moore (Ed.), *Handbook of pain and palliative care*. New York: Springer.

Lethem, J., Slade, P. D., et al. (1983). Outline of a fear-avoidance model of exaggerated pain perception-I. *Behaviour Research and Therapy, 21*(4), 401–408.

Mayer, T. G., & Gatchel, R. J. (1988). *Functional restoration for spinal disorders: The sports medicine approach*. Philadelphia: Lea & Febiger.

Mayer, T. G., Gatchel, R. J., et al. (1985). Objective assessment of spine function following industrial injury: A prospective study with comparison group and one-year follow-up. *Spine, 10*, 482–493.

Mayer, T. G., Gatchel, R. J., et al. (1987). A prospective two-year study of functional restoration in industrial low back injury. An objective assessment procedure. *JAMA: The Journal of American Medical Association, 258*(13), 1763–1767 [published erratum appears in JAMA 1988 Jan 8;259(2):220].

Mayer, T., Gatchel, R., et al. (1999). Outcomes comparison of treatment for chronic disabling work-related upper extremity disorders. *Journal of Occupational and Environmental Medicine, 41*, 761–770.

Mayer, T. G., Gatchel, R. J., et al. (2006). Postinjury rehabilitation management. In W. S. Marras & W. Karwowski (Eds.), *The occupational ergonomics handbook: Intervention, controls and applications in occupational ergonomics*. CRC: Boca Raton, FL.

McCracken, L. M., Gauntlett-Gilbert, J., et al. (2007). The role of mindfulness in a contextual cognitive-behavioral analysis of chronic pain-related suffering and disability. *Pain, 131*(1–2), 63–69.

McCrea, H., Wright, M. E., et al. (2000). Psychosocial factors influencing personal control in pain relief. *International Journal of Nursing Studies, 37*(6), 493–503.

McEwen, B. S. (1998). Protective and damaging effects of stress mediators. *The New England Journal of Medicine, 338*, 171–179.

McMahon, M. J., Gatchel, R. J., et al. (1997). Early childhood abuse in chronic spinal disorder patients. A major barrier to treatment success. *Spine, 22*(20), 2408–2415.

Melzack, R. (1993). Pain: Past, present and future. *Canadian Journal of Experimental Psychology, 47*(4), 615–629.

Melzack, R. (1999). From the gate to the neuromatrix. *Pain. Supplement, 6*, S121–126.

Melzack, R. (2005). Evolution of the neuromatrix theory of pain. *Pain Practice, 5*, 85–94.

Melzack, R., & Casey, K. L. (1968). Sensory, motivational, and central control determinants of pain: A new conceptual model. In D. Kenshalo (Ed.), *The skin senses* (pp. 423–443). Springfield: Thomas.

Melzack, R., & Wall, P. D. (1965). Pain mechanisms: A new theory. *Science, 50*, 971–979.

Nathan, P. W. (1976). The gate control theory of pain: A critical review. *Brain, 99*, 123–158.

Naylor, M. R., Seminowicz, D. A., Somers, T. J., & Keefe, F. J. (2011). Pain imaging. In R. J. Moore (Ed.), *Handbook of pain and palliative care*. New York: Springer.

Okifuji, A., Turk, D. C., et al. (1999). Clinical outcomes and economic evaluation of multidisciplinary pain centers. In A. R. Block, E. F. Kremer, & E. Fernandez (Eds.), *Handbook of pain syndromes* (pp. 169–191). Mahwah, NJ: Lawrence Erlbaum.

Palermo, Y. (2011). The art of pain: the patient's perspective of chronic pain. In R. J. Moore (Ed.), *Handbook of pain and palliative care*. New York: Springer.

Parrish, B. P., Zautra, A. J., et al. (2008). The role of positive and negative interpersonal events on daily fatigue in women with fibromyalgia, rheumatoid arthritis, and osteoarthritis. *Health Psychology, 27*(6), 694–702.

Polatin, P. B., Kinney, R. K., et al. (1993). Psychiatric illness and chronic low-back pain. The mind and the spine – Which goes first? *Spine, 18*(1), 66–71.

Reich, J., Rosenblatt, R., et al. (1983). DSM-III: A new nomenclature for classifying patients with chronic pain. *Pain, 16*, 201–206.

Roy, R. (2008). *Psychosocial interventions for chronic pain: In search of evidence*. New York: Springer.

Samwel, H. J. A., Evers, A. W. M., et al. (2006). The role of helplessness, fear of pain, and passive pain-coping in chronic pain patients. *The Clinical Journal of Pain, 22*(3), 245–251. doi:210.1097/1001.ajp.0000173019.0000172365.f0000173015.

Schmidt, R. F. (1972). The gate control theory of pain: An unlikely hypothesis. In R. Jansen, W. D. Keidel, A. Herzet, et al. (Eds.), *Pain: Basic principles, pharmacology, therapy* (pp. 57–71). Stuttgart: Thieme.

Seligman, M. E. P. (1975). *Helplessness: On depression, development and death*. San Francisco: Freeman.

Severeijns, R., Vlaeyen, J. W. S., et al. (2001). Pain catastrophizing predicts pain intensity, disability, and psychological distress independent of the level of physical impairment. *The Clinical Journal of Pain, 17*(2), 165–172.

Short, R., III, & Vetter, T. R. (2011). Acute to chronic pain: transitions in the post surgical patient. In R. J. Moore (Ed.), *Handbook of pain and palliative care*. New York: Springer.

Tan, G., Jensen, M. P., et al. (2008). Negative emotions, pain, and functioning. *Psychological Services, 5*(1), 26–35.

Tennen, H., Affleck, G., et al. (2006). Depression history and coping with chronic pain: A daily process analysis. *Health Psychology, 25*(3), 370–379.

Turk, D. C., & Monarch, E. S. (2002). Biopsychosocial approaches on chronic pain. In R. J. Gatchel & D. C. Turk (Eds.), *Psychological approaches to pain management: A practitioner's handbook* (pp. 3–29). New York: Guilford.

Turner, J. A., Jensen, M. P., et al. (2000). Do beliefs, coping, and catastrophizing independently predict functioning in patients with chronic pain? *Pain, 85*, 115–125.

Turner, J. A., Mancl, L., et al. (2006). Short- and long-term efficacy of brief cognitive-behavioral therapy for patients with chronic temporomandibular disorder pain: A randomized, controlled trial. *Pain, 121*, 181–194.

Velly, A. M., Chen, H., Ferreira, J. R., & Friction, J. R. (2011). Temporomandibular disorders and fibromyalgia. In R. J. Moore (Ed.), *Handbook of pain and palliative care*. New York: Springer.

Wall, P. D. (1989). The dorsal horn. In P. D. Wall, P. D. Wall, R. Melzack, & R. Melzack (Eds.), *Textbook of pain* (pp. 102–111). New York: Churchill Livingstone.

White, K. L., Williams, F., et al. (1961). The etiology of medical care. *The New England Journal of Medicine, 265*, 885–886.

Woodwell, D. A. (2000). *National ambulatory medical survey: 1998 Summary advanced data from vital and health statistics no. 315*. Hyattsville, MO: National Center for Health Statistics.

Part I
Communication and Pain

Chapter 2
Pain and Intercultural Communication

James Hallenbeck

Introduction

Pain is a universal experience, suffered in isolation. At the most basic level, pain serves a useful function in alerting organisms to threats to bodily integrity. In more advanced, social animals such as chimpanzees, communication regarding pain may enhance the chance for survival as others are enlisted in defense and support of the individual. In humans, communication obviously takes on far greater levels of complexity as potential responses to communicated pain are so varied and nuanced. Still, at its core communication about pain is driven by the need for assistance from others.

In this chapter, we will examine communication about chronic pain through the lens of intercultural communication. Intercultural communication as a field offers a useful perspective that may heighten awareness of common pitfalls that frequently give rise to miscommunication. I will then suggest some strategies that should minimize the risk or severity of miscommunication in the context of pain.

Much of the literature about pain communication, including work on survey instruments and pain scales, has focused on trying to determine pain severity, the qualitative characteristics of pain, and at times the veracity of pain complaints. Driving this literature is an understandable desire to characterize the underlying physiology giving rise to a pain complaint, so that therapy can most appropriately and effectively be delivered. Cross-cultural work in this vein often seeks to determine the transferability of survey instruments among cultural groups (Gaston-Johansson et al. 1990; Zatzick and Dimsdale 1990; Thomas and Rose 1991; Cleeland and Ryan 1994; Chaudakshetrin et al. 2007). This is admirable and necessary, but efforts in this vein fall short in a most basic way. Such approaches tend to perceive language and culture as barriers or veils, which must be broached in order to locate an underlying biologic reality (Cleeland and Ryan 1994). While this may be reasonable at a certain level of physiology, such reductionism neglects the fact that pain as an experience is inexorably interwoven with culture and that for humans language is essential in giving voice to such experience (Pugh 1991; Im et al. 2009; Schiavenato and Craig 2010).

Cross-cultural misunderstandings can indeed obscure formal medical diagnoses. However, it is also true is that any episode of communication about pain represents its own truth within a cultural context and such truth is correlated with but independent of biologic reality (Fruend 1990; Trnka 2007).

J. Hallenbeck, MD (✉)
Division of General Medical Disciplines, Department of Medicine,
Stanford University School of Medicine, Stanford, CA, USA

VA Palo Alto Health Care Services, Palo Alto, CA, USA

R.J. Moore (ed.), *Handbook of Pain and Palliative Care: Biobehavioral Approaches for the Life Course*,
DOI 10.1007/978-1-4419-1651-8_2, © Springer Science+Business Media, LLC 2012

This truth usually represents in part a request for some response from others within the context of a particular relationship in a particular culture. The response may be behavioral, the administration of some aid or medication, or relational, as through a demonstration of empathy (Goubert et al. 2005). For example, if a person with a history of substance abuse purposely lies about pain with a goal of getting some drug, there certainly is a problem in the episode of communication in terms of biologic veracity. However, the communication is still "truthful" or at least real in terms of being a request from one person to another for a desired response. Such a request is made in the context of a social and regulatory system that gives access to such drugs to a select few.

The emphasis in many survey instruments on severity of pain and its biologic origin is itself a cultural construct of biomedicine, which prioritizes physiologic causality over more social aspects of experience (Hahn 1995, Kleinman 1995; Fabrega 1997; Hallenbeck 2007). In any such instrument, particular aspects of pain communication are to be elicited to the exclusion of others. Survey instruments, then, represent a culturally sanctioned form of forced communication, albeit with beneficent intent, which may or may not serve the purposes of individuals experiencing pain.

High and Low Context Communication

Intercultural communication is a field of anthropology, first developed by Edward Hall (1976, 1983, 1990, 1997). Hall noted that human interactions and related communication can be broadly classified as being high or low in their cultural context. High context communication embeds large amounts of meaning within the situation or context within which communication occurs. Where people are when they are communicating, who is present, and how they position themselves relative to one another are all parts of the context in which a message is delivered, interpreted, and received. High context communication is thus *relational*. That is, a major goal of such communication is to affect in some way the relationship of those participating in it. Relational goals may include establishment or clarification of the relationship. They may also relate to a request for some change in behavior or assistance. In everyday life, courtship behavior such as dating is an example of an inherently high context encounter. Low context communication, in contrast, is concrete, situation specific, and task-oriented and involves minimal relational work. Such communication is usually straightforward and relatively unambiguous. Asking for street directions is an example of low context communication.

Hall noted that serious cross-cultural misunderstandings can occur when people using low context communication styles interact with others using high context communication styles (or where people using very different high context styles interact with one another). Different ethnic groups may prefer relatively higher or lower contextual communication styles. Certain groups, most notably those of Northern European descent, are believed to be relatively lower in contextual style than others, such as Southern Europeans or Asians (Samovar and Porter 1997). Clashes can occur among individuals from different ethnic groups, based in part on their differing communication styles in this regard. However, cross-cultural clashes can also occur within relatively homogenous ethnic groups. A case in point can be seen commonly in encounters between clinicians, acculturated to the low context world of biomedicine and the lay public, who tend to experience sickness as relational, high context events, regardless of ethnicity (Hallenbeck 2006; Hallenbeck and Periyakoil 2009). Both high and low context approaches to sickness make sense within their particular cultural framings. A scientific, physiology-driven understanding of *disease* allows for a very precise and often effective optimization of medical therapies. Low context communication includes math, computer, code, and scientific and medical language. It often works better across linguistic groups and cultures precisely because it avoids complex and confounding meanings associated with ordinary language. For instance, the use of pain scores as a means of communicating pain severity via mathematical symbols (1–10) is a low context means of communication, which offers a real advantage in this regard. A Likert scale between 1 and 10 means pretty much the same thing in all languages and cultural groups. In contrast, high context communication about sickness also makes sense in that *illness* (as opposed to a disease) almost always affects more than one person. Serious illness usually involves an alteration in the relations among closely linked individuals. The sick person becomes dependent upon others, clinicians, family members, and caregivers, for a wide range of needs. High and low context approaches to sickness make sense in their own realms; and ideally these two approaches are complementary and synergistic. However, at worst, what is risked is people talking past another and serious miscommunication.

In terms of intercultural communication, pain is a particularly interesting topic. Like all symptoms pain is by definition a subjective phenomenon. The definition of pain according to International Association for the Study of Pain (IASP) suggests the nature of the problem:

> Pain has been defined as an unpleasant sensory and emotional experience associated with actual or potential tissue damage, or described in terms of such damage. Note: The inability to communicate verbally does not negate the possibility that an individual is experiencing pain and is in need of appropriate pain-relieving treatment. Pain is always subjective (2010).

As this quote states, pain is a subjective biopsychosocial experience, which may or may not be associated with tissue damage. As a symptom, pain is unusual in its variable correlation with objective reality (tissue damage). By contrast, patients with nausea or dyspnea usually have clear objective markers associated with their symptoms. The cautionary note regarding communication points to difficulties linking subjective experiences with objective reality. One could also add that when pain *has* been communicated, it does not necessarily mean that tissue damage has occurred. When no association with tissue damage is found, what does this mean? Does it mean that such an association is present, but clinicians have missed it? Is the "unpleasant experience" being described properly in terms of pain but with no tissue damage? In this instance is the usage of the word pain takes on metaphoric implications. Or, is the person claiming pain not having an unpleasant experience and is in effect lying?

Tissue damage suggests the need for a low context approach to healing. The machine is broken and repairs are in order. Where repair is not possible, a "system override" is needed, where the brain is told to ignore the blinking red panic light. The subjective and often emotional experience of pain in contrast cries out for connection with others in hopes of finding assistance and relief or, where relief is inadequate, at least some degree of empathy and understanding and is thus high context (Biro 2010). Pain, then, is both a high and low context event, requiring both technical and relational expertise for optimal treatment.

In some conditions, common experience leaves little question as to whether tissue damage has occurred. Patients with acute and obvious wounds, burns, and broken bones rarely need to convince others of the severity or veracity of their pain. Cries of anguish and grimacing erupt spontaneously in such severe pain, even in the absence of another person. The objective reality of trauma and the subjective cry for help present as one coherent message. However, in many pain states often classified as chronic pains, there may be little correlation between objective markers of tissue damage and subjective experience of pain and suffering, even where the associated suffering is every bit as real and great (Hadjistavropoulos and Craig 1994). Curiously, one would think that it is precisely in such cases that individuals would want to communicate verbally their distress to others, if for no other reason than to compensate for the lack of physical stigmata validating their complaints. And yet, clinicians often see the exact opposite. Patients with chronic pain tend to withdraw. They do not cry out.

Acute and Chronic Pain in Evolutionary Terms

> Pain is obviously a fundamental biological property of evolved species that is replete with significant information regarding the need states of an organism and its capacity for adaptive behavior. It constitutes a hallmark of sickness and can elicit caring and nurturing. Fabrega (1997, p. 62).

Let us consider more closely the puzzle presented by the nature of pain. Why is it that when pain is most obvious, people scream the loudest and when pain is least obvious, they are often silent? Such a communication strategy makes sense in evolutionary terms, as highlighted by the experience of nonhuman, social animals. In calling out with acute injury, a social animal alerts other members of the herd of an immediate and urgent need for defense and support. Other members of the group may not only provide defense (e.g., against an attacking animal), but may be able to provide immediate pain relief (as in taking a thorn out of a foot). Both the vocal and nonverbal communication of pain and the social response of "sympathetic pain" (feeling pain or discomfort in seeing another wounded and in pain) appear instinctual and transcultural in their prevalence (Prkachin 1992; Otti et al. 2010; Williams 2002; Goubert et al. 2005; Frith 2009). By way of example, Botvinick and colleagues demonstrated through magnetic resonance imaging similar patterns of cortical stimulation in volunteers viewing facial expressions of pain as occurred in them during thermally induced pain (Botvinick et al. 2005). How then to explain the withdrawal and silence so common in many chronic pains?

Many pains characterized as "chronic" are in fact better characterized by their representing in fact or metaphorically certain types of deep tissue pain. Temporal longevity of a pain episode (acute versus chronic) is variably correlated with this type of pain for which we lack a commonly accepted word in English. Headaches offer a very good case in point. Most headaches, while temporally of a short (acute) duration, do not give rise to vocal outbursts, but rather often result in withdrawal and relative quiet typical of "chronic pain." Withdrawal in evolutionary terms would be an appropriate response to bodily damage involving certain deep tissues. In animals and in ancient times for people the best chance for survival would have been hiding out and waiting for internal healing, if possible, to occur. Others would be less likely to be of immediate assistance. Indeed, there may have been some survival benefit attached to keeping a low profile. In such situations, communication between the sick individual and other members of the herd or tribe would be less urgent. Such communication to the extent it existed would likely transmit the importance of keeping quiet and being less, rather than more visible.

While primitive people often had little to offer medically to treat conditions giving rise to such chronic [sic] pains, they were generally able to provide support, such as food, water, and shelter, to the sick individual, while they waited to heal. Following traumatic injury, after the initial, spontaneous crying out of acute pain, tissue damage is often so obvious that further evocation or communication would seen unnecessary for the purpose of enlisting ongoing support and exemption from one's usual social duties. However, for chronic pain, the opposite is the case. Precisely because there is no obvious stigmata of tissue damage, language offers a means for communicating the internal experience of pain, eliciting needed support, and justifying exemptions from social duties. Thus, while chronic pain may not provoke as immediate and guttural a cry as acute pain tends to do, if anything the need for verbal communication is far greater.

One could make the argument, based on the above, that we are "hard-wired" in our responses to acute pain. That is, we are programmed to respond viscerally to images and vocalizations of acute pain. The more horrific the image, the louder the vocalization, the more immediate and intense our instinctual response. Put simply, we are pretty good at "seeing" and empathetically responding to acute pain. In contrast, for equally valid reasons in evolutionary terms we are "color-blind" to certain "chronic" pains. We cannot "see" them and our empathetic responses to such pains are blunted.

A small study highlights the above point. In a study of "gold standard" (thought to be truthful in their pain complaints), cancer patients' clinicians and caregivers (mostly family members) spent time talking with patients in varying degrees of pain (Grossman 1991). They were not allowed to speak specifically about the pain. Patients, clinicians, and caregivers were then asked to rate the pain using a 0–10 scale. Concordance between patient-reported pain and other's assessment was then noted. The results are included in a table below.

Patients' assessments correlated with those of	0–2 Little or no pain (%)	3–6 Moderate pain (%)	7–10 Severe pain (%)
Nurse	82	51	7
House Officer	66	26	21
Oncology Fellow	70	29	27
Caregiver	79	37	13

What can be seen is that when patients had little or no pain, concordance by clinicians (nurse, house officer, oncology fellow) and caregivers (people who knew the patient well) was fairly good. However, these observers were unable to recognize more severe states of pain. These results are rather the opposite of what we might imagine were the study to be replicated with acute, traumatic pain. In acute pain we can easily imagine great concordance between subjects and observers. The study is also interesting because it dispels two common myths; that if a person just "knew" the patient better, they would be better at recognizing severe pain. Caregivers were in fact less accurate than the physicians. Another myth is that people in more sensitive, empathetic positions (nurses, caregivers) should do better than "less sensitive" task-oriented people, like physicians. In fact, nobody was very good at "seeing" the severe, chronic pain of the patient.

The problem is actually worse than this. In many cases we are not only color-blind to chronic pain, we are blind to our blindness. Because we are so good at recognizing and responding to acute pain, we come to believe we are able to recognize pain in all forms. The common resistance by clinicians to efforts to get them to repeatedly inquire about pain using pain scores, for example, can be understood not so much as objection to the notion that pain is bad and ought to be treated but rather as a deeper resistance to the apparently absurd notion that we need to ask about what should be so obvious (Biro 2010, p. 13; Young and Davidhizar 2008).[1]

High and Low Context Pain Communication

Communication regarding acute pain is relatively low in context, even when help is requested from others. The guttural cry of acute pain is straightforward, task-oriented, and works well across very divergent cultures and language groups. As noted earlier, biomedicine, as a subculture, tends to favor low context communication. Numbers, data, and images are valued over words and meaning. Fabrega, who has written extensively on the evolution of sickness and healing, notes that modern medicine has become quite skilled at alleviating most acute symptoms such as pain, but less skilled in alleviating the distress and suffering associated with chronic illness (Fabrega 1997). Chronic pain would be included among such distress. In part this undoubtedly reflects physiologically based difficulties in alleviating certain chronic conditions such as neuropathic pain. However, in part it may also be that low context, biomedical clinicians are more comfortable responding to the low context communication of those in acute pain and conversely less comfortable responding to more complex, high context communication typical of chronic pain. One could argue that greater comfort in response

---

[1] In the healthcare system within which I work pain scores have been mandated as "the fifth vital sign" for over a decade. Objections to this policy first arose based on the technical and rather trivial point that pain is a *symptom*, not a sign. In watching many case presentations by residents in training and other physicians it is extremely rare to see pain presented as a vital sign (following pulse, respiration, temperature, and blood pressure), despite this official policy. Rather, the oxygen saturation number, which is new fifth vital sign is eminently measureable, fills this role.

to acute pain communication reflects not only relatively greater efficacy of treatment and certainty of diagnosis, but also a more favorable reimbursement structures, at least in fee-for-services healthcare systems. However, such reimbursement systems are themselves a product of a society that values low context certainty and unambiguous results over high context relationships. The common aversion to patients with chronic pain goes beyond such practicalities. The inherently high context nature of interactions with individuals suffering chronic pain may be threatening for clinicians, who understandably seek clear boundaries between person and professional personae. Given current limitations in our ability to "cure" chronic pain and the common public perception that such cure is a reasonable expectation of care, clinicians may fear getting caught up in a sticky web of protracted interactions.

Let us then consider such high context communications in more detail. As has been stressed earlier, high context communication is primarily relational. However, the nature of such relationships varies from ones of the provision of basic aid or simple defense to extremely complex relationships based on empathy, mutual understanding, and even politics, enacted through mutually constructed narratives.

In discrete encounters, relational work is often interwoven with task-oriented work. Such relational work often manifests as a set of subtexts to the "text" of verbal communication, which often revolves around concrete, low context medical tasks. Common relational/high context subtexts include (among others):

- Trust
- Respect
- Obligation
- Affect (gratitude, anger, etc.) relative to the other person
- Empathy and mutual understanding
- Specialness
- Empathy and mutual understanding
- Legitimacy of pain complaint/sick role
- Power

While these subtexts are presented as discrete categories, considerable overlap exists among them. Trust, respect, and empathy, for example, overlap. Let us consider these categories in more detail and highlight them with relevant examples in pain management. For illustrative purposes we will consider here relationships between providers and patients, although these subtexts also exist in other relationships (e.g., among family members).

Trust: Trust exists relative to distrust. Trust relates to truthfulness or veracity of the pain complaint, but also to the ability of participants to abide by social contracts. Such contracts may be formally codified in written form as may be done with opioid agreements (Heit). However, the use of such agreements does not mean that true trust exists. It is often quite the opposite. Where such contracts are thought necessary almost by definition trust is questionable, at best. Indeed, where the use of such agreements is mandated by the clinician, this is more a display of differential power than a marker of trust. Still, as Heit notes, "Opioid agreements have the potential to improve the therapeutic relationship." (p. 376) While much writing, especially as relates to pain management in substance abuse, addresses the issue of trust and truthfulness of patients, trust or lack thereof is by definition a two-way street. Patients need to trust that they are respected, that clinicians have adequate competency to address their problems, and that clinicians will do so with due diligence. The "therapeutic relationship" Heit writes about to a large degree reflects an evolving, iterative, process in which trust is either built or damaged through interactions among participants. While trust/mistrust as an issue may be relatively overt, as in drug screening, more often, where mistrust exists it works as an unspoken subtext, played out as participants try to demonstrate their relative trustworthiness or question the trustworthiness of the other (Parsons et al. 2007).

Respect: Respect overlaps with trust, empathy, and an appreciation of specialness (Branch 2006). It differs somewhat from trust in that it is less tightly linked to truthfulness. Respect requires an appreciation for the other, which may exist even if and where the other is quite foreign, even though evidence suggests respect tends to grow with familiarity (Beach et al. 2006). Disrespect, conversely, may be driven either by a negative past history with an individual or a negative experience or stereotype regarding a group or class the other person is perceived as representing. Disrespect or frank prejudice may be felt and displayed toward others based on race, religion, ethnicity, gender, sexual orientation, social or professional role – or any number of factors. While mistrust and distrust may reflect stereotyping or prejudice, they may also be rooted in the personal histories of individual clinicians and patients. Evidence suggests, for example, that African-Americans may receive substandard pain management, relative to other ethnic groups (Nampiaparampil et al. 2009). The reasons for this are likely very complex. Some clinicians may associate drug-seeking behavior with certain ethnic groups such as African-Americans, based both on stereotyping and perhaps past interactions with individuals that may have suggested a link between ethnicity and drug abuse. Conversely, some African-Americans may be all too aware of a history of substandard treatment and care for African-Americans and may have experienced discrimination in seeking medical care. Such experiences on both sides can sow the seeds of distrust, which can readily manifest in shows of disrespect, which insidiously can confirm underlying distrust. Conversely, respect can be demonstrated and expressed even in initial encounters, prior to any evolution of a trusting relationship, which takes time. Indeed, in most initial clinical encounters, the demonstration of mutual respect is the cornerstone upon which strong, trusting relationships are built.

Obligation: What is a "therapeutic relationship?" A therapeutic relationship is defined as a relationship that maximizes the possibility of healing of body, mind, and spirit. In the process of creating such a relationship some sense of personal closeness or bonding between clinician and patient is inevitable, even within their professional relationship. Obligation is a term rarely used in low context cultures, but is of great importance in high context encounters. It refers to an internal drive to respond to a need in another person by doing something positive or helpful. Obligation may exist as simply relative to an ascribed role. Thus, clinicians may speak of a *professional obligation* to treat patients beneficently and to do as little harm as possible. However, obligation is also very personal, based on prior interactions among people. If previously a person responds positively and does some good for another, then the other may feel a sense of indebtedness to this person. In "returning the favor" to this person, mutual obligation is built. Such mutual obligation acts rather like a social glue binding people together. In professional relationships, obligation may or may not be engendered simply by doing one's job. Relieving a patient's pain (and in turn being thanked and paid for this service) may foster some sense of mutual obligation – or not – if such work is viewed merely as an equal trade or barter transaction. Personal obligation is more reliably fostered if and when something outside the expected role is done. Thus, for example if a clinician "goes out of the way" (beyond formal role expectations) to do something good for a patient (get a blanket, e.g., for a cold inpatient or gives a patient their personal cell phone number), then a sense of obligation is likely to be fostered.

Affect: Emotions are present in many clinical encounters as a subtext. This is readily apparent in facial expression. People smile or frown. They speak with anger or fear, or perhaps the voice and body language suggest comfort, trust, and positive feelings toward the other. This is entirely natural. As with other subtexts, in clinical encounters emotions tend to arise while addressing task-oriented work, such as clinical assessment, procedures, or information giving. Studies suggest that many physicians encountering emotions during such encounters will tend to focus on the cognitive or medical tasks at hand, rather than address the emotion directly (Suchman et al. 1997; Detmar et al. 2001). This may be because clinicians feel they are in a stronger position when dealing with technical matters, but it may also be because clinicians believe it is unprofessional (outside their role) to deal with the emotions of the other or their own feelings. Most clinicians lack formal training on how best to deal with strong emotions either in patients or themselves (Parle et al. 1997). Even simple skills such as mirroring techniques ("You seem angry [or afraid or whatever] … ") can be of help if and when strong emotions are present and need to be openly recognized and adequately discussed.

Specialness: We all want to be thought to be special in some way, which we may label "specialness." When we are in trouble or sick, as when we are in pain, the desire for recognition of our specialness grows stronger. This seems particularly so in our modern world, where healthcare is more an impersonal industry than a unique relationship between healer and patient. The need for such recognition tends to be even greater if one belongs to an underclass group, such as minority or other disenfranchised population, including chronic pain patients (Haugli et al. 2004). Such a need may also be greater where the particular illness is one that is questioned or held in low esteem in society. Patients with certain forms of chronic pain or substance abuse, and patients lacking mental capacity, as in those with retardation or dementia, are examples of such patient classes. However, most all of us feel this in our roles as patients. We want clinicians who recognize our uniqueness and importance not just as a matter of ego aggrandizement, but for very practical reasons.

Special patients get better care: Explicit recognition of specialness is a great way to display respect and to build strong relationships, although at times limits need to be placed if and when specialness spills over into entitlement. An example of such recognition might be, "I've treated many patients with your condition, but I know they are not you and that each person's situation is unique. I want to understand your situation so I can better help you (as compared to treating the disease)." Practically speaking, patients want clinicians to recognize specialness by devoting adequate allocation of time and energy to their cases. Most people are aware, I believe, that clinician time is very limited and they reasonably worry that they might be short-changed. However, as important as time is, the relative attention or energy a clinician invests in a case or encounter is just as important. Most patients can readily tell if a clinician is really focused on them and their needs or is distracted by other thoughts.

Empathy and mutual understanding: Empathy and mutual understanding arise from an existential and practical paradox. In being empathetic and understanding of the other we must appreciate that individual as a unique person and yet must also ground ourselves in some commonality of being (Goubert et al. 2005; Moore and Hallenbeck 2010). The need to be understood both at cognitive and emotional levels is a very advanced human trait. Patients living with pain, especially chronic pain, experience their pain as a part of a rich and complex narrative. Such narratives, like any good play, have various actors, heroes and villains, plot twists, and often morals. Narratives progress over time. The complexities of such stories present real challenges for patients and clinicians, given the limited time available in real-world clinical encounters. Patients, driven by a need to be understood, often work very hard to figure out how best to encapsulate their complex experiences into a few short phrases – rather like trying to tell an epic poem in haiku form. They are variably successful. Some patients actually writing out the epic in long form, in hopes the clinician will take the time to read the entire document. This is rarely a successful strategy. Often, patients use metaphor, a compressed form of speech, to try to explain themselves (Biro 2010; Scarry 1985) The use of metaphor is a high context mode of communication, in that it is based on both speaker and listener sharing a common understanding of the metaphor's meaning. For example, if a patient said, "I feel like Sisyphus. Every time I make a little progress, the rock rolls over me," this could be a very effective means of communicating frustration and a lack of progress, despite great effort. However, metaphor depends on a common understanding of implied meanings. The Sisyphus metaphor is meaningless if the listener is unfamiliar with the story of Sisyphus.

Specific to pain, Biro and others point to yet another paradox: The need to give voice to that which is unspeakable (Biro 2010). Pain is beyond words. Elaine Scarry goes further in noting that severe pain "unmakes" peoples' social worlds (Scarry 1985). And yet, for both practical reasons, discussed earlier in terms of survival value, and existential reasons there is an overwhelming drive to transcend the subjective isolation of pain. Biro and Scarry both highlight the importance of meta-phor as means to this end. The best we can do in trying to help others understand and relate to our pain is to try to invoke some common image. Metaphors often relate to external weapons, such as a knife, or violent actions, such as stabbing, shooting, burning, tearing, or crushing. Such imagery can be useful in a low context way of directing a differential diagnosis. Beyond such practicality, meta-phor works to promote at least a semblance of common understanding, which in turn works to promote empathy (Moore and Hallenbeck 2010).

Clinicians may similarly be challenged in their efforts to communicate. Time restraints are an obvious problem, limiting their ability to attend to the patient. It is difficult to communicate often alien medical narratives, stories of how certain diseases come about and how associated disease plots may unfold. Clinicians may also resort to metaphor in trying to explain complex aspects of physiol-ogy. The other great challenge clinicians experience is that they too seek and appreciate empathy and understanding, although they may feel discouraged in their professional roles to admit or display such a need. Self-disclosure by a clinician, particularly of a weakness or vulnerability can be danger-ous in an highly litigious society, and to the extent it is overly self-serving, and unprofessional (Hallenbeck 2000). However, sometimes it is precisely the trust engendered in risking self-disclosure that patients need, if a deeper relationship is to develop. How is it that we, as clinicians, communicate to patients that while we cannot really "feel" their pain, we find some resonance with their suffering, as we too have experienced pain and have suffered? (Moore and Hallenbeck 2010) Sometimes, what is most therapeutic for patients is just knowing they are working with another real-life human being, who has his or her own narrative and associated vulnerabilities and limitations.

Legitimacy: Legitimacy is really a subset of specialness, but given its importance in pain manage-ment, I have expanded on this point at this time. Legitimacy is rarely considered openly by clinicians in thinking about healthcare, but it is very important given the relative value and attention paid to certain illnesses over others. Legitimacy of various illnesses differs among cultures and shifts over time[2] (Sontag 1978; Tishelman 1991). In our current medical culture, diseases that are *visible* – either directly or via scans, are *treatable* (preferably to cure), and viewed as *independent of indi-vidual responsibility* – due to "bad luck" or genes versus bad behavior, are favored over illnesses lacking these characteristics. In terms of pain management, consider by way of contrast pain due to acute trauma, as compared to chronic pain of unclear etiology. Is there any doubt that as a society we recognize the legitimacy of the prior over the latter? Especially in many cases involving chronic pain, the subtext of patients' communication seems often to revolve around trying to establish the legitimacy of their complaint (see also Palermo 2011). Such communication and behavior may take the form of "pseudoaddiction," as Weissman put it, which may manifest through rather unusual behaviors which may be misunderstood by clinicians as evidence of addiction, when in fact they are efforts toward recognition of legitimacy, tolerance to pain medications (e.g., opioids), and the need for adequate pain relief (Weissman and Haddox 1989; Weissman 1994). Conversely, where the patient's story is suspect, the subtext for many clinicians may be a questioning of legitimacy.

Power: Power differentials exist in most social interactions. In pain management, power differentials are particularly great. Pain is a most personal experience and yet, people suffering from pain gener-ally are not "in charge" of their own care; clinicians are. Such power differentials also exist else-where in healthcare, often because special technology or skill is required to address a specific concern, as in surgery. What is unusual about pain management is that most such care is low-tech. The general public has free access to acetaminophen, aspirin, and nonsterioidals, but for most every-thing else, especially controlled substances such as opioids, they are completely dependent on clini-cians. That is, to a very large degree we must depend upon others both to recognize the legitimacy

---

[2]See Sontag on the shifting view of cancer over time from an illness that was seen not only as a death sentence, but as something overtly shameful (Sontag 1978).

of our pain and provide relief from it.[3] Power differentials generally stay in the background in clinical care unless major disputes arise. In such cases, jostling for power positions may become a subtext to clinical encounters. Clinicians may stress their authority, through clinical role, competency/expertise, and law, to be the judges of who gets what therapy. Patients who disagree with clinical decisions may stress their "patient rights" and general autonomy. They may claim discrimination and stigma. Or they may argue from the position that their pain and associated suffering are ultimately unknowable by others. The subtext often seems to read, "It is *my* pain. You cannot possibly know what this is like. Why are you in charge of my suffering?" It is true. While pain may or may not be affirmed or even legitimized, it cannot be denied. As clinicians we may have the power to deny desired medications or therapies, but we can never be completely sure in our opinions as to whether or not pain is actually present.

Paradoxically, given this, patients do have a certain power. Precisely because objective markers for pain are lacking, it is impossible to prove that someone is *not* in pain. Kleinman has noted that complaints of pain may be one of a limited set of sanctioned means of protest within ascribed sick roles in certain social and political contexts. For example in China, as Kleniman explores, complaints of pain may represent a relatively acceptable form of protest against totalitarian aspects of society (Kleinman 1994). As such, complaints of pain may in part reflect an effort of disempowered individuals to be socially acknowledged and to gain some control over their lives. Again, here we must stress that in terms of communication the issue is not whether such complaints are or are not "real." Independent of any such reality complex dynamics of power exist for both clinicians and patients.[4]

There is nothing inherently wrong with the fact that power is an issue in encounters regarding pain. However, issues of power may escalate to frank battles at the level of discourse and practice, wounding patients and clinicians alike, if the subtext is not acknowledged and addressed in some meaningful way either through the subtext or by raising the subtext to the text. As discussed further below, when a subtext, power, or any other is addressed through (or within) the subtext, this means that the clinician, who is aware of such a subtext, modifies what he or she says or does in a manner that addresses the concern of the subtext, but without drawing explicit attention to that subtext. For example, in addressing a power subtext through the subtext the clinician might state his or her understanding of expectations and responsibilities for both his or herself and the patient. "Raising the subtext to the text" might be done by calling attention to a power struggle underway and explicitly addressing power concerns. For example, a physician might state, "We are struggling with who gets to decide what medicine is best for you. I understand that only you can really appreciate how much pain you are in. However, the state says that when I write a prescription, it is on my license. So I have a professional obligation to meet certain standards of care in doing so. I don't blame you for being frustrated with this, but, yes, I am in charge of determining how much and what medicine to give you. I will do my best to listen to you and weigh your concerns in making a decision."

While the above could be expanded upon and arguably other common relational themes could also be added, hopefully the reader gets the point. While such subtexts often play a significant role in high context clinical encounters, they usually remain in the subtext, and are therefore not acknowledged.

---

[3] As a palliative care physician, who teaches pain management to physicians-in-training, I am acutely aware that should I need opioids for some pain, I am completely at the mercy of such physicians and their colleagues for relief. While I can, if need be, prescribe my own blood pressure pills and many other medications (wisely or unwisely), I cannot prescribe for myself or my family opioids or other controlled substances. I am not suggesting that this is wrong, but given the well-documented lack of general competency in primary pain management, it is worrisome and a strong motivator for me as a teacher.

[4] Scarry presents a detailed discussion of legitimacy and power in relation to torture. Her thesis is that torture is not so much about information gathering as it is an attempt by a regime whose legitimacy is threatened to bolster legitimacy through the "unmaking" or de-legitimatizing the world of the dissident through a display of power and the induction of pain. While such a discussion is far from the field of clinical care, it graphically highlights the importance of legitimacy and power in any discussion about pain (Scarry 1985).

Too often they are the proverbial "elephants in the room" that nobody recognizes or talks about. Clinicians often do not address them with patients, despite their important roles. At the end of the chapter I will give some suggestions for how to deal more skillfully with these subtexts, when they do arise.

Pain Assessment Instruments

Let us now consider pain assessment instruments in light of the above. Such instruments serve very useful functions. Well-designed instruments allow us to better understand important aspects of pain experiences, such as severity, temporal variation, qualitative aspects of pain, and the impact of pain on functioning and quality of life (McDowell 2006). Instruments help us understand not only the experience of individuals, but to compare experiences and response to therapies across groups. They may serve as helpful reminders of good questions we might otherwise forget to ask in doing a pain assessment. As mentioned briefly earlier, by formal design, pain instruments are low in context as a means of communication in their focus on specific aspects of the pain experience and their task-oriented nature – working to answer specific questions, depending on the instrument. Their low context nature offers real advantages. While language and culture may serve as barriers cross-culturally, even these barriers are open to study. One can determine which words work or do not work across cultural groups, as many studies have demonstrated. The great attraction of the numerical pain score, arguably the assessment tool lowest in its contextual framing, is precisely that numbers tend to mean the same thing in all languages. But let us consider the cost of such low context approaches. By filtering communication through a prescribed form (the instrument) certain messages get through and others do not (Schiavenato and Craig 2010). While such filtering enables standardization and consistency, it is important to recognize that any such instrument is itself a product of culture. Certain questions and answers are valued to the exclusion of others. This may be problematic to the extent that pain instruments, including visual analogue or other pain scales, become imposed on patients as the approved means of communicating, even when such cultural imposition is done with beneficent intent (de Williams et al. 2000; see also Palermo 2011). Holen et al. reported on results from an expert panel on the relative importance of ten dimensions of pain assessment in palliative care – intensity, temporal pattern, treatment and exacerbating/relieving factors, location, treatment, interference with quality of life, quality, affect, duration, beliefs, and pain history in that order (Holen 2006). Reviewed instruments commonly neglected even such highly ranked dimensions temporal variation in pain (16%). No tools addressed all top five ranked dimensions (Dy 2009). We see in this rank ordering a prioritization of more disease-specific aspects of pain such as intensity and pain location. Aspects related more to patients' life narratives (effect on quality of life, beliefs, and pain history) were ranked less important. Pointing this out is not so much a criticism of this rank order (presumably patients are rather interested in the intensity of their pain) as a comment on the inevitable filtering that occurs in the use of such instruments. Relational issues between the patient and the particular clinician working with that patient are, as far as I know, NEVER a sanctioned or queried topic with the possible exception of general patient satisfaction surveys – despite the obvious importance of therapeutic relationships in healing. Even the few quality of care measures that have been developed deal with *process* issues (changes in treatment, follow-up) or more general patient satisfaction, not the specific relationship between the patient and treating clinician beyond perhaps asking how broadly satisfied patients are (Dy 2006; Lorenz 2006).

I have posited that by definition interactions relating to pain are inherently high context and relational. Does this mean that where pain assessment tools are used that these relational aspects of communication are negated? Hardly. Patients generally try to communicate their relational needs *through* and *around* such assessments. Consider the visual analogue pain score. The overt intent of the analogue pain score (and related instruments) is to facilitate communication of severity of pain at the moment the patient is being queried. It is rather like a "snapshot" of pain severity, useful in trending pain intensity and response to therapy. While this is precisely what the clinician desires through the use of this low context metaphor, this is not necessarily all the patient wishes to communicate. Pain can be monitored as a series of snapshots, but it is experienced as a continuum. In self-assessing their situations, patients tend to project from past experience through their current state and from there, into the future. The *trend*, whether things are getting better or worse, is not just an academic measure of severity or response to therapy (although this is important) but a critical element in assessing whether further help is needed or not and indeed it is an important factor in the greater issue of suffering. If pain is becoming difficult to bear and is worsening, then the perceived need for assistance becomes greater. Standard analogue scales in and of themselves contain no method of communicating this sense of urgency. Some pain assessment forms add on a question regarding the adequacy of pain relief and good interviewers may ask if current pain relief is "adequate" or if additional help is needed, but such queries goes beyond the narrowly defined meaning of a 0–10 pain score. So what, then, do patients do, if faced with the conundrum of trying to communicate a more urgent need? Certainly, they may do so by communicating *outside* the score – by more frequent, louder, more emphatic requests, or by nonverbal behaviors suggesting more severe pain, as they often do (Schiavenato and Craig 2010). However, they may also learn to communicate *through* the pain score (de Williams et al. 2000; Knotkova et al. 2004). Through an iterative series of interactions with clinicians they may learn that reporting certain pain scores gives rise to more predictable responses from clinicians. Knowing this, transmute the metaphor, using numbers to reflect the relative urgency of response desired, rather than pain intensity. From my observations, while there is significant variability among patients in this regard scores from 0 to 3 generally mean there is little urgency, 4–6, some urgency and 7+ great urgency. Patients may even report on a "0–10 scale" scores of 12 or 15, which, while mathematically absurd, accurately reflect desired urgency of response. Patients then become acculturated to the use of the pain and in turn co-opt the pain score metaphor and use it with their own meaning for their own purposes, which are not necessarily the same as clinicians' meanings and purposes. Patients likely vary in their use of scores for this purpose and the internal thresholds they set for determining relative urgency.

Intercultural Communication Skills in Pain Management

The discussion earlier would be little more than a philosophical rambling if it did not result in some changes in clinician communication and behavior. Some suggested strategies for doing so are outlined below. In the introduction, I suggested that serious miscommunication is a risk to the extent that clinicians do not understand or respond to high context messages from patients (and families). On the flip side, skillful use of high context communication skills can promote improved understanding, a deeper "therapeutic relationship," possibly time savings, and almost certainly better patient and clinician satisfaction.

Awareness. It may seem strange, but the most important communication skill related to this topic is awareness of contextual issues when they arise and subsequent classification into low and high context categories. In everyday life, high and low context communication "happens" largely out of consciousness. While this is adequate, indeed appropriate for everyday life, it is not adequate for good clinical care provided in situations, as in pain management, where low and high context styles frequently clash. Clinicians are advised to start by cultivating awareness of the task-oriented (low context) and relational (high context) aspects of their interactions. All the subtexts listed earlier are examples of high context issues that may arise. Additional, common, basic examples of task-oriented and relational events are listed in the table below.

Task-oriented communication	Relational communication
Clinical assessment and reassessment of disease process	Introductions and greetings
Communication regarding biologically directed disease treatment – medications, injections, blocks, etc.	Inquiry regarding nonbiological aspects of personhood
Patient education regarding medical aspects of disease process	Compliments, praise, statements of respect
Healthcare process issues – setting up follow-up appointments, billing, etc.	Use of metaphor

The following, brief vignette highlights how task-oriented and relational communication might intermingle in routine office practice.

Interaction	Interpretation
"Good morning Mrs. Smith. Nice to see you." "Nice to see you, Doctor"	Greeting. Positive affect toward other. Respect
"How is your back pain today? On a scale of 0–10, how much pain do you have?"	Clinical assessment
"About a 2. Those pills you gave me really helped. Thank you"	Low context response. Praise. Gratitude
"I'm glad. I know it has been hard for you. You have really hung in there with the treatment plan"	Positive affect toward other. Empathy. Praise
"Is the pain still going down your leg?"	Clinical assessment

Of course, in real life things are more complicated, especially where negative or threatening subtexts arise. However, the basic skills of awareness and classification still serve. Having become more aware, the clinician can make conscious *choices* as to how best to respond (as compared to responding automatically or semiconsciously). Some common choices to be made are:

- Address highlight relational issues (or not)
- Expand current lines of communication or truncate them and switch to another line
- Raise subtexts to "texts" or deal with them within the subtext

Highlight relational issues: Probably the simplest thing a clinician can do is to look for opportunities to say and do things that promote positive relationships. One exercise is to observe and reflect on the percentage of time spent on task-oriented issues relative to relational issues. In many, arguably most situations the task issues are the priority and will quite appropriately take the bulk of time. However, the clinician is encouraged to increase somewhat the quantity and quality of relational comments made. Statements of respect and praise go a long way. Brief inquiries and statements regarding nonmedical aspects of a patient serve both as statements of respect, but also are evidence of the clinician's recognition of the patient's personhood. Stating explicitly your intent and obligation to do good and be helpful is encouraged. When sad or difficult emotions arise, you may wish to share them with the goal of demonstrating your caring and humanness. If, for example, a procedure does not have the desired effect, consider sharing your regret, given your desire to do good.

Expansion, truncation, and switch: In the vignette above notice where the physician expanded on the relational thread started by the patient in thanking the doctor. The physician continues on this line and offers praise in return. However, with the sentence, "You have really hung in there," this line of conversation is truncated, followed by a switch back to clinical assessment. A common error made by clinicians is to miss cues or opportunities to continue or expand on a particular thread – even where such is clearly indicated (Suchman et al. 1997).[5] The clinician may stubbornly stay on a low context thread (often clinical assessment), even where the patient has signaled a desire for a shift, as the following vignette highlights:

Physician: "On a scale of 0–10, how bad is your pain?"
Patient: "About a 9. Doctor, I don't know if I can stand it anymore. Nothing you seem to do makes any difference. When I finally get to sleep, I wish I just wouldn't wake up … "
Physician: "Uh-huh. That's too bad. Have you been doing your exercises as ordered?"

This example is a caricature, but in real life clinicians often miss cues as presented here that some expansion on a thread is needed. The patient statement at a minimum requires clarification of the ambiguous statement about "not waking up." Is this suicidality or the patient's way of communicating the severity of suffering and perhaps frustration with therapy as prescribed by this physician to date? Beyond this, the patient's statement practically begs for expansion of the relational thread. Note, the challenge to the physician; nothing *you* do makes any difference. The statement calls for at least an empathic response beyond, "Uh-huh, that's too bad." The physician may choose to raise this subtext (questioning the physician's skill and interest) to the text or may choose to address it within the subtext. An example of continuing this thread and raising the subtext might be:

I'm sorry to hear you are having such a difficult time. It sounds like you are frustrated that the therapies we've tried to date have not worked. I'm frustrated too, as I want you to feel better. I wouldn't blame you if you were upset with me (*raising the subtext to the text*) because the pills haven't worked. You need to know I'll keep trying to find something that helps. I hope you will keep trying too. Now, tell me more about not wanting to wake up. Is it that you just are tired of the pain or have you had thoughts of suicide?

One reason clinicians may fear following up on patient cues and relational issues is that they may think that by doing so, they will spend or waste precious time. However, at least one study suggests that where they ignore such cues in fact they end up spending more time (Levinson et al. 2000). This positive reframing of emotional and verbal cues may lead to increased patient satisfactory and a decrease in clinician burnout. Moreover, as the suggested response above highlights, addressing these issues need not be unduly time consuming.

Raising subtexts to texts versus addressing within the subtext: The statement above gives a another simple example of how a subtext might be raised, when the clinician says, "I would not blame you for being upset with me … ." As this example illustrates, usually the dilemma of how to deal with a subtext manifests when the subtext is negative or threatening in so way. Far too commonly, when negative subtexts arise the subtext is simply ignored, often by focusing on whatever low context, clinical issues are at hand. It is difficult to state exactly when one should raise the subtext versus dealing with it within the subtext. This depends on the context. The following general guidelines for raising the subtext are offered for consideration:

- When the subtext has become so dominant that it is difficult to make progress on other tasks and difficult to work within the subtext toward a positive outcome.
- When the raising of the subtext, even when negative, offers an opportunity for positive framing of the response (The example above offers an illustration of this – "upset-ness" gives rise to an opportunity to find common ground and a statement of caring.).
- When the clinician believes that both patient (or family) and the clinician can handle the issue raised emotionally without losing control.

---

[5]I recall a dramatic example of this in observing a new medical student practice doing a history and physical. The student was pushing through a list of questions on a "check-list." In doing the social history he asked, "Are you married?" "No, the patient replied. "My wife died six months ago." Uh-huh. Children? How many sexual partners have you had in the last year?" The patient's response begged for an empathic statement and at least a brief expansion. Continuing with the check-list – especially given the questions asked, seemed heartless, even cruel, even though this was completely unintentional.

- When such an explicit statement of a relational subtext would be culturally acceptable to the other. Raising the subtext is, somewhat paradoxically, a low-context approach to a high context problem. This may be more acceptable in some groups and for some individuals than for others.

The above suggests that as important as whether to raise a subtext is how the subtext is understood and how it is raised. At one extreme, subtexts may be raised by "taking off the gloves" and engaging directly in battle. For example, in a power dispute with a pain patient with a history of substance abuse, who is insulting the clinician, it might be tempting in anger to "get personal" in return or make an insensitive statement of power, by saying something like, "Listen, you, I'm the doctor here. You will take what I give you or you can go someplace else." Obviously, this would be a highly unprofessional response. A preferred strategy might be saying something like that posed above, which dispassionately outlines the fact that physicians write prescriptions on their licenses.

Summary

I have introduced what are likely for many new terms for particular aspects of communication. And yet we all naturally and skillfully shift from low to high context communication every day. In other words, we are already experts in many of the issues and techniques raised earlier. The difference, I hope, is that clinicians struggling in difficult encounters with patients with pain will be able to more consciously and skillfully use these concepts to improve the quality of their interactions with patients, which will in turn result in improved patient outcomes and mutual satisfaction.

References

Beach, M. C., Roter, D. L., et al. (2006). Are physicians' attitudes of respect accurately perceived by patients and associated with more positive communication behaviors? *Patient Education and Counseling, 62*(3), 347–354.

Biro, D. (2010). *The language of pain*. New York: Norton.

Botvinick, M., Jha, A. P., et al. (2005). Viewing facial expressions of pain engages cortical areas involved in the direct experience of pain. *NeuroImage, 25*(1), 312–319.

Branch, W. T., Jr. (2006). Viewpoint: Teaching respect for patients. *Academic Medicine, 81*(5), 463–467.

Chaudakshetrin, P., Prateepavanich, P., et al. (2007). Cross-cultural adaptation to the Thai language of the neuropathic pain diagnostic questionnaire (DN4). *Journal of the Medical Association of Thailand, 90*(9), 1860–1865.

Cleeland, C. S., & Ryan, K. M. (1994). Pain assessment: Global use of the Brief Pain Inventory. *Annals of the Academy of Medicine, Singapore, 23*(2), 129–138.

de Williams, A. C., Davies, H. T., & Chadury, Y. (2000). Simple pain rating scales hide complex idiosyncratic meanings. *Pain, 85*(3), 457–463.

Detmar, S. B., Muller, M. J., et al. (2001). The patient-physician relationship. Patient-physician communication during outpatient palliative treatment visits: An observational study. *The Journal of American Medical Association, 285*(10), 1351–1357.

Fabrega, H. (1997). *Evolution of sickness and healing*. Berkeley: University of California Press.

Frith, C. (2009). Role of facial expressions in social interactions. *Philosophical Transactions of the Royal Society of London. Series B, Biological Sciences, 364*(1535), 3453–3458.

Gaston-Johansson, F., Albert, M., et al. (1990). Similarities in pain descriptions of four different ethnic-culture groups. *Journal of Pain and Symptom Management, 5*(2), 94–100.

Goubert, L., Craig, K. D., et al. (2005). Facing others in pain: The effects of empathy. *Pain, 118*(3), 285–288.

Hadjistavropoulos, H. D., & Craig, K. D. (1994). Acute and chronic low back pain: Cognitive, affective, and behavioral dimensions. *Journal of Consulting and Clinical Psychology, 62*(2), 341–349.

Hahn, R. (1995). *Sickness and healing*. New Haven: Yale University Press.

Hall, E. (1976). *Beyond culture*. Garden City: Anchor.

Hall, E. (1983). *The dance of life*. Garden City, NY: Anchor.

Hall, E. (1990). *The silent language*. NY: Anchor.

Hall, E. (1997). Context and meaning. In L. Samovar & R. Porter (Eds.), *Intercultural communication* (pp. 45–54). Belmont: Wadsworth.

Hallenbeck, J. (2000). A dying patient, like me? *American Family Physician, 62*(4), 888–890.

Hallenbeck, J. (2006). High context illness and dying in a low context medical world. *The American Journal of Hospice & Palliative Care, 23*(2), 113–118.

Hallenbeck, J. (2007). Cross-cultural issues. In A. Berger, J. Shuster, & J. Von Roenn (Eds.), *Palliative care and supportive oncology* (pp. 515–525). Philadelphia: Lippincott Williams & Wilkins.

Hallenbeck, J., & Periyakoil, V. (2009). Intercultural communication in palliative care. In C. D. Kissane, B. Bulz, & P. Butow (Eds.), *Handbook of communication in oncology and palliative* (pp. 389–398). New York: Oxford University Press.

Haugli, L., Strand, E., et al. (2004). How do patients with rheumatic disease experience their relationship with their doctors? A qualitative study of experiences of stress and support in the doctor-patient relationship. *Patient Education and Counseling, 52*(2), 169–174.

Im, E. O., Lee, S. H., et al. (2009). A national online forum on ethnic differences in cancer pain experience. *Nursing Research, 58*(2), 86–94.

International Association for the Study of Pain Website. (2010).

Kleinman, A. (1994). Pain and resistance – The delegitimation and relegitimation of local worlds. In M. G. Delvechio, P. Browdwin, B. Good, & A. Kleinman (Eds.), *Pain as human experience – An anthropological perspective* (pp. 169–197). Berkeley: University of California Press.

Kleinman, A. (1995). *Writing in the margin: Discourse between anthropology and medicine*. Berkeley: University of California Press.

Knotkova, H., Crawford Clark, W., et al. (2004). What do ratings on unidimensional pain and emotion scales really mean? A multidimensional affect and pain survey (MAPS) analysis of cancer patient responses. *Journal of Pain and Symptom Management, 28*(1), 19–27.

Levinson, W., Gorawara-Bhat, R., et al. (2000). A study of patient clues and physician responses in primary care and surgical settings. *The Journal of American Medical Association, 284*(8), 1021–1027.

McDowell, I. (Ed.). (2006). Pain measurements. In: *Measuring health* (pp. 470–519). New York, Oxford University Press.

Moore, R. J., & Hallenbeck, J. (2010). Narrative empathy and how dealing with stories helps: Creating a space for empathy in culturally diverse care settings. *Journal of Pain and Symptom Management, 40*(3), 471–476.

Nampiaparampil, D., Nampiaparampil, J. X., & Harden, R. N. (2009). Pain and prejudice. *Pain Medicine, 10*(4), 716–721.

Otti, A., Guendel, H., et al. (2010). I know the pain you feel-how the human brain's default mode predicts our resonance to another's suffering. *Neuroscience, 169*(1), 143–148.

Palermo, Y. (2011). The art of pain: The patient's perspective of chronic pain. In R. J. Moore (Ed.), *Handbook of pain and palliative care*. New York: Springer.

Parle, M., Maguire, P., et al. (1997). The development of a training model to improve health professionals' skills, self-efficacy and outcome expectancies when communicating with cancer patients. *Social Science & Medicine, 44*(2), 231–240.

Parsons, S., Harding, G., et al. (2007). The influence of patients' and primary care practitioners' beliefs and expectations about chronic musculoskeletal pain on the process of care: A systematic review of qualitative studies. *The Clinical Journal of Pain, 23*(1), 91–98.

Prkachin, K. M. (1992). The consistency of facial expressions of pain: A comparison across modalities. *Pain, 51*(3), 297–306.

Pugh, J. F. (1991). The semantics of pain in Indian culture and medicine. *Culture, Medicine and Psychiatry, 15*(1), 19–43.

Samovar, L., & Porter, R. (Eds.). (1997). *Intercultural communication*. Wadsworth: Belmont.

Scarry, E. (1985). *The body in pain*. New York: Oxford University Press.

Schiavenato, M., & Craig, K. D. (2010). Pain assessment as a social transaction: Beyond the "gold standard". *The Clinical Journal of Pain, 26*(8), 667–676.

Sontag, S. (1978). *Illness as metaphor*. New York: Farrar, Straus & Giroux.

Suchman, A. L., Markakis, K., et al. (1997). A model of empathic communication in the medical interview. *The Journal of American Medical Association, 277*(8), 678–682.

Thomas, V. J., & Rose, F. D. (1991). Ethnic differences in the experience of pain. *Social Science & Medicine, 32*(9), 1063–1066.

Trnka, S. (2007). Languages of labor: Negotiating the "real" and the relational in Indo-Fijian women's expressions of physical pain. *Medical Anthropology Quarterly, 21*(4), 388–408.

Weissman, D. E. (1994). Understanding pseudoaddiction. *Journal of Pain and Symptom Management, 9*(2), 74.

Weissman, D. E., & Haddox, J. D. (1989). Opioid pseudoaddiction – An iatrogenic syndrome. *Pain, 36*(3), 363–366.

Williams, A. C. (2002). Facial expression of pain: An evolutionary account. *The Behavioral and Brain Sciences, 25*(4), 439–455; discussion 455–488.

Young, J. L., & Davidhizar, R. (2008). Attitude: Impact on pain assessment. *Journal of Practical Nursing, 58*(2), 6–10.

Zatzick, D. F., & Dimsdale, J. E. (1990). Cultural variations in response to painful stimuli. *Psychosomatic Medicine, 52*(5), 544–557.

Chapter 3
Truth Telling and Palliative Care

Lidia Schapira and David P. Steensma*

Truth is one of the most powerful therapeutic agents available to us, but we still need to develop a proper understanding of its clinical pharmacology, and to recognize optimum timing and dosage in its uses. Similarly, we need to understand the closely related metabolisms of hope and denial (Michael Simpson 1982).

Introduction

It is challenging to write about truth telling in medicine at a time in history when transparency and open access to information dominate our culture. Young adults now entering the medical profession cannot remember a time without social networks, or the era before data and instant knowledge with commentary were almost immediately available to anyone with access to the Internet. And yet the medical and nursing literature continue to debate therapeutic uses of truth, the ownership of data, and the consequences of receiving either sufficient or inadequate information to empower patients to decide their own medical fate. Our training and clinical experience in malignant hematological disorders and cancer inform our chapter and our orientation towards truth telling in medicine. Palliative care and the treatment of pain pose unique challenges in communication, given the imperative to alleviate suffering and to provide comfort. We do feel that handling difficult news and information can be approached in a systematic way and that clinicians across disciplines can benefit from a clear strategy and similar guiding principles.

In the United States and other countries with open access to technology and a firm orientation towards scientific medicine, patient autonomy usually trumps other ethical and social concerns (Schneider 1998). Patients increasingly participate in making decisions about all aspects and phases of treatment. Such involvement demands they be adequately briefed and demonstrate appropriate

---

*The authors report no relevant conflicts of interest.

L. Schapira, MD (✉)
Department of Medicine, Massachusetts General Hospital, Boston, MA, USA

Harvard Medical School, Boston, MA, USA
e-mail: lschapira@partners.org

D.P. Steensma, MD
Dana-Farber Cancer Institute, Boston, MA, USA

Department of Medicine, Brigham and Women's Hospital, Boston, MA, USA

Harvard Medical School, Boston, MA, USA

R.J. Moore (ed.), *Handbook of Pain and Palliative Care: Biobehavioral Approaches for the Life Course,*
DOI 10.1007/978-1-4419-1651-8_3, © Springer Science+Business Media, LLC 2012

understanding of benefits and risks associated with various treatment modalities. Medical students are taught to think of the doctor–patient relationship as a collaboration between partners based on mutual respect, trust, and common goals. Since this construct depends on honest disclosure, the conversation has shifted from whether or not to provide information to how best to communicate in order to preserve hope and facilitate coping. Clinicians now juggle demands to inform with their commitment to protect patients from harm that may arise from confronting dire situations. In this chapter, we examine the evidence that supports open and uncensored communication and also recognize that practice is typically informed by opinion and instinct in the context of pain and palliative care.

Patient advocacy organizations in Western countries have clearly endorsed the practice of providing information as a means to empowerment. Research confirms that access to clear information can assist patients in coping with an uncertain future and provide support for their decision. Feeling better prepared for a consultation with the specialist often allows patients and their relatives to ask more questions and improves the likelihood that more information will be exchanged in the time allotted. It is also helpful to bear in mind that many educated patients want to be informed but may still defer to experts to guide them in making decisions. While it is difficult to anticipate how medical practice will evolve, it is likely that future patients will not only read their own medical records and have the chance to review their laboratory data and surgical reports, but will also have a limited role in editing their electronic charts, thus adding their distinct voice to the narrative that contains their medical history. Indeed patients at many medical centers in the United States already have access to their charts via secure sites. So within this construct, the idea that truth and information are regulated only by physicians is likely to become obsolete. The "balance of power" in the doctor–patient relationship, which firmly tipped in favor of the physician during the late nineteenth and most of the twentieth centuries, has also decisively shifted back towards patients (Furst 1998).

We anticipate that personal health information will increasingly become available to those who wish to have it and that medical professionals will continue to need to meet the challenge of providing the interpretation, guidance, and support that will be required in the face of abundant raw data. What remains to be defined are the parameters for optimal "dosing" of such information so that it is helpful for individual patients. Colleagues who think of telling the truth as a therapeutic intervention may justly warn that confronting the data in isolation may lead to increased anxiety. Future research and innovative modes of providing emotional coaching face to face or remotely with technical assistance (via telephone or videoconference) will be indispensable to define a "new normal."

There are many ways of defining what constitutes "truth" in medical settings. Philosophers argue that truth may be buried in a communicative act and gains significance for the patient through a construction of meaning (Surbone 2006). Truth then is relative and can only be understood in the context of a person's life rather than construed as a mere recitation of medical diagnoses, interventions, and possible outcomes. This argument provides a powerful role for physicians in shaping a patient's narrative and mediating their understanding of events and possible choices and constitutes an aspect of clinical practice that many professionals find very rewarding (Surbone 2000).

Research has shown that the majority of American, Australian, and European patients wish to be informed of their specific diagnosis and prognosis, and, with guidance and support, can effectively cope with even the grimmest information (Jotkowitz et al. 2006; Bruera et al. 2000; Spiegel 1999). It bears emphasizing that this is not an approach that appeals to all individuals or cultures. Clinicians need to recognize and respect the preferences of patients and families who prefer to delegate decision-making to a designated family member and to remain "ignorant." These situations are not infrequent and demand of clinicians a significant degree of cultural humility and consideration of values that may even clash with our prevailing practices. Our advice is to document clearly who is in charge of information in the context of the family unit and to establish without any doubt that the patient clearly prefers this method of communication. For most of our patients, receiving information is the first step towards coping with difficult news and regaining control over their own destiny. Another important aspect to help patients cope successfully is to preserve and protect the family unit and important social relationships. Caregivers need and want to know about the nature of the illness especially if it is not curable, although many are not told and are consequently unprepared in the final days of life (Dahlstrand et al. 2008). An important principle guiding palliative care is to help patients and their loved ones to share feelings evoked by the new reality and to assist each other to move progressively closer to fully accepting the situation without despair (Parkes 1978). In contrast to fears about realistic discussion of a poor prognosis causing depression or emotional damage, several recent studies have demonstrated instead that honest disclosure facilitates coping, and that continued aggressive care for advanced cancer is associated with poorer quality of life, increased depression among patients, and a complicated bereavement for surviving relatives (Wright et al. 2008). Other data indicate that bereavement outcomes of surviving caregivers may be improved when good communication was present during the patient's last days and the caregivers were prepared for the eventual outcome (Hebert and Schulz 2006).

Physicians have always worried that full disclosure of difficult information and a clear rendition of a limited prognosis will lead to despair and may even hasten a patient's decline and eventual demise. Studies conducted fifty years ago suggested that doctors themselves preferred to be informed of the diagnosis and outlook if they had an incurable illness although they were not prepared to provide such information to their patients. This apparent contradiction captures a dilemma that confronts clinicians even today (Fallowfield 1997) and can be best understood by realizing that avoidance of truth telling is more commonly a symptom of the clinician's own discomfort, perhaps reflecting the doctor's own narrow emotional range (Fallowfield 1997). Evidence suggests that individual doctors' responses tend to be similar with all patients (Fallowfield 1997) and that moral judgments and decision-making is driven by automatic emotional responses (Greene et al. 2008, 2009; Greene 2003; Greene and Haidt 2002). Rather than resorting to abstract reasoning, doctors and nurses respond to moral dilemmas with "gut reactions." The interplay between emotional responses and rational constructions, shaped by genetic, cultural, and professional codes, is the focus of ongoing neuroscientific research. We expect the information that will emerge from these studies will provide new foundational arguments that capture the complex moral and practical dimensions of clinical encounters and shed light on how doctors regulate their own feelings and expressions of empathy.

It is easy to imagine that withholding certain facts may appear as a deplorable omission to some and a charitable act to others. Avoiding the truth or disclosing only very limited aspects of it (which is more common today than outright deception) could be construed as kindness but may still cause harm. If a sick person is referred for tests and prescribed treatments that fail to relieve symptoms, and then told nothing, the message conveyed is that the truth must be so horrible that it cannot be discussed and the patient may feel both isolated and anxious (Katz 1986). Minimizing or omitting important information may indeed make the patient happier in the short term but violates the patient's trust and the future credibility of the physician (Simpson 1982). The practical consequence is that it excludes the doctor from being able to provide solace in the future and patient and doctor lose the opportunity to create an enduring and therapeutic alliance.

A carefully conducted ethnographic study of patients with metastatic lung cancer treated in the Netherlands provides a framework for understanding the consequences of this collusion between doctors and patients (The et al. 2000). Well-intentioned specialists and patients regularly managed to focus on logistics of treatment, latest test results, and other quotidian issues, and repeatedly failed to address the bigger picture and ultimate likely outcome. The results were predictable: when treatments failed and time suddenly ran out, patients and their relatives were surprised and unprepared, and bereaved relatives expressed regret over much that had been left undone.

Truth is not just an item traded between doctors and patients. The same instinct to protect and minimize suffering leads some patients to lie or withhold discouraging information from their spouse, children, or caregivers. Patients may minimize their symptoms or ask few questions during office visits in order to protect or buffer their loved one. If the doctor fails to notice the cues that alert him to this behavior, he may enable the avoidance by stressing only positives and framing information in the most favorable terms.

A patient's choice to withhold information or to provide only partial and misleading information is also counterproductive. There is confirmatory evidence to support this view from recent research. A well-designed study of bone marrow transplant patients and their spousal caregivers or partners examined the repercussions of "protective buffering," a term used by social scientists to describe behaviors such as hiding discouraging information or worries in order to protect a loved one (Langer et al. 2009). The study team queried patients and their spouses at two different time points – prior to transplant, and again 50 days after – about communication and relationship satisfaction. The investigators found that both the person who wished to protect the loved one and the person who was ostensibly being protected exhibited signs of distress, and both relationship partners expressed less satisfaction in their relationship than patient and spouse/partner dyads who did not engage in such hiding.

The assumption that frank disclosure of diagnostic and prognostic information is always beneficial might be challenged on the grounds that it fails to take into consideration the patient's best interest, or the patient's ability to receive or understand such complex news. Any clinical intervention, procedural or cognitive, that is carried out only to comply with medical protocol without due consideration of the patient's capacity, preferences, or humanity violates core principles of professionalism and moral behavior. Cultural mores and practices for truth telling in the setting of an incurable illness need to be considered, as well as the patient's legal right to refuse information as long as he delegates decision making capacity to a proxy of his choice. There is never a moral justification for a blunt, compassionless, robotic "core dump" of raw information, which reflects poorly on the professional and risks emotional harm to the patient.

It is also clear that because hope is dynamic and multifaceted, it is always possible to paint a picture that is authentic yet leaves some room for hope (Renz et al. 2009). A recent study by Smith and colleagues showed that honest communication in fact helps patients to preserve hope (Smith et al. 2010). In one analysis in the pediatric oncology setting, nearly half of 194 surveyed parents of children with cancer reported that *any* communication from the physician made them feel hopeful; parents overall reported that the more they knew about prognosis, the more hopeful they felt, even when the prognosis was poor (Mack et al. 2007). These and other data support the notion that even in the most poignant or emotionally difficult circumstances, the presence of a physician with good communication skills can be an extraordinarily powerful therapeutic tool.

Information needs change over time; clinical situations as well as individual and family attitudes evolve and adjust, and doctors involved in longitudinal care learn more about what matters deeply to each patient. Doctors who hesitated to provide comprehensive prognostic information at the time of an initial consultation may find an opportune moment after an initial crisis is successfully averted or once the patient's pain is better controlled. Patients who were initially averse to learning prognostic information and elected to hear only what was required to provide consent to treatment may later spontaneously ask about their condition and prognosis. Conversely, patients who are quite near the end of life may be less inclined to seek discussion of a specific survival time. Often patients choose to obtain information by asking team members other than the physician, or by looking things up on their own. It is a mistake for physicians to assume that patients who have not been informed do not know, or that those who have been informed will act in a certain way. Likewise, patients who are simply unable to handle a difficult truth are able to employ denial as defense mechanism even after being fully informed.

Although there is virtually universal agreement today about the need to avoid intentionally giving patients incorrect information, as well as widespread concern about the dangers of supplying no information, our collective understanding of the optimal mechanisms for presenting truthful information – i.e., what to say and when – remains quite limited. Compassionate and empathetic clinicians who want to be both honest and truthful may still be uncertain in each case about the degree of detail to provide (for instance, when to provide numerical estimates of life expectancy, or to mention rare but horrendous potential complications), in what order to make that information available, and which areas deserve emphasis during the limited time available for a clinical encounter. Having a good ear and following an individual patient's cues is essential, and communication skills are clearly teachable, but intimate conversation remains an intricate and subtle art. Family members can act as facilitators of truth by asking questions, taking notes, and then debriefing after the consultation is over. They can also block the effective delivery of information, perhaps guided by protective instincts. A recent study from Australia showed that family members often prefer to deliberately leave out important facts or details in order to "soften" the information (Mitchison et al. 2011).

There are clear and useful "cognitive roadmaps" to help clinicians to deliver bad and sad news effectively and compassionately (Mitchison et al. 2011; Baile et al. 1999). For instance, it is recommended that we give a patient some warning that bad news is forthcoming without keeping the recipient either in a state of indefinite suspense (i.e., stalling) or conveying the bad news abruptly and bluntly (Baile et al. 2000). Asking the patient what he or she already knows and how much he or she wants to know is an important next step. Obtaining approval for disclosing the information comes next, followed by discussing the information in clear language with frequent stops to check the patient is not overwhelmed and is following the conversation. As events unfold, the doctor can respond to the patient's emotion and provide a clear summary of the situation and expert recommendations for how to manage the disease and formulate the best possible treatment plan.

Some physicians whose goal is to be truthful, yet who also wish to avoid bludgeoning the patient with a series of bleak particulars all at once, prefer to initially present a few simple essentials and then to let the patient and family elicit further details with questions. Other doctors have a communication style that favors a more comprehensive recitation of facts that the doctor feels are "need to know." Which style is preferred by patients is not well studied, and specific preferences for how and what information is presented may depend on factors such as patients' age, ethnicity, and level of education attainment (Maynard 2003).

There are several special circumstances regarding truth telling and disclosure that should also be considered. Patients participating in clinical trials have unique needs for truthful information, since in most studies of new approaches to cancer the participants are being put at some risk. Full understanding of the trial's purposes and mechanisms may be difficult for many patients to achieve, as a level of biological sophistication may be required, and some information about the trial or study compound may be proprietary, unpublished, or (as in the case of Phase I trials) almost absent. The amount of information that must be conveyed prior to treatment is dictated by long and wordy consent forms, which stress uncertainty and possible risks, and often crafted to protect institutions and individuals from legal action rather than truly intending to inform patients. Even with unrestricted access to information, healthcare professionals may feel confused or unprepared to provide guidance or respond to complex clinical situations and questions from patients and significant others.

Another set of challenging situations may arise when patients and doctors from different cultural backgrounds meet, which is increasingly common in the diverse and pluralistic contemporary world. The practices and expectations of doctors, patients, and family members and other caregivers are shaped by culture – not just the culture of each person's origin, but that in which the clinical encounter takes place. For example, a patient's adult son may request that his father not be told the truth – neither about the diagnosis nor details of a treatment plan (Parker et al. 2001). His request likely stems from a deeply ingrained belief that it is not in a patient's best interest to have full knowledge about a fatal diagnosis, and that families should decide how much information should filter through to the patient (McCabe et al. 2010; Blackhall et al. 1995). In Japan, for instance, families typically are the first to know a diagnosis and treatment plan (although the patient is often eventually told some basic information), while in China and Korea, families routinely make decisions on behalf of the patient without consulting the patient – a responsibility that is commonly delegated to the eldest (male) relative (Kagawa-Singer and Blackhall 2001; Uchitomi and Ymawaki 1997). Among immigrant families, varying degrees of assimilation and acculturation to the new country may result in intergenerational familial conflict about the degree to which traditional cultural expectations should be respected (Li and Chou 1997). Cultural norms may evolve relatively rapidly, as has been seen recently in Italy where autonomy is increasingly important relative to beneficence (Butow et al. 1997).

Patients with cognitive impairment, either congenital or due to a disease and its therapy, may also vary widely in their ability to understand the implications of a diagnosis and make care decisions. What to tell patients with limited mental capacity must be individualized and will typically require consultation with family members or a legal guardian. In these situations clinicians need to be very clear and straightforward in the way they present information and choices, including possible complications of the untreated illness or symptom and of the therapies offered and discussed, and to document this clearly.

Incarcerated patients lose many rights, but the right to full disclosure about diagnosis and prognosis and the right to high quality palliative care are not among them (Surbone et al. 2004). However, for security reasons, certain logistical information may need to be withheld from the patient (e.g., dates of the next planned evaluation or treatment outside of prison walls).

Regardless of the specific care setting, the primary mission of palliative care professionals is to assist and guide patients through treatment and rehabilitation until the very last moment of life. Maintaining the patient's integrity and dignity throughout the course of illness are high priorities; realistic care plans can be individualized to best match patient's personal goals. From this vantage point, truth is equated with access to whatever medical facts are available, including prognosis. It is only by truth telling that the patient can truly understand the circumstances and make the best decisions for present and future. We can only hope that future medical practice and science will support the primal role of information exchange and the need for caring and compassionate relationships that foster trust and well-being for patients and their loved ones.

References

Baile, W. F., Buckman, R., Lenzi, R., et al. (2000). SPIKES – A six step protocol for delivering bad news: Application to the patient with cancer. *The Oncologist, 5*(4), 302–311.

Baile, W. F., Kudelka, A. P., & Beale, E. A. (1999). Communication skills training in oncology. Description and preliminary outcomes of workshops on breaking bad news and managing patient reactions to illness. *Cancer, 86*(5), 887–897.

Blackhall, L. J., Murphy, S. T., & Frank, G. (1995). Ethnicity and attitudes toward patient autonomy. *The Journal of the American Medical Association, 274*, 820–825.

Bruera, E., Neumann, C. M., Mazzocato, C., et al. (2000). Attitudes and beliefs of palliative care physicians regarding communication with terminally ill patients. *Palliative Medicine, 14*(4), 287–298.

Butow, P. N., Tattersall, M. H., & Goldstein, D. (1997). Communication with cancer patients in culturally diverse societies. *Annals of the New York Academy of Sciences, 809*, 317–329.

Dahlstrand, H., Hauksdottir, A., Valdimarsdottir, U., et al. (2008). Disclosure of incurable illness to spouses: Do they want to know? A Swedish population-based follow-up study. *Journal of Clinical Oncology, 26*(20), 3372–3379.

Fallowfield, L. (1997). Truth sometimes hurts but deceit hurts more. *Annals of the New York Academy of Sciences, 809*, 525–536.

Furst, L. (1998). *Between doctors and patients: The changing balance of power*. Charlottesville, VA: The University Press of Virginia.

Greene, J. D. (2003). From neural "is" to moral "ought": What are the moral implications of neuroscientific moral psychology? *Nature Reviews. Neuroscience, 4*, 847–850.

Greene, J. D., Cushman, F. A., Stewart, L. E., Lowenberg, K., Nystrom, L. E., & Cohen, J. D. (2009). Pushing moral buttons: The interaction between personal force and intention in moral judgment. *Cognition, 111*(3), 364–371.

Greene, J., & Haidt, J. (2002). How (and where) does moral judgment work? *Trends in Cognitive Sciences, 6*(12), 517–523.

Greene, J. D., Morelli, S. A., Lowenberg, K., Nystrom, L. E., & Cohen, J. D. (2008). Cognitive load selectively interferes with utilitarian moral judgment. *Cognition, 107*, 1144–1154.

Hebert, R. S., & Schulz, R. (2006). *Journal of Palliative Medicine, 9*(5), 1164–1171.

Jotkowitz, A., Glick, S., & Gezundheit, B. (2006). Truth-telling in a culturally diverse world. *Cancer Investigation, 24*(8), 786–789.

Kagawa-Singer, M., & Blackhall, L. J. (2001). Negotiating cross-cultural issues at the end of life: "You got to go where he lives". *The Journal of the American Medical Association, 286*(23), 2993–3001.

Katz, J. (1986). *The silent world of doctor and patient.* New York, NY: The Free Press.

Langer, S. L., Brown, J. D., & Syrjala, K. L. (2009). Intrapersonal and interpersonal consequences of protective buffering among cancer patients and caregivers. *Cancer, 115*(18 Suppl), 4311–4325.

Li, S., & Chou, J. L. (1997). Communication with the cancer patient in China. *Annals of the New York Academy of Sciences, 809*, 243–248.

Linder, J. F., & Meyers, F. J. (2007). Palliative care for prison inmates: "Don't let me die in prison". *The Journal of the American Medical Association, 298*(8), 894–901.

Mack, J. W., Wolfe, J., Cok, E. F., et al. (2007). Hope and prognostic disclosure. *Journal of Clinical Oncology, 25*(35), 5636–5642.

Maynard, D. (2003). *Bad news, good news: Conversational order in everyday talk and clinical settings.* Chicago, IL: University of Chicago Press.

McCabe, M. S., Wood, W. A., & Goldberg, R. M. (2010). When the family requests withholding the diagnosis: Who owns the truth? *Journal of Oncology Practice, 6*(2), 94–96.

Mitchison, D., Butow, P., Sze, M., Aldridge, L., Hui, R., Vardy, J., Eisenbruch, M., & Iedema, R. (2011). *Goldstein D. Psychooncology Feb: Prognostic Communication preferences of migrant workers and their relatives.*

Parker, P. A., Baile, W. F., de Moor, C., et al. (2001). Breaking bad news about cancer: Patients' preferences for communication. *Journal of Clinical Oncology, 19*(7), 2049–2056.

Parkes, C. M. (1978). Psychological aspects. In C. M. Saunders (Ed.), *The management of terminal disease* (pp. 44–64). London: Edward Arnold.

Renz, M., Koeberle, D., Cerny, T., et al. (2009). Between utter despair and essential hope. *Journal of Clinical Oncology, 27*(1), 146–149.

Schneider, C. (1998). *The practice of autonomy: patients, doctors, and medical decisions.* NY: Oxford University Press.

Simpson, M. A. (1982). Therapeutic uses of truth. In E. Wilkes (Ed.), *The dying patient.* Lancaster: MYP Press.

Smith, T. J., Dow, L. A., Virago, E., et al. (2010). Giving honest information to patients with advanced cancer maintains hope. *Oncology (Williston Park)., 24*(6), 521–525.

Spiegel, D. (1999). A 43-year-old woman coping with cancer. *The Journal of the American Medical Association, 282*(4), 371–378.

Surbone, A. (2000). Truth telling. *Annals of the New York Academy of Sciences, 913*, 52–62.

Surbone, A. (2006). Telling the truth to patients with cancer: What is the truth? *The Lancet Oncology, 7*(11), 944–950.

Surbone, A., Ritossa, C., & Spagnolo, A. G. (2004). Evolution of truth-telling attitudes and practices in Italy. *Critical Reviews in Oncology/Hematology, 52*(3), 165–172.

The, A. M., Hak, T., Koeter, G., et al. (2000). Collusion in doctor-patient communication about imminent death: An ethnographic study. *BMJ, 321*(7273), 1376–1381.

Uchitomi, Y., & Ymawaki, S. (1997). Truth telling practice in cancer care in Japan. *Annals of the New York Academy of Sciences, 809*, 290–299.

Wright, A. A., Zhang, B., Ray, A., et al. (2008). Associations between end-of-life discussions, patient metnal health, medical care near death, and caregiver bereave adjustment. *The Journal of the American Medical Association, 300*(14), 1665–1673.

Chapter 4
Communication and Palliative Care: E-Health Interventions and Pain Management

Gary L. Kreps

The Symbolic Nature of Pain and Pain Management

Pain management is a major challenge for both healthcare consumers and providers. Pain is a complex biological and psychological phenomenon (Ahles et al. 1983; Nelson and Weir 2001). Physical pain and psychological pain operate together indelibly. Physical pain is a very important biological process whereby the body sends neural messages to the brain to alert human beings about dangerous abnormal bodily processes, intrusions, and threats. Pain promotes symbolic awareness to these problems and encourages attempts to identify the root causes of pain and the development of strategies for relieving these root causes. While pain serves an important alerting function, it is also a very uncomfortable phenomenon for pain sufferers, and chronic repetitive pain, in particular, can become a major problem for individuals to cope with. Effective pain management treats both the physiological and symbolic aspects of pain (Fitzmartin et al. 1995; Holland 2003; Mendenhall 2003).

Every physical cause of pain is interpreted symbolically by individuals (often in very idiosyncratic ways) as psychological pain. In essence, physical manifestations of pain are embedded in unique personal symbolic interpretations of pain. What is more, psychological interpretations of pain derive from biological reactions to physical threats as well as to our reactions to unpleasant feelings and emotions. Humans have developed the ability to mirror the physical pain phenomenon symbolically to make sense of psychological distress. Yet, physical and psychological causes of pain feel like identical phenomena to most people. It is often difficult to distinguish between physical and psychological causes of pain; they both hurt. In essence, there are many different physical and symbolic sources for pain in the modern world and pain management has become a significant issue for many people. Pain management is a high priority issue for those individuals confronting serious chronic diseases, debilitating illnesses, and intrusive mental health problems.

The interpretation of pain is very subjective and is different for each person and each unique situation. When we are fully occupied at an engrossing and stimulating activity, we may not be as aware of pain as we might be when we are trying to sleep at night. The perceptions of pain that we habituated while busy earlier in the day, often come to the forefront when there are not competing foci for our attention. Some people with recurrent pain develop the ability to tune out (habituate) the pain by focusing their mind on other thoughts. Furthermore, the same causes of pain may be perceived very differently. For one person an injection may feel excruciatingly painful, while others may barely feel

G.L. Kreps, PhD (✉)
Department of Communication, George Mason University,
4000 University Drive, MS 3D6, Fairfax, VA 22030, USA
e-mail: gkreps@gmu.edu

R.J. Moore (ed.), *Handbook of Pain and Palliative Care: Biobehavioral Approaches for the Life Course*,
DOI 10.1007/978-1-4419-1651-8_4, © Springer Science+Business Media, LLC 2012

the injection at all. Effective pain management must take these subjective interpretations of pain into account and strive to influence the ways individuals interpret their pain experiences.

While the biological process of pain is uncomfortable, the interpretation of that discomfort is modified by a variety of internal and external factors that can either intensify or de-intensify the pain experience. For example, some internal (psychological) factors that can exacerbate the experience of pain may include feelings of depression, fatigue, uncertainty, loss of control, anxiety, fear, hopelessness, and loneliness. External (environmental) factors that can exacerbate the perception of pain may include harsh lighting, unsettling noises, crowding, and jostling. All of these internal and external factors that can exacerbate the perception of pain can be moderated (to a greater or lesser extent) through verbal and nonverbal communication. There are direct links between communication and psychology, where the messages we perceive influence the meanings we create (Kreps 1996; see also Pollo and Benedetti 2011). Communication interventions to help manage pain need to be designed to minimize the meanings created that intensify the pain experience and maximize meanings that de-intensify the experience of pain.

Pharmacological and surgical interventions are common medical responses for treating pain (see also Zhao and Cope 2011). Certain medications can effectively block pain, numbing the pain response in the brain. However, many of these pain medications can be highly addictive, can numb other mental and physical processes, and can lead to a range of unpleasant side effects (such as sleep disorders, digestive problems, impotence and sexual response issues, etc.) too. Surgery is another medical intervention strategy that is often used to help correct physical abnormalities that can cause pain. Unfortunately, many surgical procedures are very invasive and can lead to additional sources of pain for patients, particularly during their, often long and uncomfortable, process of rehabilitation from surgery (see also Short and Vetter 2011; Sehgal et al. 2011). Surgical procedures can also often have unpleasant side effects (including risks of infection and long-term physical limitations) that can lead to new sources of pain and discomfort (see also Adler et al. 2011). These medical interventions are best suited for treating the physical causes of pain, but have been less successful in addressing the psychological aspects of pain. Yet it is the ability to respond effectively to the psychological aspects of pain that are critically important for long-term pain management.

Symbolic interpretations of pain, whether caused by intrusive physical phenomena or from emotional reactions to difficult situations, can be influenced by human communication since communication has a direct effect on the creation of meanings (Fitzmartin et al. 1995). Communication has been shown to help consumers cope with pain by helping them increase their understanding about the causes of pain, their unique patterns of pain incidence, and the best strategies for pain management (Berry et al. 2003; Kimberlin et al. 2004; Kreps 2004). While human interaction is probably not the best therapeutic strategy for healing physical wounds that lead to pain, supportive and informative interaction has been found to be a powerful therapeutic process for promoting active pain management and reducing symbolic feelings of pain and suffering (Novy 2004). However, access to therapeutic and informative health communication, particularly at the points in time when pain management support is most needed, is often limited for many pain sufferers. There is a tremendous need to increase access to relevant and strategic health communication to promote pain management.

Communication and the Delivery of Health Care

A large body of research has shown that effective communication between healthcare consumers and providers is a critical factor in the delivery of high quality care (see Kreps and Chapelsky Massimilla 2002; see also Hallenbeck 2011; Palermo 2011). Both healthcare consumers and providers have tremendous needs for relevant, accurate, and timely information to help them make their best health decisions and to coordinate the delivery of care. Yet, research has shown that there are numerous barriers to effective communication in the delivery of care, including limited communication skills by both consumers and providers, differential levels of health literacy, inter-cultural communication challenges, time constraints, poor access to relevant health information, political struggles and power differentials between healthcare providers and consumers, low levels of inter-professional cooperation between members of healthcare teams, and the lack of interpersonal sensitivity in healthcare interactions (Kreps 1996, 2001; Pargeon and Hailey 1999). These communication barriers that limit the delivery of effective health care also limit the effectiveness of pain management.

Effective consumer–provider communication can promote coordinated care, informed health decision making, and help reduce medical errors (Kreps and O'Hair 1995). Arora's (2003) comprehensive review of the literature showed that physicians' communicative behavior (specifically, establishing effective interpersonal relationships, facilitating active exchange of relevant health information, and encouraging patient involvement in decision making) had a positive impact on patient health outcomes. The physician and other healthcare providers can use strategic health communication to help their patients who are experiencing significant pain and discomfort by providing timely, accurate, and sensitive information to promote palliative care and relieve discomfort (Bostrom et al. 2004; Kreps 2004). Active and effective communication can help consumers and providers work together to reduce pain and suffering. Critical communication issues that enable these positive outcomes include the development of effective relational interdependence between healthcare consumers and providers, providing both consumers and providers with relevant and timely health information, establishing active channels for feedback to promote adaptation in palliative care, coordinating verbal and nonverbal communication effectively, using communication technologies to support palliative care, and using communication to promote consumer empowerment in pain and symptom management. In fact, a revealing study by Kimberlin et al. (2004) showed that the key communication strategies that cancer patients believed their care providers could use to help them manage pain included: (1) exchanging relevant health information, (2) increasing active provider–patient participation, (3) building strong provider–patient relationships, (4) overcoming time barriers, (5) addressing their concerns about pain medications, (6) enhancing appropriate involvement of family and informal caregivers in the communication process, and (7) improving coordination of care between all members of the care team. Palliative care education programs can help prepare healthcare providers to communicate with patients in ways that help promote effective pain management (Carr et al. 2003; Egbert et al. 2008; Morrison and Morrison 2006; Rogers and Todd 2000).

Strategic health communication can perform a major role in helping to manage pain. Kreps (2004) proposed a model of Communication and Symptom Management (see Fig. 4.1) that illustrates the interdependence between the patient, the patient's healthcare providers, and the patient's friends and family. This model suggests that for effective pain and symptom management there needs to be active lines of communication between these different individuals. Effective health communication enables these partners in the healthcare enterprise to share relevant symptom information about the pain experience so they can increase understanding about the causes of pain, the intensity of pain, and the intervention strategies that provide the greatest pain relief. Communication is also needed to provide critical feedback about when pain relief is needed and how effectively current pain management strategies are working. Effective communication can encourage active adaptation to the patient's changing pain management needs. Active lines of communication enable healthcare partners to cooperate in making shared decisions about pain management. Good communication can provide needed emotional support to pain sufferers and encourage coordination of efforts in the management of pain (Dobratz et al. 1991). Partners can also use their strategic communication skills to provide personal advocacy for the patient, promote physical and psychological comfort for the patient, and encourage patient self-efficacy. This chapter examines ways that electronic health (e-health) technologies can help facilitate accomplishment of these critically important communication processes.

COMMUNICATION AND SYMPTOM MANAGEMENT MODEL

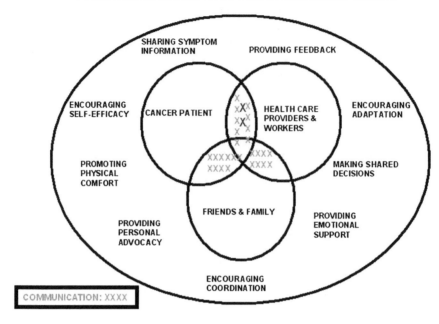

Fig. 4.1 Communication and symptom management model

The Advent of E-Health Communication

We are in the midst of an information revolution in modern society that is transforming the ways that we communicate and organize information. Nowhere is the adoption of new information technologies more evident than in the delivery of care and the promotion of health (Kreps and Neuhauser 2010; Neuhauser and Kreps 2010). There has been a rapid growth in the development and use of new health information technologies, such as electronic medical records, online support groups, and the omnipresent availability of health information via specialized web sites. This growing use of health information technologies has become known as e-health, which Eng defines as "the use of emerging information and communication technology, especially the Internet, to improve or enable health and health care" (2001, p. 1). E-health encompasses a range of overlapping disciplines that relate to the application of information, computer and communication technology to the delivery of health care and the promotion of health.

E-health communication strategies include, but are not limited to, health information on the Internet, computer assisted learning, online support groups, online collaborative communities, information tailored by computer technologies, computer-controlled in-home telephone counseling, biometric assessment and transmission, and patient–provider e-mail contact. Each of these e-health technologies has the potential for helping to promote pain management to the extent that they can provide consumers with relevant information to increase understanding of their pain experience, help consumers explore different strategies for reducing their experience of pain, coordinate the delivery of effective and timely palliative care, and provide consumers with needed social support. Question: what about liability issues? How have these been addressed?

E-health communication technologies can work in concert with other channels of communication. For example, it is advantageous for physicians to talk with their patients about health information that patients may have gathered from the Internet to help explain the information to the patients and its relevance to their health conditions. Similarly, in pain management, computerized information systems, such as web sites, the use of e-mail, and electronic patient records, can effectively supplement interpersonal communication between patients and their healthcare providers. Use of these electronic communication channels can extend the reach of interpersonal channels by providing communication access at any time day or night for feedback about the pain management needs, additional information about pain management strategies, and reinforcement for pain management requests and strategies that have been shared (Hesse et al. 2005).

E-Health Interventions and Pain Management

There have been several promising new e-health interventions developed for promoting effective pain management. Some of these interventions are designed to provide pain sufferers with more information about the pain experience and strategies for coping with pain. For example, there are now a broad range of web sites dedicated to providing both consumers and healthcare providers with education and support about pain and pain management. Some of these web sites include:

http://www.pain.com
http://www.webmd.com/pain-management
http://www.nlm.nih.gov/medlineplus/pain.html
http://www.painfoundation.org/
http://www.ampainsoc.org/

However, there is little external oversight over the accuracy, currency, completeness, and accessibility of the information provided on these web sites. Consumers must make good decisions about whether the pain management information they find on these web sites is appropriate for them and what the best strategies are for implementing these pain management recommendations. This is an ideal opportunity for supplementing web surfing with more direct communication with healthcare professionals. Doctors, nurse, pharmacists, and other health professionals can also help consumers make sense of and apply pain management information gathered on the web (Manzanec et al. 2002). Some healthcare providers and healthcare systems enable patients to consult with their providers online, making it relatively quick and easy to get help interpreting web-based information about pain management. There are also online pain consultation services and ask-a-doctor sites available such as:

http://www.painclinic.org/home-onlineconsultation.htm
http://health.answergem.com/
http://www.justanswer.com/health

The best strategy for consumers to ensure they understand and use properly the pain management information they gather online is to discuss the information with their healthcare providers (Hesse et al. 2005). A trusted healthcare professional can help them about making sense of the pain management information and advise them about the best strategies for utilizing the information for managing pain (Berry et al. 2003; Detmar et al. 2000).

A number of promising e-health interventions are designed to promote awareness and coordination in facilitating prompt response to pain incidents. For example, Wilkie et al. (2003) have introduced a computerized format for self-reporting pain assessment, *PAIN*Report*It*, that has been shown to help patients gain personal control over pain management and share real-time information about pain incidence and treatment with their providers. Computerized self-report systems like this one can promote coordination of efforts in responding quickly to severe pain incidents (Detmar et al. 2001; Huang et al. 2003).

There has been a lot of promising work on the development of online diaries for tracking pain incidence and management (Jamison et al. 2001; Peters et al. 2000; Stone et al. 2003). These electronic diary systems help patients and providers identify the unique patterns each patient experiences in pain incidence and management, as well as to report these incidents in real time. This diary data can help patients and providers predict when pain incidents are likely to occur and plan advance strategies for quick and decisive pain management interventions. Evidence suggests that these diaries are particularly useful for empowering patients (and providers) to better understand unique patterns of pain incidence and severity, as well as to develop good prevention and intervention plans to minimize pain (Marceau et al. 2007).

Other work has focused on the development of computerized assessment programs for measuring pain (Cook et al. 2004; Jamison et al. 2002). Electronic pain questionnaires have been shown to be just as accurate as paper and pencil measurement tools, yet they are more adaptive to tracking, storing, and sharing this pain information with healthcare providers who can use this information for managing pain (Jamison et al. 2006; Junker et al. 2008). The use of handheld devices has made the collection of pain information portable for consumers who experience pain at different times and different places (Newman et al. 1999; VanDenKerkhof et al. 2003). It enables efficient storage and processing of pain information, as well as the ability to share this information electronically with others.

There is a long history of using peer support groups to help people cope with serious health problems (Kreps 2001; see also Cowan 2011). The advent of online social support groups has made it easier for people to connect with others over long distances, especially when support group members may find it difficult to travel, as is the case for many people with serious health problems (Eng 2001; Ferguson 1996; Kreps and Neuhauser 2010). Several online support groups have been developed for pain sufferers, their caregivers, and their healthcare providers. For example, see:

http://www.mdjunction.com/chronic-pain
http://www.chronicpainsupport.org/
http://www.healthcentral.com/chronic-pain/support-groups.html
http://www.dailystrength.org/c/Chronic-Pain/support-group
http://www.backpainsupportgroup.com/

These online support groups allow pain sufferers (and their caregivers) to connect with others who are experiencing similar pain issues and to share relevant information and develop strategies for managing pain. The asynchronous nature of these online support groups means that group members can post messages whenever they need support or information, and do not need to wait for specific group meeting times. Evidence has suggested that the information provided on these online support groups is of very high quality and group participation provides many benefits to users (Ferguson 1996; Lindsay et al. 2009).

Telehealth information systems also have a long history of use to provide health professional advice and care to consumers in remote areas where there may be limited health services available (Kreps and Neuhauser 2010). These telehealth systems have also been used effectively to deliver pain management interventions (Appel et al. 2002; Peng et al. 2006; Pronovost et al. 2009). Research has shown that telehealth management interventions have resulted in significant improvements in both pain and depression for consumers who may not have had access to in-person care by enhancing health communication and the coordination of care (Chumbler et al. 2007; Harris et al. 2007; Peng et al. 2006).

New Directions for E-Health Interventions for Pain Management

While current e-health developments for the management of pain have been very promising, we are just at the very beginning of designing and implementing powerful computer-based intervention programs. The future is very promising for the development of smart, interactive, and comprehensive health information systems that will travel with consumers wherever they go (mobile health), automatically monitor consumer health status (real-time data capture), share relevant health information with all members of the pain management team (inter-professional coordination), and deliver pain management support to consumers when and where they need it. The integration of artificial intelligence into the design of health information systems will allow e-health programs to interact meaningfully with consumers about their pain management needs and concerns. These new smart systems e-health information systems can be tailored to provide personalized information to consumers based upon the consumers' unique experiences and information needs.

New embedded information technologies that are either worn on consumers' clothing or implanted within their bodies have the potential for continuously collecting physiological information that will enable proactive prediction of pain events and will allow early response interventions to prevent pain incidents. These imbedded information systems could be designed to deliver relevant health information to consumers, stimulate their neural pathways to minimize pain, and perhaps even administer needed pain medications to pain sufferers. The growth of nanotechnology is making smaller and less invasive embedded information technologies increasingly feasible for use as embedded health information systems to support pain management.

The development and implementation of online palliative care training systems can make help healthcare providers and consumers develop the communication competencies needed to support effective pain management. Similar health communication education programs have already been designed and implemented to train healthcare providers to communicate effectively with culturally diverse, low health literacy, and low English proficiency consumers (see http://ftp://ftp.hrsa.gov/healthliteracy/training.pdf). E-health systems that support the development and use of sensitive and strategic health communication practices to support pain management can increase both the quality of care for pain and enhance self-management of pain. Particular attention must be taken to make sure that pain management support technologies are made available and accessible to vulnerable and hard to reach populations (see Kreps et al. 2007 for an examination of strategies for making e-health applications work for under-served and vulnerable groups).

The future for the development of e-health communication interventions for promoting pain management is bright. Creative technology developers are designing new tools and programs for supporting effective health communication that will help meet the information needs of consumers who confront serious pain and the caregivers that help these consumers. Health communication technology will become a central part of effective, far-reaching, and proactive pain management.

Question: Any suggestions for how these interventions can gain assess to hard to reach and vulnerable populations?

References

Adler, B., Yarchoan, M., & Adler, J. R. (2011). Neurosurgical interventions for the control of chronic pain conditions. In R. J. Moore (Ed.), *Handbook of pain and palliative care*. New York, NY: Springer.

Ahles, T., Blanchard, E., & Ruckdeschel, J. (1983). The multidimensional nature of cancer-related pain. *Pain, 17*, 277–288.

Appel, P. R., Bleiberg, J., & Noiseux, J. (2002). Self-regulation training for chronic pain: Can it be done effectively by telemedicine? *Telemedicine Journal and E-Health, 8*, 361–368.

Arora, N. K. (2003). Interacting with cancer patients: The significance of physicians' communication behavior. *Social Science and Medicine, 57*, 791–806.

Berry, D. L., Wilkie, D. J., Thomas, C. R., Jr., & Fortner, P. (2003). Clinicians communicating with patients experiencing cancer pain. *Cancer Investigation, 21*(3), 374–381.

Bostrom, B., Sandh, M., Lundberg, D., & Fridlund, B. (2004). Cancer-related pain in palliative care: Patients' perceptions of pain management. *Journal of Advanced Nursing, 45*(4), 410–419.

Carr, E., Brockbank, K., & Barrett, R. (2003). Improving pain management through interprofessional education: Evaluation of a pilot project. *Learning in Health and Social Care, 2*(1), 6–17.

Chumbler, N. R., Mkanta, W. N., Richardson, L. C., Harris, L., Darkins, A., Kobb, R., & Ryan, P. (2007). Remote patient–provider communication and quality of life: Empirical test of a dialogic model of cancer care. *Journal of Telemedicine and Telecare, 13*, 20–25.

Cook, A. J., Roberts, D. A., Henderson, M. D., Van Winkle, L. C., Chastain, D. C., & Hamill-Ruth, R. J. (2004). Electronic pain questionnaires: A randomized crossover comparison with paper questionnaires for chronic pain assessment. *Pain, 110*, 310–317.

Cowan, P. (2011). Support groups for chronic pain. In R. J. Moore (Ed.), *Handbook of pain and palliative care*. New York, NY: Springer.

Detmar, S. B., Aaronson, N. K., Wever, L. D., Muller, M., & Schornagel, J. H. (2000). How are you feeling? Who wants to know? Patients' and oncologists' preferences for discussing health-related quality-of-life issues. *Journal of Clinical Oncology, 18*, 3295–3301.

Detmar, S. B., Muller, M. J., Wever, L. D., Schornagel, J. H., & Aaronson, N. K. (2001). Health-related quality-of-life assessments and patient-physician communication: A randomized controlled trial. *Journal of the American Medical Association, 285*(10), 1351–1357.

Dobratz, M. C., Wade, R., Herbst, L., & Ryndes, T. (1991). Pain efficacy in home hospice patients: A longitudinal study. *Cancer Nursing, 14*(1), 20–26.

Egbert, N., Sparks, L., Kreps, G. L., & Du Pré, A. (2008). Finding meaning in the journey: Methods of spiritual coping for aging cancer patients. In L. Sparks, D. O'Hair, & G. L. Kreps (Eds.), *Cancer communication and aging* (pp. 277–291). Cresskill, NJ: Hampton Press.

Eng, T. R. (2001). *The e-health landscape: A terrain map of emerging information and communication technologies in health and health care*. Princeton, NJ: The Robert Wood Johnson Foundation.

Ferguson, T. (1996). *Health online: How to find health information, support groups, and self help communities in cyberspace*. Reading, MA: Addison-Wesley.

Fitzmartin, G. M., Blum, D., & Swanton, R. (1995). Psychosocial barriers to cancer pain relief. *Cancer Practice, 3*(2), 71.

Hallenbeck, J. (2011). Pain and intercultural communication. In R. J. Moore (Ed.), *Handbook of pain and palliative care*. New York, NY: Springer.

Harris, L. M., Kreps, G. L., & Dresser, C. (2007). Health communication technology and quality of cancer care. In D. O'Hair, G. L. Kreps, & L. Sparks (Eds.), *Handbook of communication and cancer care* (pp. 59–71). Cresskill, NJ: Hampton Press.

Hesse, B. W., Nelson, D. E., Kreps, G. L., Croyle, R. T., Arora, N. K., Rimer, B. K., & Viswanath, K. (2005). Trust and sources of health information. The impact of the Internet and its implications for health care providers: Findings from the first Health Information National Trends Survey. *Archives of Internal Medicine, 165*(22), 2618–2624.

Holland, J. C. (2003). Psychological care of patients: Psycho-oncology's contribution. *Journal of Clinical Oncology, 21*(23s), 253s–265s.

Huang, H.-Y., Wilkie, D., Faan, Z. S., Berry, D., Hairabedian, D., Judge, M. K., Farber, S., & Chabal, C. (2003). Developing a computerized data collection and decision support system for cancer pain management. *CIN: Computers, Informatics, Nursing, 21*, 206–217.

Jamison, R. N., Fanciullo, G., & Baird, J. C. (2002). Introduction: Computer and information technology in the assessment and management of patients with pain. *Pain Medicine, S3*, 83–84.

Jamison, R. N., Raymond, S. A., Levine, J. G., Slawsby, E. A., Nedeljkovic, S. S., & Katz, N. P. (2001). Electronic diaries for monitoring chronic pain: 1-year validation study. *Pain, 91*, 277–285.

Jamison, R. N., Raymond, S. A., Slawsby, E. A., McHugo, G. J., & Baird, J. C. (2006). Pain assessment in patients with low back pain: Comparison of weekly recall and momentary electronic data. *The Journal of Pain, 7*, 192–199.

Junker, U., Freyhagen, R., Längler, K., Gockel, U., Schmidt, U., Tölle, T. R., Baron, R., & Kohlmann, T. (2008). Paper versus electronic rating scales for pain assessment: A prospective, randomised, cross-over validation study with 200 chronic pain patients. *Current Medical Research and Opinion, 24*, 1797–1806.

Kimberlin, C., Brushwood, D., Allen, W., Radson, A., & Wilson, E. (2004). Cancer patient and caregiver experiences: Communication and pain management issues. *Journal of Pain and Symptom Management, 26*, 566–578.

Kreps, G. L. (1996). The interface between health communication and health psychology. *Journal of Health Psychology, 1*(3), 259–260.

Kreps, G. L. (2001). The evolution and advancement of health communication inquiry. In W. B. Gudykunst (Ed.), *Communication yearbook 24* (pp. 232–254). Newbury Park, CA: Sage.

Kreps, G. L. (2004). The role of communication in cancer pain and symptom management. *Psycho-Oncology, 13*(1 Suppl), 35.

Kreps, G. L., & Chapelsky Massimilla, D. (2002). Cancer communications research and health outcomes: Review and challenge. *Communication Studies, 53*(4), 318–336.

Kreps, G. L., Gustafson, D., Salovey, P., Perocchia, R. S., Wilbright, W., Bright, M. A., & Muha, C. (2007). The NCI Digital Divide Pilot Projects: Implications for cancer education. *Journal of Cancer Education, 22*(Suppl 1), S56–S60.

Kreps, G. L., & Neuhauser, L. (2010). New directions in e-health communication: Opportunities and challenges. *Patient Education and Counseling, 78*, 329–336.

Kreps, G. L., & O'Hair, D. (Eds.). (1995). *Communication and health outcomes*. Cresskill, NJ: Hampton Press.

Lindsay, S., Smith, S., Bellaby, P., & Baker, R. (2009). The health impact of an online heart disease support group: A comparison of moderated versus unmoderated support. *Health Education Research, 24*, 646–654.

Manzanec, P., Buras, D., Hudson, J., & Montana, B. (2002). Transdisciplinary pain management. *Journal of Hospice and Palliative Nursing, 4*(4), 228–234.

Marceau, L. D., Link, C., Jamison, R. N., & Carolan, S. (2007). Electronic diaries as a tool to improve pain management: Is there any evidence? *Pain Medicine, S3*, S101–S109.

Mendenhall, M. (2003). Psychosocial aspects of pain management: A conceptual framework for social workers on pain management teams. *Social Work in Health Care, 36*(4), 35–51.

Morrison, L., & Morrison, R. S. (2006). Palliative care and pain management. *Medical Clinics of North America, 90*, 983–1004.

Nelson, W., & Weir, R. (2001). Biopsychosocial approaches to the treatment of chronic pain. *The Clinical Journal of Pain, 17*(4), 114–127.

Neuhauser, L., & Kreps, G. L. (2010). E-health communication and behavior change: Promise and performance. *Social Semiotics, 20*(1), 7–24.

Newman, M. G., Consoli, A. J., & Taylor, C. B. (1999). A palmtop computer program for the treatment of generalized anxiety disorder. *Behavior Modification, 23*, 597–619.

Novy, D. (2004). Psychological approaches for managing chronic pain. *Journal of Psychopathology and Behavioral Assessment, 26*(4), 279–288.

Palermo, Y. (2011). The art of pain: The patient's perspective of chronic pain. In R. J. Moore (Ed.), *Handbook of pain and palliative care*. New York, NY: Springer.

Pargeon, K. L., & Hailey, B. J. (1999). Barriers to effective cancer pain management. *Journal of Pain and Symptom Management, 18*, 358–368.

Peng, P. W., Stafford, M. A., Wong, D. T., & Salenieks, M. E. (2006). Use of telemedicine in chronic pain consultation: A pilot study. *The Clinical Journal of Pain, 22*, 350–352.

Peters, M. L., Sorbi, M. J., Kruise, D. A., Kerssens, J. J., & Bensing, J. M. (2000). Electronic diary assessment of pain, disability and psychological adaptation in patients differing in duration of pain. *Pain, 84*, 181–192.

Pollo, A., & Benedetti, F. (2011). Pain and the placebo/nocebo effect. In R. J. Moore (Ed.), *Handbook of pain and palliative care*. New York, NY: Springer.

Pronovost, A., Peng, P., & Kern, R. (2009). Telemedicine in the management of chronic pain: A cost analysis study. *Canadian Journal of Anesthesia, 56*, 590–596.

Rogers, M. S., & Todd, C. J. (2000). The 'right kind' of pain: Talking about symptoms in outpatient oncology consultations. *Palliative Medicine, 14*(4), 299–307.

Sehgal, N., Falco, F., Benjamin, A., Henry, J., Josephson, Y., & Manchikanti, L. (2011). Rehabilitation treatments for chronic musculoskeletal pain. In R. J. Moore (Ed.), *Handbook of pain and palliative care*. New York, NY: Springer.

Short, R., & Vetter, T. R. (2011). Acute to chronic pain: Transitions in the post surgical patient. In R. J. Moore (Ed.), *Handbook of pain and palliative care*. New York, NY: Springer.

Stone, A. A., Broderick, J. E., Schwartz, J. E., Shiffman, S. S., Litcher-Kelly, L., & Calvanese, P. (2003). Intensive momentary reporting of pain with an electronic diary: Reactivity, compliance, and patient satisfaction. *Pain, 104*, 343–351.

VanDenKerkhof, E. G., Goldstein, D. H., Lane, J., Rimmer, M. J., & Van Dijk, J. P. (2003). Using a personal digital assistant enhances gathering of patient data on an acute pain management service: A pilot study. *Canadian Journal of Anaesthesia, 50*, 368–375.

Wilkie, D. J., Judge, M. K. M., Berry, D. L., Dell, J., Zong, S., & Gilespie, R. (2003). Usability of a Computerized PAIN Report It in the general public with pain and people with cancer pain. *Journal of Pain and Symptom Management, 25*, 213–224.

Zhao, Z., & Cope, D. K. (2011). Nerve blocks, trigger points, and intrathecal therapy for chronic pain. In R. J. Moore (Ed.), *Handbook of pain and palliative care*. New York, NY: Springer.

Chapter 5
Educating Patients and Caregivers About Pain Management: What Clinicians Need to Know

Micke Brown, Amanda Crowe, and Stefanie Cousins

Introduction

Public health is primarily concerned with the health of the entire population, rather than the health of individuals. Its features include an emphasis on the promotion of health and the prevention of disease and disability; the collection and use of epidemiological data, population surveillance, and other forms of empirical quantitative assessment; a recognition of the multidimensional nature of the determinants of health; and a focus on the complex interactions of many factors – biological, behavioral, social, and environmental – in developing effective interventions (Childress et al. 2002).

The prevalence of pain is high and it exacts a tremendous toll on our society. Yet it is often missing from the public health agenda at the community, state, and federal levels.

According to the Council of State Governments (CSG), the overall goal of public health is to prevent disease or injury in a whole population – a city, state, or country, which differs from the goal of health care, which is to care for individuals. The example the Council cites for distinction is cancer. A public health approach to cancer could involve a statewide public awareness campaign about the risk factors for cancer such as smoking or sun exposure, while a healthcare approach would focus on educating individuals about such risk factors (Healthy States 2009). How does this relate to pain?

If pain was formally recognized as part of our national public health agenda, public awareness campaigns would highlight pain prevention and cover risk factors for the development of the disease of chronic pain. As an expectation rather than an option, education for the consumer, the healthcare professional, caregivers, and policy makers would be developed as a broad outreach effort. States would be looking at ways to disseminate information in a variety of venues as part of a state-based initiative, similar to efforts by the state-based offices of aging and cancer control plans.

Unfortunately, pain is not a public health priority, so the burden is on healthcare professionals, patients, and caregivers to educate and advocate for better pain management.

Successful models could be used as patient education frameworks for pain as they are ripe for repurposing. For example, the comprehensive state cancer plan model is based on collaborative effort of government agencies (CDC, NIH, and state legislatures) along with the public sector (hospitals and universities, cancer advocacy groups, and others). These plans have been in existence

M. Brown, BSN, RN (✉)
American Pain Foundation, Baltimore, MD, USA
e-mail: mbrown@painfoundation.org

A. Crowe, MA, MPH • S. Cousins, MPH
Impact Health Communications, LLC
e-mail: amanda.crowe@alumni.duke.edu; stefaniecousins@gmail.com

R.J. Moore (ed.), *Handbook of Pain and Palliative Care: Biobehavioral Approaches for the Life Course*,
DOI 10.1007/978-1-4419-1651-8_5, © Springer Science+Business Media, LLC 2012

since 1998 and are revised every 3–4 years. They provide a framework for states to assess disease burden that affect their constituents, identify and create work partnerships with researchers and others to move science into the practice setting, learn and adopt interventional strategies, evaluate program outcomes, and benchmark with other states. Yet, cancer impacts 0.4% of the U.S. population according to the American Cancer Society (ACS) estimates. The impact of pain is far greater. However, no comparable model exists to address the effect of pain on a societal level. Taking the cancer control model and adapting it into a national plan to address pain would be a powerful step in a positive direction.

Knowledge Is Power

Public and professional knowledge about pain is lacking. It has been well published since the late 1990s, that the majority of healthcare professionals' knowledge base and corresponding skill sets around the subject of pain are substandard. Little has changed in the past 20 years. Most medical, nursing, and pharmacy school curricula fail to adequately integrate pain management education into the field of required studies. Seasoned healthcare professionals are not well incentivized to improve their pain education. Fear of regulatory scrutiny over opioid prescribing practices seems to be a common deterrent for many physicians and members of the clinical team. Though the experience of pain is common and complex, academic coursework and continuing medical education remains optional.

Meanwhile, there is a general shift in our healthcare delivery system away from the traditional disease-centered model of care to one that is patient-centered, which takes into account an individual's lifestyle, personal preferences, cultural beliefs and traditions, and family. With this rise of patient-centered care and empowerment, consumers are seeking out information and are more willing to speak up and advocate on their own behalf to obtain quality care that is right for them. People living with pain, their caregivers, and the public either struggle with obtaining quality information about pain and its treatment or live in a vacuum about its impact on their life and the lives of others.

Education and active engagement in pain care and treatment helps to equip people with the skills and confidence they require to be active participants in their own care. In order to help improve patient interaction, healthcare providers should strive to enhance their clinical know-how as well as learn how to translate this information to their patients in a meaningful way.

Finding the right information and having the skills to engage in health decision making is an important step for individuals to successfully be "team players" in their pain care. Pain is a complex experience, everyone is different, and pain management and treatment must be personalized. That means what's right for one person may not be right for someone else with the same condition.

In this information age, everyone is constantly bombarded with information. While it is empowering to know that anyone can go to the next medical appointment having done some independent research, it can also be overwhelming to sift through and interpret this information while balancing it with a person's own priorities for treatment (American Pain Foundation 2009).

Educating people with pain, their caregivers, and the public helps everyone become well informed about how to weigh various treatment choices while considering personal preferences. This helps the individual feel more confident in the choices made and enhances the "buy-in" that ensures adherence to care. People who participate actively in their own care tend to report better results and higher satisfaction with their treatment choices and overall care than those who are less involved.

Over the course of a patient's journey with pain, he/she might undergo a process that leads him/her from being a passive recipient of information to one who is actively engaged in his/her own treatment. The individual becomes empowered by the resources available from healthcare providers, as well as the community of support he/she might find locally or online. Choosing to become better educated about treatment options; asking the difficult questions; and, being more assertive when making choices that affect health and well-being are essential behaviors that are more commonly seen today and expected by many clinicians as essential for shared decision making. This is especially important for people living with chronic illnesses, including persistent pain, which remains largely misunderstood and requires ongoing self-care.

This idea of shared decision making also emphasizes the ethical requirement for healthcare providers to fully inform the individual about the risks and benefits of available, multimodal treatment options, while ensuring that their patient's needs and preferences guide the decision making process (Ibid) (see also Rich 2011; Fine 2011). Living with pain is an uphill battle for many individuals, especially when pain is persistent. The challenges people face in getting their pain treated, the lack of trained specialists, and disparities in pain management underscore the need for more purposeful education and empowerment about pain.

For people with pain and their families, managing pain is challenging even under the best of circumstances. Trying to navigate a complex and often confusing healthcare system can make getting the treatment they need even more difficult. Similar to those living with other chronic illnesses, people with persistent pain face ongoing challenges in trying to deal with a health system originally built to treat acute illnesses (American Pain Foundation 2009).

A large proportion of individuals seek help from multiple providers before their pain condition is acknowledged, let alone appropriately managed. For those with disabling pain, access to pain specialists is very limited. This is due to the limited number of specialists (about 5,000 in the entire USA) and the current systems that support the training and reimbursement of specialists (American Pain Foundation 2006).

Who Is Treating Patients with Pain

Data from a national survey suggest that attitudes and practices vary substantially among the disciplines that treat chronic pain. For example, the survey, which included primary care physicians (PCPs), pain physicians, chiropractors, and acupuncturists found that:

- PCPs treat approximately 52% of people with chronic pain, pain physicians treat 2%, chiropractors treat 40%, and acupuncturists treat 7%. Of those with chronic pain seen for evaluation, the percentages subsequently treated on an ongoing basis range from 51% (PCPs) to 63% (pain physicians).
- Pain physicians prescribe long-acting opioids (e.g., methadone) and adjuvant analgesics (e.g., antidepressants, anticonvulsants) some 50–100% more often than do PCPs.
- PCPs were the least likely of the groups surveyed to be confident about managing musculoskeletal and neuropathic pain and the least likely to favor mandatory pain education for all PCPs (American Pain Foundation 2006).

As with most medical treatment for a number of chronic illnesses, pain management falls short among certain groups. In the case of pain, women, children, and older adults are at greater risk for being adversely affected by chronic pain (see also Vetter 2011; Keogh 2011; McCarberg and Cole 2011). Even those who are fortunate enough to find a qualified pain specialist may still face hurdles along the way.

Pain is treatable, and it often takes multiple tries to find the treatment that works best for each individual. It is not easy deciding whether to try a different therapy, take a new medication, undergo surgery, maintain current treatment, or discontinue treatment altogether. Being well informed is the first step. Whether you are a person living with pain, a relative, partner, friend, or a clinician, advocating for and making the best decisions about pain takes time, skill, and patience.

Making Patient Education a Priority

The role of patient education has been well established in a variety of chronic conditions, including asthma, diabetes, arthritis, and hypertension. Most of the literature related to pain education has focused on the information needs and preferences of people with cancer. This is likely to translate to people with pain from other causes. While some educational tools and strategies have been studied, particularly as they relate to improving treatment adherence, immunization rates, and other disease management issues, many activities and services to help educate and equip individuals with skills for self-care are based on practical experience and knowledge of health communications.

Patient education strategies and tools should include a variety of mediums that enhance mass population learning: in-office displays of pain-specific brochures, newsletters, videos, audiotapes, posters, content on practice or hospital web sites, use of pain notebooks or diaries, referring people to credible web sites, structured educational/coaching programs, and web-based tools. The latter require considerable more personnel and resources and are not covered here, but nonetheless are important to mention.

Building Skills and Setting Goals

Key objectives that healthcare providers can use to educate their patients may include:

- Increasing patients' and caregivers' understanding of pain.
- Delivering messages that are culturally sensitive and address disparities in care.
- Discussing treatment goals.
- Addressing the psychosocial, spiritual, and physical aspects of pain.
- Empowering individuals to self-advocate by providing tools/handouts and other tips for self-management/skills acquisition to manage chronic pain.
- Teaching the appropriate use of pain treatment options.
- Creating an environment where people can talk openly and ask questions, thereby, improving patient–provider communications.

Skills Building

For people living with persistent pain, gaining the knowledge and the skills to manage pain is integral to the process of finding pain relief. As with other chronic illnesses, people with pain need to know how to self-manage their pain.

Healthcare providers should take the time necessary to empower people with pain and their caregivers to get their life back by providing counsel on specific actions and behaviors that can alleviate pain (e.g., in some cases, stress management, therapeutic exercise or massage, keeping a pain notebook, nutrition). This should also include efforts to address depression, sleep disturbances, issues of isolation, or intimacy that tend to coexist with many pain conditions.

Translating Education to Practice

Patient education is central to improving pain management (American Cancer Society 2001; Gordon and Warde 1995). Successful education has been shown to improve outcomes and adherence to treatment protocols, and also improve and enhance patient satisfaction. For this reason, it is important to take the time to help people with pain and their caregivers become educated consumers of pain management and know how to so they can self-advocate. Sadly, too many individuals are unprepared. While certain policies, including the Joint Commission's standards for pain assessment and management, have helped drive pain education and awareness, there is still considerable room for improvement.

Because healthcare providers are a leading source of health information for the public – even in this digital age – they should be equipped to serve as health educators and make it a priority. This role should be seen as an integral part of clinical practice, especially as the public increasingly navigate their options for pain care and self-advocate.

Effectively Educating Your Patients

To effectively educate people with chronic pain, providers should strive to:

1. Recognize the barriers to effective pain treatment that might impede a balanced and complete understanding of pain and options for treatment
2. Understand what kind of information their patients are seeking and how and where they get their information (i.e., ensure their patients are consulting credible sources and be prepared to address conflicting information)
3. Integrate strategies that facilitate ongoing dialogue and information sharing, including leveraging teachable moments, skills training (how to define and accurately convey pain experience), encouraging social and psychological support, and advocating on their patients' behalf
4. Help their patients better describe their pain and how it impacts daily function and quality of life (See APF's top 10 tips for explaining your pain to others 2011; available at http://www.painfoundation.org/learn/living/top-ten-tips/)

Educational efforts may also include: information about the specific pain condition, the goals of therapy, methods for pain assessment, and appropriate use of pain treatment options – both medication and nondrug techniques.

Dispelling Myths and Identifying Other Barriers to Pain Care Is Part of Educating (or Re-educating) Public

Pain is riddled with myths and misperceptions, making the task of informing and educating affected individuals – and the public – about pain and its management that much more challenging. Misunderstandings about pain are often fueled by preconceived notions or myths (see Table 5.1).

Table 5.1 Six common pain myths

Pain is "all in your head." Although we our brains process the perception of pain, this does not mean that pain is imaginary when the source of pain is not well understood. Pain is all too real to the person who lives with it on a daily basis

Pain is just something one has to live with. Pain traditionally has been viewed as an inevitable consequence of a disease or condition. The fact is most pain can be relieved with proper pain management

Pain is a natural part of growing older. While pain is more common as we age, because conditions that cause pain (e.g., arthritis, degenerative joint diseases, cancer, shingles, osteoporosis) are more frequent in older adults, it should not be something people have to endure untreated

The best judge of pain is the physician or nurse. There is little relationship between what a physician or nurse might "guess" about their patient's pain and actual pain experience. The person with pain is the authority on the existence and severity of his/her pain. The self-report is most reliable indicator

Seeking medical care for pain is a sign of weakness. Pain carries a stigma, and many people hesitate talking about their pain and how it affects their daily life; they also do not want to be considered a "bad patient"

Use of strong pain medication leads to addiction. Many people living with pain, and even some healthcare practitioners, falsely believe that opioid pain medicines are universally addictive. As with any medication, there are risks, but these risks can be managed when these medicines are properly prescribed and taken as directed. For more information about safety issues related to opioids and other pain therapies, visit http://www. painsafe.org

Source: American Pain Foundation, *Policymaker's Guide to Understanding Pain and Its Management*

Table 5.2 Common barriers to effective pain management (National Cancer Institute 2011)

Clinician barriers

In clinical encounters with their patients, healthcare providers may have:

- Gaps in knowledge due to limited training in pain management
- Inadequate pain assessment skills
- Negative attitudes toward prescribing opioids due to side effects, concerns over tolerance, and addiction
- Apprehension prescribing opioids due to fears of regulatory scrutiny
- Belief that treating pain takes too much time and effort and may not relieve patient
- Limited or no training in providing culturally sensitive care

Patient barriers

During their contact with healthcare providers, the communication skills, psychosocial well-being, and attitudes toward pain of the person with pain may affect their ability or willingness to report pain. They may have:

- Reluctance to report pain
- Concern about distracting physicians from treatment of underlying disease
- Fear that pain is a sign that any underlying disease is worsening
- Concerns about not being a "good" patient
- Reluctance to take pain medication
- Fear of addiction or perception of being an addict (more pronounced among minority patients) (Anderson et al. 2002)
- Worries about unmanageable side effects (e.g., constipation, nausea, clouded thought)
- Concern about becoming tolerant to pain medications
- Poor adherence to prescribed analgesic regimen (Miaskowski et al. 2001)

Health system barriers

The healthcare system has fundamental barriers to effective pain management with its infrastructure, prescription reimbursement, access issues, and regulation of medication. Examples include:

- Lack of transportation to the physician or pharmacy
- Low supply or unavailability of opioids at local pharmacy
- Lack of a home caregiver to assist with administering drugs
- Limits on the number of prescriptions filled per month
- Most appropriate treatment either not reimbursed or too costly for the individual/families in need
- Restrictive regulation of controlled substances
- Problems of availability of treatment or access to it

Studies have shown these key areas can all, in some way, create obstacles for effective management of pain

So for any educational effort to be successful, it is important not only to address gaps in knowledge, but also attitudes toward pain and pain management. Stoicism, fears of opioid addiction, and cultural beliefs all affect the use of, and adherence to, pain therapies.

When educating an affected individual or caregiver about pain, it is also essential to consider the barriers that might already be hindering quality pain care. Such barriers can be contributed to the person with pain, healthcare providers, and the health system (see Table 5.2).

Understanding Health Information Seeking Can Help Guide Education Efforts

The digital boom has made the Internet a leading source for health information. A February 2011 Pew Internet & Family Life Project survey found that eight in ten Internet users look for health information online and that number continues to grow, even among the older adult population. Sixty percent of survey respondents reported that their online searches influenced treatment decisions with about 40% confirming that their search influenced the decision to seek care from a healthcare provider (Pew Internet & Family Life Project 2011).

It is important for the public to understand the quality of Internet sites and how to determine whether the information is accurate and trustworthy, since there are millions of health-related web sites catering to the growing demand for medical information. Not all web sites are created equal and some may contain false or misleading information. See APF's web site for *Top 10 Tips for Finding Quality Health Information Online*, a helpful resource for patients and families (American Pain Foundation 2009). If individuals do not have access to the Internet at home, they may be able to find a computer with online access at their local library, public university, community, and senior centers. Some of these venues hold tutorials about how to start a search. Family members, neighbors, and friends can also help research health information for them.

Understanding how and where people seek healthcare information, as well as what they want to know, is critical for healthcare providers. Awareness of these factors may help providers tailor information, advice, and suggested resources for their patients. Generally, people will use a variety of sources to obtain health information. Many rely on traditional information sources – healthcare professionals, the Internet, books, the media, friends, and family members. Remember, many studies find that healthcare professionals remain among the most trusted source of information. Individuals typically rely on other sources to supplement medical information provided by healthcare professionals.

Repetition in a variety of forms will reinforce desired messaging about content and desired behavioral changes. Studies have shown that 40–80% of the medical information patients receive is forgotten immediately and nearly half of the information retained is incorrect (Kessels 2003).

What Patients Want to Know About Persistent Pain

In general, people living with persistent pain want information or advice on:

1. How to understand their pain, specifically the cause
2. What to expect, when they might experience pain, and what it might feel like
3. Pain treatment options, including pain medication, medical or surgical treatments, and nonpharmacological approaches
4. How to cope with pain
5. How pain negatively impacts their lives physically, psychologically, and socially

6. How to connect with other people with pain to find out what their pain was like, how it has affected their lives, what they are doing to cope, what their doctors suggest in terms of pain relief, and the method of pain relief they found to be most effective
7. Where to find healthcare providers who manage pain, whom to consult, and various treatments available
8. How to describe pain (Bender et al. 2008; Anderson et al. 1979)

These preferences for pain information can also apply to people with other types of pain. APF also periodically surveys its membership and other groups of people living with pain to assess information needs.

Tools for Healthcare Providers

The following pages provide a variety of tools for healthcare providers to use in elevating pain awareness and understanding among their patients.

In-Practice and Community-Based Strategies and Tools to Educate Patients

Learning about their pain condition, what to expect and the options available for relief can empower individuals and give them a sense of control. Of course, limited provider–patient face time can make it much more difficult to cover all critical teaching points during an average clinical encounter. That is why – whenever possible – it is important for healthcare providers to look for and take advantage of teachable moments and maintain an open dialogue with their patients.

Teachable Moments

Each clinician (e.g., physician, nurse, pharmacist, social worker, or therapist) contact is an opportunity to engage in a teachable moment. Using reflective communication methods, such as Teach Back, Tell Back (Teach Back Method 2009), is one example of how to incorporate education during routine, daily contact in the clinical setting. A variety of print, audio, and video materials that are sensitive to literacy levels may be provided in clinical common areas, such as waiting rooms, rest rooms, and exam rooms. Reinforcing the content of these materials is vital during face-to-face clinic time. Incorporating interactive materials that may be used in the home environment and reviewed during office visits not only provides information often missing during periodic reviews, but also encourages involvement by the person living with pain. Moreover, these materials may be verified and reviewed by family members when necessary, and may serve as a quality improvement tool to adjust/tailor the pain treatment plan. For more information, see APF's *Targeting Chronic Pain Notebook* as one model (http://www.painfoundation.org/learn/publications/target-notebook.html).

Written Educational Materials

Printed materials in the form of waiting room posters, brochures, self-assessment and pain management checklists, and standardized instructions can help to augment and reinforce information shared during one-on-one consultations. These resources can also help to improve recall of verbal instructions.

Other useful material to offer patients include pain diaries (see APF's *Targeting Chronic Pain Notebook*, http://www.painfoundation.org/learn/publications/files/TargetNotebook.pdf), newsletters with up-to-date articles about pain (e.g., APF's *Pain Community News*, http://www.painfoundation. org/learn/publications/pain-community-news-archives.html) and pain condition fact sheets (e.g., cancer pain, musculoskeletal, neuropathic, arthritis) with pharmacologic and nonpharmacologic treatment options (see APF's *Spotlight* series on various types of pain topics at http://www.painfoundation.org/ learn). Checklists might be provided to individuals to prompt a discussion with their healthcare provider about pain management or referrals for treatment modalities beyond prescription medication.

Health Literacy

Health literacy – a person's ability to obtain, process, and understand health information and use that information to make good decisions about one's health and medical care (IOM 2004; U.S. Department of Health and Human Services 2000) – is emerging as a significant barrier to improving health status.

Since health literacy could be a barrier to understanding educational materials about pain, any information provided should be:

- Written at the eighth grade reading level or less
- Written in a style that uses minimal but accessible statistics (e.g., "33% of adults" should be written as "one out of three adults")
- Visually appealing, uncluttered, and easy to follow
- Personalized to the individual user or his/her diagnosis (e.g., space for lab results, pain notes, list of medications and dosages, etc.)
- Focused on an action and behavior rather than general awareness (e.g., steps to control pain)
- Supplemented by verbal support and instructions, which allow the provider to adapt educational points based on responses from the patient (Zirwas and Holder 2009; Aldridge 2004)

> In 2011, the new standard: PC.02.01.21 requires healthcare institutions to effectively communicate with patients when providing care, treatment, and services. The rationale states that effective patient–provider communication is necessary for patient safety. Research shows that patients with communication problems are at an increased risk of experiencing preventable adverse events, and that patients with limited English proficiency are more likely to experience adverse events than English speaking patients. Performance will be measured by evidence of oral and written communication needs, including the patient's preferred language for discussing healthcare, the need for personal devices such as hearing aids or glasses, language interpreters, communication boards, and translated or plain language materials (Joint Commission Patient-Centered Communication Standards 2011).

The average American adult cannot read above the eighth grade level (Doak et al. 1996; Winslow 2001); yet, the majority of patient education materials are written at the high school or college level. One in three American adults finds it difficult to obtain or digest medical information due to limited health literacy. Of note, many over-the-counter medication labels require a tenth grade reading level, leaving many unable to follow important dosing instructions (Doak et al. 1996; Winslow 2001).

Limited health literacy can affect a patient's ability to:

- Fill out complex forms
- Locate providers and services
- Share personal information such as health history
- Take care of oneself
- Manage a chronic disease
- Understand how to take medicines

Source: U.S. Department of Health and Human Services

Individuals most likely to experience low health literacy are older adults, racial and ethnic minorities, people with less than a high school degree or GED certificate, people with low income levels, nonnative speakers of English, and people with compromised health status.

The information healthcare professionals provide to their patients and their family members and caregivers is only as good as the recipient's ability to understand the material. Therefore, pain education messages should be developed to include materials that are appropriate for low literacy and non-English speaking populations.

Enhancing Pain Communication

Communication between people with pain and healthcare providers is a vital part of treatment. The following are several tools than can help open up lines of communication.

Keep Pain Questions Handy

Many people may not actively talk about pain. Keeping pain-related questions on hand can help to guide discussions about pain. This is especially important when evaluating individuals where pain might be suspected (e.g., those with diabetes or arthritis, pre- and postoperative follow-ups, older adults at increased risk of shingles/PHN, and degenerative diseases).

In his book *Listening to Pain*, Dr. Scott Fishman, chair and president of the American Pain Foundation, and chief of the Division of Pain Medicine and Professor of Anesthesiology at the University of California at Davis, recommends asking the following questions as part of the initial patient assessment to assist in accurately assessing pain and using the information as an opportunity for pain education (Let's Talk Pain 2010):

- Where is the location of your pain?
- What is the character of your pain?
- How and when did the pain start?
- Is the pain continuous or intermittent?
- What are the exacerbating and relieving factors of your pain? What makes it feel better or worse, including medication, rest, activity, stress, sleep, or hot showers?
- What is the effect of stress on your pain, as well as the source of stressors?
- Any sleep disturbances?
- Any ongoing medical concerns?
- How does pain affect functioning at school or work?

- How does pain affect quality of life functions, such as relationships, sex, or recreation?
- What does the patient expect from medications or other treatments in terms of analgesia or recovered functions?

People with pain should be encouraged to bring a trusted family member or friend to each appointment for support and to lower anxiety levels, but also to increase recall.

Pain Diaries and Pain Intensity Scales

Pain is a subjective experience. Not only does a person need to be able to convey his/her pain to the practitioner, it is also important to make sure caregivers understand the limits pain imposes on function, as well as related issues like depression, sleep deprivation, and intimacy. As pain is invisible to others, individuals need tools and tutorials on how to describe their pain and its impact on various aspects of their lives.

Pain diaries can help enhance communication about pain and provide opportunities for patient education during clinical contact. These can help with tracking pain intensity throughout the day, how pain impacts sleep and function, what therapies are working, etc. (see APF's *Targeting Chronic Pain Notebook*, http://www.painfoundation.org/learn/publications/files/TargetNotebook. pdf). Keeping this kind of record can also facilitate patient–provider communication. It allows the person with pain to translate a subjective pain experience in terms of its effect on function and quality of life, which are the cornerstones of treatment success. This tool also helps the clinician evaluate the pain treatment plan and adjust according to key objectives in pain care: pain reduction, prevalence of troublesome side effects, functional improvement, and impact on quality of life.

Pain intensity scales that are used in the inpatient and outpatient settings can serve as a springboard for discussion and education, especially among patients who find it difficult to accurately describe the intensity of their pain (American Pain Foundation 2008). The rating scales are just one part of the overall pain assessment, yet can help uncover the impact of pain treatment when assessed at critical points in time: at rest, during activities, best and worst times of the day, overall averages, and as patient-directed goals.

Support Groups Foster Information Sharing

Psychosocial support – through in-person support groups or online forums – can provide a nonthreatening venue for comfort, ideas, and education (Gold and McClung 2006). Group support can facilitate information sharing and affords people with pain a way to connect with others who face similar challenges, ask questions, and get advice and information on how to self-manage chronic pain.

PainAid (http://painaid.painfoundation.org), APF's free online support community, is staffed entirely by highly qualified volunteers with a range of backgrounds, all of whom either live with chronic pain or care for people who do. Topics range from illness-specific pain, traditional and complementary treatments, to depression and family matters, to financial issues such as disability and workers compensation. PainAid provides platforms for online chats as well Ask-the-Experts message boards moderated by licensed healthcare professionals and is available 24/7.

Advocate as Well as Educate

Chronic pain can be compared to other diseases like breast cancer and HIV/AIDS that were once poorly understood, lacked funding and backing. But people affected by these diseases and the healthcare providers who treated them rallied together to get the issues on the national agenda. It takes courage, perseverance, and the belief that "where there's a will, there's a way."

Despite the significant number of people who suffer with pain, the National Institutes of Health spends less than 1% of its research budget on pain studies. This small proportion of funding brings into stark reality the fact that pain is often inadequately assessed and treated, resulting in needless suffering and poor patient outcomes despite the fact that pain is one of the most common reasons patients consult a healthcare provider.

Beyond one-on-one clinical interactions with those living with pain, health professionals can and should champion the cause of better pain management by educating their colleagues and the public at large. This is an essential step to help raise awareness and understanding of pain as a public health priority.

Healthcare providers and institutions need to understand the epidemic of pain and how it is best assessed and treated. One way to do this is conduct presentations to colleagues about pain and pain management. Other strategies include adding pain materials to admission and discharge packets, posting reminders about pain and its management in elevators, and conducting in-house training for all levels of hospital employees on the effect of pain in the variety of clinical settings where they will come into contact with people experiencing pain during the course of their daily interactions. Hospitals and ambulatory care centers distribute a number of marketing materials that profile chronic pain in newsletters, brochures, and other marketing materials.

When possible, healthcare providers can conduct community education and advocacy activities. This might include speaking at health fairs, meeting with policymakers, serving as a medical expert to encourage in-depth and balanced news coverage of pain, writing a column about the prevalence of pain for the local newspaper, and encouraging patients to share their experience with pain for the benefit of others.

Leveraging Other Allied Health Professionals

Healthcare providers have numerous opportunities to help their patients take advantage of other resources. They may refer people with pain to patient navigator programs if they exist, in-house or community social workers, and other support services. Each of these options provides potential points of interaction with experts who look out for their patients' best interests, answer questions, and support others as they work to lessen their pain.

A number of resources exist to assist healthcare providers and their patients affected by pain. Social workers in the healthcare setting as well as in the community provide support services and educational resources for individuals who have questions about their treatment, need referrals for other kinds of services in the community, and feel as though they have someone looking out for their best interests.

Many healthcare facilities and hospitals now have trained health professionals who serve as patient advocates, patient navigators, and/or ombudsmen (these terms are sometimes used interchangeably). These patient advocates serve as a link between patients and their healthcare providers to help improve or maintain a high quality of care.

They can provide guidance to individuals and their family members and assist with activities like coordinating medical appointments, filling out insurance forms, connecting those in need of supportive services if employment, financial, legal, or other issues arise, or simply helping to develop a list of questions for subsequent appointments. They often help participate in conflict resolution, when needed and help interpret the patient experience during ethics committee hearings and quality improvement work groups. Patient advocates and navigators are usually social workers or nurses, but may also be chaplains or specially trained lay persons.

If a medical center or hospital does not have a patient navigator, a social worker might be able to help patients resolve difficult or confusing practical and emotional issues and point them to other resources. The Patient Advocate Foundation can also provide assistance and is available by visiting http://www.patientadvocate.org or calling 1-800-532-5274.

Summary

It has been well published since the late 1990s, that a majority of healthcare professionals' knowledge base and corresponding skill sets around the subject of pain are substandard. Little has changed in the past 20 years. Most medical, nursing, and pharmacy school curricula fail to adequately integrate pain management education into the field of required studies. Seasoned healthcare professionals are not well incentivized to improve their pain education. Fear of regulatory scrutiny over opioid prescribing practices seems to be a common deterrent for many physicians and members of the clinical team. Though the experience of pain is common and complex, academic coursework and continuing medical education remains optional.

People living with pain, their caregivers, and the public either struggle with obtaining quality information about pain and its treatment or live in a vacuum about its impact on their life and the lives of others. Education and active engagement in pain care and treatment helps to equip people with the skills and confidence they require to be active participants in their own care. In order to help improve the interaction with their patients and families, healthcare providers should strive to enhance their clinical know-how as well as learn how to translate this information to their patients in a meaningful way (see the section "Checklist" below for tips on educating patients about their pain).

Finding the right information and having the skills to engage in health decision making is an important step for individuals to successfully be "team players" in their pain care and for that care to be patient-centric. Pain is a complex experience, everyone is different, and pain management and treatment must be personalized. That means what's right for one person may not be right for someone else with the same condition. Educating people with pain, their caregivers, and the public helps everyone become well informed about how to weigh various treatment choices while considering personal preferences. This helps the individual feel more confident in the choices made and enhances the "buy-in" that heightens adherence to care. People who participate actively in their own care tend to report better results and higher satisfaction with their treatment choices and overall care than those who are less involved.

Checklist

What you can do to better educate people about pain?

In the office:

- Place educational materials such as posters and brochures in waiting rooms and exam rooms. Be sure to provide information on where people can access this information.
- Consider providing a pain-related newsletter along with other magazines in the waiting room (see archived issues of *Pain Community News* at http://www.painfoundation.org).
- Provide reminder cards for follow-up appointments, especially for those who have been prescribed chronic opioid therapy. Provide these individuals with guidance on preparing for follow-up appointments and tips for safely using opioids. APF's *Chronic Opioid Therapy: Preparing for*

Your Appointments (http://www.painfoundation.org/learn/publications/files/cot-appointments.
pdf) and *Chronic Opioid Therapy: The Dos and Don'ts to Help Avoid Problems* (http://www.
painfoundation.org/learn/publications/files/cot-dos-donts.pdf) is designed to reflect what providers want to know from their patients and can help facilitate education and quality of care.

• Ask staff to handout a brief pain questionnaire for completion before going into examination room
  and/or include pain on any health status/history forms given to your patients upon check-in.

At home:

• Provide information that people with pain and caregivers can review at home. This might include

  – Answers to commonly asked questions about pain and its management
  – Facts sheets on specific pain problems or pain-relieving techniques for self-care
  – Information on the psychosocial aspects of pain
  – Information for caregivers
  – A list of reputable online resources on pain on hand for those who want to do more research

In the community:

• Advocate for better pain management within and outside of clinic/hospital using quality management
  programs, ethics committee or pain committee. If a pain committee does not exist – start one.
• Write a column about pain and managing painful conditions for your hospital and local paper.
• Participate as an exhibitor in a health fair.
• Offer to speak to your rotary, chamber of commerce, churches, synagogues, and other places of
  worship, senior centers, support groups, etc.

More Sources for Pain Information

American Academy of Pain Management: http://www.aapainmanage.org
American Academy of Pain Medicine: http://www.painmed.org
American Pain Foundation: http://www.painfoundation.org
American Pain Society: http://www.ampainsoc.org
American Society for Pain Management Nursing: http://www.aspmn.org
Center to Advance Palliative Care: http://www.capc.org
Hospice and Palliative Nurses Association: http://www.hpna.org/
NIH Pain Consortium: http://painconsortium.nih.gov/
Pain and Palliative Care Resource Center/City of Hope: http://www.cityofhope.org/prc
Pain and Policy Studies Group/Wisconsin University: http://www.painpolicy.wisc.edu

References

Aldridge, M. D. (2004). Writing and designing readable patient education materials. *Nephrology Nursing Journal,
    31*(4), 373–377.
American Cancer Society. (2001). Try: *National Comprehensive Cancer Network and American Cancer Society.
    Cancer pain treatment guidelines for patients.* Atlanta, GA.
American Pain Foundation. (2006). *Provider prescribing patterns and perceptions: Identifying solutions to build
    consensus on opioid use in pain management – A roundtable discussion.* Retrieved December 2010 from http://
    www.painfoundation.org/learn/publications/apf-report-provider.html.

American Pain Foundation. (2008). *A reporter's guide: Covering pain and its management*. Retrieved December 2010 from http://www.painfoundation.org/learn/publications/files/reporters-guide.pdf.

American Pain Foundation. (2009). *Online health decision making guide*. Retrieved November 8, 2010 from http://www.painfoundation.org/learn/programs/health-decision-making/.

Anderson, J. L., Dodman, S., Kopelman, M., & Fleming, A. (1979). Patient information recall in a rheumatology clinic. *Rheumatology, 18*(1), 18–22.

Anderson, K. O., Richman, S. P., Hurley, J., et al. (2002). Cancer pain management among underserved minority outpatients: Perceived needs and barriers to optimal control. *Cancer, 94*(8), 2295–2304.

Bender, J. L., Hohenadel, J., Wong, J., Katz, J., Ferris, L. E., Shobbrook, C., Warr, D., & Jadad, A. R. (2008). What patients with cancer want to know about pain: A qualitative study. *Journal of Pain and Symptom Management, 35*(2), 177–187.

Childress, J. F., Faden, R. R., Gaare, R. D., Gostin, L. O., Kahn, J., Bonnie, R. J., Kass, N. E., Mastroianni, A. C., Moreno, J. D., & Nieburg, P. (2002). Public health ethics: Mapping the terrain. *The Journal of Law, Medicine & Ethics, 30*, 170–178.

Doak, C., Doak, L., & Root, J. (1996). *Teaching patients with low literacy skills*. Philadelphia, PA: JB Lippincott.

Fine, P. (2011). Recognition and resolution of ethical barriers to palliative care research. In R. J. Moore (Ed.), *Handbook of pain and palliative care*. New York, NY: Springer.

Gold, D. T., & McClung, B. (2006). Approaches to patient education: Emphasizing the long-term value of compliance and persistence. *The American Journal of Medicine, 119*(4 Suppl 1), 32S–37S.

Gordon, J. S., & Warde, D. E. (1995). Correcting patients' misconceptions about pain. *The American Journal of Nursing, 95*, 43–45.

Healthy States. (2009). Retrieved November 4, 2010 from http://www.healthystates.csg.org/Public+Health+Issues/.

Institute of Medicine. Washington, DC: National Academies Press; 2004. Health Literacy: A Prescription to End Confusion.

Joint Commission Patient-Centered Communication Standards. (2011). Retrieved December 2010 from http://www.jointcommission.org/assets/1/6/Post%20PatientCenteredCareStandardsEPs%20201006091.PDF.

Keogh, E. (2011). Sex differences in pain across the life course. In R. J. Moore (Ed.), *Handbook of pain and palliative care*. New York, NY: Springer.

Kessels, R. P. (2003). Patients' memory for medical information. *Journal of the Royal Society of Medicine, 96*(5), 219–222.

Let's Talk Pain. (2010). *Getting started: A dialogue with your patient about pain*. Retrieved April 2011 from http://www.letstalkpain.org/health_care/dialogue.html.

McCarberg, B., & Cole, B. (2011). Pain in the older person. In R. J. Moore (Ed.), *Handbook of pain and palliative care*. New York, NY: Springer.

Miaskowski, C., Dodd, M. J., West, C., et al. (2001). Lack of adherence with the analgesic regimen: A significant barrier to effective cancer pain management. *Journal of Clinical Oncology, 19*(23), 4275–4279.

National Cancer Institute. (2011). *Highlights of pain management*. Retrieved April 8, 2011 from http://www.cancer.gov/cancertopics/pdq/supportivecare/pain/HealthProfessional.

Pew Internet & Family Life Project. (2011). *Health topics*. Retrieved April 7, 2011 from http://www.pewinternet.org/~/media//Files/Reports/2011/PIP_HealthTopics.pdf.

Rich, B. A. (2011). The delineation and explication of palliative options of last resort. In R. J. Moore (Ed.), *Handbook of pain and palliative care*. New York, NY: Springer.

Teach Back Method. (2009). Retrieved December 2010 from http://www.nchealthliteracy.org/toolkit/tool5.pdf.

U.S. Department of Health and Human Services. (2000). *Healthy people 2010*. Washington, DC: U.S. Government Printing Office. (Originally developed for Ratzan, S. C., & Parker, R. M. (2000). Introduction. In C. R. Selden, M. Zorn, S. C. Ratzan, & R. M. Parker (Eds.), *National Library of medicine current bibliographies in medicine: Health literacy*. NLM Pub. No. CBM 2000-1. Bethesda, MD: National Institutes of Health, U.S. Department of Health and Human Services)

Vetter, T. R. (2011). Pediatric chronic pain. In R. J. Moore (Ed.), *Handbook of pain and palliative care*. New York, NY: Springer.

Winslow, E. H. (2001). Patient education materials: Can patients read them, or are they ending up in the trash? *The American Journal of Nursing, 101*(10), 33–38.

Zirwas, M. J., & Holder, J. L. (2009). Patient education strategies in dermatology part 2. *The Journal of Clinical Aesthetic Dermatology, 2*(12), 28–34.

Part II
Assessment

Chapter 6
Pain Assessment Tools in Palliative Cancer Care

**Marianne Jensen Hjermstad, Dagny Faxvaag Haugen,
Michael I. Bennett, and Stein Kaasa**

Pain in Cancer

Pain is among the frequently occurring and most feared symptoms in patients with advanced cancer. About 90% of cancer patients experience pain at some point during their illness (Caraceni and Portenoy 1999). A review on cancer pain presented pooled prevalence rates ranging from 33% after curative treatment to 64% in patients having advanced disease, with one-third overall rating their pain as moderate or severe (van den Beuken-van Everdingen et al. 2007). These unacceptably high prevalence rates exist in spite of great medical, pharmacological, and technological advances, supplemented by the increased interest in pain assessment methods. Although pain relief is usually achieved by using the World Health Organization (WHO) guidelines for cancer pain management (WHO Guidelines 1996), we also know that many patients with advanced disease are expected to develop pain syndromes that can vary in complexity, some which are difficult to treat (Fainsinger and Nekolaichuk 2008). Regardless of whether the pain originates from the cancer disease, treatment, late effects, comorbidities, or disease progression, or is aggravated because of genetic predispositions (Sloan and Zhao 2006) or mutations (Mok et al. 2009), psychosocial factors or existential issues, a continuous monitoring of pain and other symptoms should be conducted in all stages of the cancer disease to guide symptom management, individualize treatment, and improve clinical research (Kaasa et al. 2008; Hjermstad et al. 2009).

M.J. Hjermstad, RN, MPH, PhD, Associate Professor (✉)
Regional Center for Excellence in Palliative Care Department of Oncology,
Oslo University Hospital, Box 4956, Nydalen 0424 Oslo, Norway

European Palliative Care Research Centre, Norwegian University of Science and Technology, Trondheim, Norway
e-mail: m.j.hjermstad@medisin.uio.no

D.F. Haugen, MPH, PhD
European Palliative Care Research Centre, Norwegian University of Science and Technology, Trondheim, Norway

Regional Centre of Excellence for Palliative Care, Western Norway,
Haukeland University Hospital, Bergen, Norway

M.I. Bennett, MD, Professor
Leeds Institute of Health Sciences, University of Leeds, Leeds, UK

S. Kaasa, MD, PhD, Professor
The Cancer Department, Trondheim University Hospital, Trondheim, Norway

European Palliative Care Research Centre, Norwegian University of Science and Technology, Trondheim, Norway

R.J. Moore (ed.), *Handbook of Pain and Palliative Care: Biobehavioral Approaches for the Life Course*,
DOI 10.1007/978-1-4419-1651-8_6, © Springer Science+Business Media, LLC 2012

Pain due to cancer is a complex symptom that may negatively affect life in general and the consequences may be viewed differently by patients and physicians (Velikova et al. 2008), thereby accentuating the need for subjective reports (Cleeland 2007). However, the plethora of assessment tools developed during the last 2 decades does not seem to overcome the single most important barrier to optimal pain management, namely the lack of systematic assessment of pain as part of the daily clinical routine in oncology settings (Caraceni et al. 2005; Kaasa et al. 2008; Meuser et al. 2001; Patrick et al. 2003; Von Roenn et al. 1993). Inappropriate use of opioids due to barriers on the part of patients, physicians, the society, and institutions may also explain the inadequacy in pain relief (Maltoni 2008; Thomas 2007). Furthermore a review on pain assessment in clinical studies has shown that validated pain tools were not always appropriately used in the trials (Caraceni et al. 2005).

Complex pain management is associated with a number of factors such as neuropathic pain (NP) (Bennett et al. 2007; Mercadante et al. 2009), breakthrough pain (BTP) (Haugen et al. 2010; Hwang et al. 2003; Portenoy et al. 1999), initial pain intensity (Fainsinger et al. 2009), psychological distress (Fainsinger and Nekolaichuk 2008; Hwang et al. 2002; Lawlor et al. 1997), cognitive function (Fainsinger et al. 2005; Hanks et al. 2000; Mercadante et al. 2000a), etc. This means that it may be difficult to predict the likelihood of pain relief for a given patient, in particular because there is no universally accepted and consensus based classification system to group patients according to these associated variables. This lack of a standardized approach to pain classification and assessment also makes it difficult to compare research results from pain trials in cancer. In fact, the lack of homogeneous standard methods for assessment and classification of cancer pain in palliative cancer treatment is particularly evident in controlled clinical trials (Caraceni et al. 2006; Caraceni and Weinstein 2001; Fainsinger et al. 2010).

This shortcoming becomes evident when looking at the cancer pain literature that most often reports pain prevalence rates without describing other medical and patient-related variables that may be associated with the pain experience (Fainsinger et al. 2005; Caraceni et al. 2006; Caraceni 2001).

Another complicating factor that relates to the management of cancer pain and the use of results from pain trials is the vast heterogeneity in study samples from general and palliative oncology populations (Boisvert and Cohen 1995; Borgsteede et al. 2006; Fainsinger and Nekolaichuk 2008; Kaasa et al. 2006; Currow et al. 2009). There is still no universally accepted framework defining the most relevant variables to classify a palliative care cancer population, although this has been called for by researchers and scientific associations since the 1970s (Arner and Arner 1985; Bruera et al. 1989; Foley 2004; Ventafridda and Caraceni 1991). The need to improve the international classification and assessment was also emphasized in the recently updated opioid guidelines for cancer pain from the EAPC (European Association for Palliative Care) (Caraceni et al. 2011).

Thus, as can be inferred from the above, the overall concept of "cancer pain" does not suffice to classify or assess the different pain characteristics due to a number of different factors (tumor related, etiologic, pathophysiologic, anatomic, treatment related, etc.) that need to be properly assessed to optimize cancer pain management.

Classification of Cancer Pain

Definition and Intent

The intention of a cancer pain classification system is to improve pain management (Hjermstad et al. 2009; Fainsinger et al. 2005; Knudsen et al. 2009). Through a standardized and systematic description it is possible to perform a grouping of patients according to agreed upon characteristics of the disease, the pain, and the patient thereby controlling for the variability of the samples studied. These

Table 6.1 Main contents of the three formal, validated pain classification systems (ECS-CP, CPPS, IASP)*

The Edmonton classification system for cancer pain (ECS-CP)	The cancer pain prognostic scale	Classification of chronic pain of the international association for the study of pain (IASP)
Pain mechanism	Mixed pain	Regions involved (axis I)
Incident pain	Worst pain severity	Systems involved (axis II)
Psychological distress	Daily opioid dose	Temporal characteristics (axis III)
Addictive behavior	Emotional well-being	Pain intensity/time since onset of pain (axis IV)
Cognitive function		Aetiology (axis V)

*Printed with permission from the Knudsen et al. (2009)

groups may help in predicting the likelihood of successful pain treatment or in the identification of the approximately 20% of cancer patients who are less likely to respond to standard treatment.

Originally, classification was a method originating from biology for the grouping or categorization of living organisms (http://en.wikipedia.org.wiki.classification. Classification), which also refers to the principles underlying the classification. The ICD-10 classification of diseases (International Classification of Diseases. http://www.who.int.classifications.icd.en) is an example of a widely used system for grouping or classifying different types of diseases, corresponding to the TNM classification, the common language for describing oncology patients (Piccirillo and Feinstein 1996). A similar standardized, consensus-based approach to pain classification is not in widespread use, despite the development of the International Association for the Study of Pain (IASP) (International Association for the Study of Pain 1994) classification system and the Edmonton Classification System for Cancer Pain (ECS-CP) (Fainsinger and Nekolaichuk 2008; Fainsinger et al. 2005; Bruera et al. 1989, 1991; Nekolaichuk et al. 2005) (Table 6.1).

Agreed upon definitions are of the utmost importance for description of patient cohorts in clinical studies, in clinical practice, and in order to understand for whom specific guidelines are developed. This is also necessary for making comparisons across studies and for drawing conclusions about medication or other treatment options. Stringent definitions of patient characteristics and observations are required to identify to which class or subclass the patient belongs (Cherny and Portenoy 2004; Hempel 1961).

The need for an internationally accepted classification system for cancer pain with a common language for use both in research and in clinical practice has been recognized in reviews, studies, and editorials (Caraceni and Portenoy 1999; Fainsinger and Nekolaichuk 2008; Kaasa et al. 2008; Mercadante et al. 2000b; Kaasa 2010). In order to succeed in being a frequently used tool in clinical practice, the system must be regarded as relevant, short, and applicable according to the given situation, i.e., prediction of pain relief. A major challenge, however, particularly so in palliative care, is that the system needs to be brief and sufficiently comprehensive. Items to consider include the clinical characteristics of the pain, the relationship to underlying pathological processes and pain mechanisms (i.e., visceral, neuropathic, idiopathic), other domains such as localization, as well as patient-related factors (i.e., socio-demographic factors, cognitive function, history of addiction, etc.).

Classification Systems for Cancer Pain

A review on cancer pain classification systems (Knudsen et al. 2009) identified three tools judged to be relevant for pain classification, all in the form of treatment evaluation tools. None of these were systematically developed or validated: The Opioid Escalation Index (OEI) is a classification system of opioid responsiveness used in the original (Mercadante et al. 1994), as well as in subsequent studies by the developers (Mercadante 1998; Mercadante et al. 2000a, b). The OEI is a measure of the patient's opioid requirement combined with the level of pain intensity. Another system by the same author presented six prognostic groups for the likelihood of pain relief after pain treatment with NSAIDs and opioids (Mercadante et al. 1992). The factors included were number of days until achieving pain relief, the presence of incident pain, and the required dose of opioids. However, these scales were based on a retrospective grouping of patients after specific treatment regimens, thereby not providing a universal framework for cancer pain classification. The third of the nonvalidated systems, developed in 1994 (Cleeland et al. 1994), could be viewed as a treatment appropriateness evaluation tool, rather than a classification system. It compared the patient's self-reported peak pain intensity with the most potent analgesic drug that was prescribed to the patient.

The review identified three classification systems that were labeled as formal systems. These tools encompass a set of domains and items which constitute a defined or standardized classification system intended for use across studies (Knudsen et al. 2009) and the tools were systematically developed and partially validated: the IASP Classification of Chronic Pain (International Association for the Study of Pain 1994; Bonica 1979), the Cancer Pain Prognostic Scale (CPPS) (Hwang et al. 2002), and the ECS-CP (Fainsinger and Nekolaichuk 2008; Fainsinger et al. 2005; Bruera et al. 1989, 1991; Nekolaichuk et al. 2005).

The IASP list of pain terms was first published in 1979 (Bonica 1979), later revised and extended twice (International Association for the Study of Pain 1994) as a result of expert opinions and clinical experience. In the IASP Classification of Chronic Pain for malignant and nonmalignant chronic pain syndromes, each clinical pain syndrome is assigned a code number based on five areas: (1) anatomical site, (2) organ systems of which abnormal functioning produces pain, (3) temporal characteristics, (4) pain intensity and time since debut, and (5) pain etiology. This provides important information about difficult malignant and chronic pain syndromes primarily based on physician's examinations with pain intensity and duration being the only factors based on patients' own report. The systematic literature review (Knudsen et al. 2009) identified only one clinical study in which the IASP system was used (Grond et al. 1996).

The same review identified only one study employing the CPPS: the original development study (Hwang et al. 2002). The CPPS is basically an index score, primarily based on self-report, that is used to dichotomize patients into good or poor prognosis for pain relief. The score is based on four domains: worst pain severity on an 11-point NRS scale (0–10), emotional well-being from the FACT-G (Functional Assessment of Cancer Therapy Scale) (Cella et al. 1993), daily oral opioid dose >60 mg, and the presence of mixed pain.

The ECS-CP, however, has gone through several, stepwise and systematic validation studies, and has recently been subject to a large, international validation study suggesting that the ECS-CP can predict pain complexity in a variety of countries and palliative care settings (Fainsinger et al. 2010). In the first version of the ECS-CP, called the Edmonton Staging System (ESS), patients with advanced cancer were classified as having a good, intermediate, or poor prognosis for successful pain treatment, based on their scores on seven domains: mechanism of pain, incident pain, previous opioid exposure, cognitive function, psychological distress, opioid tolerance, and past history of drug or alcohol abuse (Bruera et al. 1989). A subsequent study led to a dichotomization of the groups, good or bad prognosis for pain control (Bruera et al. 1995), while two of the factors, cognitive function and previous opioid consumption, were removed as they were not found to be independent predictors for achieving pain control.

In a later, regional multicentre study, aiming to test inter-rater reliability and predictive validity evidence, cognitive function was reintroduced based on expert opinions and literature reviews while tolerance was excluded due to interpretational difficulties (Fainsinger et al. 2005). The next validation study (Nekolaichuk et al. 2005) was performed to gather construct validity evidence to develop consensus definitions and to develop and evaluate the administration manual (Fainsinger et al. 2008). Input from national and international expert reviews by means of the Delphi techniques (Hasson et al. 2000) led to some revisions, with five domains (mechanism of pain, incident pain, addictive behavior, psychological distress, cognitive status) being included in the renamed ECS-CP.

As can be inferred from this section, only one of the classification tools, the ECS-CP, has been used in more than one study, and has been subject to several revisions based on international validation studies, expert opinions, and formal construct validation (Fainsinger et al. 2010; Kaasa 2010).

The Present Recommendations for Cancer Pain Classification

In September 2009, an international expert meeting was arranged in Milan, Italy aiming to reach a consensus on how to assess and classify cancer pain (Kaasa et al. 2011). Meeting participants represented a wide range of disciplines (e.g., oncology, neurology, epidemiology, psychology, biostatistics, palliative care, public health, anesthesiology, and nursing) and were selected on the basis of their research and clinical expertise in cancer pain assessment and classification.

The panel was also representative of international research groups addressing cancer pain assessment and classification like the EPCRC (European Palliative Care Research Collaborative), a pan-European, EU funded translational research program (European Palliative Care Research Collaborative (EPCRC). http://www.epcrc.org/), PROMIS (Patient-Reported Outcomes Measurement Information System. http://www.nihpromis.org/default.aspx), IMMPACT (Initiative on Methods, Measurement and Pain Assessment in Clinical Trials. http://www.immpact.org/), CPOR-SG (Cancer Pain Outcome Research Study Group) (Apolone et al. 2006), and several associations involved in oncology and pain like the IASP (International Association for the Study of Pain. http://www.iasp-pain.org), ASCO (American Society of Clinical Oncology. http://www.asco.org/), ESMO (European Society for Medical Oncology) (European Association for Palliative Care (EAPC). http://www.eapcnet.org/), AIOM (Associazione Italiana di Oncologia Medica. http://www.aiom.it/), EORTC (European Organisation for the Research and Treatment of Cancer. http://www.eortc.be/), EAPC (European Association for Palliative Care. http://www.eapcnet.org/), SICP (Società Italiana Cura Palliativ. http://www.sicp.it/) and of international regulatory and health authorities, EMA (European Medicines Agency. http://www.ema.europa.eu/) and the WHO (World Health Organization. http://www.who.int/).

The expert panel suggested using the ECS-CP classification system as the template and international standard for assessment and classification of cancer pain (Kaasa et al. 2011). This is due to the stepwise and iterative process of development that has been followed in the development of the ECS-CP (Fainsinger and Nekolaichuk 2008; Fainsinger et al. 2005; Bruera et al. 1989, 1991; Nekolaichuk et al. 2005), which has also been the framework for instrument development within the EPCRC (Kaasa et al. 2008; European Palliative Care Research Collaborative (EPCRC). http://www. epcrc.org/) and other organizations (Patient-Reported Outcomes Measurement Information System (PROMIS). http://www.nihpromis.org/default.aspx; European Organisation for Research and Treatment of Cancer (EORTC). http://www.eortc.be/) with standardized procedures consisting of empirical data collection, literature reviews, expert consensus surveys, and patient focus groups and surveys (Kaasa et al. 2008; Hjermstad et al. 2009).

Furthermore, the ECS-CP is the only classification system that has been used in clinical work, albeit somewhat limited, because of the ongoing work both in Canada and internationally, with a large ECS-CP validation study led by the Canadian group (Fainsinger et al. 2010) and the multicenter study conducted by the EPCRC, the EPCRC-CSA (European Palliative Care Research Collaborative (EPCRC). http://www.epcrc.org/). The present version of the ECS-CP that has been launched under the acronym CPACS (Cancer Pain Assessment and Classification System) (Kaasa et al. 2010) contains four of the domains that have been identified by experts as important for pain assessment in palliative care (Hjermstad et al. 2008; Holen et al. 2006), namely, *pain intensity*, *pain mechanism* (± *neuropathic pain*), *BTP*, and *psychological distress*. However, based on forthcoming international clinical and validation studies, the content may be revised and developed further, as part of any dynamic tool development process in the twenty-first century (Kaasa et al. 2011).

Assessment of Cancer Pain

While the previous section emphasized the need for systematic consensus-based classification systems to optimize treatment and focused on the recent, promising progress in this respect, this section is devoted to the assessment of cancer pain in palliative care. A thorough assessment is crucial for a valid classification system as well as for day-to-day clinical management of pain.

Definitions and Concepts

Per definition, assessment is a synonym to estimation: the determination of importance, size, or value in various areas (http://www.merriam-webster.com/dictionary/symptom). Thus, pain assessment may be based on patients' self-report obtained by answering single or multiple items (questions) that cover one or more pain domains.

A domain or dimension is the distinguished part of an abstract or physical space where something exists, is performed, or is valid (http://www.merriam-webster.com/dictionary/domain). In relation to cancer pain, pain intensity and BTP are domains of the pain symptom. For example, pain experts have recommended that cancer pain assessment comprises at least five key domains: pain intensity, temporal pattern, exacerbating/relieving factors, localization, and interference (Hjermstad et al. 2008; Holen et al. 2006).

An item is an entry in a list or one object in a collection of objects (http://www.merriam-webster.com/dictionary/item). In relation to measurement theory, it is based on the idea that the probability of getting an item correct is a function of a latent trait or ability. Thus, items for assessment of the various pain domains must be selected on the basis of their ability to serve as indicators of the specific pain domain, i.e., intensity, pain quality, BTP, etc., particularly so in clinical work. To enhance the clinical utility, the answer categories, time windows, and number of response options should be easily comprehensible and perceived as clinically relevant, once again a prerequisite for a correct classification.

Methods for Pain Assessment

Pain assessment may be based on information registered in the patients' charts, proxy ratings, or observer-based scores by nurses or physicians if the patient is unable to respond verbally or in writing, due to trauma or different impairments. However, studies have shown that the correlation between patient-rated and observer-rated pain intensity decreased with increasing pain levels on a numerical rating scale from 0 to 10 (Ahlers et al. 2008; Banos et al. 1989). Thus, due to the subjective nature of the pain experience that is strongly influenced by individual variables (psychological, emotional, cultural, etc.), information on pain needs to be elicited directly from the patient whenever possible (Kaasa et al. 2008; Hjermstad et al. 2008) and then be combined with clinical findings and supplementary examinations. The use of subjective assessments, however, accentuates the importance of using a standardized assessment system to enhance the possibility to validly describe, quantify, and monitor pain at a given point or over time (Kaasa et al. 2008; Hjermstad et al. 2009).

Pain assessment has traditionally been performed by paper- and pencil-based questionnaires of various lengths for self-report, checklists of variable length, or in the form of interviews using closed or open-ended questions. Various mechanical or plastic devices, graphical charts, drawings, etc., are also used, but less often (Jensen 2003). The rapid technological development, however, now opens

Table 6.2 Criteria for the ideal symptom assessment tool for self-report

Characteristics	Requirements
Acceptable	Easy and quick to complete, for patients and clinicians
	Perceived as clinically useful, for patients and clinicians
	Easy and quick to score
Comprehensive with relevant content	Comprehensive symptom assessment, prevalence, severity and distress
	Relevant and sufficient for decision making, targeted, relevant timeframe
	Applicable for research
Flexible	Adaptive to changes and development
	Applicable in various formats (paper, electronic, plastic)
User-friendly	Brief, easy to understand, easy to score appealing lay-out
	Unequivocal questions and answers
Psychometrically sound	Reliability: precise, reproducible, stable, repeatable, good internal consistency
	Validity: measures what's intended, appropriate, meaningful and useful for a specific purpose
	• Sufficient face and content validity
	• Sufficient criterion validity (concurrent and predictive)
	• Sufficient construct validity (discriminative and convergent)
	Accuracy: correlates well with similar tools
	Sensitivity: identifying present symptoms
	Specificity: excluding symptoms that are not present
	Responsiveness: detects with-in patient changes over time

for pain registration by different electronic devices (palms, laptops, cell phones, direct web entries, etc.) that may facilitate the transfer of information from the patients' charts to the bedside, yield immediate summated or index scores, and be readily available for any clinical or research purposes. It should be remembered, however, that these methods do not enhance the validity and clinical utility of the assessments per se, which are dependent on the format and selection of the questions that are presented to the patients.

Psychometric Requirements and Tool Development

All pain measures, regardless of mode of administration, must possess the necessary psychometric properties to provide reliable results. The psychometric properties encompass *reliability* issues; how consistently and reproducibly the instrument measures a symptom, different aspects of *validity;* if the instrument really measures what it purports to measure (*face, content, criterion, construct validity*), as well as sufficient sensitivity and specificity (Table 6.2). Ideally, pain assessment should be brief, precise, multidimensional, and specifically targeted to the patient population. There should also be a balance between the aspects of validity and brevity, especially so in frail patients. Furthermore, it should be remembered that even if a tool fulfills the statistical tests with respect to psychometric properties, it does not necessarily mean that it is valid for all populations in all situations, from diagnosis to the last stage of the disease. A systematic review examining 21 tools concluded that there is no ideal tool for general symptom assessment in cancer, based on the evaluation of psychometric properties, content, intended population, and practicality (Kirkova et al. 2006), a conclusion that also pertains to pain assessment tools.

A major problem in relation to cancer pain assessment, in general oncology as well as in palliative care, is the abundance of tools, poorly defined concepts, huge variations in the answer options, and ambiguity in the interpretation of scores, which in turn creates confusion and prohibits comparison across studies. A review showed that 24 different adjectives were used to anchor the extreme scale values in 54 studies aiming to compare unidimensional scales for assessment of pain intensity (Hjermstad et al. 2011). Whether the variability in anchors and response options directly influences the numerical scores is a question that needs to be empirically tested, but also something that in itself calls for a standardization of assessment methods. A review on the contents of pain assessment tools, covering the period from 1966 to 2003 (Holen et al. 2006), showed that 80 different tools assessing pain by one or more items were used for self-report of pain in palliative cancer care. A subsequent follow-up review identified 11 new pain assessment tools developed for use in palliative care in the next 4 years (Hjermstad et al. 2008). Of these 11, 9 were multidimensional, and 3 of the 5 highest ranked domains in Holen's review (Holen et al. 2006): *intensity* (rank 1), *treatment/relief/exacerbation* (rank 3), and *localization* (rank 4) were included in seven, six, and five of the tools, respectively. Only one, an ad hoc inventory for clinical practice, included all five dimensions (Gutgsell et al. 2003).

Another problem that is related to the steady flow of new tools is the fact that many tools are developed to examine a small and specific area of interest, i.e., pain beliefs, information, prescription routines, etc. (Hjermstad et al. 2008). This limits the usefulness of the tools that are used only once or maybe in a very limited number of studies (Hjermstad et al. 2008). Consequently, there is often a need for additional instruments in clinical studies to obtain a detailed pain assessment, which in turn increases the burden on patient and staff. The instrument package may be perceived as cumbersome by both parties, which may reduce the use, compliance, and validity, and the "vicious circle" of unsystematic symptom assessment is complete. Furthermore, many new tools have been developed without adhering to the recommended guidelines for tool development to ensure adequate psychometric properties, such as the internationally accepted EORTC methodology (Sprangers et al. 1998). Only 2 of 11 instruments identified in a review were extensively validated or cross-culturally tested (Hjermstad et al. 2008). To meet the methodological requirements for development of symptom tools, the work of the EPCRC has been conducted in a systematic, stepwise manner with systematic literature reviews, expert opinions, patient input, empirical testing and validation, and international consensus processes, as previously described in detail (Kaasa et al. 2008; Hjermstad et al. 2009; Haugen and Kaasa 2010; European Palliative Care Research Collaborative (EPCRC). http://www.epcrc.org/). This process has been followed in the development of other assessment tools as well, e.g., within the PROMIS (Patient-Reported Outcomes Measurement Information System (PROMIS). http://www.nihpromis.org/default.aspx) and the EORTC (European Organisation for Research and Treatment of Cancer (EORTC). http://www.eortc.be/).

In order to optimize pain assessment, clear definitions and conceptualizations of the relevant domains to be included are necessary, as strongly emphasized in the NIH consensus statement on pain, depression, and fatigue some years ago (Consensus Development Program and National Institutes of Health 2002). The clinical relevance and face validity are key aspects for clinical use and standardization, and despite patients' involvement in tool development being emphasized (Food and Drug Administration 2006; Burgers et al. 2004; DeWalt et al. 2007), this step is often bypassed in the development of new tools. An example of the conceptual framework used to ensure a uniform use of concepts in the development process within the EPCRC is displayed in Fig. 6.1.

Pain Assessment Tools in Palliative Cancer Care

Many comprehensive symptom tools and symptom distress tools like the 31-item Rotterdam Symptom Checklist (RSCL) (de Haes et al. 1990), the 13-item core version of the MDASI (M. D. Anderson Symptom Inventory) (Cleeland et al. 2000), and the 32-item Memorial Symptom

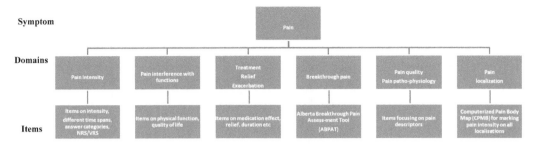

Fig. 6.1 The conceptual framework used for assessment of pain in the EPCRC data collection study The figure displays the structural framework used by the EPCRC (European Palliative Care Research Collaborative (EPCRC). http://www. epcrc.org/) with the overall symptom *pain*, being divided into different domains: i.e., *intensity, breakthrough pain* which are assessed by several *items*

Assessment Scale Short Form (MSAS-SF) (Chang et al. 2000) contain one or more items on pain (Table 6.3). Together with self-reporting tools on general QoL or health-related QoL such as the SF-36 (Ware 1993), the EORTC QLQ-C30 (Aaronson et al. 1993), the shorter version EORTC QLQ PAL-15 for palliative care patients (Groenvold et al. 2006), the FLIC (Schipper et al. 1984) and the FACT-G (Cella et al. 1993), these are in frequent use in cancer (Victorson et al. 2008). All these inventories contain highly prevalent symptoms like pain, depression, nausea, and fatigue, and the items are most often scored on verbal rating scales (VRS) with 4–6 answer categories with different time frames (Table 6.3). The pain items may be in the form of single item scores, form multi-item pain scales, or be part of summated symptom index scores. Depending on the actual tool, the intensity, frequency, and impact of symptoms on various functions may be assessed.

Generally speaking, however, QoL tools, general symptom checklists, or distress inventories are less well suited for close clinical follow-up, assessment of fluctuating symptoms such as pain, and monitoring of treatment effect. This is first and foremost related to the time frame, which most often refers to the past week, up to the past 4 weeks (Table 6.3), but also to the fact that some arithmetic may be necessary to calculate clinically meaningful scores for items and scales, limiting the usefulness of the tools in daily clinical practice. Because pain intensity probably is the most clinically relevant dimension of the pain experience, one should be cautious to use combination scores to guide treatment, without specifically monitoring pain intensity per se. Combining pain intensity scores with, e.g., pain interference may be less relevant in clinical settings as it may obscure the actual scores of each domain (Jensen 2003; Fayers et al. 2011). Research has shown that patients may not be able to distinguish between functional impairment due to pain and impairment that is due to other causes (Stenseth et al. 2007).

Nevertheless, it is important to remember that a complex pain experience requires a multidimensional assessment. Well-validated instruments like the Brief Pain Inventory (BPI) (Daut et al. 1983) or the McGill Short Form questionnaire (Melzack 1987) are recommended for a more comprehensive, multidimensional pain assessment in cancer (Kaasa et al. 2008; Jensen 2003; Caraceni et al. 2002). Both tools are specific pain tools (Table 6.3), are frequently used in cancer clinical trials and follow-up studies, and have been translated into and validated in several languages.

The BPI (Daut et al. 1983) was designed to assess pain intensity and to what extent pain interferes with normal activity. The intensity scale contains four items measuring worst and least pain during the past 24 h, and average and present pain intensity, all scored on NRS-11 (Table 6.3). Pain interference is assessed in relation to seven areas of daily life (general activity, mood, walking ability, normal work, relations with other persons, sleep, enjoyment of life). However, studies using the BPI have observed that the BPI interference scores are higher in patients with deteriorated functional performance compared to patients with close to normal functional performance, regardless of the

Table 6.3 Description and content of frequently used multidimensional tools used for assessment of pain in palliative cancer care

Name of tool[a]	Author, pub yr	Pain dimensions in tool[b]	No of pain items	Uni-dimensional pain or pain scale	Scale, answer categories for pain items in tool	Time line for pain items
General symptom tools						
ESAS	Bruera et al. (1989)	Int			NRS-11; i.e., 0 *no pain – 10 worst possible pain*	Right now
MDASI	Cleeland et al. (2000)	Int	1	Uni	NRS-11: *0 not present – 10 as bad as you can imagine* according to question	During the past week
MSAS-SF	Chang et al. (2000)	Int, Treat, + pain syndromes	1	Uni	Presence of symptom:, dichotomous Y/N Frequency: VRS-4: 1 *rarely–4 almost constantly* Severity: VRS-4: 1 *slight – 4 very severe* Distress: VRS-5: 0 *not at all – 4 very much*	During the past week
Quality of life tools						
EORTC QLQ-C30	Aaronson et al. (1993)	Int, inf	2	Pain scale	VRS-4, 1: *"not at all" – 4: very much*	During the past week
EORTC QLQ-PAL 15	Groenvold et al. (2006)	Int, inf	2	Pain scale	VRS-4, 1: *"not at all" – 4: very much*	During the past week
FACT-G	Cella et al. (1993)	Int	1	Single item	VRS-5, 0: *"not at all" – 4: very much*	Past 7 days
FLIC	Schipper et al. (1984)	Inf, Bel	2			
SF-36	Ware (1993)	Int, inf	2	Bodily pain scales		Last week

Pain tools						
BPI-SF	Daut et al. (1983)	Int, Loc, Inf, Treat, Qual	15	Intensity scales, 4 items	Int: NRS-11: *0 no pain – 10 pain as bad as you can imagine* Loc: body map Inf: related to seven areas: general activity, mood, walking ability, normal work, relations with other persons, sleep, enjoyment of life, NRS-11, anchors depending on area	Int: worst and least pain past 24 h + average and present
SF-MPQ	Melzack (1987)	Int, Loc, Qual, Temp	23	3 scales: affective, sensory, total	Scales: VRS-4: *0 none – 3 severe* Int: VAS 100 mm: *no pain – worst possible pain*, PPI: VRS-5: *0 no pain – 5 excruciating*	Int: past week, present

[a]Tool abbreviations: *ESAS* Edmonton symptom assessment scale; *MDASI* M. D. Anderson symptom inventory; *MSAS-SF* memorial symptom assessment schedule short form; *EORTC QLQ-C30* European organisation for research and treatment of cancer quality-of-life questionnaire; *EORTC QLQ-PAL 15* EORTC questionnaire for palliative care; *FACT-G* functional assessment of cancer therapy scale; *FLIC* functional living index-cancer; *SF-36* medical outcome study 36-item short form health survey; *BPI-SF* brief pain inventory; *SF-MPQ*: Mc Gill pain questionnaire; *PPI* present pain intensity

[b]Abbreviations for dimensions: *Treat* effects of treatment; *Aff* pain affect; *Bel* pain beliefs; *Dur* duration; *Hist* pain history; *Inf* pain interference; *Int* pain intensity; *Loc* pain location; *Qual* pain quality; *Rel* pain relief and exacerbating/relieving factors; *Temp* temporal pattern

pain intensity scores, and that the interference items do not function optimally from a psychometric point of view (Holen et al. 2008; Radbruch et al. 1999).

The McGill Pain Questionnaire (MPQ) (Melzack 1975) is a measure of the subjective pain experience, across sensory, affective, and evaluative dimensions of pain. It has been found to discriminate well between acute and chronic pain and to be sensitive enough to detect differences in pain relief. However, it uses 78 words to describe pain quality and requires at least 5–10 min to complete. Thus, the shorter version (SF-MPQ) (Melzack 1987) is a more efficient measure of pain for clinical assessment and research purposes, well validated in various patient populations (Grafton et al. 2005; Melzack and Katz 2001) and is widely used in cancer clinical settings. The SF-MPQ consists of 15 descriptors (11 sensory; 4 affective) which are rated on an intensity scale as 0=none, 1=mild, 2=moderate, or 3=severe. Three pain scores are derived from the sum of the intensity rank values of the words chosen for sensory, affective, and total descriptors, respectively. The SF-MPQ also includes the Present Pain Intensity (PPI) index of the standard MPQ and a visual analogue scale (VAS) for assessment of pain intensity (Table 6.3).

The Edmonton Symptom Assessment Scale (ESAS) (Bruera et al. 1991) is probably the most frequently used and well-known self-reporting tool for assessment of symptoms in palliative care (Nekolaichuk et al. 2008). It has been validated in different samples and nationalities and against other instruments like the FACT-G (Cella et al. 1993) and the MSAS (Chang et al. 2000). The ESAS consists of the nine frequent cancer symptoms (pain, nausea, tiredness, etc.) (plus an optional tenth) that are scored on a Numerical Rating Scale (NRS-11) (0=not at all, no symptom, best, 10=worst possible) with a time frame referring to the present situation (now) (Table 6.3). Most studies demonstrate high compliance (Nekolaichuk et al. 2008), although qualitative research has shown that patients report difficulties in relation to terminology and numerical rating assignments, implying that more extensive validation and modifications of the tool may be necessary (Nekolaichuk et al. 2008; Watanabe et al. 2009). However, the tool is easy to score, yields immediate results, and is probably most effective for immediate screening of clinical symptoms.

Reviews and recommendations agree on the use of single-item unidimensional tools, such as Numerical Rating Scales (NRS), VRS, and VAS, for assessment of pain intensity in clinical settings (Jensen 2003; Breivik et al. 2008; Caraceni et al. 2002; Dworkin et al. 2005). Among the unidimensional tools, the VAS is by far the most frequently used scale (Caraceni et al. 2005; Jensen 2003). The NRS and the VAS are shown to be more powerful in detecting changes in pain intensity than a VRS (Kaasa et al. 2010; Jensen 2003; Breivik et al. 2008; Caraceni et al. 2002), but frail, elderly patients and the cognitively impaired may have difficulties interpreting the VAS (Jensen 2003; Caraceni et al. 2002; Chibnall and Tait 2001). A short description of unidimensional scales is presented in Table 6.4.

To ensure a uniform way of assessing pain, the expert group from the Milan meeting proposed that similar methods for cancer pain assessment should be used whenever possible, both in clinical practice and in clinical research (Kaasa et al. 2010). However, this does not preclude specific considerations with respect to the actual patient population. On the one hand, it is obvious that certain population characteristics have to be considered, such as age, frailty, literacy level, cognitive impairment, etc. For example, the higher number of errors on the VASs with increasing age and other impairments makes this scale less applicable in the cognitively impaired, as documented in the literature (Jensen 2003; Caraceni et al. 2002; Chibnall and Tait 2001). This is also in line with a recent letter based on a study comparing NRS and VRS, emphasizing the need to be selective in the use of scales for clinical use (Ripamonti and Brunelli 2009). However, because the psychometric properties largely depend on certain basic characteristics, the selection of scales is better guided by specific consensus-based recommendations rather than left to the judgment of the individual clinicians. This also means that the same methodology (scale, wording, time frame, and format) should be applied when assessing pain over time in the same patient population.

Table 6.4 Properties of numerical rating scale, verbal rating scale and visual rating scale

Numerical rating scale – NRS	Commonly from 0 to 10 (NRS-11) or 1–10 (NRS-10)
	Usually, only the two extreme categories are labeled, e.g., "no pain at all" and "worst imaginable pain"
	NRS may be called a VNRS/VNS when the scale is explained or shown on paper to the patient who responds by indicating a number
Verbal rating scale – VRS	Ordered categorical scale with each response option consisting of adjectives. For different levels of pain intensity, "no pain," "mild pain," "moderate pain," "severe pain," "extreme pain," and the "most intense pain imaginable" form a 6-category VRS scale (VRS-6)
	VRS scales are commonly of lengths 4–7. The adjectives are scored by assigning numbers (0–6) to each response option
	The scale may also be called VPS (verbal pain scale), VDS (verbal descriptor scale) or SDS (simple descriptor scale)
Bipolar – VRS	A VRS that goes from, e.g., "very much worse" to "very much better"
	Usually with a central neutral option (e.g., "no change"), but may also have no neutral option thereby forcing decisions by using an even number of response options. Bipolar scales, therefore, usually have 3, 5, or 7 options
Visual analogue scale – VAS	Consists of a straight line, usually 0–100 mm, with the extreme categories labeled as for NRS. The distance measured from the "no pain" end to the patient's mark is the VAS score
	Often graduated with labeled marks indicating tens (10, 20, 30, etc) or with unlabelled marks for the units

Pain Intensity

Pain intensity is probably the most studied dimension of the pain experience regardless of disease and this dimension is included in almost all pain and symptom assessment tools (Hjermstad et al. 2011). Pain intensity was also regarded as the most important and relevant dimension for pain assessment by both cancer pain experts and cancer patients (Hjermstad et al. 2008; Holen et al. 2006).

Furthermore, pain intensity has a high clinical relevance and is an important determinant for selection of treatment choices and urgency. Pain intensity is an important outcome for monitoring treatment effect if assessed in a valid manner with a standardized methodology. One study showed that hourly pain intensity ratings on an NRS-11 in 8 h corresponded well with patients' average 8-h pain intensity scores, indicating that both present and average pain intensity scores have high clinical relevance (Caraceni et al. 2010b). The level of pain intensity is shown to interfere with functional capacity and negatively impact on the quality of life in patients (Chow et al. 2006). One study found that higher pain intensity scores on an NRS-11 were significantly associated with BTP, somatic pain, younger age, and decreased function (Caraceni and Portenoy 1999), while others have reported that higher initial pain intensity ratings were predicted by neuropathic, bone, mixed, and incident pain presence in palliative cancer patients upon admittance to a specialized palliative care unit (Stromgren et al. 2004). The level of pain intensity at the initial assessment has also been shown to be a significant predictor of the complexity of cancer pain management and the time needed to obtain stable pain control (Fainsinger et al. 2009).

Simple, repeated ratings of pain intensity with specified time intervals have been demonstrated as valid measures for evaluation of pain changes (Jensen 2003; Breivik et al. 2008; Caraceni et al. 2002). A recent study supplemented the standard 24-h pain intensity rating with rating of the most severe PI last 24 h to specifically address pain exacerbations (Brunelli et al. 2010), at the same time comparing the usefulness of different unidimensional scales for these purposes. Results showed that pain intensity was an appropriate outcome for evaluations of cancer pain exacerbations, and that patients used the simple NRS-11 more appropriately than VRSs. Thus, repeated and standardized assessments of pain intensity by unidimensional rating scales are feasible in most settings, and an important clinical outcome.

Breakthrough Pain

The temporal aspect of the pain experience is an important part of any pain assessment (Foley 2004; Hjermstad et al. 2008; Holen et al. 2006). The reported prevalence rates of BTP in cancer patients range from 40 to 80%, a variation that is due to different definitions, settings, patient populations, and assessment methods (Haugen et al. 2010; Mercadante et al. 2010).

Most often BTP is defined in relation to an adequately controlled background pain, e.g., as "a transitory exacerbation of pain that occurs on a background of otherwise stable pain in a patient receiving chronic opioid therapy" according to the widely used definition by Portenoy and Hagen (1990). However, other definitions focus on "episodic flares of pain" regardless of whether or not the baseline pain is controlled (Svendsen et al. 2005), or "episodic pain of varying intensity on a pain free-background" (Swanwick et al. 2001).

The temporal variation of pain is rarely included in the plethora of pain assessment tools that are used in cancer, and if so, simply assessing temporal fluctuations does not cover all aspects of BTP. Treatment of BTP represents a major clinical challenge. Studies show that patients report a median of four BTP episodes each day that many of these are associated with movement and often last less than 30 min (Swanwick et al. 2001; Zeppetella et al. 2001). Thus, a detailed history of the temporal pattern and all related factors is necessary to make an optimal treatment plan. For example, the EAPC recommendation suggested that the following dimensions of BTP should be assessed: *Intensity* (onset and peak intensity), *temporal aspects* (frequency, onset, duration, relation of episode to administration of drugs, onset of effect), *location, pain quality, treatment-related factors* (precipitating, alleviating and preventing factors, predictability, use of analgesics), *interference* and *relation* (to background pain) (Mercadante et al. 2002b).

A recent review on cancer BTP revealed that there is no international consensus concerning the definition of cancer BTP, nor any classification system or well-validated assessment tools (Haugen et al. 2010). Ten specific BTP assessment tools were identified, nine were intended for self-report by patients, while seven of these nine had been used in one study only. None of the identified tools covered all the suggested domains. Furthermore, only two were partially validated, showing that the validation of specific BTP tools is scarce. One tool, the Alberta Breakthrough Pain Assessment Tool (ABPAT), was developed through a Delphi process and patient think-aloud interviews (Hagen et al. 2008). The first version of the ABPAT was primarily intended for research purposes, but was included in a large international multicenter symptom study (EPCRC-CSA) (European Palliative Care Research Collaborative (EPCRC). http://www.epcrc.org/) as a first step to further clinical validation.

The review by Haugen et al. (Haugen et al. 2010) in line with others (Mercadante et al. 2002b; Hagen et al. 2008; Bennett 2010) concluded that a consensus-based agreement on the terminology for temporal factors and BTP is urgently needed (Haugen et al. 2010; Mercadante et al. 2002b; Hagen et al. 2008). In this respect it is promising that there is strong concurrence on key dimensions across the published recommendations on the assessment of BTP (Mercadante et al. 2002b; Bennett et al. 2005a; Davies et al. 2009), as shown in Table 6.5.

Neuropathic Pain

NP has been defined as "pain resulting from a lesion, damage, or dysfunction of the somatosensory nervous system" (International Association for the Study of Pain 1994) and has recently been redefined as "Pain arising as a direct consequence of a lesion or disease affecting the somatosensory system" (Treede et al. 2008). Cancer-related NP is a frequent condition associated with the

Table 6.5 Recommendations for assessment of cancer breakthrough pain*

Name of tool	First author, pub yr	Recommended dimensions[1]	Scale, answer categories
Report from consensus conference of an expert working group	Mercadante et al. (2002a, b)	Int: onset and peak intensity Temp: frequency, onset, duration, relation of episode to administration of drugs, onset of effect Loc: location Qual Treat: precipitating, alleviating, and preventing factors, predictability, use of analgesics Inf: (use brief pain inventory), psychological symptoms Rel + Pathophysiology	Int: VAS, NRS, VRS (should be used for frequent, repeated measurements during a BTP episode) Inf: brief pain inventory, beck depression inventory, beck anxiety inventory, performance status measures (ECOG, Karnofsky)
Consensus panel recommendations	Bennett et al. (2005a)	Int: severity Temp: frequency, onset, time to peak severity, duration Loc: location Qual: character Treat: precipitating factors/events, predictability, analgesia Inf: impact (functional status and quality of life), analgesia, activities of daily living, adverse effects, aberrant drug-related behavior Rel	Int: NRS, VAS, Wong-Baker FACES pain rating scale Treat/Inf: following initiation or changes in the management of BTP, patients should be reassessed using the "four as" of chronic pain medicine: analgesia, activities of daily living, adverse effects, and aberrant drug-related behavior Inf: brief pain inventory, pain diary pain assessment and education tool of the national pain education council may be helpful
Recommendations of a task group	Davies et al. (2009)	Int Temp: onset, frequency, duration Loc Qual Treat: exacerbating/relieving factors, treatment-related factors Inf + Pathophysiology, +etiology	Standard pain scales (NRS, VRS) to determine response to treatment

*Table adapted from Haugen et al. (2010), with permission from author

cancer disease and its treatment and represents a significant clinical challenge. Thus, a specific assessment of the intensity and characterization of the pain, including patients' descriptions of the pain quality, is crucial for optimal treatment, as emphasized in the EMA guidelines (Guideline on clinical medicinal products intended for the treatment of neuropathic pain. http://www.ema.europa.eu/). Pain quality was defined as one of the prioritized domains in the cancer pain expert surveys (Hjermstad et al. 2008; Holen et al. 2006) and is also included in the dimension *pain mechanism* (NP) of the CPACS (Kaasa et al. 2011).

The special characteristics and treatment challenges of NP have led to the development of screening tools which can be completed during clinician interview or by self-report. Some tools contain clinical examination items which necessitate clinician administration but all of them contain verbal descriptors of the pain experience and pain quality (Bennett et al. 2007).

An ongoing EPCRC literature review on NP has identified 11 different tools specifically developed for assessment of NP. Of these, eight are screening tools designed to help identify NP: DN-4 (Douleur Neuropathique en 4 questions) (Bouhassira et al. 2005), the ID-Pain (Portenoy 2006), the Leeds Assessment of Neuropathic Symptoms and Signs (LANSS) (Bennett 2001), the S-LANSS for self-report (Bennett et al. 2005b), Neuropathic Pain Questionnaire (NPQ) 12-item version (Krause and Backonja 2003) and the substantially shorter 3-item NPQ-SF (Backonja and Krause 2003), painDetect (Freynhagen et al. 2006), and the StEP (Standardized Evaluation of Pain) (Scholz et al. 2009) (Table 6.6).

The remaining three are measurement tools designed to assess the intensity of symptoms: the Neuropathic Pain Scale (NPS) (Galer and Jensen 1997), the NPSI (Neuropathic Pain Symptom Inventory) (Bouhassira et al. 2004), and the Pain Quality Assessment Scale (PQAS) that was developed as an extension of the NPS containing additional items on pain quality (Jensen et al. 2006).

An expanded and revised version of the SF-MPQ (Melzack 1987) has also been developed by adding symptoms relevant to NP and by modifying the response format to a 0–10 numerical rating scale (Dworkin et al. 2009). The objective was to develop a single measure of the major symptoms of both neuropathic and nonneuropathic pain for use in studies and clinical trials, as a response to the EFNS (European Federation of Neurological Societies) guidelines for the assessment of NP claiming that neither MPQ nor SF-MPQ is specifically designed to assess NP despite assessing sensory and affective dimensions of pain (Cruccu et al. 2010).

All of the instruments (Table 6.6) have demonstrated good psychometric properties in the validation studies but exact compliance rates were not reported. None of these NP tools were initially developed or validated for use in cancer, although patients with malignancies were included in the validation study of the LANSS and in a separate small study of cancer patients, with classification rates similar to those in the original development study (Potter et al. 2003). The majority of the NP tools were developed in order to differentiate NP from nociceptive pain with different degrees of specificity and sensitivity. It has been hypothesized that NP may indicate reduced response to analgesia and a more negative impact on daily living and quality of life than nociceptive pain (Cleeland et al. 2010), the latter, which is due to tissue damage (fractures, sprains, burns, etc.), tends to be episodic and typically resolves when the tissue damage heals. Thus, there is a call for good quality studies on incidence, prevalence, severity, and time course of NP and cancer, as well as on the direct impact on the patient's quality of life has been called for (Lema et al. 2010).

A tabulation (Bennett et al. 2007) of 17 pain descriptors that were shared by five of the instruments in Table 6.6 (LANSS, DN4, NPQ, painDetect, ID Pain) showed that eight were included in two or more tools, while five, *numbness, electrical pain, pain evoked by light touching, pricking/tingling, hot/burning pain*, were included in four, the last two also in the StEP (Cruccu and Truini 2009). This means that a number of descriptors were unique to one instrument, e.g., changes in skin color (LANSS), squeezing, and overwhelming pain (NPQ).

Nevertheless, the assessment of NP requires standardization in order to clinically phenotype pain etiologies that have been shown in animal models to be partially driven by neuropathic mechanisms, and this is particularly true in cancer pain (Kerba et al. 2010). It seems likely that results from further clinical testing and the common features across tools may constitute the basis for a future standardized assessment of NP (Bennett et al. 2007) including the incidence, prevalence, and severity of NP, and clinical and demographic factors associated with this. Better diagnostic tools may also aid in the work towards a better classification of cancer-related neuropathic syndromes in order to improve treatment (Lema et al. 2010).

Table 6.6 Content and characteristics of assessment tools for neuropathic pain (NP)

Tool name, author	Number, type of items	Clinical exam	Administration mode	Adjectives to describe the pain	Scale, answer categories	Time line	Tool objective
Screening tools							
LANSS, Bennett (2001)	7 items; sensory descriptors related to the skin: 4 Temporal: 1 Clinical testing: 2	Yes	No	Unpleasant skin sensation (prickling/tingling), different look (mottled/red/pink skin), skin sensitive to touch, bursting/sudden pain, hot/burning skin, allodynia, altered pin-prick threshold	Dichotomous; Y/N, values for Y/N differ for each item. Summary score >12 indicates NP mechanisms	Last week	A simple clinical tool to distinguish NP symptoms from symptoms of nociceptive pain
NPQ, Krause and Backonja (2003)	12 items, sensory descriptors/ sensitivity: 10 Affective items: 2	No	Self-report	Numb, burning, sensitive, shooting, electrical, tingling, squeezing, freezing, unpleasant, overwhelming, increased pain by touch, by weather changes	NRS 0-100, 0: *no*+descriptor *pain*, 100: *the most*+descriptor for *pain imaginable*	Usual pain	Screening tool for NP based on pain quality descriptors
NPQ-SF, Backonja and Krause (2003)	3 items All sensory	No	Self-report	Numb, tingling, increased pain by touch	As above	Usual pain	Determine minimum no. of NPQ-items sufficient to predict NP vs. non-NP with same accuracy
DN4, Bouhassira et al. (2005)	10 items; sensory descriptors: 7 Sensory, clinical examination items: 3	Yes, 3 items[a]	Self-report, 7 items[a]	Burning, cold, electric shocks, tingling, pins and needles, numbness, itching, hypoesthesia to touch, to prick, increased pain with brushing	Dichotomous Y/N, present/absent	Not specified	Clinician-administered tool[a] for comparing NP and non-NP
S-LANSS, Bennett et al. (2005b)	9 items; localization, body map drawing: 1 Pain intensity: 1 Diff. pain qualities: 6 Temporal: 1	No	Self-report	Prickling/tingling, mottled/red/ pink skin, sensitive skin, bursting/sudden pain, hot/ burning, allodynia, numb/tender	Pain intensity: NRS-11, *0: none – 10 severe pain* Other: dichotomous; Y/N, values for Y/N differ for each item. Summary score >12 indicates NP mechanisms	Last week	Use of self report to identify NP as distinct from nociceptive pain
ID-Pain, Portenoy (2006)	6 items; sensory descriptors: 5 Localization: 1, related to pain in the joints	No	Self-report	Pins and needles, hot/burning, numb, electrical, increased pain with light touch+localization limited to joints	Dichotomous; Y/N, transformed to 0/1: higher scores indicate NP component	Last week	Screening tool to differentiate NP from nociceptive pain, not assessing pain intensity

(continued)

Table 6.6 (continued)

Tool name, author	Number, type of items	Clinical exam	Administration mode	Adjectives to describe the pain	Scale, answer categories	Time line	Tool objective
Pain detect, Freynhagen et al. (2006)	9 items, sensory descriptors: 7, Radiation: 1, Temporal: 1	No	Self-report, paper-and pencil+palm version	Numb, burning, tingling, pain evoked by touch, heat/cold, light pressure, electrical, fluctuation, radiation	VRS-5 *0: never – 5: very strongly.* Score >19 indicates 90% with NP components	Not specified	Screening tool for NP in chronic low back pain that discriminates NP and non-NP
StEP Scholz et al. (2009)	46 items explored by 16 questions+39 exams explored by 23 tests	Yes	Structured interview+ standardized bedside examination (23 tests)	Throbbing, pounding, pulsating, shooting, radiating, cramping, squeezing, stabbing, sharp, aching, dull, painful pins, and needles, stinging, burning, hot+dysesthesia	Intensity: NRS-11, *0: no pain – 10 maximum imaginable pain*	Present	Screening tool for chronic pain that aims to distinguish between pain subtypes/etiologies
Measurement tools							
NPS, Galer and Jensen (1997)	10 items; average intensity: 1, intensity of deep vs. surface: 1 Diff. pain qualities: 7 Temporal aspect: 1	No	Self-report	Intense, sharp, hot/burning, dull, cold, sensitive, itchy, unpleasant, deep vs. surface, temporal aspect	Temporal: 3 point categorical scale Other: NRS-11, *0: no pain or not+descriptor-* 10: *the most+descriptor imaginable*	Average pain	Assessment of distinct pain qualities in NP, assessment of treatment outcomes
NPSI, Bouhassira et al. (2004)	12 items, Diff. pain qualities: 10 Duration: 2	No	Self-report	Burning, squeezing, pressure, duration of spontaneous pain, electric shocks, stabbing, frequency of pain "attacks," increased pain with brushing, pressure, contact with something cold, pins/needles, tingling	NRS-11, *0: no+descriptor or no pain – 10: the worst+descriptor imaginable or worst pain imaginable* total intensity score: of first 5 items	Average last 24 h	Evaluation of the different NP symptoms
PQAS, Jensen et al. (2006)	20 items; average intensity: 1, intensity of deep: vs. surface: 1 Diff. pain qualities: 17 Temporal aspect: 1	No	Self-report	Same as the NPS plus tender, shooting, numb, electrical, tingling, cramping, radiating, throbbing, aching, heavy	NRS-11, scale as above. Categories as in NPS	Average pain last week	Improve assessment of neuropathic pain by adding pain quality items to the NPS, that are also useful for non-neuropathic pain

DN-4 Douleur Neuropathique en 4 questions; *LANSS* leeds assessment of neuropathic symptoms and signs; *S-LANSS* for self report; *NPQ* neuropathic pain questionnaire; *NPQ-SF* neuropathic pain questionnaire short form; *NPS* neuropathic pain scale; *NPSI* neuropathic pain symptom inventory; *PQAS* pain quality assessment scale

[a]Developed as a clinical tool to be administered through patient interview, self-report of the seven descriptor items have shown similar results

The Present Recommendations for Cancer Pain Assessment

The most important message in relation to cancer pain assessment, in palliative care as well as in oncology, is to discontinue the flow of new pain assessment tools by adhering to well-validated instruments using a standardized methodology. Furthermore, it is necessary to agree on the specific measures that should be used for assessment of the specific domains of the cancer pain experience.

The recommendations from the consensus meeting in Milan (Kaasa et al. 2011) suggested that the following three domains are the most relevant pain outcomes in clinical practice and in research: *pain intensity*, *pain relief*, and the *temporal pattern of pain*.

In relation to assessment of *pain intensity*, the present recommendation is to employ the NRS-11 with standard endpoints taken from the BPI (0: *No pain* – 10: *Pain as bad as you can imagine*) (Kaasa et al. 2011). Choosing the NRS is based on documentation in the literature, previous consensus based recommendations for cancer pain assessment, the brevity and ease of use of the scale, and the fact that the NRS is intuitively easy to comprehend across cultures with little bias demonstrated in specific groups (elderly, impaired, illiterate, etc.) (Jensen 2003; Breivik et al. 2008; Hjermstad et al. 2011; Caraceni et al. 2002; Dworkin et al. 2005).

For clinical monitoring of pain, the actual wording of the prompt question and the appropriate time frame is crucial. The following two clinically relevant time frames were proposed depending upon the purpose of the assessment: (a) *average pain intensity during the last 24 h* and (b) *average pain intensity during the last week*. This does not mean that other time frames and prompts are not to be used, e.g., *worst pain* and *least pain* that may be highly relevant in pain studies. However, average pain intensity in the last 24 h and last week is proposed as the minimum assessment.

If changes in pain over time or pain relief from medication are to be monitored, pain intensity is also proposed as the primary outcome with the same wording and time frames as described earlier. The difference between the initial and subsequent assessments should be evaluated, with specific emphasis on baseline pain intensity. Generally speaking, a 30% reduction in pain intensity on the NRS-11 is regarded as a clinically meaningful change, but it should be remembered that the percentage takes on different numerical values depending on the baseline values (Farrar et al. 2009). For example, a 30% reduction of an initial pain score of 7–10 corresponds to a value of 3, whereas a 30% reduction of a score at the lower end of the NRS (1–3) refers to a value of 1 (Kaasa et al. 2011).

In relation to *BTP*, the review by Haugen et al. concluded that the ideal BTP assessment tool should include the following domains: *number of different BTPs*, relation *to background pain*, *intensity, temporal factors* (frequency, onset, duration, course, relationship to fixed analgesic dose), *localization* (body map), *treatment-related factors* (exacerbation/relief), *precipitating factors/ predictability*, *response and satisfaction with treatment*, and *interference* (with activities and QoL) (Haugen et al. 2010). This is in line with the recommendations from the Milan meeting (Kaasa et al. 2011), BTP being one of the core domains in the CPACS classification system, and a recent paper indicating that BTP should be monitored using a longitudinal design (Mercadante et al. 2010). Furthermore, the need for standardization of BTP assessment was emphasized, in line with the call for a common and agreed upon terminology, in a recent editorial in pain (Bennett 2010).

Pain mechanism (neuropathic vs. nociceptive pain) was also defined as one of the core domains of the CPACS at the Milan consensus conference (Kaasa et al. 2011) building on the ECS-CP (Fainsinger and Nekolaichuk 2008; Fainsinger et al. 2005; Bruera et al. 1989, 1991; Nekolaichuk et al. 2005). While the NP part of the ECS-CP is a clinical diagnosis based on clinicians' judgment, a screening tool could be an important asset to improve the diagnosis, if proven good enough. Thus, it is important to agree on a simple, reliable, and valid measure to assess the major characteristics of both neuropathic and nociceptive pain in order to distinguish the two. Future work should strive for standardized and consensus-based assessment methods in line with the recent recommendations (Bennett 2010; Lema et al. 2010; Kerba et al. 2010).

Conclusion

The tremendous interest in symptom assessment in general and cancer pain measurement in particular has been to the benefit of both patients and science. However, we have now reached a point when we should join efforts and continue on a common path. The continuous flow of new tools with different definitions and nomenclature is unlikely to improve the standard of cancer pain assessment. However, the ongoing international and collaborative work striving for consensus, as well as the recent recommendations, is promising. It is time to welcome all consensus-based approaches aiming to standardize and facilitate the assessment of the subjective pain experience in order to improve cancer pain management and promote research.

References

Aaronson, N. K., Ahmedzai, S., Bergman, B., et al. (1993). The European Organization for Research and Treatment of Cancer QLQ-C30: A quality-of-life instrument for use in international clinical trials in oncology. *Journal of the National Cancer Institute, 85*, 365–376.

Ahlers, S. J. G. M., van Gulik, L., van der Veen, A. M., et al. (2008). Comparison of different pain scoring systems in critically ill patients in a general ICU. *Critical Care, 12*(1), R15.

Apolone, G., Bertetto, O., Caraceni, A., et al. (2006). Pain in cancer. An outcome research project to evaluate the epidemiology, the quality and the effects of pain treatment in cancer patients. *Health and Quality of Life Outcomes, 4*, 7.

Arner, S., & Arner, B. (1985). Differential effects of epidural morphine in the treatment of cancer-related pain. *Acta Anaesthesiologica Scandinavica, 29*, 32–36.

Backonja, M. M., & Krause, S. J. (2003). Neuropathic pain questionnaire – short form. *The Clinical Journal of Pain, 19*, 315–316.

Banos, J. E., Bosch, F., Canellas, M., et al. (1989). Acceptability of visual analogue scales in the clinical setting: A comparison with verbal rating scales in postoperative pain. *Methods and Findings in Experimental and Clinical Pharmacology, 11*, 123–127.

Bennett, M. (2001). The LANSS pain scale: The Leeds assessment of neuropathic symptoms and signs. *Pain, 92*, 147–157.

Bennett, M. I. (2010). Cancer pain terminology: Time to develop a taxonomy that promotes good clinical practice and allows research to progress. *Pain, 149*, 426–427.

Bennett, M. I., Attal, N., Backonja, M. M., et al. (2007). Using screening tools to identify neuropathic pain. *Pain, 127*, 199–203.

Bennett, D., Burton, A. W., Fishman, S., et al. (2005a). Consensus panel recommendations for the assessment and management of breakthrough pain. Part 2: Management. *Pharmacy and Therapeutics, 30*, 354–361.

Bennett, M. I., Smith, B. H., Torrance, N., & Potter, J. (2005b). The S-LANSS score for identifying pain of predominantly neuropathic origin: Validation for use in clinical and postal research. *The Journal of Pain, 6*, 149–158.

Boisvert, M., & Cohen, S. R. (1995). Opioid use in advanced malignant disease: Why do different centers use vastly different doses? A plea for standardized reporting. *Journal of Pain and Symptom Management, 10*, 632–638.

Bonica, J. J. (1979). The need of a taxonomy. *Pain, 6*, 247–248.

Borgsteede, S. D., Deliens, L., Francke, A. L., et al. (2006). Defining the patient population: One of the problems for palliative care research. *Palliative Medicine, 20*, 63–68.

Bouhassira, D., Attal, N., Alchaar, H., et al. (2005). Comparison of pain syndromes associated with nervous or somatic lesions and development of a new neuropathic pain diagnostic questionnaire (DN4). *Pain, 114*, 29–36.

Bouhassira, D., Attal, N., Fermanian, J., et al. (2004). Development and validation of the neuropathic pain symptom inventory. *Pain, 108*, 248–257.

Breivik, H., Borchgrevink, P. C., Allen, S. M., et al. (2008). Assessment of pain. *British Journal of Anaesthesia, 101*(1), 17–24.

Bruera, E., Kuehn, N., Miller, M. J., et al. (1991). The Edmonton Symptom Assessment System (ESAS): A simple method for the assessment of palliative care patients. *Journal of Palliative Care, 7*, 6–9.

Bruera, E., Macmillan, K., Hanson, J., & MacDonald, R. N. (1989). The Edmonton staging system for cancer pain: Preliminary report. *Pain, 37*, 203–209.

Bruera, E., Schoeller, T., Wenk, R., et al. (1995). A prospective multicenter assessment of the Edmonton staging system for cancer pain. *Journal of Pain and Symptom Management, 10*, 348–355.

Brunelli, C., Zecca, E., Martini, C., et al. (2010). Comparison of numerical and verbal rating scales to measure pain exacerbations in patients with chronic cancer pain. *Health and Quality of Life Outcomes, 8,* 42.

Burgers, J. S., Fervers, B., Haugh, M., et al. (2004). International assessment of the quality of clinical practice guidelines in oncology using the appraisal of guidelines and research and evaluation instrument. *Journal of Clinical Oncology, 22,* 2000–2007.

Caraceni, A. (2001). Evaluation and assessment of cancer pain and cancer pain treatment. *Acta Anaesthesiologica Scandinavica, 45*(9), 1067–1075.

Caraceni, A., Brunelli, C., Martini, C., et al. (2005). Cancer pain assessment in clinical trials. A review of the literature (1999–2002). *Journal of Pain and Symptom Management, 29*(5), 507–519.

Caraceni, A., Brunelli, C., Martini, C., et al. (2006). Enhancing the quality of controlled clinical trials in cancer pain first requires that pain assessment methods are appropriately understood and used. *British Journal of Cancer, 8,* 1121.

Caraceni, A., Cherny, N., Fainsinger, R., et al. (2002). Pain measurement tools and methods in clinical research in palliative care: Recommendations of an Expert Working Group of the European Association of Palliative Care. *Journal of Pain and Symptom Management, 23,* 239–255.

Caraceni, A., Hanks, G., Kaasa, S., & on behalf of the European Association for Palliative Care. (2011). Evidence-based guidelines for the use of opioid analgesics in the treatment of cancer pain: The 2011 EAPC recommendations (2011). In press, Lancet Oncology.

Caraceni, A., & Portenoy, R. K. (1999). An international survey of cancer pain characteristics and syndromes. IASP Task Force on Cancer Pain. International Association for the Study of Pain. *Pain, 82,* 263–274.

Caraceni, A., & Weinstein, S. M. (2001). Classification of cancer pain syndromes. *Oncology (Williston Park), 15,* 1627–40; 1642.

Caraceni, A., Zecca, E., Martini, C., et al. (2010b). The validity of average 8-h pain intensity assessment in cancer patients. *European Journal of Pain, 14,* 441–445.

Cella, D. F., Tulsky, D. S., Gray, G., et al. (1993). The Functional Assessment of Cancer Therapy scale: Development and validation of the general measure. *Journal of Clinical Oncology, 11,* 570–579.

Chang, V. T., Hwang, S. S., Feuerman, M., et al. (2000). The memorial symptom assessment scale short form (MSAS-SF). *Cancer, 89,* 1162–1171.

Cherny, N., & Portenoy, R. K. (2004). Cancer pain: Principles of assessment and syndromes. In P. D. Wall & R. Melzack (Eds.), *Textbook of pain* (pp. 787–823). London: Churchill Livingstone.

Chibnall, J. T., & Tait, R. C. (2001). Pain assessment in cognitively impaired and unimpaired older adults: A comparison of four scales. *Pain, 92,* 173–186.

Chow, E., Doyle, M., Li, K., et al. (2006). Mild, moderate, or severe pain categorized by patients with cancer with bone metastases. *Journal of Palliative Medicine, 9,* 850–854.

Cleeland, C. S. (2007). Symptom burden: Multiple symptoms and their impact as patient-reported outcomes. *Journal of the National Cancer Institute. Monographs, 37,* 16–21.

Cleeland, C. S., Farrar, J. T., & Hausheer, F. H. (2010). Assessment of cancer-related neuropathy and neuropathic pain. *The Oncologist, 15*(Suppl 2), 13–18.

Cleeland, C. S., Gonin, R., Hatfield, A. K., et al. (1994). Pain and its treatment in outpatients with metastatic cancer. *The New England Journal of Medicine, 330,* 592–596.

Cleeland, C. S., Mendoza, T. R., Wang, X. S., et al. (2000). Assessing symptom distress in cancer patients: The M.D. Anderson Symptom Inventory. *Cancer, 89,* 1634–1646.

NIH Consensus Development Program, National Institutes of Health. (2002). NIH State-of-the-Science Statement on symptom management in cancer: Pain, depression, and fatigue. *NIH Consensus and State-of-the-Science Statements, 19,* 1–29.

Cruccu, G., Sommer, C., Anand, P., et al. (2010). EFNS guidelines on neuropathic pain assessment: Revised 2009. *European Journal of Neurology, 17,* 1010–1018.

Cruccu, G., & Truini, A. (2009). Tools for assessing neuropathic pain. *PLoS Medicine, 6,* e1000045.

Currow, D. C., Wheeler, J. L., Glare, P. A., et al. (2009). A framework for generalizability in palliative care. *Journal of Pain and Symptom Management, 37*(3), 373–386.

Daut, R. L., Cleeland, C. S., & Flanery, R. C. (1983). Development of the Wisconsin brief pain questionnaire to assess pain in cancer and other diseases. *Pain, 17,* 197–210.

Davies, A. N., Dickman, A., Reid, C., et al. (2009). The management of cancer-related breakthrough pain: Recommendations of a task group of the Science Committee of the Association for Palliative Medicine of Great Britain and Ireland. *European Journal of Pain, 13,* 331–338.

de Haes, J. C., van Knippenberg, F. C., & Neijt, J. P. (1990). Measuring psychological and physical distress in cancer patients: Structure and application of the Rotterdam Symptom Checklist. *British Journal of Cancer, 62,* 1034–1038.

DeWalt, D. A., Rothrock, N., Yount, S., & Stone, A. A. (2007). Evaluation of item candidates: The PROMIS qualitative item review. *Medical Care, 45,* S12–S21.

Dworkin, R. H., Turk, D. C., Farrar, J. T., et al. (2005). Core outcome measures for chronic pain clinical trials: IMMPACT recommendations. *Pain, 113,* 9–19.

Dworkin, R. H., Turk, D. C., Revicki, D. A., et al. (2009). Development and initial validation of an expanded and revised version of the Short-form McGill Pain Questionnaire (SF-MPQ-2). *Pain, 144*, 35–42.

Fainsinger, R. L. (2008). Global warming in the palliative care research environment: Adapting to change. *Palliative Medicine, 22*, 328–335.

Fainsinger, R. L., Fairchild, A., Nekolaichuk, C., et al. (2009). Is pain intensity a predictor of the complexity of cancer pain management? *Journal of Clinical Oncology, 27*, 585–590.

Fainsinger, R. L., & Nekolaichuk, C. L. (2008). A "TNM" classification system for cancer pain: The Edmonton Classification System for Cancer Pain (ECS-CP). *Supportive Care in Cancer, 16*, 547–555.

Fainsinger, R., Nekolaichuk, C., & Lawlor, P. (2010). An international multicenter validation study of a pain classification system for cancer patients. *European Journal of Cancer*. doi: 10.1016/j.ejca.2010.07.019.

Fainsinger, R. L., Nekolaichuk, C. L., Lawlor, P. G., & Neumann, C. M. (2008). Edmonton classification system for cancer pain (ECS-CP). *Journal of Pain and Symptom Management, 29*(3), 224–237.

Fainsinger, R. L., Nekolaichuk, C. L., Lawlor, P. G., et al. (2005). A multicenter study of the revised Edmonton Staging System for classifying cancer pain in advanced cancer patients. *Journal of Pain and Symptom Management, 29*, 224–237.

Farrar, J. T., Pritchett, Y. L., Robinson, M., et al. (2009). The clinical importance of changes in the 0 to 10 numeric rating scale for worst, least, and average pain intensity: Analyses of data from clinical trials of Duloxetine in pain disorders. *The Journal of Pain, 11*(2), 109–118.

Fayers, P. M., Hjermstad, M. J., Klepstad, P., et al. (2011). The dimensionality of pain: Palliative and chronic pain patients differ in their reports of pain intensity and interference. *Pain, 152*, 1608–1620.

Foley, K. M. (2004). Acute and chronic cancer pain syndromes. In D. Doyle, G. W. C. Hanks, & N. MacDonald (Eds.), *Oxford textbook of palliative medicine* (pp. 298–316). New York: Oxford University Press.

Food and Drug Administration. (2006). Guidance for Industry. *Patient-reported outcome measures: Use in medical product development to support labeling claims*. US Food and Drug administration website. Retrieved, from http://www.fda.gov/cder/guidance/5460dft.pdf. Accessed February 5, 2011.

Freynhagen, R., Baron, R., Gockel, U., & Tolle, T. R. (2006). painDETECT: A new screening questionnaire to identify neuropathic components in patients with back pain. *Current Medical Research and Opinion, 22*, 1911–1920.

Galer, B. S., & Jensen, M. P. (1997). Development and preliminary validation of a pain measure specific to neuropathic pain: The Neuropathic Pain Scale. *Neurology, 48*, 332–338.

Grafton, K. V., Foster, N. E., & Wright, C. C. (2005). Test-retest reliability of the short-form McGill pain questionnaire: Assessment of intraclass correlation coefficients and limits of agreement in patients with osteoarthritis. *The Clinical Journal of Pain, 21*, 73–82.

Groenvold, M., Petersen, M. A., Aaronson, N. K., et al. (2006). EORTC QLQ-C15-PAL: The new standard in the assessment of health-related quality of life in advanced cancer? *Palliative Medicine, 20*, 59–61.

Grond, S., Zech, D., Diefenbach, C., et al. (1996). Assessment of cancer pain: A prospective evaluation in 2266 cancer patients referred to a pain service. *Pain, 64*, 107–114.

Gutgsell, T., Walsh, D., Zhukovsky, D. S., et al. (2003). A prospective study of the pathophysiology and clinical characteristics of pain in a palliative medicine population. *The American Journal of Hospice & Palliative Care, 20*, 140–148.

Hagen, N. A., Stiles, C., Nekolaichuk, C., et al. (2008). The Alberta breakthrough pain assessment tool for cancer patients: A validation study using a delphi process and patient think-aloud interviews. *Journal of Pain and Symptom Management, 35*, 136–152.

Hanks, G., Portenoy, R. K., MacDonald, N., et al. (2000). Difficult pain problems. In D. Doyle, G. Hanks, & N. MacDonald (Eds.), *Oxford textbook of palliative medicine* (pp. 454–477). Oxford: Oxford University Press.

Hasson, F., Keeney, S., & McKenna, H. (2000). Research guidelines for the Delphi survey technique. *Journal of Advanced Nursing, 32*, 1008–1015.

Haugen, D. F., Hjermstad, M. J., Hagen, N. A., et al. (2010). Assessment and classification of cancer breakthrough pain. A systematic literature review. *Pain, 149*, 476–482.

Haugen, D. F., & Kaasa, S. (2010). Update on the EPCRC project on pain, depression and fatigue. *European Journal of Palliative care, 17*(3), 136–140.

Hempel, C. G. (1961). Introduction to the problems of taxonomy. In J. Zubin (Ed.), *Field studies in the mental disorders* (pp. 3–22). New York: Grune and Stratton.

Hjermstad, M. J., Fainsinger, R., & Kaasa, S. (2009). Assessment and classification of cancer pain. *Current Opinion in Supportive and Palliative Care, 3*, 24–30.

Hjermstad, M. J., Fayers, P. M., Haugen, D. F., & Loge, J. H. (2011). Studies comparing numerical rating scales, verbal rating scales and visual analogue scales for assessment of pain intensity – a systematic review. *Journal of Pain and Symptom Management, 41*, 1073–1093.

Hjermstad, M. J., Gibbins, J., Haugen, D. F., et al. (2008). Pain assessment tools in palliative care: An urgent need for consensus. *Palliative Medicine, 22*(8), 895–903.

Holen, J. C., Hjermstad, M. J., Loge, J. H., et al. (2006). Pain assessment tools: Is the content appropriate for use in palliative care? *Journal of Pain and Symptom Management, 32*, 567–580.

Holen, J. C., Lydersen, S., Klepstad, P., et al. (2008). The brief pain inventory: Pain's interference with functions is different in cancer pain compared with noncancer chronic pain. *The Clinical Journal of Pain, 24*, 219–225.

Hwang, S. S., Chang, V. T., Fairclough, D. L., & Kasimis, B. (2002). Development of a cancer pain prognostic scale. *Journal of Pain and Symptom Management, 24*, 366–378.

Hwang, S. S., Chang, V. T., & Kasimis, B. (2003). Cancer breakthrough pain characteristics and responses to treatment at a VA medical center. *Pain, 101*, 55–64.

International Association for the Study of Pain. (1994). *International classification of chronic pain*. Seattle: IASP Press.

Jensen, M. P. (2003). The validity and reliability of pain measures in adults with cancer. *The Journal of Pain, 4*, 2–21.

Jensen, M. P., Gammaitoni, A. R., Olaleye, D. O., et al. (2006). The pain quality assessment scale: Assessment of pain quality in carpal tunnel syndrome. *The Journal of Pain, 7*, 823–832.

Kaasa, S. (2008). Palliative care research: Time to intensify international collaboration. *Palliative Medicine, 22*, 301–302.

Kaasa, S. (2010). An international multicenter study of a pain classification system for cancer patients. *European Journal of Cancer*. doi: 10.1016/j.ejca.2010.07.019. Editorial, 16, 2865–2866.

Kaasa, S., Apolone, G., Klepstad, P., et al. (2011). Expert conference on cancer pain assessment and classification, the need for international consensus: Working proposals on international standards (2011). Accepted for publication, BMJ Supportive and Palliative Care.

Kaasa, S., Hjermstad, M. J., & Loge, J. H. (2006). Methodological and structural challenges in palliative care research: How have we fared in the last decades? *Palliative Medicine, 20*, 727–734.

Kaasa, S., Loge, J. H., Fayers, P., et al. (2008). Symptom assessment in palliative care: A need for international collaboration. *Journal of Clinical Oncology, 26*, 3867–3873.

Kerba, M., Wu, J., Duan, Q., et al. (2010). Neuropathic pain features in bone metastases patients referred for palliative radiotherapy. *Journal of Clinical Oncology, 28*, 4892–4897.

Kirkova, J., Davis, M. P., Walsh, D., et al. (2006). Cancer symptom assessment instruments: A systematic review. *Journal of Clinical Oncology, 24*, 1459–1473.

Knudsen, A. K., Aass, N., Fainsinger, R., et al. (2009). Classification of pain in cancer patients – a systematic literature review. *Palliative Medicine, 23*, 295–308.

Krause, S. J., & Backonja, M. M. (2003). Development of a neuropathic pain questionnaire. *The Clinical Journal of Pain, 19*, 306–314.

Lawlor, P., Walker, P., Bruera, E., & Mitchell, S. (1997). Severe opioid toxicity and somatization of psychosocial distress in a cancer patient with a background of chemical dependence. *Journal of Pain and Symptom Management, 13*, 356–361.

Lema, M. J., Foley, K. M., & Hausheer, F. H. (2010). Types and epidemiology of cancer -related neuropathic pain: The intersection of cancer pain and neuropathic pain. *The Oncologist, 15*(suppl), 3–8.

Maltoni, M. (2008). Opioids, pain, and fear. *Annals of Oncology, 19*, 5–7.

Melzack, R. (1975). The McGill pain questionnaire: Major properties and scoring methods. *Pain, 1*, 277–299.

Melzack, R. (1987). The short-form McGill pain questionnaire. *Pain, 30*, 191–197.

Melzack, R., & Katz, J. (2001). The McGill pain questionnaire: Appraisal and current status. In D. C. Turk & R. Melzack (Eds.), *Handbook of pain assessment* (pp. 35–52). London: Guilford Press.

Mercadante, S. (1998). Opioid responsiveness in patients with advanced head and neck cancer. *Supportive Care in Cancer, 6*, 482–485.

Mercadante, S., Armata, M., & Salvaggio, L. (1994). Pain characteristics of advanced lung cancer patients referred to a palliative care service. *Pain, 59*, 141–145.

Mercadante, S., Casuccio, A., Pumo, S., & Fulfaro, F. (2000a). Factors influencing the opioid response in advanced cancer patients with pain followed at home: The effects of age and gender. *Supportive Care in Cancer, 8*, 123–130.

Mercadante, S., Casuccio, A., Pumo, S., & Fulfaro, F. (2000b). Opioid responsiveness-primary diagnosis relationship in advanced cancer patients followed at home. *Journal of Pain and Symptom Management, 20*, 27–34.

Mercadante, S., Fulfaro, F., & Casuccio, A. (2002a). Pain mechanisms involved and outcome in advanced cancer patients with possible indications for celiac plexus block and superior hypogastric plexus block. *Tumori, 88*, 243–245.

Mercadante, S., Gebbia, V., David, F., et al. (2009). Tools for identifying cancer pain of predominantly neuropathic origin and opioid responsiveness in cancer patients. *The Journal of Pain, 10*, 594–600.

Mercadante, S., Maddaloni, S., Roccella, S., & Salvaggio, L. (1992). Predictive factors in advanced cancer pain treated only by analgesics. *Pain, 50*, 151–155.

Mercadante, S., Radbruch, L., Caraceni, A., et al. (2002b). Episodic (breakthrough) pain: Consensus conference of an expert working group of the European Association for Palliative Care. *Cancer, 94*, 832–839.

Mercadante, S., Zagonel, V., Breda, E., et al. (2010). Breakthrough pain in oncology: A longitudinal study. *Journal of Pain and Symptom Management, 40*, 183–190.

Meuser, T., Pietruck, C., Radbruch, L., et al. (2001). Symptoms during cancer pain treatment following WHO-guidelines: A longitudinal follow-up study of symptom prevalence, severity and etiology. *Pain, 93*, 247–257.

Mok, T. S., Wu, Y. L., Thongprasert, S., et al. (2009). Gefitinib or carboplatin-paclitaxel in pulmonary adenocarcinoma. *The New England Journal of Medicine, 361*, 947–957.

Nekolaichuk, C. L., Fainsinger, R. L., & Lawlor, P. G. (2005). A validation study of a pain classification system for advanced cancer patients using content experts: The Edmonton Classification System for Cancer Pain. *Palliative Medicine, 19*, 466–476.

Nekolaichuk, C., Watanabe, S., & Beaumont, C. (2008). The Edmonton symptom assessment system: A 15-year retrospective review of validation studies (1991–2006). *Palliative Medicine, 22*, 111–122.

Patrick, D. L., Ferketich, S. L., Frame, P. S., et al. (2003). National Institutes of Health State-of-the-Science Conference Statement: Symptom management in cancer: Pain, depression, and fatigue, July 15-17, 2002. *Journal of the National Cancer Institute, 95*, 1110–1117.

Piccirillo, J. F., & Feinstein, A. R. (1996). Clinical symptoms and comorbidity: Significance for the prognostic classification of cancer. *Cancer, 77*, 834–842.

Portenoy, R. K. (2006). Development and testing of a neuropathic pain screening questionnaire: ID pain. *Current Medical Research and Opinion, 22*, 1555–1565.

Portenoy, R. K., & Hagen, N. A. (1990). Breakthrough pain: Definition, prevalence and characteristics. *Pain, 41*, 273–281.

Portenoy, R. K., Payne, D., & Jacobsen, P. (1999). Breakthrough pain: Characteristics and impact in patients with cancer pain. *Pain, 81*, 129–134.

Potter, J., Higginson, I. J., Scadding, J. W., & Quigley, C. (2003). Identifying neuropathic pain in patients with head and neck cancer: Use of the leeds assessment of neuropathic symptoms and signs scale. *Journal of the Royal Society of Medicine, 96*, 379–383.

Radbruch, L., Loick, G., Kiencke, P., et al. (1999). Validation of the German version of the brief pain inventory. *Journal of Pain and Symptom Management, 18*, 180–187.

Ripamonti, C. I., & Brunelli, C. (2009). Comparison between numerical rating scale and six-level verbal rating scale in cancer patients with pain: A preliminary report. *Supportive Care in Cancer, 17*, 1433–1434.

Schipper, H., Clinch, J., McMurray, A., & Levitt, M. (1984). Measuring the quality of life of cancer patients: The functional living index-cancer: Development and validation. *Journal of Clinical Oncology, 2*, 472–483.

Scholz, J., Mannion, R. J., Hord, D. E., et al. (2009). A novel tool for the assessment of pain: Validation in low back pain. *PLoS Medicine, 6*, e1000047.

Sloan, J. A., & Zhao, C. X. (2006). Genetics and quality of life. *Current Problems in Cancer, 30*, 255–260.

Sprangers, M. A., Cull, A., & Groenvold, M. (1998). *EORTC Quality of Life Study Group: Guidelines for developing questionnaire modules*. Brussels: EORTC.

Stenseth, G., Bjornes, M., Kaasa, S., & Klepstad, P. (2007). Can cancer patients assess the influence of pain on functions? A randomised, controlled study of the pain interference items in the Brief Pain Inventory. *BMC Palliative Care, 6*, 2.

Stromgren, A. S., Groenvold, M., Petersen, M. A., et al. (2004). Pain characteristics and treatment outcome for advanced cancer patients during the first week of specialized palliative care. *Journal of Pain and Symptom Management, 27*, 104–113.

Svendsen, K. B., Andersen, S., Arnason, S., et al. (2005). Breakthrough pain in malignant and non-malignant diseases: A review of prevalence, characteristics and mechanisms. *European Journal of Pain, 9*, 195–206.

Swanwick, M., Haworth, M., & Lennard, R. F. (2001). The prevalence of episodic pain in cancer: A survey of hospice patients on admission. *Palliative Medicine, 15*, 9–18.

Thomas, J. (2007). Optimizing opioid management in palliative care. *Journal of Palliative Medicine, 10*(Suppl 1), S1–S18.

Treede, R. D., Jensen, T. S., Campbell, J. N., et al. (2008). Neuropathic pain: Redefinition and a grading system for clinical and research purposes. *Neurology, 70*, 1630–1635.

van den Beuken-van Everdingen, M. H., de Rijke, J. M., Kessels, A. G., et al. (2007). Prevalence of pain in patients with cancer: A systematic review of the past 40 years. *Annals of Oncology, 18*, 1437–1449.

Velikova, G., Awad, N., Coles-Gale, R., et al. (2008). The clinical value of quality of life assessment in oncology practice-a qualitative study of patient and physician views. *Psycho-Oncology, 17*, 690–698.

Ventafridda, V., & Caraceni, A. (1991). Cancer pain classification: A controversial issue. *Pain, 46*, 1–2.

Victorson, D., Barocas, J., Song, J., & Cella, D. (2008). Reliability across studies from the functional assessment of cancer therapy-general (FACT-G) and its subscales: A reliability generalization. *Quality of Life Research, 17*, 1137–1146.

Von Roenn, J. H., Cleeland, C. S., Gonin, R., et al. (1993). Physician attitudes and practice in cancer pain management. A survey from the Eastern Cooperative Oncology Group. *Annals of Internal Medicine, 119*, 121–126.

Ware, J. E. (1993). *SF 36 health survey manual and interpretation guide*. Boston: New England Medical Center.

Watanabe, S., Nekolaichuk, C., Beaumont, C., & Mawani, A. (2009). The Edmonton symptom assessment system – what do patients think? *Supportive Care in Cancer, 17*, 675–683.

WHO Guidelines. (1996). *Cancer pain relief*. Geneva: World Health Organization.

Zeppetella, G., O'Doherty, C. A., & Collins, S. (2001). Prevalence and characteristics of breakthrough pain in patients with non-malignant terminal disease admitted to a hospice. *Palliative Medicine, 15*(3), 243–246.

Chapter 7
Quality Indicators for Pain in Palliative Care

Sydney Dy and Hsien Seow

Introduction

Despite strong evidence that interventions can greatly improve pain management for persons with advanced cancer, these advances have not been completely translated into clinical practice. Routine quality measurement is one potential solution that can improve the delivery of pain interventions. A quality indicator or quality measure is *an agreed-upon process or outcome measure that is used to assess quality of care,* specified with a numerator and denominator to indicate the intended population, recommended care, and exclusions.

$$\text{Quality indicator} = \frac{\text{\# patients who received the specified intervention}}{\text{\# patients for whom the intervention was indicated}}$$

Quality indicators are population-level measures expressed using rates, as opposed to a measurement tool such as a pain visual analog scale, which is used to collect data at the individual patient level. For example, while a patient's pain could be assessed with a visual analog scale, the corresponding quality indicator could also measure the rate of pain screening on an entire hospital unit. Indicators also specify data elements and instructions for data collection, timing, and descriptions of data analysis and reporting. They are intended to be used routinely, can provide feedback to guide short-term quality improvement or longer-term restructuring of care, and generally draw on administrative data, medical records, or data collected directly from patients and families (e.g., via survey).

Quality indicators can be classified as pertaining to structure (the environment in which health care is provided), process (how health care is provided), and outcome (the consequences of health care) (Donabedian 1988). Accurately measuring care for comparing quality or as a baseline for quality improvement interventions requires quality indicators that are supported by experts and research evidence, scientifically valid and useful, and feasible to implement (Campbell et al. 2002). Indicators' validity depends on the validity of the measurement of pain or the associated outcome, including the instrument used and the completeness of documentation. For example, for a pain indicator that applies only to severe pain, if pain is documented only for half of patients, the denominator (patients

S. Dy, MD, MSc, (✉)
Johns Hopkins University, Rm 609, 624 N Broadway, Baltimore, MD 21205, Norway

H. Seow, PhD
McMaster University, Juravinski Cancer Center 699 Concession Street 4th Floor, Room 4-229 Hamilton, Ontario, L8V 5C2, Norway

R.J. Moore (ed.), *Handbook of Pain and Palliative Care: Biobehavioral Approaches for the Life Course,*
DOI 10.1007/978-1-4419-1651-8_7, © Springer Science+Business Media, LLC 2012

with severe pain) will be incomplete and the generalizability of the quality data will be limited. Indicators should also be feasible to efficiently extract from existing data sources or obtain from patients or families and reliable when assessed by different abstractors or methods. Ideally, indicator results should also be associated with health outcomes valued by patients and families.

This chapter reviews frameworks for quality indicators in palliative care relevant to pain management, key palliative care quality indicators sets addressing pain, and palliative care research applying pain quality indicators. The chapter concludes by discussing barriers to developing and applying palliative care quality indicators in pain and future research directions.

Frameworks for Quality Indicators in Palliative Care

Due to the need to address deficits in palliative and end-of-life care, several seminal US initiatives have aimed to develop frameworks for quality indicators in palliative care. First, the National Consensus Project (NCP) (National Consensus Project 2004) helped defined broad clinical domains for palliative care, based on professional consensus from five major US palliative care organizations. Specifically, the domains of quality palliative care include: structure and processes of care; physical aspects of care; psychological and psychiatric aspects of care; social aspects of care; spiritual, religious and existential aspects of care; cultural aspects of care; care of the imminently dying patient; and ethical and legal aspects of care. The guidelines are applicable to specialist-level palliative care delivered in a range of treatment settings, as well as to the work of providers in primary treatment settings where palliative approaches to care are integrated into daily clinical practice.

Based on the NCP domains, the National Quality Forum (NQF) endorsed a Palliative Care Framework (National Quality Forum 2006) to develop a set of preferred practices related to palliative and hospice care. They identified and endorsed 38 preferred practices as suitable for implementation by palliative care and hospice programs across many practice settings. The framework aimed to lay the foundation for the development of performance measures for evaluating these programs.

There are many challenges in translating the broad domains defined by these projects into measurable aspects of care, and in evaluating them for feasibility, reliability, and validity. Unlike some clinical areas (e.g., cardiovascular care), there are few randomized trials to support evidence-based quality indicators in palliative care. Quality measurement often depends on aspects of care that may be uncommonly or inconsistently documented, such as reports of pain and when pain medications were administered. Defining the population or denominator where indicators apply may also be problematic in palliative care, since some aspects of palliative care should begin at diagnosis of a chronic illness.

Two projects have focused on expanding these frameworks to make them more applicable to quality indicators, one focusing on end-of-life cancer care (Seow et al. 2009a, b) and one on hospice (Carolinas Center for Medical Excellence 2008). Both projects also have relevance for the development and application of palliative care quality indicators in general. Both built on the previous initiatives described above, updated reviews of existing indicators and data sources, and obtained input from experts.

Figure 7.1 displays the framework for assessing cancer quality indicators for end-of-life care, as defined in the National Cancer Institute (NCI) cancer continuum of care (Epstein and Street 2007). Yet even though the framework is defined as end-of-life, end-of-life issues may also be relevant from the time of diagnosis, as in the consensus documents on palliative care. Some quality domains particularly relevant at the end-of-life, such as pain and fatigue, also apply throughout the entire spectrum of care. Isolating issues for a particular disease or a particular point in the disease trajectory is difficult and often impractical. Therefore the framework is purposefully broad so as to include the range of issues cancer patients might face at the end of life, while not neglecting patients with comorbidities or those facing these issues at other points in the disease continuum. The framework should also be applicable, with modifications, to a more general palliative care population.

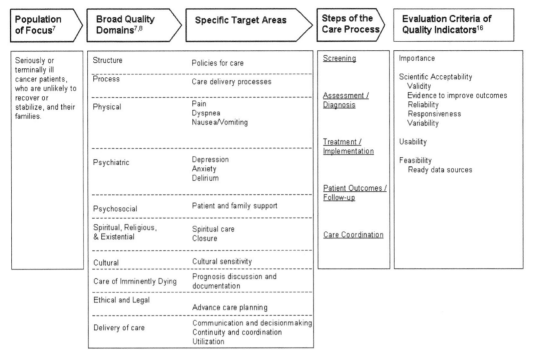

Population of Focus[7]	Broad Quality Domains[7,8]	Specific Target Areas	Steps of the Care Process	Evaluation Criteria of Quality Indicators[16]
Seriously or terminally ill cancer patients, who are unlikely to recover or stabilize, and their families.	Structure	Policies for care	Screening	Importance
	Process	Care delivery processes		Scientific Acceptability Validity Evidence to improve outcomes Reliability Responsiveness Variability
	Physical	Pain Dyspnea Nausea/Vomiting	Assessment / Diagnosis	
	Psychiatric	Depression Anxiety Delirium	Treatment / Implementation	Usability Feasibility Ready data sources
	Psychosocial	Patient and family support	Patient Outcomes / Follow-up	
	Spiritual, Religious, & Existential	Spiritual care Closure	Care Coordination	
	Cultural	Cultural sensitivity		
	Care of Imminently Dying	Prognosis discussion and documentation		
	Ethical and Legal	Advance care planning		
	Delivery of care	Communication and decisionmaking Continuity and coordination Utilization		

Fig. 7.1 Framework for developing and assessing quality indicators for cancer care at the end-of-life

The framework identifies five steps for developing and assessing a quality indicators, defining the (1) population of focus; (2) broad quality domains; (3) specific target areas; (4) steps of the care process; and (5) evaluation criteria of quality indicators. Put differently, the first step identifies *who* to measure, steps 2–4 identify *what* to measure, and step 5 assesses *how well* the indicator works. The framework also addresses a broad range of quality indicators, system-level issues (general structure and processes of care) as well as person-level concerns (e.g., pain management). In areas where few quality indicators exist, the framework can also help guide indicator development, whereas in areas where indicators exist but are not widespread, the framework can help to identify barriers and facilitate implementation and adoption. Each of the steps in the framework is briefly summarized below.

Population of Focus: The framework's first step defines the relevant population and denominator for end-of-life quality indicators. As such, a critical first step in using this framework for a particular domain or project would be to specify an appropriate and definable population and setting for measurement. For example, the population of focus might include all patients from the time of cancer diagnosis when measuring quality of communication, but only include patients at high risk of dying (such as those with widely metastatic disease and poor function or individuals no longer eligible for chemotherapy) when measuring receipt of hospice care.

Broad Quality Domains: The framework builds on the broad domains of quality palliative care endorsed by the NCP and NQF, which have been widely recognized and circulated.

Specific Target Areas: Within each broad domain of quality end-of-life cancer care, there exist specific *target areas* for indicators of quality end-of-life care.

Steps of the Care Process and Outcomes: Quality indicators may also target a specific step in the care process or a specific patient outcome. The framework adapted the process steps developed by the QA (Quality Assessment) Tools project and applied in the Cancer-Quality-ASSIST project to develop quality indicators for supportive cancer care, described in more detail later in this chapter

(Lorenz et al. 2009). Steps include *screening*, *assessment / diagnosis* (more detailed evaluation of those with a positive screen), *treatment / implementation*, and *follow-up* (whether the provider checks on the impact of the intervention). In addition, the expert panel suggested adding *care coordination* due to the multidisciplinary and multisite nature of cancer care. Quality indicators may also focus on transitions between steps, such as the time between diagnosis and treatment, and transfer of information and care responsibilities between different types of providers and settings. Considering these steps can help contextualize quality measurement and provide a clearer portrait of end-of-life care delivery, helping to identify when documentation will occur and by whom.

Evaluation Criteria of Quality Indicators: The framework's final step sets criteria for evaluating the quality indicators' appropriateness for use for quality improvement and accountability. The framework adapted and expanded upon the current NQF criteria used to evaluate quality indicators: importance, scientific acceptability, usability, and feasibility (National Quality Forum 2008). The first criterion, *importance*, denotes whether an indicator addresses a critical component in care, affects outcomes, and has room for improvement. *Scientific acceptability* includes the concepts of validity and reliability. The concept of *feasibility* depends on the availability of quality data that can be obtained or extracted without undue burden, and *usability* applies to how the results of the indicator can be applied to improve care.

Although many indicators are currently available, much more coordination, rigorous evaluation, further development and supporting evidence are needed to advance the field and make quality indicators an accepted part of measuring the quality of palliative care. The proposed framework aims to facilitate the development, assessment, and implementation of quality indicators specific to cancer end-of-life care, but can be adapted for palliative care quality indicators in general. Using this framework, we can more consistently and effectively measure and improve the quality of palliative care. Indicator developers can also use this framework to build indicators that are scientifically acceptable and valid and reflect the broad and specific dimensions of palliative care, and expand the evidence to support their widespread use. The framework may also inform quality programs seeking to choose indicators and policymakers searching for priority areas where further evidence is needed. Ultimately, frameworks for quality indicator development and implementation can also help to refine effective and efficient ways to use indicators to evaluate and improve pain management and palliative care.

Key Quality Indicator Sets in Palliative Care and Pain

Within the past decade, additional research on the development and characteristics of quality indicators for palliative care and pain has been conducted. Quality indicator sets relevant to palliative care can be derived from administrative claims data, medical records, and/or patient surveys. With the exception of claims data-based indicator sets (since there is no information on pain in claims), palliative care indicator sets all include pain indicators. Pain quality indicators can be used for a variety of purposes, including benchmarking the level of quality of care; identifying areas of care in need of improvement; or evaluating the success of quality improvement projects. Some indicator sets focus on cancer care, some on specific settings (such as hospice or intensive care unit care), and some are more general. Others are limited to palliative care and still others include palliative care-relevant indicators as part of a larger set.

Several recent reviews have summarized available palliative care quality indicators. A systematic review of palliative care quality indicators (Pasman et al. 2009) included 16 eligible publications and identified 142 quality indicators, covering all but one domain (cultural aspects) of palliative care.

Within the domain of physical aspects of care, 44 unique quality indicators were identified, of which 16 were specifically for pain. All quality indicators included had numerators and denominators that were defined or could be directly deduced from the description, or provided a performance standard for the population. The palliative care quality indicators' sets included various patient groups (e.g., cancer, elderly people) and specific health settings (e.g., nursing home, home, intensive care unit), and most indicator sets meeting the eligibility criteria were from the United States (US). In another review, the PEACE (Palliative Care Quality Measurement Project) addressed quality indicators and associated measurement instruments relevant to palliative care, with a focus on hospice (Carolinas Center for Medical Excellence 2008) and another systematic review focused on measures relevant to cancer end-of-life care (Lorenz et al. 2006).

Since these reviews were conducted, a number of other palliative care quality indicator projects have been completed with content relevant to pain management, and some of the projects cited in these reviews have also recently undergone additional development. These indicator sets are compiled through various data collection methods, including medical record reviews and patient surveys; in different populations, including cancer-specific and nonspecific indicators sets; and in various settings, including inpatient and outpatient care and hospice. Some of the indicator sets cited in previous reviews, and many newer indicator sets, have now been evaluated for feasibility, reliability, and/or validity (see e.g., Dy et al. 2010; Walling et al. 2010; Fine et al. 2010). Select indicator sets are summarized in Tables 7.1 and 7.2 and below.

Two main indicator sets and a recent survey instrument address palliative care for cancer pain. Lorenz et al. developed a medical record-review-based set of cancer-specific, process-level, quality indicators for inpatient and outpatient settings through a series of systematic reviews and a multidisciplinary expert panel consensus process, resulting in 15 pain indicators (Lorenz et al. 2009). The 15 cancer-specific quality indicators for pain addressed the stages of care in the framework and various clinical issues including routine inpatient and outpatient screening, pain education, pharmacological management (including side effects prophylaxis), timely follow-up, continuity of medications, and radiotherapy for bone metastases and spinal cord compression. These indicators were then evaluated through testing in a total sample of 356 advanced cancer patients in two clinical settings, resulting in a set of 41 indicators which met criteria for feasibility, reliability, and validity; 10 of the 15 pain indicators met these criteria (Table 7.3).

The American Society for Clinical Oncology (ASCO) Quality Oncology Practice Initiative (QOPI) (http://qopi.asco.org) (Jacobson et al. 2008) is intended for use in outpatient oncology clinical practice. It is also being applied in large oncology practices, academic settings, and fellowship programs. QOPI is based on clinical practice guidelines and is regularly updated, and includes a number of palliative care indicators, including pain assessment, treatment, and follow-up. For general hospitalized populations, a palliative care benchmarking project from the University Health Consortium (UHC) addressing inpatient care in palliative care patients includes indicators relevant to pain, such as screening (Twaddle et al. 2007). An indicator set for the vulnerable elderly (ACOVE) including palliative care indicators (Lorenz et al. 2007) has also recently been evaluated, with similar pain indicators and results (Walling et al. 2010). An indicator set for palliative care in the intensive care unit setting also includes indicators for regular pain screening and adequate pain management (Nelson et al. 2006).

For hospice care, the National Hospice and Palliative Care Organization (NHPCO) has developed an indicator for timely treatment of pain in hospice (Ryndes et al. 2000). The PEACE (Palliative Care Quality Measurement Project) conducted further pilot testing on selected measures in a set of hospices, including some pain measures (Carolinas Center for Medical Excellence 2008). Finally, the Cancer Pain Practice Index (Fine et al. 2010; Herr et al. 2010) was specifically developed for cancer pain in older adults in hospice programs, using a process of reviewing clinical guidelines and expert review. The resulting 11-indicator tool is comprehensive and efficient and had good interrater reliability (Fine et al. 2010; Herr et al. 2010).

Collectively, these indicators address the general conceptual areas of pain screening, including use of numeric scales; detailed assessment and diagnosis; treatment of pain and common painful complications; and follow-up and outcomes, including pain relief and satisfaction.

Table 7.1 Selected quality indicator sets relevant to palliative care that include pain (cancer-specific)

Set	Description	Relevant domains	Evaluation	References
American Society of Clinical Oncology (ASCO) Quality Oncology Practice Initiative (QOPI)	Outpatient oncology (EOL part of larger measurement set) In routine use	Pain, dyspnea, communication/decision-making, utilization (Dana-Farber indicators), chemotherapy decision-making, nausea/vomiting (chemo), anemia	Community oncology practices	Jacobson et al. (2008), McNiff, Personal communication. Summary of QOPI Measures, Spring 2008
Cancer quality-ASSIST	Outpatient and hospital	Pain, dyspnea, delirium, insomnia, fatigue, nausea/vomiting, advance care planning	Reviewed for validity by expert panel, and for feasibility, validity, and reliability with professional chart abstraction	Dy et al. (2010)
Japanese end-of-life cancer quality indicators		Pain, dyspnea, delirium, oral care, decision-making/preferences/communication, psychosocial care, distress, religion	None	Miyashita et al. (2008)
QA tools (cancer)	Outpatient	Pain	Limited for pain	Lorenz et al. (2006)

Table 7.2 Selected quality indicator sets relevant to palliative care that include pain (noncancer-specific)

Set	Description	Relevant domains	Evaluation	References
University Health System Consortium (UHC)	Hospital Revised 2007	Pain, dyspnea, communication/prognosis, psychosocial, coordination (discharge planning)	Multicenter evaluation 2004 and 2007, ongoing	Twaddle et al. (2007), UHC personal communication
VHA	Intensive care	Pain, communication/decision-making, psychosocial, spiritual	Multicenter evaluation ongoing	Nelson et al. (2006)
National Hospice and Palliative Care Organization (NHPCO) National Data Set (NDS)	Hospice In routine use	Pain, comprehensive after-death survey of caregivers*	Evaluation with hospice-collected data	Ryndes et al. (2000), Connor et al. (2005)
Palliative Care Quality Measures Project (PEACE)	Builds on National Association for Home Care and Hospice (NAHC) and NHPCO measurement projects	Pain, dyspnea, depression/anxiety, nausea, constipation, psychosocial needs, spiritual needs, preparation for death, care planning, adverse events	Evaluation with hospice-collected data	Carolinas Center for Medical Excellence (2008)
RWJF Critical Care Workgroup	Intensive care	Patient and family-centered communication and decision-making, communication within team and with patients/family, continuity, psychosocial support, symptom management, spiritual support	None	Mularski et al. (2006a, b)
ACOVE (Assessing Care of Vulnerable Elders) Pain, ACOVE End of Life	Outpatient, hospital	Pain, dyspnea, nausea/vomiting, communication/decision-making/care planning, psychosocial, continuity, spiritual	Limited to date; ongoing with professional chart abstraction	Lorenz et al. (2006, 2007), Etzioni et al. (2007)
PCPI: Physician Consortium for Performance Improvement (American Medical Association)	Ambulatory care	Pain, advance care planning	None	AMA (2010)

Table 7.3 Cancer quality-ASSIST project: summary list of core quality indicators for pain after feasibility, reliability, and validity testing (process measures; cancer specific) (Dy et al. 2010)

Quality indicator	Stage of illness
If a cancer patient has a cancer-related outpatient visit, then there should be screening for the presence or absence and intensity of pain using a numeric pain score, because pain is common and often undertreated, and pain identification is required to initiate treatment	Screening and prevention
If a cancer patient is admitted to a hospital, then there should be screening for the presence or absence of pain	Screening and prevention
If a patient with cancer pain is started on a long-acting opioid formulation, then a short-acting opioid formulation for breakthrough pain should also be provided, because intermittent worsening of pain is common, and breakthrough medications can improve overall pain control	Symptomatic management
If a patient with cancer pain is started on chronic opioid treatment, then he or she should be offered either a prescription or nonprescription bowel regimen within 24 h or there should be documented contraindication to a bowel regimen, because opioid analgesics frequently cause constipation that may cause discomfort	Symptomatic management
If a patient's outpatient cancer pain regimen is changed, then there should be an assessment of the effectiveness of treatment at or before the next outpatient visit with that provider or at another cancer-related outpatient visit, because pain regimens often need to be adjusted or changed to achieve pain relief with the least amount of side effects	Symptomatic management
If a patient has advanced cancer and receives radiation treatment for painful bone metastases, then he or she should be offered single-fraction radiation or there should be documentation of a contraindication to single-fraction treatment, because single-fraction radiation is of equal efficacy and may be less burdensome for patients and families when they are facing the consequences of late-stage cancer	Symptomatic management
If a cancer patient has new neurologic symptoms or findings on physical examination consistent with spinal cord compression, then he or she should be treated with steroids as soon as possible, but within 24 h or a contraindication to steroids should be documented, because treatment can prevent or slow paralysis	Follow-up
If a cancer patient has new neurologic symptoms or findings on physical examination consistent with spinal cord compression, then a whole-spine magnetic resonance imaging (MRI) scan or myelography should be performed as soon as possible, but within 24 h or there should be documentation of why an MRI scan was not appropriate, because spinal cord compression is common in cancer patients and paralysis can be prevented	Follow-up
If a cancer patient has confirmation of spinal cord compression on radiologic examination, then radiotherapy or surgical decompression should be initiated within 24 h or a contraindication for such therapy should be documented, because paralysis can be prevented with these treatments	Follow-up
If a cancer patient is treated for spinal cord compression, then there should be follow-up of neurologic symptoms and signs within 1 week after treatment is completed, because symptoms can progress despite treatment and further treatment to prevent paralysis may be needed	Follow-up

Selected Palliative Care Research Applying Pain Quality Indicators

A number of the quality indicator sets described above have been evaluated across a variety of clinical and outpatient settings. Results for selected pain indicators from these sets in the areas of screening, assessment, treatment, and follow-up are described below.

Screening: Screening indicators address routine pain assessment using numeric or nonspecific scales in inpatient, intensive care, outpatient, and unspecified settings. Screening to determine who may have pain is a necessary first step both in the effective management of pain and in the proper conduct of research and quality improvement (Swarm et al. 2007; Lorenz et al. 2006). Without regular screening, many patients with significant pain do not have pain documented in the medical record and do not receive adequate analgesia (Rhodes et al. 2001). Effective measurement begins with patient self-report: without asking the patient, clinicians' assessments of pain are usually inaccurate. One study found little correlation between physician and nurse assessments of cancer patients' pain and patient reports of pain; correlation was lowest for patients with severe pain (Grossman et al. 1991). Discrepancies between patients and physicians in perceptions of pain severity are also predictive of inadequate management (Cleeland et al. 1994). As described in Chapter 45, a large number of well-evaluated pain assessment tools are available.

Results of testing are available for several pain indicators. A relatively high number of eligible cases met the UHC indicator in the inpatient setting for regular assessment (mean 96%) and use of a numeric pain scale (mean 85%). Results for the inpatient ASSIST pain indicator were similar (Twaddle et al. 2007; Dy et al. 2010). Results for an outpatient ASSIST screening indicator were somewhat lower (79% in one setting) (Dy et al. 2010). VHA, Inc., a cooperative of nonprofit hospitals, evaluated a measure of more frequent screening (q 4 h) in an ICU setting, which was met in 87% of cases (Nelson et al. 2006). A QOPI indicator of whether pain was assessed on the last community oncology visit prior to death found that 56% of records met the measure on an initial evaluation; 69% met the measure in a second round 6 months later, and there was substantial variation among practices (range, 30–90%) (Jacobson et al. 2008).

Treatment: Treatment indicators include having a pain plan of care, and the use of a bowel regimen in patients receiving opioids. UHC includes an indicator on regular prophylaxis of opioid-induced constipation, which indicated a mean of 59% (median 59%, 20–93%) of patients who were placed on opioids were provided with a prophylactic bowel regimen (Twaddle et al. 2007). The results from an ASSIST indicator on the same issue were similar (Dy et al. 2010).

Follow-up/outcome : Follow-up/outcome indicators include whether patients with changes in a pain regimen had follow-up to determine effectiveness, whether those with pain were made comfortable or had a decrease in pain scores, and patient and family measures of satisfaction with pain treatment. An ASSIST indicator of whether reassessment was done on the next outpatient visit after an outpatient cancer pain regimen was changed was met 97% of the time (Dy et al. 2010). In the 2004 UHC measures, pain relief or reduction within 48 h of hospitalization was met in a mean of 76% (median 78%, range 46–92%) of patients with pain. The VHA measure of optimal pain management (percentage of 4-h intervals in the ICU with pain score <3 on a 0–10 scale) was met in 85% of cases (Nelson et al. 2006). Cancer Care Ontario (CCO) instituted a measure of satisfaction with pain treatment among outpatients with cancer: 70% of patients reported complete and 25% partial satisfaction with pain treatment (Lorenz et al. 2006).

In summary, across all domains of cancer pain management, from screening to follow-up, quality indicators have now been developed and evaluated in a variety of settings. Although further research is needed to refine these indicators and evaluate associations with improved outcomes, in a recent consensus conference, experts agreed that these indicators are now ready for widespread clinical and policy implementation (Seow et al. 2009a, b).

Challenges in Quality Indicator Development and Implementation

Although much progress has been made in developing and implementing quality indicators for pain, quality indicators for pain are still not yet widely implemented and rarely go beyond screening and documentation of pain scores. Barriers to broader and effective implementation of pain quality measures include challenges with feasibility of abstracting data on pain, data quality, and the lack of evidence of associations between quality measurement and improved outcomes. Research has shown that pain assessment by itself may not lead to improved outcomes (Mularski et al. 2006a, b). As a consequence, the steps of comprehensive assessment, treatment, and follow-up may not occur. A comprehensive assessment of a patient who screens positive for pain is critical, and there are many barriers to effective assessment, such as underestimating the impact of pain by patients, fear of consequences of pain management such as addiction, and lack of knowledge. Beyond initial screening and documentation, the extent that pain relief and reassessment occurs is still unclear. Quality indicators for pain should not just focus on the level of pain, but also on the extent to which pain has been successfully relieved. Moreover, despite a wide proliferation of pain assessment tools, quality indicators for pain beyond screening are not widely used, mainly due to lack of evidence. Pain relief as an outcome also needs to be linked to care processes, to better understand how to achieve quality improvement in this domain.

Categorizing quality indicators by the steps in the care process may also aid in the identification of steps in the care pathway where improvements can be made. For example, the Cancer Quality-ASSIST evaluation addressed a broader range of indicators in identifying patients with pain (e.g., pain screening), treatment (e.g., using short-acting opioids for patients on long-acting medications), and follow-up (e.g., reassessment after treatment in the outpatient setting). However, many indicators do not meet the criteria for feasibility, reliability, and/or reliability, often due to inconsistent or unstructured medical record documentation (e.g., the etiology of pain or the lack of adequate documentation of the impact of pain on functional status). Indeed, simply documenting that key processes occur and incorporating this documentation into the flow of clinical care is still an important barrier for many quality indicators, not just pain.

Instead documentation of processes should be kept simple, as in the Cancer Pain Practice Index (Fine et al. 2010). Care teams must assess pain as a first step, using well-validated and feasible tools such as a visual analog scale or the Edmonton Symptom Assessment System (Schulman-Green et al. 2010), followed by reassessment. New quality reporting initiatives, such as the Physician Consortium on Performance Improvement and developing Center for Medicare and Medicaid Services (CMS) and Joint Commission programs emphasizing pain management as part of quality assessment and public reporting, will provide incentives and standardization for use of these quality measures.

EMRs, worksheets, or templates may aid in consistent and improved documentation and reporting. Some measures require patient-reported outcomes, which should also be documented in the medical record. Making measurement part of the standard of care will require incentives or structures for better assessment and documentation. Although applying indicators across different settings, with different structures and resources, is challenging, the development of a measurement toolbox that includes an efficient and clear set of pain indicators could help standardize measurement and improve reporting (Seow et al. 2009a, b).

Other limitations to current pain indicators include the fact that pain measures generally exclude those who cannot report their pain, which is problematic in vulnerable populations with a high percentage of nonverbal patients, such as the seriously or terminally ill or nursing home populations (see also Fine 2011). In addition, patients with some degree of cognitive impairment or sedation may also be excluded from pain measures, even though many of these patients are actually able to report their pain (Ferrell et al. 1995). Variable exclusion of these patients limits the utility of pain assessment measures for comparisons across populations, between facilities, and/or over time. Even for patients who can report their pain, pain scores abstracted from the medical record for indicators may not be accurate. One recent research study found that pain scores recorded in medical records did not correlate well with symptom scores obtained directly from patients (Lorenz et al 2009).

There has also been limited measure development in children, although some guidelines are available, such as a position paper on end-of-life pain management for the child with cancer (Hooke et al. 2002). Measurement of pain outcomes is even more important in vulnerable populations. Studies have shown that adults with dementia receive less pain medication than those who are cognitively intact (see also Kovach 2011). Untreated pain can also lead to more adverse outcomes, such as delirium (Morrison et al. 2003). The use of surrogates for pain measurement, retrospective pain measurement, methods to account for missing data or different methods of assessment within a population, and exclusion of some patients from the denominator are all important issues in vulnerable populations where assessment is not possible for everyone or varies among patients.

Future Directions in Developing Pain Quality Indicators in Palliative Care

Ultimately, pain relief as an outcome needs to be linked to care processes, to better understand how to achieve quality improvement in this domain. Quality indicator efforts are challenged to balance between measuring process and outcomes, and balancing between documenting that a process has occurred with whether the process was done well. In the context of pain, where the study of indicators is better developed, demonstrating the relationships between processes and outcomes and documenting outcomes is now needed, including how pain indicators link to improved patient outcomes.

To overcome documentation and reporting challenges, pain indicators need to be easily documented and incorporated into workflow processes. Furthermore, pain indicators need to be incorporated into the design of the oncology record or EMR, whenever possible, to ensure feasible reporting. One solution, both for improving quality measurement and for improving the information available to both patients and providers, is routine collection of patient-reported outcomes (PROs) to add to the clinical encounter and medical record. Recent studies show that routine collection of patient-reported outcome data may help in identifying areas of concern and monitoring patients (Schulman-Green et al. 2010). Incorporating PROs requires demonstrating benefits to providers and payors and showing patients that the data they provide will enhance their care. Information technology (e.g., EMRs) can provide a number of benefits for incorporating PRO assessment. In particular, PROs can be disassociated from the provider–patient encounter, allowing for more frequent monitoring; PRO data collection can be more easily tailored to patient needs, and used across a variety of clinical settings.

Two clear limitations of current pain quality indicators are the focus on the physical aspects of pain and the lack of coordination with other palliative care domains. In the Cancer Quality-ASSIST project, less quantitative pain issues such as the etiology of pain or pain education could not be reliably extracted from the medical records due to a lack of structured documentation. Similarly, less tangible issues, such as psychosocial and cultural differences in the experience of pain, are even more challenging to abstract from records and are inconsistently assessed and documented. Clearly, pain is often associated with other issues, such as depression, quality of life, and spiritual distress, and quality pain assessment should be linked to these issues. However, these issues are underdocumented, and abstraction of physician documentation has historically been unreliable for these types of issues due to variations in language used and wording in the medical records. Although very important in ensuring quality care, providers' responses to pain scores, such as whether an appropriate evaluation was done for a patient in severe pain, are complex and difficult to abstract reliably with uni-dimensional indicators. More complex documentation systems, algorithms, or other technology for translating documentation into quality evaluations will likely be needed for more comprehensive quality evaluation for multidimensional issues such as provider responses, cultural assessment and competency, and psychosocial care.

Finally, although patient-centered measures of pain management, such as questions about satisfaction with pain, may address some of these issues, these measures may not correlate well with objective measures of pain management. Additional research is needed to deconstruct what other elements may also contribute to patients' and families' responses to these questions. Patient and family-centered outcomes are a cornerstone of palliative care. Indicators need to incorporate direct input from patients and a family in process and outcome measures, such as the impact of patient preferences and cultural issues and barriers that impact pain management.

Conclusions

In summary, quality indicators for palliative care and pain differ from other quality indicators in a variety of ways. Palliative care indicators may be supported less by high quality research evidence (e.g., large clinical trials), and more by expert consensus and demonstration that their use improves outcomes. Patient-reported outcomes are necessary to measure care, and administrative data or medical records are often incomplete in their current forms for all but a few screening indicators. Although developing measures for improving palliative care remains challenging, the urgency to include better measures also intensifies as patient outcomes at the end-of-life continue at suboptimal levels despite improvement efforts. Although pain may have the most evidence to support treatment and well-developed quality indicators of any domain in palliative care, uncontrolled pain in palliative care is still a common issue.

Therefore, for pain, where multiple reasonable measures are now available across settings and populations, quality measurement for pain can and should be completed to determine where quality of care needs to be improved (Seow et al. 2009a, b). Choosing the best measure may actually be less important than measuring and reporting consistently in a manner that can be standardized and compared across settings (Seow et al. 2009a, b). Future research in this field should also focus on the development of better and more reliable methods to improve quality and to collect additional data from patients that accurately reflect their pain and experiences. Only through measuring the quality of care for pain management can we better determine what systems and providers most need to improve, accurately document the impact on patients and families, and evaluate the impact of quality improvement interventions.

References

American Medical Association (AMA). (2010). *Physician Consortium for Performance Improvement (PCPI). Consortium Measures, 2010.* Retrieved, from http://www.ama-assn.org, December 31, 2010.

Campbell, S. M., Braspenning, J., Hutchinson, A., & Marshall, M. (2002). Research methods used in developing and applying quality indicators in primary care. *Quality & Safety in Health Care, 11*, 358–364.

Carolinas Center for Medical Excellence. (2008). *Palliative Care Quality Measurement Project (PEACE).* Retrieved, from http://www.thecarolinascenter.org/default.aspx?pageid=24, October 11, 2011.

Cleeland, C. S., Gonin, R., Hatfield, A. K., Edmonson, J. H., Blum, R. H., Stewart, J. A., et al. (1994). Pain and its treatment in outpatients with metastatic cancer. *The New England Journal of Medicine, 330*, 592–596.

Connor, S. R., Teno, J., Spence, C., & Smith, N. (2005). Family evaluation of hospice care: results from voluntary submission of data via website. *Journal of Pain and Symptom Management, 30*(1), 9–17.

Donabedian, A. (1988). The quality of care. How can it be assessed? *The Journal of the American Medical Association, 260*(12), 1743–1748.

Dy, S. M., Lorenz, K. A., ONeill, S., Asch, S. M., Walling, A. M., Tisnado, D., et al. (2010). Cancer quality-ASSIST supportive oncology quality indicator set: Feasibility, reliability, and validity testing. *Cancer, 116*(13), 3267–3275.

Epstein, R. M., & Street, R. L., Jr. (2007). Chapter 4: Key communication tasks and outcomes: The cancer care continuum. In R. M. Epstein, R. L. Street Jr., R. M. Epstein, R. L. Street Jr., R. M. Epstein, & R. L. Street Jr. (Eds.), *Patient-centered communication in cancer care: Promoting healing and reducing suffering* (pp. 68–88). Bethesda: National Cancer Institute, NIH Publication No. 07-6225.

Etzioni, S., Chodosh, J., Ferrell, B. A., & MacLean, C. H. (2007). Quality indicators for pain management in vulnerable elders. *Journal of the American Geriatrics Society, 55*(Suppl 2), S403–S408.

Ferrell, B. A., Ferrell, B. R., & Rivera, L. (1995). Pain in cognitively impaired nursing home patients. *Journal of Pain and Symptom Management, 10*, 591–598.

Fine, P. (2011). Recognition and resolution of ethical barriers to palliative care research. In R. J. Moore (Ed.), *Handbook of pain and palliative care.* New York: Springer.

Fine, P., Herr, K., Titler, M., Sanders, S., Cavanaugh, J., Swegle, J., Forcucci, C., Tang, X., Lane, K., & Reyes, J. (2010). The cancer pain practice index: A measure of evidence-based practice adherence for cancer pain management in older adults in hospice care. *Journal of Pain and Symptom Management, 39*(5), 791–802.

Grossman, S. A., Sheidler, V. R., Swedeen, K., Mucenski, J., & Piantadosi, S. (1991). Correlation of patient and caregiver ratings of cancer pain. *Journal of Pain and Symptom Management, 6*, 53–57.

Herr, K., Titler, M., Fine, P., Sanders, S., Cavanaugh, J., Swegle, J., Forcucci, C., & Tang, X. (2010). Assessing and treating pain in hospices: Current state of evidence-based practices. *Journal of Pain and Symptom Management, 39*(5), 803–819.

Hooke, C., Hellsten, M. B., Stutzer, C., & Forte, K. (2002). Pain management for the child with cancer in end-of-life care: APON position paper. *Journal of Pediatric Oncology Nursing, 19*, 43–47.

Jacobson, J. O., Neuss, M. N., McNiff, K. K., Kadlubek, P., Thacker, L. R. 2nd, Song, F., et al. (2008). Improvement in oncology practice performance through voluntary participation in the Quality Oncology Practice Initiative. *Journal of Clinical Oncology, 26*, 1893–1898.

Kovach, C. R. (2011). Assessing pain and unmet needs in patients with advanced dementia: The role of the serial trial intervention (STI). In R. J. Moore (Ed.), *Handbook of pain and palliative care*. New York: Springer.

Lorenz, K. A., Dy, S. M., Naeim, A., Walling, A. M., Sanati, H., Smith, P., et al. (2009). Quality measures for supportive cancer care: The cancer quality-ASSIST (assessing symptoms side effects and indicators of supportive treatment) project. *Journal of Pain and Symptom Management, 37*(6), 943–964.

Lorenz, K. A., Lynn, J., Dy, S., Wilkinson, A., Mularski, R. A., Shugarman, L., et al. (2006). Quality measures for symptoms and advance care planning in cancer: A systematic review. *Journal of Clinical Oncology, 24*, 4933–4938.

Lorenz, K. A., Rosenfeld, K., & Wenger, N. (2007). Quality indicators for palliative and end-of-life care in vulnerable elders. *Journal of the American Geriatrics Society, 55*(Suppl 2), S318–S326.

Miyashita, M., Nakamura, A., Morita, T., & Bito, S. (2008). Identification of quality indicators of end-of-life cancer care from medical chart review using a modified Delphi method in Japan. *The American Journal of Hospice & Palliative Care, 25*, 33–38.

Morrison, R. S., Magaziner, J., Gilbert, M., Koval, K. J., McLaughlin, M. A., Orosz, G., et al. (2003). Relationship between pain and opioid analgesics on the development of delirium following hip fracture. *Journal of Gerontology Series A: Biological Sciences and Medical Sciences, 58*, 76–81.

Mularski, R. A., Curtis, J. R., Billings, J. A., Burt, R., Byock, I., Fuhrman, C. et al. (2006a). Proposed quality measures for palliative care in the critically ill: A consensus from the Robert Wood Johnson Foundation Critical Care Workgroup. *Critical Care Medicine, 34*(11), S404–S411.

Mularski, R. A., White-Chu, F., Overbay, D., Miller, L. Asch, S.M., Ganzini, L. (2006b). Measuring pain as the 5th vital sign does not improve quality of pain management. *Journal of General Internal Medicine, 21*, 607–612.

National Consensus Project for Quality Palliative Care. (2004). *Clinical practice guidelines for quality palliative care*. Pittsburgh: National Consensus Project for Quality Palliative Care.

National Quality Forum. (2006). *A national framework and preferred practices for palliative and hospice care quality*. Washington: National Quality Forum.

National Quality Forum. (2008). *Measure evaluation criteria*. Washington: National Quality Forum.

Nelson, J. E., Mulkerin, C. M., Adams, L. L., Pronovost, P. J. (2006). Improving comfort and communication in the ICU: A practical new tool for palliative care performance measurement and feedback. *Quality & Safety in Health Care, 15*, 264–271.

Pasman, H. R., Brandt, H. E., Deliens, L., & Francke, A. L. (2009). Quality indicators for palliative care: A systematic review. *Journal of Pain and Symptom Management, 38*(1), 145–156.

Rhodes, D. J., Koshy, R. C., Waterfield, W. C., Wu, A. W., & Grossman, S. A. (2001). Feasibility of quantitative pain assessment in outpatient oncology practice. *Journal of Clinical Oncology, 19*, 501–508.

Ryndes, T., Connor, S., Cody, C., et al. (2000). *Report on the alpha and beta pilots of end result outcome measures constructed by the outcomes forum: A joint effort of the National Hospice and Palliative Care Organization and the National Hospice Work Group*. Retrieved, from http://www.nhpco.org/, October 10, 2011.

Schulman-Green, D., Cherlin, E. J., McCorkle, R., Carlson, M. D., Pace, K. B., Neigh, J. et al. (2010). Benefits and challenges in use of a standardized symptom assessment instrument in hospice. *Journal of Palliative Medicine, 13*, 155–159.

Seow, H., Snyder, C. F., Mularski, R. A., Shugarman, L. R., Kutner, J. S., Lorenz, K. A., Wu, A. W., & Dy, S. M. (2009a). A framework for assessing quality indicators for cancer care at the end of life. *Journal of Pain and Symptom Management, 38*(6), 903–912.

Seow, H., Snyder, C. F., Shugarman, L. R., Mularski, R. A., Kutner, J. S., Lorenz, K. A., Wu, A. W., & Dy, S. M. (2009b). Developing quality indicators for cancer end-of-life care: Proceedings from a national symposium. *Cancer, 115*, 3820–3829.

Swarm, R., Anghelescu, D. L., Benedetti, C., Blinderman, C. D., Boston, B., Cleeland, C., et al. (2007). National comprehensive cancer network (NCCN). Adult cancer pain. *Journal of the National Comprehensive Cancer Network, 5*(8), 726–751.

Twaddle, M. L., Maxwell, T. L., Cassell, B., et al. (2007). Palliative care benchmarks from academic medical centers. *Journal of Palliative Medicine, 10*, 86–98.

Walling, A. M., Asch, S. M., Lorenz, K. A., Roth, C. P., Barry, T., Kahn, K. L., & Wenger, N. S. (2010). The quality of care provided to hospitalized patients at the end of life. *Archives of Internal Medicine, 170*(12), 1057–1063.

Chapter 8
Palliative Care Clinical Trials: Generalizability and Applicability in Hospice and Palliative Care Practice

David C. Currow and Amy P. Abernethy

History of Evidence-Based Practice

There has been a rapid development of the evidence base for clinical practice and service delivery in the last half century. All clinical disciplines have benefitted from the process of evolving data that can underpin many key clinical decisions on a daily basis. The aim of this chapter is to outline key parameters unique to palliative care to aid generalizability and applicability in day-to-day practice and policy.

Although that evidence has been increasingly available (and accessible) across this period of time, the proposal to systematically find, evaluate and apply the best level of evidence to the full range of decisions required in health care (from service planning to whether an antibiotic should be used for upper respiratory tract infections) is relatively new and really only dates over the last 2 decades. The explicit categorization of evidence into a hierarchy is likewise a relatively new innovation allowing more robust studies of a higher level of evidence to build directly on existing less robust evidence. This allows for an easier way for clinicians and policy makers to apply knowledge, but also allows researchers to deliberately design studies to improve the quality of evidence available.

Although evidence has been used to methodically build the basis for practice over more than two centuries, there were few attempts to apply systematically the same level of rigor to all decisions in health care and to strive to improve the level of evidence until relatively recently. Clinicians and health planners the world over had used evidence but often in a piecemeal way. Researchers had generated evidence but perhaps without considering the specific gaps in knowledge that their work could help to close.

A central task of evidence-based medicine is to relate available evidence which has been generated in a research setting to the patient seen clinically or the service setting – the application of

D.C. Currow, BMed, MPH, FRACP (✉)
Discipline, Palliative and Supportive Services, Flinders University,
Bedford Park, Adelaide, SA 5042, Australia
e-mail: david.currow@flinders.edu.au

A.P. Abernethy, MD
Discipline, Palliative and Supportive Services, Flinders University,
Bedford Park, Adelaide, SA 5042, Australia

Department of Medicine, Division of Medical Oncology, Duke University Medical Centre,
Durham, NC, USA

R.J. Moore (ed.), *Handbook of Pain and Palliative Care: Biobehavioral Approaches for the Life Course*,
DOI 10.1007/978-1-4419-1651-8_8, © Springer Science+Business Media, LLC 2012

generalizable knowledge (Sackett and Rosenberg 1995; Jordhøy et al. 2002). Generalizability of study findings is whether or not the results will hold for all combinations of the elements (external validity); applicability of findings is whether or not the results will hold for a particular combination of factors for which the results are to be used. Generalizability is therefore a property of the study, and applicability is the way a clinical decision or policy maker uses the knowledge.

Aggregating evidence can help develop population-wide evidence-based clinical guidelines. This aggregation may bring data together in systematic reviews or in meta-analyses. Such a process brings together (generally) more than one clinician or researcher to systematically collect the literature and explicitly include studies for the review. More than anything, when well done, such data can aid clinicians' abilities to confidently and rapidly decide whether or not a reported intervention is applicable in the setting for a patient or the clinical setting in which they practice. Perceived barriers include a long history of poor recruitment to trials (overcome by multisite trials), the frailty of the population (overcome by careful trial design with the shortest possible census point and ensuring that participant burden is minimized), the sense of vulnerability for patients being approached to participate in research relating to the quality of their care (overcome by careful, ethically sound trial design that relates directly to their clinical care) and clinician gate keeping (probably the most difficult issue to address effectively on a day-to-day basis in hospice and palliative care).

The Genesis of Hospice and Palliative Care as a Discipline

Although estimates and claims differ, publically funded end-of-life services are, like evidence-based practice, relatively new and so hospice and palliative care services have been developing in tandem. For a number of reasons the evidence base for hospice, palliative and supportive care has developed relatively slowly. Clinical and health services research has lagged behind many other clinical disciplines. In part, this can be attributed to the fact that the early days of hospice and palliative care was derived largely from a counter-culture (Clarke 2000). Not only did that allow models of care to develop locally, but also took the performance of those services towards very different measures when compared with the rest of the health system. By definition, this may also have reduced the perceived need to generalize findings from one locally developed service to another.

In major health systems around the world, palliative care is now recognized as a specialty in its own right – the United Kingdom, Australia, Canada, the United States of America and India. Such recognition also demands levels of academic rigor of the discipline that will drive, to some degree, improving the evidence base for practice and its routine uptake. Adopting key standards of evidence and how these should be incorporated into practice becomes an imperative rather than an option. It requires:

– A critical evaluation of decision-making.
– Identifying obstacles to translating research evidence into clinical practice (Abernethy and Currow 2008).
– Overcoming identified obstacles.
– Further research efforts to drive the development of quality evidence.

One challenge that is more specific to hospice and palliative care studies is the need to evaluate better nonpharmacological interventions including complementary care. Designing and competing for funding for such studies is potentially more difficult than an industry-sponsored phase III study comparing standard care to a new medication. Ethically, all such interventions should be evaluated as rigorously as any other new approach to care, especially given the fact that the population for whom care is being provided is so vulnerable and any unexpected, untoward effects will be magnified for the individual patient.

For pharmacological interventions, the medications used in hospice and palliative care are mostly off-patent, relatively inexpensive, and (by the nature of the practice) used for a relatively short period of time. Whether rigorous studies should be done in hospice and palliative care is still debated, with the argument being in favor of patients who were being provided palliative care had the same rights to the best level of evidence defining net clinical benefit as anyone else in the health system. Net clinical benefit encompasses both the therapeutic effect and any toxicity in quantifiable (and therefore reproducible) ways. It can therefore be argued that hospice and palliative care patients have a greater need to have the net clinical benefit carefully evaluated given their progressive frailty and increasing polypharmacy as their disease progresses (Currow et al. 2007).

Every aspect of palliative care service provision is assessable by rigorously designed, adequately powered randomized trials. Pharmacological studies should cover the full spectrum of symptom control. Nonpharmacological studies should cover symptom control as well as interventions offered to emotional support, social support and addressing issues of sexuality. Every intervention that is offered in hospice and palliative care should be provided to patients and their families on the basis of a continued commitment to developing and implementing new evidence.

The other source of phase III studies is the development of new medications – either whole classes of medications or medications with more efficacious profiles – more predictable benefit or less toxicity. In hospice and palliative care, there have been few new classes of medications limiting pharmaceutical company involvement in sponsoring phase II or phase III studies. Instead, the sector has relied heavily on studies of medications that have no commercial attraction for the industry. In reality, the sector has a handful of industry-sponsored studies looking at new formulations of delivery systems that can be covered by patent for existing medications and an occasional new class of medication.

Competitive funding agencies are beginning to invest in this research, but the ability to adapt excellent phase III study designs to this patient population has taken time and effort (Abernethy et al. 2010; Currow et al. 2006). Such studies can and should be done, but they require a greater investment because they require screening a larger number of potential participants to generate successful enrolment and ways of allowing for dropout from the study unrelated to the intervention itself without compromising the integrity of the study. On the positive side, given that such studies are seeking a robust clinical difference between arms, the sample sizes for rigorously designed, adequately powered studies can be surprisingly small.

The Available Evidence Base in Hospice and Palliative Care

There is a strong evidence base despite repeated assertions that there is little or no evidence to underpin clinical practice or service design. A rapidly evolving evidence base needs to be taken up into practice with high quality trials being done to support quality evidence in the discipline including adequately powered randomized controlled trials (Tieman et al. 2008). The evidence base for hospice and palliative care has grown more rapidly than new clinical knowledge overall. The quality and level of evidence also appear to be improving systematically.

Evidence into Practice

It is difficult to get uptake of new evidence into practice in any discipline. Hospice and palliative care is probably no better or worse than any other clinical specialty. There are a range of responses to new evidence – ultra-early adopters through those who simply refuse to adopt high level evidence even when it is directly applicable to the patient(s) they treat. Changing the behaviour of established practitioners is never easy, and few approaches have been shown predictably to deliver sustained uptake (O'Brien et al. 2007).

Ultimately how is new evidence evaluated and adopted into practice? Critical appraisal relies on the assessment of both internal and external validity. It relies on the ability of researchers to adequately and accurately describe their work and the setting in which the study was performed. At the same time, the person reading the research requires an ability to apply the information to the setting in which they are working and the patient population that they serve.

Having generated new evidence, there is still the problem of getting the highest quality of evidence into practice. Most people working in hospice and palliative care were trained in an era before evidence-based practice was taught, and critical appraisal will have been something that has been learnt on the job. The critique of new information is therefore limited in the discipline despite structured approaches to making expert commentary available in a format where the critical appraisal has been formally undertaken (Abernethy and Arnold 2006).

Clinicians need to use critical appraisal skills for an individual patient to:

– Evaluate the evidence.
– Apply the evidence appropriately to their clinical populations.
– Make more clinically relevant decisions.

The overarching purposes of evidence-based medicine is improving quality of care at a population level and this is therefore also one of its key challenges (Bakitas et al. 2006; Borgsteede et al. 2006). In turn, population-level clinical guidelines or consensus best practice statements only become meaningful when they are applied rigorously to practice.

What Research Concepts Do Palliative Medicine Clinicians Need to Understand to Generalize Research Findings into Practice?

EBP, the application of EBM principles and methods to daily clinical decision-making, encourages clinicians and health service planners to find the best evidence available to them from wherever it can be sourced. The core skills are a series of sequential steps: ask; find; appraise; act; and evaluate. There are key definitions that need to be understood in order to optimize the use of data in the literature (Craig et al. 2001).

Definitions needed include:

Internal validity: this refers to the quality of study design and, in the case of interventional studies, increases confidence in the ability to infer cause (the independent variable(s)) and effect (on the dependent variable).

External validity/generalizability: the extent to which the findings of a study can be applied to another patient, population or setting of care.

Applicability: the ability to apply the findings to a patient/group of patients in the broadest terms (Jordhoy et al. 2003).

Will this person react the same way to the intervention for the same net clinical benefit?

Effect size: the magnitude of benefit attributed to an intervention, a construct that is independent of sample size. Effect size should be the benefit over and above any placebo effect or the benefit seen in standard practice in studies evaluating new interventions.

Both generalizability and applicability require knowing the population (or patients) and the setting of the original study (a responsibility of the person reporting the research). Applicability requires the clinician applying the evidence to answer the question, "Would this individual patient have been eligible for the study under consideration?"

Poor generalizability poses a problem for effective uptake of research findings. Inability to relate the findings of studies to patients at hand, particularly where patients present with complex or co-morbid conditions as in palliative care, significantly impedes the uptake of new knowledge into practice (Francke et al. 2008; Tinetti et al. 2004). Data derived from one sub-population in order to inform decisions about a different sub-population is likely to be limited even in apparently homogeneous populations. For example, in a meta-analysis of data from 141 trials, Dhruva and Redberg found that participants in cardiovascular studies used by the Centers for Medicare and Medicaid Services (CMS) for coverage determinations differed significantly from the clinical populations to which these funding decisions would apply (Dhruva and Redberg 2008). Another study of randomized controlled trials in high-impact general medical journals found that exclusion criteria defining participant populations are often not reported clearly or justified. For example upper limits of age for participation set arbitrarily in clinical trials directly limit the applicability of the results to daily clinical practice (Van Spall et al. 2007).

Hospice and Palliative Care as a Referral-Based Speciality

It could be argued that people admitted to a coronary care unit are a relatively homogeneous population in comparison to people referred to hospice or palliative care services. In cardiology, people with significant cardiac pathology are almost certain to be referred to coronary care. When new interventions are evaluated (accepting the quality of the study design and adequate power calculations) a multisite study in coronary care units is likely to generate evidence that can be rapidly applied across the sector with confidence.

By contrast, people with a life-limiting illness have approximately a one in two chance of being referred to specialist hospice or palliative care services at best. For some diseases, this rate may be far lower. Even such a limitation would not be largely unnoticeable if the *same* 50% of the population was referred to hospice and palliative care services, but this is not the case. Local referral patterns have often developed on the basis of relationships between clinicians rather than on the basis of the complexity of needs for patients or their caregivers. This is a pivotal concept then in deciding how to generalize new evidence in palliative care studies because it is likely that the study population and the population to whom the findings are to be applied *are* different.

In hospice and palliative care, referral to services and resource utilization are not well predicted by diagnosis or prognosis (Lidstone et al. 2003). Simple categorization by diagnosis, severity of disease or estimated prognosis will not predict the complexity of needs of the population referred to specialist services (Waller et al. 2010). In hospice and palliative care, diversity in the characteristics of service models utilized and patient populations referred limit the ability to apply new knowledge (Franks et al. 2000; Gott et al. 2001; Currow et al. 2004; Rosenwax et al. 2005). Wide national and local variations (Addington-Hall et al. 1998; Bestall et al. 2004) are in part due to differences in health system structures, resources and clinical relationships (Currow et al. 2009; Wheeler et al. 2011). This diversity of hospice and palliative care service models creates barriers to the translation of best evidence into practice with rigorously designed and executed studies (Green 2006; Foley 2003). "Usual practice" pharmacological and nonpharmacological therapies also differ widely between services and health systems, at times because best evidence has not been applied. Clinical sub-populations differ in life expectancy, functional status, and the prevalence, nature and severity of co-morbidities. Ultimately, practicing clinicians cannot apply a study's results to a "real-world" patient or setting – the specific contribution of evidence-based practice.

There are therefore two key additional questions in the process of generalizability that is either absent or a minor consideration for most other clinical disciplines but is paramount in hospice and palliative care:

– Would the population reported in the study be referred to the palliative care service to which the results are being applied?
– Would the person to whom the results are being applied have been referred to the clinical study being reported?

Difficulties in this generalizing step may introduce bias, and even error, into the translation of hospice and palliative care research evidence into practice or policy.

Current Tools to Help Aid Evidence into Practice: Methodological Checklists

To date, the process of evaluating evidence for uptake into practice or policy has been built around an evaluation of the methodologies used in the execution of the study. Largely, these tools help to explore key facets of internal validity for researchers, clinicians and policy makers to aid design, reporting and interpretation. Relevant examples include:

– AGREE (*A*ppraisal of *G*uidelines for *Re*search and *E*valuation), for assessing the quality of observational studies (Brouwers et al. 2010).
– CONSORT (*Con*solidated *S*tandards *o*f *R*eporting *T*rials) for randomized clinical trials (Schulz et al. 2010).
– MOOSE (*M*eta-Analysis *o*f *O*bservational *S*tudies in *E*pidemiology) (Stroup et al. 2000).
– QUORUM (Quality of Reporting of Meta-Analyses) (Clarke 2000).
– STARD (*Sta*ndards for *R*eporting of *D*iagnostic Accuracy) for diagnostic studies (Bossuyt et al. 2003).
– STROBE (*St*rengthening the *R*eporting of *Ob*servational Studies in *E*pidemiology), which pertains to case–control, cohort, and cross-sectional studies (von Elm et al. 2007).

Discipline-Specific Checklists

To complement aids to evaluate internal validity, there is the need to create discipline-specific checklists that can help to evaluate external validity or generalizability.

How easily could any of us describe our service's key attributes to a colleague in another country, region or even within the same city? How easily can we define which people are referred to our services from the denominator of all those who could be referred? It can be argued that hospice and palliative care additionally requires a discipline-based tool to allow two key characteristics to be defined:

– The service.
– The patients referred to that service.

Such an approach directly complements the methodology-based checklists of internal validity.

The key characteristics of a service and the population that they serve need to be captured in a simple and succinct checklist. Such a process draws directly on the iterative processes that have underpinned the development of checklists such as CONSORT. By focusing on descriptors of services and populations served, it is likely that there can be improved application of research findings. Such descriptors need to be supported with agreed definitions.

In other disciplines, there do not appear to be any discipline-specific tools to aid evaluation of external validity. For some disciplines, this is probably of little import (coronary care, surgical care of acute appendicitis) but highly relevant to other disciplines that share similar characteristics – referral-dependent, differing models of care, a wide range of care settings and key outcomes still being debated. Services such as rehabilitation, mental health and geriatrics probably fit this category. This process should allow researchers to easily describe the populations included in their studies and the model of service delivery. In turn, that would help clinicians and policy makers to identify rapidly the ways in which to apply best the findings of relevant research studies. This may facilitate matching between new evidence and its application in day-to-day practice.

Defining succinctly and accurately the setting in which the research was conducted (service and patient characteristics) by the researcher and the setting in which it will be applied by the end user (clinician or health planner) requires a discipline-specific approach to evidence-based care (in contrast to the methodologically based approach that has underpinned the process of systematic evaluation of studies until now). Two sides contribute to the process of generalizing research findings into practice. The first is the ability of researchers to describe the population that they are studying in the context of the service(s) from which these people are drawn. Finding ways to standardize this description in a systematized way will help researchers to reproducibly describe the work that they are undertaking. Likewise, for clinicians a simple process of identifying a common language may make the process of translation into practice far easier.

Systemic Reasons for Progressing this Work

Without a stronger framework to compare like with like, or to highlight differences between research and clinical sites, hospice and palliative care services are unlikely to be able to adequately:

- Complete effectively for limited health funding.
- Develop guidelines, outcome measures and consensus best practice statements.
- Ensure people with greatest needs are those who access services (Lidstone et al. 2003; Higginson and Addington-Hall 1999).

A Framework with Which to Approach Generalizability in Hospice and Palliative Care

A brief systematic checklist that creates a reproducible framework for describing generalizability is likely to aid researchers as they succinctly describe the population and setting in which the study has been conducted, and help end-users such as clinicians and health planners as they seek to apply the findings. This requires a list of study domains that define meaningfully key variations in services and the populations that they serve.

Five domains have been identified as being of benefit to this process. Ideally these domains will be incorporated in the design of data collection during the study. By using the same domains in reporting the study, it is also hoped that end-users will get used to the format to allow for rapid interpretation of new results. Such a process may directly aid communication between researchers and clinicians as they seek jointly to improve services. The domains include issues defined around:

- Patients and caregivers.
- Health professionals.
- Service structure.

Table 8.1 Pivotal fields for applying findings from different types of research in hospice and palliative care research to the local environment

| | | Domain | | Service | | |
		Individual participant's demographics	Caregiver	Clinical population referred	Descriptors	Funding
Study	Healthy volunteer	X				
	Efficacy randomized controlled trial (RCT)	X		X		
	Other clinical intervention trials including effectiveness RCTs	X		X	X	X
	Health services research (including intervention trials)	X	X	X	X	X
	Cohort studies	X	±	X	X	X
	Qualitative	X		X	±	±
	Best supportive care	X	X	X	X	X

- Jurisdictional health and social policies.
- The outcome measure in the.

In order to simplify these processes, clinicians or policy makers should read a paper and frame the research question that is being asked. From there, the reader should decide the best methodology to answer that question and the population who can best answer it. Having determined the population, consider the key fields in order to best understand the issue (Table 8.1). From there, what are the particular domains that need to be reported in order to aid an understanding of applicability. At the same time, in order to optimally apply new knowledge, the reader must be able to define his or her own service in the same domains in order to look at the comparability of the setting in which the evidence was generated and the setting to which the evidence will be applied.

Different populations and study designs will be described most effectively by using the domains that apply directly to them (Table 8.1). For example, a pharmacokinetic study of a medication used in palliative care using healthy volunteers does not need to reflect the health or social system in which the study is conducted. Studies focusing on interventions to support caregivers more effectively will rely heavily on social service funding and models of care together with basic demographics of the caregivers. Unless some other way of accessing caregivers is available, the characteristics of patients referred to the specialist hospice or palliative care service is still very important to report.

In the light of a review of what is actually published in palliative care research, a series of sub-domains is proposed that covers the key descriptors of services and populations to aid in the application of new research. This work, like the development of the CONSORT statement, is an evolution but represents the fields that are most likely to be of value to researchers, clinicians and policy makers (Table 8.2).

Applying the Process

There is one more crucial application of this process. When "best supportive care" is used as a comparator arm in oncology clinical trials, there is wide variation in what is meant by the term and what is offered in the trial setting in clinical practice (Cherny et al. 2009). These variations are seen

Table 8.2 Checklist to improve the ability of clinicians and service planners to apply hospice or palliative care research to their setting

Domain		Sub-domain	Measure	Population... ...Reported in this study	...In my service
Patient's demographics		Age	Mean (standard deviation		
		Gender	SD, median, range)		
		Socio-economic indices	Percentage		
			A nationally accepted index		
		Ethnicity	Country of birth (to highlight groups with known poorer access)		
Caregiver#		Caregiver availability	Percentage of patients without an identified caregiver		
Service	Clinical population referred	Life-limiting illness	Cancer/noncancer		
		Performance status	AKPS* or ECOG**		
		Time from referral until death	Mean (SD), median (range)		
	Descriptors	Study setting	Inpatient, community, outpatient, combination		
		Basis for referral	Prognosis ± diagnosis ± needs		
Health and social policy		Health care funding mechanisms	Universal coverage, user pays, etc.		
Research		Primary outcome measure in study	Study outcome measures validated in the target hospice or palliative care population	Yes/no	

*Australian Modified Karnofsky Performance Status
** Eastern Cooperative Oncology Group functional status

between studies, between sites in studies and potentially even within sites in the clinical study context. This checklist can help to describe the key characteristics of the population seen and the services delivered to trial participants. More importantly, this checklist may also be a way of helping researchers to standardize more easily the best supportive care that is offered in clinical trials.

Conclusion

Hospice and palliative care services around the world are based on referral from other clinical services. Because of a lack of standardization in who should be referred, populations ultimately referred can differ widely. These variations are amplified because the actual service to which people are referred may be structured in many different ways even within the same health system's funding model. Describing key characteristics of patients and caregivers, and the service to which they are referred in the context of their health system may help researchers describe their work, and clinicians and policy makers apply the findings in a more informed way. Facilitating uptake of research is a key to improving the quality of care that is given across the whole population. Such a discipline-specific process complements methodological checklists such as CONSORT.

References

Abernethy, A. P., & Arnold, R. M. (2006). PC-FACS: A real-time evidence resource for busy palliative care clinicians. *Journal of Palliative Medicine, 9*(1), 24–28.

Abernethy, A. P., Basch, E., Bull, J., Cleeland, C. S., Currow, D. C., Fairclough, D., et al. (2010). A strategy to advance the evidence base in palliative medicine: Formation of a Palliative Care Research Cooperative group. *Journal of Palliative Medicine, 13*(12), 1407–1413.

Abernethy, A. P., & Currow, D. C. (2008). Culture and financing influence palliative care services, study populations, and generalizability of research findings [letter]. *Journal of Palliative Medicine, 11*(2), 146.

Addington-Hall, J., Altmann, D., & McCarthy, M. (1998). Which terminally ill cancer patients receive hospice in-patient care? *Social Science & Medicine, 46*, 1011–1016.

Bakitas, M. A., Lyons, K. D., Dixon, J., & Ahles, T. A. (2006). Palliative care program effectiveness research: Developing rigor in sampling design, conduct, and reporting. *Journal of Pain and Symptom Management, 31*, 270–284.

Bestall, J. C., Ahmed, N., Ahmedzai, S. H., Payne S.A., Noble B., Clark D. (2004). Access and referral to specialist palliative care: Patients' and professionals' experiences. *International Journal of Palliative Nursing, 10*, 381–389.

Borgsteede, S. D., Deliens, L., Francke, A. L., Stalman W. A., Willems D. L., Van Eijk J. T., et al. (2006). Defining the patient population: One of the problems for palliative care research. *Palliative Medicine, 20*, 63–68.

Bossuyt, P. M., Reitsma, J. B., Bruns, D. E., Gatsonis C. A., Glasziou P. P., Irwig L. M., et al. (2003). Towards complete and accurate reporting of studies of diagnostic accuracy: The STARD initiative. *Clinical Chemistry, 49*(1), 1–6.

Brouwers, M. C., Kho, M. E., Browman, G. P., Burgers J.S., Cluzeau F., Feder G., et al. (2010). Development of the AGREE II, part 1: Performance, usefulness and areas for improvement. *Canadian Medical Association journal, 182*(10), 1045–1052.

Cherny, N., Strasser, F., Abernethy, A. P., Sapir, R., Currow, D. C., & Zafar, S. Y. (2009). Improving the methodologic and ethical validity of best supportive care studies in oncology: Lessons from a systematic review. *Journal of Clinical Oncology, 27*(32), 5476–5486.

Clarke, M. (2000). The QUORUM statement. *Lancet, 355*(9205), 756–757.

Craig, J. C., Irwig, L. M., & Stockler, M. R. (2001). Evidence based medicine: Useful tools for decision making. *The Medical Journal of Australia, 174*, 248–253.

Currow, D. C., Abernethy, A. P., & Fazekas, B. S. (2004). Palliative needs of whole populations: A comprehensive population approach to determining need. *Palliative Medicine, 18*, 239–247.

Currow, D. C., Abernethy, A. P., Shelby-James, T., & Phillips, P. A. (2006). Patient and service impacts of conducting a large palliative care clinical trial. *Palliative Medicine, 20*(8), 735–743.

Currow, D. C., Stevenson, J. P., Abernethy, A. P., Plummer, J., & Shelby-James, T. M. (2007). Prescribing in palliative care as death approaches. *Journal of the American Geriatrics Society, 55*(4), 590–595.

Currow, D. C., Wheeler, J., Glare, P., Kaasa S., Abernethy A. P. (2009). A framework for generalizability in palliative care. *Journal of Pain and Symptom Management, 37*, 373–386.

Dhruva, S. S., & Redberg, R. F. (2008). Variations between clinical trial participants and Medicare beneficiaries in evidence used for Medicare national coverage decisions. *Archives of Internal Medicine, 168*(2), 136–140.

Foley, K. M. (2003). Advancing palliative care in the United States. *Palliative Medicine, 17*(2), 89–91.

Francke, A., Smit, M., de Veer, A., Mistiaen P. (2008). Factors influencing the implementation of clinical guidelines for health care professionals: A systematic meta-review. *BMC Medical Informatics and Decision Making, 8*(1), 38.

Franks, P. J., Salisbury, C., Bosanquet, N., Wilkinson E. K., Kite S., Naysmith A., et al. (2000). The level of need for palliative care: A systematic review of the literature. *Palliative Medicine, 14*, 93–104.

Gott, M. C., Ahmedzai, S. H., & Wood, C. (2001). How many inpatients at an acute hospital have palliative care needs? Comparing the perspectives of medical and nursing staff. *Palliative Medicine, 15*, 451–460.

Green, L. W. (2006). Glasgow RE evaluating the relevance, generalization, and applicability of research: Issues in external validation and translation methodology. *Evaluation & the Health Professions, 29*, 126–152.

Higginson, I. J., & Addington-Hall, J. M. (1999). Palliative care needs to be provided on basis of need rather than diagnosis [letter]. *British Medical Journal, 318*, 123.

Jordhøy, M. S., Fayers, P. M., Ahlner-Elmqvist, M., Kaasa S. (2002). Lack of concealment may lead to selection bias in cluster randomized trials of palliative care. *Palliative Medicine, 16*(1), 43–49.

Jordhoy, M. S., Saltvedt, I., Fayers, P., Loge J. H., Ahlner-Elmqvist M., Kaasa S. (2003). Which cancer patients die in nursing homes? Quality of life, medical and sociodemographic characteristics. *Palliative Medicine, 17*, 433–444.

Lidstone, V., Butters, E., Seed, P. T., Sinnott C., Beynon T., Richards M. (2003). Symptoms and concerns amongst cancer outpatients: Identifying the need for specialist palliative care. *Palliative Medicine, 17*, 588–595.

O'Brien, M. A., Rogers, S., Jamtvedt, G., Oxman, A. D., Odgaard-Jensen, J., Kristoffersen, D. T., et al. (2007). Educational outreach visits: Effects on professional practice and health care outcomes. *Cochrane Database of Systematic Reviews, (4)*, CD000409. doi: 10.1002/14651858.CD000409.pub2.

Rosenwax, L. K., McNamara, B., Blackmore, A. M., & Holman, C. D. (2005). Estimating the size of a potential palliative care population. *Palliative Medicine, 19*, 556–562.

Sackett, D. L., & Rosenberg, W. M. (1995). On the need for evidence-based medicine. *Journal of Public Health Medicine, 17*(3), 330–334.

Schulz, K. F., Altman, D. G., Moher, D., & For the CONSORT Group. (2010). CONSORT 2010 Statement: Updated guidelines for reporting parallel group randomized trials. *Annals of Internal Medicine, 152*, 726–732.

Stroup, D. F., Berlin, J. A., Morton, S. C., Olkin I., Williamson D. G., Rennie D., et al. (2000). Meta-analysis of observational studies in epidemiology (MOOSE) group. *The Journal of the American Medical Association, 283*(15), 2008–2012.

Tieman, J., Sladek, R., & Currow, D. C. (2008). Changes in the quantity and level of evidence of palliative and hospice care literature: The last century. *Journal of Clinical Oncology, 26*(35), 5679–5683.

Tinetti, M. E., Bogardus, S. T., Jr., & Agostini, J. V. (2004). Potential pitfalls of disease-specific guidelines for patients with multiple conditions. *The New England Journal of Medicine, 351*(27), 2870–2874.

Van Spall, H. G. C., Toren, A., Kiss, A., Fowler R. A. (2007). Eligibility criteria of randomized controlled trials published in high-impact general medical journals: A systematic sampling review. *The Journal of the American Medical Association, 297*(11), 1233–1240.

von Elm, E., Altman, D. G., Egger, M., et al. (2007). STROBE initiative. Strengthening the reporting of observational studies in epidemiology (STROBE) statement: Guidelines for reporting observational studies. *British Medical Journal, 335*(7624), 806–808.

Waller, A., Girgis, A., Johnson, C., Mitchell, G., Yates, P., Kristjanson, L., Tattersall, M., et al. (2010). Facilitating needs based cancer care for people with a chronic disease: Evaluation of an intervention using a multi-centre interrupted time series design. *BMC Palliative Care, 9*:2.

Wheeler, J. L., Green, A., Tieman, J. J., Abernethy, A. P., Currow, D. C. (2011). Characteristics of palliative care studies reported in the specialized literature. J Pain Symptom Manage. [Accepted 12 July 2011].

Chapter 9
Dynamic Pain Assessment: An Application of Clinical Infometrics to Personalized Pain Treatment and Management

Chih-Hung Chang

Introduction

Pain is a major public health problem. It is highly prevalent, affecting 100 million Americans each year. Pain is also costly, both in human and economic terms. It is often unreported, untreated, or undertreated, resulting in diminished physical, psychological, and social well-being. It is the most common complaint of people seeking medical treatment (Schappert 1992), placing an immense economic burden on the health care system.

Accurate assessment of complex and multidimensional pain is undoubtedly a challenging but necessary first step to its optimal treatment and management. The availability and accessibility of such pain information to physicians is critical when making clinical decisions in concert with their patients. The availability of an integrated psychometrics-driven and informatics-assisted pain measurement-to-treatment-to-management system can provide an environment to accurately and conveniently capture, analyze, and present easy-to-use pain data to facilitate optimal pain treatment, thus increasing satisfaction, reducing costs, and ultimately improving an individual's quality of care and quality of life.

Modern psychometrics, e.g., item response theory (IRT) (Chang and Reeve 2005; Hambleton et al. 1991), offers promise for the development of a clinically relevant, culturally sensitive, and psychometrically sound assessment tool. Advanced informatics, e.g., information and communications technology (ICT) (Christensen et al. 2007; United Nations 2003), can potentially improve the mobility, efficiency, and accuracy of clinical and self-reported data collection and reporting. Unfortunately, their integrative use has either not been fully implemented or reached the desired levels of potential benefits each offers in clinical research and practice.

It is viable to harness the advances and innovations in psychometrics and informatics for the development of a practically useful pain assessment, treatment, and management system. The successful execution of the measurement-to-management approach can lessen the complexity of pain assessment, help eliminate cultural or language barriers, and make it easily transferrable to other symptoms, conditions, and clinical settings.

C.-H. Chang, Ph.D (✉)
Buehler Center on Aging, Health and Society, Northwestern University
Feinberg School of Medicine, Chicago, IL, USA

Department of Medicine, Division of General Internal Medicine,
Northwestern University Feinberg School of Medicine, Chicago, IL, USA

Robert H. Lurie Comprehensive Cancer Center of Northwestern University, Chicago, IL, USA

R.J. Moore (ed.), *Handbook of Pain and Palliative Care: Biobehavioral Approaches for the Life Course*,
DOI 10.1007/978-1-4419-1651-8_9, © Springer Science+Business Media, LLC 2012

The Need for Integrated Methods to Improve Pain Outcomes

Pain has Significant Health, Economic, and Societal Impacts

Each year 75 million Americans suffer from chronic pain and over 30 million of them are under-treated. Additionally, 25 million Americans experience acute pain from injuries or surgeries (see also Short and Vetter 2011). Pain correlates with a long list of ailments impacting health and quality of life (Gallagher et al. 2000; Mantyselka et al. 2003; Ohayon and Schatzberg 2003; Spiegel et al. 1994). Pain also takes an enormous toll on families and caregivers, depresses work productivity (Stewart et al. 2003), and places a tremendous economic burden on the healthcare system (Gibson and Weiner 2005; Raj 2004; Ferrell et al. 1990) (see also May 2011). The high prevalence and substantial impact of pain in older adults also make it a pressing issue as the population ages (Fox et al. 1999; Landi et al. 2001; Whelan et al. 2004) (see also Cole and McCarberg 2011).

Accurate Pain Assessment Is Critical to Its Optimal Treatment

Pain is subjective, multidimensional, and complex to measure (Ahles et al. 1983; McGuire 1992). Incomplete assessment (under or inaccurate reporting) of pain has been described as a significant barrier to its relief (Von Roenn et al. 1993). Accurate and continuous pain assessment plays a vital role in the provision of critical data to screen and identify a patient's medical problem, facilitate patient–physician communication, guide the selection of optimal treatment options, monitor treatment progress, and evaluate treatment outcomes over time (see also Hjermstad et al. 2011; Kovach 2011; Seow and Dy 2011). Efficient and cost-effective pain management also relies heavily on readily available data from reliable and valid self-report questionnaires (Gatchel and Turk 1996; Jamison 1996a, b; Karoly and Jensen 1987; Keefe 2000).

The Need for Culturally Sensitive Pain Assessment Still Exists

Cross-cultural variation in reporting pain experience has been observed in clinical settings. The lack of shared meaning or understanding of pain among patients and clinicians appears to contribute to ineffective treatment. Racial and ethnic minorities are at risk for inadequate access to pain care (Bonham 2001; Anderson et al. 2009) (see also Green 2011). The growing ethnic diversity of the U.S. population also underscores the significance of, and the need for, linguistically appropriate and culturally sensitive pain measures for those who primary language is not English, but few measures in English have been properly translated and validated.

Current Pain Assessment Tools Have Limitations for Clinical Use

Despite their widespread use, paper-and-pencil-based pain assessment tools have limitations (Jamison et al. 2001; Litt et al. 1998; Stone et al. 2003; Straka et al. 1997). One practical concern is that the pain data collected by this method are often not readily available for clinicians to analyze and interpret at the point of service due to the time-consuming data entry process. Although numerous electronic pain tools are currently available, their clinical usefulness is also restricted in some ways (Jamison et al. 2002). One significant barrier has to do with the complexity of the interface for patients to navigate efficiently, particularly for those who are not technically competent. In order to streamline the processes and improve these tools to obtain good pain information that can lead to better clinical outcomes, it demands a more advanced and effective method for pain data acquisition and reporting.

Psychometrics and Informatics Together Offer Practical Solutions and Improvements

Modern Psychometrics Enhances Assessment

IRT, developed and commonly used in educational and psychological measurement, holds great promise to improve clinical outcome assessment. It has become increasingly popular in health and medical sciences because it provides more adaptable and effective methods of scale construction, analysis, and scoring (see Chang and Reeve (2005)). IRT can help operationally define the multidimensional, subjective pain experience with measurable characteristics and improve its assessment quality. IRT can also help to establish measures that are clinically relevant, cultural-sensitive, and age-appropriate to allow for more meaningful between-group comparisons.

Advanced Informatics Improves on Traditional Methods

Computerized tools that utilize ICT offer promise, if properly designed, as they can provide a better means to allow a patient's pain data to be reliably self-reported and recorded from multiple front-end devices, securely transmitted and stored in a back-end server, and properly summarized and accessible during the clinical encounter. The use of a dynamic display (e.g., 3-dimensional representation of the human body) in a portable Tablet or touch-screen computer permits a variety of user-friendly data entry elements and formats (e.g., varying colors to indicate pain intensity) (Jamison et al. 2002; Anon 1986; Chang et al. 2007; Sakauye 2005; Rodriguez 2001). Interactive programs can ask patients a series of distinct yet related questions to instantaneously get a much more complete picture of their symptoms (e.g., pain), which is often unattainable from the traditional paper-and-pencil-based assessments.

An Integrative Psychometrics-Informatics Approach Improve Processes and Outcomes

For clinical information such as self-reported pain to be used effectively in clinical care, the assessment tools must be not only clinically relevant and psychometrically sound, but also be user-friendly, culturally appropriate, and easily accessible to permit patients to accurately report their current conditions. The information then must be summarized and easily interpretable to facilitate patient–physician communications about the clinical issues to ensure the development and delivery of adequate and culturally appropriate care. Psychometrics and informatics each offers unique yet complimentary features and can be integrated and work synergistically together to capitalize the potential improvements and practical benefits. Integrated psychometrics–informatics tools hold much promise to facilitate physician–patient–family communications, optimize treatment choices, and improve symptom and disease management. These practical solutions and promising enhancements towards personalized pain care merit further exploration and evaluation.

Frameworks and Conceptual Models

Multidimensional Pain

Pain has been defined by the International Association for the Study on Pain Subcommittee on Taxonomy as "an unpleasant sensory and emotional experience associated with actual or potential tissue damage or described in terms of such damage." (Anon 1986) Pain is a multidimensional experience with many contributing and interacting biological/pathobiological mechanisms (see Fig. 9.1). These mechanisms may be nociceptive, peripheral neurogenic, central, affective/cognitive or may relate to output systems such as the motor and autonomic nervous system (see also Al-Chaer 2011). However, pain is also a subjective experience (see also Gatchel et al. 2011; Palermo 2011).

The Conceptual STATE Care Process Model

The STATE model has four steps in the care cycle: (1) Screening; (2) Tailored Assessment; (3) Treatment; and (4) Evaluation (see Fig. 9.2). At the beginning of a medical consultation, a patient is often being asked a set of predefined screening questions, in addition to vital signs, so that a preliminary assessment of his/her current health status can be established (Screening step). When the specific clinical care needs are detected, a more comprehensive assessment tailored to those identified needs will then be conducted for a deeper level of evaluation (Tailored Assessment step). After a thorough assessment of clinical problems, clinicians can discuss treatment options with their patients and come up with most appropriate treatment plans (Treatment step). Outcomes-based evaluation will then be conducted to determine whether the treatments have impacts and/or benefits to patients and whether the goals of treatment have been achieved (Evaluation step).

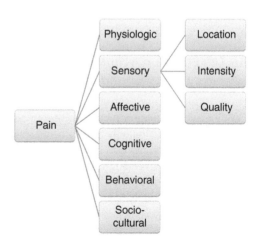

Fig. 9.1 Multidimensional pain experience

Fig. 9.2 The STATE model

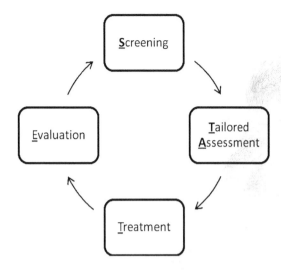

Fig. 9.3 Clinical infometrics

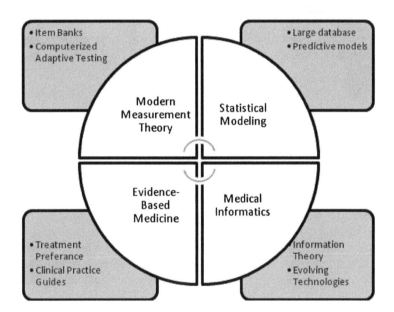

The Field of "Clinical Infometrics"

Clinical Infometrics (Chang et al. 2007), as we define it, is a synthesis of measurement sciences, evidence-based medicine, statistical modeling, and informatics that allows research findings to guide clinical decision making in nearly real time (see Fig. 9.3). It is purported to integrate methodologies and technologies to collect multidimensional patient-reported outcomes information and make immediate comparisons against population-based data and practice guidelines to offer clinical guidance for optimal treatment outcomes. The system has four key components: (1) a modern measurement theory component that administers tailored assessments; (2) a statistical modeling component that develops predictive models from large databases; (3) an evidence-based medicine component that combines clinical experience and practice guidelines; and (4) an informatics component that deals with the resources, devices, and methods required to optimize the acquisition, storage, retrieval and use of information.

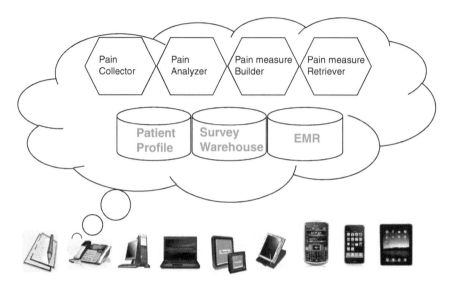

Fig. 9.4 The dynamic pain assessment system architecture

The Dynamic Pain Assessment System Architecture

The dynamic pain assessment system is designed to be multifunctional that can serve as a data collector, analyzer, builder, and retriever within a single system. Users can choose their preferred and accessible front-end devices (e.g., telephone, Tablet PC, Smartphone) to interact with the back-end server system (see Fig. 9.4). For instance, a patient can enter data via regular phone and a clinical staff can enter other data via Internet concurrently through an integrated multitasking environment. The data can be securely transmitted, processed, stored, and retrieved for additional statistical analysis or summary reporting via wire and wireless communication technologies.

The Design of the Dynamic Pain Assessment System

Item Bank Development

In order to develop a comprehensive yet practically useful item bank for pain assessment, treatment, and management, we need to adjudicate and reconcile domains or priority areas identified in the existing multidimensional pain frameworks. It is also crucial that we carefully define what are to be measured and include a sufficient pool of items to cover the latent continuum of that pain domain. IRT-based models can then be used to assess the psychometric properties of the measure and identify items that might perform differently across different groups (e.g., male vs. female) or different types of pain.

Computerized Adaptive Testing Platform

To make dynamic pain assessment a reality, all item parameters must be calibrated to a common metric using IRT and the items in the pool should span the full range of trait levels in the population. A dynamic pain assessment program can be designed to administer the pain care items according to an iterative algorithm consisting of administering an item, estimating a person's latent trait level, and selecting the next best item from an item bank to administer until some predetermined, discipline appropriate, stopping rule is met (e.g., minimal standard error, content coverage, or maximum scale length). Test administration needs to be standardized so that each patient has a comparable experience (e.g., standardized screen layout) when using Internet-connected computers to eliminate potential bias. Ultimately, the dynamic pain assessment system can be designed as a multipurpose assessment program that has the capability to store pain items, administer adaptive tests, and generate a report with the list of topics needed for attention.

Conclusions and Implications

Dynamic Pain Assessment Addresses Pain Measurement Issues

Modern psychometrics, i.e., IRT, offers sound and improved methods for scale construction, analysis, and scoring. Accurate and comprehensive assessment of pain is the foundation for its understanding and subsequent treatment. The development of the dynamic pain assessment measure utilizes IRT to ensure its comprehensiveness, appropriateness, and cultural sensitivity. It also allows a patient to report their pain from a single sensation to a comprehensive, multidimensional, and holistic experience.

Dynamic Pain Assessment Utilizes Informatics to Develop a Platform Best Suited for Use in Diverse Patients

Advanced informatics provides software and hardware improvement necessary in the design of a customized and scalable system. A well-designed portable, hand-held platform can provide an excellent low-stress pain assessment option, with particular applicability for older adults who are unsuited to more intrusive diagnostic procedures. Dynamic pain assessment is designed to address most of these significant issues, if not all, thus providing a significant advance beyond pain assessment methods currently in use. It is especially important to design something useful for the elderly population, who may suffer from reduced mobility and cognitive deficits.

Dynamic Pain Assessment Addresses Cultural Disparities in Pain Care

Studies have shown that culture, race, and ethnicity influence how adults experience and report pain (Bonham 2001; Anderson et al. 2009). The population is becoming more diverse and more attention will need to be paid to the linguistic/cultural factors that influence the experience of pain (Sakauye 2005; Rodriguez 2001; Nguyen et al. 2005; Portenoy et al. 2004). One significant innovation of the dynamic pain assessment system is to ensure that the measure and platform are culturally and linguistically accessible to the growing population of older and more diverse patients. The culturally appropriate tool will facilitate communication between clinicians and patients, especially those who may have difficultly giving clear verbal accounts.

Dynamic Pain Assessment Uses a Team Science Approach to Maximize Multidisciplinary Expertise

The development, design, and implementation of the dynamic pain assessment system that is clinically relevant, culturally sensitive, psychometrically sound, and user-friendly would demand a multidisciplinary team with unique and complimentary experiences in clinical pain assessment and management, geriatrics, psychometrics, mobile technology, and human computer interface design. Such combination of these knowledge and skills provides the basis for the development and deployment of a much-needed and enhanced pain assessment and management system that is not currently available in clinical settings.

In summary, the dynamic pain assessment approach represents a paradigm shift in harnessing multidisciplinary psychometrics–informatics innovations to create a class of reliable, novel, easy-to-use, noninvasive assessment and management tool that is transferrable to other health care settings and sites, populations and clinical conditions. It is feasible to design a software-based dynamic pain assessment system to allow for easy integration and installation on existing devices at primary care providers offices and can run anywhere, on any device, and allow an individual to report their pain characteristics easily and accurately and communicate their experience of pain to care providers in a timely manner. Successful implementation will result in a fully functional system for use in large-scale clinical research, practice, and trials. When universally adopted and thorough validated, this system can effectively improve clinical care generally and pain care specifically.

References

United Nations. (2003). *Economic and Social Commission for Western Asia. Information and Communications Technology Division. Review of information and communications technology and development* (p. v). New York: United Nations.

Ahles, T. A., Blanchard, E. B., & Ruckdeschel, J. C. (1983). The multidimensional nature of cancer-related pain. *Pain, 17*(3), 277–288.

Al-Chaer, E. (2011). Neuroanatomy of pain and pain pathways. In R. J. Moore (Ed.), *Handbook of pain and palliative care*. New York: Springer.

Anderson, K. O., Green, C. R., & Payne, R. (2009). Racial and ethnic disparities in pain: Causes and consequences of unequal care. *The Journal of Pain, 10*(12), 1187–1204.

Anon. (1986). Classification of chronic pain. Descriptions of chronic pain syndromes and definitions of pain terms. Prepared by the International Association for the Study of Pain, Subcommittee on Taxonomy. *Pain Suppl, 3*, S1–S226.

Bonham, V. L. (2001). Race, ethnicity, and pain treatment: Striving to understand the causes and solutions to the disparities in pain treatment. *The Journal of Law, Medicine & Ethics, 29*(1), 52–68.

Chang, C. H., Boni-Saenz, A. A., Durazo-Arvizu, R. A., Desharnais, S., Lau, D. T., & Emanuel, L. L. (2007). A system for interactive assessment and management in palliative care. *Journal of Pain and Symptom Management, 33*(6), 745–755.

Chang, C.-H., & Reeve, B. B. (2005). Item response theory and its applications to patient-reported outcomes measurement. *Evaluation & the Health Professions, 28*(3), 1–19.

Christensen, M., Remler, D., & National Bureau of Economic Research. (2007). Information and communications technology in chronic disease care why is adoption so slow and is slower better? *NBER working paper series working paper 13078*. Cambridge: National Bureau of Economic Research. Retrieved, from http://papers.nber.org/papers/w13078.

Cole, B., & McCarberg, W. (2011). Pain in the older person. In R. J. Moore (Ed.), *Handbook of pain and palliative care*. New York: Springer.

Ferrell, B. A., Ferrell, B. R., & Osterweil, D. (1990). Pain in the nursing home. *Journal of the American Geriatrics Society, 38*(4), 409–414.

Fox, P. L., Raina, P., & Jadad, A. R. (1999). Prevalence and treatment of pain in older adults in nursing homes and other long-term care institutions: A systematic review. *Canadian Medical Association journal, 160*(3), 329–333.

Gallagher, R. M., Verma, S., & Mossey, J. (2000). Chronic pain. Sources of late-life pain and risk factors for disability. *Geriatrics, 55*(9), 40–44; 47.

Gatchel, R. J., Haggard, R., Thomas, C., & Howard, K. J. (2011). A biopsychosocial approach to understanding chronic pain and disability. In R. J. Moore (Ed.), *Handbook of pain and palliative care*. New York: Springer.

Gatchel, R. J., & Turk, D. C. (1996). *Psychological approaches to pain management: A practitioner's handbook*. New York: Guilford Press.

Gibson, S. J., & Weiner, D. K. (2005). *Pain in older persons*. Seattle: IASP Press.

Green, C. (2011). Disparities in pain management and palliative care. In R. J. Moore (Ed.), *Handbook of pain and palliative care*. New York: Springer.

Hambleton, R. K., Swaminathan, H., & Rogers, H. J. (1991). *Fundamentals of item response theory*. Newbury Park: Sage.

Hjermstad, M., Faxvaag Haugen, D., Michael Bennett, I., & Kaasa, S. (2011). Pain assessment tools in palliative care and cancer. In R. J. Moore (Ed.), *Handbook of pain and palliative care*. New York: Springer.

Jamison, R. N. (1996a). *Learning to master your chronic pain*. Sarasota: Professional Resource Press.

Jamison, R. N. (1996b). *Mastering chronic pain: A professional's guide to behavioral treatment*. Sarasota: Professional Resource Press.

Jamison, R. N., Gracely, R. H., Raymond, S. A., et al. (2002). Comparative study of electronic vs. paper VAS ratings: A randomized, crossover trial using healthy volunteers. *Pain, 99*(1–2), 341–347.

Jamison, R. N., Raymond, S. A., Levine, J. G., Slawsby, E. A., Nedeljkovic, S. S., & Katz, N. P. (2001). Electronic diaries for monitoring chronic pain: 1-year validation study. *Pain, 91*(3), 277–285.

Karoly, P., & Jensen, M. P. (1987). *Multimethod assessment of chronic pain* (1st ed.). Oxford: Pergamon Press.

Keefe, F. (2000). Self-report of pain: Issues and opportunities. In A. A. Stone, C. A. Bachrach, J. B. Jobe, H. S. Kurtzman, & V. S. Cain (Eds.), *The science of self-report: Implications for research and practice* (pp. 17–37). Mahwah: Lawrence Erlbaum.

Kovach, C. (2011). Assessing pain and unmet needs in patients with advanced dementia: The role of the serial trial intervention (STI). In R. J. Moore (Ed.), *Handbook of pain and palliative care*. New York: Springer.

Landi, F., Onder, G., Cesari, M., et al. (2001). Pain management in frail, community-living elderly patients. *Archives of Internal Medicine, 161*(22), 2721–2724.

Litt, M. D., Cooney, N. L., & Morse, P. (1998). Ecological momentary assessment (EMA) with treated alcoholics: Methodological problems and potential solutions. *Health Psychology, 17*(1), 48–52.

Mantyselka, P. T., Turunen, J. H., Ahonen, R. S., & Kumpusalo, E. A. (2003). Chronic pain and poor self-rated health. *The Journal of the American Medical Association, 290*(18), 2435–2442.

May, S. (2011). Chronic low back pain. In R. J. Moore (Ed.), *Handbook of pain and palliative care*. New York: Springer.

McGuire, D. B. (1992). Comprehensive and multidimensional assessment and measurement of pain. *Journal of Pain and Symptom Management, 7*(5), 312–319.

Nguyen, M., Ugarte, C., Fuller, I., Haas, G., & Portenoy, R. K. (2005). Access to care for chronic pain: Racial and ethnic differences. *The Journal of Pain, 6*(5), 301–314.

Ohayon, M. M., & Schatzberg, A. F. (2003). Using chronic pain to predict depressive morbidity in the general population. *Archives of General Psychiatry, 60*(1), 39–47.

Palermo, Y. (2011). The art of pain: The patient's perspective of chronic pain. In R. J. Moore (Ed.), *Handbook of pain and palliative care*. New York: Springer.

Portenoy, R. K., Ugarte, C., Fuller, I., & Haas, G. (2004). Population-based survey of pain in the United States: Differences among white, African American, and Hispanic subjects. *The Journal of Pain, 5*(6), 317–328.

Raj, P. P. (2004). The prevalence of chronic pain in the United States remains high, imposing a large economic burden on patients and society. *Pain Practice, 4*(Suppl 1), S1–S3.

Rodriguez, C. S. (2001). Pain measurement in the elderly: A review. *Pain Management Nursing, 2*(2), 38–46.

Sakauye, K. (2005). Cultural influences on pain management in the elderly. *Comprehensive Therapy, 31*(1), 78–82.

Schappert, S. M. (1992). National ambulatory medical care survey: 1989 summary. *Vital Health Statistics Series 13, 110*, 1–80.

Seow, H., & Dy, S. (2011). Quality indicators for pain in palliative care. In R. J. Moore (Ed.), *Handbook of pain and palliative care*. New York: Springer.

Short, R., & Vetter, T. (2011). Acute to chronic pain: Transitions in the post surgical patient. In R. J. Moore (Ed.), *Handbook of pain and palliative care*. New York: Springer.

Spiegel, D., Sands, S., & Koopman, C. (1994). Pain and depression in patients with cancer. *Cancer, 74*(9), 2570–2578.

Stewart, W. F., Ricci, J. A., Chee, E., & Morganstein, D. (2003). Lost productive work time costs from health conditions in the United States: Results from the American Productivity Audit. *Journal of Occupational and Environmental Medicine, 45*(12), 1234–1246.

Stone, A. A., Shiffman, S., Schwartz, J. E., Broderick, J. E., & Hufford, M. R. (2003). Patient compliance with paper and electronic diaries. *Controlled Clinical Trials, 24*(2), 182–199.

Straka, R. J., Fish, J. T., Benson, S. R., & Suh, J. T. (1997). Patient self-reporting of compliance does not correspond with electronic monitoring: An evaluation using isosorbide dinitrate as a model drug. *Pharmacotherapy, 17*(1), 126–132.

Von Roenn, J. H., Cleeland, C. S., Gonin, R., Hatfield, A. K., & Pandya, K. J. (1993). Physician attitudes and practice in cancer pain management. A survey from the Eastern Cooperative Oncology Group. *Annals of Internal Medicine, 119*(2), 121–126.

Whelan, C. T., Jin, L., & Meltzer, D. (2004). Pain and satisfaction with pain control in hospitalized medical patients: No such thing as low risk. *Archives of Internal Medicine, 164*(2), 175–180.

Chapter 10
Assessing Pain and Unmet Need in Patients with Advanced Dementia: The Role of the Serial Trial Intervention (STI)

Christine R. Kovach

Introduction

Chronic pain is a problem for many older adults, with prevalence estimates ranging from 25 to 86% (Fries et al. 2001; AGS Panel on Persistent Pain in Older Persons 2002; Herr 2002). Older adults with dementia do not differ in prevalence of conditions associated with pain (Proctor and Hirdes 2001). One study of long-term care residents with dementia found pain prevalence of 21% (Williams et al. 2005). Common nociceptive pain conditions in older adults include orthopedic conditions such as fracture, osteoarthritis, gout, tendonitis, and skin lesions. Neuropathic pain may arise from herpetic neuralgia, spinal conditions, central post stroke pain, trigeminal neuralgia, and peripheral neuropathies. Other common conditions that may cause both nociceptive and neuropathic pain include chronic low back pain, malignancy, and conditions associated with vascular compromise (Hadjistavropoulos et al. 2007).

Unresolved physical pain is linked to numerous negative sequelae including sleep disturbances, decreased socialization, malnutrition, agitation, depression, impaired immune function, impaired ambulation, increased morbidity, increased health care use and costs, and increased mortality (Chang et al. 1995; Ferrell 1995; Liebeskind 1991; Moss 1997; Won et al. 1999).

Multiple studies have found that people with cognitive impairment report less pain in response to noxious stimuli than cognitively intact older adults (Fisher-Morris and Gellatly 1997; Scherder et al. 1999; Hindley et al. 1995). While peripheral nociceptive responses appear to be intact, one possible explanation for decreased pain response is that neurodegenerative changes and deterioration of neurotransmitter systems may affect how nociceptive information is transmitted to the somatosensory cortex (Price 2000).

There is increasing evidence that the decreased report of pain in people with dementia may reflect the individual's decreased ability to cognitively process painful sensations or to experience pain as threatening, rather than merely indicating a reduced sensitivity to pain (Chow 2000; Tsai and Chang 2004; Schuler et al. 2004). Benedetti et al. (1999) found no difference in stimulus detection but higher levels of pain tolerance in those with dementia compared to cognitively intact subjects. Another study found that people with cognitive impairment report less pain affect and suffering and indicated that pain had less effect on daily physical and mental functioning than those who were cognitively intact (Scherder et al. 1999). Porter et al. (1996) found that people with dementia

C.R. Kovach, PhD, RN, FAAN (✉)
Self-Management Science Center, University of Wisconsin-Milwaukee College of Nursing,
Cunningham Hall 1921 East Hartford Avenue, Milwaukee, WI, 53201-0413, USA
e-mail: ckovach@uwm.edu

R.J. Moore (ed.), *Handbook of Pain and Palliative Care: Biobehavioral Approaches for the Life Course*,
DOI 10.1007/978-1-4419-1651-8_10, © Springer Science+Business Media, LLC 2012

experienced lower heart rate increase in preparation for the pain of venipuncture but higher heart rate increases following the venipuncture than cognitively intact controls. These findings support the notion that the emotional component of pain may be diminished but that the actual physical sensation of pain is not altered. Areas of the brain such as the thalamic and intralaminar nuclei that play an important role in the motivational-affective processing of pain are severely compromised in Alzheimer's disease (Rub et al. 2002). The primary sensory areas, in contrast are relatively preserved (Dickson 2001).

People with dementia receive less assessment and treatment for pain than older adults who are cognitively intact (Morrison and Siu 2000; Martin et al. 2005). Reasons for poor management of pain in people with dementia include failure to recognize symptoms of pain, changes in the person's ability to accurately self-report pain, caregiver misconceptions, and biases against the demented person by medical professionals (Herr and Decker 2004).

Challenges of Pain Assessment

Evidence from several studies suggests that people with mild cognitive impairment can still provide reasonably accurate verbal reports of pain. Tools such as the Verbal Descriptor Scale, Numerical Rating Scales, and Faces Pain Scale have adequate reliability and validity and can be used for self-report of pain in those with cognitive impairment (Feldt 2000; Scherder and Bouma 2000; Closs et al. 2004). Self-report has traditionally been preferred for mild dementia because behavioral observations of pain vary considerably depending on factors such as the training and biases of the observer, who is present during the observation, whether the person is at rest or engaged in activity, and the timing of the observation period (Hadjistavropoulos et al. 2007). However, Scherder et al. (2005) point out that most self-report scales measure intensity and not the affective components of pain and suggest that both self-report and observational scales be used to target both the sensory and affective aspects of pain.

As dementia progresses the use of self-report tools becomes less valid and reliable, and proxy report or behavioral observations are used to assess pain. Behavioral observations are preferred to proxy report because multiple studies have found that family and professional caregivers grossly underestimate pain in people with dementia (Horgas and Dunn 2001; Cohen-Mansfield and Lipson 2002). Since people with advanced dementia have difficulty reporting their own pain, nurses and family caregivers often have to make judgments about pain based on behaviors. When assessing these behavioral cues, changes may be subtle. Consistent caregivers who are educated to regularly look for pain behaviors are vital in this regard since they are more apt to notice subtle changes (Kovach et al. 2000). Behaviors commonly associated with pain are listed in Table 10.1.

Behavioral Assessment of Pain in Dementia:

Table 10.1 Common pain behaviors

Body part cues	Tense muscles, pulling away when touched, rubbing or holding a body part, shifting weight when seated, protecting a part of the body when moving
Change in activity	Restless body movement, agitation, combative/angry, exiting behavior, withdrawing or becoming quiet, resisting care, aggression, an increase or decrease in activity
Change in function	Changes in mobility, decreased or increased sleep, increased confusion, decreased appetite, increased physical dependence, a change in social interaction, slow movement
Vocal	Crying, moaning, nonspecific verbal perseveration, a specific verbal confirmation of pain
Other	Facial grimacing, change in respirations

The five behavioral observation tools with the strongest psychometric properties are the DS-DAT (Discomfort Scale for Dementia of the Alzheimer's Type), CNPI (Checklist of Nonverbal Pain Indicators), NOPPAIN (Noncommunicative patient's pain assessment instrument), PACSLAC (pain assessment checklist for seniors with limited ability to communicate), and the Doloplus 2 (Herr et al. 2006).

Use of a formal pain observation tool coupled with a formal protocol for assessment and treatment is recommended in this population because health care professionals have the tendency to under-identify behavior changes and the need for additional physical assessment. In a study of 155 nursing home residents with advanced dementia, we found that sensitivity, or probability of identifying a real behavior change, was generally low for the staff nurses, ranging between 35 and 65% for the different types of behaviors. Also, additional assessment was felt to be needed for 51% of residents by the staff nurse and for 73% of residents by an expert advanced practice nurse (Kovach et al. 2011).

In a study of comorbid problems developing in nursing home residents with advanced dementia, we found a high prevalence of pain and delayed identification of multiple comorbid problems. Over the 6 weeks of data collection, 34 of 65 residents (52%) experienced new pain or exacerbations of chronic pain (musculoskeletal = 20; cancer pain = 4; gastrointestinal pain = 1). Of the 149 new physical problems that developed over 6 weeks, there were additional problems that may have been associated with pain or other uncomfortable symptoms (urinary tract infection = 10; pneumonia = 9; skin infection = 9; nausea, vomiting, diarrhea = 8; constipation = 6; skin infection = 6; leg edema = 5; upper respiratory infection = 5; conjunctivitis = 1) (Kovach et al. 2010). The days from symptom presentation to diagnosis ranged from <1 to 29 days (median = 4). In this study, a 1 unit decrease in nurse assessment skill was associated with a 54% increase in the time to identify new physical problems ($p < 0.001$). Residents without specific physical symptoms had 127% longer times to have their new physical problems identified ($p = 0.009$).

One critical problem associated with the underassessment and undertreatment of pain in this population are the difficulties distinguishing pain from other etiologies. We will report here two case studies from the nursing home study of comorbid problems that highlight how treatment can go awry.

Case A

A 97-year-old severely demented female on day 1 of data collection was yelling out with movement during care activities or transfer from the bed to wheelchair. She had been in the nursing home 9 months, was nonambulatory, had limited ability to verbally communicate, and her bilateral knee pain was well controlled with scheduled hydrocodone/acetaminophen. She also received scheduled lorazepam for anxiety. Multiple nurse assessments revealed full range of motion to her lower extremities and she denied pain. In addition to yelling, "help me," "No, No No" or "ooh, ooh ooh," when approached or moved, she began to be resistive to care and looked very frightened when approached. The staff interpreted this change in behavior as anxiety and responded by approaching care slowly and explaining what was being done and the reason for the care. She was provided positive verbal feedback every time she was "cooperative with cares" and was frequently reassured that "she will be all right and not fall" when transferred. On day 13 of data collection, when asked if she had pain she responded "yes" and touched her upper left leg. She was treated with her scheduled hydrocodone/ acetaminophen and positive reinforcement for being cooperative. On day 21, the timing of her scheduled hydrocodone/acetaminophen and lorazepam were changed to 1 h before morning care was delivered, even though she was again denying any pain. On day 22, when asked about pain she pointed to her left leg and when the right leg was touched she yells out. On day 23, an X-ray revealed a left intertrochanteric fracture.

Case B

A 91-year-old moderately demented female with a pleasant demeanor, and persistently smiling countenance had been in the nursing home 57 months, was ambulatory, and retained the ability to verbally communicate regarding her back pain. Her back pain was well controlled with scheduled acetaminophen and as needed tramadol. On day 8 she verbally complained about hemorrhoid pain and was treated with medication and a supportive cushion. She presented on day 11 of data collection with a clear change in condition. Though she continued to smile, she became withdrawn, refused meals, and spit out her medications, including her oral analgesics. This behavior continued and she started "spitting out yellow phlegm." Multiple checks of vital signs were normal, she was afebrile, her lungs were clear, and she had no cough. On day 14 she fell and on day 15 she was restless all night, was spitting up larger amounts of "yellow phlegm." While continuing to smile, she began to grab staff clothing and jab at them. On day 18, she complained of fatigue, refused to open her mouth and did not complain of pain. A nurse looked into her mouth and multiple "pus pockets" were noted. She was started on an antibiotic. On day 19 she complained of "hurting all over" was very restless and stated "I can't swallow." Her daughter ordered hospice care and all scheduled medications were discontinued. On day 22, she was seen by a dentist who diagnosed an acute abscess of the mandibular anterior area that was tender to the touch. She was started on antibiotic and opioid injections, clonazepam orally disintegrating tablets and viscous lidocaine for the jawline. On day 23, she was much weaker and on day 25, she died.

In Case A the resident's behavioral symptoms were misinterpreted as anxiety and paranoia rather than as the symptom of pain. Caregivers inadvertently treated her anxiety rather than discovering the etiology underlying the behavior. Her history of anxiety probably contributed to this misinterpretation as well as her inability to verbally communicate. Since she had a history of bilateral knee pain, staff focused on physical assessments on the knees and may not have been alarmed by some pain behaviors associated with movement. Since the pain behaviors were present on the first day of data collection it is still unclear how long she had pain from the hip fracture. It was not until day 22 when she clearly pointed to her left leg when asked about pain and yelled out when touched that an X-ray was ordered. This case highlights some of the challenges in weighing the physical discomfort, psychological stress, and costs of diagnostic tests for people with advanced dementia against the potential for identifying and treating conditions that will improve comfort and quality of life.

In Case B, the staff were able to identify an abrupt change in condition. However, pretty clear cues such as stopping eating, refusing medications, and spitting up yellow phlegm were not followed up with a thorough enough assessment. Assessments focused on possible respiratory or urinary tract infections and no one looked into her mouth until 1 week after the symptoms started. This case also highlights how the tendency for older adults to have a blunted fever response complicates the diagnosis of infection. The resident's pleasant demeanor and persistently smiling countenance may have also contributed to the delayed diagnosis. Research has shown that those residents with more disruptive behaviors such as calling out verbally and physical agitation receive more assessment and treatment than those who are more passive and quiet (Kovach et al. 2006a, b). This case also points to the fact that just because a demented person can consistently verbally communicate some symptom such as back and hemorrhoid pain. Clinicians and caregivers cannot assume that verbal communication will occur for other pain etiologies.

Differentiation of Pain from Other Etiologies: Use of the Serial Trial Intervention (STI)

Since behaviors associated with pain in people with dementia may also indicate other physical or psychosocial unmet needs, the use of a differential assessment and treatment protocol can help to identify the person's unmet need and target treatment more appropriately. The Serial Trial Intervention (STI), developed by our team, was designed for this purpose. The STI is designed to help people in the middle or late stages of dementia. For these people who may be losing their verbal skills and cannot tell you there is a problem, changes in behavior are the only indications that something is wrong. Failure to meet their needs can also have many negative consequences including discomfort for the person, agitated behavior, hospitalizations, resistiveness to care, staff frustration, and death. The STI will be described followed by research results testing use of the STI.

The five steps of the STI are listed in Fig. 10.1. Following identification of behavior change, two levels of targeted assessment and treatment are used. If those steps are not successful in uncovering the problem and successfully treating the person, analgesics and possibly a psychotropic medication are used during Steps 3, 4 and 5. The STI allows assessments and treatments to be customized to the

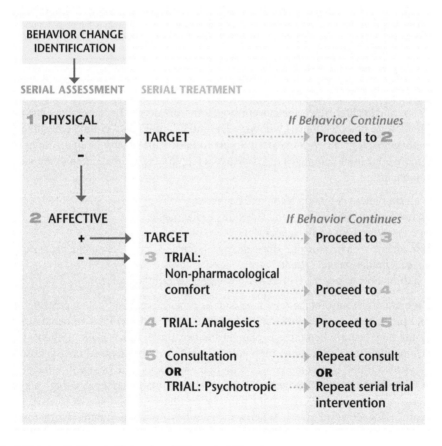

Fig. 10.1 ©Christine R. Kovach, University of Wisconsin-Milwaukee

Table 10.2 Description of steps of the serial trial intervention

Identify *behavioral symptoms* by using an explicit schedule and procedures for the nurse and ancillary staff. When a resident exhibits changes in behavior that are not effectively treated through basic care provided by the ancillary staff the STI is initiated by the nurse. The STI process is stopped when behavioral symptoms decrease by 50% or more. Continued movement through steps of the STI is based on results of assessments and decreases in symptoms by less than 50% in time frames that have been established for specified treatments. If the behavioral symptom continues after completing all five steps, the process is repeated.

STI Step1 Perform *physical needs assessment* that focuses on conditions associated with discomfort. If assessment is positive, a *targeted intervention* is implemented or the appropriate discipline is consulted to begin treatment. If the assessment is negative, or if treatment fails to decrease symptoms by at least 50%, the nurse moves to the next step

STI Step 2 Perform *affective needs assessment* that focuses on needs of people with dementia: (a) environmental stress threshold not exceeded (Wahl and Weisman 2003); (b) balance between sensory stimulating and sensory calming activity throughout the day (Kovach et al. 2004); (c) receipt of meaningful human interaction each day (Taft et al. 1997). If assessment is positive, a *targeted intervention* is implemented or the appropriate discipline is consulted to begin treatment. If the assessment is negative, or if treatment fails to decrease symptoms by at least 50%, the nurse moves to the next step

STI Step 3 Administer a *trial of nonpharmacological comfort treatment(s)*. Treatments used are tailored to the person and the situation, and are based on a list of psychosocial and environmental treatments that have been associated with decreasing agitated behaviors. If a trial of nonpharmacological comfort treatment(s) does not ameliorate behaviors in a time frame likely to show outcomes, the nurse should move to step 4

STI Step 4 Administer a *trial of analgesics* by either administering the prescribed "as needed" (i.e., pro re nata [prn]) analgesic or obtaining orders to escalate a current analgesic. If there is not a response to a trial course of analgesics, consider consultation regarding further escalation or proceed to the next step

STI Step 5 Consult with other disciplines or practitioners (i.e., the nurse practitioner, physician, hospice, geropsychiatry). A *trial of prescribed psychotropic drug* may be administered in this step, if the behavior continues and the nurse and prescriber carefully considers alternatives and weighs the potential for side affects against the comfort needs of the resident

2006 The Author. Copyright held by Christine Kovach

individual's specific health history and current symptoms and needs. Because many nurses working in nursing homes are practical nurses who have had more limited background education in assessment and pathophysiology, providing extra training to these staff or setting up a system in which a nurse with more education completes assessments is recommended. The main components of our training program are:

- Educate all staff about dementia, pain, and behaviors.
- Teach comprehensive physical assessment skills to the nurses.
- Enhance pain assessment and management.
- Teach assessment of environmental stressors, psychological and social unmet needs, and the need for balanced stimulation and retreat.
- Instruct staff on how to use the STI (http://www.ageandcommunity.org/).

We recommend assessing for both pain as well as other changes in behavior using an explicit schedule and procedures for the nurse and ancillary staff to follow. Passive behaviors are often overlooked and may occur when there is pain or another unmet need (Colling 2000). Changes in eating, sleeping, and functional status may indicate pain or other physical or psychosocial problems. We have also found that some people with dementia who have pain will attempt to get out of bed, out of their chair, or off the unit. We have labeled this behavior "exiting" and believe it may be an attempt to get away from their pain. When the person's pain is treated, the exiting behavior ceases (Kovach et al. 2000). When a resident has a change in behavior that is not effectively treated through basic care provided by the ancillary staff, the STI should be initiated by the nurse. Steps of the STI are outlined in Table 10.2 and Fig. 10.1. Continued movement through steps of the STI is based on the results of assessments and failure of symptoms to improve within a reasonable time frame for that treatment. For example, one would expect to see positive response to an analgesic within a shorter time frame than an antibiotic or an antidepressant. Responses to non-pharmacological comfort interventions such as repositioning, distraction, or massage can be evaluated in shorter time frames. If the symptoms continue after completing all five steps, the process is repeated.

Step 1: Physical Assessment

The Step 1 physical needs assessment should focus on conditions associated with pain as well as common conditions seen in this age group. Knowing the resident's clinical history can also aid in targeting the assessment. Common infections in this population are pneumonia, urinary tract infections, and skin and soft tissue infections (Gavazzi and Krause 2002). Undertreated or untreated musculoskeletal or neuropathic pain is frequently uncovered during this physical assessment. In our training program at the University of Wisconsin-Milwaukee, in additional to teaching registered and practical nurses assessment of musculoskeletal pain and common infections, we emphasize training nurses in the assessment of neuropathic pain, symptoms of arterial and venous insufficiency, abnormal lung sounds, and common skin disorders. If the assessment is positive, a targeted intervention is implemented or the appropriate health care provider is consulted to decide on a possible treatment. Since the care of those with advanced illness involves considering the benefits and risks of treatment in light of overall goals of an individual, it is not expected that each new physical assessment change will be treated.

Step 2: Assessing Environmental Stress

Dementia decreases the threshold for tolerating stress from the environment (Hall and Buckwalter 1987; Lawton 1986, See also Stoney 2011). Response to excessive environmental stress is agitation and decreased function (Beck et al. 2002). Environmental stress may come from auditory, visual, tactile, taste, or olfactory stimuli. As outlined in Table 10.1, Step 2 includes an assessment of environmental stress, including whether there is a balance between sensory-stimulating and sensory-calming activity throughout the day, and whether the person has received therapeutic human interaction each day.

People with dementia are also vulnerable to both under stimulation and stimulus inundation (Kovach 2000; Kovach and Schlidt 2001; Kovach and Wells 2002). In a randomized controlled trial with 78 participants, nursing home residents with dementia who received an intervention that controlled the person's daily activity schedule so that there was a balance between the person's high-arousal and low-arousal states had significantly less agitation than the control group (Kovach et al. 2004).

Step 2 of the STI also directs the nurse to determine if each person is receiving at least 10 min of meaningful human interaction a minimum of 2 times each day. For the purpose of meeting an individual's need for meaningful human interaction, we stipulate that the one-on-one interaction must have the central purpose of making a therapeutic human connection. Chatting calmly with the person while providing a bath may be quite therapeutic. However, this would not meet the requirement since the central purpose is not to make a therapeutic human connection. Examples of therapeutic human connections are socializing, providing a hand massage, and reminiscing. Individual

Table 10.3 Psychosocial and environmental treatments associated with decreasing agitated and pain behaviors in people with dementia

Nonpharmacolgical treatments	
Providing a rummage box	Exercise group
Assisting person up to wheelchair	Ambulating with staff
Cooking group	Providing a basket of laundry for the person to fold
Scrubbing vegetables	1:1 visiting/therapeutic communication
Reminiscence activity	Reading poetry
Providing magazines to browse	Doing a spiritual intervention
Aromatherapy	Pet therapy
Music therapy	Baking bread
Holding a "coffee club"	Gardening
Art activity	Changing environment/move to a different room
Watching television	Watching a bird aviary or fish tank
Viewing a film	Providing a quiet environment/quiet time
Cueing/redirecting	Hugging
Massaging hands or feet	Providing a warm foot soak
Providing a sweater or blanket	Providing fluids
Providing a snack	Assisting person to the bathroom
Providing time for a nap	Providing personal hygiene assistance
Applying a heating pad	

Note: many of these items listed take less than 10 min to complete

preferences are determined whenever possible and needed interactions are "ordered" by the nurse and completion is recorded along with other treatments given in the medical record.

Step 3: Nonpharmacological Comfort Treatments

In Step 3 a trial of nonpharmacological comfort treatments, tailored to the individual and the situation, is given to the patient. We provide staff with the list of common psychosocial and environmental treatments (see also Table 10.3). These treatments have been empirically or anecdotally associated with decreasing agitated and pain behaviors, are low cost, and most can be completed in 10 min or less. All of these nonpharmacological comfort interventions require additional testing for efficacy.

Step 4: Administration of Analgesics

Step 4 involves the administration of the resident's prescribed "as needed" (i.e., *pro re nata [prn]*) analgesic, or obtaining orders to escalate a current analgesic. If there is not a response to a trial course of analgesics, nurses are encouraged to consult with the prescriber or supervisor regarding the need for further escalation of analgesic drug or dose. Step 5 involves consulting with other disciplines or practitioners (e.g., nurse practitioner, physician, hospice, geropsychiatry) and possibly administering a trial of a prescribed psychotropic drug. The potential side effects of psychotropic drugs must be weighed against using alternative nonpharmacological treatments and attaining comfort for the resident. A consensus statement on treatment options for dementia-related symptoms of severe agitation and aggression, published in 2008, provides a helpful overview of potential risks and indications for use (Salzman et al. 2008).

In a randomized controlled trial, with blinded data collectors, the group of residents receiving care using the STI ($n = 57$) had less discomfort ($F = 9.64$ ($p < 0.001$) df (2,109)) and were more likely to resolve behavioral symptoms (Fisher's $p = 0.002$) than control group participants ($n = 57$). In total, 93% of the participants who received the STI had improvement in behavioral symptoms of 50% or more as recorded by the nurse. Also, the treatment group received more physical assessment ($Z = 8.051$, $p < 0.001$), affective assessment ($Z = 7.518$, $p < 0.001$), and pharmacological intervention ($Z = 4.383$, $p < 0.001$) than the control group. There was not a statistically significant difference between the groups in the use of nonpharmacological interventions ($Z = 1.045$, $p = 0.296$). In addition, nurses using the STI displayed more persistence in assessing and treating than control nurses ($Z = 7.014$, $p < 0.001$) (Kovach et al. 2006a, b).

The behaviors that were most frequently initiated in the STI were nonspecific vocalizations, combative and resistive behaviors, restless body movement, and specific verbal complaints. Examples of verbal complaints were specific complaints of hunger, thirst, pain, or the need for assistance. Most of the participants had more than one behavioral symptom ($n = 30$, 53%). Twenty participants had two symptoms, nine had three, and one patient had four symptoms that led to initiating the STI (Mean $= 1.75$ behaviors per participants, SD $= 0.80$). The behaviors that initiated the STI in this sample may also represent symptoms that got noticed or were considered problematic by the staff.

Of the 32 verbal participants in this study (i.e., nonspecific vocalizations or specific verbal complaint), 17 also had nonverbal behaviors (53%). Of that 17, only 1 stated a specific verbal complaint (6%). In contrast, of the 15 verbal participants who did not have nonverbal behaviors, 8 (53%) were able to verbally communicate a specific complaint. These results are consistent with other research findings that behaviors are a way to express unmet need when verbal communication skills are lost (Beck and Vogelpohl 1999; Mahoney et al. 1999; Weiner et al. 1999; Feldt 2000; Kovach et al. 2001).

Use of each component of the intervention was examined. As a result of Step 1 assessment, 49 positive physical assessment findings were found in 23 of the 57 treatment group participants (40%). Changes in activity, musculoskeletal and urinary tract problems were the most frequent behaviors observed. Four urinary tract infections and three cases of pneumonia were diagnosed based on assessment findings. One person had both pneumonia and a urinary tract infection.

Only 7 of the 23 people with a positive assessment finding received a targeted intervention in Step 1 (30%). Four of the six participants with infections were given antibiotics. The literature is equivocal on whether antibiotics for people with advanced dementia improve comfort or prolong survival (Hurley et al. 1993; van der Steen et al. 2002). Seven participants displayed clear signs or symptoms of pain. This included specific verbal complaint of pain, pain or stiffness during movement, symptoms of peripheral neuropathy, and rubbing of body parts during the physical assessment. Only two of these participants received analgesics as a part of the Step 1 intervention and nonpharmacological comfort interventions were not used. Four received analgesics finally at Step 4 and 1 was not given an analgesic for symptoms of knee stiffness while standing.

Of the 39 participants who had their affective needs assessed in Step 2, 13 (33%) had a positive finding indicating either too much environmental stress ($n = 10$), an imbalance in the pacing of sensory stimulating and sensory calming activity (excessive stimulation $= 2$; not enough stimulation $= 1$) or too little meaningful human interaction ($n = 2$). Of the 13 participants with a positive affective assessment, 11 (85%) received one or more targeted treatments.

Step 3, of the nonpharmacological intervention trial, was given to 29 participants. Therapeutic communication and verbal cueing were the most frequently used nonpharmacological interventions. A trial of analgesics was given to 20 participants and three of these participants received a second escalation of analgesics. The majority of analgesics given were nonnarcotics (20 of 26 new prescriptions). Five individuals received a trial of psychotropic medication and five participants were forwarded for consultation.

When testing the efficacy of multicomponent interventions, it is difficult to discern the effect of specific components on outcomes. To begin to understand the contribution of each component, we calculated the percentage of participants who received treatment at each step of the STI including those that showed improvement in behavioral symptoms of 50% or more as recorded by the nurse. Targeted treatments given in response to positive physical assessment findings were followed by improvements in behavior for 6 of 7 patients treated (85.7%). Step 2 targeted treatments for affective needs yielded improvement in behavioral symptoms for 8 of 11 treated (73%). Trials of nonpharmacological treatments were perceived to be effective for 18 of 29 participants (62.1%). Nonpharmacological treatments were effective for many in Steps 1 and 3 and carried fewer potential side effects (Michocki 2001). Trials of analgesics were perceived to be highly effective, yielding an improvement in behavioral symptoms for 75% (15 of 20) of participants. Most analgesics given were either short-acting nonnarcotics or drugs that combine an opioid with acetaminophen. The continued reliance of prescribers on acetaminophen and nonsteroidal anti-inflammatory (NSAIDs) should be questioned because the analgesic ceiling for acetaminophen limits the number of tablets an individual can take before significantly increasing the risk of liver damage (Doyle and Woodruff 2004). In 2011, the Food and Drug Administration (FDA) announced that it was asking drug companies to limit the amount of acetaminophen in all prescription products that combine the drug with other medications to no more than 325 mg per tablet or capsule. Sandra Kweder of the FDA said, "Overdose from prescription combination products containing acetaminophen account for nearly half of all cases of acetaminophen-related liver failure in the United States, many of which result in liver transplant or death" (Stein 2011). Also long-acting opioids are recommended for chronic pain to maintain serum levels, and decrease breakthrough pain and intermittent sedation (American Pain Society 1997; Joranson et al. 2000).

A trial of psychotropic medication was followed by improvement in behavioral symptoms for 4 participants (80%), and 2 of the 5 who received additional care following consultation (40%) had improvement. In addition to the serious side effects associated with some psychotropic drugs, use of these medications may decrease the person's capacity to display behavioral symptoms that can communicate pain or another unmet need. The perceived effectiveness of each of the five steps of the STI for a portion of the sample suggests that a multidimensional approach is preferable to simply using a pain scale to identity and pain.

Those participants who were vocals (e.g., complaining, yelling, moaning, specific verbal complaint) received more care than those who expressed symptoms through nonvocal behaviors. Those with vocal symptoms averaged assessment of 6.1 body systems (SD = 3.1) compared to 4.6 (SD = 2.9) for the nonvocal (t (54) = −1.68, one-tailed p = 0.049). Vocal residents were also more likely to receive a new pharmacological interventions (phi correlation coefficient for nominal 2 × 2 contingency = 0.241, p = 0.035), but there was not a difference in use of nonpharmacological interventions between vocal and nonvocal groups. These findings seem to indicate that people who are more vocal get more noticed.

Challenges and Barriers

The American Pain Society has recommended that pain be regarded as the fifth vital sign. Conducting pain assessment with vital signs may not be feasible in many long-term care settings that measure vital signs infrequently. Results of a Delphi survey indicate that one sample of experienced long-term care staff perceived optimum frequency for pain assessment as only "on admission" followed by "as needed dependent on medical diagnosis and/or condition" (Molony et al. 2005). Pain assessment is impeded by a lack of utilization of pain assessment tools, lack of understanding of pain behaviors, and a lack of routinized assessment for pain and behavior. There is also a need for family caregivers to have in-depth knowledge and a strategy for implementing basic pain assessment in at-risk community dwelling residents with dementia.

Research suggests that there is often a disconnect between the patient's subjective experience of pain, their reporting of pain, and assessment findings and pain treatment by clinicians. McCaffery et al. (2000) found that nurses' personal opinions about the patient's pain were stronger determinants of opioid dose than documented assessments. One study by the Veterans Health Administration found that measuring pain as the fifth vital sign did not improve quality of pain management. Patients with substantial pain documented by the fifth vital sign often had inadequate pain management (Mularski et al. 2006). Lack of communication and trust between physicians and nurses also impedes treatment (Kaasalainen et al. 2007; Cunningham 2006). Bowers et al. (2001) found that a consequence of nurses perceived time constraints was forgoing the "should-do" to complete the "must-do" work. If pain management is thought of as "should-do" work, as suggested in a study of nurse decision making (Kaasalainen et al. 2007), pain treatment will be inadequate.

Treatment is also impeded by prescribing practices. There continues to be a reluctance to administer opioids to people with dementia and a reliance on short-acting analgesics for chronic pain (Kaasalainen et al. 2007; Kovach et al. 2006b; See also Hallenbeck 2011; See also Palermo 2011). Heightened scrutiny by the U.S. Drug Enforcement Administration's (DEA) of prescribing practices in nursing homes across America may also be delaying and impeding treatment. The Controlled Substances Act requires physicians to write out, sign, and fax prescription for all pain medications, instead of allowing nursing home nurses to take verbal or verbal telephone direction from physicians to order and administer medication, as is done in hospitals (Rannazzisi 2010). U.S. Senator Herb Kohl, Chairman of the Special Committee on Aging, remarked "The hours it may take for a nursing home to fully comply with DEA regulations can feel like an eternity to an elderly nursing home resident who is waiting for relief from excruciating pain. It is safe to say that most laws are created to prevent suffering. In the case of the DEA's recent crackdown of nursing homes, it appears that the law exacerbates it" (United States Senate Special Committee on Aging 2010).

Recommendations and Conclusion

Deficits in recognizing behavior change, identifying behavior change as a symptom of pain, assessment skill, and lack of knowledge of an array of therapeutic interventions are associated with inadequate pain management of people with dementia. Competence of staff needs to be improved through training, through requiring that more registered nurses provide care in nursing homes, and through the wide-scale transfer of empirically validated interventions such as the STI to clinical care provided in the nursing home. This intervention is not costly, is replicable and effective and has been associated with no serious side effects. The diffusion of this intervention into practice, particularly in poor-performing homes, will not be far-reaching without organized efforts such as federal implementation programs.

Additional research is needed to provide similar systems for assessment and treatment to community dwelling people with dementia and for use in acute care situations. There is a lack of understanding of the degree to which health disparities and access to care issues are potential contributors to inadequate pain assessment and management in this population.

Research to develop new analgesics that are safe and effective, particularly to treat musculoskeletal and neuropathic pain, is needed. There is also a need to expand the repertoire of nonpharmacological interventions that are effective and that are used to treat common pain ailments.

In conclusion, while improvements in the recognition and treatment of pain in older adults with dementia have occurred, there remains need for substantial improvements. Efforts need to target continuing education, research, and public policy change.

References

American Geriatrics Society Panel on Persistent Pain in Older Persons. (2002). The management of persistent pain in older persons. *Journal of the American Geriatrics Society, 50*, 1–20.

American Pain Society. (1997). The use of opioids for the treatment of chronic pain. A consensus statement from the American Academy of Pain Medicine and the American Pain Society. *The Clinical Journal of Pain, 13*, 6–8.

Beck, C. K., Vogelpohl, T. S. (1999). Problematic vocalizations in institutionalized individuals with dementia. *J Gerontol Nurs, 25*, 17–26; quiz 48, 51.

Beck, C. K., Vogelpohl, T. S., Rasin, J. H., Uriri, J. T., O'Sullivan, P., Walls, R., Phillips, R., & Baldwin, B. (2002). Effects of behavioral interventions on disruptive behavior and affect in demented nursing home residents. *Nursing Research, 51*(4), 219–228.

Benedetti, F., Vighetti, S., Ricco, C., Lagna, E., Bergamasco, B., Pinessi, L., & Rainero, I. (1999). Pain threshold and tolerance in Alzheimer's disease. *Pain, 80*(1–2), 377–382.

Bowers, B. J., Lauring, C., & Jacobson, N. (2001). How nurses manage time and work in long-term care facilities. *Journal of Advanced Nursing, 33*(4), 484–491.

Chang, R. W., Dunlop, D., Gibbs, J., & Hughes, S. (1995). The determinants of walking velocity in the elderly. An evaluation using regression trees. *Arthritis and Rheumatism, 38*(3), 343–350.

Chow, T. W. (2000). Personality in frontal lobe disorder Psychiatry. *Reports, 2*(5), 446–451.

Closs, S. J., Barr, B., Briggs, M., Cash, K., & Seers, K. (2004). A comparison of five pain assessment scales for nursing home residents with varying degrees of cognitive impairment. *Journal of Pain and Symptom Management, 27*, 196–205.

Cohen-Mansfield, J., & Lipson, S. (2002). Pain in cognitively impaired nursing home residents: How well are physicians diagnosing it? *Journal of the American Geriatrics Society, 50*(6), 1039–1044.

Colling, K. B. (2000). A taxonomy of passive behaviors in people with Alzheimer's disease. *Journal of Nursing Scholarship, 32*, 239–244.

Cunningham, C. (2006). Determining whether to give pain relief to people with dementia: The impact of verbal and written communication on the decision to administer "as required" analgesia to people with dementia in care homes. *Alzheimer's Care Quarterly, 7*(2), 95–103.

Dickson, D. W. (2001). Neuropathology of Alzheimer's disease and other dementias. *Clinics in Geriatric Medicine, 17*, 209–228.

Doyle, D., & Woodruff, R. (2004). *The IAHPC manual of palliative care*. Houston: International Association for Hospice and Palliative Care.

Feldt, K. S. (2000). The checklist of nonverbal pain indicators (CNPI). *Pain Management Nursing, 1*(1), 13–21.

Ferrell, B. A. (1995). Pain evaluation and management in the nursing home. *Annals of Internal Medicine, 123*(9), 681–687.

Fisher-Morris, M., & Gellatly, A. (1997). The experience and expression of pain in Alzheimer's patients. *Age and Ageing, 26*, 497–500.

Fries, B. E., Simon, S. E., Morris, J. N., Flodstrom, C., & Bookstein, F. L. (2001). Pain in US nursing homes: Validating a pain scale for the minimum data set. *Gerontologist, 41*(2), 173–179.

Gavazzi, G., & Krause, K. H. (2002). Ageing and infection. *The Lancet Infectious Diseases, 2*, 659–666.

Hadjistavropoulos, T., Keela, H., Turk, D. C., Fine, P. G., Dworkin, R. H., Helme, R., Jackson, K., et al. (2007). An interdisciplinary expert consensus statement on assessment of pain in older persons. *The Clinical Journal of Pain, 23*, S1–S43.

Hall, G. R., & Buckwalter, K. C. (1987). Progressively lowered stress threshold: A conceptual model for care of adults with Alzheimer's disease. *Archives of Psychiatric Nursing, 1*(6), 399–406.

Hallenbeck, J. (2011). Pain and intercultural communication. In R. J. Moore (Ed.), *Handbook of pain and palliative care*. New York: Springer.

Herr, K. (2002). Pain assessment in cognitively impaired older adults. *The American Journal of Nursing, 102*, 65–67.

Herr, K., Bjoro, K., & Decker, S. (2006). Tools for assessment of pain in nonverbal older adults with dementia: A state of the science review. *Journal of Pain and Symptom Management, 31*(2), 170–192.

Herr, K., & Decker, S. (2004). Assessment of pain in older adults with severe cognitive impairment. *Annals of Long Term Care, 12*(4), 46–52.

Hindley, N. J., Jobst, K. A., King, E., Barnetson, L., Smith, A., & Haigh, A. M. (1995). High acceptability and low morbidity of diagnostic lumbar puncture in elderly subjects of mixed cognitive status. *Acta Neurologica Scandinavica, 91*, 405–411.

Horgas, A. L., & Dunn, K. (2001). Pain in nursing home residents. Comparison of residents' self-report and nursing assistants' perceptions. Incongruencies exist in resident and caregiver reports of pain; therefore, pain management education is needed to prevent suffering. *Journal of Gerontological Nursing, 27*(3), 44–53.

Hurley, A. C., Volicer, B., Mahoney, M. A., & Volicer, L. (1993). Palliative fever management in Alzheimer patients: Quality plus fiscal responsibility. *Advances in Nursing Science, 16*, 21–32.

Joranson, D. E., Ryan, K. M., Gilson, A. M., & Dahl, J. L. (2000). Trends in medical use and abuse of opioid analgesics. *The Journal of the American Medical Association, 283*, 1710–1714.

Kaasalainen, S., Coker, E., Dolovich, L., Papaioannou, A., Hadjistavropoulos, T., Emil, A., & Ploeg, J. (2007). Pain management decision making among long-term care physicians and nurses. *Western Journal of Nursing Research, 29*(5), 561–580.

Kovach, C. R. (2000). Sensoristasis and imbalance in persons with dementia. *Journal of Nursing Scholarship, 32*(4), 379–384.

Kovach, C. R., Cashin, J. R., & Sauer, L. (2006a). Deconstruction of a complex tailored intervention to assess and treat discomfort of people with advanced dementia. *Journal of Advanced Nursing, 55*(6), 678–688.

Kovach, C. R., Griffie, J., Muchka, S., Noonan, P. E., & Weissman, D. E. (2000). Nurses' perceptions of pain assessment and treatment in the cognitively impaired. *Clinical Nurse Specialist, 14*(5), 215–220.

Kovach, C. R., Logan, B., Joosse, L., & Noonan, P. E. (2011). Failure to identify behavioral symptoms of people with dementia and the need for follow-up physical assessment. *Research in Gerontological Nursing, 18*, 1–5.

Kovach, C. R., Logan, B., Noonan, P. E., Schlidt, A. M., Smerz, J., Simpson, M., & Wells, T. (2006b). Effects of the serial trial intervention on discomfort and behavior in demented nursing home residents. *American Journal of Alzheimer's Disease and Other Dementias, 21*(3), 147–155.

Kovach, C. R., Logan, B. R., Simpson, M. R., & Reynolds, S. A. (2010). Factors associated with time to identify physical problems of nursing home residents with dementia. *American Journal of Alzheimer's Disease and Other Dementias, 25*(4), 317–323.

Kovach, C. R., Noonan, P. E., Griffie, J., Muchka, S., & Weissman, D. E. (2001). Use of the assessment of discomfort in dementia protocol. *Applied Nursing Research, 14*, 193–200.

Kovach, C. R., & Schlidt, A. M. (2001). The agitation activity interface of people with dementia in long-term care. *American Journal of Alzheimer's Disease and Other Dementias, 16*(4), 240–246.

Kovach, C. R., Taneli, Y., Dohearty, P., Schlidt, A. M., Cashin, S., & Silva-Smith, A. L. (2004). Effect of the BACE (Balancing Activity Controls Excesses) intervention on agitation of people with dementia. *Gerontologist, 44*(6), 797–806.

Kovach, C. R., & Wells, T. (2002). Pacing of activity as a predictor of agitation for people with dementia in acute care. *Journal of Gerontological Nursing, 28*(1), 28–35.

Lawton, M. P. (1986). *Environment and aging*. Albany: Center for the Study of Aging.

Liebeskind, J. C. (1991). Pain can kill. *Pain, 44*(1), 3–4.

Mahoney, E. K., Hurley, A. C., Volicer, L., Bell, M., Gianotis, P., Hartshorn, M., Lane, P., Lesperance, R., Macdonald, S., Novakoff, L., Rheaume, Y., Timms, R., & Warden, V. (1999). Development and testing of the resistiveness to care scale. *Research in Nursing & Health, 22*, 27–38.

Martin, R., Williams, J., Hadjistavropoulos, T., Hadjistavropoulos, H. D., & MacLean, M. (2005). A qualitative investigation of seniors' and caregivers' views on pain assessment and management. *Canadian Journal of Nursing Research, 37*(2), 142–164.

McCaffery, M., Ferrell, B. R., & Pasero, C. (2000). Nurses' personal opinions about patients' pain and their effect on recorded assessments and titration of opioid doses. *Pain Management Nursing, 1*, 79–87.

Michocki, R. J. (2001). Polypharmacy and principles of drug therapy. In A. M. Adelman & M. P. Daly (Eds.), *20 common problems in geristrics*. New York: McGraw-Hill Publishers.

Molony, S. L., Kobayashi, M., Holleran, E. A., & Mezey, M. (2005). Assessing pain as a fifth vital sign in long-term care facilities: Recommendations from the field. *Journal of Gerontological Nursing, 31*(3), 16–24.

Morrison, R. S., & Siu, A. L. (2000). A comparison of pain and its treatment in advanced dementia and cognitively intact patients with hip fracture. *Journal of Pain and Symptom Management, 19*, 240–248.

Moss, P. (1997). Negotiating spaces in home environments: Older women living with arthritis. *Social Science & Medicine, 45*(1), 23–33.

Mularski, R. A., White-Chu, F., Overbay, D., Miller, L., Asch, S. M., & Ganzini, L. (2006). Measuring pain as the 5th vital sign does not improve quality of pain management. *Journal of General Internal Medicine, 21*(6), 607–612.

Palermo, Y. (2011). The art of pain: The patient's perspective of chronic pain. In R. J. Moore (Ed.), *Handbook of pain and palliative care*. New York: Springer.

Porter, F. L., Malhotra, K. M., Wolf, C. M., Morris, J. C., Miller, J. P., & Smith, M. C. (1996). Dementia and response to pain in the elderly. *Pain, 68*(2–3), 413–421.

Price, D. D. (2000). Psychological and neural mechanisms of the affective dimension of pain. *Science, 288*, 1769–1772.

Proctor, W., & Hirdes, J. (2001). Pain and cognitive status among nursing home residents in Canada. *Pain Research & Management, 6*, 119–125.

Rannazzisi, J. (2010). *Statement of before the Special Committee on Aging United States entitled, "The war on drugs meets the war on pain: Nursing home patients caught in the crossfire" presented on March 24, 2010*. Retrieved October 4, 2010, from http://www.justice.gov/dea/speeches/100324_rannazzis_hearing.PDF.

Rub, U., Del Tredici, K., Del Turco, D., & Braak, H. (2002). The intralaminar nuclei assigned to the medial pain system and other components of this system are early and progressively affected by the Alzheimer's disease-related cytoskeletal pathology. *Journal of Chemical Neuroanatomy, 23*, 279–290.

Salzman, C., Jeste, D. V., Meyer, R. E., Cohen-Mansfield, J., Cummings, J., Grossberg, G. T., Jarvik, L., Kraemer, H. C., Lebowitz, B. D., Maslow, K., Pollock, B. G., Raskind, M., Schultz, S. K., Wang, P., Zito, J. M., & Zubenko, G. S. (2008). Elderly patients with dementia-related symptoms of severe agitation and aggression: Consensus statement on treatment options, clinical trials methodology, and policy. *The Journal of Clinical Psychiatry, 69*(6), 889–898.

Scherder, E., & Bouma, A. (2000). Visual analogue scales for pain assessment in Alzheimer's disease. *Gerontology, 46*, 47–53.

Scherder, E., Bouma, A., Borkent, M., & Rahman, O. (1999). Alzheimer patients report less pain intensity and pain affect than non-demented elderly. *Psychiatry, 62*(3), 265–272.

Scherder, E., Oosterman, J., Swaab, D., Herr, K., Ooms, M., Ribbe, M., Sergeant, J., Pickering, G., & Benedetti, F. (2005). Recent developments in pain in dementia. *British Medical Journal, 330*, 461–464.

Schuler, M., Njoo, N., Hestermann, M., Oster, P., & Hauer, K. (2004). Acute and chronic pain in geriatrics: Clinical characteristics of pain and the influence of cognition. *Pain Medicine, 5*(3), 253–262.

Stein, R. (2011). *FDA targets acetaminophen amounts delivered in prescription painkillers.* The Washington Post. Retrieved January 18, 2011, from http://www.washingtonpost.com/wp-dyn/content/article/2011/01/13/AR2011011306675.html.

Stoney, C. (2011). Stress and pain. In R. J. Moore (Ed.), *Handbook of pain and palliative care.* New York: Springer.

Taft, L.B., Fazio, S., Seman, D., & Stansell, J. (1997). A psychosocial model of dementia care: theoretical and empirical support. *Archives of Psychiatric Nursing 11*(1), 13–20.

Tsai, P. F., Chang, J. Y. (2004). Assessment of pain in elders with dementia. *Medsurg Nurs, 13*(6):364–369; 390

United States Senate Special Committee on Aging. (2010). *U.S. Sen. Kohl: Examines effects of DEA crackdown on nursing home delivery of pain medication* [Press release]. Retrieved October 4, 2010, from http://aging.senate.gov/record.cfm?id=323379.

Van der steen, J. T., Ooms, M. E., Van der wal, G., Ribbe, M. W. (2002). Pneumonia: The demented patient's best friend Discomfort after starting or withholding antibiotic treatment. *J Am Geriatr Soc, 50*, 1681–1688.

Wahl, H. & Weisman, G.D. (2003). Environmental gerontology at the start of the new millennium: reflections on its historical, empirical 616–627.

Weiner, D., Peterson, B., & Keefe, F. (1999). Chronic pain-associated behaviors in the nursing home: Resident versus caregiver perceptions. *Pain, 80*, 577–588.

Williams, C., Zimmerman, S., Sloan, P., & Reed, P. (2005). Characteristics associated with pain in long-term care residents with dementia. *Gerontologist, 45*, 68–73.

Won, A., Lapane, K., Gambassi, G., Bernabei, R., Mor, V., & Lipsitz, L. A. (1999). Correlates and management of nonmalignant pain in the nursing home. SAGE Study Group. Systematic assessment of geriatric drug use via epidemiology. *Journal of the American Geriatrics Society, 47*(8), 936–942.

Part III
Common Pain Conditions

Chapter 11
Pediatric Chronic Pain

Thomas R. Vetter

Introduction

Pediatric chronic pain has extensive and frequently sustained detrimental effects on the health, development and quality of life of young people, with an attendant adverse impact on all those invested in their well-being (Gold et al. 2009; Vetter 2008). It has long been appreciated that the optimal management of pediatric chronic pain addresses its equally important biological, psychological, and social components (Kozlowska et al. 2008; Varni et al. 1995; Zeltzer et al. 1997a). Nevertheless, despite significant advances in its management, pediatric chronic pain remains underdiagnosed, undertreated, and misunderstood (Walker 2008). In addition to the marked developmental continuum across the pediatric age range, this discrepancy is largely due to the complexity and diversity of pediatric chronic pain and resulting clinical disconnect between its biomedical and psychosocial elements (Eccleston and Clinch 2007).

This discussion will first present two theoretical models whose tenets and constructs form the basis and justification for a biopsychosocial approach to the management of pediatric chronic pain. The utility and perhaps the necessity of incorporating pediatric health-related quality as a multidimensional clinical measure will in turn be examined. Published biopsychosocial data on the types of pediatric patients who are typically referred to a pediatric pain medicine clinic will then be reviewed. Qualitative survey data on the pediatric chronic pain experience and its attendant personal narrative will also be reviewed in further support of its biopsychosocial nature. Finally, against the backdrop of the overall goal of multidisciplinary pediatric pain management, a brief synopsis of currently available evidence-based best practices, including biomedical and psychosocial modalities, will be provided. Potential areas for future research will lastly be highlighted. Of note, for the sake of brevity, this discussion will focus on the older child and adolescent and not include the neonate.

A Multidimensional Biobehavioral Model of Pediatric Pain

Current thinking considers chronic pain to be a multidimensional construct that includes biological, psychological, and social components (Turk and Flor 1999; Turk and Monarch 2002). A multidimensional Biobehavioral Model of Pediatric Pain (Fig. 11.1) (Varni 1995; Varni et al. 1995) was

T.R. Vetter, MD, MPH (✉)
Division of Pain Medicine, Department of Anesthesiology, University of Alabama School
of Medicine, 619 South 19th Street, JT-862, Birmingham, AL 35249-6810, USA
e-mail: tvetter@uab.edu

R.J. Moore (ed.), *Handbook of Pain and Palliative Care: Biobehavioral Approaches for the Life Course*,
DOI 10.1007/978-1-4419-1651-8_11, © Springer Science+Business Media, LLC 2012

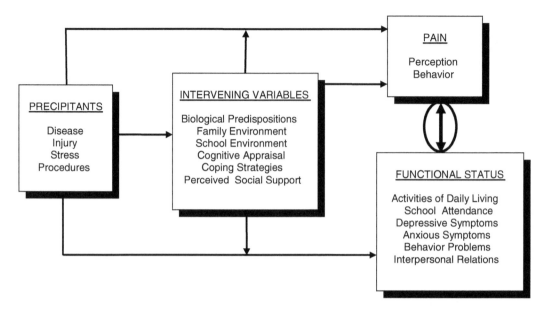

Fig. 11.1 A hypothesized multidimensional biobehavioral model of pediatric pain developed to account for the complex and individual pediatric chronic pain experience. Adapted from Varni et al. (1996b), p. 180. © 1996 by Plenum Publishing. Reprinted with permission

developed in an attempt to account for the frequently observed variability in pediatric pain perception, pain behavior, and functional status in children with ostensibly a comparable disease, injury, or procedural burden (Varni et al. 1996b). This multidimensional biobehavioral (biopsychosocial) model was predicated on there being a number of potentially modifiable precipitants and intervening factors that contribute to pediatric pain perception and a child's associated functional status and health-related quality of life (Varni 1995; Varni et al. 1995). It was likewise hypothesized that a bidirectional relationship and effect exist between pain perception and pain behavior and functional status. As Varni et al. (1996b) noted:

> This theoretical framework is further delineated into pain antecedents, which have a causal role in pain onset or exacerbate pain intensity, pain concomitants (e.g., depression, anxiety), which occur only during a painful episode and which may be reciprocal, and pain consequences, which persist beyond pain relief and include long-term psychological, social, and physical disability (p. 516).

The validity of this multidimensional Biobehavioral Model of Pediatric Pain was examined in children and adolescents with symptomatic juvenile idiopathic arthritis (JIA) and a variety of other pediatric rheumatic diseases (Sawyer et al. 2004, 2005; von Weiss et al. 2002). A strong negative relationship was observed between children's self-reported pain intensity with JIA and their self-reported health-related quality of life, including various aspects of functional status (Sawyer et al. 2005). In contrast, effective pain coping strategies in children with JIA have a significant positive effect on the physical, emotional, and social functioning domains that comprise their health-related quality of life (Sawyer et al. 2004). Fewer daily environmental hassles and greater social support from classmates and parents were significant predictors of less adjustment problems and depression in children with a pediatric rheumatic disease (von Weiss et al. 2002).

Since the initial proposal of Varni's biobehavioral (biopsychosocial) model, data have been published supporting that the school environment is an additional key intervening variable in the interrelationship of pediatric pain, its precipitants, and resulting functional status (Fig. 11.1) (Kashikar-Zuck et al. 2007; Logan et al. 2008b, 2009). When this Biobehavioral Model of Pediatric Pain was also applied in a predominantly African-American sample of adolescents residing in an urban school system, a significant relationship was observed between anxiety and psychosocial stress and the experience of headache and abdominal pain (White and Farrell 2006). Of note, the Biobehavioral Model of Pediatric Pain is commensurate with the ongoing commitment of the American Academy of Pediatrics (AAP) to the prevention, early detection, and management of behavioral, developmental, and social problems as a priority in present pediatric practice (American Academy of Pediatrics 2001).

The Family Stress Model

In an effort to optimize contemporary pediatric healthcare, attention has also been focused by the AAP on the greater compositional diversity and functional dynamics of the contemporary American family (Schor 2003). The Family Stress Model (Conger et al. 2000) implicitly guided the AAP in generating its current *Family Pediatrics: Report of the Task Force on the Family* (Schor 2003). The Family Stress Model (Fig. 11.2) is predicated upon the intrinsic interrelationship between socioeconomic status, family processes, and human development. The model acknowledges the strong correlation between lower socioeconomic status (with its attendant economic hardships) and disparities in the cognitive, social, emotional, and physical health and well-being of children, adolescents, and young adults (Conger et al. 2000; Conger and Donnellan 2007). In addressing the resulting detrimental clinical outcomes, the Family Stress Model seeks to identify the biological, psychological, and social resources vs. vulnerabilities that may reduce or intensify the economic stress process (Conger et al. 2000).

The Family Stress Model is quite germane to understanding the pediatric chronic pain experience, given that family, parental, and situational factors are widely held to play a major integrative role in the natural history of pediatric chronic illness and specifically, the development and perpetuation of chronic pain (Fig. 11.3) (Chambers 2003; Chambers et al. 2002; McGrath and Hillier 2003; Palermo and Chambers 2005). Moreover, contending with a child who is suffering from a chronic medical condition, especially one that is associated with chronic pain and disability, is also a potent parental and family stressor (Eccleston et al. 2004; Jordan 2005). A survey of 533 parents of chronically ill children revealed 45% of them to have health-related quality-of-life impairment, across the domains of sleep, social functioning, daily activities, vitality, positive emotions, and depressive emotions – supporting the need for a family-centered approach in pediatrics (Hatzmann et al. 2008).

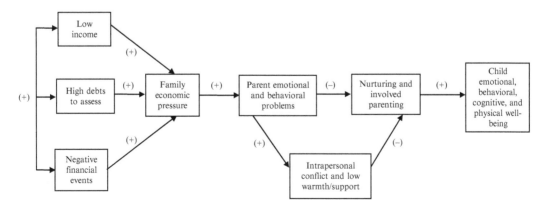

Fig. 11.2 The family stress model applied by the American Academy of Pediatrics *Task Force on the Family* and germane to the pediatric chronic pain experience. From Conger and Donnellan (2007), p. 180. Reprinted, with permission, from the Annual Review of Psychology, Vol. 58. © 2007 by Annual Reviews www.annualreviews.org

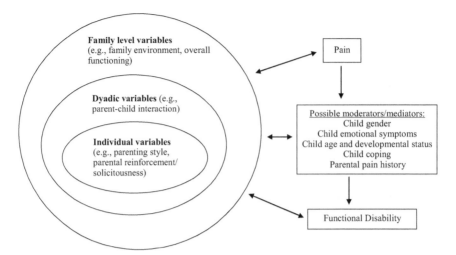

Fig. 11.3 Integrative model of parent and family factors in pediatric chronic pain and its associated disability. From Palermo and Chambers (2005), p. 3. © 2007 by International Association for the Study of Pain. Reprinted with permission from the Elsevier B.V

An effective biopsychosocial approach to pediatric pain is also commensurate with the family-centered pediatric healthcare model that has also been promulgated by the AAP (2003).

Current Consensus on the Factors Associated with Pediatric Chronic Pain and Disability

Pediatric chronic pain can have a widespread impact on many aspects of daily living for patients and their families. The actual prevalence of pain and disability in the pediatric populations is not known. The majority of children who do report pain do not tend to show extensive distress and disability. Recent evidence suggests that pediatric patients of all ages, including the extremely premature neonates, are all capable of experiencing pain and subsequent disability as a result of tissue injury, medical illnesses, therapeutic and diagnostic procedures, trauma, and surgery (Davies et al. 2010; Lago et al. 2009; Roth-Isigkeit et al. 2005). Moreover, given the lack of assessment and barriers to treatment of pediatric pain, a minority of youth report pain and disability, including associated depression and maladaptive coping. These issues tend to be more pronounced in younger age groups and in groups with long term, chronic illness. Similar to other studies, sex differences in pain reporting have been observed, with girls tending to report pain in greater numbers than boys (Eccleston and Clinch 2007; see also, Keogh 2011).

A recent Delphi poll of professionals with a specific interest in chronic pain in children and adolescents was undertaken to reach a consensus as to the factors associated with pediatric chronic pain and disability (Miro et al. 2007). Factors deemed most important by these stakeholders in the development of chronic pain included: (1) child's psychological characteristics: the child's tendency to somaticize, depressed personality, and anxious personality; (2) parent's psychological characteristics: parental emotional instability; (3) characteristics of the pain experience: suffering from constant pain, and a family history of chronic pain; (4) characteristics of pain management: an excessive use of healthcare services for the child pain complaints, an inappropriate consumption of medicines to relieve the pain, doctor searching for the pain problem without finding anything wrong, and a low compliance with the healthcare professionals' recommendations; (5) psychological factors related to the child's pain experience: catastrophic thinking of the child and parents about the child's pain, child's negative expectations about the course of her or his pain problems, and the presence of positive reinforcements in response to the child's pain behaviors; and (6) a stressful environment (e.g., due to family difficulties, problems at school) (Miro et al. 2007). By the same token, the consensus factors considered by these stakeholders to be most important in the development of a disability include: (1) child's psychological characteristics: the tendency to somaticize, and a depressed personality; (2) parents' psychological characteristics: high anxiety; (3) psychological factors related to the child's pain experience: pain-related fear avoidance (child's and parents' catastrophic thinking about the child's pain, and child's avoidance behaviors due to the fear of experiencing more pain), child's beliefs about her or his being disabled by the pain, and pain modeling factors (parents' avoidance behaviors due to the fear of experiencing more pain, parents' belief that pain incapacitates, and parents' own disability because of pain); and (4) parents' ability to deal with her or his child's pain (Miro et al. 2007).

Health-Related Quality of Life and Pediatric Chronic Pain

Pediatric chronic pain is a complex and individual and social experience (Graumlich et al. 2001; Malaty et al. 2005; Schechter et al. 2003). It is often difficult for patients and their parents to fully describe the impact of the experience and meaning of chronic pain using only self-reported or observational unidimensional pain intensity scales (Gaffney et al. 2003; Stevens 1994). As noted above, chronic pain has a substantial adverse impact on children and adolescents, resulting in significantly worse physical functioning, psychological functioning, social functioning, in addition to lower satisfaction with life and poorer self-perceived health status (Merlijn et al. 2006; Palermo 2000).

In contrast to more conventional physiologic, laboratory, and radiological assessments of disease, the measurement of health-related quality of life (HRQoL) can provide equally important insight into these adverse effects of pediatric chronic disease, especially those associated with pain and disability (Eiser and Morse 2001b, c; Guyatt et al. 1993; Vetter 2007). Sequentially assessing HRQoL can also provide clinicians, their patients, and their parents with additional information about the longitudinal effectiveness of a chronic pain treatment regimen and assist in point-of-service clinical decision-making (Drotar 2004a; Varni et al. 2005; Vetter 2007).

Health-related quality of life has become a central issue in the effective assessment, treatment, and management of pediatric chronic diseases, and it has been posited that the measurement of HRQoL should be routine in pediatric outcomes research and clinical practice (Eiser 2004; Palermo et al. 2008; Parsons and Mayer 2004). The Pediatric Initiative on Methods, Measurement, and Pain Assessment in Clinical Trials (PedIMMPACT) has recently recommended that investigators conducting pediatric clinical trials in chronic and recurrent pain should consider assessing outcomes in pain intensity; physical functioning; emotional functioning; role functioning; symptoms and adverse events; global judgment of satisfaction with treatment; sleep; and economic factors (McGrath et al. 2008).

Nevertheless, the measurement of HRQoL in pediatric research and clinical practice has remained limited as compared to its measurement in the adult population (Clarke and Eiser 2004; Varni et al. 2005). Conceptual and methodological issues have hindered the routine assessment of HRQoL in chronically ill children and adolescents, including those suffering from chronic pain (De Civita et al. 2005; Drotar 2004a; Matza et al. 2004). One fundamental issue is the central yet complex role of child development and the associated dynamic social and psychological contexts in which a child or adolescent perceives health vs. disease (Forrest et al. 2003). Specifically, parents, siblings, and peers, as well as the classroom setting and the community, can all play an important role in the self-perceived HRQoL of a child or adolescent (Matza et al. 2004; Palermo 2000).

These methodological challenges can be overcome, however, if sufficient consideration is given to the choice of an age-appropriate pediatric HRQoL instrument (Drotar 2004b; Eiser and Morse 2001b; Landgraf and Abetz 1996; Vetter 2007). The use of an adult generic HRQoL measure (e.g., 36-Item Short-Form Health Survey, SF-36) should be avoided in chronic diseases of childhood due to its likely failure to tap important pediatric health domains and its response burden (Eiser and Morse 2001c). A parental proxy assessment of a younger child's HRQoL is a viable alternative. However, children 8–11 years of age appear to report significantly lower HRQoL than their parents (Theunissen et al. 1998). Therefore, whenever possible, in addition to those of a parental proxy, the pediatric patient's own health perceptions should also be elicited (Eiser and Morse 2001a). If the health survey instrument is appropriately structured, a child as young as 4 years of age can provide meaningful, even if only concrete insight into their self-perceived health status, including their experience of pain. More subjective or abstract health domains can be self-reported by individuals 8 years of age and older (Eiser et al. 2000; Matza et al. 2004; Vetter 2007).

Previous pediatric studies have also observed an imperfect concordance or cross-informant variance in patient self-reported health-related quality vs. parent proxy-reported health-related quality (Knight et al. 2003). This discordance has been observed not only in healthy subjects (Cremeens et al. 2006), and in a community adolescent sample (Waters et al. 2003), but also in patients specifically with functional abdominal pain (Youssef et al. 2006), cancer (Varni et al. 2002; see also Ransom et al. 2011), and sickle cell pain (Panepinto et al. 2005). Nevertheless, despite the attendant methodological challenges, the assessment of HRQoL represents a vital element of pediatric outcomes research (Palermo et al. 2008).

The Biopsychosocial Characteristics of Pediatric Chronic Pain Patients: Additional Barriers to Its Effective Management

A consistent clinical profile has been observed over the last decade among patients referred to four tertiary-care multidisciplinary, pediatric pain medicine clinics (Eccleston et al. 2004; Kashikar-Zuck et al. 2001; Logan et al. 2009; Vetter 2008). All four cohorts were likely fraught with selection bias due to referral patterns, and cancer-related pain was conspicuously absent in these published study samples. Nevertheless, collectively, they still offer important insight into the biopsychosocial characteristics of pediatric chronic pain.

In a group of 73 patients presenting to a pediatric pain medicine clinic, most were adolescents, Caucasian (90%), female (78%), and 45% had pain of greater than 24 months duration. While many reported more than one pain location, back pain (18%), abdominal pain (16%), limb pain (15%), and myofascial pain (15%) were the most common primary types of pain. Most patients reported at least mild to moderate levels of depression, and approximately 15% of the patients reported severe levels of depressive symptoms. Based upon the Functional Disability Inventory (FDI), approximately 75% of study subjects self-reported moderate to high levels of functional disability (FDI score > 10), including disruption in psychosocial functioning (Kashikar-Zuck et al. 2001).

In a second group of 80 pediatric patients with chronic pain who were referred for assessment at a specialized tertiary care chronic pain management service, the majority (71%) were girls, with a mean age of 14.5 years, whose pain had persisted for an average of 3.9 years. Using a chronic pain syndrome diagnostic system (rather than more conventional ICD-9 coding) (Malleson and Clinch 2003), four conditions were most common: complex regional pain syndrome (CRPS) type 1 (26%), juvenile widespread idiopathic musculoskeletal pain (24%), recurrent abdominal pain (12%), and low back pain (12%). Based upon their responses on a battery of previously validated questionnaires, these adolescents frequently reported clinically significant levels of disability (85%), depression (31%), and anxiety (50%), and their parents reported similarly frequent high levels of depression

(40%), anxiety (60%), and parenting stress (66%). Multiple regression analyses revealed that the strongest predictors of this adolescent emotional distress were the extent to which the adolescents catastrophize and seek social support to cope with the pain (Eccleston et al. 2004).

A third such cohort of 100 pediatric pain patients were predominantly adolescent (median age of 14 years) females (68%), whose median duration of chronic pain was 16 months. Low back pain (14%), myofascial pain or fibromyalgia (14%), abdominal pain (12%), and headache (8%) were most predominant. A substantial proportion of these patients exhibited evidence on psychological testing of clinically significant anxiety (63%) and/or depression (84%) at the time of their initial evaluation. The mean initial patient self-reported and parent proxy-reported health-related quality of life scores (PedsQL Total Score) were also significantly lower than the PedsQL Total Score values previously observed in pediatric rheumatology, pediatric migraine, and pediatric cancer patients being treated in single subspecialty clinics (Vetter 2008). This is not surprising given that such anesthesiology-based, multidisciplinary pediatric chronic pain medicine programs appear to often function as "the court of last resort" for particularly clinically enigmatic and challenging patients and families. This phenomenon was reflected in the rather low self-reported parent healthcare satisfaction with previous, ostensibly inadequately effective chronic pain-related treatment (Vetter 2008). Such intense chronic pain-related symptoms and disability mandate a robust multidisciplinary care team approach, which focuses on both the biological, psychological, and social pathology and needs of the pediatric patient and the family.

A fourth published sample of 217 patients, who presented for initial evaluation of chronic or recurrent functional (i.e., nonmalignant) pain symptoms at a similar tertiary pediatric chronic pain outpatient clinic within a large urban children's hospital, were primarily female (80%) and Caucasian (93%), with a 22-month mean duration of pain. Based upon responses on the Child Depression Inventory (CDI), only moderate levels of depressive symptoms were observed overall, with just 20% of the sample falling in the at-risk or clinically significant range of depressive symptoms. Nevertheless depressive symptoms strongly correlated with a variety of school functioning indicators, supporting the study hypothesis that depressive symptoms play a key role in influencing the degree of school impairment in adolescents with chronic pain (Logan et al. 2009).

It bears worth noting that data indicate that such adolescents presenting for evaluation and treatment of chronic pain may minimize self-reported psychological distress due to a social desirability response bias (Logan et al. 2008a). Furthermore, it has been previously observed that adolescent pain patients may infrequently exhibit diagnosable levels of depression, but that depressive symptoms, even at sub-clinical levels, may be clinically significant because they indicate poorer emotional coping resources (Eccleston et al. 2004). Given the findings in this and previous studies that show depressive symptoms are associated with functional disabilities in the presence of chronic pain, even sub-clinical levels of depressive symptoms deserve greater attention and represent a potentially important targets for treatments aimed at functional restoration and rehabilitation rather than simply a reduction in pain intensity (Logan et al. 2009). Thus, formal psychological assessment for depression, as well as anxiety, using a conventional scoring tool and/or a patient interview (Holmbeck et al. 2008; Kazdin 2005; Rudolph and Lambet 2007; Southam-Gerow and Chorpita 2007), should be part and parcel of the initial and the ongoing evaluation of the pediatric chronic pain patient.

The Effects of Race and Ethnicity on Pediatric Chronic Pain

Race is a social category based on similar ancestry and physical characteristics, while ethnicity is based also on shared behavior and culture (Edwards et al. 2001). It is widely accepted that racial and ethnic disparities in pediatric health and healthcare are extensive, pervasive, and persistent

(Flores 2010; see also Green 2011). Although racial and ethnic healthcare disparities existing among adults with chronic pain are well documented (Anderson et al. 2009), published epidemiological data on pediatric chronic pain have been drawn almost exclusively from nonminority, middle-class populations outside the United States (Vetter 2011). Furthermore, little attention has been focused on race, ethnicity, socioeconomics, and the social environment as likely causal factors in the onset, persistence, and impact of pediatric chronic pain (Fortier et al. 2009; Schwartz et al. 2007).

The Qualitative Nature of Pediatric Chronic Pain and the Patient's Personal Narrative

Because of the innately subjective and hence qualitative nature of pediatric chronic pain, research attention has also recently focused on collecting complementary data from semi-structured, qualitative patient interviews and patients' personal narratives to gain a better understanding of the impact of pain-associated functioning limitations on children's lives and the strategies they develop to try to continue functioning.

A mixed-methods approach was applied in a group of 45 children (71% female, 64% Caucasian, mean age of 14.7 years), who presented a tertiary university-based pediatric pain clinic suffering predominantly from headache, myofascial pain, and/or functional neurovisceral pain disorder (Meldrum et al. 2008). Analysis of the data derived from standardized questionnaires and semi-structured interviews identified three distinct functioning distinct patterns or groups of functional limitation and coping strategies, which were designated as Adaptive (29%), Passive (29%), and Stressed (58%). These three groups did not differ significantly in demographics or clinical pain characteristics. Distinct differences emerged. Adaptive children continued to participate in many activities, often because of more effective use of distraction and of other independently developed strategies to continue functioning. The adaptive children were also more likely to realize that focusing on pain would heighten their perception of pain. Passive children had already given up most activities, tended to use passive distraction when in pain, and were more likely to feel isolated and different from peers. Stressed children described themselves as continuing to function, but were highly focused on their pain and the difficulties of daily living with it. Parent ratings of their child's global health on the Child Health Questionnaire (CHQ PF50) also differed significantly across the groups; with the Adaptive group exhibiting higher CHQ PF50 scores and thus better perceived global health than the Passive group. Child self-report total scores Social Anxiety Scale for Children (SASC) also differed significantly across the groups, with the Stressed group reporting higher SASC scores and higher overall social anxiety than the Passive group (Meldrum et al. 2008).

While likely not practical in routine clinical practice, the use of patient narrative in clinical therapy and research (i.e., "narrative medicine") can provide valuable insight into the human pain experience (Carr et al. 2005; see also Morris 2011). Such a narrative method has recently been used to better understand the impact of chronic or recurrent pain on children within the context of their own lives and experiences, specifically, in 53 children (68% female; 68% Caucasian, mean age 14.2 years), who presented a tertiary university-based pediatric pain clinic suffering predominantly from headaches, functional neurovisceral pain disorder, and/or myofascial pain (Meldrum et al. 2009). Based upon a 30–90 min, semi-structured life history interview at home prior to their first pain clinic visit and a follow-up interview at 6–12 months post-intake, five common themes of the children's chronic pain experience emerged (Table 11.1).

Using narrative methodology similar to the seminal adult work on narrative by Frank (1995), six major, richly detailed descriptive pediatric chronic pain narratives, with unique characters and plotlines were in turn identified (Table 11.2). These narratives are consonant with previously published studies (Aasland et al. 1997; Hunfeld et al. 2002a; Mulvaney et al. 2006). These findings

Table 11.1 The common themes of children's chronic pain experience (Meldrum et al. 2009)

Theme: frequent patient expression
The choice to hide pain from parents and friends: "I don't want to be a sob story"
A sense of isolation and difference from peers and classmates: "I'm different and everybody stares and stuff"
Pain as an obstacle to personal activities and goals: "It keeps me from doing a lot of things I like"
Fears about how pain will affect the future: "I'm scared I might always have this problem"
Perceived lack of physician understanding: "I think about why it's called the medical practice"

Table 11.2 The pediatric chronic pain narratives: characters and plotlines (Meldrum et al. 2009)

The character	The plotline
The constant patient	The medical narrative
The invalid	Defeated by the pain
The weary soldier	Fighting constant stress
The stoic	"Pushing through" the pain
The positive thinker	One step at a time
The decision-maker	The major rewrite

validate the conventional clinical belief that patient isolation, changed self-perception, activity limitations, concerns about barriers to future goals, and lack of medical validation are vital to children's perception of the biopsychosocial impact of chronic pain on their lives (Meldrum et al. 2009).

The Pragmatic Goal of Pediatric Chronic Pain Management

The more pragmatic goal of pediatric chronic pain management is the timely return of a patient to as normal and functional a life as possible – with an associated improvement in health-related quality of life – while at the same time reducing the attendant stress on the parents and other family members (Bennett et al. 2000; Hunfeld et al. 2001, 2002b; Palermo 2000; Varni et al. 1996a). Indeed, at the time of their initial evaluation, patients and their parents naturally seek the complete elimination of the child or adolescent's presenting pain. Yet, this clinical outcome is unfortunately often unobtainable, with upwards of 48 and 30% of pediatric patients reporting persistent pain at 1- and 2-year follow-up, respectively (Perquin et al. 2003). Moreover, youngsters with chronic pain often go on to experience chronic pain as young adults. In a longitudinal study of a cohort of children 8, 11, and 14 years of age, suffering from chronic headache or chronic back pain, 59% of the females and 39% of the males reported similar pain at 21, 24, and 27 years of age (Brattberg 2004).

A Synopsis of Biomedical and Psychosocial Modalities in Pediatric Management

The effective assessment, treatment, and management of the myriad of chronic pain conditions that afflict children and adolescents are a very complex clinical endeavor (Zeltzer et al. 1997b, c). The management of pediatric chronic pain and its attendant patient disability and family dysfunction optimally follows a multidimensional and multidisciplinary approach (Schechter et al. 2003), which is specifically tailored to the identified medical, psychological, and social needs of each patient and family (Bennett et al. 2000; Bursch et al. 1998). Any such comprehensive pediatric pain management algorithm calls for an interdisciplinary approach that includes rehabilitation, as well as psychosocial therapies, and when indicated, analgesic and adjuvant medications, an increasing use of complementary and alternative methods, and interventional techniques (Knotkova and Pappagallo 2007).

While an extensive review of available modalities is beyond the scope of this chapter, a brief integrative synopsis is provided. For more in-depth coverage, the reader is referred to available general therapeutic reviews (Chambliss et al. 2002) and comprehensive textbooks (Finley 2006; McClain and Suresh 2010; Walco and Goldschneider 2008), as well as focused reviews on pediatric chronic headache (Hershey et al. 2006, 2007; Lewis 2009; Winner 2008), musculoskeletal pain (Clinch and Eccleston 2009; Connelly and Schanberg 2006; Malleson and Clinch 2003), fibromyalgia (Buskila 2009), neuropathic pain (Walco et al. 2010), and abdominal pain (American Academy of Pediatrics 2005; Berger et al. 2007).

Biomedical Modalities: Analgesic Medications

Due to an unfavorable risk–benefit ratio (i.e., an inadequate economic return to justify the cost of required additional clinical trials and potential medical liability), pharmaceutical companies in the United States and the European Union have infrequently sought regulatory approval of their novel analgesics or adjuncts for use in the pediatric chronic pain population (Breitkreutz 2008; Li et al. 2007; Manolis and Pons 2009). This phenomenon has resulted in common pediatric off-label medication use (Benjamin et al. 2006; Milne and Bruss 2008; Roberts et al. 2003). Despite greater recent studies and labeling changes of pediatric medications (e.g., the FDA Pediatric Exclusivity Program) (Benjamin et al. 2009), the majority of pediatric outpatient visits involve off-label prescribing across all medication categories, with off-label prescribing more frequent for younger children and those receiving care from specialist pediatricians (Bazzano et al. 2009).

Even in adults, many current analgesic medications (including notably gabapentin and amitriptyline) are used off-label, with clinicians relying upon at best small-scale investigator-initiated trials in deciding whether to prescribe a medication (Chen et al. 2009; Radley et al. 2006). Rationale polypharmacy, based upon mechanistic stratification (Beydoun and Backonja 2003) and a stepped care approach (Kroenke et al. 2009), is typically applied in adults with chronic pain, with the goal of maximizing clinical benefit and minimizing side effects (Varrassi et al. 2010). A similar patient-individualized, trial-and-error strategy is also typically applied in children and adolescents with chronic pain. More preclinical, clinical, and translational (population) studies are needed to improve the efficacy of combination drug therapy that has become an integral part of a comprehensive approach to the management of chronic pain in adult and pediatric pain populations (Mao et al. 2011).

Tramadol

The routine use of tramadol warrants consideration in pediatric chronic pain (Bozkurt 2005). When given postoperatively as a single 1 or 2 mg/kg oral dose in children between the ages of 7 and 16 years, tramadol has demonstrated a narcotic dose-sparing effect, with a minimal adverse side effect profile (Finkel et al. 2002). An open-label, multicenter trial of the safety profile and analgesic efficacy of tramadol in 7–16-year olds for the treatment of painful conditions lasting up to 30 days found that tramadol 1–2 mg/kg orally every 4–6 h (maximal dose of 8 mg/kg/day, not to exceed 400 mg/day) to be a safe and effective analgesic in this patient population (Rose et al. 2003).

Tramadol must be converted by the cytochrome P450 2D6 (CYP2D6) isoenzyme to its active metabolite, *O*-demethyl tramadol (M1), to provide analgesia (Grond and Sablotzki 2004). Of note, CYP2D6 metabolizes approximately 25% of current drugs, including some commonly prescribed

Table 11.3 Myths and obstacles to prescribing opioids for pediatric chronic pain (Friedrichsdorf and Kang 2007)

Parents
- Fear of giving up
- Misconceptions of opioids as "too strong for children"
- Fear of side effects
- Worry their child will become "addicted" to pain medications
- Cultural or religious beliefs

Healthcare providers
- Lack of sufficient education regarding managing pain
- Misconceptions about frequency and severity of side effects, such as respiratory depression
- Worries that opioids will shorten life expectancy
- Concerns that escalating opioid doses will increase the likelihood of tolerance, and thus make pain control more difficult as the disease progresses

antidepressants (e.g., fluoxetine, paroxetine, all of the tricyclic antidepressants [TCAs]) and opioids (e.g., codeine, hydrocodone, and methadone) (Caraco 2004; Weinshilboum 2003). CYP2D6 activity ranges considerably within a general population and among different ethnic groups, with ultrarapid metabolizers, extensive (normal) metabolizers, intermediate metabolizers, and poor metabolizers (Gardiner and Begg 2006; Zhou 2009a, b). Because of this genetic polymorphism, large inter-individual variation in the enzyme activity exists, with 1.5–10% of Caucasians, 1.9–7.3% of African-Americans, 1.8–19% of Africans, 0–2–4.8% of Asians, and 2.2–6.6% of Hispanics lacking sufficient CYP2D6 enzymatic activity and thus being poor metabolizers of its substrates (Bernard et al. 2006; Zhou et al. 2009). This inability to metabolize via CYP2D6 is one factor that also contributes to inadequate pain management across ethnically diverse patient populations.

The effect of CYP2D6 activity in drug metabolism is further complicated by the activity of a drug itself on CYP2D6, as CYP2D6 inhibitors may make extensive (normal) metabolizers act like intermediate metabolizers or poor metabolizers. Thus, the co-administration of tramadol and a number of medications, including methadone, any of the TCAs, duloxetine, and many of the selective serotonin reuptake inhibitors (SSRIs), can result in seizures, due to inhibition of CYP2D6 and the accumulation of tramadol, or serotonin syndrome (Sansone and Sansone 2009; Tashakori and Afshari 2010), even at their recommended doses.

Transdermal Fentanyl

A number of myths and obstacles, including fears of addiction or diversion, continue to hamper the prescription of opioids for pediatric cancer pain (Friedrichsdorf and Kang 2007) and for chronic nonmalignant (noncancer) pain that is refractory to other analgesics (Table 11.3) (McGrath and Ruskin 2007). Whereas most adults actively seek pain relief, children may cope with pain by withdrawing, rather than crying or asking for medication. Once routine, pediatric intramuscular injections are fortunately now less common, for their use prompts many children to not complain of pain for fear that the nurse's answer to their pain would be a dreaded analgesic injection ("a shot"). Nevertheless, children often believe they deserve their pain as punishment for something they did wrong (Rice 1996). Children and adolescents have widely variable individual pain perceptions of similar conditions, often resulting in widely different analgesic needs. While these differences are likely based on a combination of past experiences, culture, and genetics (Brislin and Rose 2005), additional insight is needed as to how best to assess and to address these predilections (Kraemer and Rose 2009).

While transdermal fentanyl has been used for pediatric cancer pain and palliative care (Collins et al. 1999; Finkel et al. 2005; Zernikow et al. 2007), this unique drug delivery system also has a place in the management of noncancer pain. A recently introduced transdermal fentanyl patch with a lower drug release rate of 12.5 μg/h has made it more applicable in the pediatric population (Zernikow et al. 2009). However, while observational clinical and pharmacokinetic studies have been published, at this time, no pediatric randomized or controlled cohort studies have been reported (Zernikow et al. 2007).

Tricyclic Antidepressants

Despite a paucity of published randomized controlled trials, the TCAs are widely prescribed for a variety of pediatric chronic pain conditions. The TCAs are frequently used as the first-line drug of choice for pediatric chronic pain. Pain relief is often seen at lower doses (75 mg in adults) than required for the treatment of depression or generalized anxiety (Bryson and Wilde 1996). However, the TCAs have a relatively narrow therapeutic margin. An electrocardiogram (ECG) should be obtained in all patients prior to initiating a TCA to rule out Wolf-Parkinson-White (WPW) and a prolonged QT syndrome, heart rhythm disorders that can potentially cause a fast, chaotic heartbeat and are contraindications to the use of a TCA. A repeat ECG is indicated at a TCA dose of greater than 1 mg/kg/day. The TCAs are metabolized primarily by the CYP2D6 isoenzyme, with amitriptyline metabolized to nortriptyline, and imipramine metabolized to desipramine. The secondary amine TCAs (nortriptyline and imipramine) are less sedating than the tertiary amine TCAs (amitriptyline and imipramine), which often determine clinical preference. The usual starting dose of a TCA is 10 mg/day (0.15 mg/kg/day), with an analgesic target dose of 1 mg/kg/day. Nortriptyline is commercially available as a liquid solution (10 mg/5 mL), facilitating its weight-based dosing in children. The TCAs are equipotent, which facilitates conversion from one agent to another (e.g., nortriptyline in lieu of amitriptyline for less sedation).

As noted above, genetic polymorphism of the CYP2D6 enzyme exists, with some patients being poor (slow) metabolizers of the TCAs (Bernard et al. 2006; Zhou et al. 2009). Therefore, a plasma TCA level should be obtained when a dose of 0.5 mg/kg/day is reached, and if the plasma TCA level is within the therapeutic reference range (100–250 ng/mL for amitriptyline and nortriptyline or 50–150 ng/mL for nortriptyline alone) (Lexi-Comp 2010; Wilson 2003), the daily dose should not be further increased. The parent molecule and its metabolite are additive in therapeutic effect but also toxicity. While the TCAs are often discounted as being excessively side effect prone, the newer serontonin-norepinephrine reuptake inhibitors (SNRIs) like venlafaxine (Effexor®), duloxetine (Cymbalta®), and milnacipran (Savella®) have a similar dose-dependent anticholinergic (muscarinic receptor antagonist) side effect profile (Kong and Irwin 2009; Kroenke et al. 2009; Verdu et al. 2008).

Antiepileptic Drugs

Based upon available adult studies (Hauser et al. 2009; Wiffen et al. 2005), gabapentin (Neurontin®) is a potential and promising pediatric analgesic adjuvant. Gabapentin is FDA-approved as an adjunctive therapy in the treatment of partial seizures in pediatric patients 3 years of age and older. Gabapentin is commercially available as a 100 mg capsule and a liquid solution (250 mg/5 mL), facilitating its weight-based dosing in children. In adults an initial gabapentin dose of 300 mg every 8 h, titrated as indicated in 100–300 mg increments up to 600–1,200 mg every 8 h, appears optimal. Extrapolating from adult studies and applying an ideal adult body weight of 60–70 kg, an initial pediatric oral dose of 5 mg/kg every 8 h, titrated slowly up to 20 mg/kg every 8 h, appears reasonable. This gabapentin dose is commensurate with that for the treatment of pediatric epilepsy and has supportive pediatric pharmacokinetic data, with a therapeutic plasma level of 5–15 μg/mL

(Haig et al. 2001; Holmes 1997; Hwang and Kim 2008). Of note, plasma gabapentin levels can be readily obtained, whereas plasma pregabalin (Lyrica®) levels are not commercially available. Gabapentin is eliminated from the systemic circulation by renal excretion as unchanged drug and is not appreciably metabolized in humans. As in adults, reduced gabapentin doses are mandated in patients 12 years of age or older with renal dysfunction. Gabapentin should not be used in children less than 12 years old with compromised renal function.

While gabapentin has the greatest clinical track record of use for pediatric chronic pain conditions (albeit completely off-label), published data also support the use of at least two other antiepileptic drugs. Topiramate (Topamax®) has been shown to be more effective than placebo for the prophylaxis of pediatric migraine (Cruz et al. 2009; Lakshmi et al. 2007; Lewis et al. 2009; Winner et al. 2005). While its reported use for pediatric chronic pain is very limited (Lalwani et al. 2005), oxcarbazepine (Trileptal®) has gained acceptance for pediatric epilepsy (Chung and Eiland 2008; Franzoni et al. 2009; Kothare et al. 2006; Pina-Garza et al. 2005). While hyponatremia is less commonly observed in children and adolescents than in adults taking oxcarbazepine, nevertheless, serum sodium levels should be monitored with its use.

Psychosocial Modalities

Individual and/or family therapy, especially using a cognitive-behavioral or coping-skills model, has been shown to be effective in treating a broad-spectrum of common pediatric chronic pain conditions (Eccleston et al. 2003, 2009), including, specifically, headache (Andrasik and Schwartz 2006; Holroyd and Drew 2006; Powers and Andrasik 2005; Rosen 2008), fibromyalgia (Degotardi et al. 2006; Kashikar-Zuck et al. 2005), recurrent abdominal pain (Duarte et al. 2006; Huertas-Ceballos et al. 2008; Levy et al. 2010; Robins et al. 2005), and CRPS (Lee et al. 2002).

Nevertheless, it is vital to recognize that these psychological therapies may not be readily available due to geographic location, or an affordable option for many families of children and adolescents with chronic pain, and that many parents and children may be quite resistant to any such treatment recommendation that seems to imply that the pain is somehow "not real" or "all in my head" (Meldrum et al. 2009). One potential way to circumvent these financial constraints and geographic proximity is to utilize an Internet-based delivery method (Long and Palermo 2009). This method has been shown to have some efficacy in pediatric cancer patients and in pediatric pain populations (see also Quintana and Jane, this volume). When compared to a wait-list control regimen, Internet delivery of family cognitive behavioral therapy was shown to be more efficacious in reducing pain intensity and improving functional disability in a group of 48 older children and adolescents, aged 11–17 years, with chronic headache, abdominal, or musculoskeletal pain and associated functional disability (Palermo et al. 2009). Similar greater benefit was observed in 65 adolescents headache patients who received two different self-help training programs (multimodal cognitive-behavioral training and applied relaxation) presented via the Internet as compared to a conventional educational intervention (Trautmann and Kroner-Herwig 2010).

Conclusions

It has long been appreciated that the optimal management of pediatric chronic pain addresses its equally important biological, psychological, and social components (Kozlowska et al. 2008; Varni et al. 1995). There is thus a substantial body of literature to support a multidisciplinary, biopsychosocial approach to pediatric chronic pain (Simons et al. 2010a). While considerable attention has been focused on the psychological and social components, greater insight is needed into the complex interaction between a child or adolescent with chronic pain and the home, school, and other elements of the social environment (Forgeron et al. 2010; Logan and Scharff 2005; Simons et al. 2010b).

Applying Varni's now classic multidimensional Biobehavioral Model of Pediatric Pain (Varni 1995; Varni et al. 1995), as well as other health behavior models (e.g., the Health Belief Model), additional clinical, methodological and other research attention continues to be focused on consistently determining and in turn longitudinally addressing the presence of comorbid mood disorders, the strength of a pediatric patient's coping mechanisms, the presence of pain-promoting vs. pain-reducing parental behaviors, and preexisting parental pain and disability, all of which appear to be valid prognosticators of eventual patient outcome (Brace et al. 2000; Chambers et al. 2002; Gauntlett-Gilbert and Eccleston 2007; Kashikar-Zuck et al. 2001; Lynch et al. 2006; Peterson and Palermo 2004; Simons et al. 2008, 2010a).

There is also a need for additional research that explores whether the parent–child agreement vs. discordance on health-related quality of life is dependent on additional factors such as the proxy's relationship to child (i.e., mother vs. father), the mental health of the parent, and different disease types or pain conditions (e.g., headache vs. abdominal pain vs. low back pain) (Cremeens et al. 2006). Lastly, additional attention needs to be focused on the interrelationship between patient/parent satisfaction with pain treatment, adherence to or compliance with a multimodal pediatric chronic pain treatment plan, and resulting health-related quality of life as a patient-reported outcome (Knight et al. 2003; McGrath et al. 2008; Simons et al. 2010a).

As noted above, pediatric chronic pain research has historically relied largely upon patients sampled from subspecialty clinical practices (Claar et al. 2008; Palermo 2009; Walco et al. 2009), resulting in innate selection bias and thus questionable external validity (Bornhoft et al. 2006; Estellat et al. 2009; Juni et al. 2001; Rothwell 2005). Racial and ethnic disparities clearly exist in the prevalence and treatment of adult chronic pain in the United States (Green et al. 2003; Nguyen et al. 2005; Portenoy et al. 2004; Riley et al. 2002), but little such epidemiological data have been published about the pediatric population in the United States (Vetter 2011). While ethnic differences in the perception, experience, and impact of adult pain have received growing attention in recent years (Edwards et al. 2005; Riley et al. 2002), greater attention now needs to be focused on race, ethnicity, socioeconomics, and the social environment as causal factors in the onset, persistence, and characteristics of pediatric chronic pain (Fortier et al. 2009).

One other promising but still to be fully developed area is the application of complementary and alternative medicine (CAM) therapy for pediatric chronic pain (Tsao 2006). The last decade has witnessed a growing body of literature on the use of CAM modalities for a variety of pediatric chronic diseases (e.g., cancer, rheumatoid arthritis, and cystic fibrosis), including those associated with pain and disability (Tsao and Zeltzer 2005). In a recent survey of predominantly female adolescents presenting to a single, multidisciplinary, tertiary clinic specializing in pediatric chronic pain, the most popular CAM therapies were biofeedback, yoga, and hypnosis; the least popular were art therapy and energy healing, with craniosacral, acupuncture, and massage being intermediate (Tsao et al. 2007). These survey data are commensurate with previously reported, more generalized pediatric CAM practice patterns (Lin et al. 2005). Despite the common yet erroneous perception that an aversion for needles makes acupuncture less likely to be tolerated in children (Kemper et al. 2000), there is evidence supporting the use of acupuncture in the pediatric population, including for chronic pain conditions (Jindal et al. 2008; Kundu and Berman 2007). The use of acupuncture for pediatric pain is a long-standing practice in Eastern cultures, yet despite growing interest in the West, there has been relatively little systematic research on acupuncture for pediatric chronic pain (Waterhouse et al. 2009). Thus, large-scale randomized controlled trials are needed to further address the safety, effectiveness, and acceptability of acupuncture in children and adolescents (Kundu and Berman 2007; Libonate et al. 2008).

References

Aasland, A., Flato, B., & Vandvik, I. H. (1997). Psychosocial factors in children with idiopathic musculoskeletal pain: A prospective, longitudinal study. *Acta Paediatrica, 86*(7), 740–746.

American Academy of Pediatrics. (2001). The new morbidity revisited: A renewed commitment to the psychosocial aspects of pediatric care. Committee on Psychosocial Aspects of Child and Family Health. *Pediatrics, 108*(5), 1227–1230.

American Academy of Pediatrics. (2003). Family-centered care and the pediatrician's role. *Pediatrics, 112*(3 Pt 1), 691–697.

American Academy of Pediatrics. (2005). Chronic abdominal pain in children. *Pediatrics, 115*(3), e370–e381.

Anderson, K. O., Green, C. R., & Payne, R. (2009). Racial and ethnic disparities in pain: Causes and consequences of unequal care. *The Journal of Pain, 10*(12), 1187–1204.

Andrasik, F., & Schwartz, M. S. (2006). Behavioral assessment and treatment of pediatric headache. *Behavior Modification, 30*(1), 93–113.

Bazzano, A. T., Mangione-Smith, R., Schonlau, M., Suttorp, M. J., & Brook, R. H. (2009). Off-label prescribing to children in the United States outpatient setting. *Academic Pediatrics, 9*(2), 81–88.

Benjamin, D. K., Jr., Smith, P. B., Murphy, M. D., Roberts, R., Mathis, L., Avant, D., et al. (2006). Peer-reviewed publication of clinical trials completed for pediatric exclusivity. *Journal of the American Medical Association, 296*(10), 1266–1273.

Benjamin, D. K., Jr., Smith, P. B., Sun, M. J., Murphy, M. D., Avant, D., Mathis, L., et al. (2009). Safety and transparency of pediatric drug trials. *Archives of Pediatrics & Adolescent Medicine, 163*(12), 1080–1086.

Bennett, S. M., Huntsman, E., & Lilley, C. M. (2000). Parent perceptions of the impact of chronic pain in children and adolescents. *Children's Health Care, 29*(3), 147–159.

Berger, M. Y., Gieteling, M. J., & Benninga, M. A. (2007). Chronic abdominal pain in children. *British Medical Journal, 334*(7601), 997–1002.

Bernard, S., Neville, K. A., Nguyen, A. T., & Flockhart, D. A. (2006). Interethnic differences in genetic polymorphisms of CYP2D6 in the U.S population: Clinical implications. *The Oncologist, 11*(2), 126–135.

Beydoun, A., & Backonja, M. M. (2003). Mechanistic stratification of antineuralgic agents. *Journal of Pain and Symptom Management, 25*(5 Suppl), S18–S30.

Bornhoft, G., Maxion-Bergemann, S., Wolf, U., Kienle, G. S., Michalsen, A., Vollmar, H. C., et al. (2006). Checklist for the qualitative evaluation of clinical studies with particular focus on external validity and model validity. *BMC Medical Research Methodology, 6*, 56.

Bozkurt, P. (2005). Use of tramadol in children. Paediatric Anaesthesia, 15(12), 1041–1047.

Brace, M. J., Scott Smith, M., McCauley, E., & Sherry, D. D. (2000). Family reinforcement of illness behavior: A comparison of adolescents with chronic fatigue syndrome, juvenile arthritis, and healthy controls. *Journal of Developmental and Behavioral Pediatrics, 21*(5), 332–339.

Brattberg, G. (2004). Do pain problems in young school children persist into early adulthood? A 13-year follow-up. *European Journal of Pain, 8*(3), 187–199.

Breitkreutz, J. (2008). European perspectives on pediatric formulations. *Clinical Therapeutics, 30*(11), 2146–2154.

Brislin, R. P., & Rose, J. B. (2005). Pediatric acute pain management. *Anesthesiology Clinics of North America, 23*(4), 789–814.

Bryson, H. M., & Wilde, M. I. (1996). Amitriptyline: A review of its pharmacological properties and therapeutic use in chronic pain states. *Drugs & Aging, 8*(6), 459–476.

Bursch, B., Walco, G. A., & Zeltzer, L. (1998). Clinical assessment and management of chronic pain and pain-associated disability syndrome. *Journal of Developmental and Behavioral Pediatrics, 19*(1), 45–53.

Buskila, D. (2009). Pediatric fibromyalgia. *Rheumatic Diseases Clinics of North America, 35*(2), 253–261.

Caraco, Y. (2004). Genes and the response to drugs. *The New England Journal of Medicine, 351*(27), 2867–2869.

Carr, D. B., Loeser, J. D., & Morris, D. B. (2005). *Narrative, pain, and suffering.* Seattle: IASP Press.

Chambers, C. T. (2003). The role of family factors in pediatric pain. In P. J. McGrath & G. A. Finley (Eds.), *Pediatric pain: Biological and social context* (pp. 99–103). Seattle: IASP Press.

Chambers, C. T., Craig, K. D., & Bennett, S. M. (2002). The impact of maternal behavior on children's pain experiences: An experimental analysis. *Journal of Pediatric Psychology, 27*(3), 293–301.

Chambliss, C. R., Heggen, J., Copelan, D. N., & Pettignano, R. (2002). The assessment and management of chronic pain in children. *Paediatric Drugs, 4*(11), 737–746.

Chen, D. T., Wynia, M. K., Moloney, R. M., & Alexander, G. C. (2009). U.S. physician knowledge of the FDA-approved indications and evidence base for commonly prescribed drugs: Results of a national survey. *Pharmacoepidemiology and Drug Safety, 18*(11), 1094–1100.

Chung, A. M., & Eiland, L. S. (2008). Use of second-generation antiepileptic drugs in the pediatric population. *Paediatric Drugs, 10*(4), 217–254.

Claar, R. L., Baber, K. F., Simons, L. E., Logan, D. E., & Walker, L. S. (2008). Pain coping profiles in adolescents with chronic pain. *Pain, 140*(2), 368–375.

Clarke, S. A., & Eiser, C. (2004). The measurement of health-related quality of life (QOL) in paediatric clinical trials: A systematic review. *Health and Quality of Life Outcomes, 2*, 66.

Clinch, J., & Eccleston, C. (2009). Chronic musculoskeletal pain in children: Assessment and management. *Rheumatology (Oxford, England), 48*(5), 466–474.

Collins, J. J., Dunkel, I. J., Gupta, S. K., Inturrisi, C. E., Lapin, J., Palmer, L. N., et al. (1999). Transdermal fentanyl in children with cancer pain: Feasibility, tolerability, and pharmacokinetic correlates. *The Journal of Pediatrics, 134*(3), 319–323.

Conger, K. J., Rueter, M. A., & Conger, R. D. (2000). The role of economic pressure in the lives of parents and their adolescents: The family stress model. In L. J. Crockeet & R. J. Silbereisen (Eds.), *Negotiating adolescence in times of social change* (pp. 201–233). Cambridge: Cambridge University Press.

Conger, R. D., & Donnellan, M. B. (2007). An Interactionist perspective on the socioeconomic context of human development. *Annual Review of Psychology, 58*, 175–199.

Connelly, M., & Schanberg, L. (2006). Latest developments in the assessment and management of chronic musculoskeletal pain syndromes in children. *Current Opinion in Rheumatology, 18*(5), 496–502.

Cremeens, J., Eiser, C., & Blades, M. (2006). Factors influencing agreement between child self-report and parent proxy-reports on the Pediatric Quality of Life Inventory 4.0 (PedsQL) generic core scales. *Health and Quality of Life Outcomes, 4*, 58.

Cruz, M. J., Valencia, I., Legido, A., Kothare, S. V., Khurana, D. S., Yum, S., et al. (2009). Efficacy and tolerability of topiramate in pediatric migraine. *Pediatric Neurology, 41*(3), 167–170.

Davies, E. H., Ollivier, C. M., & Saint Raymond, A. (2010). Paediatric investigation plans for pain: Painfully slow! *European Journal of Clinical Pharmacology, 66*(11), 1091–1097.

De Civita, M., Regier, D., Alamgir, A. H., Anis, A. H., Fitzgerald, M. J., & Marra, C. A. (2005). Evaluating health-related quality-of-life studies in paediatric populations: Some conceptual, methodological and developmental considerations and recent applications. *PharmacoEconomics, 23*(7), 659–685.

Degotardi, P. J., Klass, E. S., Rosenberg, B. S., Fox, D. G., Gallelli, K. A., & Gottlieb, B. S. (2006). Development and evaluation of a cognitive-behavioral intervention for juvenile fibromyalgia. *Journal of Pediatric Psychology, 31*(7), 714–723.

Drotar, D. (2004a). Measuring child health: Scientific questions, challenges, and recommendations. *Ambulatory Pediatrics, 4*(4 Suppl), 353–357.

Drotar, D. (2004b). Validating measures of pediatric health status, functional status, and health-related quality of life: Key methodological challenges and strategies. *Ambulatory Pediatrics, 4*(4 Suppl), 358–364.

Duarte, M. A., Penna, F. J., Andrade, E. M., Cancela, C. S., Neto, J. C., & Barbosa, T. F. (2006). Treatment of nonorganic recurrent abdominal pain: Cognitive-behavioral family intervention. *Journal of Pediatric Gastroenterology and Nutrition, 43*(1), 59–64.

Eccleston, C., & Clinch, J. (2007). Adolescent chronic pain and disability: A review of the current evidence in assessment and treatment. *Paediatrics & Child Health, 12*(2), 117–120.

Eccleston, C., Crombez, G., Scotford, A., Clinch, J., & Connell, H. (2004). Adolescent chronic pain: Patterns and predictors of emotional distress in adolescents with chronic pain and their parents. *Pain, 108*(3), 221–229.

Eccleston, C., Malleson, P. N., Clinch, J., Connell, H., & Sourbut, C. (2003). Chronic pain in adolescents: Evaluation of a programme of interdisciplinary cognitive behaviour therapy. *Archives of Disease in Childhood, 88*(10), 881–885.

Eccleston, C., Palermo, T. M., Williams, A. C., Lewandowski, A., & Morley, S. (2009). Psychological therapies for the management of chronic and recurrent pain in children and adolescents. *Cochrane Database Systemic Reviews,* (2), CD003968.

Edwards, C. L., Fillingim, R. B., & Keefe, F. (2001). Race, ethnicity and pain. *Pain, 94*(2), 133–137.

Edwards, R. R., Moric, M., Husfeldt, B., Buvanendran, A., & Ivankovich, O. (2005). Ethnic similarities and differences in the chronic pain experience: A comparison of African American, Hispanic, and white patients. *Pain Medicine, 6*(1), 88–98.

Eiser, C. (2004). Use of quality of life measures in clinical trials. *Ambulatory Pediatrics, 4*(4), 395–399.

Eiser, C., Mohay, H., & Morse, R. (2000). The measurement of quality of life in young children. *Child: Care, Health and Development, 26*(5), 401–414.

Eiser, C., & Morse, R. (2001a). Can parents rate their child's health-related quality of life? Results of a systematic review. *Quality of Life Research, 10*(4), 347–357.

Eiser, C., & Morse, R. (2001b). The measurement of quality of life in children: Past and future perspectives. *Journal of Developmental and Behavioral Pediatrics, 22*(4), 248–256.

Eiser, C., & Morse, R. (2001c). Quality-of-life measures in chronic diseases of childhood. *Health Technology Assessment, 5*(4), 1–157.

Estellat, C., Torgerson, D. J., & Ravaud, P. (2009). How to perform a critical analysis of a randomised controlled trial. *Best Practice & Research. Clinical Rheumatology, 23*(2), 291–303.

Finkel, J. C., Finley, A., Greco, C., Weisman, S. J., & Zeltzer, L. (2005). Transdermal fentanyl in the management of children with chronic severe pain: Results from an international study. *Cancer, 104*(12), 2847–2857.

Finkel, J. C., Rose, J. B., Schmitz, M. L., Birmingham, P. K., Ulma, G. A., Gunter, J. B., et al. (2002). An evaluation of the efficacy and tolerability of oral tramadol hydrochloride tablets for the treatment of postsurgical pain in children. *Anesthesia and Analgesia, 94*(6), 1469–1473.

Finley, G. A. (Ed.). (2006). *Bringing pain relief to children: Treatment approaches.* New York: Humana Press.

Flores, G. (2010). Technical report – Racial and ethnic disparities in the health and health care of children. *Pediatrics, 125*(4), e979–e1020.

Forgeron, P. A., King, S., Stinson, J. N., McGrath, P. J., MacDonald, A. J., & Chambers, C. T. (2010). Social functioning and peer relationships in children and adolescents with chronic pain: A systematic review. *Pain Research & Management, 15*(1), 27–41.

Forrest, C. B., Shipman, S. A., Dougherty, D., & Miller, M. R. (2003). Outcomes research in pediatric settings: Recent trends and future directions. *Pediatrics, 111*(1), 171–178.

Fortier, M. A., Anderson, C. T., & Kain, Z. N. (2009). Ethnicity matters in the assessment and treatment of children's pain. *Pediatrics, 124*(1), 378–380.

Frank, A. W. (1995). *The wounded storyteller: Body, illness, and ethics.* Chicago: University of Chicago Press.

Franzoni, E., Gentile, V., Pellicciari, A., Garone, C., Iero, L., Gualandi, S., et al. (2009). Prospective study on long-term treatment with oxcarbazepine in pediatric epilepsy. *Journal of Neurology, 256*(9), 1527–1532.

Friedrichsdorf, S. J., & Kang, T. I. (2007). The management of pain in children with life-limiting illnesses. *Pediatric Clinics of North America, 54*(5), 645–672.

Gaffney, A., McGrath, P. A., & Dick, B. (2003). Measuring pain in children: Developemental and instrument issues. In N. L. Schechter, C. B. Berde, & M. Yaster (Eds.), *Pain in infants, children, and adolescents* (2nd ed., pp. 128–141). Philadelphia: Lippincott Williams & Wilkins.

Gardiner, S. J., & Begg, E. J. (2006). Pharmacogenetics, drug-metabolizing enzymes, and clinical practice. *Pharmacological Reviews, 58*(3), 521–590.

Gauntlett-Gilbert, J., & Eccleston, C. (2007). Disability in adolescents with chronic pain: Patterns and predictors across different domains of functioning. *Pain, 131*(1–2), 132–141.

Gold, J. I., Yetwin, A. K., Mahrer, N. E., Carson, M. C., Griffin, A. T., Palmer, S. N., et al. (2009). Pediatric chronic pain and health-related quality of life. *Journal of Pediatric Nursing, 24*(2), 141–150.

Graumlich, S. E., Powers, S. W., Byars, K. C., Schwarber, L. A., Mitchell, M. J., & Kalinyak, K. A. (2001). Multidimensional assessment of pain in pediatric sickle cell disease. *Journal of Pediatric Psychology, 26*(4), 203–214.

Green, C. (2011). Disparities in pain management and palliative care. In R. J. Moore (Ed.), *Handbook of pain and palliative care: Biobehavioral approaches for the life course.* New York: Springer.

Green, C. R., Baker, T. A., Smith, E. M., & Sato, Y. (2003). The effect of race in older adults presenting for chronic pain management: A comparative study of black and white Americans. *The Journal of Pain, 4*(2), 82–90.

Grond, S., & Sablotzki, A. (2004). Clinical pharmacology of tramadol. *Clinical Pharmacokinetics, 43*(13), 879–923.

Guyatt, G. H., Feeny, D. H., & Patrick, D. L. (1993). Measuring health-related quality of life. *Annals of Internal Medicine, 118*(8), 622–629.

Haig, G. M., Bockbrader, H. N., Wesche, D. L., Boellner, S. W., Ouellet, D., Brown, R. R., et al. (2001). Single-dose gabapentin pharmacokinetics and safety in healthy infants and children. *The Journal of Clinical Pharmacology, 41*(5), 507–514.

Hatzmann, J., Heymans, H. S., Ferrer-i-Carbonell, A., van Praag, B. M., & Grootenhuis, M. A. (2008). Hidden consequences of success in pediatrics: Parental health-related quality of life – results from the Care Project. *Pediatrics, 122*(5), e1030–e1038.

Hauser, W., Bernardy, K., Uceyler, N., & Sommer, C. (2009). Treatment of fibromyalgia syndrome with gabapentin and pregabalin – A meta-analysis of randomized controlled trials. *Pain, 145*(1–2), 69–81.

Hershey, A. D., Kabbouche, M. A., & Powers, S. W. (2006). Chronic daily headaches in children. *Current Pain and Headache Reports, 10*(5), 370–376.

Hershey, A. D., Winner, P., Kabbouche, M. A., & Powers, S. W. (2007). Headaches. *Current Opinion in Pediatrics, 19*(6), 663–669.

Holmbeck, G. N., Thill, A. W., Bachanas, P., Garber, J., Miller, K. B., Abad, M., Holmbeck, G. N., Thill, A. W., Bachanas, P., Garber, J., Miller, K. B., Abad, M., et al. (2008). Evidence-based assessment in pediatric psychology: Measures of psychosocial adjustment and psychopathology. *Journal of Pediatric Psychology, 33*(9), 958–980. discussion 952–981.

Holmes, G. L. (1997). Gabapentin for treatment of epilepsy in children. *Seminars in Pediatric Neurology, 4*(3), 244–250.

Holroyd, K. A., & Drew, J. B. (2006). Behavioral approaches to the treatment of migraine. *Seminars in Neurology, 26*(2), 199–207.

Huertas-Ceballos, A., Logan, S., Bennett, C., & Macarthur, C. (2008). Psychosocial interventions for recurrent abdominal pain (RAP) and irritable bowel syndrome (IBS) in childhood. *Cochrane Database Systemic Reviews,* (1), CD003014.

Hunfeld, J. A., Perquin, C. W., Bertina, W., Hazebroek-Kampschreur, A. J. M., van Suijlekom-Smit, L. W. A., Koes, B. W., et al. (2002a). Stability of pain parameters and pain-related quality of life in adolescents with persistent pain: A three-year follow-up. *The Clinical Journal of Pain, 18*(2), 99–106.

Hunfeld, J. A., Perquin, C. W., Duivenvoorden, H. J., Hazebroek-Kampschreur, A. A., Passchier, J., van Suijlekom-Smit, L. W., et al. (2001). Chronic pain and its impact on quality of life in adolescents and their families. *Journal of Pediatric Psychology, 26*(3), 145–153.

Hunfeld, J. A., Perquin, C. W., Hazebroek-Kampschreur, A. J. M., Passchier, J., van Suijlekom-Smit, L. W. A., & van der Wouden, J. C. (2002b). Physically unexplained chronic pain and its impact on children and their families: The mother's perception. *Psychology and Psychotherapy, 75*(Pt 3), 251–260.

Hwang, H., & Kim, K. J. (2008). New antiepileptic drugs in pediatric epilepsy. *Brain & Development, 30*(9), 549–555.

Jindal, V., Ge, A., & Mansky, P. J. (2008). Safety and efficacy of acupuncture in children: A review of the evidence. *Journal of Pediatric Hematology/Oncology, 30*(6), 431–442.

Jordan, A. (2005). The impact of pediatric chronic pain on the family. *Pediatric pain letter: Commentaries on pain in infants, children, and adolescents.* Retrieved September 6, 2010, from http://pediatric-pain.ca/ppl/issues/v7n1_2005/v7n1_jordan.pdf.

Juni, P., Altman, D. G., & Egger, M. (2001). Systematic reviews in health care: Assessing the quality of controlled clinical trials. *British Medical Journal, 323*(7303), 42–46.

Kashikar-Zuck, S., Goldschneider, K. R., Powers, S. W., Vaught, M. H., & Hershey, A. D. (2001). Depression and functional disability in chronic pediatric pain. *The Clinical Journal of Pain, 17*(4), 341–349.

Kashikar-Zuck, S., Lynch, A. M., Graham, T. B., Swain, N. F., Mullen, S. M., & Noll, R. B. (2007). Social functioning and peer relationships of adolescents with juvenile fibromyalgia syndrome. *Arthritis and Rheumatism, 57*(3), 474–480.

Kashikar-Zuck, S., Swain, N. F., Jones, B. A., & Graham, T. B. (2005). Efficacy of cognitive-behavioral intervention for juvenile primary fibromyalgia syndrome. *The Journal of Rheumatology, 32*(8), 1594–1602.

Kazdin, A. E. (2005). Evidence-based assessment for children and adolescents: Issues in measurement development and clinical application. *Journal of Clinical Child and Adolescent Psychology, 34*(3), 548–558.

Kemper, K. J., Sarah, R., Silver-Highfield, E., Xiarhos, E., Barnes, L., & Berde, C. (2000). On pins and needles? Pediatric pain patients' experience with acupuncture. *Pediatrics, 105*(4 Pt 2), 941–947.

Keogh, E. (2011). Sex differences in pain across the life course. In R. J. Moore (Ed.), *Handbook of pain and palliative care: Biobehavioral approaches for the life course.* New York: Springer.

Knight, T. S., Burwinkle, T. M., & Varni, J. W. (2003). Heath-related quality of life. In E. J. Sobo & P. S. Kurtin (Eds.), *Child health services research: Application, innovations, and insights* (pp. 209–241). San Francisco: Jossey-Bass.

Knotkova, H., & Pappagallo, M. (2007). Adjuvant analgesics. *The Medical Clinics of North America, 91*(1), 113–124.

Kong, V. K., & Irwin, M. G. (2009). Adjuvant analgesics in neuropathic pain. *European Journal of Anaesthesiology, 26*(2), 96–100.

Kothare, S. V., Mostofi, N., Khurana, D. S., Mohsem, B., Melvin, J. J., Hardison, H. H., et al. (2006). Oxcarbazepine therapy in very young children: A single-center clinical experience. *Pediatric Neurology, 35*(3), 173–176.

Kozlowska, K., Rose, D., Khan, R., Kram, S., Lane, L., & Collins, J. (2008). A conceptual model and practice framework for managing chronic pain in children and adolescents. *Harvard Review of Psychiatry, 16*(2), 136–150.

Kraemer, F. W., & Rose, J. B. (2009). Pharmacologic management of acute pediatric pain. *Anesthesiology Clinics, 27*(2), 241–268.

Kroenke, K., Krebs, E. E., & Bair, M. J. (2009). Pharmacotherapy of chronic pain: A synthesis of recommendations from systematic reviews. *General Hospital Psychiatry, 31*(3), 206–219.

Kundu, A., & Berman, B. (2007). Acupuncture for pediatric pain and symptom management. *Pediatric Clinics of North America, 54*(6), 885–889.

Lago, P., Garetti, E., Merazzi, D., Pieragostini, L., Ancora, G., Pirelli, A., et al. (2009). Guidelines for procedural pain in the newborn. *Acta Paediatrica, 98*(6), 932–939.

Lakshmi, C. V., Singhi, P., Malhi, P., & Ray, M. (2007). Topiramate in the prophylaxis of pediatric migraine: A double-blind placebo-controlled trial. *Journal of Child Neurology, 22*(7), 829–835.

Lalwani, K., Shoham, A., Koh, J. L., & McGraw, T. (2005). Use of oxcarbazepine to treat a pediatric patient with resistant complex regional pain syndrome. *The Journal of Pain, 6*(10), 704–706.

Landgraf, J. M., & Abetz, L. (1996). Measuring health outcomes in pediatric populations: Issues in psychometrics and application. In B. Spilker (Ed.), *Quality of life and pharmacoeconomics in clinical trials* (2nd ed., pp. 793–802). Philadelphia: Lippincott-Raven Publishers.

Lee, B. H., Scharff, L., Sethna, N. F., McCarthy, C. F., Scott-Sutherland, J., Shea, A. M., et al. (2002). Physical therapy and cognitive-behavioral treatment for complex regional pain syndromes. *The Journal of Pediatrics, 141*(1), 135–140.

Levy, R. L., Langer, S. L., Walker, L. S., Romano, J. M., Christie, D. L., Youssef, N., et al. (2010). Cognitive-behavioral therapy for children with functional abdominal pain and their parents decreases pain and other symptoms. *The American Journal of Gastroenterology, 105*(4), 946–956.

Lewis, D. (2009). Pediatric migraine. *Neurologic Clinics, 27*(2), 481–501.

Lewis, D., Winner, P., Saper, J., Ness, S., Polverejan, E., Wang, S., et al. (2009). Randomized, double-blind, placebo-controlled study to evaluate the efficacy and safety of topiramate for migraine prevention in pediatric subjects 12 to 17 years of age. *Pediatrics, 123*(3), 924–934.

Lexi-Comp. (2010). Amitriptyline. *Merck maunal online medical libraries* Retrieved September 6, 2010, from http://www.merck.com/mmpe/print/lexicomp/amitriptyline.html.

Li, J. S., Eisenstein, E. L., Grabowski, H. G., Reid, E. D., Mangum, B., Schulman, K. A., et al. (2007). Economic return of clinical trials performed under the pediatric exclusivity program. *Journal of the American Medical Association, 297*(5), 480–488.

Libonate, J., Evans, S., & Tsao, J. C. (2008). Efficacy of acupuncture for health conditions in children: A review. *Scientific World Journal, 8*, 670–682.

Lin, Y. C., Lee, A. C., Kemper, K. J., & Berde, C. B. (2005). Use of complementary and alternative medicine in pediatric pain management service: A survey. *Pain Medicine, 6*(6), 452–458.

Logan, D. E., Claar, R. L., & Scharff, L. (2008a). Social desirability response bias and self-report of psychological distress in pediatric chronic pain patients. *Pain, 136*(3), 366–372.

Logan, D. E., & Scharff, L. (2005). Relationships between family and parent characteristics and functional abilities in children with recurrent pain syndromes: An investigation of moderating effects on the pathway from pain to disability. *Journal of Pediatric Psychology, 30*(8), 698–707.

Logan, D. E., Simons, L. E., & Kaczynski, K. J. (2009). School functioning in adolescents with chronic pain: The role of depressive symptoms in school impairment. *Journal of Pediatric Psychology, 34*(8), 882–892.

Logan, D. E., Simons, L. E., Stein, M. J., & Chastain, L. (2008b). School impairment in adolescents with chronic pain. *The Journal of Pain, 9*(5), 407–416.

Long, A. C., & Palermo, T. M. (2009). Brief report: Web-based management of adolescent chronic pain: Development and usability testing of an online family cognitive behavioral therapy program. *Journal of Pediatric Psychology, 34*(5), 511–516.

Lynch, A. M., Kashikar-Zuck, S., Goldschneider, K. R., & Jones, B. A. (2006). Psychosocial risks for disability in children with chronic back pain. *The Journal of Pain, 7*(4), 244–251.

Malaty, H. M., Abudayyeh, S., O'Malley, K. J., Wilsey, M. J., Fraley, K., Gilger, M. A., et al. (2005). Development of a multidimensional measure for recurrent abdominal pain in children: Population-based studies in three settings. *Pediatrics, 115*(2), e210–e215.

Malleson, P., & Clinch, J. (2003). Pain syndromes in children. *Current Opinion in Rheumatology, 15*(5), 572–580.

Manolis, E., & Pons, G. (2009). Proposals for model-based paediatric medicinal development within the current European Union regulatory framework. *British Journal of Clinical Pharmacology, 68*(4), 493–501.

Mao, J., Gold, M. S., & Backonja, M. M. (2011). Combination drug therapy for chronic pain: A call for more clinical studies. *The Journal of Pain, 12*(2), 157–166.

Matza, L. S., Swensen, A. R., Flood, E. M., Secnik, K., & Leidy, N. K. (2004). Assessment of health-related quality of life in children: A review of conceptual, methodological, and regulatory issues. *Value in Health, 7*(1), 79–92.

McClain, B. C., & Suresh, S. (Eds.). (2010). *Handbook of pediatric chronic pain: Current science and integrative practice*. New York: Springer.

McGrath, P. A., & Hillier, L. M. (2003). Modifying the psychological factors that intensify chidren's pain and prolong disability. In N. L. Schechter, C. B. Berde, & M. Yaster (Eds.), *Pain in infants, children, and adolescents* (2nd ed., pp. 85–104). Philadelphia: Lippincott Williams & Wilkins.

McGrath, P. A., & Ruskin, D. A. (2007). Caring for children with chronic pain: Ethical considerations. *Paediatric Anaesthesia, 17*(6), 505–508.

McGrath, P. J., Walco, G. A., Turk, D. C., Dworkin, R. H., Brown, M. T., Davidson, K., et al. (2008). Core outcome domains and measures for pediatric acute and chronic/recurrent pain clinical trials: PedIMMPACT recommendations. *The Journal of Pain, 9*(9), 771–783.

Meldrum, M. L., Tsao, J. C., & Zeltzer, L. K. (2008). "Just be in pain and just move on": Functioning limitations and strategies in the lives of children with chronic pain. *Journal of Pain Management, 1*(2), 131–141.

Meldrum, M. L., Tsao, J. C., & Zeltzer, L. K. (2009). "I can't be what I want to be": Children's narratives of chronic pain experiences and treatment outcomes. *Pain Medicine, 10*(6), 1018–1034.

Merlijn, V. P. B. M., Hunfeld, J. A. M., van der Wouden, J. C., Hazebroek-Kampschreur, A. A. J. M., Passchier, J., & Koes, B. W. (2006). Factors related to the quality of life in adolescents with chronic pain. *The Clinical Journal of Pain, 22*(3), 306–315.

Milne, C. P., & Bruss, J. B. (2008). The economics of pediatric formulation development for off-patent drugs. *Clinical Therapeutics, 30*(11), 2133–2145.

Miro, J., Huguet, A., & Nieto, R. (2007). Predictive factors of chronic pediatric pain and disability: A Delphi poll. *The Journal of Pain, 8*(10), 774–792.

Morris, D. B. (2011). Narrative and pain: Towards an integrative model. In R. J. Moore (Ed.), *Handbook of pain and palliative care: Biobehavioral approaches for the life course*. New York: Springer.

Mulvaney, S., Lambert, E. W., Garber, J., & Walker, L. S. (2006). Trajectories of symptoms and impairment for pediatric patients with functional abdominal pain: A 5-year longitudinal study. *Journal of the American Academy of Child and Adolescent Psychiatry, 45*(6), 737–744.

Nguyen, M., Ugarte, C., Fuller, I., Haas, G., & Portenoy, R. K. (2005). Access to care for chronic pain: Racial and ethnic differences. *The Journal of Pain, 6*(5), 301–314.

Palermo, T. M. (2000). Impact of recurrent and chronic pain on child and family daily functioning: A critical review of the literature. *Journal of Developmental and Behavioral Pediatrics, 21*(1), 58–69.

Palermo, T. M. (2009). Assessment of chronic pain in children: Current status and emerging topics. *Pain Research & Management, 14*(1), 21–26.

Palermo, T. M., & Chambers, C. T. (2005). Parent and family factors in pediatric chronic pain and disability: An integrative approach. *Pain, 119*(1–3), 1–4.

Palermo, T. M., Long, A. C., Lewandowski, A. S., Drotar, D., Quittner, A. L., & Walker, L. S. (2008). Evidence-based assessment of health-related quality of life and functional impairment in pediatric psychology. *Journal of Pediatric Psychology, 33*(9), 983–996.

Palermo, T. M., Wilson, A. C., Peters, M., Lewandowski, A., & Somhegyi, H. (2009). Randomized controlled trial of an Internet-delivered family cognitive-behavioral therapy intervention for children and adolescents with chronic pain. *Pain, 146*(1–2), 205–213.

Panepinto, J. A., O'Mahar, K. M., DeBaun, M. R., Loberiza, F. R., & Scott, J. P. (2005). Health-related quality of life in children with sickle cell disease: Child and parent perception. *British Journal of Haematology, 130*(3), 437–444.

Parsons, S. K., & Mayer, D. K. (2004). Health-related quality of life assessment in hematologic disease. *Hematology/Oncology Clinics of North America, 18*(6), 1235–1248.

Perquin, C. W., Hunfeld, J. A., Hazebroek-Kampschreur, A. A., van Suijlekom-Smit, L. A., Passchier, J., Koes, B. W., et al. (2003). The natural course of chronic benign pain in childhood and adolescence: A two-year population-based follow-up study. *European Journal of Pain, 7*(6), 551–559.

Peterson, C. C., & Palermo, T. M. (2004). Parental reinforcement of recurrent pain: The moderating impact of child depression and anxiety on functional disability. *Journal of Pediatric Psychology, 29*(5), 331–341.

Pina-Garza, J. E., Espinoza, R., Nordli, D., Bennett, D. A., Spirito, S., Stites, T. E., et al. (2005). Oxcarbazepine adjunctive therapy in infants and young children with partial seizures. *Neurology, 65*(9), 1370–1375.

Portenoy, R. K., Ugarte, C., Fuller, I., & Haas, G. (2004). Population-based survey of pain in the United States: Differences among white, African American, and Hispanic subjects. *The Journal of Pain, 5*(6), 317–328.

Powers, S. W., & Andrasik, F. (2005). Biobehavioral treatment, disability, and psychological effects of pediatric headache. *Pediatric Annals, 34*(6), 461–465.

Radley, D. C., Finkelstein, S. N., & Stafford, R. S. (2006). Off-label prescribing among office-based physicians. *Archives of Internal Medicine, 166*(9), 1021–1026.

Ransom, S., Pearman, T. P., Philip, E., & Anwar, D. (2011). Adult cancer-related pain. In R. J. Moore (Ed.), *Handbook of pain and palliative care: Biobehavioral approaches for the life course*. New York: Springer.

Rice, L. J. (1996). Pain management in children. *Canadian Journal of Anaesthesia, 43*(5 Pt 2), R155–R162.

Riley, J. L., III, Wade, J. B., Myers, C. D., Sheffield, D., Papas, R. K., & Price, D. D. (2002). Racial/ethnic differences in the experience of chronic pain. *Pain, 100*(3), 291–298.

Roberts, R., Rodriguez, W., Murphy, D., & Crescenzi, T. (2003). Pediatric drug labeling: Improving the safety and efficacy of pediatric therapies. *Journal of the American Medical Association, 290*(7), 905–911.

Robins, P. M., Smith, S. M., Glutting, J. J., & Bishop, C. T. (2005). A randomized controlled trial of a cognitive-behavioral family intervention for pediatric recurrent abdominal pain. *Journal of Pediatric Psychology, 30*(5), 397–408.

Rose, J. B., Finkel, J. C., Arquedas-Mohs, A., Himelstein, B. P., Schreiner, M., & Medve, R. A. (2003). Oral tramadol for the treatment of pain of 7–30 days' duration in children. *Anesthesia and Analgesia, 96*(1), 78–81.

Rosen, N. L. (2008). Psychological issues in the evaluation and treatment of tension-type headache. *Current Pain and Headache Reports, 12*(6), 425–432.

Roth-Isigkeit, A., Thyen, U., Stoven, H., Schwarzenberger, J., & Schmucker, P. (2005). Pain among children and adolescents: Restrictions in daily living and triggering factors. *Pediatrics, 115*(2), e152–e162.

Rothwell, P. M. (2005). External validity of randomised controlled trials: "to whom do the results of this trial apply?". *The Lancet, 365*(9453), 82–93.

Rudolph, K. D., & Lambet, S. F. (2007). Child and adoescent depression. In E. J. Mash & R. A. Barkley (Eds.), *Assessment of childhood disorders* (4th ed., pp. 213–252). New York: The Guilford Press.

Sansone, R. A., & Sansone, L. A. (2009). Tramadol: Seizures, serotonin syndrome, and coadministered antidepressants. *Psychiatry (Edgmont), 6*(4), 17–21.

Sawyer, M. G., Carbone, J. A., Whitham, J. N., Roberton, D. M., Taplin, J. E., Varni, J. W., et al. (2005). The relationship between health-related quality of life, pain, and coping strategies in juvenile arthritis – A one year prospective study. *Quality of Life Research, 14*(6), 1585–1598.

Sawyer, M. G., Whitham, J. N., Roberton, D. M., Taplin, J. E., Varni, J. W., & Baghurst, P. A. (2004). The relationship between health-related quality of life, pain and coping strategies in juvenile idiopathic arthritis. *Rheumatology, 43*(3), 325–330.

Schechter, N. L., Berde, C. B., & Yaster, M. (2003). Pain in infants, children, and adolescents: An overview. In N. L. Schechter, C. B. Berde, & M. Yaster (Eds.), *Pain in infants, children, and adolescents* (2nd ed., pp. 3–18). Philadelphia: Lippincott Williams & Wilkins.

Schor, E. L. (2003). Family pediatrics: Report of the task force on the family. *Pediatrics, 111*(6 Pt 2), 1541–1571.

Schwartz, L. A., Radcliffe, J., & Barakat, L. P. (2007). The development of a culturally sensitive pediatric pain management intervention for African American adolescents with sickle cell disease. *Children's Health Care, 36*(3), 267–283.

Simons, L. E., Claar, R. L., & Logan, D. L. (2008). Chronic pain in adolescence: Parental responses, adolescent coping, and their impact on adolescent's pain behaviors. *Journal of Pediatric Psychology, 33*(8), 894–904.

Simons, L. E., Logan, D. E., Chastain, L., & Cerullo, M. (2010a). Engagement in multidisciplinary interventions for pediatric chronic pain: Parental expectations, barriers, and child outcomes. *The Clinical Journal of Pain, 26*(4), 291–299.

Simons, L. E., Logan, D. E., Chastain, L., & Stein, M. (2010b). The relation of social functioning to school impairment among adolescents with chronic pain. *The Clinical Journal of Pain, 26*(1), 16–22.

Southam-Gerow, M. A., & Chorpita, B. F. (2007). Anxiety in children and adolescents. In E. J. Mash & R. A. Barkley (Eds.), *Assessment of childhood disorders* (4th ed., pp. 347–397). New York: The Guilford Press.

Stevens, B. (1994). Pain assessment in children: Birth through adolescence. *Child and Adolescent Clinics of North America, 6*, 725–743.

Tashakori, A., & Afshari, R. (2010). Tramadol overdose as a cause of serotonin syndrome: A case series. *Clinical Toxicology (Philadelphia), 48*(4), 337–341.

Theunissen, N. C., Vogels, T. G., Koopman, H. M., Verrips, G. H., Zwinderman, K. A., Verloove-Vanhorick, S. P., et al. (1998). The proxy problem: Child report versus parent report in health-related quality of life research. *Quality of Life Research, 7*(5), 387–397.

Trautmann, E., & Kroner-Herwig, B. (2010). A randomized controlled trial of Internet-based self-help training for recurrent headache in childhood and adolescence. *Behaviour Research and Therapy, 48*(1), 28–37.

Tsao, J. C. (2006). CAM for pediatric pain: What is state-of-the-research? *Evidence-Based Complementary and Alternative Medicine, 3*(1), 143–144.

Tsao, J. C., Meldrum, M., Kim, S. C., Jacob, M. C., & Zeltzer, L. K. (2007). Treatment preferences for CAM in children with chronic pain. *Evidence-Based Complementary and Alternative Medicine, 4*(3), 367–374.

Tsao, J. C., & Zeltzer, L. K. (2005). Complementary and alternative medicine approaches for pediatric pain: A review of the state-of-the-science. *Evidence-Based Complementary and Alternative Medicine, 2*(2), 149–159.

Turk, D. C., & Flor, H. (1999). Chronic pain: A biobehavioral perspective. In R. J. Gatchel & D. C. Turk (Eds.), *Psychosocial factors in pain: Critical perspectives* (pp. 18–34). New York: The Guilford Press.

Turk, D. C., & Monarch, E. S. (2002). Chronic biopsychosocial perspective on chronic pain. In D. C. Turk & R. J. Gatchel (Eds.), *Psychological approaches to pain management: A practitioner's handbook* (2nd ed., pp. 3–29). New York: Guilford Press.

Varni, J. W. (1995). Pediatric pain: A decade biobehavioral perspective. *Behavioral Therapist, 18*, 65–70.

Varni, J. W., Blount, R. L., Waldron, S. A., & Smith, A. J. (1995). Management of pain and distress. In M. C. Roberts (Ed.), *Handbook of pediatric psychology* (2nd ed., pp. 105–123). New York: The Guilford Press.

Varni, J. W., Burwinkle, T. M., Katz, E. R., Meeske, K., & Dickinson, P. (2002). The PedsQL in pediatric cancer: Reliability and validity of the Pediatric Quality of Life Inventory Generic Core Scales, Multidimensional Fatigue Scale, and Cancer Module. *Cancer, 94*(7), 2090–2106.

Varni, J. W., Burwinkle, T. M., & Lane, M. M. (2005). Health-related quality of life measurement in pediatric clinical practice: An appraisal and precept for future research and application. *Health and Quality of Life Outcomes, 3*(1), 34.

Varni, J. W., Rapoff, M. A., Waldron, S. A., Gragg, R. A., Bernstein, B. H., & Lindsley, C. B. (1996a). Chronic pain and emotional distress in children and adolescents. *Journal of Developmental and Behavioral Pediatrics, 17*(3), 154–161.

Varni, J. W., Rapoff, M. A., Waldron, S. A., Gragg, R. A., Bernstein, B. H., & Lindsley, C. B. (1996b). Effects of perceived stress on pediatric chronic pain. *Journal of Behavioral Medicine, 19*(6), 515–528.

Varrassi, G., Muller-Schwefe, G., Pergolizzi, J., Oronska, A., Morlion, B., Mavrocordatos, P., et al. (2010). Pharmacological treatment of chronic pain – The need for CHANGE. *Current Medical Research and Opinion, 26*(5), 1231–1245.

Verdu, B., Decosterd, I., Buclin, T., Stiefel, F., & Berney, A. (2008). Antidepressants for the treatment of chronic pain. *Drugs, 68*(18), 2611–2632.

Vetter, T. R. (2007). A primer on health-related quality of life in chronic pain medicine. *Anesthesia and Analgesia, 104*(3), 703–718.

Vetter, T. R. (2008). A clinical profile of a cohort of patients referred to an anesthesiology-based pediatric chronic pain medicine program. *Anesthesia and Analgesia, 106*(3), 786–794.

Vetter, T. R. (2011). Demographics of chronic pain in children. In B. C. McClain & S. Suresh (Eds.), *Handbook of pediatric chronic pain: Current science and integrative practice* (1st ed.). New York: Springer.

von Weiss, R. T., Rapoff, M. A., Varni, J. W., Lindsley, C. B., Olson, N. Y., Madson, K. L., et al. (2002). Daily hassles and social support as predictors of adjustment in children with pediatric rheumatic disease. *Journal of Pediatric Psychology, 27*(2), 155–165.

Walco, G. A., Dworkin, R. H., Krane, E. J., LeBel, A. A., & Treede, R. D. (2010). Neuropathic pain in children: Special considerations. *Mayo Clinic Proceedings, 85*(3 Suppl), S33–S41.

Walco, G. A., & Goldschneider, K. R. (Eds.). (2008). *Pain in children: A practical guide for primary care* (1st ed.). New York: Humana Press.

Walco, G. A., Rozelman, H., & Maroof, D. A. (2009). The assessment and management of chronic and recurrent pain in adolescents. In W. T. O'Donohue (Ed.), *Behavioral approaches to chronic disease in adolescence: A guide to integrative care* (pp. 163–175). New York: Springer.

Walker, S. M. (2008). Pain in children: Recent advances and ongoing challenges. *British Journal of Anaesthesia, 101*(1), 101–110.

Waterhouse, M., Tsao, J. C., & Zeltzer, L. K. (2009). Commentary on the use of acupuncture in chronic pediatric pain. *Journal of Developmental and Behavioral Pediatrics, 30*(1), 69–71.

Waters, E., Stewart-Brown, S., & Fitzpatrick, R. (2003). Agreement between adolescent self-report and parent reports of health and well-being: Results of an epidemiological study. *Child: Care, Health and Development, 29*(6), 501–509.

Weinshilboum, R. (2003). Inheritance and drug response. *The New England Journal of Medicine, 348*(6), 529–537.

White, K. S., & Farrell, A. D. (2006). Anxiety and psychosocial stress as predictors of headache and abdominal pain in urban early adolescents. *Journal of Pediatric Psychology, 31*(6), 582–596.

Wiffen, P. J., McQuay, H. J., Edwards, J. E., & Moore, R. A. (2005). Gabapentin for acute and chronic pain. *Cochrane Database Syst Rev,* (3), CD005452.

Wilson, J. F. (2003). Survey of reference ranges and clinical measurements for psychoactive drugs in serum. *Therapeutic Drug Monitoring, 25*(2), 243–247.

Winner, P. (2008). Pediatric headache. *Current Opinion in Neurology, 21*(3), 316–322.

Winner, P., Pearlman, E. M., Linder, S. L., Jordan, D. M., Fisher, A. C., & Hulihan, J. (2005). Topiramate for migraine prevention in children: A randomized, double-blind, placebo-controlled trial. *Headache, 45*(10), 1304–1312.

Youssef, N. N., Murphy, T. G., Langseder, A. L., & Rosh, J. R. (2006). Quality of life for children with functional abdominal pain: A comparison study of patients' and parents' perceptions. *Pediatrics, 117*(1), 54–59.

Zeltzer, L. K., Bursch, B., & Walco, G. (1997a). Pain responsiveness and chronic pain: A psychobiological perspective. *Journal of Developmental and Behavioral Pediatrics, 18*(6), 413–422.

Zeltzer, L. K., Bush, J. P., Chen, E., & Riveral, A. (1997b). A psychobiologic approach to pediatric pain: Part I. History, physiology, and assessment strategies. *Current Problems in Pediatrics, 27*(6), 225–253.

Zeltzer, L. K., Bush, J. P., Chen, E., & Riveral, A. (1997c). A psychobiologic approach to pediatric pain: Part II. Prevention and treatment. *Current Problems in Pediatrics, 27*(7), 264–284.

Zernikow, B., Michel, E., & Anderson, B. (2007). Transdermal fentanyl in childhood and adolescence: A comprehensive literature review. *The Journal of Pain, 8*(3), 187–207.

Zernikow, B., Michel, E., Craig, F., & Anderson, B. J. (2009). Pediatric palliative care: Use of opioids for the management of pain. *Paediatric Drugs, 11*(2), 129–151.

Zhou, S. F. (2009a). Polymorphism of human cytochrome P450 2D6 and its clinical significance: Part I. *Clinical Pharmacokinetics, 48*(11), 689–723.

Zhou, S. F. (2009b). Polymorphism of human cytochrome P450 2D6 and its clinical significance: Part II. *Clinical Pharmacokinetics, 48*(12), 761–804.

Zhou, S. F., Liu, J. P., & Chowbay, B. (2009). Polymorphism of human cytochrome P450 enzymes and its clinical impact. *Drug Metabolism Reviews, 41*(2), 89–295.

Chapter 12
Pain in the Older Person

Bill H. McCarberg and B. Eliot Cole

By the year 2030, there well be 70 million Americans 65 years or older (20% of the US population) (Centers for Disease Control and Prevention 2001). The chronic conditions associated with older adults such as osteoarthritis, atherosclerosis, cancer, and diabetes are likely to contribute to the already escalating costs. About one-third of total US health care costs, $300 billion, are spent on older adults. In this population, pain is the most common symptom noted when consulting a physician (Otis and McGeeney 2001). The most frequently reported source of pain in one study was lower back pain (40%), arthritis (24%), previous fractures (14%), and neuropathies (11%) (Ferrel et al. 1990). Another study of long-term care residents found 45–80% had substantial pain from musculoskeletal origin that affected their functional status and quality of life (Helm and Gibson 1999). Almost half of older adults and 20% of those reporting no limitations in activities of daily living claim limited ability to walk one-quarter of a mile due to pain and fatigue (Hardy et al. 2010).

Pain is not a normal part of aging. Yet many conditions that commonly occur or worsen with aging also produce pain: diabetic peripheral neuropathy, postherpetic neuralgia, osteoarthritis, and cancer related pain, etc. Poor pain management can lead to deconditioning, gait disturbances, and falls. These can cause pain and aggravate preexisting pain. The cognitively impaired elderly are even more at risk. In a study by Won, 74% of a demented, elderly long-term care population suffered from inadequately treated pain (Won et al. 1999). Despite these patients being institutionalized and under the care of health professionals, the high prevalence of pain was overlooked, in part because identifying pain requires special assessment skills not used by many long-term care facilities. Depression, anxiety, decreased socialization, sleep disturbance, impaired ambulation, and increased health care use have all been found to be associated with the presence of pain in older people (Parmelee et al. 1991).

Some of the best information on pain management in older populations comes from data generated in nursing homes and home care populations. Nursing homes vary greatly in the amount of formal or informal health care they may provide and differ dramatically from state to state and within states. Twenty thousand nursing homes provide care for almost two million older persons in the United States. Nursing homes account for more than twice as many beds compared to acute care hospitals and more than three times as many facilities with residents who are typically poor and

B.H. McCarberg, MD (✉)
University of California at San Diego School Medicine,
San Diego, CA, USA
e-mail: bill.h.mccarberg@kp.org

B.E. Cole, MD
Shoals Hospital Senior Care Center, Muscle Shoals, AL, USA

R.J. Moore (ed.), *Handbook of Pain and Palliative Care: Biobehavioral Approaches for the Life Course*,
DOI 10.1007/978-1-4419-1651-8_12, © Springer Science+Business Media, LLC 2012

disabled. It has been estimated that for every resident in a nursing home, there are three more with similar disabilities living at home or other long-term care facilities (Ouslander et al. 1997).

Elderly persons also present with multiple medical problems, many of which are irreversible, and cure is rare. The spectrum of complaints, manifestations of distress, and differential diagnosis are often different in elderly persons. The implications of functional impairment can be profound, and recovery from illness is often less dramatic and slower to occur. Despite this, relief of discomfort and disability modification can often be achieved. Without adequate awareness of the nuances of elderly patients' pain management, care is less than optimal.

For example, osteoarthritis is the most common painful disorder in older individuals with over 80% of people older than 75 having symptomatic osteoarthritis, and 80% over the age of 50 have radiologic evidence of osteoarthritis (Sharma 2001).Despite the prevalence and suffering precipitated by pain, it often remains under reported and under treated especially in the elderly. The incidence of under treatment of pain in older patients ranges from 25 to 50% in adult communities (Ferrell 1991). It ranges from 45 to 80% in nursing homes (Ferrell et al. 1990), and as high as 85% in long-term care facilities (Mobily and Herr 1996).

Multiple reasons for inadequate care have been cited in the literature. Older adults often express that pain is inevitable and that the treatment is worse than the symptom. They fear underlying causes, such as cancer, and the side effects of the analgesics. Health care providers lack adequate education in pain management and some believe, mistakenly, that older patients have a higher pain tolerance. Treatment is also often withheld because of concerns about falling, diminished cognition, addiction, and constipation. The elder patient may contribute to this problem by failing to report when pain is present. In one study, up to 56% of health symptoms are regularly underreported in our aging population (Ferrell 1995). In this chapter, we highlight issues related to pain in older patients.

Neurophysiology of Aging

Excitatory and inhibitory mechanisms in the nervous system exert differential effects contributing to the experience of pain and depend on complex communications among many neural systems. The effects of age on the human brain are known to be extensive, involving changes in structure, neurochemistry, and function (Hunskaar et al. 1985). Cellular and neurochemical substrates change thereby altering the pain sensation (nociception). There is strong evidence of a progressive, age-related loss of serontonergic and noradrenergic neurons in the dorsal horn suggesting impairment of the pain inhibitory system (Ko et al. 1997; Iwata et al. 2002). Peripheral nerves decrease with age, both unmyelinated and myelinated, and increasing age shows signs of related damage or degeneration of sensory fibers (Knox et al. 1989; Kakigi 1987).

There are so many integrated processes involved in pain, it is difficult to determine what effects these changes have. An increased pain threshold has been shown with age. Decreased acuity for pain may place older people at a greater risk of tissue damage (Birren and Schroots 1995). Age is not associated with substantive functional change over much of the pain stimulus–response curve (Chakour et al. 1996). Increasing pain reports with age occur when stimuli are intense or persist for longer periods.

It is widely believed that elderly persons do not experience pain with the same intensity as a younger population and this is not borne out in the literature (Mobily and Herr 1996). Nerves that have been injured by trauma or disease can become more sensitive. Older persons are more likely to have slow resolution of peripheral sensitization despite tissue healing leading to prolonged pain states not seen in younger populations. Under circumstances where pain is likely to persist, older people are especially vulnerable to the negative impacts of pain.

Assessment

There are many diagnostic challenges in assessing pain in the elder person. Aggressive testing or implementation of complicated treatment is less important than providing comfort and effective symptom management for many patients (Ferrell 1996). Incomplete medical records and unavailability of consultants often hamper initial assessment. Diagnostic laboratories, radiographs, or other resources common in ambulatory settings may not be available because of lack of convenient transportation. Testing or consultations disrupt the frail elderly's schedules, resulting in missed medication and meals.

Pain descriptor may not be accurate, the location and onset of the pain may not be precise or remembered. A diagnosis of neuropathic pain may be missed if the signs and symptoms of neural dysfunction are not recognized. Neuropathic pain (diabetic peripheral neuropathy, post herpetic neuralgia, etc.) may arise from many neurologic levels, manifesting with negative neurosensory symptoms, such as loss of sensation, or with positive sensory symptoms such as paresthesia, hyperalgesia, dyesthesia, or allodynia. Elderly persons in long-term care settings can present unique challenges to pain assessment with as many as 50% of the residents likely to have significant cognitive impairment and psychological illness (Ferrell 1995).

Nociceptive pain (arthritis, surgery, fracture, etc.) usually relates to known pathology, is more precisely localized, and pain levels often represent level of tissue damage. There can be considerable overlap in the symptoms between neuropathic and nociceptive pain. The symptoms that are more suggestive of neuropathy include burning, electrical sensations, sharp, stabbing, shooting, knife-like, numbness, and pins/needles often with a sudden paroxysmal pattern.

Commonly used tools for measuring pain – for example, the Visual Analog Scale (VAS), the McGill Pain Questionnaire (MPQ), and the Verbal Descriptor Scales (VDS) – are reliable and valid measures of pain, especially nociceptive pain.

Two scales developed specifically to assess neuropathic pain include:

- Neuropathic Pain Scale (NPS): Galer and Jensen (1997) includes two items that assess the global dimensions of pain intensity and pain unpleasantness, and eight items that assess specific qualities of NP. An eleventh item assesses the temporal sequence of pain.
- Leeds assessment of neuropathic symptoms and signs (LANSS) (Bennett 2001) Pain Scale: a seven-point scale based on an analysis of sensory description and bedside examination of sensory dysfunction. An advantage of using the LANSS is that it provides immediate information in clinical settings.

Mood, physical functioning, pain-coping strategies, and social support can have a significant impact on both the patient's ability to adjust to pain and the effectiveness of treatment. Depression has been associated with the pain of postherpetic neuralgia, spinal cord injury, and HIV-AIDs. A number of psychological assessment tools are available, including the Beck Depression Inventory (Beck et al. 1961), the Pain Disability Index (Pollard 1984), and the Coping Strategies Questionnaire (Rosenstiel and Keefe 1983).

Incomplete medical records, failure to disclose use of alcohol or recreational drugs, lack of appropriate diagnostic tests, and undisclosed medications may complicate initial assessment in older adults. Loss of vision, hearing, and cognitive impairments contribute to the difficulty. Even patients with moderate cognitive impairment can provide useful and reliable information if the provider is patient and allows adequate time. Concrete questions with yes or no responses are helpful. Pain can wax and wane, making frequent assessments more valid than relying on patient memory. Observing patient behavior and obtaining information from family or other caregivers can be valuable sources of information when the patient lacks optimal communication skills (see also Kovach 2011). At times an analgesic medication trial may provide useful information. Providing comfort, maintaining cognitive function, and effective symptom management is more important than aggressive testing for a definitive diagnosis, especially near the end of life (Bennett 2001).

Self-Management: What Can Older Adults Do to Manage Their Own Pain?

Since age cannot be controlled, as adults grow older, additional strategies may be used to lessen the severity and frequency of pain. These approaches range from weight stabilization (after weight loss if necessary), smoking cessation, maintenance of blood sugar in the normal range (if diabetic to prevent worsening of diabetic peripheral neuropathy related pain), correction of abnormal physiological markers (e.g., lipids predisposing one to increased risk of cardiovascular and cerebrovascular disease), treatment of depression, daily exercise program, proper nutrition, adequate sleep, and daily cognitive activity. While controlled studies do not absolutely establish that these approaches significantly prevent or reduce pain, from a common sense perspective it seems reasonable to provide patients with information that helps them maximize their potential, better anticipate painful circumstances, use proper body mechanics to limit or prevent injury, and to optimize overall fitness and health status.

Being overweight (along with depression and smoking) is an independent predictor associated with an increased likelihood of incident pain (Shi et al. 2010). Overweight and obese twins may be more likely to report low back pain, tension-type or migraine headache, fibromyalgia, abdominal pain, and chronic widespread pain than normal-weight twins after adjustment for age, gender, and depression; mechanisms underlying these relationships are likely diverse and multifactorial, with the associations partially explained by familial and sociodemographic factors, and depression (Wright et al. 2010). A nearly twofold increase has been found in the probability of chronic pain among elderly people with abdominal obesity that was independent of the other components of metabolic syndrome, high sensitivity C-reactive protein (hsCRP), established surrogate markers for insulin resistance, depression, anxiety, and the presence of painful co-morbid conditions (Ray et al. 2010). Taken together, these studies suggest that there may be potential benefit from programs combining training in weight management and pain management (Somers et al. 2010).

Elevations in serum lipids are known to be a significant risk factor for coronary artery disease (CAD); the association between hyperlipidemia and CAD in older men and women has been shown in epidemiologic studies. Dietary modification is considered an essential part of an overall strategy to reduce cardiovascular risk. Cardiac rehabilitation and exercise training programs improve plasma lipids levels and reduce the prevalence of metabolic syndrome (Aslam et al. 2009).

Due to muscle weakness, reduced aerobic capacity, and limited flexibility of joints and muscles, range of motion, strengthening, and aerobic exercises are recommended for patients with osteoarthritis (Allegrante and Marks 2003). Fibromyalgia literature supports the notion that tailored exercise reduces symptoms and improves fitness; the therapeutic alliance between healthcare provider and patient is enhanced if both understand the potential physiologic obstacles to exercise and the benefits of exercise for the condition (Jones and Liptan 2009). Exercise is effective for the management of chronic lower back pain for up to 1 year after treatment and for fibromyalgia for up to 6 months although there is conflicting evidence about which exercise program is effective for chronic lower back pain; evidence of exercise effectiveness is limited for chronic neck pain, soft tissue shoulder disorders, and lateral epicondylitis (Mior 2001). Older patients who have CAD typically have markedly reduced exercise capacity and overall physical function; exercise training programs significantly improve exercise capacity and overall fitness (Aslam et al. 2009).

Not every approach has to be "high tech" or "cutting edge" to give someone with pain a bit of relief. With respect to self-management of acute lower back pain, the Kaiser health plan recommends to its members that ice be applied immediately, medication be taken as directed, and that good posture and body positions be maintained (The Permanente Medical Group and Inc 2003).

Additionally, sitting with legs extended in a bathtub or on the floor, engaging in prolonged chair sitting, and sitting in a chair without the use of a towel roll to keep the back in a neutral position is discouraged. Little, simple things can make a real difference.

Red Flags: When Must Older Adults Seek Out Medical Attention

Medical attention should be immediately sought for any acute pain that has not been previously evaluated, especially for chest pain and severe ("worst in lifetime") headaches. In some cases, "new" pain is acute recognition of persistent pain, making it difficult to determine when to seek medical care. Whenever pain limits performance of activities of daily living, interferes with appetite and sleep, or contributes to anxiety and depression, proper medical evaluation is warranted.

So-called "red flags" for lower back pain include gradual onset of back pain, age greater than 50 years, thoracic back pain, pain lasting longer than 6 weeks, history of trauma, fever/chills/night sweats, unintentional weight loss, pain worse with recumbency, pain worse at night, unrelenting pain despite supratherapeutic doses of analgesics, history of malignancy and/or immunosuppression, recent procedure causing bacteremia, and/or intravenous drug use. Physical finding of fever, hypotension, extreme hypertension, pale/ashen appearance, pulsatile abdominal mass, peripheral pulse amplitude differentials, spinous process tenderness, focal neurologic signs, and acute urinary retention all suggest serious potential pathology (Winters et al. 2006).

"Red flags" for headache include sudden onset, worsening pattern, headache with systemic illness, presence of focal neurologic signs or symptoms, papilledema, triggered by cough/exertion, during pregnancy or postpartum, and those occurring with cancer, Lyme disease, and HIV infections (Lipton et al. 2004). Underlying mechanisms include subarachnoid or subdural hemorrhage, mass lesion, meningitis/encephalitis, arteriovenous malformation, cortical vein or cranial sinus thrombosis, carotid artery dissection, pituitary apoplexy, metastasis, and opportunistic infection (Lipton et al. 2004).

Transitions: How to Manage Pain During Transitions in Care Settings over Time

Aspects of the psychosocial environment are thought to be associated with a higher likelihood of reporting pain, particularly chronic pain; these aspects may especially be potential risk factors for future development of musculoskeletal pain according to some (Blyth et al. 2007). Transition from one level of care to another or from one venue to another is one of many psychosocial stressors facing older people. Commonly, older people are relocated from their homes of many decades to the homes of their adult children, to assisted living facilities, and skilled care units when their partner dies. While such change is intended to be in the best interest of the survivor, it is a significant disruption for most people. Older people must occasionally enter hospitals due to new onset of illness and/or complications from existing conditions. For some, the level of care needed requires admission to a tertiary care facility far away from their homes.

Transition from one level of care to another or from one environment to another also creates opportunities for affected patients to "slip through the cracks." This is not deliberate on the part of healthcare providers, but often reflects poor communication during transitions (e.g., patients not able to express themselves, failure of caregivers to give thorough report, lack of comprehensiveness in transfer documents), complicated by processes used in different care facilities. Moving from the community into a skilled care facility, rehabilitation program, acute care hospital, palliative care program, and hospice create challenges for patients and their caregivers.

Pain Management at the End of Life

Contrary to the desired and idealized death at home, most Americans die in hospitals wishing to be free of distressing symptoms, having the opportunity to communicate with others, and believing their needs will be attended to by healthcare providers knowledgeable about end-of-life care (Pantilat 2002). It is critical for caregivers to communicate clearly about treatment options and to create opportunities for patients and provide input (see also Wachholtz and Makowski 2011; Kovach 2011; Fine 2011; Hallenbeck 2011).

Those coming to the end of their lives in skilled care facilities often face considerable hardship as nursing home staff provide care for more diverse, frail, and complex dying residents, hampered by persistent staff shortages, high staff turnover, and inadequate reimbursement to provide high-quality, end-of-life care (Pantilat 2002). Most clinicians, nurses, and aides do not receive formal training in palliative care during their training and lack necessary skills. This is further complicated by the general lack of physician and/or advanced mid-level practitioner presence in such facilities as primary care providers self-select for in- or out-patient care, creating an inevitable loss of longitudinal awareness of patients beyond their immediate needs.

To better care for older people throughout their lives, healthcare providers at all levels need more education about the likelihood of pain and its management, consistent approaches for the control of pain, integration of pain and symptom management into an overall palliative focus as lives conclude, use of medical documentation systems accessible to caregivers in more than one facility, and need to keep plans of care up-to-date as patients move from one venue to another. Wherever possible, institutional pain relief nurses, champions, or educators should be utilized to advocate for patients regardless of care setting, and to serve as fixed assets within facilities to educate and mentor others in best practices for pain management and end-of-life care. Adherence to recognized national standards and implementation of institutional policies declaring pain assessment and management to be essential aspects of care, making pain management methods more consistent within facilities while simultaneously recognizing the need to individualize care based upon unique circumstances will do much to improve pain across the remaining life span of older people.

Predictions for a Potentially Painful Future

As noted in the beginning of this chapter, America is growing older. Americans are living longer. Growing older, however, is not linearly related to pain, but growing older does give someone the opportunity to experience painful life events and disease processes. Sadly, many assume that older people must experience more pain as a direct function of aging and thus take a minimalistic approach to pain control.

Recent demographic trends suggest that in the future there will be fewer in the pool of workers in the marketplace, with many older Americans opting to work longer as their skills are needed or their economic circumstances dictate that they must keep working. This will create pressure on healthcare professionals to keep older people functioning in the workplace longer, while longer life expectancy will mean that more people will be living painfully. Unless pain is managed effectively, and addressed as early as possible, excessive utilization of finite resources may occur.

Summary

The US population is growing older and is living longer. While age does not cause pain directly, it gives opportunity for painful conditions to develop. Growing older is not for the faint of heart, but there is nothing we can do to stop it from happening. Pain must never be discounted as part of aging. Future practitioners must not make the erroneous assumption that older people do or do not have pain as a class, but make individual assessments leading to treatment decisions based upon the mechanism of pain generation. While there is certainly no universal strategy for managing pain, many common approaches can be used to effectively manage symptoms and treat those living with persistent pain. Armed with facts about the aging process and the occurrence of pain in the older person, required by accreditation bodies to do more for older people in pain, and greater commitment to provide pain relief should translate into older patients in pain receiving enhanced scrutiny, more thorough assessment, and lifelong management of their pain regardless of venue of care or underlying disease state.

References

Allegrante, J. P., & Marks, R. (2003). Self-efficacy in management of osteoarthritis. *Rheumatic Diseases Clinics of North America, 29*, 747–768.

Aslam, F., Haque, A., Lee, L. E., & Foody, J. (2009). Hyperlipidemia in older adults. *Clinics in Geriatric Medicine, 25*, 591–606.

Beck, A. T., Ward, C., & Mendelson, M. (1961). Beck Depression Inventory (BDI). *Archives of General Psychiatry, 4*, 561–571.

Bennett, M. (2001). The LANSS Pain Scale: the Leeds assessment of neuropathic symptoms and signs. *Pain, 92*, 147–157.

Birren, J. E., & Schroots, J. F. (1995). History, concepts, and theory in the psychology of aging. In J. E. Birren & K. W. Schaie (Eds.), *Handbook of the psychology of aging* (4th ed.). San Diego: Academic.

Blyth, F. M., Macfarlane, G. J., & Nicholas, M. K. (2007). The contribution of psychosocial factors to the development of chronic pain: The key to better outcomes for patients? *Pain, 129*, 8–11.

Centers for Disease Control and Prevention. (2001). Healthy aging: preventing disease and improving quality of life among older Americans. Atlanta: CDC. Retrieved January 7, 2002, from www.cdc.gov/nccdphp/aag-aging.htm

Chakour, M., Gibson, S. J., Bradbeer, M., & Helme, R. D. (1996). The effect of age on A delta and C fibre thermal pain perception. *Pain, 64*, 143–152.

Ferrel, B. A., Ferrel, B. R., & Osterweil, D. (1990). Pain in the nursing home. *Journal of American Geriatrics Society, 38*, 409–414.

Ferrell, B. A. (1991). Pain management in elderly people. *Journal of the American Geriatrics Society, 39*, 64–73.

Ferrell, B. A. (1995). Pain evaluation and management in the nursing home. *Annals of Internal Medicine, 123*, 681–687.

Ferrell, B. A. (1996). Overview of aging and pain. In B. A. Ferrell & B. R. Ferrell (Eds.), *Pain in the elderly*. Seattle: IASP Press.

Ferrell, B. A., Ferrell, B. R., & Osterweil, D. (1990). Pain in the nursing home. *Journal of the American Geriatrics Society, 38*, 409–414.

Fine, P. (2011). Recognition and resolution of ethical barriers to palliative care research. In R. J. Moore (Ed.), *Handbook of Pain and Palliative Care: Biobehavioral Approaches for the Life Course*. New York: Springer.

Galer, B., & Jensen, M. (1997). Development and preliminary validation of a pain measure specific to neuropathic pain. The neuropathic pain scale. *Neurology, 48*, 332–338.

Hallenbeck, J. (2011). Pain and intercultural communication. In R. J. Moore (Ed.), *Handbook of Pain and Palliative Care: Biobehavioral Approaches for the Life Course*. New York: Springer.

Hardy, S. E., McGur, D. J., & Studenski, S. A. (2010). *Journal of the American Geriatrics Society, 58*, 539–544.

Helm, R. D., & Gibson, S. J. (1999). Pain in older people. In I. K. Crombie, P. R. Croft, S. J. Linton, et al. (Eds.), *Epidemiology of pain*. Seattle: IASP Press.

Hunskaar, S., Fasmer, O. B., & Hole, K. (1985). Acetylsalicylic acid, paracetamol and morphine inhibit behavioral responses to intrathecally administered substance P or capsaicin. *Life Sciences, 37*, 1835–1841.

Iwata, K., Fukuoka, T., Kondo, E., Tsuboi, Y., Tashiro, A., Noguchi, K., et al. (2002). Plastic changes in nociceptive transmission of the rat spinal cord with advancing age. *Journal of Neurophysiology, 87*(2), 1086–1093.

Jones, K. D., & Liptan, G. L. (2009). Exercise interventions in fibromyalgia: clinical applications from the evidence. *Rheumatic Diseases Clinics of North America, 35*, 373–391.

Kakigi, R. (1987). The effect of aging on somatosensory evoked potentials following stimulation of the posterior tibial nerve in man. *Electroencephalography and Clinical Neurophysiology, 68*, 227–286.

Knox, C. A., Kokmen, E., & Dyck, P. J. (1989). Morphometric alteration of rat myelinated fibres with aging. *Journal of Neuropathology and Experimental Neurology, 48*(2), 119–139.

Ko, M. L., King, M. A., Gordon, T. L., & Crisp, T. (1997). The effects of aging on spinal neurochemistry in the rat. *Brain Research Bulletin, 42*(2), 95–98.

Kovach, C. R. (2011). Assessing pain and unmet needs in patients with advanced dementia: The role of the serial trial intervention (STI). In R. J. Moore (Ed.), *Handbook of Pain and Palliative Care: Biobehavioral Approaches for the Life Course*. New York: Springer.

Lipton, R. B., Bigal, M. E., Steiner, T. J., Silberstein, S. D., & Olesen, J. (2004). Classification of primary headaches. *Neurology, 63*, 427–435.

Mior, S. (2001). Exercise in the treatment of chronic pain. *The Clinical Journal of Pain, 17*(4 suppl), S77–S85.

Mobily, P., & Herr, K. (1996). Barriers to managing resident's pain. *Contemporary Long Term Care, 19*, 60A–60B.

Otis, J. A. D., & McGeeney, B. (2001). Managing pain in the elderly. *Clinical Geriatrics, 9*, 82–88.

Ouslander, J. G., Osterweil, D., & Morley, J. (1997). *Medical care in the nursing home* (2nd ed.). New York: McGraw-Hill.

Pantilat, S. Z. (2002). End-of-life care for the hospitalized patient. *The Medical Clinics of North America, 86*, 749–770.

Parmelee, P. A., Katz, I. R., & Lawton, M. P. (1991). The relation of pain to depression among institutionalized aged. *Journal of Gerontology, 46*, 15–21.

Pollard, C. A. (1984). Preliminary validity study of the pain disability index. *Perceptual and Motor Skills, 59*(3), 974.

Ray, L., Lipton, R. B., Zimmerman, M. E., Katz, M. J., Derby, C.A. (2010). Mechanisms of association between obesity and chronic pain in the elderly. Pain. doi:10.1016/j.pain.2010.08.043; in press.

Rosenstiel, A. K., & Keefe, F. J. (1983). The use of coping strategies in chronic low back pain patients: relationship to patient characteristics and current adjustment. *Pain, 17*(1), 33–44.

Sharma, L. (2001). Epidemiology of osteoarthritis. In R. W. Moskowitz, O. S. Howell, R. D. Altman, et al. (Eds.), *Osteoarthritis: diagnosis and medical/surgical management* (3rd ed.). Philadelphia: W.B. Saunders.

Shi, Y., Wooten, W. M., Roberts, R. O., & Warner, D. O. (2010). Modifiable risk factors for incidence of pain in older adults. *Pain, 151*, 366–371.

Somers, T. J., Wren, A. A., Keefe, F. J. (2010). Understanding chronic pain in older adults: Abdominal fat is where it is at. Pain. 2011;152(1):53–9.

The Permanente Medical Group, Inc. (2003). Self-management for acute lower back pain. Regional Health Education 90815 (Revised 7-05).

Wachholtz, A., & Makowski, S. (2011). Spiritual dimensions of pain and suffering. In R. J. Moore (Ed.), *Handbook of Pain and Palliative Care: Biobehavioral Approaches for the Life Course*. New York: Springer.

Winters, M. E., Kluetz, P., & Zilberstein, J. (2006). Back pain emergencies. *The Medical Clinics of North America, 90*(3), 505–523.

Won, A., Lapane, K., Gambassi, G., et al. (1999). Correlates and management of nonmalignant pain in the nursing home. *Journal of the American Geriatrics Society, 47*, 936–942.

Wright, L. J., Schur, E., Noonan, C., Ahumada, S., Buchwald, D., & Afari, N. (2010). Chronic pain, overweight, and obesity: findings from a Community-Based Twin Registry. *The Journal of Pain, 11*(7), 628–635.

Chapter 13
Pain After Traumatic Brain Injury

Jason K. Ough and Devi E. Nampiaparampil

Introduction

The annual incidence of TBI in the United States has been estimated at approximately 1.7 million cases. This figure does not account for patients evaluated at military or Veterans Affairs (VA) hospitals (Faul et al. 2010). Recent American military data shows that nearly a quarter of soldiers wounded in recent conflicts have sustained a TBI (Blyth and Bazarian 2010). European data estimates that the annual incidence of TBI is as high as 500 per 100,000 population (Maas et al. 2007). These numbers may underestimate the problem, however, since they do not account for the countless people with TBI who remain undiagnosed perhaps because they do not present to medical settings. TBI is at least 10 times more common than spinal cord injury (Khan et al. 2003). It is the most common cause of death and disability in trauma patients (Berry et al. 2010).

TBI exacts a physical, mental, and emotional toll – not only on patients and their families, but also on the medical system and society as a whole. Pain in the TBI population is significant and can affect cognition, emotion, and function, which can thereby negatively affect rehabilitation and interfere with recovery (Bohnen and Jolles 1992). Knowledge of the epidemiology, pathophysiology, and diagnosis of TBI and its sequelae is important for complete understanding of this condition and is crucial for thorough recovery and reintegration into the community. In this chapter, we will address these aspects of care.

Epidemiology

In 1995, the CDC, in the *Guidelines for Surveillance of Central Nervous System Injury*, defined TBI as: "craniocerebral trauma, specifically, an occurrence of injury to the head (arising from blunt or penetrating trauma or from acceleration-deceleration forces) that is associated with any of these

J.K. Ough, MD (✉)
Department of Anesthesiology, New York University Langone Medical Center,
NYU School of Medicine, New York, NY, USA
e-mail: jkough@gmail.com

D.E. Nampiaparampil, MD
Department of Anesthesiology, New York University Langone Medical Center,
NYU School of Medicine, New York, NY, USA

Department of Rehabilitation Medicine, NYU School of Medicine, New York, NY, USA

Department of Veterans Affairs New York Harbor Health Care System, New York, NY, USA

R.J. Moore (ed.), *Handbook of Pain and Palliative Care: Biobehavioral Approaches for the Life Course*,   177
DOI 10.1007/978-1-4419-1651-8_13, © Springer Science+Business Media, LLC 2012

occurrences attributable to the injury: decreased level of consciousness, amnesia, other neurologic or neuropsychological abnormalities, skull fracture, diagnosed intracranial lesions, or death (Corrigan 2010; Thurman et al. 1995b)."

The World Health Organization (WHO) adopted a similar definition in their report on neurotrauma and defined TBI as "an occurrence of injury to the head with at least one of the following: observed or self-reported loss of consciousness (LOC) or amnesia due to head trauma, neurologic or neuropsychological changes or diagnoses of skull fracture or intracranial lesions that can be attributed to head trauma, or an occurrence of death resulting from trauma with head injury or TBI listed in the sequence of conditions that resulted in death (Thurman et al. 1995a)." The WHO further specifies that TBI cases must arise from blunt or penetrating trauma, or acceleration–deceleration forces. It excludes other head injuries including lacerations, facial fractures, metabolic or infectious encephalopathies, neoplasms, strokes, and intracerebral hemorrhage not due to trauma (Thurman et al. 1995a).

The hallmark diagnostic features of TBI include head injury associated with alterations in consciousness or amnesia. However, many authors continue to define TBI in various manners (including patients with concussion injury or using the terms head injury and brain injury interchangeably), which leads to ambiguity in both the clinical and research settings.

It has been estimated that 275,000 hospitalizations for nonfatal TBI occur annually in the United States (Faul et al. 2010). The overall annual incidence of TBI in the United States is reported to be 506.4 cases per 100,000 population, with emergency department visits comprising nearly 80% of these cases (Faul et al. 2010; Corrigan et al. 2010). These figures may be underestimates, however, as it is believed that up to 40% of patients with mild TBI do not seek medical care, and 25% do not even report their injuries to a health care provider (Sosin et al. 1996). The reported incidence of TBI is higher in developing countries, and this has been attributed to an increased rate of motor vehicle injuries (Corrigan et al. 2010).

The incidence of TBI is not evenly distributed among all age groups or across gender. An Australian review by Khan et al. in 2003 reported that the incidence of TBI peaked in the 15–35-year-old age group, and males were 3–4 times more likely to suffer from TBI than females. This may be a reflection of potentially preventable risk-taking behavior (Khan et al. 2003).

Determining the lifetime prevalence of TBI can also be challenging. Two birth cohort studies (one in Finland and one in New Zealand) have investigated the lifetime prevalence of TBI. The Finnish investigators retrospectively reviewed the hospital records and death certificates of 12,000 residents born in 1966. They found that, by age 35, approximately 3.8% of the cohort had at least 1 hospitalization for TBI (Winqvist et al. 2007b). The average annual incidence of TBI was 118 cases per 100,000 population (Winqvist et al. 2007b). They also calculated that at age 34 the prevalence of TBI with residual sequelae from injury was 269 cases per 100,000 population (Winqvist et al. 2007b). The New Zealand study authors utilized prospective interviews to collect data and included concussive head injuries in the definition of TBI (McKinlay et al. 2008). They reported that by age 25, there was a 31.6% prevalence of TBI that required medical care (McKinlay et al. 2008). Other retrospective studies have estimated lifetime prevalence rates for TBI to range between 5.7 and 8.5% (Anstey et al. 2004; Silver et al. 2001).

Mortality

TBI may decrease life expectancy (Masel and DeWitt 2010). CDC data shows that an estimated 52,000 patients with TBI in the United States die annually (Faul et al. 2010). This represents 3.5% of all cases of TBI. In the United States, TBI is a contributing factor in nearly one-third of all injury-related deaths (Faul et al. 2010). On the other hand, a European review in 2005 reported an average

TBI mortality rate of 15 deaths per 100,000 cases per year, or approximately 6.4% of total new cases per year (Tagliaferri et al. 2006; Svestkova et al. 2010).

Costs of TBI: Direct and Indirect Costs

Corrigan et al. reported that total lifetime costs of all TBI cases in the year 2000 were over $60 billion, with productivity losses of over $50 billion (Corrigan et al. 2010). The lifetime cost per person for TBI has been estimated at nearly $45,000, with the highest costs being among men aged 25–44 years old (Corrigan et al. 2010).

Among patients injured in motor vehicle collisions, those with TBI have a lower probability of returning to work and are at increased risk of having prolonged disability (Bazarian et al. 2005). Rimel et al. reported an unemployment rate of 34% among patients with minor head injury (Rimel et al. 1981a).

Common Causes of TBI in Different Populations

The most common causes of TBI across all age groups in the United States listed in order of prevalence are falls, motor vehicle collisions, being struck by or against an object, and assault (Faul et al. 2010). Data from the CDC shows that falls are by far the leading cause of TBI in the United States and are most frequent in those under the age of 4 or over the age of 75 (Faul et al. 2010) (Fig. 13.1). Most emergency department visits and hospitalizations for TBI are related to falls, and from the years 2002 to 2006, there has been an increase in fall-related TBI in children under the age of 14 and adults over the age of 65 (Faul et al. 2010). Motor vehicle-related injury is the most common cause of TBI in the 15–24-year-old age group and has the highest TBI-associated mortality (Faul et al. 2010; Thurman et al. 1999).

The cause of TBI in pediatric populations varies by age. Inflicted TBI is a major cause of TBI in infants and is often associated with severe diffuse injury as well as hypoxic–ischemic injury

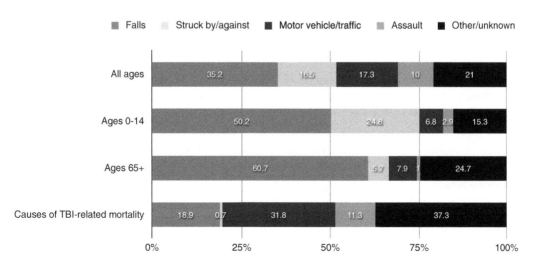

Fig. 13.1 Common causes of traumatic brain injury (Faul et al. 2010)

frequently due to delays in treatment (Barlow et al. 2005; Keenan et al. 2006). The outcomes in these patients are generally worse than in other forms of TBI. Falls are the primary cause of brain injury in toddlers (Giza et al. 2007). A younger age correlates with the presence of subdural hematomas and diffuse cerebral edema, while contusions are less common (Giza et al. 2007). Motor vehicle accidents become more prevalent in older children and adolescents (Giza et al. 2007). Sports-related head injuries are common in adolescents and young adults and represent a unique type of repetitive mild injury that can have cumulative effects (Matser et al. 1999; Collins et al. 1999).

In the United States, three major risk factors for TBI are age, gender, and insurance status. Persons under 4 years of age or over 65 years of age are at increased risk of developing TBI, as are males, who are twice as likely as females to sustain TBI. In terms of insurance status, uninsured patients had nearly twice the risk of sustaining TBI compared to those with private insurance (Faul et al. 2010; Langlois et al. 2003; Selassie et al. 2004).

Alcohol use has been involved in a high percentage of TBI cases (Bell and Sandell 1998). Corrigan reported that between 36 and 51% of all patients who sustain a TBI are intoxicated from alcohol at the time of injury (Corrigan 1995). Winqvist et al. reported that alcohol use in parents increased the childhood risk of TBI. They also stated that adolescent use of alcohol increased the risk of adult TBI, and TBI related to alcohol use increased the risk of repeated brain injury (Winqvist et al. 2006, 2007a, b).

Prevention of TBI

Proper education and safety regarding high-risk behaviors can limit the incidence of TBI. By identifying populations and persons at high risk for TBI, appropriate prevention measures can be instituted. Most experts on the prevention of TBI recommend utilizing protective gear such as seatbelts while in motor vehicles, and helmets while bicycling or riding motorcycles. Participants and coaches for high-impact sports are urged to exercise caution and judgment (Cassidy et al. 2004). Alcohol has also been noted to play a role in increasing risk of TBI, and education about its use and abuse may also be helpful in the prevention of TBI.

Methods of Classification

The various definitions of TBI have complicated the surveillance and collection of epidemiologic data, and ambiguity exists with respect to classification of TBI. There are several different methods and scales available to measure the severity of TBI (Table 13.1). In general, most systems broadly define three categories of TBI: mild, moderate, and severe. Criteria used to categorize these patients include Glasgow Coma Scale (GCS) score, Abbreviated Injury Severity Scale (AISS), duration of

Table 13.1 Classification of traumatic brain injury (Blyth and Bazarian 2010; Corrigan et al. 2010)

Criteria	Mild TBI	Moderate TBI	Severe TBI
Glasgow coma scale	13–15	9–12	8 or less
Abbreviated injury severity scale	1–2	3	4–6
Loss of consciousness	0–30 min	30 min–24 h	More than 24 h
Posttraumatic amnesia	0–1 day	1–7 days	More than 7 days
Imaging findings[a]	Usually normal	Dependent on mechanism and location of injury	Dependent on mechanism and location of injury

[a]Noncontrast head CT is the imaging study of choice for acute head injury

LOC, and duration of posttraumatic amnesia (Corrigan et al. 2010). Within some of these scales, there exists even further variation, including initial GCS score plus GCS at 24 h postinjury vs. lowest overall GCS score within 24 h of injury (Hoffman et al. 2007).

Mild TBI

Mild TBI comprises nearly 90% of all head injuries and approximately 75–85% of all forms of TBI (Khan et al. 2003; Thornhill et al. 2000). Mild brain injury is the most frequently studied of the three broad categories of TBI. Most studies define mild TBI as the presence of an initial GCS score of 13–15 with potential LOC of less than 30 min (Blyth and Bazarian 2010; Lahz and Bryant 1996; Uomoto and Esselman 1993). Other studies have alternatively included measurements such as LOC at time of trauma (Lahz and Bryant 1996) or duration of LOC less than 20 min with concurrent hospitalization of less than 48 h (Rimel et al. 1981b).

The CDC provides a standard definition of mild TBI, which states: "Mild TBI is an injury to the head (arising from blunt trauma or acceleration or deceleration forces) that results in 1 or more of the following: any period of confusion, disorientation, or impaired consciousness; any dysfunction of memory around the time of injury; LOC lasting less than 30 min; or the onset of observed signs or symptoms of neurological or neuropsychological dysfunction (National Center for Injury Prevention and Control 2003)."

Moderate and Severe TBI

Moderate TBI has been defined as a GCS score of 9–12, and severe TBI as a GCS score of 3–8 (Rimel et al. 1982). Some authors group moderate and severe TBI together, with various criteria such as a GCS score of 12 or less, greater than 30 min in a coma, or greater than 24 h of posttraumatic amnesia (Lahz and Bryant 1996; Walker et al. 2005). One study categorized general severe head injury as duration of LOC greater than 24 h, with concomitant cerebral contusion or intracerebral hemorrhage (Jensen and Nielsen 1990).

Mechanism of Injury and Pathologic Features

The mechanism of TBI is typically due to external blunt or penetrating trauma to the head, skull, dura, or brain (Kennedy et al. 2007). Other mechanisms include acceleration–deceleration injury (i.e., whiplash) or coup-contrecoup injury, which may lead to trauma without an actual external force of impact (Kennedy et al. 2007). TBI caused by blast injury (seen most often in military patients) is caused by brain over- or under-pressurization, which causes ultrastructural and biochemical alterations, most commonly in air-filled organs or at air–liquid interfaces (Kennedy et al. 2007; DePalma et al. 2005). The most vulnerable sites to blast injury are the tympanic membranes and the lungs. Military body armor has made great strides in protecting soldiers from penetrating injury, but it does not protect against the barotrauma of blast injury. Central nervous system damage due to blast injury may primarily occur as a result of diffuse axonal injury or due to acute gas embolism from pulmonary injury (DePalma et al. 2005).

Diffuse axonal injury, resulting from axonal strain, is the primary pathologic feature of TBI (Lux 2007). Increasing amounts of diffuse axonal injury generally correlate with increasing severity of TBI (Lux 2007). These injuries may eventually develop into pathologic neurophysiologic changes, such as altered levels of neurotransmitters, impaired axonal transport, synaptic loss, and disruption of neuronal circuits (Lux 2007; DeKosky et al. 2010). In some cases of mild TBI, axonal injury may be reversible, which may explain the complete or near-complete recovery (Lux 2007).

Other pathologic mechanisms of TBI are cerebral contusions, mechanical tissue damage, synaptic loss and neuronal dysfunction, and even ischemia (Khan et al. 2003; Lux 2007; DeKosky et al. 2010; Bryant 2008). The injuries may be due to immediate damage or secondary injury in the days immediately following the trauma (Khan et al. 2003). The anatomic distribution of injuries tends to involve the frontal and anterior temporal lobes (Lux 2007).

Mild TBI may be characterized by contusion and mild edema, leading to variable chronic cognitive or neuropsychiatric impairment (DeKosky et al. 2010). Mild repetitive TBI may result in alterations of the axonal and cytoskeletal structures, leading to abnormal protein aggregations and neurofibrillary tangles (DeKosky et al. 2010). Severe TBI may result in chronic impairment of neuronal homeostasis as well as protein aggregation (DeKosky et al. 2010).

Diagnosis of TBI

The CDC and WHO definitions of TBI may be interpreted broadly, and thus may lead to overdiagnosis of TBI. A more clinically oriented assessment of TBI may involve taking a full history and physical, reviewing laboratory results, and possibly obtaining imaging studies such as MRI or CT. MRI has been shown to be more sensitive than CT at identifying TBI but is not necessary or sufficient for the diagnosis (Lux 2007). These studies, as well as other tests including electroencephalography, are frequently normal or nonspecific (Andary et al. 1993). Understanding a patient's cognitive functioning prior to injury is an essential aspect of assessing TBI, and for this reason, neuropsychological assessment may be more clinically appropriate for evaluating TBI (Andary et al. 1993). Full classification of the severity of TBI is performed by using one of the metrics previously described (GCS, AISS, duration of LOC).

Signs and Symptoms of TBI

TBI typically presents with symptoms characteristic of a postconcussive state, including cognitive problems (difficulties with memory, attention, and concentration, slowed cognitive processing speed), physical problems (fatigue, headache, sleep disturbances), and affective problems (anxiety, depression) (Kennedy et al. 2007; Lux 2007; Bryant 2008). Current evidence favors both organic and psychological factors in contributing to the symptoms of TBI (Bryant 2008).

Treatment of TBI and Its Sequelae

There are a wide variety of complications and comorbidities associated with TBI, including cognitive, physical, and emotional or social difficulties (Table 13.2). Mild TBI generally has a good prognosis, and most patients can expect to make a significant recovery (Warden 2006). Patients with mild TBI and cognitive and behavioral changes often experience recovery in as few as 4–12 weeks, or up to 3–6 months after injury (Khan et al. 2003; Kennedy et al. 2007; Mooney et al. 2005).

Table 13.2 Common complications and comorbidities of traumatic brain injury, based on injury severity (Nampiaparampil 2008)

Mild TBI
Cognitive deficits
Attention
Memory
Calculation
Judgment
Insight
Reasoning
Sensory deficits
Sight
Hearing
Touch
Communication difficulties
Language expression
Comprehension
Social difficulties
Compassion
Interpersonal social awareness
Mental health problems
Depression
Anxiety
Personality changes
Aggression/irritability
Social inappropriateness
Sleep disturbance
Vertigo/dizziness
Moderate to severe TBI (includes above list)
Abnormal states of consciousness
Speech/swallow deficits
Cranial neuropathies
Paresis/paralysis
Seizure disorders
Movement disorders
Complications of prolonged bed rest

In a 2010 article, Cernich et al. provide a comprehensive, evidence-based review of cognitive rehabilitation of TBI. The authors recommend neuropsychological assessment to identify cognitive deficits (Cernich et al. 2010). Physical, occupational, and speech therapy were also recommended (Cernich et al. 2010). Pharmacological treatment may include psychostimulant medications such as methylphenidate (and to a lesser extent, cholinesterase inhibitors and dopaminergic agents) to help TBI patients that have attention or memory deficits, or impairment of executive function (Cernich et al. 2010).

Treatment includes both patient and family education, as well as psychological support. Inpatient rehabilitation is not usually needed for mild TBI, but may be required for more severe cases. Approximately 10–15% of patients with mild TBI report long-term symptoms associated with a persistent postconcussive syndrome (Khan et al. 2003). Some explanations for persistent symptoms include premorbid cognitive or psychiatric conditions that may complicate recovery, underestimation of injury severity, or financial or legal incentives for secondary gain (Mooney et al. 2005). Although most patients with mild TBI do not require chronic care, those who report persistent cognitive, emotional, and behavioral difficulties often do (Jennekens et al. 2010). There also appears to be a correlation between the length of time since the initial trauma and an increased need for care (Jennekens et al. 2010).

Predictors of Mortality and Prognosis

Increased age has been shown to have correlation with mortality and functional outcome in TBI (Gomez et al. 2000). Gender has also been shown to play a role. Male gender is associated with a higher risk of TBI. Female gender is associated with poorer functional outcomes following severe TBI (Lingsma et al. 2010). Ethnicity correlates with mortality after TBI. One study has shown that Asian patients with moderate to severe TBI have a higher mortality rate than African-American or white patients (Berry et al. 2010). Other studies have also noted that the greater the degree of clinical injury severity, the poorer the prognosis (Lingsma et al. 2010).

In general, patients with severe TBI tend to have poor outcomes, and nearly half of this population dies within 2 h of the injury (DeWall 2010). Willemse et al. conducted a review of prospective cohort studies in order to identify predictors for ongoing long-term (>1 year) disability following TBI, and found strong associations between older age, substance abuse, unemployment before the injury, and increased severity of disability at the time of discharge from rehabilitation (Willemse-van Son et al. 2009).

Special Populations: Pediatric

In the pediatric population, three original studies evaluated chronic pain as an outcome of TBI. Necajauskaite et al. conducted a cross-sectional study in Lithuania of children who had experienced a single mild TBI. The children were studied 1–5 years after the trauma. 47.1% reported headache prior to the trauma and 70.6% of the children had headache immediately after the trauma. 62.7% experienced chronic headache. In the children who had preexisting headache, there was a significant increase in the frequency of headaches after the trauma. 45.3% of the patients with mild TBI reported the presence of headaches 1–7 days per month. 29.7% stated that the headache was triggered by irregular sleep (Necajauskaite et al. 2005).

Overweg-Plandsoen et al. studied posttraumatic headache in the pediatric population in the Netherlands and found a prevalence of 45.5% (Overweg-Plandsoen et al. 1999). Lanzi et al. investigated the clinical characteristics of headache after brain injury in the Italian pediatric population. Twelve to 18 months after the trauma, 29.7% of the children reported chronic headache. In 41.5% of the patients, there appeared to be no correlation between the location of the head injury and the site of the headache. The study also reported that two of the pediatric subjects with preexisting diagnoses of migraines had remission of their headache symptoms after the trauma (Lanzi et al. 1985).

Timonen et al. noted that persons with TBI before the age of 15 were at higher risk for psychiatric hospitalization by age 31, and that males with both a psychiatric disorder and childhood history of TBI were at higher risk of having criminal activity (Timonen et al. 2002). McKinlay et al. reported that persons with TBI before the age of 5 were at increased risk of later developing attention-deficit/hyperactivity disorder, oppositional-defiant behavior, conduct disorder, substance abuse, and mood disorders (McKinlay et al. 2009).

Special Populations: Geriatric

According to the CDC, adults who are 75 years of age and older have the highest rates of hospitalization and death due to TBI (Faul et al. 2010). Falls are the most common cause of TBI in the geriatric population (Faul et al. 2010). The diagnosis of TBI may be complicated by various other comorbidities that are common in this population. Older patients typically have a higher prevalence of physical deconditioning. They may also have multiple medical comorbidities and polypharmacy. Each of these factors may confound the diagnosis and treatment of TBI in this population. Bhullar et al. performed a retrospective chart review of patients with TBI after blunt trauma and found that there was no significant difference in mortality between adults 65 and 80 years of age, and those above 80 years of age (Bhullar et al. 2010).

Special Populations: Military

TBI among soldiers has been a major concern since World War I (when it was referred to as "shell shock"). In 1992, Congress formed the Defense and Veterans Brain Injury Center (DVBIC) to bring TBI care and research to the forefront of the military health care system (Jones et al. 2007; Schwab et al. 2007). The DVBIC has pioneered developments in the field of TBI care. Physicians at the Walter Reed Army Medical Center developed a screening process for TBI in the military population, which includes an initial interview and evaluation of cognitive function (Schwab et al. 2007). Those patients that are identified as having severe TBI are medically stabilized and transferred to an intensive rehabilitation center (Schwab et al. 2007).

Recently, TBI has increased in prominence within the military population. It is referred to as "the signature injury of the Iraq and Afghanistan conflicts (Jones et al. 2007; Hoge et al. 2008)." It has been estimated that approximately 20–25% of soldiers wounded in these recent conflicts have mild TBI, whereas the head injury rate was cited as less than 15% during the Vietnam War (Blyth and Bazarian 2010; Hoge et al. 2008; Okie 2005). Some have attributed this increase to the technological advances made in body armor and helmets, which are protecting soldiers from previously fatal injuries, and which may be artificially increasing the rate of TBI (Hoge et al. 2008; Okie 2005). In the military population with TBI, approximately 88% sustained closed TBI and 12% incurred penetrating TBI (Schwab et al. 2007). Of all cases of TBI in soldiers in this most recent conflict, 56% of cases were moderate or severe (Schwab et al. 2007).

Typically, these soldiers develop TBI following a blast injury, which causes rapid pressure shifts that can produce concussion or contusion. Up to 25% of people with severe blast injuries die as a result (Okie 2005). Survivors of these injuries who experience TBI may have persistent postconcussive symptoms such as headache and/or problems with memory or concentration (Hoge et al. 2008).

In 2008, Hoge et al. conducted a survey of 2,525 U.S. Army Infantry soldiers returning from a year-long deployment to Iraq, and reported that 15.2% of soldiers surveyed had sustained a mild TBI, defined as an injury with LOC or altered mental status (Hoge et al. 2008). They also reported that soldiers with mild TBI were more likely to be young, male, and junior in rank (Hoge et al. 2008). The authors then compared this cohort with mild TBI to those who reported other injuries. They found that 71.2% of the mild TBI group met criteria for posttraumatic stress disorder (PTSD), whereas only 16.2% of those with other injuries (excluding mild TBI) met the same criteria for PTSD (Hoge et al. 2008). It was also noted that, compared to the non-TBI group, the mild TBI group was more likely to report poor health, missed workdays, increased medical visits, and other physical and psychological complaints, including headache (Hoge et al. 2008). However, after adjusting for PTSD and depression, there was no longer a significant association between mild TBI and most of the aforementioned complaints (Hoge et al. 2008). This implies that these two conditions may be significant mediators of many of the physical and psychological problems associated with TBI (Hoge et al. 2008).

Special Populations: Disability and Litigation

Patients with TBI may have a higher prevalence of disability than the general population. In one sample group of patients with mild TBI, nearly three-quarters reported disability associated with TBI (Mooney et al. 2005). The probability of disability related to TBI increases with age and is higher in women (Langlois et al. 2006). Data from 2003 reported an estimated 43.3% of hospitalized TBI survivors in the United States had injury-related disability 1 year after trauma (Selassie et al. 2008). The prevalence of Americans living with a disability related to TBI has been estimated to be 3.2 million (Corrigan et al. 2010; Zaloshnja et al. 2008).

In a European review, Tagliaferri et al. reported that persistent problems following severe TBI were described in selected studies, and included changes in employment, physical complaints, memory problems, and neuropsychological problems (Tagliaferri et al. 2006).

Chronic Pain After TBI

In a 2008 meta-analysis, Nampiaparampil reported that chronic pain is a common complication of TBI, independent of psychological disorders such as PTSD or depression (Nampiaparampil 2008). Described as a constant pain of at least 6 months' duration, chronic pain has been reported by over half of all TBI patients (Lahz and Bryant 1996). Painful conditions are prevalent among patients with TBI and may include headaches, musculoskeletal conditions, complex regional pain syndrome (CRPS), spasticity, heterotopic ossification, and neuropathic pain (Lahz and Bryant 1996; Sherman et al. 2006).

Evaluating pain in patients with TBI can be complicated because of the higher prevalence of cognitive impairments in this population (Gellman et al. 1992). Interestingly, chronic pain was reported in 75.3% of mild TBI patients, 32.1% of severe TBI patients, and 43.1% of military TBI patients (Nampiaparampil 2008). It has been hypothesized that this disparity exists due to the fact that the more severely injured patients have an increased degree of cognitive impairment, which leads to decreased self-monitoring and reporting of pain (Young 2007). Bryant et al. noted that TBI patients generally manage chronic pain differently than do those without brain injury (Bryant et al. 1999).

One study reported that 95% of patients with mild TBI complained of pain that interfered with activities of daily living as opposed to 22% of patients with moderate or severe TBI (Andary et al. 1993). Another study found that over 85% of TBI patients with chronic pain reported pain on a daily basis (Lahz and Bryant 1996). Overall, studies have found that nearly three-quarters of all patients with TBI report some level of pain at 1 year postinjury, and over half of these patients report interference with activities of daily living (Hoffman et al. 2007).

In all cases, it has been emphasized that a complete, biopsychosocial approach be taken to evaluate the patient with TBI and chronic pain. Both conditions have overlapping symptoms such as pain behaviors, sleep disturbances, chronic fatigue, anxiety, and depression (Andary et al. 1993). Mistakenly identifying certain chronic pain symptoms as a consequence of brain injury may lead to improper or inadequate treatment (Uomoto and Esselman 1993). Failure to treat pain adequately in this population may eventually complicate rehabilitation and compromise recovery, as well as have a negative emotional impact on the individual (Sherman et al. 2006). However, effective treatment and prevention of chronic pain problems in this population may lower the incidence of disability (Uomoto and Esselman 1993).

Posttraumatic Headache/Postconcussion Syndrome

Headache is the most common pain complaint in all TBI patients (with a reported incidence of 57.8%), and much of the research on TBI and pain has been focused on posttraumatic headache (Nampiaparampil 2008). In fact, headache is the most common sequelae of closed head injury, as well as the most common presenting symptom of mild TBI (Lane and Arciniegas 2002; Tyrer and Lievesley 2003). The prevalence of headache associated with TBI is as high as 57.8% (Nampiaparampil 2008). Patients with mild TBI reported a higher incidence of headaches (89%) than did patients with moderate or severe TBI (18%) (Uomoto and Esselman 1993).

Posttraumatic headache is a distinct classification, defined by the International Headache Society (IHS) as a headache that begins within 14 days of regaining consciousness after TBI (Walker et al. 2005). The IHS further categorizes posttraumatic headache by severity of injury: significant head trauma vs. minor head trauma, but it does not define the etiology of the headache (Branca and Lake 2004). Posttraumatic headache is defined as chronic when it persists for over 8 weeks postinjury (Branca and Lake 2004).

It is clinically impossible to differentiate posttraumatic headache from chronically recurrent headache, which may be present in TBI patients who had preinjury headaches (Jensen and Nielsen 1990). Posttraumatic headache is generally poorly characterized, and many TBI patients chronically complain of different types of headaches simultaneously (Young 2007; Sherman et al. 2006). Usually, these headaches are classified as migraines, are secondary to musculoskeletal complaints, or are related to rebound from analgesics (Sherman et al. 2006; Branca and Lake 2004).

A related condition is postconcussion syndrome, a term which is sometimes used interchangeably with posttraumatic headache, and which has been described as occurring after a head injury with LOC. It includes cognitive symptoms (memory loss and poor concentration), affective symptoms (depression and anxiety, irritability), and somatic symptoms (headache, dizziness, nausea, fatigue) (Kay et al. 1971; Smith-Seemiller et al. 2003). Many of these symptoms overlap in patients with chronic pain conditions who do not have TBI.

Headache pain has not been found to correlate with injury severity (Hoffman et al. 2007). Treatment of posttraumatic headache is similar to treatment of headache in nontraumatic settings, and includes oral medications such as muscle relaxants, SSRIs, and anticonvulsants (Ivanhoe and Hartman 2004).

Other Pain Syndromes

Patients with TBI can also have other pain symptoms related to the initial trauma, or as a result of the TBI or its treatment. This population is at increased risk to develop other chronic pain syndromes as well. Some of these syndromes include conditions which are common in the general population such as musculoskeletal complaints. These patients are also more likely to develop less common syndromes such as CRPS and heterotopic ossification.

Uomoto et al. identified other local chronic pain complaints among TBI patients, including neck and shoulder pain, and back pain. These complaints were identified more frequently in the mild TBI group, as compared to the moderate or severe groups (Uomoto and Esselman 1993). Leung et al. noted that the prevalence of shoulder pain in patients with TBI, for example, was 62% (Leung et al. 2007).

Myofascial Pain Syndrome

Myofascial pain syndrome is one of the most common causes of posttraumatic pain, and the most common affected muscles in patients with TBI are splenius cervicus, semispinalis capitis, suboccipital muscles, trapezius, sternocleidomastoid, temporalis, masseters, occipitalfrontalis, and pterygoids (Ivanhoe and Hartman 2004). Trigger points may be identified in any of these muscles, and may be treated with injection. Myofascial pain may also contribute to the development of posttraumatic headache (Ivanhoe and Hartman 2004).

Complex Regional Pain Syndrome

CRPS type I, formerly referred to as reflex sympathetic dystrophy, is characterized by pain out of proportion to injury, as well as vascular and sudomotor changes in the affected limb. A study of 100 patients with TBI admitted to an acute brain injury unit found that the overall incidence of CRPS in this population was 12% based on clinical exam and imaging findings (Gellman et al. 1992). The mean onset of symptoms was within 4 months of injury (Ivanhoe and Hartman 2004).

Since CRPS may have a subtle presentation initially, the study authors recommend that a high suspicion be maintained in any patient with TBI and spasticity or hyperalgesia of an upper extremity (Gellman et al. 1996).

Spasticity

Unlike headache, spasticity of the limbs is more common in severe TBI patients than in patients with mild TBI. Spasticity of the limbs may result from loss of upper motor neuron control and may lead to joint contractures and, eventually, cause pain and limit mobility (Sherman et al. 2006; Gellman et al. 1996). These contractures can also interfere with proper rehabilitation and treatment (Sherman et al. 2006). The most commonly affected areas of the upper extremity are the shoulder, elbow, and wrist (Gellman et al. 1996). Treatment for spasticity includes medications such as muscle relaxants that may be administered orally or intrathecally via an implantable pump. Nerve blocks utilizing local anesthetics or botulinum toxin have also been used to treat spasticity (Ivanhoe and Hartman 2004).

Heterotopic Ossification

Heterotopic ossification is abnormal formation of bone in the soft tissue typically surrounding joints. The incidence after TBI has been reported as low as 11% and as high as 75%, depending on the study (Gellman et al. 1996). Garland et al. reviewed nearly 500 patients with head injury, and found clinically significant heterotopic ossification in 11% of patients, with 53% of these cases being in the upper extremity (Garland et al. 1980). Risk factors for the development of heterotopic ossification include prolonged coma and spasticity, both common conditions in patients with TBI (Ivanhoe and Hartman 2004). Bone scans are the ideal diagnostic study, and treatment includes nonsteroidal anti-inflammatory drugs, bisphosphonates, and surgical resection (Ivanhoe and Hartman 2004).

Biopsychosocial Factors/Comorbidities

Biopsychosocial factors are of critical importance, particularly in the mild TBI population. Many patients require significant support in coping with their condition. Some patients, due to the nature of their injury, may have difficulties with communication and expressing their symptoms. Others may face challenges in the changes to their social structure and interpersonal relationships. Difficulties with activities of daily living and work-related functioning are also significant factors that can affect the long-term treatment and prognosis of individuals in this population.

Mood disorders are common in the TBI population and are a well-documented result of brain injury (Branca and Lake 2004). Psychiatric illnesses develop more often in patients with TBI as compared to noninjured patients (Deb et al. 1999). Deb et al. found a significantly higher rate of depression and anxiety in TBI patients compared to the general population, and Viguier et al. reported that depression, anxiety, and cognitive dysfunction were more prevalent in the population with TBI vs. the population without brain injury (Deb et al. 1999; Viguier et al. 2001). Hoffman et al. found that risk factors for pain at 1 year postinjury included being female and nonwhite, and the presence of depression during rehabilitation (Hoffman et al. 2007). Tyrer et al. reported that the prevalence of depression following TBI varied from 5 to 25%, depending on the population (Tyrer and Lievesley 2003). Depression has been shown to be a strong predictor of disability following head injury (Tyrer and Lievesley 2003).

Koponen et al. reported the results of a study that evaluated the presence of psychiatric disorders in TBI patients during a 30-year follow-up and found that 48.3% had an Axis I disorder that began after the brain injury (Koponen et al. 2002). The most common disorders were major depression (26.7%), alcohol abuse or dependence (11.7%), and panic disorder (8.3%) (Koponen et al. 2002). The authors also found that 23.3% of the study group had at least one personality disorder (most commonly avoidant, paranoid, or schizoid) (Koponen et al. 2002).

Bryant et al. found that 27% of patients with TBI had symptoms of PTSD (Bryant et al. 1999). It was also noted that TBI patients with chronic pain were more likely to exhibit PTSD symptoms (Bryant et al. 1999). TBI patients that report high levels of both pain and PTSD symptoms also tend to report higher levels of affective disturbances and mood disorders (Tyrer and Lievesley 2003). Hoge et al. noted that both PTSD and depression contribute to the relationship of mild TBI and physical health problems (Hoge et al. 2008).

Compared to patients with moderate or severe TBI, patients with mild TBI are at greater risk of developing PTSD (Warden 2006). This may be due to the fact that mild TBI causes some degree of cognitive dysfunction, which creates difficulty for patients in terms of coping strategies, leading to an increased incidence or severity of PTSD (Bryant 2008). It is possible that certain symptoms routinely attributed to mild TBI may in fact be secondary to PTSD, and that PTSD, in turn, may itself compound mild TBI (Bryant 2008). Unfortunately, there does not appear to be a universally accepted method of differentiating between mild TBI-related symptoms vs. PTSD-related symptoms (Bryant 2008).

In all cases, the psychological character of the patient before the injury plays a large role in defining the ability and extent to which the patient is able to cope and adapt to life postinjury (Iezzi et al. 2007). Most patients with TBI do not return to their baseline preinjury status (Branca and Lake 2004). The gold standard for assessing patients after brain injury is comprehensive neurocognitive testing (Branca and Lake 2004).

The stress and distress of pursuing litigation in the setting of TBI has also been shown to lead to increased and more persistent pain symptoms, disability, and overall poor prognosis for full recovery (at least for the duration of the litigation) (Iezzi et al. 2007).

TBI is also associated with sleep disorders. In a survey of 452 patients with TBI, Ouellet et al. reported that 50.2% of those surveyed reported symptoms of insomnia (Ouellet et al. 2006). Fichtenberg et al. noted that the rates of sleep disturbances following TBI ranged from 36 to 70% depending on the study (Fichtenberg et al. 2000). The authors also found a strong correlation between insomnia and depression among patients with TBI (Fichtenberg et al. 2000).

Treatment Strategies for Pain After TBI

Treatment in the acute phase for pain in the TBI population includes medications such as nonsteroidal anti-inflammatory drugs, opiates, and other drugs such as ketamine. Optimal treatment usually requires combinations of different classes of oral medications in order to minimize side effects (Tyrer and Lievesley 2003). Medications with anticholinergic or sedating effects should probably be avoided if possible, since they may worsen the cognitive dysfunction already experienced by patients with TBI (Lux 2007).

Assessment of TBI patients with chronic pain should include complete physical and psychological evaluations, ideally in a multidisciplinary setting (Tyrer and Lievesley 2003). Nearly all classes of oral medications have been used, including opioids, NSAIDs, muscle relaxants, psychostimulants, anticonvulsants, and antidepressants (Tyrer and Lievesley 2003). Opioids should be started at low dose in short-acting formulation and titrated upward until pain is controlled or limited by adverse effects (Tyrer and Lievesley 2003).

There should also be emphasis on recovery of cognitive function in this population, beginning with a thorough neuropsychological assessment to identify the cognitive functions most in need of rehabilitation (Cernich et al. 2010; Sherman et al. 2006). Cognitive impairment may negatively impact recovery if patients are unable to adhere to recommendations (Sherman et al. 2006). Physical, occupational, and speech therapy are also recommended as part of a complete treatment regimen (Cernich et al. 2010).

Areas of Ongoing Research: Biomarkers

In 2007, the National Institute of Neurological Disorders and Stroke conducted a workshop in order to develop a reliable classification system for TBI (Saatman et al. 2008). One of the topics discussed was the utility of biomarkers, in the serum or CSF, as a tool for the diagnosis and classification of TBI, as well as a prognostic tool (Saatman et al. 2008). A study by Redell et al. examined circulating microRNAs in the plasma of patients with TBI (Redell et al. 2010). Levels of these microRNAs have been found to be altered in certain diseases, and the investigators reported that levels of specific microRNA markers were found to be elevated in TBI (Redell et al. 2010). Several studies have investigated the role of S-100B (a protein found in glial cells) in the serum of both adult and pediatric TBI patients, and it has been shown that serum levels are significantly higher in patients with intracranial pathology (Hallén et al. 2010; Herrmann et al. 2001).

Areas of Ongoing Research: Disparities Research

Gary et al. performed a literature review to examine racial and ethnic differences in postinjury outcomes following TBI. The authors noted that African-Americans and Hispanics have a higher incidence of TBI as compared to whites, and found that African-American and Hispanic patients with TBI were more likely to have worse outcomes and less likely to receive treatment than white patients (Gary et al. 2009). However, when Berry et al. reviewed moderate to severe TBI cases in the Los Angeles County Trauma System over a 7-year period, they found that only Asians were at a higher risk of death, when compared to African-Americans, Hispanics, and whites (Berry et al. 2010).

The causes for these disparities are the subject of much debate and are likely multifactorial, including cultural traditions and attitudes of the patient, language barriers, inherent bias in the health care system, and differences in access to health care (Gary et al. 2009).

Conclusion

TBI is an issue of universal significance. It imposes deleterious effects on patients, their families, and society as a whole. The heterogeneity in diagnostic criteria complicates the accurate diagnosis of the condition and the reliable collection of epidemiological data. This, in turn, makes it difficult to investigate the morbidity and mortality of TBI and to evaluate the efficacy of different treatment approaches. Continued research in this field may lead to discoveries that can dramatically improve the diagnosis, treatment, and ultimately prevention of this potentially devastating condition.

Once the diagnosis of TBI becomes more streamlined, it will be easier to develop predictive models for brain injury. This will also allow us to identify markers for the development of different types of brain injury and then identify treatments aimed at those targets.

References

Andary, M. T., Vincent, F., & Esselman, P. C. (1993). Chronic pain following head injury. *Physical Medicine and Rehabilitation Clinics, 4*(1), 141–150.

Anstey, K. J., Butterworth, P., Jorm, A. F., Christensen, H., Rodgers, B., & Windsor, T. D. (2004). A population survey found an association between self-reports of traumatic brain injury and increased psychiatric symptoms. *Journal of Clinical Epidemiology, 57*(11), 1202–1209.

Barlow, K. M., Thomson, E., Johnson, D., & Minnis, R. A. (2005). Late neurologic and cognitive sequelae of inflicted traumatic brain injury in infancy. *Pediatrics, 116*, e174–e185.

Bazarian, J. J., McClung, J., Shah, M. N., Cheng, Y., Flesher, W., & Kraus, J. (2005). Mild traumatic brain injury in the United States, 1998–2000. *Brain Injury, 19*, 85–91.

Bell, K. R., & Sandell, M. E. (1998). Brain Injury rehabilitation. Post acute rehabilitation and community integration. *Archives of Physical Medicine and Rehabilitation, 79*, S21–S25.

Berry, C., Ley, E. J., Mirocha, J., & Salim, A. (2010). Race affects mortality after moderate to severe traumatic brain injury. *The Journal of Surgical Research, 163*(2), 303–308.

Bhullar, I. S., Roberts, E. E., Brown, L., & Lipei, H. (2010). The effect of age on blunt traumatic brain-injured patients. *American Surgeon, 76*(9), 966–968.

Blyth, B. J., & Bazarian, J. J. (2010). Traumatic alterations in consciousness: Traumatic brain injury. *Emergency Medicine Clinics of North America, 28*, 571–594.

Bohnen, N., & Jolles, J. (1992). Neurobehavioral aspects of post concussive symptoms after mild head injury. *The Journal of Nervous and Mental Disease, 180*, 183–192.

Branca, B., & Lake, A. E. (2004). Psychological and neuropsychological integration in multidisciplinary pain management after TBI. *The Journal of Head Trauma Rehabilitation, 19*(1), 40–57.

Bryant, R. A. (2008). Disentangling mild traumatic brain injury and stress reactions. *The New England Journal of Medicine, 358*(5), 525–527.

Bryant, R. A., Marosszeky, J. E., Crooks, J., et al. (1999). Interaction of posttraumatic stress disorder and chronic pain following traumatic brain injury. *The Journal of Head Trauma Rehabilitation, 14*(6), 588–594.

Cassidy, J. D., Carroll, L. J., Peloso, P. M., et al. (2004). Incidence, risk factors and prevention of mild traumatic brain injury: Results of the WHO Collaborating Centre Task Force on Mild Traumatic Brain Injury. *Journal of Rehabilitation Medicine, 36*, 28–60.

Cernich, A. N., Kurtz, S. M., Mordecai, K. L., & Ryan, P. B. (2010). Cognitive rehabilitation in traumatic brain injury. *Current Treatment Options in Neurology, 12*(5), 412–423.

Collins, M. W., Grindel, S. H., Lovell, M. R., et al. (1999). Relationship between concussion and neuropsychological performance in college football players. *The Journal of the American Medical Association, 282*, 964–970.

Corrigan, J. D. (1995). Substance abuse as a mediating factor in outcome from traumatic brain injury. *Archives of Physical Medicine and Rehabilitation, 76*(4), 302–309.

Corrigan, J. D., Selassie, A. W., & Orman, J. A. (2010). The epidemiology of traumatic brain injury. *The Journal of Head Trauma Rehabilitation, 25*(2), 72–80.

Deb, S., Lyons, I., Koutzoukis, C., et al. (1999). Rate of psychiatric illness 1 year after traumatic brain injury. *American Journal of Psychiatry, 156*(3), 374–378.

DeKosky, S. T., Ikonomovic, M. D., & Gandy, S. (2010). Traumatic brain injury – football, warfare, and long-term effects. *The New England Journal of Medicine, 363*(14), 1293–1296.

DePalma, R. G., Burris, D. G., Champion, H. R., & Hodgson, M. J. (2005). Blast injuries. *The New England Journal of Medicine, 352*(13), 1335–1342.

DeWall, J. (2010). The ABCs of TBI evidence-based guidelines for adult traumatic brain injury care. *The Journal of Emergency Medicine Services, 35*, 54–61.

Faul, M., Xu, L., Wald, M. M., & Coronado, V. G. (2010). *Traumatic brain injury in the United States: Emergency department visits, hospitalizations and deaths 2002–2006*. Atlanta: Centers for Disease Control and Prevention, National Center for Injury Prevention and Control.

Fichtenberg, N. L., Millis, S. R., Mann, N. R., et al. (2000). Factors associated with insomnia among post-acute traumatic brain injury survivors. *Brain Injury, 14*(7), 659–667.

Garland, D. E., Blum, C. E., & Waters, R. L. (1980). Periarticular ossification in head-injured adults. *The Journal of Bone and Joint Surgery, 62*, 1143–1146.

Gary, K. W., Arango-Lasprilla, J. C., & Stevens, L. F. (2009). Do racial/ethnic differences exist in post-injury outcomes after TBI? A comprehensive review of the literature. *Brain Injury, 23*(10), 775–789.

Gellman, H., Keenan, M. E., & Botte, M. J. (1996). Recognition and management of upper extremity pain syndromes in the patient with brain injury. *The Journal of Head Trauma Rehabilitation, 11*(4), 23–30.

Gellman, H., Keenan, M. E., Stone, L., et al. (1992). Reflex sympathetic dystrophy in brain-injured patients. *Pain, 51*(3), 307–311.

Giza, C. C., Mink, R. B., & Madikians, A. (2007). Pediatric traumatic brain injury: Not just little adults. *Current Opinion in Critical Care, 13*, 143–152.

Gomez, P. A., Lobato, R. D., Boto, G. R., et al. (2000). Age and outcome after severe head injury. *Acta Neurochir (Wien), 142*, 373–381.

Hallén, M., Karlsson, M., Carlhed, R., et al. (2010). S-100B in serum and urine after traumatic head injury in children. *Journal of Trauma, 69*(2), 284–289.

Herrmann, M., Curio, N., Jost, S., et al. (2001). Release of biochemical markers of damage to neuronal and glial brain tissue is associated with short and long term neuropsychological outcome after traumatic brain injury. *Journal of Neurology Neurosurgery Psychiatry, 70*(1), 95–100.

Hoffman, J. M., Pagulayan, K. F., Zawaideh, N., et al. (2007). Understanding pain after traumatic brain injury: Impact on community participation. *American Journal of Physical Medicine & Rehabilitation, 86*(12), 962–969.

Hoge, C. W., McGurk, D., Thomas, J. L., et al. (2008). Mild traumatic brain injury in U.S. Soldiers returning from Iraq. *The New England Journal of Medicine, 358*(5), 453–463.

Iezzi, T., Duckworth, M. P., Mercer, V., & Vuong, L. (2007). Chronic pain and head injury following motor vehicle collisions: A double whammy or different sides of a coin. *Psychology, Health & Medicine, 12*(2), 197–212.

Ivanhoe, C. B., & Hartman, E. T. (2004). Clinical caveats on medical assessment and treatment of pain after TBI. *The Journal of Head Trauma Rehabilitation, 19*(1), 29–39.

Jennekens, N., de Casterlé, B. D., & Dobbels, F. (2010). A systematic review of care needs of people with traumatic brain injury (TBI) on a cognitive, emotional and behavioural level. *Journal of Clinical Nursing, 19*(9–10), 1198–1206.

Jensen, O. K., & Nielsen, F. F. (1990). The influence of sex and pre-traumatic headache on the incidence and severity of headache after head injury. *Cephalalgia, 10*, 285–293.

Jones, E., Fear, N. T., & Wessely, S. (2007). Shell shock and mild traumatic brain injury: A historical review. *American Journal of Psychiatry, 164*(11), 1641–1645.

Kay, D. W., Kerr, T. A., & Lassman, L. P. (1971). Brain trauma and the postconcussional syndrome. *Lancet, 13*, 1052–1055.

Keenan, H. T., Runyan, D. K., & Nocera, M. (2006). Child outcomes and family characteristics 1 year after severe inflicted or noninflicted traumatic brain injury. *Pediatrics, 117*, 317–324.

Kennedy, J. E., Jaffee, M. S., Leskin, G. A., et al. (2007). Posttraumatic stress disorder and posttraumatic stress disorder-like symptoms and mild traumatic brain injury. *Journal of Rehabilitation Research and Development, 44*(7), 895–919.

Khan, F., Baguley, I. J., & Cameron, I. D. (2003). Rehabilitation after traumatic brain injury. *The Medical Journal of Australia, 178*(6), 290–295.

Koponen, S., Taiminen, T., Portin, R., et al. (2002). Axis I and II psychiatric disorders after traumatic brain injury: A 30-year follow-up study. *American Journal of Psychiatry, 159*(8), 1315–1321.

Lahz, S., & Bryant, R. A. (1996). Incidence of chronic pain following traumatic brain injury. *Arch Phys Med Rehab, 77*(9), 889–891.

Lane, J. C., & Arciniegas, D. B. (2002). Posttraumatic headache. *Current Treatment Options in Neurology, 4*(1), 89–104.

Langlois, J. A., Kegler, S. R., Butler, J. A., et al. (2003). Traumatic brain injury-related hospital discharges: Results from a 14-state surveillance system, 1997. *MMWR Surveillance Summaries, 52*(4), 1–20.

Langlois, J. A., Rutland-Brown, W., & Thomas, K. E. (2006). *Traumatic brain injury in the United States: Emergency department visits, hospitalizations, and deaths*. Atlanta: Centers for Disease Control and Prevention, National Center for Injury Prevention and Control.

Lanzi, G., Balotti, U., Borgatti, R., et al. (1985). Late post-traumatic headache in pediatric age. *Cephalalgia, 5,* 211–215.

Leung, J., Moseley, A., Fereday, S., et al. (2007). The prevalence and characteristics of shoulder pain after traumatic brain injury. *Clinical Rehabilitation, 21*(2), 171–181.

Lingsma, H. F., Roozenbeek, B., Steyerberg, E. W., et al. (2010). Early prognosis in traumatic brain injury: From prophecies to predictions. *Lancet Neurology, 9*(5), 543–554.

Lux, W. E. (2007). A neuropsychiatric perspective on traumatic brain injury. *Journal of Rehabilitation Research and Development, 44*(7), 951–961.

Maas, A. I., Marmarou, A., Murray, G. D., Teasdale, G. M., & Steyerberg, E. W. (2007). Prognosis and clinical trial design in traumatic brain injury: The IMPACT study. *Journal of Neurotrauma, 24,* 232–238.

Masel, B. E., & DeWitt, D. S. (2010). Traumatic brain injury: A disease process, not an event. *Journal of Neurotrauma, 27*(8), 1529–1540.

Matser, E. J., Kessels, A. G., Lezak, M. D., et al. (1999). Neuropsychological impairment in amateur soccer players. *The Journal of the American Medical Association, 282,* 971–973.

McKinlay, A., Grace, R. C., Horwood, L. J., Ridder, E. M., MacFarlane, M. R., & Fergusson, D. M. (2008). Prevalence of traumatic brain injury among children, adolescents and young adults: Prospective evidence from a birth cohort. *Brain Injury, 22*(2), 175–181.

McKinlay, A., Grace, R. C., Horwood, L. J., et al. (2009). Adolescent psychiatric symptoms following preschool childhood mild traumatic brain injury: Evidence from a birth cohort. *The Journal of Head Trauma Rehabilitation, 24*(3), 221–227.

Mooney, G., Speed, J., & Sheppard, S. (2005). Factors related to recovery after mild traumatic brain injury. *Brain Injury, 19*(12), 975–987.

Nampiaparampil, D. E. (2008). Prevalence of chronic pain after traumatic brain injury: A systematic review. *The Journal of the American Medical Association, 300*(6), 711–719.

National Center for Injury Prevention and Control. (2003). *Report to congress on mild traumatic brain injury in the United States: Steps to prevent a serious public health problem.* Atlanta: Centers for Disease Control and Prevention.

Necajauskaite, O., Endziniene, M., & Jurieniene, K. (2005). Prevalence, clinical features, and accompanying signs of post-traumatic headache in children. *Medicine (Kaunas), 41*(2), 100–108.

Okie, S. (2005). Traumatic brain injury in the war zone. *The New England Journal of Medicine, 352*(20), 2043–2047.

Ouellet, M. C., Beaulieu-Bonneau, S., & Morin, C. M. (2006). Insomnia in patients with traumatic brain injury: Frequency, characteristics, and risk factors. *The Journal of Head Trauma Rehabilitation, 21*(3), 199–212.

Overweg-Plandsoen, W. C. G., Kodde, A., van Straaten, M., et al. (1999). Mild closed head injury in children compared to traumatic fractured bone; neurobehavioral sequelae in daily life 2 years after the accident. *Neuropediatrics, 158,* 249–252.

Redell, J.B., Moore, A.N., Ward, N.H., et al. (2010). Human traumatic brain injury alters plasma microRNA levels. *J Neurotraum, 27*(12), 2147–56.

Rimel, R. W., Giordani, B., Barth, J. T., Boll, T. J., & Jane, J. A. (1981a). Disability caused by minor head injury. *Neurosurgery, 9,* 221–228.

Rimel, R. W., Giordani, B., Barth, J. T., Boll, T. J., & Jane, J. A. (1981b). Disability caused by minor head injury. *Neurosurgery, 9*(3), 221–228.

Rimel, R. W., Giordani, B., Barth, J. T., & Jane, J. A. (1982). Moderate head injury: Completing the clinical spectrum of brain trauma. *Neurosurgery, 11,* 344–351.

Saatman, K. E., Duhaime, A. C., Bullock, R., et al. (2008). Classification of traumatic brain injury for targeted therapies. *Journal of Neurotrauma, 25,* 719–738.

Schwab, K. A., Warden, D., Lux, W. E., Shupenko, L. A., & Zitnay, G. (2007). Defense and veterans brain injury center: Peacetime and wartime missions. *Journal of Rehabilitation Research and Development, 44*(7), xiii–xxi.

Selassie, A. W., Pickelsimer, E. E., Frazier, L., Jr., et al. (2004). The effect of insurance status, race, and gender on emergency department disposition of persons with traumatic brain injury. *The American Journal of Emergency Medicine, 22,* 465–473.

Selassie, A. W., Zaloshnja, E., Langlois, J. A., et al. (2008). Incidence of long-term disability following traumatic brain injury hospitalization in the United States. *The Journal of Head Trauma Rehabilitation, 23*(2), 123–131.

Sherman, K. B., Goldberg, M., & Bell, K. R. (2006). Traumatic brain injury and pain. *Physical Medicine and Rehabilitation Clinics, 17*(2), 473–490.

Silver, J., Kramer, R., Greenwald, S., & Weissman, M. (2001). The association between head injuries and psychiatric disorders: Findings from the New Haven NIMH Epidemiologic Catchment Area Study. *Brain Injury, 15*(11), 935–945.

Smith-Seemiller, L., Fow, N. R., Kant, R., & Franzen, M. D. (2003). Presence of post-concussion syndrome symptoms in patients with chronic pain vs mild traumatic brain injury. *Brain Injury, 17*(3), 199–206.

Sosin, D. M., Sniezek, J. E., & Thurman, D. J. (1996). Incidence of mild and moderate brain injury in the United States, 1991. *Brain Injury, 10*(1), 47–54.

Svetstkova, O., Angerova, Y., Sladkova, P., Bickenbach, J.E., & Raggi, A. (2010). Functioning and disability in traumatic brain injury. Disabil Rehabil, 32, Suppl 1, S68–77.

Tagliaferri, F., Compagnone, C., Korsic, M., & Servadei, F. (2006). A systematic review of brain injury epidemiology in Europe. *Acta Neurochir (Wien), 148*, 255–268.

Thornhill, S., Teasdale, G. M., Murray, G. D., et al. (2000). Disability in young people and adults one year after head injury: Prospective cohort study. *British Medical Journal, 320*, 1631–1635.

Thurman, D. J., Alverson, C., Dunn, K. A., Guerrero, J., & Sniezek, J. E. (1999). Traumatic brain injury in the United States: A public health perspective. *The Journal of Head Trauma Rehabilitation, 14*, 602–615.

Thurman, D. J., Kraus, J. F., & Romer, C. J. (1995a). *Standards for surveillance of neurotrauma.* Geneva: World Health Organization.

Thurman, D. J., Sniezek, J. E., Johnson, D., et al. (1995b). *Guidelines for surveillance of central nervous system injury.* Atlanta: Centers for Disease Control and Prevention, US Department of Health and Human Services.

Timonen, M., Miettunen, J., Hakko, H., et al. (2002). The association of preceding traumatic brain injury with mental disorders, alcoholism and criminality: The northern Finland 1966 birth cohort study. *Psychiatry Research, 113*(3), 217–226.

Tyrer, S., & Lievesley, A. (2003). Pain following traumatic brain injury: Assessment and management. *Neuropsychological Rehabilitation, 13*(1), 189–210.

Uomoto, J. M., & Esselman, P. C. (1993). Traumatic brain injury and chronic pain: Differential types and rates by head injury severity. *Arch Phys Med Rehab, 74*(1), 61–64.

Viguier, D., Dellatolas, G., Gasquet, I., et al. (2001). A psychological assessment of adolescent and young adult inpatients after traumatic brain injury. *Brain Injury, 15*(3), 263–271.

Walker, W. C., Seel, R. T., Curtiss, G., & Warden, D. L. (2005). Headache after moderate and severe traumatic brain injury: A longitudinal analysis. *The Archieves of Physical Medicne Rehabiliatation, 86*(9), 1793–1800.

Warden, D. (2006). Military TBI during the Iraq and Afghanistan wars. *The Journal of Head Trauma Rehabilitation, 21*(5), 398–402.

Willemse-van Son, A. H., Ribbers, G. M., Hop, W. C., et al. (2009). Community integration following moderate to severe traumatic brain injury: A longitudinal investigation. *Journal of Rehabilitation Medicine, 41*, 521–527.

Winqvist, S., Jokelainen, J., Luukinen, H., et al. (2006). Adolescents' drinking habits predict later occurrence of traumatic brain injury: 35-year follow-up of the northern Finland 1966 birth cohort. *The Journal of Adolescent Health, 39*(2), 275.e1–275.e7.

Winqvist, S., Jokelainen, J., Luukinen, H., et al. (2007a). Parental alcohol misuse is a powerful predictor for the risk of traumatic brain injury in childhood. *Brain Injury, 21*(10), 1079–1085.

Winqvist, S., Lehtilahti, M., Jokelainen, J., Hillbom, M., & Luukinen, H. (2007b). Traumatic brain injuries in children and young adults: A birth cohort study from northern Finland. *Neuroepidemiology, 29*(1/2), 136–142.

Young, J. A. (2007). Pain and traumatic brain injury. *Physical Medicine and Rehabilitation Clinics, 18*(1), 145–163.

Zaloshnja, E., Miller, T., Langlois, J. A., & Selassie, A. W. (2008). Prevalence of long-term disability from traumatic brain injury in the civilian population of the United States, 2005. *The Journal of Head Trauma Rehabilitation, 23*(6), 394–400.

Chapter 14
Pain in the Battlefield Injured

Anthony Dragovich and Steven P. Cohen

Introduction

War is a reality of human existence with no foreseeable end. Since the Bronze age, when Sargon the Great conquered all of Mesopotamia producing the world's first military dictatorship, civilizations have waged wars against each other (Gabriel and Metz 2007). Yet amid all the carnage and suffering, many advances have been made in areas as diverse as science, politics, and medicine. Modern warfare is no exception. In the past, high disease rates decimated entire armies. Today nonbattle injuries (NBI) and the chronic pain conditions that recur (collectively referred to as NBI) are the leading cause of hospital admissions and evacuation from theater. In addition, improved body armor, forward-deployed medical care, and rapid evacuation to more sophisticated treatment centers have resulted in nearly 90% of wounded service members surviving their initial injury (Callander and Hebert 2006). These factors translate to an increase in the wounded-in-action (WIA) to killed-in-action (KIA) ratios from 3:1 in Vietnam to 7:1 in Operations Iraqi (OIF) and Enduring Freedom (OEF) (The War et al. 2007; Goldberg 2010). However, this success is also the source of many current medical challenges. In this chapter, we describe battle and nonbattle injury patterns, our current pain management and treatment paradigms with a specific emphasis of pain in polytrauma patients and chronic low back pain (LBP) in battlefield injured populations and in veterans. We conclude with a discussion of future directions to enhance the management of pain in battlefield injured patient populations.

Polytrauma and Battle Injury

The majority of patients in the current wars have sustained injuries or been exposed to explosive forces that would have been fatal in previous conflicts. Training, tactics, and protective gear are predominantly responsible for the increased survival rate and distribution of wounds (Bellamy 1995; Carey 1996; Goldberg 2010). Excellent body armor, timely frontline support from unit medics, and

A. Dragovich, MD (✉)
Pain Medicine at Womack Army Medical Center, Ft. Bragg, NC, USA
e-mail: Anthony.Dragovich@us.army.mil

S.P. Cohen, MD
Uniformed Services University of the Health Sciences, Bethesda, MD, USA

Department of Anesthesiology, Johns Hopkins School of Medicine, New York, NY, USA

R.J. Moore (ed.), *Handbook of Pain and Palliative Care: Biobehavioral Approaches for the Life Course*,
DOI 10.1007/978-1-4419-1651-8_14, © Springer Science+Business Media, LLC 2012

Table 14.1 Reported addiction rates in the general population

References	Addiction rate, article type
Ives et al. (2006)	32%, prospective survey
Adams et al. (2006)	4.9%, prospective registry
Fishbain et al. (1992)	18.9%, systematic review
Portenoy and Foley (1986)	5%, case series

a rapid, efficient evacuation system have dramatically improved survival rates and WIA:KIA ratios since the Vietnam War. Indeed the ability to prevent morbidity and death from polytrauma including fatal head, chest, and abdominal wounds is also a key factor in our current medical success. Polytrauma is defined as trauma to several body areas organ systems. This trauma occurs at the same time and one of more of the injuries is life threatening. Clearly, no amount of medical care can undo a fatal injury. The only solution is protection and primary prevention of polytrauma as risk mitigation accomplished through improved body armor, vehicles, and technological advancement, especially in the realm of remote frequency jamming.

The predominant threat in the present conflicts in OIF (Operation Iraq Freedom) and OEF (in Afghanistan) is from improvised explosive devices (IEDs), which account for approximately two-thirds of all battle-related injuries. In descending order, the three leading causes of polytrauma in OIF are from explosions (IEDs), gunshot wounds, and rocket-propelled grenades (OTSG). However, despite improvements in protective equipment, the distribution pattern of survivable injuries has remained virtually unchanged since WWII. Specifically, upper and lower extremity injuries including brain TBI (traumatic brain injury), limb loss, burns blindness, fractures, abdominal injuries, and chest wounds continue to account for approximately 70% of all nonfatal battlefield injuries (Islinger et al. 2000; Zouris et al. 2006; Macgregor et al. 2010). This underscores the fact that the majority of fatal injuries primarily involve the head, chest, and/or abdomen. If these injuries can be reduced or prevented, survival rates will increase in parallel.

Blast Injuries

Blast injuries are typically characterized by an enormous explosive force resulting in severe extremity wounds, predominantly due to fragmentation (Islinger et al. 2000; Ramasamy et al. 2009). Without body armor, these injuries would carry high mortality rates. Moreover, many more extremity injuries would be fatal without the quick, competent medical care provided by medical corpsmen. Their ability to stop catastrophic hemorrhaging with pressure dressings and tourniquets is another key aspect of improved survival rates. From the time of injury through recovery and rehabilitation, the main challenge for all members of the multidisciplinary team of clinicians who treat these patients is how to maximize their mental and physical capabilities while minimizing pain and suffering.

Acute Pain Management

The treatment of battlefield pain is largely a function of the type and acuity of injury, the stability of the patient, the level (formerly known as echelon) of care, and the availability of resources (Table 14.1). The chain of casualty evacuation is built upon levels or echelons of care (now known as "roles"), which were developed during the Civil War and improved during WWII to facilitate the rapid evacuation of wounded service members to increasingly sophisticated treatment centers based on their specific medical condition and needs (Blansfiled 1999). To maximize efficiency and ensure the continued availability of resources, healthcare providers at each level provide no more care than necessary to either focus on rehabilitation as a strategy to return the soldier to duty, or to safely evacuate the casualty to the next highest role. For first echelon treatment, pain management consists of parenteral morphine, nonsteroidal anti-inflammatory drugs (NSAIDs), or acetaminophen, which some units dispense to individual soldiers as part of "wound packs" (Wedmore et al. 2005). COX-2 inhibitors possess the advantage of having minimal inhibitory effects on platelet function, which can prolong or expedite bleeding. One theoretical concern over the use of NSAIDs is an increased risk of renal failure in dehydrated and hypovolemic soldiers (Nakahura et al. 1998). This risk is mitigated by the young age, and lack of concomitant medical problems and medication usage in most deployed soldiers. Acetaminophen may be marginally safer than other NSAIDs, but it is also generally less effective as an analgesic and is largely devoid of anti-inflammatory properties (Towheed et al. 2006).

Morphine is the gold standard analgesic used for battlefield pain control, having been first administered orally in the War of 1812 and parenterally in the U.S. Civil War. Intramuscular (IM) morphine can be given on the battlefield or battalion aid station (BAS), ideally by a medical corpsman, or alternatively by a buddy, or the soldier himself. Although IM administration generally provides rapid and reliable analgesia, the liabilities of this delivery mode include variable absorption during shock and with lower extremity wounds, and the risk of infection. Intravenous administration is more reliable than IM use, but is often impractical and requires specialized equipment and trained personnel (Jowitt and Knight 1983). The U.S. military is currently investigating the feasibility of providing transmucosal fentanyl citrate in "wound packs" to small, highly disciplined units that tend to operate independently without the benefit of an organized, medical support system (e.g. Special Forces) (Black and Mcmanus 2009). The pharmacokinetics of transmucosal delivery are comparable to IM administration, with therapeutic blood levels being reached within 10–15 min, and peak plasma concentration occurring about 20 min after administration (Fine and Streisand 1998). Depending on the formulation, between 25 and 50% of transmucosal fentanyl is absorbed via the oral or buccal mucosa, with another 15–25% being slowly absorbed through the gastrointestinal tract. The pharmacokinetics of transmucosal fentanyl also appear to be independent of age, unaffected by multiple dose regimens, and less prone to hemodynamic variations (Egan et al. 2000; Kharasch et al. 2004). This may make it an ideal agent for battlefield analgesia. Kotwal et al. recently reported using high dose (1,600 µg) oral transmucosal fentanyl citrate to treat 27 soldiers with acute orthopedic injuries in an out-of-hospital setting in OIF (Kotwal et al. 2004). Excellent pain relief without the need for additional analgesia was reported in 19 patients, with minor, self-limiting side effects occurring in eight soldiers. In one patient who received a repeat dose of fentanyl followed by subsequent intravenous opioids, hypoventilation requiring reversal with naloxone occurred 4 h postadministration. Other rapidly acting analgesics that may someday be used in lieu of parenteral opioids include intranasal butorphanol, intranasal ketamine, and fentanyl buccal tablets (Davis 2010).

Second echelon medical treatment facilities include mobile field surgical teams and forward surgical teams (FST), whose providers include surgeons, anesthetists, and nurses. The primary functions of FSTs are resuscitation and stabilization. Pain control at this level of care generally involves oral opioids, nonopioid analgesics, and intravenous opioids, which can be safely monitored by nurses and other trained personnel. Patient-controlled analgesia may also be used at these facilities as resources dictate.

Combat support hospitals (CSH), which have fully replaced mobile army surgical hospitals or MASH units in the U.S. military, represent the backbone of forward-deployed medical care. Care at these units generally includes a wide array of medical and surgical specialists some of whom may possess training in pain management. Since the U.S. and allied militaries do not currently classify anesthesiologists and most other physicians by subspecialty training, having a pain management specialist serving downrange in a forward-deployed area is a serendipitous endeavor. However, this may soon change, as both the U.S. Army and Navy have appointed pain management consultants to their respective Surgeon Generals. Recommendations from the Army Surgeon General's (2010) pain medicine task force stated that a provider trained in pain management should be assigned to each CSHs. However, at the present time, these recommendations have not been adopted.

Table 14.2 Advantages of peripheral nerve catheters for war injuries

Can provide anesthesia for repeat surgery or wound debridement
Can provide excellent, limb-specific analgesia
Stable hemodynamics
Minimal side effects
Reduced need for opioid and other analgesics
Improved alertness
Requires only simple, easily transportable equipment

Care at third echelon military treatment facilities includes intensive care units and medical wards, which may administer continuous infusions of opioid and nonopioid (e.g. ketamine and epidural infusions of local anesthetics) analgesics for acute and subacute injuries. When pain management-trained anesthesiologists are deployed to CSH, more advanced interventions such as sympathetic and paravertebral blocks may be performed. Recently, anesthesiologists have also begun to employ peripheral nerve catheters for intermediate-term pain control (Buckenmaier et al. 2005, 2006). In addition to providing safe and titratable pain relief, peripheral nerve catheters also can be used for anesthesia in patients requiring repeat surgery or wound debridement (Table 14.2). With proper maintenance and monitoring, tunneled peripheral nerve catheters can be reliably used for up to 3 weeks or longer postplacement. The main factors limiting the routine use of peripheral nerve block catheters are the speed of evacuation, variability in training levels of medical personnel, and theoretical concerns about masking compartment syndrome. Compartment syndrome may result in permanent nerve and muscle damage (Wall et al. 2010).

To a lesser degree, care at this level focuses on reducing the long-term sequelae of acute injury. Recently, the U.S. military has attempted to reduce the incidence of chronic pain following trauma or surgery by the preventive use of neuropathic pain medications such as gabapentin. When used preemptively before surgical procedures associated with a high incidence of severe acute and chronic postsurgical pain, gabapentin, pregabalin, and similar drugs used to treat neuropathic pain have been shown to reduce perioperative pain and opioid requirements, and decrease the incidence of chronic postsurgical pain (Fassoulaki et al. 2001, 2002; Hurley et al. 2006). At fourth and fifth echelon treatment centers, acute and chronic pain management is also similar to the care received in civilian trauma centers and pain management clinics, respectively.

Emerging developments in the acute pain management of combat casualties, especially the polytrauma patient, also require additional evaluation (Malchow and Black 2008). There is a lack of randomized, controlled studies with long-term outcomes. That said, there is a growing body of evidence that suggests that early and effective use of analgesia is associated with improved short-term outcomes including a decreased incidence of thromboembolic events (Tuman et al. 1991; Sorenson and Pace 1992), decreased pulmonary complications (Wu et al. 2006), shortened ICU and hospital stays (Liu et al. 1995), and a diminished catabolic stress response marked by absent tachycardia, decreased oxygen consumption, and the avoidance of immunosuppression (Desborough 2000; Schricker et al. 2004). Whether these short-term effects will actually translate into better long-term benefits is yet another area ripe for clinical investigation.

Acute Pain

There is considerable evidence that acute pain intensity is a strong predictor for the development of chronic pain (Kelhet et al. 2006; see also Short and Vetter 2011). Research studies and clinical experience both support the hypothesis that chronic pain develops in association with a hypervigilant state that is initiated by a traumatic event and reinforced by prolonged acute pain (De Kock 2009, see also Vetter 2011). A predisposition toward the development of hypervigilance varies in terms of the type of trauma, the length of exposure, genetic susceptibility, age, gender, and related factors. Thus, the intensity and duration of the inciting traumatic event must overcome an "unknown" threshold such that the hypervigilant state develops, thereby creating the biobehavioral environment where acute pain can become chronic. However, once a hypervigilant state exists, biobehavioral factors including fear, anxiety, and perceptual amplification, which are associated with the patient's hypervigilance, become barriers to effective pain control and relief. Early and effective pain relief (e.g. pharmacologic) in association with psychological therapies (e.g. cognitive behavioral therapy) have been shown to decrease acute pain, thereby preventing acute pain patient from reaching the hypervigilance threshold, and making that biobehavioral transition from acute pain to chronic pain (De Kock 2009, see also Short and Vetter 2011). Holbrock et al. found an association between morphine use and the decreased development of post-traumatic stress disorder (PTSD) (Holbrook et al. 2010). Aggressive pain management is key to the prevention of the transition from acute pain to long-term chronic pain states and psychological morbidity (De Kock 2009; see also Short and Vetter 2011).

Despite this need, a multidisciplinary team that includes a psychologist or psychiatrist is not included in the military table of organization and equipment (MTOE). The MTOE is the document that regulates staffing for all deployed military units including the CSHs. One psychiatrist is assigned to the CSH, but they are a limited resource. Their primary role as part of the multidisciplinary team is the diagnosis and treatment of psychiatric diseases (e.g. intractable depression, suicidal ideation, generalized anxiety disorder, etc.). The psychiatrist can serve as a consult to assist with pain treatment. However, due to the rapid evacuation from the CSH and operational tempo, they are frequently unable to provide treatment before the patient is evacuated. Training of the multidisciplinary team in the treatment of fear, uncertainty, and anxiety by all clinical staff is a critical component for the combat environment and care (Newcomer et al. 2010). In our practice at Fort Bragg, we found that the nursing staff was able to effectively improve patient's anxiety and pain levels by teaching them to use and teach guided imagery, distraction, and relaxation techniques in conjunction with prescribed medication or pain relief procedures.

Multidisciplinary pain care includes psychotherapies (e.g. cognitive behavioral therapy; see also Donovan et al. 2011) that focus on the treatment of depression, fear, and anxiety with the goal of improving the patients' sense of control and is one method that has been shown to lessen the biological pain that the patient experiences. The development of an acute pain treatment regimen that is designed to lessen biological pain often presents a clinical conundrum. Every acute pain management strategy requires a basal analgesic regimen. Currently, only opioids and local anesthetic nerve blockade provide adequate analgesia and can be used as the primary analgesic. Many other classes of medications such as N-methyl-D-aspartate (NMDA) receptor antagonists, alpha-2 receptor agonists, NSAIDs, sodium channel blockers, anticonvulsants, and presynaptic calcium channel blockers can be used as adjunctive pain medications, but none either alone or in combination can provide analgesia comparable to opioids and nerve blocks. Therefore, either opioids or local anesthetic nerve blockade should form the centerpiece of any analgesic plan, with adjunctive medications used to augment the primary analgesic. In the case of local anesthetics, augmentation by adjunctive pain medications provides additional pain relief at the cost of increased medication-related side effects. Conversely, if opioids are the base analgesic, adjunctive medications can actually decrease many opioid-related side effects due to synergy and opioid sparing effects (Pal et al. 1997).

Opioids in the Treatment of Pain in the Battlefield Injured: Pros and Cons

Opioid analgesia is a key pillar to universal effective pain management in the current and future theater of war yet; despite the potential for adverse events, opioid-centered analgesia remains the primary base analgesic for acute pain management. Opioids are effective for all types of pain if used in the appropriate dose regimen, though neuropathic pain syndromes generally require higher doses, and this issue needs to be factored into the short- and long-term treatment plan and communicated to the patient (Ballantyne and Shin 2008). Other advantages of opioid analgesics include physician familiarity and the absence of end-organ toxicity. That said, opioid-centered analgesia has many adverse and well-known side effects including: respiratory depression, sedation, nausea, vomiting, bowel dysfunction, abuse, and addiction (Trescot et al. 2006). Some of the lesser-known side effects of intermediate or long-term opioid use include immunosuppression, hyperalgesia, increased bone mass demineralization, and anabolic hormonal suppression (Daniel 2002; Page 2005; Angst and Clark 2006). Collectively, these adverse effects are likely to have a negative long-term impact on polytrauma patients who are at greater risk for the development of long-term chronic pain syndromes.

The observed discrepancy in addiction rates as described in Table 14.1 is primarily due to variations in definition. The Diagnostic and Statistical Manual for Mental Disorders (DSM IV) does not have a definition for prescription drug misuse or addiction. The DSM IV only has a definition that is applicable to prescription drug abuse. Studies have employed a variety of definitions, from the clear-cut definition of abuse as defined in the DSM IV to the more liberal definitions such as "aberrant drug-related behaviors" or the subjective provider impression of misuse (Starrels et al. 2010). As a consequence, the current rate of opioid abuse, misuse, or addiction in the active duty U.S. military population is currently unknown.

Most wounded soldiers are treated with opioids for an extended period of time during the acute and convalescent phases after their injury. To date, however, this population has not been screened for opioid or other substance abuse risk factors *prior* to the initiation of opioid therapy. The military does not monitor substance abuse history unless a soldier is referred to the Army Substance Abuse Program (ASAP) for the treatment of substance addiction or abuse. This includes soldiers who enlisted in the military with prior substance abuse histories. The military medical community has recognized that opioid abuse, misuse, and addiction present clear risks to individual soldiers and military combat strength. There is also additional evidence that shows that male gender, low socioeconomic status (SES), genetic factors, family background/environment may also play a role in an individual's susceptibility for substance abuse disorders (Hall et al. 2008). The military population has some notable differences compared to the civilian population which include the predominantly young age, male sex, disposition for risk-taking behaviors, post-traumatic cognitive deficits, and the high prevalence of PTSD. While the current rate of opioid abuse, misuse, and addiction in the active duty military is not known, multiple initiatives at the local and national level have been undertaken to create and evaluate evidence-based best practices that balance the morale of the warfighter and medical necessities of appropriate pain treatment vs. the real individual and collective risk of pain medication, specifically opioid, abuse, or misuse (Chou et al. 2009; Benzon et al. 2010).

Alternatives to Opioid Analgesia

One alternative to opioid analgesia is the local anesthetic nerve blockage. Local anesthetic nerve blockade is the only other pain treatment modality capable of providing effective basal analgesia as part of an effective acute pain management strategy. Local anesthetic nerve blockade is commonly referred to as regional anesthesia, and is typically performed by placement of a catheter in either the epidural space or near a large peripheral nerve or nerve plexus by the anesthesiologist.

Studies have also shown improved patient outcomes and fewer adverse events with regional anesthesia (Guinard et al. 1992; Grass 1993). Improved outcome measures include decreased ICU and hospital stays (Yeager et al. 1987; Tuman et al. 1991); (Rawal et al. 1984), decreased cardiovascular mortality (Yeager et al. 1987; Tuman et al. 1991), decreased pulmonary dysfunction

(Rawal et al. 1984; Guinard et al. 1992), earlier return of bowel function (Rawal et al. 1984), decreased neuroendocrine stress (Yeager et al. 1987), decreased infection rate (Yeager et al. 1987), and decreased mortality (Wu et al. 2004, 2006). Wu et al., in an analysis of the Medicare claims database from 1997 to 2001 involving 3,501 patients, revealed a significantly lower odds of death ratio at 7 and 30 days postoperatively for patients who received a postoperative epidural (Wu et al. 2006). At this time, insufficient evidence exists that can determine if regional anesthesia can prevent or lessen the development of chronic pain including phantom limb pain (PLP). Five prospective studies evaluated perioperative epidural and regional nerve blocks to prevent the development of PLP (Bach et al. 1988; Elizaga et al. 1994; Jahangir et al. 1994; Pinzur et al. 1996; Nikolajsen et al. 1997). Although all studies found improved short-term pain relief, only Jahangiri et al. reported a decrease in PLP at 6 and 12 months postoperatively (Jahangir et al. 1994). The other five studies were equivocal. Animal studies also show that it is possible to inhibit the development of long-term chronic pain states; but human studies designed to decrease the incidence of postamputation PLP show mixed results (Manchikanti and Singh 2004; Rooney et al. 2007) (see also Foell and Flor 2011). What these retrospective and short-term studies show is that regional anesthesia can provide physiologic and cognitive benefits. Additional long-term prospective human studies are required to confirm these effects.

Regional anesthesia is also the only modality that can control pain without cognitive or physiologic side effects. Effective regional anesthesia enables wounded service members to avoid the sequelae of untreated acute pain, prevent the transition of the transition of acute pain to chronic pain, and prevent the known dose-related side effects of opioids (Buckenmaier et al. 2005, 2006; Malchow and Black 2008). However, regional anesthesia is not without risks. Major risks include local anesthetic toxicity and nerve injury (Auroy et al. 2002). The incidence of nerve injury varies widely and ranges from 0.2 to 2% (Stan et al. 1995; Faccenda and Finucane 2001), which can be reduced even further with the use of image-guided ultrasound, or peripheral nerve stimulation. The incidence of seizures secondary to local anesthetic toxicity with a peripheral nerve catheter is approximately 1 in 1,000, compared to 1 in 8,000 for epidural catheters (Auroy et al. 2002). The incidence of cardiac arrest from local anesthetic toxicity is 1 in 10,000 and 1 in 7,000 for epidural and peripheral nerve blocks, respectively (Auroy et al. 2002). Other risks of regional anesthesia include pneumothorax, diaphragmatic paralysis secondary to phrenic nerve block for upper extremity blocks, inadvertent spinal anesthesia, epidural hematoma, bleeding, allergic reactions, and infection (Auroy et al. 2002; Greensmith and Murray 2006).

In summary, additional research is needed to determine the best pain treatment strategies in the polytrauma patient. Untreated acute pain has detrimental immediate physiologic effects that have the potential to adversely affect long-term outcomes, including the development of PTSD and the transition to other chronic pain syndromes (Saxe et al. 2001; Hoge et al. 2004; De Kock 2009; see also Short and Vetter 2011; Donovan et al. 2011). The best treatment regimen, however, is still a matter of controversy. This controversy will not be resolved without conducting large-scale, clinical prospective trials.

Nonbattle Injuries (NBI)

A recent epidemiological study by Cohen et al. (2005) showed that among medically evacuated soldiers from OIF treated in pain clinics in level IV military treatment centers, injuries incurred during combat missions accounted for only 17% of cases. Over half of the patients presented with LBP, and the majority were diagnosed with lumbosacral radiculopathy. In descending order, the most commonly utilized treatments were NSAIDs, short-acting opioids, physical therapy, anticonvulsants, and epidural steroid injections (ESI). In those soldiers in whom disposition data were available, only 2% returned to duty with their unit. Multiple reasons contribute this low return to duty rate including more severe disease that necessitated evacuation to level IV treatment, the logistical difficulty of returning to the war zone from a level IV MTF, and a decreased desire to return to the war zone once a soldier is in the United States (Cohen et al. 2005).

Johnson et al. performed a retrospective review of American military patients evacuated out of theater during the first 4 months of Operation Iraqi Freedom (OIF) (Johnson et al. 2005). A total of 1,236 patients were evacuated: there were 256 battle casualties (20.7%), 510 injuries (41.3%), and 470 disease patients (38.0%). The patients included 1,123 males (91%) and 113 females (9%). Battle casualties were predominately male, 252 men (98%) vs. 4 women (2%). Injuries and medical diseases including pregnancy were the primary cause of evacuation for women. However, the dominant cause of attrition among female soldiers is still disease and injury (e.g. falls) rather than combat wounds which is supported by the fact that 2% of all battle fatalities are female. Hope et al. in an epidemiologic study found similar on duty causes of injuries with falls being the most common between the sexes (need citation). Sex differences in pain have also been reported (see also Keogh 2011). Women had longer average hospital stays for injuries of similar severity. This is an important area for future research. A full review of sex differences and injury patterns in the battlefield injured has not been performed to date.

There is some evidence that chronic pain may persist in war veterans presenting with NBI. A cohort study conducted by Gironda et al. found that 47% of 793 OIF and OEF veterans reported at least some degree of pain during their initial visit to a veteran's administration hospital (Gironda et al. 2006). Among these patients, 59% rated their pain as at least "moderate." In descending order, the most common pain complaints were back pain (46%), leg pain (31%), arm pain (8%), and neck pain (6%). In large-scale studies performed in Gulf War veterans, the prevalence rate of chronic, diffuse pain symptomatology has ranged from 7% (Fukuda et al. 1998) to 45% in more recently studies (Kang et al. 2009). Other recent studies show that at least a portion of somatic symptoms in veterans may be due to concomitant psychopathology (e.g. PTSD) or other Axis I disorders (Amin et al. 2010). In a population-based survey of 3,682 Gulf War veterans and military combat nonparticipants, Barrett et al. (2002) found a strong association with PTSD and poor physical health symptoms. Over 95% of the 53 soldiers with PTSD experienced musculoskeletal symptoms, as compared to less than 50% of former soldiers without PTSD. The strong association between chronic pain and Axis I disorders indicate that chronic pain is a causative factor in the development of the psychiatric disorders including depression and anxiety (Fishbain 1999). Fishbain in a review of comorbid psychiatric disorders and chronic pain patients reported that over 94% of chronic pain patients have at least one associated comorbid axis I diagnosis (Fishbain 1999). Moreover, once a psychiatric disorder is manifest the treatment of the underlying pain condition is more complex and the long-term prognosis is worse. Therefore, early aggressive pain treatment as prevention is likely to improve clinical outcomes.

The low return-to-duty rate reported by Cohen et al. and the high prevalence of persistent pain in veterans have led some experts to advocate early and aggressive treatment of acute or recurrent chronic pain conditions in forward-deployed pain clinics. White and Cohen reported data on 126 soldiers and other Department of Defense beneficiaries who were treated over 1 year in the first pain treatment center established within a theater of combat operations (White and Cohen 2007). Similar to the data reported in fourth-level military treatment facilities (Cohen et al. 2005), the most common diagnosis was radiculopathy, which accounted for approximately two-thirds of all new consults. The next most common diagnoses were thoracic pain, groin pain, nonradicular leg pain, and axial LBP. Not surprisingly, the most frequently performed procedures were ESI, trigger point injections, intra-articular facet blocks, and inguinal area nerve blocks. The return-to-duty rate in this study was an impressive 95%, which represents a dramatic improvement over the 2% return-to-duty rate reported by Cohen et al. in an earlier study in a similar patient population (Cohen et al. 2005). Of note, all seven patients medically evacuated to the continental United States were male patients with groin pain. Groin pain can be difficult to treat and has a high association with psychological comorbidities.

Although the stark differences in return-to-duty rates also support aggressive pain management in forward-deployed areas; several confounding factors contribute to the large discrepancy in return-to-theater rates (Cohen et al. 2005; Johnson et al. 2005). These include: a higher percentage of secondary gain issues among soldiers treated at fourth-level MTF, more concomitant psychopathology in those soldiers already medically evacuated out of theater, and more stringent selection criteria in the latter study (Elkayam et al. 1996; Fishbain 1999; Barrett et al. 2002). Specifically, soldiers who were treated "in theater" may have been more motivated to remain with their units, more likely to be mission-essential personnel whose commanders requested treatment, and more likely to have conditions amenable to treatment and rapid recovery. Dragovich and Trainer in a recent epidemiological study also reported similar results. Between December 2008 and June 2009, 31 patients with either radicular or axial LBP were treated with interventional therapies at Ibn Sina Hospital in Baghdad, Iraq. The return-to-duty rate in this study was 97% (Dragovich and Trainer 2011).

In summary, pain management in the battlefield setting is fraught with a unique set of challenges almost unimaginable in civilian pain treatment facilities. Given the wide variations in medical resources and personnel, there is actually no "optimal" pain treatment for war injuries. Instead, treatment should be individually tailored based on a patient's injury, hemodynamic condition, available resources, and the ability to adequately monitor treatment response. In modern warfare, the most common cause of soldier attrition are acute and recurrent nonbattle-related injuries, similar to those encountered in civilian pain treatment facilities and primary care offices. Recent evidence also suggests that the high return-to-unit rates observed in recent studies can be obtained through the deployment of aggressive pain management capabilities in mature theaters of operation.

Pain Conditions Encountered

Low Back Pain (LBP)

LBP is the most common presenting symptom likely to be encountered by the pain practitioner deployed to CSH. This is not surprising considering the repetitive stress of the previous training, heavy loads services members must carry, frequent transportation over rough terrain in military vehicles with stiff suspensions, heavy individual body armor (IBA) requiring abnormal posture that is worn for hours at a time, sleep deprivation, and the high degree of psychophysiological stressors faced by soldiers deployed to combat zones. A recent 5-year longitudinal cohort study conducted by Carragee and Cohen in 154 special operation U.S. Army reservists with no prior history of back pain, 84 and 64% reported mild and moderate LBP, respectively, when surveyed monthly after drill weekend (Carragee and Cohen Spine 2009). In deployed combat soldiers on duty 24 h/day, the authors estimated that the annual incidence of LBP would be higher. Among the various causes of LBP, radiculopathy from nerve root irritation may be the most commonly encountered condition. Compared to axial LBP, lumbosacral radiculopathy is generally associated with a more favorable prognosis (Carragee 2005).

The mainstay of interventional treatment for lumbar radiculopathy (sciatica) is ESI. ESI exert their beneficial effects by virtue of their anti-inflammatory properties, inhibition of the enzyme phospholipase A2, a critical enzyme necessary for the production of prostaglandins, suppression of ectopic discharges from injured neurons, and a reduction of capillary permeability (McLain et al. 2005). Although ESIs have been successfully used to treat axial back pain, the ideal candidates for treatment are those patients with pain of greater than 6 months duration, leg pain, increased back pain, young age, intermittent pain, and the absence of concomitant spinal stenosis (Benzon 1986; Butterman 2004). The use of fluoroscopic guidance is highly recommended for interlaminar ESI, and is necessary for transforaminal epidural steroid injections (TFESI). Even in experienced hands, the technical failure rate for "blind" ESI ranges from approximately 10% in the lumbar region to upwards of 50% for blinded cervical ESI (Renfrew et al. 1991; Fredman et al. 1999; Stitz and Sommer 1999; Stojanovic et al. 2002). Studies also show that only about 26% of blindly performed interlaminar ESI reached the targeted area of pathology in patients with previous back surgery (Fredman et al. 1999). TFESIs are technically more challenging than interlaminar ESI. However this intervention may provide additional clinical benefit since the medication is directly deposited over the affected nerve root, resulting in a higher incidence of ventral epidural spread, which is where the inciting disc pathology lies. In a recent comparative study, superior outcomes were found for TFESI compared to interlaminar ESI (Schaufele et al. 2006).

Patients who may have a diagnosis of radicular pain should receive CT scans of the appropriate spine area. Whereas MRI is the gold standard for imaging soft tissue and disc anatomy, these are not readily available in forward-deployed areas. In comparison to MRI, CT scans are approximately 90% sensitive and 70% specific in detecting disc pathology (Foristall and Marsh 1988). In comparison to drugs used to treat neuropathic pain such as gabapentin and amitriptyline, the advantages of ESI in combat-deployed service members include the speed of onset of treatment (e.g. 48–72 h) and the absence of central nervous system depressant effects such as lethargy, fatigue, and cognitive dysfunction. In addition, although ESIs are considered by many to be the best nonsurgical interventional therapy for radicular pain, controversy still exists regarding their long-term efficacy (Carette et al. 1997; Rozenberg et al. 1999; Riew et al. 2006).

Lumbar zygapophysial (a.k.a. facetogenic or facet pain) joint pain accounts for between 10 and 15% of patients with chronic axial LBP (Cohen and Raja 2007). The typical pattern of presentation is a dull aching pain, often bilateral, that radiates from the low back into the buttocks and posterolateral thighs. Less frequently, facetogenic pain is referred into the lower leg or groin. Whereas the history and physical exam can be suggestive of facet joint pain, an analgesic response to fluoroscopically guided low-volume diagnostic blocks of either the zygapophysial joints themselves or the medial branches that innervate them, is the gold standard for diagnosis (Bogduk 1997).

The interventional treatment of facetogenic pain consists of either intra-articular injections with corticosteroid, which may benefit a small number of patients with an acute inflammatory component, or more frequently radiofrequency denervation of the medial branch nerves that innervate the painful joints. For both treatments, there is conflicting evidence regarding the efficacy of this treatment (Cohen and Raja 2007). Moreover, due to the inherent risks of transportation and the lack of radiofrequency capability, a combination of diagnostic and therapeutic intraarticular facet injections are usually recommended in theater. In patients with radiological evidence of an acute inflammatory process, intra-articular corticosteroids may afford up to 3 months of excellent pain relief (Pneumaticos et al. 2006; Cohen and Raja 2007). These procedures can be repeated every 3 months, or the patient may be treated with radiofrequency denervation of the medial branches to provide intermediate term (6–18 months) pain relief. Radiofrequency denervation can only be performed at certain Army CSH or at a third- or fourth-level MTF.

Sacroiliac (SI) joint pain is also a frequent source of chronic axial LBP, accounting for roughly 15–20% of cases (Cohen 2005). Compared to other causes of back pain such as facet arthropathy and degenerative disc disease, SI joint is more likely to result from a specific inciting event such as a fall, motor vehicle accident, or parachute jump. Variation in age has also been observed in clinical studies. For example, unlike elderly patients who are more likely to have intra-articular pathology, the primary pain generator in younger patients with documented SI joint pain tends to be extra-articular (i.e. secondary to pathology in the surrounding ligaments or muscles). The typical presentation of SI joint pain is a unilateral aching pain in the low back or buttock with myriad possible referral patterns. The pain is typically reproduced with palpation and can often be reproduced with provocative maneuvers such as Patrick's or Gaenslen's tests (Hoppenfeld 1976). In patients with SI joint pain, multiple studies have demonstrated good intermediate- to long-term pain relief lasting up to 6 months with intra- or periarticular injections done with corticosteroid and local anesthetic. Previous studies have demonstrated that radiographic guidance is necessary to achieve accurate placement in or around the joint (Rosenberg et al. 2000). In patients who obtain significant but short-term pain relief from SI joint blocks, longer duration relief can often be obtained with radiofrequency ablation of the L4 and L5 primary dosal rami and S1–3 lateral branches (Cohen and Abdi 2003). Since predisposing factors such as leg length discrepancy or pelvic obliquity often contribute to a painful SI joint, physical therapy can be helpful in alleviating and preventing recurrent pain.

Another consequence is the development of myofascial pain of the low back. Myofascial pain accounts for over 80% of acute back pain episodes, and nearly 20% of patients with chronic axial back pain (Long et al. 1996). The inordinate degree of strain placed on soft tissue structures from Kevlar, body armor, and heavy gear, the development of ligamentous injury, muscle strains, trigger points, and frank spasm is particularly burdensome for combat units. Frequently, muscle spasm is superimposed on a more acute, underlying condition. The hallmark of treatment of myofascial pain is physical therapy where the aim is to identify and treat the underlying cause(s), and also pharmacotherapy. In individuals with acute back pain, the strongest evidence exists for the use of muscle relaxants and NSAIDs for the treatment and prevention of this type of pain. For chronic spine pain, systematic evidence-based reviews have determined that tricyclic antidepressants may provide significant pain relief and functional improvement, though the effect size is small and many patients will exhibit treatment-limited side effects (Cohen and Argoff 2008). When discrete bands of contracted muscle are palpable, trigger point injections done with local anesthetic can provide excellent relief.

Spinal stenosis and degenerative disc disease are also other common causes of LBP, with a higher incidence in the elder population. Whereas ESI can sometimes provide pain relief for these conditions, the benefit is often incomplete and transient. Less frequent sources of back pain and/or leg pain that should be ruled out include osteomyelitis, vertebral fractures, acute herpes zoster, and acute or worsening spondylolisthesis (Koes et al. 2006).

Cervical Spine Pain

Approximately 16–22% of adults suffer from chronic neck pain, with the condition having a higher prevalence in women than men (Guez et al. 2002). In one recent review, the annual prevalence rate of neck pain was estimated to be between 30 and 50% (Guez et al. 2002). Among patients with chronic neck pain, approximately 30% report a history of neck injury, which is often the result of a whiplash-associated disorder (e.g. motor vehicle accident) (Guez et al. 2003; see also Sterling 2011). In military pain clinics, neck pain and cervicogenic headaches also account for about 10–15% of NBI (Cohen et al. 2005; White and Cohen 2007).

There are numerous predisposing factors for neck pain in soldiers including prolonged static loads (from Kevlar), abnormal postures (e.g. secondary to body armor, or the position(s) assumed by snipers), work-related stress, and full-force exertion. In patients with acute neck or upper thoracic pain, the etiology is likely to be myofascial in origin. In chronic axial neck pain that occurs insidiously or in response to whiplash-associated injury, the facet joints are the most common pain generators (Aprill and Bogduk 1992; Manchikanti et al. 2002). Myofascial pain can be treated with muscle relaxants, NSAID, tricyclic antidepressants, short-term duty modification, and trigger point injections. For cervical facetogenic pain, intra-articular steroids can provide intermediate-term relief in a subset of patients with an acute inflammatory process. In patients with injection-confirmed cervical zygapophysial joint pain who do not respond to intra-articular steroids, radiofrequency denervation can provide intermediate-term benefit, but may require evacuation to a third- or fourth-level MTF.

Cervical radiculopathy typically manifests as neck pain radiating down an arm(s) in a dermatomal distribution, sometimes accompanied by weakness and sensory changes. Although history and physical exam (e.g. Spurling's test) can be suggestive, the diagnosis is usually confirmed by radiological imaging. Similar to lumbar radicular pain, symptoms of cervical radiculopathy are generally responsive to cervical ESI. Yet, due to reports of death and paralysis, cervical TFESI are not recommended in a medically austere environment (Baker et al. 2003). Other possible causes of cervicogenic headaches that may be amenable to injection therapy include atlantooccipital and atlantoaxial joint pain. Occipital neuralgia is another frequent cause of occipital headaches that is best diagnosed and treated with injections containing local anesthetic and corticosteroid (Vanelderen et al. 2010).

Nonradicular Leg Pain

Collectively, causes of nonradicular leg pain (e.g. piriformis syndrome, plantar fascitis, and greater trochanteric bursitis) account for approximately 10% of pain clinic visits from NBI. Many of these conditions tend to be associated with overuse of the affected body part. Piriformis syndrome tends to present as unilateral buttock pain, and depending on the extent of sciatic nerve involvement, extension into the lower leg. A diagnosis of piriformis syndrome is predicated on a positive response to fluoroscopically guided intramuscular injection confirmed by contrast injection, which can sometimes be facilitated with the use of a nerve stimulator to identify the adjacent sciatic nerve. In addition to their diagnostic utility, these injections can also be therapeutic.

Trochanteric bursitis (TB) is a clinical diagnosis characterized by the association of lateral hip pain, tenderness to palpation, and pain provocation by various movements. Sometimes called "pseudosciatica," TB can radiate into the distal thigh, but rarely extends below the knee. Risk factors for TB include co-existing lumbar spine pathology, gait and postural abnormalities, leg length discrepancy, female gender, and old age (Segal et al. 2007). It is important to note that a majority of patients clinically diagnosed with TB have no radiological evidence of bursa inflammation. In these patients, the true pain generator is often tendonitis, muscle tears, or trigger points (Kingzett-Taylor et al. 1999; Bird et al. 2001). Although studies have found that less than half of all trochanteric bursa injections performed without fluoroscopic guidance end up intra-bursal (Cohen and Narvaez 2005); no difference in outcomes were observed between fluoroscopically guided and landmark-guided (i.e. "blind") trochanteric bursa injections (Cohen et al. 2009). In one epidemiological study, patients who received a trochanteric bursa corticosteroid injection had almost a threefold higher rate of long-term recovery compared to those patients who did not receive an injection (Lievense et al. 2005). These procedures may be safely and effectively administered at Level I treatment centers.

Plantar fasciitis has a lifetime prevalence of almost 10% in the general population. This condition also tends to be very common in soldiers. Risk factors include excessive walking or running, especially in the early morning and on uneven surfaces, increased load-bearing associated with heavy gear; having flat feet or high arches; being overweight; and being middle age, or older age. Conservative treatment includes rest, night splints and/or orthotics, stretching exercises, and NSAIDs. Corticosteroid injections have also been shown to relieve plantar fasciitis symptoms (Tatli and Kapasi 2009).

Less Common Pain Complaints

Nonradicular arm pain is less frequently encountered than nonradicular leg pain. Aside from complex regional pain syndrome, which is rarely encountered in soldiers at third-level MTF, other causes of nonradicular arm pain include medial and lateral epicondylitis (a.k.a. tennis elbow), tendonitis, bursitis, and carpal tunnel syndrome. Injection of any of these overuse inflammatory conditions with corticosteroid and local anesthetic may result in significant pain relief and functional improvement. Since these injections tend to be targeted by palpation and landmarks, they can be done in the field without fluoroscopic guidance. In the absence of qualified personnel, topical NSAIDs (diclofenac, ibuprofen, ketoprofen, and piroxicam) have been shown in multiple controlled studies to provide significant pain relief and functional benefit in the absence of systemic side effects (Moore and Tramer 1998).

Lastly, male groin pain, female pelvic pain, and abdominal pain of unknown etiology are the least likely pain conditions to improve with interventional therapy available in theater. Common to all these conditions is the diagnostic dilemma that each poses, the lack of any reliable pharmacological or interventional treatments, and the high prevalence of coexisting psychopathology that often accompanies these disorders. In the observational study by White and Cohen, 7 of 8 patients who presented with groin pain (postherniorrhaphy pain, ilioinguinal/iliohypogastric neuralgia, and genitofemoral neuralgia) required medical evacuation out of theater (White and Cohen 2007). When a surgical scar is present, scar injections with corticosteroid and local anesthetic may afford pain relief by virtue of releasing an entrapped nerve(s) and/or suppressing ectopic discharges from injured neurons. Even in soldiers who will require medical evacuation, short-term relief may be obtained with nerve blocks performed with long-acting local anesthetics and corticosteroids. Since the majority of these blocks tend to be landmark-guided, fluoroscopy is generally not necessary, although ultrasound has been used to better target individual nerves (Eichenberger et al. 2006). In addition to interventional treatments, pharmacological therapy including antidepressants and membrane stabilizers may also provide significant benefit in select individuals (Crowell and Jones 2004; Levy 2007).

Conclusions

Polytrauma patients represent the ultimate challenge to military medical care from the time of initial injury, through transport, recovery, and rehabilitation. In modern warfare, the most common cause of soldier attrition is not battle-related injuries, but rather acute and recurrent NBI similar to those encountered in civilian pain clinics. Although recent evidence indicates that higher return-to-unit rates can be obtained with forward-deployed interventional pain management capabilities, this is not always practical (White and Cohen 2007). Pain management in the battlefield setting is fraught with a unique and often dynamic set of challenges. Given the wide variations in risks, time constraints, medical resources, and personnel, there is no "optimal" pain treatment for NBI. Optimal treatment should include a multidisciplinary approach tailored to eliminate or neutralize the underlying problem(s), prevent recurrences, address aggravating factors such as co-existing psychopathology, and facilitate a rapid return to baseline functional capacity.

The management of polytrauma battle injuries is a resource-intensive endeavor from the time of injury onset through rehabilitation. Beginning with unit medics, through evacuation and treatment at FST and CSH, these patients stress our ability to provide optimal pain management. Early postinjury, life-saving measures take precedence over pain control. Yet, these two objectives need not be mutually exclusive. As the patient transitions through the recovery process, pain control in general, and certain techniques in particular, may lead to improved long-term outcomes.

Our conflicts have created a fertile field of research opportunities. Serious knowledge gaps exist from the basic science level, through clinic practice to health systems management. Until well-designed studies can be conducted at every level of care, individual patients will continue to be treated in a heterogeneous fashion without any reliable correlation between the cost of treatment and clinical outcomes.

References

Adams, E., Breiner, S., et al. (2006). A comparison of the abuse liability of tramadol, NSAIDs, and hydrocodone in patients with chronic pain. *Journal of Pain and Symptom Management, 31*, 465–476.

Amin, M., Parisi, J., et al. (2010). War-related illness symptoms among operation Iraqi freedom/operation enduring freedom returnees. *Military Medicine, 175*(3), 155–157.

Angst, M., & Clark, J. (2006). Opioid-induced hyperalgesia: A qualitative systematic review. *Anesthesiology, 104*, 570–587.

Aprill, C., & Bogduk, N. (1992). The prevalence of cervical zygapophyseal joint pain. A first approximation. *Spine, 17*, 744–747.

Army Surgeon General's pain medicine task force. Retrieved February 10, 2010, from http://www.armymedicine. army.mil/reports/reports.html

Auroy, Y., Benhamou, D., et al. (2002). Major complications of regional anesthesia in France: The SOS Regional Anesthesia Hotline Service. *Anesthesiology, 97*, 1274–1280.

Bach, S., Noreng, M., et al. (1988). Phantom limb pain in amputees during the first 12 months following limb amputation, after preoperative lumbar epidural blockade. *Pain, 33*, 297–301.

Baker, R., Dreyfuss, P., et al. (2003). Cervical transforaminal injection of corticosteroids into a radicular artery: A possible mechanism for spinal cord injury. *Pain, 103*, 211–215.

Ballantyne, J., & Shin, N. (2008). Efficacy of opioids for chronic pain: A review of the evidence. *The Clinical Journal of Pain, 24*, 469–478.

Barrett, D., Doebbeling, C., et al. (2002). Posttraumatic stress disorder and self-reported physical health status among U.S. Military personnel serving during the Gulf War period: A population-based study. *Psychosomatics, 43*, 195–205.

Bellamy, R. (1995). Combat trauma overview. In R. Zaitchuk & R. F. Bellamy (Eds.), *Textbook of military medicine. Part IV: Anesthesia and perioperative care of the combat casualty* (pp. 1–42). Falls Church: Office of the Surgeon General.

Benzon, H. (1986). Epidural steroid injections for low back pain and lumbosacal radiculopathy. *Pain, 24*, 277–295.

Benzon, H., Connis, R., et al. (2010). Practice guidelines for chronic pain management: An updated report by the American Society of Anesthesiologists Task Force on Chronic Pain Management and the American Society of Regional Anesthesia and Pain Medicine. *Anesthesiology, 112*(4), 810–833.

Bird, P., Oakley, S., et al. (2001). Prospective evaluation of magnetic resonance imaging and physical examination findings in patients with greater trochanteric pain syndrome. *Arthritis and Rheumatism, 44*, 2138–2145.

Black, IH., & McManus, J. (2009). Pain management in current combat operations. *Prehosp Emerg Care.* Apr-Jun;*13*(2), 223–227.

Blansfiled, J. (1999). The origins of casualty evacuation and Echelons of care: Lessons learned from the American Civil War. *International Journal of Emergency Nursing, 5*, 5–9.

Bogduk, N. (1997). International Spinal Injection Society guidelines for the performance of spinal injection procedures. Part 1: Zygapophysial joint blocks. *The Clinical Journal of Pain, 13*, 285–302.

Buckenmaier, C., McKnight, G., et al. (2005). Continuous peripheral nerve block for battlefield anesthesia and evacuation. *Regional Anesthesia and Pain Medicine, 30*, 202–205.

Buckenmaier, C., Shields, C., et al. (2006). Continuous peripheral nerve block in combat casualties receiving low-molecular weight heparin. *British Journal of Anaesthesia, 97*, 874–877.

Butterman, G. (2004). Treatment of lumbar disc herniation: Epidural steroid injection compared with discetomy. A prospective, randomized study. *Journal of Bone and Joint Surgery, 86A*, 670–679.

Callander, B., & Hebert, A. (2006). The 90 percent solution. *Air Force Magazine Online.* Retrieved October 23, 2010, Available at: http://www.afa.org/magazine/oct2006/1006solution.asp.

Carragee, EJ., & Cohen SP. (2009). Lifetime asymptomatic for back pain: the validity of self-report measures in soldiers. *Spine (Phila Pa 1976).* Apr 20;*34*(9):978–983.

Carette, S., Leclaire, R., et al. (1997). Epidural corticosteroid injections for sciatica due to herniated nucleus pulposus. *The New England Journal of Medicine, 336*, 1634–1640.

Carey, M. (1996). Analysis of wounds incurred by U.S. Army Seventh Corps personnel treated in Corps hospitals during Operation Desert Storm, February 20 to March 10, 1991. *The Journal of Trauma, 40*, S165–S169.

Carragee, E. (2005). Clinical practice. Persistent low back pain. *The New England Journal of Medicine, 352*, 1891–1898.

Chou, R., Fanciullo, G., et al. (2009). Clinical guidelines for the use of chronic opioid therapy in chronic noncancer pain. *The Journal of Pain, 10*(2), 113–130.

Cohen, SP., Argoff, CE., & Carragee EJ. (2008). Management of low back pain. *BMJ.* Dec 22;337:a2718. doi: 10.1136/bmj.a2718.

Cohen, S. (2005). Sacroiliac joint pain: A comprehensive review of anatomy, diagnosis, and treatment. *Anesthesia and Analgesia, 101*, 1440–1453.

Cohen, S., & Abdi, S. (2003). Lateral branch blocks as a treatment for sacroiliac joint pain: A pilot study. *Regional Anesthesia and Pain Medicine, 28*, 113–119.

Cohen, S., Griffith, S., et al. (2005). Presentation, diagnosis, mechanisms of injury, and treatment of soldiers injured in Operation Iraqi Freedom: An epidemiological study conducted at two military pain management centers. *Anesthesia and Analgesia, 101*, 1098–1103.

Cohen, SP., Narvaez, JC., Lebovits, AH., Stojanovic, MP. (2005). Corticosteroid injections for trochanteric bursitis: is fluoroscopy necessary? A pilot study. *Br J Anaesth*. Jan;*94*(1), 100–6. Epub 2004 Oct 29.

Cohen, S., & Raja, S. (2007). Pathogenesis, diagnosis, and treatment of lumbar zygapophysial (facet) joint pain. *Anesthesiology, 106*, 591–614.

Crowell, MD., Jones, MP., Harris, LA., Dineen, TN., Schettler, VA., Olden, KW. (2004). Antidepressants in the treatment of irritable bowel syndrome and visceral pain syndromes. *Curr Opin Investig Drugs*. 2004 Jul;*5*(7), 736–42. Review.

Daniel, H. (2002). Hypogonadism in men consuming sustained-action oral opioids. *The Journal of Pain, 3*, 377–384.

Davis, M. (2010). Recent development in therapeutics for breakthrough pain. *Expert Review of Neurotherapeutics, 10*, 757–773.

De Kock, M. (2009). Expanding our horizons: Transition of acute pain to persistent pain and establishment of chronic postsurgical pain services. *Anesthesiology, 111*, 461–463.

Desborough, J. (2000). The stress response to trauma and surgery. *British Journal of Anaesthesia, 85*, 109–117.

Donovan, K. A., Thompson, L. M. A., & Jacobsen, P. B. (2011). Pain, depression and anxiety in cancer. In R. J. Moore (Ed.), *Handbook of pain and palliative care: Biobehavioral approaches for the life course*. New York: Springer.

Dragovich, A., & Trainer, RJ. A report of 3 soldiers returned to full duty after lumbar radiofrequency facet denervation in a theater of war. *Pain Med*. 2011 Apr;*12*(4), 679–81. doi: 10.1111/j.1526-4637.2010.01041.x. Epub 2011 Jan 11.

Egan, T., Sharma, A., et al. (2000). Multiple dose pharmacokinetics of oral transmucosal fentanyl citrate in healthy volunteers. *Anesthesiology, 92*, 665–673.

Eichenberger, U., Greher, M., et al. (2006). Ultrasound-guided blocks of the ilioinguinal and iliohypogastric nerve: Accuracy of a selective new technique confirmed by anatomical dissection. *British Journal of Anaesthesia, 97*, 238–243.

Elizaga, A., Smith, D., et al. (1994). Continuous regional analgesia by intraneural block: Effect on postoperative opioid requirements and phantom limb pain following amputation. *Journal of Rehabilitation Research and Development, 1994*, 179–187.

Elkayam, O., Ben Itzhak, S., et al. (1996). Multidisciplinary approach to chronic back pain: Prognostic elements of the outcome. *Clinical and Experimental Rheumatology, 14*(3), 281–288.

Faccenda, K., & Finucane, B. (2001). Complications of regional anaesthesia. Incidence and prevention. *Drug Safety, 24*, 413–442.

Fassoulaki, A., Patris, K., et al. (2002). The analgesic effect of gabapentin and mexiletine after breast surgery for cancer. *Anesthesia and Analgesia, 95*, 985–991.

Fassoulaki, A., Sarantopoulos, C., et al. (2001). Regional block and mexiletine: The effect on pain after cancer breast surgery. *Regional Anesthesia and Pain Medicine, 26*, 223–228.

Fine, P., & Streisand, J. (1998). A review of oral transmucosal fentanyl citrate: Potent, rapid and noninvasive opioid analgesia. *Journal of Palliative Medicine, 1*, 55–63.

Fishbain, D. A. (1999). Approaches to treatment decisions for psychiatric comorbidity in the management of the chronic pain patient. *Medical Clinics of North America, 83*(3), 737–760, vii.

Fishbain, D. A., Rosomoff, H., et al. (1992). Drug abuse, dependence, and addiction in chronic pain patients. *The Clinical Journal of Pain, 8*, 77–85.

Foell, J., & Flor, H. (2011). Phantom limb pain. In R. J. Moore (Ed.), *Handbook of pain and palliative care: Biobehavioral approaches for the life course*. New York: Springer.

Fredman, B., Nun, M., et al. (1999). Epidural steroids for treating "failed back surgery syndrome": Is fluoroscopy really necessary? *Anesthesia and Analgesia, 88*, 367–372.

Fukuda, K., Nisenbaum, R., et al. (1998). Chronic multisymptom illness affecting Air Force veterans of the Gulf War. *Journal of American Medical Association, 280*, 981–988.

Gabriel, R., Metz, K. (2007). A short history of war: The evolution of warfare and weapons. In Proceeding of the Read Mil Strat Strategic Studies Institute. Carlisle Barracks: US Army War College.

Gironda, R., Clark, M., et al. (2006). Pain among veterans of Operations Enduring Freedom and Iraqi Freedom. *Pain Medicine, 7*, 339–343.

Goldberg, M. (2010). Death and injury rates of U.S. military personnel in Iraq. *Military Medicine, 175*, 220–226.

Grass, J. (1993). Surgical outcome: Regional anesthesia and analgesia versus general anesthesia. *Anesthesia Review, 20*, 117–125.

Greensmith, J., & Murray, W. (2006). Complications of regional anesthesia. *Current Opinion in Anaesthesiology, 19*, 531–537.

Guez, M., Hildingsson, C., et al. (2002). The prevalence of neck pain: A population-based study from northern Sweden. *Acta Orthopaedica Scandinavica, 73*, 455–459.

Guez, M., Hildingsson, C., et al. (2003). Chronic neck pain of traumatic and non-traumatic origin: A population-based study. *Acta Orthopaedica Scandinavica, 74*, 576–579.

Guinard, J., Mavrocordatos, P., et al. (1992). A randomized comparison of intravenous versus lumbar and thoracic epidural fentanyl for analgesia after thoracotomy. *Anesthesiology, 77*, 1108–1115.

Hall, A., Logan, J., et al. (2008). Patterns of abuse among unintentional pharmaceutical overdose fatalities. *Journal of American Medical Association, 300*, 2613–2620.

Hoge, C., Castro, C., et al. (2004). Combat duty in Iraq and Afghanistan, mental health problems, and barriers to care. *The New England Journal of Medicine, 351*, 13–22.

Holbrook, T., Galarneau, M., et al. (2010). Morphine use after combat injury in Iraq and post traumatic stress disorder. *The New England Journal of Medicine, 362*, 110–117.

Hoppenfeld, S. (1976). *Physical examination of the spine and extremities* (pp. 261–262). New Jersey: Prentice-Hall.

Hurley, R., Cohen, S., et al. (2006). The analgesic effects of perioperative gabapentin on postoperative pain: A meta-analysis. *Regional Anesthesia and Pain Medicine, 31*, 237–247.

Islinger, R., Kuklo, T., et al. (2000). A review of orthopedic injuries in three recent U.S. military conflicts. *Military Medicine, 165*, 463–465.

Ives, T., Chelminski, P., et al. (2006). Predictors of opioid misuse in patients with chronic pain: A prospective cohort study. *BMC Health Services Research, 4*, 46.

Jahangir, M., Bradley, J., et al. (1994). Prevention of phantom pain after major lower limb amputation by epidural infusion of diamorphine, clonidine and bupivacaine. *Annals of the Royal College of Surgeons of England, 76*, 324–326.

Johnson, B., Carmack, D., et al. (2005). Operation Iraqi Freedom: The Landstuhl Region Medical Center experience. *The Journal of Foot and Ankle Surgery, 44*, 177–183.

Jowitt, M., & Knight, R. (1983). Anaesthesia during the Falklands campaign. The land battles. *Anaesthesia, 38*, 776–783.

Kang, H., Li, B., et al. (2009). Health of US veterans of 1991 Gulf War: A follow-up survey in 10 years. *Journal of Occupational and Environmental Medicine, 51*, 401–410.

Kelhet, H., Jensen, T., et al. (2006). Persistent post surgical pain: Risk factors and prevention. *Lancet, 367*, 1618–1625.

Keogh, E. (2011). Sex differences in pain across the life course. In R. J. Moore (Ed.), *Handbook of pain and palliative care: Biobehavioral approaches for the life course*. New York: Springer.

Kharasch, E., Hoffer, C., et al. (2004). Influence of age on the pharmacokinetics and pharmacodynamics of oral transmucosal fentanyl citrate. *Anesthesiology, 101*, 738–743.

Kingzett-Taylor, A., Tirman, P., et al. (1999). Tendinosis and tears of gluteus medius and minimus muscles as a cause of hip pain: MR imaging findings. *AJR American Journal of Roentgenology, 173*, 1123–1126.

Koes, B., van Tulder, M., et al. (2006). Diagnosis and treatment of low back pain. *British Medical Journal, 332*, 332.

Kotwal, R., O'Connor, K., et al. (2004). A novel pain management strategy for combat casualty care. *Annals of Emergency Medicine, 44*, 121–127.

Lievense, A., Bierma-Zeinstra, S., et al. (2005). Prognosis of trochanteric pain in primary care. *British Journal of General Practice, 55*, 199–204.

Liu, S., Carpenter, R., et al. (1995). Effects of perioperative analgesic technique on rate of recovery after colon surgery. *Anesthesiology, 83*, 757–765.

Long, D., BenDebba, M., et al. (1996). Persistent back pain and sciatica in the United States: Patient characteristics. *Journal of Spinal Disorders, 9*, 40–58.

Malchow, R., & Black, I. (2008). The evolution of pain management in the critically ill trauma patient: Emerging concepts from the global war on terrorism. *Critical Care Medicine, 36*, S346–S357.

Manchikanti, L., & Singh, V. (2004). Managing phantom pain. *Pain Physician, 7*, 365–375.

Manchikanti, L., Singh, V., et al. (2002). Prevalence of cervical facet joint pain in chronic neck pain. *Pain Physician, 5*, 243–249.

McLain, R., Kapural, L., et al. (2005). Epidural steroid therapy for back and leg pain: Mechanisms of action and efficacy. *The Spine Journal, 5*(2), 191–201.

Nakahura, T., Griswold, W., et al. (1998). Nonsteroidal anti-inflammatory drug use in adolescence. *The Journal of Adolescent Health, 23*, 307–310.

Newcomer, K., Shelerud, R., et al. (2010). Anxiety levels, fear-avoidance beliefs, and disability levels at baseline and at 1 year among subjects with acute and chronic low back pain. *Physical Medicine and Rehabilitation, 2*, 514–520.

Nikolajsen, L., Ilkjaer, S., et al. (1997). Randomised trial of epidural bupivacaine and morphine in prevention of stump and phantom pain in lower-limb amputation. *Lancet, 350*, 1353–1357.

OTSG Office of the Surgeon General. Available at: http://armymedicine@army.mil. Retrieved October 23, 2010.

Page, G. (2005). Immunologic effects of opioids in the presence or absence of pain. *Journal of Pain and Symptom Management, 29*, S25–S31.

Pal, S., Cortiella, J., et al. (1997). Adjunctive methods of pain control in burns. *Burns, 23*, 404–412.

Pinzur, M., Garla, P., et al. (1996). Continuous postoperative infusion of a regional anaesthetic after an amputation of the lower extremity. *Journal of Bone and Joint Surgery, 79*, 1752–1753.

Pneumaticos, S., Chatziioannou, S., et al. (2006). Low back pain: Prediction of short-term outcome of facet joint injection with bone scintigraphy. *Radiology, 238*, 693–698.

Portenoy, R., & Foley, K. (1986). Chronic use of opioid analgesics in non-malignant pain: Report of 38 cases. *Pain, 25*, 171–186.

Ramasamy, A., Hill, A., et al. (2009). Improvised explosive devices: Pathophysiology, injury profiles and current medical management. *Journal of the Royal Army Medical Corps, 155*, 265–272.

Rawal, N., Sjostrand, U., et al. (1984). Comparison of intramuscular and epidural morphine for postoperative analgesia in the grossly obese: Influence on postoperative ambulation and pulmonary function. *Anesthesia and Analgesia, 63*, 583–592.

Renfrew, D., Moore, T., et al. (1991). Correct placement of epidural steroid injections: Fluoroscopic guidance and contrast administration. *American Journal of Neuroradiology, 12*, 1003–1007.

Riew, K., Park, J., et al. (2006). Nerve root blocks in the treatment of lumbar radicular pain. A minimum five-year follow-up. *Journal of Bone and Joint Surgery, 88*, 1722–1725.

Rooney, B., Crown, E., et al. (2007). Preemptive analgesia with lidocaine prevents failed back surgery syndrome. *Experimental Neurology, 204*, 589–596.

Rosenberg, J., Quint, T., et al. (2000). Computerized tomographic localization of clinically-guided sacroiliac joint injections. *The Clinical Journal of Pain, 16*, 18–21.

Rozenberg, S., Dubourg, G., et al. (1999). Efficacy of epidural steroids in low back pain and sciatica. A critical appraisal by a French task force of randomized trials. *Revue du Rhumatisme, 66*, 79–85.

Saxe, G., Stoddard, F., et al. (2001). Relationship between acute morphine and the course of PTSD in children with burns. *Journal of the American Academy of Child and Adolescent Psychiatry, 40*, 915–921.

Schaufele, M., Hatch, L., et al. (2006). Interlaminar versus transforaminal epidural injections for the treatment of symptomatic lumbar intervertebral disc herniations. *Pain Physician, 9*, 361–366.

Schricker, T., Meterissian, S., et al. (2004). Postoperative protein sparing with epidural analgesia and hypocaloric dextrose. *Annals of Surgery, 240*, 916–921.

Segal, N., Felson, D., et al. (2007). Greater trochanteric pain syndrome: Epidemiology and associated factors. *Archives of Physical Medicine and Rehabilitation, 88*, 988–992.

Short, R., & Vetter, T. R. (2011). Acute to chronic pain: transitions in the post surgical patient. In R. J. Moore (Ed.), *Handbook of pain and palliative care: Biobehavioral approaches for the life course*. New York: Springer.

Sorenson, R., & Pace, N. (1992). Anesthetic techniques during surgical repair of femoral neck fractures. A meta-analysis. *Anesthesiology, 77*, 1095–1104.

Stan, T., Krantz, M., et al. (1995). The incidence of neurovascular complications following axilliary brachial plexus block using a transarterial approach. A prospective study of 1,000 consecutive patients. *Regional Anesthesia, 20*, 486–492.

Starrels, J., Becker, W., et al. (2010). Systematic review: Treatment agreements and urine drug testing to reduce opioid misuse in patients with chronic pain. *Annals of Internal Medicine, 152*, 712–720.

Sterling, M. (2011). Pain, Whiplash disorder and traffic safety. In R. J. Moore (Ed.), *Handbook of pain and palliative care: Biobehavioral approaches for the life course*. New York: Springer.

Stitz, M., & Sommer, H. (1999). Accuracy of blind versus fluoroscopically guided caudal epidural injections. *Spine, 24*, 1371–1376.

Stojanovic, M., Vu, T., et al. (2002). The role of fluoroscopy in cervical epidural steroid injections: An analysis of contrast dispersal patterns. *Spine, 27*, 509–514.

Tatli, Y., & Kapasi, S. (2009). The real risks of steroid injection for plantar fasciitis, with a review of conservative therapies. *Current Reviews in Musculoskeletal Medicine, 2*, 3–9.

The War List (2007). Available at: http://ptsd.combat.blogspot.com/2007/03/war-list-oefoif-statistics.html.

Towheed, T., Maxwell, L., et al. (2006). Acetaminophen for osteoarthritis. *Cochrane Database Systemic Review, 25*, CD004257.

Trescot, A., Boswell, M., et al. (2006). Opioid guidelines in the management of chronic non-cancer pain. *Pain Physician, 9*, 1–39.

Tuman, K., McCarthy, R., et al. (1991). Effects of epidural anesthesia and analgesia on coagulation and outcome after major vascular surgery. *Anesthesia and Analgesia, 73*, 696–704.

Vanelderen, P., Lataster, A., et al. (2010). Occipital neuralgia. *Pain Practice, 10*(2), 137–144.

Vetter, T. R. (2011). Pediatric chronic pain. In R. J. Moore (Ed.), *Handbook of pain and palliative care: Biobehavioral approaches for the life course*. New York: Springer.

Wall, C., Lynch, J., et al. (2010). Clinical practice guidelines for the management of acute limb compartment syndrome following trauma. *ANZ Journal of Surgery, 80*, 151–156.

Wedmore, I., Johnson, T., et al. (2005). Pain management in the wilderness and operational setting. *Emergency Medicine Clinics of North America, 23*, 585–601.

White, R., & Cohen, S. (2007). Return-to-duty rates among coalition forces treated in a forward-deployed pain treatment center: A prospective observational study. *Anesthesiology, 107*, 1003–1008.

Wu, C., Hurley, R., et al. (2004). Effect of postoperative epidural analgesia on morbidity and mortality following surgery in medicare patients. *Regional Anesthesia and Pain Medicine, 29*, 525–533.

Wu, C., Sapirstein, A., et al. (2006). Effect of postoperative epidural analgesia on morbidity and mortality after lung resection in Medicare patients. *Journal of Clinical Anesthesia, 18*, 515–520.

Yeager, M., Glass, D., et al. (1987). Epidural anesthesia and analgesia in high-risk surgical patients. *Anesthesiology, 66*, 729–736.

Zouris, J., Walker, G., et al. (2006). Wounding patterns for U.S. Marines and sailors during Operation Iraqi Freedom, major combat phase. *Military Medicine, 171*, 246–252.

Chapter 15
Pain, Whiplash Disorder and Traffic Safety

Michele Sterling

"It's only whiplash. Aren't you over it yet" (Trotter 2009).

Introduction

Whiplash-associated disorders (WAD) are a common, disabling and costly condition that occur usually as a consequence of a motor vehicle crash (MVC). Whilst the figures vary depending on the cohort studied, current understanding is that up to 50% of people who experience a whiplash injury will never fully recover (Carroll et al. 2008) and up to 30% will remain moderately to severely disabled by their condition (Rebbeck et al. 2006b; Sterling et al. 2006). The associated costs secondary to whiplash injury, which include medical care, disability, lost work productivity as well as personal costs are substantial. Claims for personal injury after whiplash cost in the United Kingdom are more than £3 billion per year (Joslin et al. 2004), while data from the United States are even more staggering with costs reaching $230 billion US dollars per annum (Blincoe et al. 2002). In Australia, whiplash injury accounts for the vast majority of submitted claims as well as the greatest incurred costs in the Queensland compulsory third party scheme (MAIC 2009). In this state, the economic costs related to whiplash injury are substantial and exceeded $500 million from 1994 to 2001 (MAIC 2002), and in New South Wales in the period 1989–1998 there were 50,000 whiplash claims costing ~$1.5 billion (NSW 1999).

There is some evidence to suggest that the incidence of whiplash injury may differ between countries (Holm et al. 2008). Some data indicate that the annual cumulative incidence of hospital visits due to whiplash injury in traffic collisions has increased during the past 30 years (Holm et al. 2008). The reasons for this increase are not clear but may be due to changes in health-seeking behaviours (Holm et al. 2008). The aim of this chapter is to outline the physiological and psychological manifestations of whiplash as well as discuss the role that stress symptoms may play in the presentation and outcomes following whiplash injury. The implications for management as well as future directions for research will be discussed.

M. Sterling, PhD (✉)
Centre of National Research on Disability and Rehabilitation Medicine (CONROD), The University of Qld, Herston, QLD, Australia
e-mail: m.sterling@uq.edu.au

R.J. Moore (ed.), *Handbook of Pain and Palliative Care: Biobehavioral Approaches for the Life Course*, DOI 10.1007/978-1-4419-1651-8_15, © Springer Science+Business Media, LLC 2012

Symptoms of Whiplash-Associated Disorders

Symptoms following whiplash injury can be diverse in nature. The predominant symptom is neck pain and it is present in almost all patients (Stovner 1996), with some patients also reporting neck stiffness (Sterner and Gerdle 2004). In addition, headache has been reported in 50–90% of patients, shoulder and arm pain in 40–70% of patients and back pain (thoracic and/or lumbar regions) in 35% of injured people (Radanov et al. 1995; Sterling et al. 2002a; Stovner 1996). Paraesthesia and/or anaesthesia, usually in the upper limbs, presents in up to 20% of patients (Sterner and Gerdle 2004). Apart from pain, other common symptoms include dizziness, visual and auditory disturbances, temporomandibular joint pain, photophobia and fatigue (Sterner and Gerdle 2004; Stovner 1996; Treleaven et al. 2003).

The onset of symptoms may occur immediately or, in many patients, may be delayed for up to 12–15 h (Hildingsson and Toolanen 1990; Sterner and Gerdle 2004). Recent systematic review data indicate that up to 50% of injured people will not have fully recovered 1 year post injury (Carroll et al. 2008). Prospective studies that have followed whiplash-injured people from soon after injury to either recovery or the development of chronic symptoms indicate that rapid improvement occurs in the first 3 months with little if any change after this period (Kamper et al. 2008; Sterling et al. 2010).

Evidence for Biological Changes as a Basis for Ongoing Pain Following Whiplash Injury

Whiplash is one of the most debated and controversial painful musculoskeletal conditions. This is in part due to the often compensable nature of the injury and that a precise pathoanatomical diagnosis is not usually achievable, at least with current imaging techniques. Whiplash has had a tumultuous history since Harold Crowe first coined the term in 1928, a term he later regretted (Crowe 1964). Many have argued about the legitimacy of the condition with some even maintaining that it is a condition of deception, folly and greed (Malleson 2002) and others that it is merely symptom "amplification" (Ferrari 2001). In recent times, perhaps co-incidentally but in parallel with the growth in empirical literature about whiplash, critics have become less vocal. There is now substantial data available demonstrating the presence of biological changes in various body systems in individuals with WAD.

Evidence for Peripheral Pathology

The determination of specific injured neck structures associated with a whiplash injury remains difficult and most likely due to the insensitivity of current imaging technologies (Ronnen et al. 1996; Steinberg et al. 2005). This is not to say that such injuries do not occur. When evidence is taken together from bioengineering studies identifying the potential for lesions to occur (Yoganandan et al. 2002), and cadaveric studies where clear lesions are demonstrated in non-survivors of a MVC (Taylor and Taylor 1996), there is reasonable justification for the presence of pathoanatomical lesions in at least some of the injured people (Bogduk 2002). Damaged structures may include zygapophyseal joints, intervertebral discs, synovial folds, vertebral bodies and nerve tissue (including dorsal root ganglia, spinal cord or brainstem) (Uhrenholt et al. 2002).

Clinical studies provide additional support for the findings of potential structural lesions from both bioengineering and cadaveric studies. Lord et al. (1996a) linked zygapophyseal arthropathy with chronic WAD by achieving substantial pain relief in some patients with persistent pain following a whiplash injury using placebo-controlled zygapophyseal joint blocks. The zygapophyseal joint may also be vulnerable due to the orientation of the articular surfaces that allow movement coupling and compressive forces during the trauma (Sizer et al. 2004). In addition, gender differences have also been observed where females may be more at risk of zygapophyseal joint damage due to decreased cartilage thickness on the articular surfaces (Yoganandan et al. 2003). This may be one possible explanation for the higher number of females who present with persistent whiplash symptoms.

Findings from clinical studies also implicate injury to peripheral nerve tissue. Clinical tests designed to provoke upper quadrant peripheral nerve structures have demonstrated the presence of apparently mechanosensitive nerve tissue (Ide et al. 2001; Sterling et al. 2002b) and mechanically hyperalgesic nerve trunks have been shown to be a feature of chronic whiplash (Greening et al. 2005; Sterling et al. 2002b). Studies utilizing quantitative electromyography have also demonstrated abnormalities suggestive of neural injury; particularly involving the lower cervical segments (Chu et al. 2005; Steinberg et al. 2005).

Magnetic resonance imaging (MRI) and functional MRI (fMRI) have further shown lesions of the cranio-cervical regions in participants with chronic whiplash (Johansson 2006; Kaale et al. 2005; Krakenes et al. 2002, 2003). These findings have been controversial with some studies showing similar "lesions" that are also present in asymptomatic individuals leading to questions as to whether such changes are actually the result of the MVC trauma (Pfirrmann et al. 2001; Roy et al. 2004).

Motor and Muscles Changes

More recent MRI data have shown structural muscle changes in the form of fatty infiltration in the neck muscles of females with chronic WAD (Elliott et al. 2006, 2009). The muscle changes are not present in asymptomatic individuals nor in those with idiopathic or non-traumatic neck pain (Elliott et al. 2008) and are not related to symptom duration or body mass index (Elliott et al. 2006). In prospective investigations, preliminary data indicate that the muscle changes occur within a few weeks of injury, are present only in participants with poor recovery and are not associated with a lack of neck movement (Elliott et al. 2010, 2011). Whilst the precise mechanisms underlying these changes are not clear, the findings do suggest that some yet undefined processes may underlie those whose condition does not resolve, and this issue requires further investigation.

There is also clear evidence of changes in neuromuscular control. Individuals who have experienced a whiplash injury are known to have impaired neck strength, which is apparent around all axes (Lindstrom et al. 2011). Changes in muscle strength are also accompanied by alterations in muscle strategies. Data suggest that the presence of neck pain is associated with alterations in task-related modulation of neck muscle activity so that motor control of the cervical spine is achieved by alternative, presumably less efficient, combinations of muscle synergistic activities. For example, altered performance on a task of upper cervical flexion has been shown to be a feature of whiplash-induced neck pain (Jull 2000; Sterling et al. 2003b) and is also present in other neck pain disorders such as idiopathic neck pain (Falla et al. 2004) and cervicogenic headache (Jull et al. 2002). In this test, individuals with neck pain perform the simple movement of upper cervical flexion with markedly different muscle activity than people without neck pain, in that there is much greater activity in the superficial neck muscles (Falla et al. 2004). These changes are thought to represent disturbed neuromuscular control (Falla et al. 2004).

Longitudinal data demonstrate that neuromuscular control changes are apparent from very soon after injury (Nederhand et al. 2002; Sterling et al. 2003b) with greater deficits in those reporting higher levels of pain and disability (Sterling et al. 2003b). Sterling et al. (2003b, 2006) observed that the disturbed motor patterns persisted, not only in those with ongoing chronic symptoms but also in those with lesser symptoms and those who reported full recovery with this phenomena persisting up to 2 years post injury. These persisting deficits in muscle control may leave recovered individuals more vulnerable to future episodes of neck pain but this proposal needs to be substantiated with further investigation (Sterling et al. 2006). Altered patterns of muscle recruitment are not unique to whiplash and identical changes have also been observed in neck pain of insidious onset (idiopathic neck pain) (Jull et al. 2004; Nederhand et al. 2002; Woodhouse and Vasseljen 2008). These findings suggest that the driver of such motor changes may be more due to the nociceptive input rather than the injury itself.

Dysfunction of sensorimotor control is also a feature of both acute and chronic WAD. Greater joint re-positioning errors have been found in patients with chronic WAD and also in those within weeks of their injury, and with moderate/severe severe pain and disability (Sterling et al. 2003b; Treleaven et al. 2003). Loss of balance and disturbed neck influenced eye movement control are present in chronic WAD (Treleaven et al. 2005a, b) but their presence in the acute stage of the injury has not been adequately investigated. Some data indicate that smooth pursuit eye movements may be unaffected in acute WAD patients (Kongsted et al. 2008a). Sensorimotor disturbances are greater in patients who also report dizziness in association with their neck pain (Treleaven et al. 2005a, b).

Most of the documented motor deficits (movement loss, altered neuromuscular control) seem to be present in whiplash-injured individuals irrespective of reported pain and disability levels and rate or level of recovery (Sterling et al. 2003b). Additionally, apart from cervical movement loss, motor deficits do not appear to have a predictive capacity (Kongsted et al. 2008a; Sterling et al. 2005). Furthermore, treatment directed at rehabilitating motor dysfunction and improving general movement shows only modest effects on reported pain and disability levels (Jull et al. 2007; Stewart et al. 2007). Together these findings suggest that motor deficits, although present, may not play a key role in the development and maintenance of chronic or persistent symptoms following whiplash injury. This is not to say that management approaches directed at improving motor dysfunction should not be provided to patients with whiplash. Rather the identification of motor deficits alone may not equip the clinician with useful information to either gauge prognosis or potential responsiveness to physical interventions.

Changes in Nociceptive Processing

Regardless of the specific structures involved, following injury and ensuing inflammation, a cascade of events occurs in the periphery, spinal cord and supraspinal nervous centres leading to upregulation of nociceptive processes. These changes have the potential to amplify the individual's pain experience. Even if identification of injured peripheral (neck) structures was easily achieved, it remains unclear whether it would improve management directions and outcomes as the correlation between objective findings and pain and disability is well known to be equivocal in whiplash (Elliott et al. 2009; Ichihara et al. 2009). Rather recent calls have been made for greater consideration of underlying pain processes that contribute to the condition in question, as this may enable the direction of the most appropriate intervention strategies (Haanpaa et al. 2009). There has now been much research demonstrating indirect evidence via sensory testing and other methods of altered pain processes as contributing factors to the clinical presentation, outcome and response to treatment of WAD.

There is now overwhelming data demonstrating the presence of sensory disturbances in patients with chronic WAD. These include decreased pain thresholds to various stimuli including mechanical pressure (Koelbaek-Johansen et al. 1999; Sterling et al. 2003a), thermal stimulation (Sterling et al. 2003a), electrical stimulation (Sheather-Reid and Cohen 1998) and vibration (Moog et al. 2002). Decreased pain thresholds or sensory hypersensitivity have been demonstrated both locally over the neck as well as at more distal or remote sites such as the upper and lower limbs where there is clearly no tissue damage. The absence of tissue damage at the site of testing suggests that a central sensitization of nociceptive pathways was the cause of the pain hypersensitivity.

These findings have been confirmed via studies assessing sensory responses following induced muscle pain with injection of hypertonic saline. Following injection to supraspinatus and tibialis anterior muscles, patients with WAD reported higher pain scores, longer duration of pain and larger areas of local and referred pain compared with healthy controls (Koelbaek-Johansen et al. 1999). Several patients also reported pain spreading to the whole leg and on the contralateral side, which was not the case in healthy subjects. These data suggest that pain hypersensitivity is not limited to the injured and surrounding areas (primary and secondary hyperalgesia), but may be generalized to the whole central nervous system. The extensive spread of referred pain is strongly suggestive for central hyperexcitability, possibly involving dis-inhibitory processes and expansion of receptive fields (Curatolo and Sterling 2011).

Augmented central nociceptive processing may occur anywhere along the neural pathways and the location of the hyperexcitability cannot be determined from these studies. Nevertheless, some studies have utilized the nociceptive withdrawal reflex to analyze spinal cord hyperexcitability. Patients with chronic WAD displayed lower reflex thresholds than healthy subjects (Banic et al. 2004; Sterling et al. 2008). These findings provide objective electrophysiological evidence for generalized spinal cord hyperexcitability. Sterling et al. (2008) addressed the question of the relationship between parameters of central hypersensitivity and psychological factors. While there was a weak correlation between catastrophizing and cold pain thresholds, spinal excitability as assessed by the nociceptive withdrawal reflex did not correlate significantly with either catastrophizing or psychological distress. A more recent investigation on 300 healthy volunteers found no impact of depression, anxiety and catastrophizing on the nociceptive withdrawal reflex, indicating that spinal cord excitability is little or not affected by descending psychological influences (Neziri et al. 2010).

The sensory disturbances observed in chronic WAD are in fact present from soon after injury. In the acute phase post injury, local cervical mechanical hyperalgesia (decreased pressure pain thresholds) is found in both individuals with lower and higher levels of pain and disability (Kasch et al. 2001; Sterling et al. 2004). This local hyperalgesia tends to resolve within a few months in individuals with good and fair recovery but persists unchanged in those who report ongoing moderate to severe symptom levels 6 months to 2–3 years post accident (Sterling et al. 2003b). In contrast to local hyperalgesia, which occurs in the acute stage irrespective of pain and disability levels, the presence of generalized hyperalgesia has been shown to be more apparent in those individuals reporting higher pain and disability (Sterling et al. 2004) and subsequent poor recovery (Sterling et al. 2003b). In addition to mechanical hyperalgesia, both cold and heat hyperalgesia are features in individuals with higher symptom levels and poor functional recovery (Sterling et al. 2003b). Most studies have explored the presence of positive sensory signs or sensory hypersensitivity. Recently, the presence of negative sensory responses or widespread hypoaesthesia (or elevated detection thresholds) occurring concurrently with hypersensitivity have also been found in patients with acute WAD (Chien et al. 2008). Similar to findings of sensory hypersensitivity, the hypoaesthetic changes were widespread and occurred in response to a variety of stimuli including vibration, thermal and electrical stimulation (Chien et al. 2008). Whilst they occurred in the majority of participants in the acute injury stage (3–4 weeks), the hypoaesthesia persisted only in those initially classified as at high risk of poor recovery (higher pain and disability and sensory hypersensitivity) (Chien et al. 2010). Considering these findings of both positive and negative sensory changes to various stimuli that are widespread and generalized throughout various body locations infers that disturbances in both excitatory and inhibitory central nervous system processes are at play.

Importantly, some of the sensory phenomena demonstrate capacity to predict individuals at risk of poor recovery. In particular, the early presence of cold hyperalgesia is emerging as a consistent prognostic factor for WAD. Initial studies demonstrated that in addition to initial moderate pain, decreased neck movement, older age and posttraumatic stress symptoms, cold hyperalgesia predicted higher levels of pain and disability at both 6 months and 2–3 years post injury (Sterling et al. 2005, 2006). Cold pain tolerance measured using the cold pressor test has also shown predictive capacity (Kasch et al. 2005). More recently it has been shown that when injured people are classified based on the presence of moderate or greater initial pain and sensory hypersensitivity, 86% of those deemed at high risk of poor recovery did indeed develop persistent symptoms at 6 months post injury (Chien et al. 2010). Further research using trajectory modelling has validated cold hyperalgesia as a predictor of a clinical pathway to chronic WAD (Sterling et al. 2009).

Whilst sensory hypersensitivity is thought to reflect augmented central pain processes, the precise underlying mechanisms are not clear. A recent prospective study investigating the nociceptive withdrawal reflex from acute to chronic WAD showed a different picture to what is seen for sensory hypersensitivity (Sterling 2010). Lowered reflex thresholds indicative of spinal cord hyperexcitability were found to be present at 3 weeks post injury in all whiplash subgroups irrespective of the extent of recovery. However by 6 months post injury, lowered reflex thresholds persisted only in those with moderate/severe symptoms having resolved in those who recovered or reported lesser symptoms at this time point. In contrast, generalized sensory hypersensitivity (pressure and cold) was only ever present in those with persistent moderate/severe symptoms and remained unchanged throughout the study period. This suggests different mechanisms underlie sensory hypersensitivity and NFR responses or at least that sensory hypersensitivity does not appear to be solely due to spinal processes.

In summary, current evidence would suggest that some central nervous system pain processes are augmented from soon after injury in those individuals who do not recover but go on to develop chronic moderate to severe pain and disability. The reasons as to why this group manifest more profound changes in pain processes is not clear but there are numerous possibilities including but not limited to: the nature, extent and duration of the original injury providing peripheral nociceptive input to the CNS (Rang et al. 1991), stress-related responses (McLean et al. 2005), psychological augmentation (Wand et al. 2010), poorer health prior to the injury (Wynne-Jones et al. 2006) or a genetic predisposition (Hocking et al. 2010). Irrespective of the cause of the changes, the data indicate that consideration of these processes in the early management of WAD will be required.

Stress System Responses

In addition to subjecting soft tissues to a biomechanical strain, an MVC event is also an acute stressor which activates physiological stress response systems (see also Stoney 2011). In recent times, models have been put forward that link stress system responses (McLean et al. 2005) and sympathetic nervous system activation (Passatore and Roatta 2006) and the various physiological changes seen in WAD including both sensory and motor manifestations.

There is some evidence available indicating autonomic disturbances are present in chronic WAD. Impaired peripheral vasoconstrictor responses have been demonstrated in both acute and chronic whiplash (Sterling et al. 2003a) but the relationship of these changes to the clinical presentation of whiplash or outcomes following injury are not clear. Gaab et al. (2005) showed reduced reactivity of the hypothalamic–pituitary adrenal axis, a closely interacting system to the autonomic system, in a small sample of participants with chronic WAD. Autonomic nervous system dysfunction has been found to be present in other painful musculoskeletal conditions such as chronic low back pain (Gockel et al. 2008), fibromyalgia (Martinez-Lavin 2007) and cervicobrachialgia (Greening et al. 2003). Individuals with posttraumatic stress disorder (PTSD) also show evidence of autonomic and HPA dysfunction (Ehlert et al. 2001) which may have some relevance for WAD where recently it was shown that a significant proportion of injured people also have symptoms of posttraumatic stress (Sterling et al. 2010).

One key component of the adrenergic system is the catechol O-methyltransferase (COMT) enzyme. COMT is the primary enzyme that degrades catecholamines, including adrenaline, noradrenaline and dopamine. Variants of the COMT gene have been associated with experimental pain sensitivity (Diatchenko et al. 2005) and with vulnerability to both chronic pain (Diatchenko et al. 2005) and anxiety disorders (Woo et al. 2002). McLean et al. (2011) recently showed that individuals with acute whiplash injury and with a COMT pain vulnerable genotype reported more severe neck pain, headache and dizziness as well as more dissociative symptoms in the immediate post-injury period in the emergency department. These individuals also estimated that they would take longer to recover both physically and emotionally (McLean et al. 2011). Whilst this study was cross-sectional in design and evaluated only patients with acute whiplash, its findings are interesting and if replicated in larger cohort studies could have important implications for the consideration of the development of chronic whiplash pain.

In summary, investigation of stress system responses and their role on both non-recovery and the clinical presentation of WAD is in its infancy. Nevertheless, due to the traumatic nature of its onset, this may be an important factor to be considered in this condition.

Psychological Features of Whiplash

The psychological presentation of whiplash can be as equally diverse as the physical presentation, with some individuals showing marked distress and others seeming resilient to the injury (Sterling et al. 2003c, 2010). Psychological factors such as high levels of pain catastrophizing (Sullivan et al. 2002), fear of movement (Vangronsveld et al. 2008), lower pain self-efficacy (Bunketorp-Kall et al. 2007) and distress (Carstensen et al. 2008) have been shown to associated with more pain and disability in acute WAD. Depressive symptoms are also a common feature of acute whiplash injury (Phillips et al. 2010) and may be associated with prior mental health problems and poorer general health (Phillips et al. 2010), as well as poor post-injury adjustment (Kivioja et al. 2004). The role of coping styles or strategies in either the prevention or development of WAD is unclear. Some data indicate that a palliative reaction (e.g., seeking palliative relief of symptoms such as distraction, smoking or drinking) was associated with longer symptom duration (Buitenhuis et al. 2003; Carroll et al. 2006). In contrast, Kivioja et al. (2005) found no evidence that different coping styles in the early stage of injury influenced the outcome at 1 year post accident. The different cohort inception times of these studies may account for differences in findings indicating that coping strategies may vary depending on the stage of the condition and this requires further investigation.

Different psychological factors may be involved in the aetiology and development of chronic whiplash pain when compared to other painful musculoskeletal conditions (Sterling et al. 2003c). For example, the role of fear of movement or kinesiophobia seems to be a less important factor in whiplash (Sterling et al. 2005) than in low back pain (Vlaeyen et al. 1995; see also May 2011). One possible explanation for the possible limited role of kinesiophobia in whiplash could be that anxiety-related factors play a more prominent role than in low back pain (Buitenhuis et al. 2011). Because neck pain starts or is attributed to an often stressful MVC, this distinguishes it from most cases of low back pain and could give rise to more or different forms of anxiety. The sudden, traumatic onset could also lead to stronger somatic beliefs and related fears regarding recovery (Buitenhuis et al. 2011).

The effect of the psychological stress surrounding the crash itself as opposed to or in addition to distress about neck pain complaints may have a significant influence on outcome. PTSD is a common sequelae of severe injuries following an MVC (Kuch et al. 1994). Yet, it is only recently that evidence has emerged that it may also play a role in less severe road accident injuries including whiplash. A recent prospective cohort study of 155 participants identified three distinct trajectories for posttraumatic stress measured using the Posttraumatic stress disorder Diagnostic Scale (PDS). These were: (1) Resilient: mild symptoms throughout the 12-month study period (40%), (2) Recovering: initial moderate symptoms declining to mild levels by 3 months (43%), and (3) Chronic moderate–severe: persistent moderate/severe symptoms throughout 12 months (17%) (Sterling et al. 2010). Furthermore, this study demonstrated that 22% of the cohort had a probable diagnosis of PTSD at 3 months post MVC with this figure dropping slightly to 17% by 12 months post injury (Sterling et al. 2010). This is the first study to demonstrate that the incidence of PTSD in WAD is similar to that identified for more serious traumatic motor vehicle injury, such as following hospital admission and traumatic brain injury (O'Donnell et al. 2003). It also showed that the persistent moderate/severe symptom trajectory was quadratic in shape indicating some symptom decrease before worsening over time. Some studies have shown an overall decline in PTSD symptoms over time whilst others have shown an increase in symptoms (O'Donnell et al. 2007). It is likely that individuals who follow this trajectory will require specific psychological interventions to prevent this course. However, such management approaches are often not provided to people with whiplash (Cote et al. 2005; Sterling et al. 2005). These findings indicate the need for additional psychological evaluation of these patients (Forbes et al. 2007) and clinicians should be aware of this factor in their assessment of whiplash-injured people.

Relationships and Interactions Between Biological and Psychological Factors

The presence of sensory hypersensitivity and psychological distress co-exist in individuals with whiplash, particularly those with moderate to severe symptoms (Sterling et al. 2005). For this reason some have argued that the sensory changes may reflect psychological factors and their associated influence on nociceptive processing (Wand et al. 2010). It would be worthwhile to have some idea of these relationships as this may provide information on how best to target or integrate different management approaches.

There does appear to be some relationship between psychological factors and sensory disturbance. Sterling et al. (2008) demonstrated moderate associations between pain thresholds (pressure and cold) at some sites, particularly at more remote sites such as in the lower limb, and both psychological distress (GHQ-28) and catastrophization (Pain Catastrophizing Scale – PCS) in individuals with chronic WAD. Similar results have been found in acute WAD, where cold pain threshold and catastrophization show moderate correlations (Rivest et al. 2010). Notably, there appears to be no relationship between psychological factors and the intensity of electrical stimulation required to elicit a flexor withdrawal response in biceps femoris neither in patients with chronic whiplash (Sterling et al. 2008) nor in healthy controls (Neziri et al. 2010). These findings indicate that psychological factors may play a role in central hyperexcitability. However, they do not support the assumption that psychological factors are the only or main factors responsible for central hyperexcitability in whiplash patients. In particular, spinal cord hyperexcitability appears not to be affected, at least significantly, by psychological factors.

The relationships between sensory changes and posttraumatic stress symptoms have also been explored. Sterling and Kenardy (2006) showed that the early presence of sensory hypersensitivity (mechanical and cold hyperalgesia) was associated with persistent posttraumatic stress symptoms but that this relationship was mediated by initial pain and disability levels (in this case, Neck Disability Index scores). These finding suggest that the link between sensory hypersensitivity and posttraumatic stress symptoms is influenced by the level of pain and disability. The relationships between sensory hypersensitivity, pain and disability and posttraumatic stress has been corroborated in a recent study. Using trajectory modelling analyses, distinct trajectories or clinical pathways for both pain and disability and posttraumatic stress were identified (Sterling et al. 2010). Interestingly, cold hyperalgesia (cold pain thresholds of less than 13°C) predicted membership to both more severe pain and disability trajectories and PTSD trajectories (Sterling et al. 2009). This suggests common mechanisms may underlie the development of chronic pain and PTSD symptoms following whiplash injury. Additionally, dual analyses revealed that the developmental trajectories of pain and disability and PTSD were mostly in synchrony (for additional studies on Chronic pain and disability, See also Gatchel et al. 2011). For example, individuals are more likely to show higher pain/disability and higher PTSD symptoms or low pain/disability and low PTSD symptoms rather than contradictory membership to say low pain/disability and high PTSD (Sterling et al. 2009). Together the findings of these studies suggest close relationships between reported pain/disability levels, posttraumatic stress symptoms and the sensory presentation of WAD and that all factors should be considered in the assessment and management of WAD.

Thus it appears that psychological factors such as distress, catastrophization and posttraumatic stress symptoms show some association with sensory hypersensitivity in chronic whiplash. However this relationship is not consistent for all modalities, measures or at all body sites tested and may be mediated by levels of pain and disability. This would suggest that psychological factors are not the only or main factors responsible for central hyperexcitability in whiplash patients. Central hyperexcitability after whiplash is therefore a complex phenomenon that probably involves both neurobiological changes as well as psychological factors.

There has been less investigation of relationships between motor dysfunction and psychological factors in WAD. Research and clinical practice in this area tends to view motor dysfunction as a physiological change with exercise being the optimal way to address such dysfunctions (Jull et al. 2008). However, some have proposed a relationship between stress responses (sympathetic activation) and motor changes following whiplash injury (Passatore and Roatta 2006), thus suggesting that interventions aimed at attenuating psychological responses may have an effect on the movement and motor function of the patient with WAD. Basic laboratory studies have shown that adrenaline exerts a weakening effect on slow twitch muscle fibres which has implications for the tonic capacity of postural type neck muscles (Roatta et al. 2008). Sympathetic activation also reduces the sensitivity of muscle spindles to muscle length changes, especially in jaw and neck muscles (Hellstrom et al. 2005) which implies that the quality of proprioceptive information on muscle length changes is reduced, which should negatively impact on feedback correction of movements and the ability of the motor system to correct perturbations.

Clinical research studies have also indicated relationships between psychological factors and motor function in WAD. A recent study used ecological monetary assessment methods via electronic diary monitoring and activity data from accelerometers to explore within-person relationships between physical and psychological factors. It was shown that trauma-related avoidance symptoms at one point during the day were associated with reduced activity later in the day but that the same relationship did not exist for fear of pain and activity (Sterling and Chadwick 2010). The promotion of activity is advocated for the management of WAD (TRACsa 2008) and thus it would seem important to identify processes associated with decreased activity that may be amenable to behavioural interventions.

Future Directions

The past 15 years in particular have seen a rapid growth in research and consequently knowledge of WAD. We now know that whiplash can be a remarkably complex condition in some individuals with disturbances in nociceptive processing, motor and postural control as well as psychological distress clearly evident. However, this improved understanding of the condition is yet to be translated to improved health outcomes for injured people or in a significant reduction in costs.

A recent Cochrane review of conservative management for WAD included 21 studies evaluating a broad variety of conservative treatment approaches for acute and sub-acute whiplash (Verhagen et al. 2007). Interventions were divided into passive (such as rest, immobilization, ultrasound, etc.) and active interventions (such as exercises, act as usual approach, etc.) and were compared with no treatment, a placebo or each other. Only eight studies were deemed to be of a high quality. The authors reported that data pooling was not possible due to clinical and statistical heterogeneity and that whilst individual studies demonstrated effectiveness of one treatment over another, the comparisons were varied and results inconsistent. Their conclusions were that the evidence neither supports nor refutes the effectiveness of either passive or active treatments to relieve the symptoms of WAD, Grades I or II (Verhagen et al. 2007).

On closer inspection of data from randomized controlled trials included in the above-mentioned reviews, despite a particular intervention for acute WAD showing efficacy, a significant proportion of injured people still go on to develop chronic pain and disability (Provinciali et al. 1996; Rosenfeld et al. 2000, 2003, 2006). For example in the study by Provinciali et al. (1996), approximately 18% of participants were worse or only reported minimal improvement following a multimodal treatment intervention. In the study by Rosenfeld et al. (2006), 48% of participants receiving an active exercise intervention still reported greater than low pain levels following the treatment intervention. Additionally, there is evidence available to indicate that the introduction of evidence-based clinical guidelines for the management of WAD (based on the promotion of activity as discussed above) did not improve either health outcomes for injured people or decrease costs (Rebbeck et al. 2006a). Thus, the current advocated approach is clearly not a panacea for whiplash.

The clinical picture is similar for chronic WAD. Two recent RCTs of different exercise approaches showed only modest effects on pain and disability (Jull et al. 2007; Stewart et al. 2007). The only intervention with clear evidence of efficacy is radio-frequency neurotomy, an invasive technique that can only be used on a highly select patient group who have clear zygapophyseal joint involvement (Lord et al. 1996b). Thus, this approach is also not the answer for all whiplash-injured people.

The emerging multifactorial nature of WAD also suggests that while the current guidelines may benefit some whiplash patients, they are likely to be inadequate for the management of those with a more complex condition including both marked physical impairment and psychological distress. More recent clinical guidelines have recognized this and have attempted to include recommendations for the identification of factors such as sensory disturbance and psychological distress, although they fall short of recommending what treatment should be provided to those with this clinical presentation (MAA 2007). The now greater understanding of the physical and psychological characteristics of the condition offers an opportunity to guide the future development of improved evidence-based management approaches in the acute/sub-acute stage of injury, with an eye towards the prevention of chronic WAD.

There also seems to be several obvious areas where trials of intervention are urgently required. The first of these would be the clear lack of trials investigating pharmacotherapy for whiplash at both the acute and chronic stages. There is now convincing evidence of augmented central nociceptive processing that is present soon after injury (Sterling et al. 2003b), persists in and predicts those individuals who have poor functional recovery (Sterling et al. 2005) and is associated with non-responsiveness to standard physical rehabilitation approaches (Jull et al. 2007). Other conditions showing similar phenomena, for example fibromyalgia(FMS), have undergone extensive investigation as to the effects of various pharmacotherapies to the extent that some medications are now approved by the USA FDA for use in this condition (Rao 2009; see also Velly et al. 2011).

There are also a far greater number of trials investigating pharmacotherapy for low back pain (Chou and Huffman 2007) (see also May 2011) than for whiplash. Furthermore, initially higher levels of pain and/or disability are the most consistent predictors of poor health outcomes following whiplash injury (Carroll et al. 2008; Kamper et al. 2008; Walton et al. 2009). Guidelines for acute pain management advocate the importance of early pain relief following injury (Macintyre et al. 2010) yet whiplash guidelines do not make this a priority of treatment as there are no high-quality trials available on which to base recommendations (MAA 2007; TRACsa 2008). In addition to pain, posttraumatic stress is also common in people with whiplash (Sterling et al. 2010). There is emerging evidence that administration of an opiate (Holbrook et al. 2010) and beta blockers (Strawn and Geracioti 2008) administered very soon after a traumatic injury can prevent the development of PTSD and these may also be novel approaches in the management of patients with acute whiplash and symptoms of posttraumatic stress. Thus trials of pharmacotherapy for whiplash should be a research priority.

There is now available a large volume of research on the psychological sequelae of whiplash injury. In contrast, there are few treatment trials of psychological interventions or combined psychological and physical management approaches for WAD. Again this is in contrast to the data available in other musculoskeletal conditions such as low back pain. Some whiplash studies have combined a cognitive behavioural type of approach delivered by a physiotherapist in conjunction with an exercise program (Soderlund and Lindberg 2001; Stewart et al. 2007) making it difficult to tease out the relative efficacy of both components. Few studies have investigated the effects of a psychological-based intervention delivered by a clinical psychologist. In view of recent findings of the presence of PTSD symptoms in some patients with whiplash (Buitenhuis et al. 2006; Sterling et al. 2010), it would seem important that future studies investigate the effectiveness of treatment that also target PTSD. Effective treatments, such as trauma-focused CBT, exist for the management of PTSD and preliminary data indicate that PTSD treatment may potentially have an effect not only on PTSD symptoms but also on pain and disability (Jenewein et al. 2009). This would also seem to be an area ripe for research where there is much supporting evidence on which to base a case for such trials.

Most clinical guidelines recommend the provision of education and advice as part of the management of WAD (MAA 2007; Moore et al. 2005; TRACsa 2008). Individual studies have investigated various educational approaches such as the provision of information pamphlets (Kongsted et al. 2008b) or educational videos (Oliveira et al. 2006) but when taken together in a systematic review, the results are disappointing in that there was moderate evidence of no difference on pain and disability for various forms of advice focusing on return to activity (Haines et al. 2009). Thus it would seem we are no closer to understanding the most effective education to provide to whiplash-injured people and the most effective way to deliver that advice. Since the provision of education and advice forms the mainstay of most management approaches albeit physical or psychological then it would seem a priority that further investigation of this area is required.

Most exercise approaches to both acute and chronic whiplash have delivered only modest effects (Jull et al. 2007; Rosenfeld et al. 2006; Stewart et al. 2007). Some studies have investigated approaches that whilst efficacious for non-traumatic neck pain, have provided disappointing results when translation to the whiplash condition is attempted (Jull et al. 2007). In this study, it was shown that those participants with higher levels of pain and disability and sensory hypersensitivity indicative of augmented central nociceptive processing responded poorly to an intensive 10-week program of specific exercise. It may be that more creative approaches to physical rehabilitation are required for whiplash, particularly for those with a more complex clinical presentation. The whiplash subgroup with sensory hypersensitivity also show sympathetic nervous system and motor disturbances (Sterling et al. 2003a, b) that are similar to features of complex regional pain syndrome type 1 (CRPS) (Rijn et al. 2007). Altered central representation of perceptual, motor and autonomic systems has been implicated as possible mechanisms underlying the pain of CRPS (Moseley 2006). Treatment approaches which broadly aim to restore altered cortical representation such as graded motor imagery and mirror visual feedback have been shown to decrease pain and disability associated with CRPS (Daly and Bialocerkowski 2009) and sensory discrimination training can also decrease pain and disability of CRPS (Moseley and Wiech 2009). The similarities of the manifestations of CRPS and complex whiplash suggest that investigation of such approaches is warranted.

Conclusions

As discussed in this chapter, there is growing evidence of both complex biological and psychological manifestations of WAD and these factors likely contribute to the significant chronicity rate and recalcitrance to treatment associated with this condition. It is becoming clear that a biobehavioural approach that considers all aspects of an individual's presentation will be necessary if gains are to be made in the management of this condition. There is still much work to be done, particularly in the development and testing of new and innovative intervention approaches.

References

Banic, B., Petersen-Felix, S., Andersen, O., Radanov, B., Villiger, P., Arendt-Nielsen, L., et al. (2004). Evidence for spinal cord hypersensitivity in chronic pain after whiplash injury and in fibromyalgia. *Pain, 107* (1–2), 7–15.

Blincoe, L., Seay, A., Zaloshnja, E., Miller, T., Romano, E., Luchter, S., et al. (2002). *Economic impact of motor vehicle crashes 2000.* Washington: Department of Transportation (US), National Highway Traffic Safety Administration (NHTSA).

Bogduk, N. (2002). Point of view. *Spine, 27*(17), 1940–1941.

Buitenhuis, J., DeJong, J., Jaspers, J., & Groothoff, J. (2006). Relationship between posttraumatic stress disorder symptoms and the course of whiplash complaints. *Journal of Psychosomatic Research, 61*(3), 681–689.

Buitenhuis, J., deJong, P., Jaspers, J., & Kenardy, J. (2011). Psychological aspects of whiplash associated disorders. In M. Sterling & J. Kenardy (Eds.), *Whiplash: Evidence-base for clinical practice.* Australia: Elsevier.

Buitenhuis, J., Spanjer, J., & Fidler, V. (2003). Recovery from acute whiplash – The role of coping styles. *Spine, 28*(9), 896–901.

Bunketorp-Kall, L., Andersson, G., & Asker, B. (2007). The impact of subacute whiplash-associated disorders on functional self-efficacy: A cohort study. *International Journal of Rehabilitation Research, 30*(3), 221–226.

Carroll, L., Cassidy, D., & Cote, P. (2006). The role of pain coping strategies in prognosis after whiplash injury: Passive coping predicts slowed recovery. *Pain, 124*(1–2), 18–26.

Carroll, L., Holm, L., Hogg-Johnson, S., Cote, P., Cassidy, D., Haldeman, S., et al. (2008). Course and prognostic factors for neck pain in Whiplash-Associated Disorders (WAD). Results of the bone and joint decade 2000–2010 task force on neck pain and its associated disorders. *Spine, 33*(42), 583–592.

Carstensen, T., Frostholm, L., Oernboel, E., Kongsted, A., Kasch, H., Jensen, T., et al. (2008). Post-trauma ratings of pre-collision pain and psychological distress predict poor outcome following acute whiplash trauma: A 12-month follow-up study. *Pain, 139*(2), 248–259.

Chien, A., Eliav, E., & Sterling, M. (2008). Hypoaesthesia occurs in acute whiplash irrespective of pain and disability levels and the presence of sensory hypersensitivity. *The Clinical Journal of Pain, 24*(9), 759–766.

Chien, A., Eliav, E., & Sterling, M. (2010). The development of sensory hypoaesthesia following whiplash injury. *The Clinical Journal of Pain, 26*, 722–728.

Chou, R., & Huffman, L. (2007). Medications for acute and chronic low back pain: A review of the evidence for an American Pain Society/American College of Physicians clinical practice guideline. *Annals of Internal Medicine, 147*(7), 505–514.

Chu, J., Eun, S., & Schwartz, J. (2005). Quantitative motor unit action potentials (QUAMP) in whiplash patients with neck and upper limb pain. *Electromyography and Clinical Neurophysiology, 45*(6), 323–328.

Cote, P., Hogg-Johnson, S., Cassidy, D., Carroll, L., Frank, J., & Bombardier, C. (2005). Initial patterns of clinical care and recovery from whiplash injuries. *Archives of Internal Medicine, 165*, 2257–2263.

Crowe, H. (1964). A new diagnostic sign in neck injuries. *California Medicine, 100*, 12–13.

Curatolo, M., & Sterling, M. (2011). Pain-processing mechanisms in whiplash associated disorders. In M. Sterling & J. Kenardy (Eds.), *Whiplash: Evidence-base for clinical practice.* Australia: Elsevier.

Daly, E., & Bialocerkowski, A. (2009). Does evidence support physiotherapy management of adult Complex Regional Pain Syndrome Type One? A systematic review. *European Journal of Pain, 13*(4), 339–353.

Diatchenko, L., Slade, G., Nackley, A., Bhalang, K., Sigurdsson, A., Belfer, I., et al. (2005). Genetic basis for individual variations in pain perception and the development of a chronic pain condition. *Human Molecular Genetics, 14*, 135–143.

Ehlert, U., Gaab, J., & Heinrichs, M. (2001). Psychoneuroendocrinological contributions to the etiology of depression, posttraumatic stress disorder, and stress-related bodily disorders: the role of the hypothalamus-pituitary-adrenal axis. *Biological Psychiatry, 57*, 141–152.

Elliott, J., Jull, G., Noteboom, T., Darnell, R., Galloway, G., & Gibbon, W. (2006). Fatty infiltration in the cervical extensor muscles in persistent whiplash associated disorders: An MRI analysis. *Spine, 31*(22), E847–E851.

Elliott, J., Jull, G., Sterling, M., Noteboom, T., Darnell, R., & Galloway, G. (2008). Fatty infiltrate in the cervical extensor muscles is not a feature of chronic insidious onset neck pain. *Clinical Radiology, 63*(6), 681–687.

Elliott, J., O'Leary, S., Sterling, M., Hendrikz, J., Pedler, A., & Jull, G. (2010). MRI findings of fatty infiltrate in the cervical flexors in chronic whiplash. *Spine, 35*(9), 948–954.

Elliott, J., et al. (2011). The temporal development of fatty infiltrates in the neck muscles following whiplash injury: an association with pain and posttraumatic stress. *Plos One, 6*(6), e21194.

Elliott, J., Sterling, M., Noteboom, T., Treleaven, J., Galloway, G., & Jull, G. (2009). The clinical presentation of chronic whiplash and the relationship to findings of MRI fatty infiltrates in the cervical extensor musculature: A preliminary investigation. *European Spine Journal, 18*(9), 1371–1378.

Falla, D., Jull, G., & Hodges, P. (2004). Neck pain patients demonstrate reduced EMG activity of the deep cervical flexor muscles during performance of the cranio-cervical flexion test. *Spine, 29*(19), 2108–2114.

Ferrari, R. (2001). Whiplash and symptom amplification. *Pain, 89*, 293–294.

Forbes, D., Creamer, M., Phelps, A., Bryant, R., McFarlane, A., Devilly, G., et al. (2007). Australian guidelines for the treatment of adults with acute stress disorder and posttraumatic stress disorder. *The Australian and New Zealand Journal of Psychiatry, 41*, 637–648.

Gaab, J., Baumann, S., Budnoik, A., Gmunder, H., Hottinger, N., & Ehlert, U. (2005). Reduced reactivity and ehnanced negative feedback sensitivity of the hypothalamus-pituitary-adrenal axis in chronic whiplash associated disorders. *Pain, 119*, 219–224.

Gatchel, R. J., Haggard, R., Thomas, C., & Howard, K. J. (2011). A biopsychosocial approach to understanding chronic pain and disability. In R. J. Moore (Ed.), *Handbook of pain and palliative care: Biobehavioral approaches for the life course*. New York: Springer.

Gockel, M., Lindholm, H., Niemisto, L., & Hurri, H. (2008). Perceived disability but not pain is connected with autonomic nervous system function among people with chronic low back pain. *Journal of Rehabilitation Medicine, 40*, 355–358.

Greening, J., Dilley, A., & Lynn, B. (2005). In vivo study of nerve movement and mechanosensitivity of the median nerve in whiplash and non-specific arm pain patients. *Pain, 115*(3), 248–253.

Greening, J., Lynn, B., & Leary, R. (2003). Sensory and autonomic function in the hands of patients with non-specific arm pain (NSAP) and asymptomatic office workers. *Pain, 104*, 275–281.

Haanpaa, M., Backonja, M., Bennett, M., Bouhassira, D., Cruccu, G., Hansson, P., et al. (2009). Assessment of neuropathic pain in primary care. *The American Journal of Medicine, 122*(10S), S13–S21.

Haines, T., Gross, A., Burnie, S., Goldsmith, C., & Perry, J. (2009). Patient education for neck pain with or without radiculopathy. *Cochrane Database of Systematic Reviews,* (4), CD005106.

Hellstrom, F., Roatta, S., Thunberg, J., Passatore, M., & Djupsjobacka, M. (2005). Responses of muscle spindles in feline dorsal neck muscles to electrical stimulation of the cervical sympathetic nerve. *Experimental Brain Research, 165*, 328–342.

Hildingsson, C., & Toolanen, G. (1990). Outcome after soft-tissue injury of the cervical spine: A prospective study of 93 car-accident victims. *Acta Orthopaedica Scandinavica, 61*(4), 357–359.

Hocking, L., Smith, B., Jones, G., Reid, D., Strachan, D., & Macfarlane, G. (2010). Genetic variation in the beta2-adrenergic receptor but not catecholamine-O-methyltransferase predisposes to chronic pain: Results from the 1958 British Birth Cohort Study. *Pain, 149*(1), 143–151.

Holbrook, T., Galarneau, M., Dye, J., Quinn, K., & Dougherty, A. (2010). Morphine use after combat injury in Iraq and post-traumatic stress disorder. *The New England Journal of Medicine, 362*(2), 110–117.

Holm, L., Carroll, L., Cassidy, D., Hogg-Johnson, S., Cote, P., Guzman, J., et al. (2008). The burden and determinants of neck pain in whiplash-associated disorders after traffic collisions. *Spine, 33*(4S), S52.

Ichihara, D., Okado, E., Chiba, K., Toyama, Y., Fujiwara, H., & Momoshima, S. (2009). Longitudinal magnetic resonance imaging study on whiplash injury patients: Minimum 10-year follow-up. *Journal of Orthopaedic Science, 14*(5), 602–610.

Ide, M., Ide, J., Yamaga, M., & Takagi, K. (2001). Symptoms and signs of irritation of the brachial plexus in whiplash injuries. *The Journal of Bone and Joint Surgery (Br), 83*, 226–229.

Jenewein, J., Wittmann, L., Moergeli, H., Creutzig, J., & Schnyder, U. (2009). Mutual influence of PTSD symptoms and chronic pain among injred accident survivors: A longitudinal study. *Journal of Traumatic Stress, 22*(6), 540–548.

Johansson, B. (2006). Whiplash injuries can be visible by functional magnetic resonance imaging. *Pain Research and Management, 11*(3), 197–199.

Joslin, C., Khan, S., & Bannister, G. (2004). Long-term disability after neck injury. A comparative study. *Journal of Bone and Joint Surgery, 86*(7), 1032–1034.

Jull, G. (2000). Deep cervical flexor muscle dysfunction in whiplash. *Journal of Musculoskeletal Pain, 8*(1/2), 143–154.

Jull, G., et al. (2002). *A randomised controlled trial of physiotherapy management for cervicogenic headache. Spine, 27*(17), 1835–1843.

Jull, G., Kristjansson, E., & Dall'Alba, P. (2004). Impairment in the cervical flexors: A comparison of whiplash and insidious onset neck pain patients. *Manual Therapy, 9*(2), 89–94.

Jull, G., Sterling, M., Falla, D., Treleaven, J., & O'Leary, S. (2008). *Whiplash, headache and neck pain: Research based directions for physical therapies*. Edinburgh: Elsevier.

Jull, G., Sterling, M., Kenardy, J., & Beller, E. (2007). Does the presence of sensory hypersensitivity influence outcomes of physical rehabilitation for chronic whiplash? – A preliminary RCT. *Pain, 129*(2), 28–34.

Kaale, B., Krakenes, J., Albrektsen, G., & Webster, K. (2005). WAD impairment rating: Neck Disability Index score according to severity of MRI findings of ligaments and membranes in the upper cervical spine. *Journal of Neurotrauma, 4*, 466–475.

Kamper, S., Rebbeck, T., Maher, C., McAuley, J., & Sterling, M. (2008). Course and prognostic factors of whiplash: A systematic review and meta-analysis. *Pain, 138*(3), 617–629.

Kasch, H., Qerama, E., Bach, F., & Jensen, T. (2005). Reduced cold pressor pain tolerance in non-recovered whiplash patients: A 1 year prospective study. *European Journal of Pain, 9*(5), 561–569.

Kasch, H., Stengaard-Pedersen, K., Arendt-Nielsen, L., & Staehelin Jensen, T. (2001). Pain thresholds and tenderness in neck and head following acute whiplash injury: A prospective study. *Cephalalgia, 21*, 189–197.

Kivioja, J., Jensen, I., & Lindgren, U. (2005). Early coping strategies do not influence the prognosis after whiplash injuries. *Injury, 36*, 935–940.

Kivioja, J., Sjalin, M., & Lindgren, U. (2004). Psychiatric morbidity in patients with chronic whiplash associated disorder. *Spine, 29*(11), 1235–1239.

Koelbaek-Johansen, M., Graven-Nielsen, T., Schou-Olesen, A., & Arendt-Nielsen, L. (1999). Muscular hyperalgesia and referred pain in chronic whiplash syndrome. *Pain, 83*, 229–234.

Kongsted, A., Leboeuf-Yde, C., Korsholm, L., & Bendix, T. (2008a). Are altered smooth pursuit eye movements related to chronic pain and disability following whiplash injuries? A prospective trial with one-year follow-up. *Clinical Rehabilitation, 22*, 469–479.

Kongsted, A., Qerama, E., Kasch, H., Bach, F., Korsholm, L., Jensen, T., et al. (2008b). Education of patients after whiplash injury: Is oral advice any better than a pamphlett? *Spine, 33*(22), E843–E848.

Krakenes, J., Kaale, B., Moen, G., Nordli, H., Gilhus, N., & Rorvik, J. (2002). MRI assessment of the alar ligaments in the late stage of whiplash injury – a study of structural abnormalities and observer agreement. *Neuroradiology, 44*(7), 617–624.

Krakenes, J., Kaale, B., Moen, G., Nordli, H., Gilhus, N., & Rorvik, J. (2003). MRI of the tectorial and posterior atlanto-occipital membranes in the late stage of whiplash injury. *Neuroradiology, 44*(6), 637–644.

Kuch, K., Cox, B., Evans, R., & Shulman, I. (1994). Phobias, panic and pain in 55 survivors of road vehicle accidents. *Journal of Anxiety Disorders, 8*(2), 181–187.

Lindstrom, R., Schomacher, J., Farina, D., Rechter, L., & Falla, D. (2011). Association between neck muscle coactivation, pain, and strength in women with neck pain. *Manual Therapy, 16*(1), 80–86.

Lord, S., Barnsley, L., Wallis, B., & Bogduk, N. (1996a). Chronic cervical zygapophysial joint pain after whiplash: A placebo-controlled prevalence study including commentary by Derby R Jr. *Spine, 21*(15), 1737–1745.

Lord, S., Barnsley, L., Wallis, B., McDonald, G., & Bogduk, N. (1996b). Percutaneous radiofrequency neurotomy for chronic cervical zygapophyseal joint pain. *The New England Journal of Medicine, 335*(23), 1721–1726.

MAA. (2007). *Guidelines for the management of whiplash associated disorders*. Sydney: Motor Accident Authority (NSW). www.maa.nsw.gov.au.

Macintyre, P., Scott, D., Schug, S., Visser, E., & Walker, S. (2010). *Acute pain management: Scientific evidence*. Melbourne: ANZVA & FPM.

MAIC. (2002). *Whiplash – Review of CTP Queensland data to 31 Dec 2001*. Brisbane: MAIC.

MAIC. (2009). *Annual report*. Brisbane.

Malleson, A. (2002). *Whiplash and other useful illnesses*. Quebec: McGill-Queen's University Press.

Martinez-Lavin, M. (2007). Stree, the stress response system, and fibromyalgia. *Arthritis Research & Therapy, 9*(4), 216–223.

May, S. (2011). Chronic low back pain. In R. J. Moore (Ed.), *Handbook of pain and palliative care: Biobehavioral approaches for the life course*. New York: Springer.

McLean, S., Clauw, D., Abelson, J., & Liberzon, I. (2005). The development of persistent pain and psychological morbidity after motor vehicle collision: Intergrating the potential rle of stress response systems into a biopsychosocial model. *Psychosomatic Medicine, 67*, 783–790.

McLean, S., Diatchenko, L., Lee, M., Swor, R., Domeier, R., Jones, J., et al. (2011). Catechol O-methyltransferase haplotype predicts immediate musculoskeletal neck pain and psychological symptoms after motor vehicle collision. *The Journal of Pain, 12*(1), 101–107.

Moog, M., Quintner, J., Hall, T., & Zusman, M. (2002). The late whiplash syndrome: A psychophysical study. *European Journal of Pain, 6*(4), 283–294.

Moore, A., Jackson, A., Jordan, J., Hammersley, S., Hill, J., Mercer, C., et al. (2005). *Clinical guidelines for the physiotherapy management of Whiplash associated disorder*. London: The Chartered Society of Physiotherapy.

Moseley, G. (2006). Graded motor imagery for pathologic pain: A randomized controlled trial. *Neurology, 67*, 2129–2134.

Moseley, G., & Wiech, K. (2009). The effect of tactile discrimination training is enhanced when patients watch the reflected image of their unaffected limb during training. *Pain, 144*(3), 314–319.

Nederhand, M., Hermens, H., Ijzerman, M., Turk, D., & Zilvold, G. (2002). Cervical muscle dysfunction in chronic whiplash associated disorder grade 2. The relevance of trauma. *Spine, 27*(10), 1056–1061.

Neziri, A., Andersen, O., Petersen-Felix, S., Radanov, B., Dichenson, A., Scaramozzino, P., et al. (2010). The nociceptive withdrawal reflex: Normative values of thresholds and reflex receptive fields. *European Journal of Pain, 14*(2), 134–141.

NSW, M. (1999). *Whiplash and the NSW motor accidents scheme. statistical information paper No. 7*. Sydney.

O'Donnell, M., Creamer, M., Bryant, R., Schnyder, U., & Shalev, A. (2003). Posttraumatic disorders following injury: An empirical and methodological review. *Clinical Psychology Review, 23*, 587–603.

O'Donnell, M., Elliott, P., Lau, W., & Creamer, M. (2007). PTSD symptom trajectories: From early to chronic response. *Behaviour Research and Therapy, 45*, 601–606.

Oliveira, A., Gevirtz, R., & Hubbard, R. (2006). A psycho-educational video used in the emergency department provides effective treatment for whiplash injuries. *Spine, 31*(15), 1652–1657.

Passatore, M., & Roatta, S. (2006). Influence of sympathetic nervous system on sensorimotor function: Whiplash associated disorders (WAD) as a model. *European Journal of Applied Physiology, 98*(5), 423–449.

Pfirrmann, C., Binkert, C., & Zanetti, M. (2001). MR morphology of alar ligaments and occipitoatlantoaxial joints: Study in 50 asymptomatic subjects. *Radiology, 218*, 133–137.

Phillips, L., Carroll, L., Cassidy, D., & Cote, P. (2010). Whiplash-associated disorders: Who gets depressed? Who stays depressed? *European Spine Journal, 19*(6), 945–956.

Provinciali, L., Baroni, M., Illuminati, L., & Ceravolo, M. (1996). Multimodal treatment to prevent the late whiplash syndrome. *Scandinavian Journal of Rehabilitation Medicine, 28*(2), 105–111.

Radanov, B., Sturzenegger, M., & Di Stefano, G. (1995). Long-term outcome after whiplash injury. A 2-year follow-up considering features of injury mechanism and somatic, radiologic, and psychological findings. *Medicine, 74*(5), 281–297.

Rang, H., Bevan, S., & Dray, A. (1991). Chemical activation of nociceptive peripheral neurones. *British Medical Bulletin, 47*, 534–548.

Rao, S. (2009). Current progress in the pharmacological therapy of fibromyalgia. *Expert Opinion on Investigational Drugs, 18*(10), 1479–1493.

Rebbeck, T., Maher, C., & Refshauge, K. (2006a). Evaluating two implementation strategies for whiplash guidelines in physiotherapy: A cluster randomised trial. *The Australian Journal of Physiotherapy, 52*(3), 165–174.

Rebbeck, T., Sindhausen, D., & Cameron, I. (2006b). A prospective cohort study of health outcomes following whiplash associated disorders in an Australian population. *Injury Prevention, 12*, 86–93.

Rijn, M., Marinus, J., Putter, H., & van Hilten, J. (2007). Onset and progression of dystonia in complex regional pain syndrome. *Pain, 130*, 287–293.

Rivest, K., Cote, J., Dumas, J.-P., Sterling, M., & deSerres, S. (2010). Relationships between pain thresholds, catastrophizing and gender in acute whiplash injury. *Manual Therapy, 15*, 154–159.

Roatta, S., Arendt-Nielsen, L., & Farina, D. (2008). Sympathetic-induced changes in discharge rate and spike-triggered average twitch torque of low-threshold motor units in humans. *The Journal of Physiology, 586*, 5561–5574.

Ronnen, J., de Korte, P., & Brink, P. (1996). Acute whiplash injury: Is there a role for MR imaging. *Radiology, 201*, 93–96.

Rosenfeld, M., Gunnarsson, R., & Borenstein, P. (2000). Early intervention in whiplash-associated disorders. A comparison of two protocols. *Spine, 25*, 1782–1787.

Rosenfeld, M., Seferiadis, A., Carllson, J., & Gunnarsson, R. (2003). Active intervention in patients with whiplash associated disorders improves long-term prognosis: A randomised controlled clinical trial. *Spine, 28*(22), 2491–2498.

Rosenfeld, M., Seferiadis, A., & Gunnarsson, R. (2006). Active involvement and intervention in patients exposed to whiplash trauma in automobile crashes reduces costs. *Spine, 31*(16), 1799–1804.

Roy, S., Hol, P., & Laerum, L. (2004). Pitfalls of magnetic resonance imaging of alar ligament. *Neuroradiology, 46*, 392–398.

Sheather-Reid, R., & Cohen, M. (1998). Psychophysical evidence for a neuropathic component of chronic neck pain. *Pain, 75*, 341–347.

Sizer, P., Poorbaugh, K., & Phelps, V. (2004). Whiplash associated disorders: Pathomechanics, diagnosis and management. *Pain Practice, 4*(3), 249–266.

Soderlund, A., & Lindberg, P. (2001). Cognit ive behavioural components in physiotherapy management of chronic whiplash associated disorders (WAD) – A randomised group study. *Physiotherapy Theory and Practice, 17,* 229–238.

Steinberg, E., Ovadia, D., Nissan, M., Menahem, A., & Dekel, S. (2005). Whiplash injury: Is there a role for electromyographic studies. *Archives of Orthopaedic and Trauma Surgery, 125*(1), 46–50.

Sterling, M. (2010). Differential development of sensory hypersensitity and spinal cord hyperexcitability following whiplash injury. *Pain, 150*(3), 501–506.

Sterling, M., & Chadwick, B. (2010). Psychological processes in daily life with chronic Whiplash: Relations of posttraumatic stress symptoms and fear-of-pain to hourly pain and uptime. *The Clinical Journal of Pain, 26*(7), 573–582.

Sterling, M., Hendrikz, J., & Kenardy, J. (2009). Developmental trajectories of pain and disability and posttraumatic stress symptoms following whiplash injury. In *Paper presented at the Australian Spine society annual meeting,* Brisbane.

Sterling, M., Hendrikz, J., & Kenardy, J. (2010). Developmental trajectories of pain/disability and PTSD symptoms following whiplash injury. *Pain, 150*(1), 22–28.

Sterling, M., Jull, G., & Kenardy, J. (2006). Physical and psychological predictors of outcome following whiplash injury maintain predictive capacity at long term follow-up. *Pain, 122,* 102–108.

Sterling, M., Jull, G., Vicenzino, B., & Kenardy, J. (2003a). Sensory hypersensitivity occurs soon after whiplash injury and is associated with poor recovery. *Pain, 104,* 509–517.

Sterling, M., Jull, G., Vicenzino, B., & Kenardy, J. (2004). Characterisation of acute whiplash associated disorders. *Spine, 29*(2), 182–188.

Sterling, M., Jull, G., Vicenzino, B., Kenardy, J., & Darnell, R. (2005). Physical and psychological factors predict outcome following whiplash injury. *Pain, 114,* 141–148.

Sterling, M., Jull, G., Vizenzino, B., Kenardy, J., & Darnell, R. (2003b). Development of motor system dysfunction following whiplash injury. *Pain, 103,* 65–73.

Sterling, M., & Kenardy, J. (2006). The relationship between sensory and sympathetic nervous system changes and acute posttraumatic stress following whiplash injury – a prospective study. *Journal of Psychosomatic Research, 60,* 387–393.

Sterling, M., Kenardy, J., Jull, G., & Vicenzino, B. (2003c). The development of psychological changes following whiplash injury. *Pain, 106*(3), 481–489.

Sterling, M., Pettiford, C., Hodkinson, E., & Curatolo, M. (2008). Psychological factors are related to some sensory pain thresholds but not nociceptive flexion reflex threshold in chronic whiplash. *The Clinical Journal of Pain, 24*(2), 124–130.

Sterling, M., Treleaven, J., Edwards, S., & Jull, G. (2002a). Pressure pain thresholds in chronic whiplash associated disorder: Further evidence of altered central pain processing. *Journal of Musculoskeletal Pain, 10*(3), 69–81.

Sterling, M., Treleaven, J., & Jull, G. (2002b). Responses to a clinical test of mechanical provocation of nerve tissue in whiplash associated disorders. *Manual Therapy, 7*(2), 89–94.

Sterner, Y., & Gerdle, B. (2004). Acute and chronic whiplash disorders – A review. *Journal of Rehabilitation Medicine, 2004*(36), 193–210.

Stewart, M., Maher, C., Refshauge, K., Herbert, R., Bogduk, N., & Nicholas, M. (2007). Randomised controlled trial of exercise for chronic whiplash associated disorders. *Pain, 128*(1–2), 59–68.

Stoney, C. (2011). Stress and pain. In R. J. Moore (Ed.), *Handbook of pain and palliative care: Biobehavioral approaches for the life course.* New York: Springer.

Stovner, L. (1996). The nosologic status of the whiplash syndrome: A critical review based on a methadological approach. *Spine, 21*(23), 2735–2746.

Strawn, J., & Geracioti, T. (2008). Noradrenergic dysfunction and the psychopharmacology of posttraumatic stress disorder. *Depression and Anxiety, 25*(3), 260–271.

Sullivan, M., Stanish, W., Sullivan, M., & Tripp, D. (2002). Differential predictors of pain and disability in patients with whiplash injury. *Pain Research and Management, 7*(2), 68–74.

Taylor, J., & Taylor, M. (1996). Cervical spinal injuries: An autopsy study of 109 blunt injuries. *Journal of Musculoskeletal Pain, 4*(4), 61–79.

TRACsa. (2008). *A clinical pathway for best practice management of acute and chronic whiplash-associated disorders.* Adelaide: South Australian Centre for Trauma and Injury Recovery.

Treleaven, J., Jull, G., & Low Choy, N. (2005a). Standing balance in persistent whiplash: A comparison between subjects with and without dizziness. *Journal of Rehabilitation Medicine, 37,* 224–229.

Treleaven, J., Jull, G., & LowChoy, N. (2005b). Smooth pursuit neck torsion test in whiplash associated disorders: Relationship to self-eports of neck pain and disability, dizziness and anxiety. *Journal of Rehabilitation Medicine, 37,* 219–223.

Treleaven, J., Jull, G., & Sterling, M. (2003). Dizziness and unsteadiness following whiplash injury – Characteristic features and relationship with cervical joint position error. *Journal of Rehabilitation, 34,* 1–8.

Trotter, K. (2009). *It's only whiplash. Aren't you over it yet,* ISBN: 1451534647.

Uhrenholt, L., Grunnet-Nilsson, N., & Hartvigsen, J. (2002). Cervical spine lesions after road traffic accidents. A systematic review. *Spine, 27*(17), 1934–1941.

Vangronsveld, K., Peters, M., Goosens, M., & Vlaeyen, J. (2008). The influence of fear of movement and pain catastrophizing on daily pain and disability in individuals with acute whiplash injury: A daily diary study. *Pain, 139*(2), 449–457.

Velly, A. M., Chen, H., Ferreira, J. R., & Friction, J. R. (2011). Temporomandibular disorders and fibromyalgia. In R. J. Moore (Ed.), *Handbook of pain and palliative care: Biobehavioral approaches for the life course*. New York: Springer.

Verhagen, A., Scholten-Peeters, G., van Wijngaarden, S., de Bie, R., & Bierma-Zeinstra, S. (2007). Conservative treatments for whiplash. *Cochrane Database of Systematic Reviews*, (2), CD003338.

Vlaeyen, J., Kole-Snijders, A., & Boeren, R. (1995). Fear of movement/reinjury in chronic low back pain patients and its relation to behavioural performance. *Pain, 1995*(62), 363–372.

Walton, D., Pretty, J., MacDermid, J., & Teasell, R. (2009). Risk factors for persistent problems following whiplash injury: Results of a systematic review and meta-analysis. *Journal of Orthopaedic & Sports Physical Therapy, 39*(5), 334–350.

Wand, B., O'Connell, N., & Parkitny, L. (2010). Letter to the Editor: Depression may contribute to the sensory changes in whiplash patients? *Manual Therapy, 15*(3): p. E1.

Woo, J., Yoon, K., & Yu, B. (2002). Catechol *O*-methyltransferase genetic polymorphism in panic disorder. *The American Journal of Psychiatry, 159*, 1785–1787.

Woodhouse, A., & Vasseljen, O. (2008). Altered motor control patterns in whiplash and chronic neck pain. *BMC Musculoskeletal Disorders, 9*, 90.

Wynne-Jones, G., Jones, G., Wiles, N., Silman, A., & Macfarlane, G. (2006). Predicting new onset of widespread pain following a motor vehicle collision. *Journal of Rheumatology, 33*, 968–974.

Yoganandan, N., Knowles, S., Maiman, D., & Pintar, F. (2003). Anatomic study of the morphology of the human cervical facet joint. *Spine, 28*, 2317–2323.

Yoganandan, N., Pintar, F., & Cusick, J. (2002). Biomechanical analyses of whiplash injuries using an experimental model. *Accident Analysis and Prevention, 34*, 663–671.

Chapter 16
Chronic Low Back Pain

Stephen May

Introduction

Chronic low back pain (CLBP) is a common problem in the general population and in those seeking healthcare. Though different definitions have been used in the past, in general it refers to back pain that has persisted for 3 months or more. The numbers of the adult population who experience back pain in any year or over their lifetime are considerable. The proportion with chronic or persistent symptoms is much larger than has been thought in the past; though many of those with persistent symptoms are not particularly disabled and are functioning reasonably normally. Furthermore many who do recover from an acute episode of back pain will have a recurrence in the following year; so for many the experience of back pain is persistent or episodic. Many individuals with back pain do not seek healthcare, but because the problem is so prevalent in the general population the numbers who do seek care are enormous, and one of the chief reasons that patients consult physicians. Again because the numbers are so large this makes back pain one of the costliest health problems for direct and indirect costs.

It is generally recognised that making a structural diagnosis for back pain from the clinical presentation in the majority of individuals is not possible; though this is possible with specialist injection-based technology. Because of this the term nonspecific low back pain has come to be widely used for the majority of people with back pain. Neurophysiological and psychosocial issues have been highlighted as being associated with chronic pain, but these appear not to be relevant to the majority of those with CLBP. But from the epidemiological evidence and the evidence relating to barriers for recovery for this group it is clear that those with CLBP are a difficult group for whom to seek effective management.

There are numerous potential treatments for those who do seek care. Some guidelines exist for this group, and there are also numerous systematic reviews that have been published evaluating the efficacy treatments that might be used. Exercises and talking therapies are probably the most commonly recommended interventions by guidelines and are supported by most systematic reviews. However, self-management commonly occurs in this group. This chapter will explore these issues in more detail that are relevant to an understanding of CLBP; and in particular explore the impact, characteristics and management options for those with CLBP.

S. May, MD (✉)
Sheffield Hallam University, Collegiate Crescent Campus, Sheffield, UK S10 2BP
e-mail: s.may@shu.ac.uk

R.J. Moore (ed.), *Handbook of Pain and Palliative Care: Biobehavioral Approaches for the Life Course*, 231
DOI 10.1007/978-1-4419-1651-8_16, © Springer Science+Business Media, LLC 2012

The Size of the Problem

Back pain is an extremely common symptom, which affects sizeable proportions of both the adolescent and adult population. At some point in their life between a half and three-quarters of all adults will experience back pain. About 40% of adults will have an episode of back pain in any 1 year, and about 15–20% of the adult population are experiencing back pain at any one point in time (Croft et al. 1997; Cassidy et al. 1998; Hillman et al. 1996; Leboeuf-Yde et al. 1996; Linton et al. 1998; McKinnon et al. 1997; Waxman et al. 2000; Hoy et al. 2010). The figures are similar from European, North American and low and middle-income countries (Hoy et al. 2010).

It used to be commonly stated that the CLBP population was relatively small, representing only about 7–8% of the back pain population; and that for the majority of those with back pain the prognosis was good (Waddell 1987, 1994; Evans and Richards 1996). However, modern epidemiological studies have demonstrated that the natural history of low back pain is not so optimistic. Croft et al. (1998) tracked 463 patients who attended their GP with recent onset back pain; they found the majority attended the GP only once; about a third attended the GP again within 3 months, and only 8% saw the GP on multiple occasions for the back pain in the following year. They also monitored symptoms and both at 3 months and at 1 year about 70–80% of the cohort reported back pain with or without disability. Clearly attendance at the GP is not a proxy measure of symptom duration. Furthermore, between 3 months and 1 year there was little improvement in the numbers still reporting symptoms. This study suggests that the CLBP population is much larger than was previously thought.

Several aspects of this study have been replicated in numerous other epidemiological cohorts with a 1-year follow-up. The development of chronic symptoms has been reported in 36–48% of different cohorts (Linton et al. 1998; Hillman et al. 1996; Waxman et al. 2000; Szpalski et al. 1995; Thomas et al. 1999). Furthermore similarly to the study by Croft et al. (1998) additional studies have also found that while natural history is good up until 3 months, with decreasing prevalence rates, at around 3 months this plateaus out and prevalence rates at 3 months and 1 year are very similar (Klenerman et al. 1995; Thomas et al. 1999). These studies have recruited participants in primary care, but also from the general population; the findings were very similar. It is clear from these studies then that about 40–50% of the back pain population develop persistent or chronic back pain.

Furthermore, the recurrence rate in those who do recover is substantial. Another episode was reported by between 55 and 76% in a number of cohorts in the follow-up year (Linton et al. 1998; Brown et al. 1998; Torrptsova et al. 1995; Klenerman et al. 1995). The strongest known risk factor for developing back pain is a history of a previous episode (Croft et al. 1997; Smedley et al. 1997; Shekelle 1997). Put differently: "Low back pain should be viewed as a chronic problem with an untidy pattern of grumbling symptoms and periods of relative freedom from pain and disability interspersed with acute episodes, exacerbations, and recurrences" (Croft et al. 1998).

Several systematic reviews on the natural history of back pain have reinforced a similar message, that about 40–50% of individuals with acute back pain will still have symptoms at 3 months, after which there is little further improvement, and about 60–70% of those who "recover" from an episode have another episode in the following year (Abbott and Mercer 2002; Pengel et al. 2003; Hestbaek et al. 2003). Because back pain is rarely fatal, unlike cancer or cardiovascular problems, it is often seen as a relatively trivial health problem (Hoy et al. 2010). However the global burden of back pain has been estimated to be 2.5 million Disability-Adjusted Life Years, which is a summary measure that quantifies affects of mortality and morbidity against an ideal picture in which the population is free of disease. CLBP represents 0.09% of the overall burden of disease in the world (Hoy et al. 2010).

Healthcare for Low Back Pain

Thus the epidemiology of back pain demonstrates it is an extremely common problem in the general population, and therefore a common cause for visiting healthcare professionals. In fact not everyone with back pain sees a physician, chiropractor, osteopath, physical therapist, or other healthcare professional. However, because it is such a widespread problem the numbers who attend for this problem are vast, making it one of the most common reasons for visiting the general practitioner. In fact it has been found that only about 40% of those with back pain in the general population actually seek care because of it (Dodd et al. 1997; Walsh et al. 1992; McKinnon et al. 1997; Santos-Eggimann et al. 2000). Waddell (1994) estimated that of 16.5 million people who had back pain in the UK in 1993, 18–42% consulted their GP, 10% attended a hospital outpatient department, 6% were seen by physical therapists in the NHS, and another 8% by private therapists, with only 0.14% going to surgery. Obviously the exact distribution will vary between countries, and it is known that surgery rates in the USA were five times the UK rate (Cherkin et al. 1994). But because the numbers in the general population who have low back pain are so large the healthcare costs are enormous.

Although many individuals with CLBP do not seek healthcare those with longer duration pain, higher intensity of pain, higher levels of functional disability and psychological affects tend to be more likely to seek healthcare (Hillman et al. 1996; Blyth et al. 2005; Jzelenberg and Burdoff 2004; Lim et al. 2006; Walker et al. 2004). These are all factors that are associated with a poor prognosis. In effect what this means is that those who do seek care are, by their very nature, likely be patients who will be resistant to improvement and difficult to treat.

Direct healthcare costs for low back pain in the UK were estimated at £1,632 million (Maniadakis and Gray 2000); and in the USA at between $8 and 18 billion (Shekelle et al. 1995). However, most estimates suggest that the medical costs of back pain are considerably smaller than the indirect, societal costs related to compensation, workplace losses or informal care. Total societal costs in the USA have been estimated at $75–100 billion (Frymoyer and Cats-Baril 1991), and at £5–10 billion in the UK (Maniadakis and Gray 2000). These costs have risen in the last 2 decades, with the increase in high technology imaging, such as magnetic resonance imaging, and high technology interventions, such as surgery. These increases have been most marked in the USA, but it appears that more interventions of these types have not resulted in better outcomes, in terms of less disability (Deyo et al. 2009). In fact it has been calculated that back pain is more costly than any other disease for which an economic analysis is available. Back pain is more costly than coronary heart disease, and more costly than the combined costs of rheumatoid arthritis, respiratory infections, Alzheimer's disease, stroke, diabetes, arthritis, multiple sclerosis, thrombosis and embolism, depression, diabetes, ischaemia and epilepsy (Maniadakis and Gray 2000). A minority of patients consume the majority of these costs, with those at the chronic and more disabled end of the spectrum associated with considerably higher costs (Wenig et al. 2009). In other words, about 15% of the back pain population account for about 70% of total costs (Webster and Snook 1994; Williams et al. 1998; Linton et al. 1998).

To summarise, it is clear from a number of epidemiological studies conducted in the general population and in those in healthcare that the numbers with CLBP are much greater than initially thought. The prevalence of CLBP used to be put at around 7–8% of the back pain population, but numerous studies have now made clear that the prevalence rate of those with persistent back pain is more in the region of 40–50%. Furthermore for those who do recover quickly recurrence is extremely common, affecting about 40% of the back pain population. Moreover, even though not everyone seeks care, because of the high numbers experiencing pain in the general population back pain impacts heavily on direct and indirect healthcare and societal costs.

What Causes Low Back Pain?

There are two positions about the source of low back pain. The term "nonspecific low back pain" has been in use for several decades, which indicates lack of diagnostic clarity about the true source of symptoms. However, some argue that a specific source of symptoms can be determined in the majority using intra-articular injections (Bogduk et al. 1996). Furthermore, the invasive nature of these procedures, the stringent methodologies required, their availability and the high levels of technical requirements make this treatment unsuitable for the majority of patients. For several decades the term "nonspecific low back pain" has been in circulation; a term which highlights the difficulty of determining the exact patho-anatomical source of these symptoms (Spitzer et al. 1987; CSAG 1994; Bigos et al. 1994). From a clinical perspective, identifying specific sources of back pain has generally not been proven. Furthermore, what has not been demonstrated is a link between specific diagnoses and the optimal treatment for that specific diagnosis. So to date the value of making specific diagnoses on the whole has not been demonstrated.

It should be emphasised that this discussion does not relate to serious spinal pathologies, such as cancer, infection, fractures or cauda equina syndrome, which are recognised through so-called "red flag" features during the history taking. These conditions are rare, perhaps no more than 1–2% of the back pain population (McGuirk et al. 2001), but need to be ruled out from usual care, and generally require urgent onward referral to a specialist. Also excluded from the nonspecific back pain population are those with radicular pain or sciatica. These patients are recognised by the distribution of referred symptoms, and accompanying neurological changes and dural signs. These patients may benefit from conservative care, but some will not and surgery maybe a consideration for some of this group.

However, alternative ways to classify the back pain population have been suggested that are based on clinical presentations. Numerous classification systems now exist, and it is not the task of this chapter to describe them; a systematic review listed 32 classification systems for back pain (McCarthy et al. 2004), and several more have been developed since then. The most commonly used classification systems are based on symptom responses to exercises or movements. Many of these classification systems use exercises to induce symptom changes in patients. The most scientifically evaluated of these is the clinical phenomenon of centralisation, which is the abolition of distal symptoms in response to repeated movements, followed by the abolition of any remaining back pain (McKenzie and May 2003). An associated phenomenon is that of directional preference exercises. This is the use of repeated exercises, such as extension or flexion exercises, to induce centralisation or a decrease and improvement in symptoms or recovery of lost movement (McKenzie and May 2003). Although the same terms are not necessarily used, numerous classification systems use a similar response to movements or positions to determine management strategies in patients with back pain.

In a systematic review, centralisation was found to be present in 52% of 325 patients with CLBP (Aina et al. 2004). The clinical response was associated with good outcomes in both the short and long term (Aina et al. 2004); and this positive prognostic indicator was confirmed in another recent systematic review (Chorti et al. 2009). In a randomised controlled trial in which 312 patients were assessed for directional preference at baseline for inclusion in the trial, 74% were determined to have a positive response to one direction of movement (Long et al. 2004). They were then randomised to receiving their directional preference exercises, opposite exercises, or nonspecific exercises. The 2-week outcome demonstrated significantly better results for the directional preference exercise group over the alternate interventions for all outcomes. The short-term outcome was necessary as the ethical review board who approved the study wanted the patients who were worse or no better at 2 weeks to be offered the chance to cross-over to receive directional preference exercises (Long et al. 2008). When this happened minimal and clinically unimportant changes turned into statistically significant outcomes across all measures. The patients in this trial had a range of acute to chronic problems, but 53% were chronic. In a secondary analysis of the directional preference subgroup patients with chronic symptoms still reported significant improvements, though significantly less than patients with acute symptoms (Long et al. 2007). In other words, there are a substantial proportion of those with CLBP who will respond well to directional preference exercises.

Biopsychosocial Concept of Low Back Pain

Alongside the vagaries of diagnosis it has come to be recognised that some patients' pain drivers do not relate to specific pathology, but rather are related to neurophysiological, psychological or social issues. The term central sensitisation relates to changes that may occur in the pain processing mechanism within the central nervous system that might lead to reduced pain thresholds, increased response to afferent input, heightened responses to stimuli and spontaneous generation of nociceptive activity (Johnson 1997; Siddall and Cousins 1997; Cousins 1994). The net result of this is that pain may be generated without any source of symptoms in the structures of the back itself, but due to a fault within the central nervous system.

An additional potential driver of chronic pain and disability comes from so-called "yellow flags". These are psychological factors that have been shown to be risk factors for the development of chronic pain (Linton 2000). Issues highlighted as relevant here have been depression, anxiety, passive coping strategies, catastrophising about symptoms, somatisation, fearful of movement and activity (termed fear-avoidance), low levels of self-efficacy, and a more externalised health locus of control (Linton 2000; see also Donovan et al. 2011). The common theme with these responses to pain is inappropriate beliefs and behaviours to the presence of pain. These inappropriate responses can escalate into chronic disability, physical deconditioning, and social disengagement (Bortz 1984; Waddell and Main 1998) (see also Gatchel et al. 2011).

Besides "yellow flags", which are unhelpful thoughts, feeling or behaviours, other work-related and social factors have been proposed as potential barriers to recovery. "Blue flags" relate to work-related factors that might interfere with a return to normal function and role activity. These are such issues as the following: high physical job demand, low expectation of return to work, low job satisfaction, low social support, and perception of stress at work. "Black flags" relate to contextual or social issues, such as misunderstanding between key players, compensation problems, social isolation, process delays, and unhelpful policies (Kendall et al. 2009). "Orange flags" have recently been proposed as significant psychological problems, not simply inappropriate beliefs, which mean that the back pain is not the clinical problem of most importance (Main et al. 2005).

There is quite strong evidence to verify the role of all these issues in the development and maintenance of chronic back pain, especially in the development of chronic symptoms and chronic disability; with more limited evidence to suggest that these factors might have a role in the development of symptoms initially (Linton 2000). What has not been fully explored is the epidemiology of these issues; as made clear earlier the prevalence rate of CLP in the general population is far larger than those who seek care. The data discussed previously would suggest that these barriers to recovery are relevant only in a relative minority of this population.

Several ways of exploring this question, which this paragraph will do, would suggest that these barriers to recovery are not relevant to the majority of individuals with CLBP. In 94 CLBP patients questioned about the effect of back pain on their function only 8% indicated interruption of normal activities due to the pain (McGorry et al. 2000). Waddell (1994) estimated that of 16.5 million people in the United Kingdom who had low back pain the preceding year only 18–42% actually attended their primary care physician, with much smaller numbers seeing other health professionals.

Similar proportions of the low back pain population who seek care have been found in more recent studies (Dodd et al. 1997; Hillman et al. 1996). Another perspective on this issue is in the way people categorise their level of disability with CLBP. Although 10–35% of individuals within these studies have categorised themselves with high levels of disability; 60–70% rated their disability as low whether they had low or high intensity of pain (von Korff et al. 1992; Klapow et al. 1993; Cassidy et al. 1998). In an Australian population-based survey of over 2,000 adults the point, annual and lifetime prevalence was reported as 26, 68 and 79% respectively (Walker et al. 2004). Of those reporting symptoms in the last 6 months again the majority reported low-intensity/low disability (43%), compared to high intensity/low disability (11%), or high disability (10.5%). StarT Back is a screening tool for trying to discern the risk of chronic disability in patients with low back pain. In their initial work to validate the tool Hill et al. (2008, 2010) found again a minority (25%) were at high risk of developing chronic disability, whereas the majority were at low (40%) or moderate risk (35%) of chronic disability.

These different ways of looking at the same issue about the extent of disability and chronic pain syndrome characteristics amongst those with long-lasting back pain would suggest that actually the majority of individuals with these problems do not have the neurophysiological or psychosocial barriers identified earlier. Many individuals with long-lasting back pain are functioning and working normally, are not generally seeking healthcare, are in fact self-managing, and are not burdened with changes to their central nervous system or excessive psychosocial problems. Therefore, to characterise and label everyone with chronic pain simply because of the persistence of their symptoms is clearly not warranted. For those patients who do seek care, all patients with CLBP should be assessed in the normal way, as if they might respond to normal conservative care. As suggested earlier passive types of coping strategies appear to make patients more likely to develop chronic pain and disability. This would indicate that active, patient-centred management strategies are most relevant in their effective care.

What Are Effective Treatments for Chronic Low Back Pain?

The treatment options for patients and clinicians for CLBP are overwhelming. One review on the topic identified 60 pharmaceutical products, 100 named techniques in chiropractic, physical therapy, osteopathy and massage therapies, 20 different exercise programmes, 26 different passive physical modalities, 9 educational and psychological approaches, and 20 different injection therapies (Haldeman and Dagenais 2008). On top of these are an array of invasive surgical approaches, lifestyle products, such as braces, beds, and ergonomic aides, and also a variety of complementary and alternative medical approaches. This is a simplified partial inventory of treatment options, but with over 200 possible treatment options, and over 20 clinician types that could be considered when seeking treatment for CLBP, the choice is potentially bewildering. Most guidelines and systematic reviews, as seen below, do not support a myriad of treatment options, but rather a limited range of interventions that might potentially be effective.

Because of the prevalence and impact of CLBP it has been suggested that this has spawned a rapidly expanding range of tests and treatments, which have not been adequately evaluated and has lead to use of poorly validated tools, with uncertain efficacy and safety, and increasing complication rates and marketing abuses (Deyo et al. 2009). In the USA between 1994 and 2004 use of lumbar spine MR imaging and lumbar epidural injection rates quadrupled, opioid prescription doubled, and fusion rates for degenerative spine conditions went up nearly five times (Deyo et al. 2009). Yet MRI in seven randomised controlled trials was not associated with an advantage in subsequent outcomes, the efficacy of spinal injections is limited, opioid use may paradoxically increase sensitivity to pain, and higher spine surgery rates may be associated with worse outcomes (Deyo et al. 2009).

Obviously this increase in healthcare input and therefore expense might be justified if improved outcomes, in terms of patient pain and function levels were improved. But this review highlighted the fact that during this rise in tests and treatments work disability attributed to musculoskeletal disorders rose from a fifth to a quarter of all disabilities.

As seen from the epidemiological evidence reviewed earlier CLBP is a difficult clinical entity to treat. Once back pain has been present for 3 months or so there appears to be limited further improvement up to a year after onset. It is unclear how much intervention at this point impacts the presence of low back pain. The most comprehensive evidence regarding the management of CLBP is derived from systematic reviews of randomised controlled trials. These systematic reviews in turn are used to make recommendations in national and international guidelines.

Few evidence-based guidelines have been published on the management of CLBP, and while there are some inconsistencies between them, there is also clear overlap (van Tulder 2008). All recent guidelines for CLBP recommend exercises. According to the NICE Guidelines (2009) published in the UK patients are encouraged to take an active approach to back pain, and be provided with advice and information to encourage self-management. Weak analgesics or non-steroidal anti-inflammatory drugs can be considered, but the side effects should be born in mind. If interventions are to be used then exercises, manipulation or acupuncture were recommended, but if there is limited response to one of these and still high levels of disability or distress then a combined physical and psychological programme is recommended. Passive interventions, such as electrotherapy or traction were not recommended. The CLIP guidelines from Canada recommended for chronic back pain, with a high level of scientific evidence, exercises, behavioural therapy, and multidisciplinary programmes (Rossignol et al. 2007). They found moderate evidence for back school in the work place; and low evidence for massage, non-steroidal anti-inflammatory drugs, McKenzie exercises, acupuncture, and some other drug-based therapies. There was high or moderate evidence that bed rest, traction, injection therapy and TENS were not recommended (Rossignol et al. 2007).

Guidelines from The American College of Physicians and the American Pain Society made a number of recommendations related to diagnosis and treatment (Chou et al. 2007). These included, a focussed history and physical examination, and using this to classify patients as nonspecific low back pain, radiculopathy or serious spinal pathology. Furthermore there was a lack of necessity or value in including routine imaging studies in the examination, unless there was a clear reason from the history that further tests were required. These were strong recommendations with moderate quality evidence. Patients should be advised to remain active and provided with information about effective self-care options; this was a strong recommendation, with moderate evidence. Self-care options could include short courses of non-steroidal anti-inflammatory drugs. In addition for CLBP they recommended exercise prescription, multidisciplinary rehabilitation, acupuncture, massage, manipulation, yoga, and cognitive behavioural therapy (Chou et al. 2007). This was a weak recommendation, with moderate quality evidence.

The European guidelines identified the fact that CLBP is not a diagnosis, but rather a symptom with varying presentations, and therefore identifying prognostic factors was essential. For most therapeutic interventions the effect sizes are modest, but they recommended exercise therapy, cognitive behavioural therapy, multidisciplinary treatment, and brief educational interventions; and also possible use of back schools and manipulation (Airaksinen et al. 2004). All guidelines are consistent in their rejection of the use of bed rest and passive physical modality treatments for CLBP.

In a critical review of 17 international guidelines, which used evidence-linked recommendations published from 1994 to 2002, exercises and, to a lesser extent and somewhat ambiguously, back school were the most consistently recommended interventions (Arnau et al. 2006). Out of six guidelines that were relevant to CLBP four recommended use of exercises, with no other intervention being so consistently supported. However it was also concluded that there were weaknesses in the guideline developments, and the methods of development of most of the guidelines should have been more rigorous, explicit and better explained.

In a review that did not include many trials, the calculated effect sizes for acupuncture, behavioural therapy, exercise therapy and non-steroidal anti-inflammatory drugs were 0.61, 0.57, 0.52 and 0.61, respectively (Keller et al. 2007). These are moderate effect sizes only. Van Tulder et al. (2000a, b) reviewed existing systematic reviews for a range of conservative treatments for CLBP. They found there was strong evidence, meaning generally consistent findings from multiple high-quality RCTs, only for exercise, multidisciplinary pain treatment programmes for patients with long-lasting severe CLBP, and manual therapy for short-term pain relief only.

May (2010) in a recent review about self-management for CLBP and osteoarthritis reviewed the evidence for education programmes and exercise for CLBP in 10 and 18 systematic reviews respectively, with the latter being just those published since 2000, and in fact two more being published since then (Swinkels et al. 2009; van Middelkoop et al. 2010). The conclusion was that advice and education were deemed useful only if they formed part of an exercise programme, though back schools were of limited value by themselves, except in an occupational setting. Exercise was supported by all 20 systematic reviews, and was deemed to be effective both short and long term, and be effective at reducing sick leave in the follow-up year. No particular exercise programme appeared to be more effective, but McKenzie, strengthening, stabilisation, stretching and aerobic exercises and yoga were all supported by one or more reviews. The evidence for manual therapy since 2000 is less clear. Two reviews came to similar conclusions, one with 39 trials (Assendelft et al. 2003), and another with 69 trials (Bronfort et al. 2004) concluded that it is better than placebo treatment or general practitioner care, but no better than other active treatments.

Given the Biopsychosocial Concept of Pain Are Biopsychosocial Interventions More Effective?

As seen from the review above there is some support for cognitive behavioural therapy, and this has become the preferred approach by some clinicians for CLBP. This makes sense in terms of the biopsychosocial concept of pain outlined earlier, but the evidence for this approach over other active treatment approaches is generally unproven. A systematic review in 2000 (van Tulder et al. 2000a, b) found that there was strong evidence that behavioural treatment was more effective than waiting-list controls and no treatment; but that the addition of behavioural treatment had no additional effect to other active treatment programmes. Since then a number of further randomised controlled trials have produced similar results; that the addition of behavioural treatment to active treatment, or in a comparison between active treatment and behavioural therapy there is little important difference in outcomes (Hay et al. 2005; George et al. 2008; Smeets et al. 2008; Dufour et al. 2010), or that behavioural treatment is only better than a no further treatment control group after an initial active management consultation (Lamb et al. 2010).

Thus the evidence would suggest that although the cognitive behavioural approach might appear to be the logical approach for this potentially difficult patient group, this approach brings no better outcomes than any approach that uses an active treatment approach. In most of these studies the control group were performing an exercise programme, and some receiving manual therapy, but both would likely be receiving communication, support, and information from the clinician. Although not directly stated as being cognitive behavioural therapy, it might be suggested that an informed, positive, and patient-centred management strategy is delivering such an intervention without being titled as such. Might this be the vital part of the behavioural treatment approach – what most clinicians would rate to be a core component of their clinical interaction? There is generally consistent evidence to support the value of exercise therapy for patients with CLBP; and some support for encouraging this active role of the patient in their self-management.

Some common features of successful programmes for chronic back problems have been suggested (Linton 1998). These were as follows:

- Adopt a multidimensional perspective to the problem, which includes consideration of psychosocial aspects
- Conduct a thorough but "low tech" examination
- Communicate findings of the examination to the patient, and issues about the problem and what they can do about it
- Emphasise self-management of the problem, and make clear that what they do is vital to the recovery process
- Reduce any unfounded fears and anxieties about pain and movement ("hurt does not mean harm")
- Make clear recommendations about keeping active and starting a graded exercises programme
- Avoid "medicalising" the problem, "high tech" investigations, long-term sick leave, and advice to "take it easy"

The Role of Self-Management

Certain facts thus stand out about the CLBP experience. It is clearly extremely common, with limited further improvement in prevalence rates between 3 and 12 months. Although the evidence is not overwhelming there is more support for active interventions such as exercise, and the use of "talking therapies" with cognitive behavioural treatments or advice and information about back care.

If healthcare services are not to be overwhelmed by this potentially massive demand upon heath care resources, practitioners must promote and encourage supported self-management of back pain problems by the patients themselves. Many individuals with back pain do not enter the healthcare system, but for those who do self-care should be encouraged, educated, empowered and facilitated. This might involve low levels of limited periods of self-medication in the early stages with analgesics and/or non-steroidal anti-inflammatory drugs alongside relevant advice and encouragement towards self-management. This will also involve encouraging and advising about an active patient-centred strategy to maintain function and activity. This is bound to involve the regular use of exercises; though the exact type of exercise programme might depend on patient preferences, but also upon a thorough mechanical evaluation to determine if the patient might respond best to directional preference or some other type of exercise programme.

As seen from epidemiological evidence about those seeking healthcare, self-management is clearly happening in the general population. In large population-based studies of individuals with knee and back pain taking medication, rest, use of hot and cold packs and exercise were the most common self-management strategies used (Albert et al. 2008; Blyth et al. 2005). In small qualitative studies involving patients with CLBP, participants have talked about the self-evident need to be involved in the management of the problem themselves, wanting information from clinicians about what they can to help themselves, and preferring management strategies in which they were involved (May 2001, 2007; Skelton et al. 1996; Borkan et al. 1995; von Korff et al. 1994). Strategies that were most commonly used were exercises and use of postural modifications. In a systematic review of patient expectations about management of back pain advice about self-management was considered important, and lack of such information was a source of dissatisfaction (Verbeek et al. 2004).

In a huge cohort of standardised outcome data that collected baseline and follow-up information on patient characteristics, interventions and outcomes on 22,019 patients with multiple site musculoskeletal problems, certain variables were associated with functional status at discharge (Deutscher et al. 2009). Amongst other findings better outcomes were associated with patient compliance with self-exercise, and the application of exercise in treatment; whereas worse outcomes were associated with the use of passive modalities. This standardised outcome data confirm findings from systematic reviews that exercise-based management strategies are most effective. This also echoes findings regarding "yellow flags". If poor levels of self-efficacy or fear avoidance, for instance, are associated with poorer outcomes, then interventions that encourage self-efficacy or reduce fear avoidance should be encouraged.

Although self-management of CLBP is both desirable and feasible there are certain barriers, relating to clinicians and to patients, which exist to its implementation. There may be a lack of congruence in perceptions between patients and clinicians about what the patients want from a consultation (Cooper et al. 2009; Woolf et al. 2004; Blakeman et al. 2006; Lansbury 2000; Potts et al. 1984; Wilson et al. 2006). Clinicians might fail to give the appropriate advice and not understand the patients' desire for self-management advice, and information about the problem and its prognosis. From the patients' perspective, depression and low levels of self-efficacy can be barriers to self-management (Axford et al. 2008; Damush et al. 2008; Krein et al. 2007). It has also been shown that a degree of acceptance of the chronic pain problem is a prerequisite for adopting self-management strategies (May 2007; McCracken 1998). Therefore depression may need to be addressed, self-efficacy should be promoted, and realistic information needs to be given about prognosis and natural history. Regarding self-efficacy, which is the individual's belief in their ability to undertake activities; this is a key determinant of activity levels and therefore individuals' ability to self-manage. Higher levels of self-efficacy have been linked with higher levels of functioning, and vice versa; thus a higher level of self-efficacy is both a cause and a result of increased activity and function (Krein et al. 2007; McAuley et al. 2003, 2006; Rejeski et al. 2001). Patients also identify problems with on-going self-management, despite recognising that in principle it is important to their problem (May 2001, 2007). Furthermore some patients have misconceptions about the management of chronic back pain, which do not align with a self-management model (Morris 2004; Goubert et al. 2004; Keen et al. 1999; Klaber-Moffett et al. 2000). For instance, some individuals consider bed-rest and "taking it easy" as relevant management options.

Thus issues around self-management are complex, and not surprisingly a range of perspectives are found. From a healthcare resources perspective, encouraging self-management activity is clearly essential. From a patient perspective, many individuals are doing this, sometimes needing support; however a minority of patients are very demanding and appear to consume the majority of the costs of back pain. From a clinician's perspective, the imperative for self-management should be focussed on directing strategies towards patient-centred care that revolves around exercises and advice.

Future Directions in the Care of Chronic Back Pain

Present guidelines and the way randomised controlled trials are conducted tend to imply that the CLBP population is homogenous in its management needs. Mostly guidelines subgroup the back population very crudely into serious spinal pathology, nerve root problems, or nonspecific back pain, which make up the majority at about 85% of the back pain population. This is neither very illuminating, nor does it help determine future management, which is usually described in a simplistic and generalised way without emphasising individual variability. Equally randomised trials generally make no attempt to select specific treatments for specific patients, but make the assumption that all patients are the same, and will respond or not regardless of whether the treatment is appropriate for the individual patient.

As this chapter has sought to demonstrate, those with chronic back pain demonstrate a range of characteristics regarding disability, healthcare seeking, work status, activity limitation, and so on. The therapeutic nihilism sometimes encountered towards this group should be tempered with the recognition that though many might be poor responders, many might also do well with patient-centred active care. The chapter has also demonstrated the on-going work that has highlighted the importance of sub-classification of back pain in general, and demonstrated that within the nonspecific back pain popula-tion there are clear subgroups likely to respond to different management approaches. These attempts to recognise the heterogeneity of the back pain population, and the need for different approaches for different subgroups is probably the most important advance that can be made in the management of this group. For instance, symptom responses to repeated movements to identify directional preference exercise programmes, and attempts to identify those at greatest risk of chronic disability and channel their management in an appropriate way, appear to be two positive ways forward.

As demonstrated in this chapter, the epidemiology of back pain makes cautionary reading for those with a simplistic answer to the problem. Back pain is with us to stay; the vast sums spent on treating, researching and analysing the problem over the last few decades have not affected inci-dence or prevalence in any way. The impact on the general population and on healthcare services is huge, but increasing investment in care, though generating large profits for some providers, has not really improved outcomes for patients on the whole. So the other aspect of care that has been stressed in this chapter is the emphasis on self-management, and the de-medicalisation of the problem. This is the only realistic way to avert ever rising costs from imaging studies, excessive conservative and surgical treatments and indirect healthcare costs.

Self-management is not about abandoning patients without help. It will involve advice and infor-mation, for instance about the importance of activity, or the possible benefit of limited self-medication. It will involve patient activity and their involvement in an exercise programme. It might involve a limited treatment programme, but with the emphasis on their own control and self-efficacy in terms of dealing with the problem. Healthcare professionals need to be supporting and empower-ing patients to be able to self-manage, not undermining them by encouraging belief sets in, generally irrelevant imaging studies, passive treatment programmes, and "cure-all" solutions.

Conclusions

Low back pain is extremely common amongst the general population; with about half the back pain population experiencing another episode in the following year, or the persistence of symptoms for many months. There appears to be little further improvement between 3 months and a year. Only about 40% of the general population with low back pain seek healthcare, but because the prevalence rate is so high this constitutes a very high consultation rate. The cost of low back pain is vast, but mostly related to the size of the problem, and to indirect rather than direct healthcare costs. Many individuals with CLBP are functioning normally, are at work, and are self managing. It is also clear that a small minority of patients absorb the majority of costs.

Patients who consult with the problem should be encouraged to remain active, and at work, and provided with information to facilitate self-management. This will include a thorough history and physical examination to rule out the very rare cases of serious spinal pathology, and to distinguish nonspecific low back pain from specific causes of back pain, such as sciatica or spinal stenosis. The majority of individuals will present with nonspecific low back pain, and should be reassured about the benign, but potentially protracted course of such an episode. A short course of medication, such as a non-opioid analgesic or a non-steroidal anti-inflammatory drug can be recommended, but long-term use (given the side effects) should be avoided.

Numerous treatments are available for this problem, but guidelines and systematic reviews have been reasonably consistent about what they endorse. Exercise programmes, with an educational component appeared to be the most effective. There was some support for manual therapy and acu-puncture, but this was less consistent; and the limited ability of these interventions to encourage self-management should also be born in mind.

References

Abbott, J. H., & Mercer, S. R. (2002). The natural history of acute low back pain. *New Zealand Journal of Physiotherapy, 30*, 8–16.

Aina, A., May, S., & Clare, H. (2004). The centralization phenomenon of spinal symptoms – A systematic review. *Manual Therapy, 9*, 134–143.

Airaksinen, O., Brox, J. I., Cedraschi, C., Hildebrant, J., Klaber-Moffett, J., Kovacs, F., et al. (2004). European guidelines for the management of chronic non-specific low back pain. http://www.backpaineurope.org/web/html/evidence.html.

Albert, S. M., Musa, D., Kwoh, C. K., Hanlon, J. T., & Silverman, M. (2008). Self-care and professionally guided care in osteoarthritis. Racial differences in a population-based sample. *Journal of Aging and Health, 20*, 198–216.

Arnau, J. M., Vallano, A., Lopez, A., Pellise, F., Delgado, M. J., & Prat, N. (2006). A critical review of guidelines for low back pain treatment. *European Spine Journal, 15*, 543–553.

Assendelft, W. J. J., Morton, S. C., Yu, E. I., Suttorp, M. J., & Shekelle, P. G. (2003). Spinal manipulative therapy for low back pain. *Annals of Internal Medicine, 138*, 871–881.

Axford, J., Heron, C., Ross, F., & Victor, C. R. (2008). Management of knee osteoarthritis in primary care: Pain and depression are the major obstacles. *Journal of Psychosomatic Research, 64*, 461–467.

Bigos, S. J., Braen, G. R., Brown, K., Deyo, R., Haldeman, S., Hart, J.L., et al. (1994). Acute Low Back Problems in Adults. Clinical Practice Guideline No. 14. AHCPR Publication No. 95-0642. Rockville, MD: Agency for Health Care Policy and Research, Public Health Service, US. Department of Health and Human Services. December 1994.

Blakeman, T., Macdonald, W., Bower, P., Gately, C., & Chew-Graham, C. (2006). A qualitative study of GPs' attitudes to self-management of chronic disease. *British Journal of General Practice, 56*, 407–414.

Blyth, F. M., March, L. M., Nicholas, M. K., & Cousins, M. J. (2005). Self-management of chronic pain: A population based study. *Pain, 113*, 285–292.

Bogduk, N., Derby, R., Aprill, C., Lord, S., & Schwarzer, A. (1996). Precision diagnosis of spinal pain. In J. N. Campbell (Ed.), *Pain 1996 – An updated review*. Seattle: IASP.

Borkan, J., Reis, S., Hermoni, D., & Biderman, A. (1995). Talking about the pain: A patient-centred study of low back pain in primary care. *Social Science & Medicine, 40*, 977–988.

Bortz, W. M. (1984). The disuse syndrome. *Western Journal of Medicine, 141*, 691–694.

Bronfort, G., Haas, M., Evans, R. L., & Bouter, L. M. (2004). Efficacy of spinal manipulation and mobilization for low back pain and neck pain: A systematic review and best evidence synthesis. *The Spine Journal, 4*, 335–356.

Brown, J. J., Wells, G. A., Trottier, A. J., Bonneau, J., & Ferris, B. (1998). Back pain in a large Canadian police force. *Spine, 23*, 821–827.

Cassidy, J. D., Carroll, L. J., & Cote, P. (1998). The Saskatchewan health and back pain survey. The prevalence of low back pain and related disability in Saskatchewan adults. *Spine, 23*, 1860–1867.

Cherkin, D. C., Deyo, R. A., Loeser, J. D., Bush, T., & Waddell, G. (1994). An international comparison of back surgery rates. *Spine, 19*, 1201–1206.

Chorti, A. G., Chortis, A. G., Strimpakos, N., McCarthy, C. J., & Lamb, S. E. (2009). The prognostic value of symptom responses in the conservative management of spinal pain. A systematic review. *Spine, 34*, 2686–2699.

Chou, R., Qaseem, A., Snow, V., Casey, D., Cross, J. T., Shekelle, P., et al. (2007). Diagnosis and treatment of low back pain: A joint clinical practice guideline from the American College of Physicians and the American Pain Society. *Annals of Internal Medicine, 147*, 478–491.

Cooper, K., Smith, B. H., & Hancock, E. (2009). Patients' perceptions of self-management of chronic low back pain: Evidence for enhancing patient education and support. *Physiotherapy, 95*, 43–50.

Cousins, M. (1994). Acute and postoperative pain. In P. D. Wall & R. Melzack (Eds.), *Textbook of pain* (3rd ed.). Edinburgh: Churchill Livingstone.

Croft, P. R., Macfarlane, G. J., Papageoorgiou, A. C., Thomas, E., & Silman, A. J. (1998). Outcome of low back pain in general practice: A prospective study. *British Medical Journal, 316*, 1356–1359.

Croft, P. R., Papageorgiou, A., & McNally, R. (1997). *Low back pain – Health care needs assessment*. Oxford: Radcliffe Medical Press.

CSAG. (1994). *Clinical standards advisory group: Back pain*. London: HMSO.

Damush, T., Wu, J., Bair, M. J., Suthermand, J. M., & Kroenke, K. (2008). Self-management practices among primary care patients with musculoskeletal pain and depression. *Journal of Behavioral Medicine, 31*, 301–307.

Deutscher, D., Horn, S. D., Dickstein, R., Hart, D. L., Smout, R. J., Gutvirtz, M., & Ariel, I. (2009). Associations between treatment processes. Patient, characteristics, and outcome in physical therapy practice. *Archives of Physical Medicine and Rehabilitation, 90*, 1349–1362.

Deyo, R. A., Mirza, S. K., Turner, J. A., & Martin, B. I. (2009). Overtreating chronic back pain: Time to back off? *Journal of the American Board of Family Medicine, 22*, 62–68.

Dodd, T., et al., (1997). *The prevalence of back pain in Great Britain in 1996.* London: The Stationery Office.

Donovan, K. A., Thompson, L. M. A., & Jacobsen, P. B. (2011). Pain, depression and anxiety in cancer. In R. J. Moore (Ed.), *Handbook of pain and palliative care: Biobehavioral approaches for the life course.* New York: Springer.

Dufour, N., Thamsborg, G., Oefeldt, A., Lundsgaard, C., & Stender, S. (2010). Treatment of chronic low back pain. A randomized, clinical trial comparing group-based multidisciplinary biopyschosocial rehabilitation and intensive individual therapist-assisted back muscle strengthening exercises. *Spine, 35,* 469–476.

Evans, G., & Richards, S. H. (1996). *Low back pain: An evaluation of therapeutic interventions.* Bristol: University of Bristol.

Frymoyer, J. W., & Cats-Baril, W. L. (1991). An overview of the incidences and costs of low back pain. *The Orthopedic Clinics of North America, 22,* 263–271.

Gatchel, R. J., Haggard, R., Thomas, C., & Howard, K. J. (2011). A biopsychosocial approach to understanding chronic pain and disability. In R. J. Moore (Ed.), *Handbook of pain and palliative care: Biobehavioral approaches for the life course.* New York: Springer.

George, S. Z., Zeppieri, G., Al, C., Cere, M. R., Borut, M. S., Hodges, M. J., et al. (2008). A randomized trial of behavioural physical therapy interventions for acute and sub-acute low back pain. *Pain, 140,* 145–157.

Goubert, L., Crombez, G., & de Bourdeaudhuij, I. (2004). Low back pain, disability and back pan myths in a community sample: Prevalence and interrelationship. *European Journal of Pain, 8,* 35–394.

Haldeman, S., & Dagenais, S. (2008). A supermarket approach to the evidence-informed management of chronic low back pain. *The Spine Journal, 8,* 1–7.

Hay, E. M., Mullis, R., Lewis, M., Vohora, K., Main, C. J., Watson, P., et al. (2005). Comparison of physical treatments versus a brief pain-management programme for back pain in primary care: A randomised clinical trial in physiotherapy practice. *Lancet, 365,* 2024–2030.

Hestbaek, L., Leboeuf-Yde, C., & Manniche, C. (2003). Low back pain: What is the long-term course? A review of studies of general patient populations. *European Spine Journal, 12,* 149–165.

Hill, J. C., Dunn, K. M., Lewis, M., Mullis, R., Main, C. J., & Foster, N. E., et al. (2008). A primary care back pain screening tool: Identifying patient subgroups for initial treatment. *Arthritis & Rheumatism, 59,* 632–641.

Hill, J. C., Dunn, K. M., Main, C. J., & Hay, E. M. (2010). Subgrouping low back pain: A comparison of the STarT Back Tool with the Orebro Musculoskeletal Pain Screening Questionnaire. *European Journal of Pain, 14*(1), 83–89.

Hillman, M., Wright, A., Rajaratnam, G., Tennant, A., & Chamberlain, M. A. (1996). Prevalence of low back pain in the community: Implications for service provision in Bradford, UK. *Journal of Epidemiology & Community Health, 50,* 347–352.

Hoy, D., Lyn, M., Brooks, P., Woolf, A., Blyth, F., & Vos, T., et al. (2010). Measuring the global burden of low back pain. *Best Practice & Research Clinical Rheumatology, 24,* 155–165.

Johnson, M. I. (1997). The physiology of the sensory dimensions of clinical pain. *Physiotherapy, 83,* 526–536.

Jzelenberg, W. I., & Burdorf, A. (2004). Patterns of care for low back pain in a working population. *Spine, 29,* 1362–1368.

Keen, S., Dowell, A.C., Hurst, K., Moffett, J.K., Tovey, P., & Williams, R. (1999). Individuals with low back pain: how do they view physical activity? *Family Practice, 16,* 39–45.

Keller, A., Hayden, J., Bombardier, C., & van Tulder, M. (2007). Effect sizes of non-surgical treatments of non-specific low-back pain. *European Spine Journal, 16,* 1776–1788.

Kendall, N. A. S., Burton, A. K., Main, C. J., & Watson, P. J. (2009). *Tackling musculoskeletal problems: A guide for the clinic and workplace – identifying obstacles using the psychosocial flags framework.* London: Stationery Office.

Klaber-Moffett, J. A., Newbronner, E., Waddell, G., Croucher, K., & Spear, S. (2000). Public perceptions about low back pain and its management: A gap between expectations and reality? *Health Expectations, 3,* 161–168.

Klapow, J. C., Slater, M. A., Patterson, T. L., Doctor, J. N., Atkinson, J. H., & Garfin, S. R. (1993). An empirical evaluation of multidimensional clinical outcome in chronic low back pain patients. *Pain, 55,* 107–118.

Klenerman, L., Slade, P. D., Stanley, I. M., Pennie, B., Reilly, J.P., Atchinson, L.E., et al. (1995). The predication of chronicity in patients with an acute attack of low back pain in a general practice setting. *Spine, 20,* 478–484.

Krein, S. L., Heisler, M., Piette, J. D., Butchart, A., & Kerr, E. A. (2007). Overcoming the influence of chronic pain on older patients' difficulty with recommended self-management activities. *Gerontologist, 47,* 61–68.

Lamb, S. E., Hansen, Z., Lall, R., Castelnuovo, E., Withers, E. J., & Nichols, V., et al. (2010). Group cognitive behavioural treatment for low-back pain in primary care: A randomised controlled trial and cost effectiveness analysis. *Lancet, 375,* 916–923.

Lansbury, G. (2000). Chronic pain management: A qualitative study of elderly people's preferred coping strategies and barriers to management. *Disability & Rehabilitation, 22,* 14.

Leboeuf-Yde, C., Klougart, N., & Lauritzen, T. (1996). How common is low back pain in the Nordic population? Data from a recent study on a middle-aged general Danish population and four surveys previously conducted in the Nordic countries. *Spine, 21,* 1518–1526.

Lim, K. L., Jacobs, P., & Klarenbach, S. (2006). A population-based analysis of healthcare utilization of persons with back disorders. *Spine, 31*, 212–218.

Linton, S. J. (1998). The socioeconomic impact of chronic back pain: Is anyone benefiting? *Pain, 75*, 163–168.

Linton, S. J. (2000). A review of psychological risk factors in back and neck pain. *Spine, 25*, 1148–1156.

Linton, S. J., Hellsing, A. L., & Hallden, K. (1998). A population-based study of spinal pain among 35-45-year-old individuals. *Spine, 23*, 1457–1463.

Long, A., Donelson, R., & Fung, T. (2004). Does it matter which exercise? A randomized control trial of exercises for low back pain. *Spine, 29*, 2593–2602.

Long, A., Donelson, R., Fung, T., & Spratt, K. (2007). Are acute, chronic, back-pain only, and sciatica-with neural-deficit valid low back pain subgroups? Not for most patients. *The Spine Journal, 7*, 63S–64S.

Long, A., May, S., & Fung, T. (2008). Specific directional exercises for patients with low back pain: A case series. *Physiotherapy Canada, 60*, 307–317.

Main, C. J., Philips, C. J., & Watson, P. J. (2005). Secondary prevention in healthcare and occupational settings in musculoskeletal conditions (focusing on low back pain). In I. Z. Schultz & R. J. Gatchel (Eds.), *Handbook of complex occupational disability claims: Early risk identification, intervention and prevention.* New York: Springer.

Maniadakis, N., & Gray, A. (2000). The economic burden of back pain in the UK. *Pain, 84*, 95–103.

May, S. (2001). Patient satisfaction with management of back pain. Part 2: An explorative, qualitative study into patients' satisfaction with physiotherapy. *Physiotherapy, 87*, 10–20.

May, S. (2007). Patients' attitudes and beliefs about back pain and its management after physiotherapy for low back pain. *Physiotherapy Research International, 12*, 126–135.

May, S. (2010). Self-management of chronic low back pain and osteoarthritis. *Nature Reviews Rheumatology, 6*, 199–209.

McAuley, E., Jerome, G. J., Elavsky, S., Marquez, D. X., & Ramsey, S. N. (2003). Predicting long-term maintenance of physical activity in older adults. *Preventive Medicine, 37*, 110–118.

McAuley, E., Konopack, J. F., Morris, K. S., Motl, R. W., Ho, L., & Doerksen, S. E., et al. (2006). Physical activity and functional limitations in older women: Influence of self-efficacy. *Journal of Gerontology, 61B*, 270–277.

McCarthy, C. J., Arnall, F. A., Strimpakos, N., Freemont, A., & Oldham, J. A. (2004). The biopsychosocial classification of non-specific low back pain: A systematic review. *Physical Therapy Reviews, 9*, 17–30.

McCracken, L. M. (1998). Learning to live with the pain: Acceptance of pain predicts adjustment in persons with chronic pain. *Pain, 74*, 21–27.

McGorry, R. W., Webster, B. S., Snook, S. H., & Hsiang, S. M. (2000). The relation between pain intensity, disability, and the episodic nature of chronic and recurrent low back pain. *Spine, 25*, 834–841.

McGuirk, B., King, W., Govind, J., Lowry, J., & Bogduk, N. (2001). Safety, efficacy, and cost effectiveness of evidence-based guidelines for the management of acute low back pain in primary care. *Spine, 26*, 2615–2622.

McKenzie, R., & May, S. (2003). *The lumbar spine: Mechanical diagnosis and therapy* (2nd ed.). New Zealand: Spinal Publications.

McKinnon, M. E., Vickers, M. R., Ruddock, V. M., Townsend, J., & Meade, T. W. (1997). Community studies of the health service implications of low back pain. *Spine, 22*, 2161–2166.

Morris, A. L. (2004). Patients' perspectives on self-management following a back rehabilitation programme. *Musculoskeletal Care, 2*, 165–179.

NICE Guidelines. (2009). *Early management of persistent non-specific low back pain.* London: National Institute for Health and Clinical Excellence.

Pengel, L. H. M., Herbert, R. D., Maher, C. G., & Refshauge, K. M. (2003). Acute low back pain: Systematic review of its prognosis. *British Medical Journal, 327*, 323–325.

Potts, M., Weinberger, M., & Brandt, K. D. (1984). Views of patients and providers regarding the importance of various aspects of an arthritis treatment program. *Journal of Rheumatology, 11*, 71–75.

Rejeski, W. J., Miller, M. E., Foy, C., Messier, S., & Rapp, S. (2001). Self-efficacy and the progression of functional limitations and self-reported disability in older adults with knee pain. *Journal of Gerontology, 56B*, S216–S265.

Rossignol, M., Arsenault, B., Dionne, C., Poitras, S., Tousignant, M., & Truchon, M., et al. (2007). *Clinic on low-back pain in interdisciplinary practice (CLIP) guidelines.* Montreal: Direction de sante publique. Agence de la santé at des servise sociaux de Montreal.

Santos-Eggimann, B., Wietlisbach, V., Rickenbach, M., Paccaud, F., & Gutzwiller, F. (2000). One-year prevalence of low back pain in two Swiss regions. *Spine, 25*, 2473–2479.

Shekelle, P. (1997). The epidemiology of low back pain. In L. G. F. Giles & K. P. Singer (Eds.), *Low back pain.* Oxford: Butterworth Heinemann.

Shekelle, P. G., Markovitch, M., & Louie, R. (1995). Comparing the costs between provider types of episodes of back pain care. *Spine, 20*, 221–227.

Siddall, P. J., & Cousins, M. J. (1997). Spine update. Spinal pain mechanisms. *Spine, 22*, 98–104.

Skelton, A. M., Murphy, E. A., Murphy, R. J. L., & O'Dowd, T. C. (1996). Patients' views of low back and its management in general practice. *British Journal of General Practice, 46*, 153–156.

Smedley, J., Egger, P., Cooper, C., & Coggon, D. (1997). Prospective cohort study of predictors of incident low back pain in nurses. *British Medical Journal, 314*, 1225–1228.

Smeets, R. J. E. M., Vlaeyen, J. W. S., Hidding, A., Kester, A. D. M., van der Heijden, G. J. M. G., & Knottnerus, J. A. (2008). Chronic low back pain: Physical training, graded activity with problem solving training, or both ? The one-year post-treatment results of a randomized controlled trial. *Pain, 134*, 263–276.

Spitzer, W.O., Skovron, M.L., Salmi, L.R., Cassidy, J.D., Duranceau, J., Suissa, S., et al. (1987). Scientific approach to the activity assessment and management of activity-related spinal disorders. *Spine, 12*(7), S1–S55.

Swinkels, A., Cochrane, K., Burt, A., Johnson, L., Lunn, T., & Rees, A. S. (2009). Exercise interventions for non-specific low back pain: An overview of systematic reviews. *Physical Therapy Reviews, 14*, 247–259.

Szpalski, M., Nordin, M., Skovron, M. L., Melot, C., & Cukier, D. (1995). Health care utilisation for low back pain in Belgium. *Spine, 20*, 431–442.

Thomas, E., Silman, A. J., Croft, P. R., Papageorgiou, A. C., Jayson, M. I. V., & Macfarlane, G. J. (1999). Predicting who develops chronic low back pain in primary care: A prospective study. *British Medical Journal, 318*(7199), 1662–1667.

Torrptsova, N. V., Benevolenskaya, L. I., Karyakin, A. N., Sergeev, I. L., & Erdesz, S. (1995). "Cross-sectional" study of low back pain among workers at an industrial enterprise in Russia. *Spine, 20*, 328–332.

van Middelkoop, M., Rubinstein, S. M., Kuijpers, T., Verhagen, A. P., Ostelo, R., & Koes, B. W., et al. (2010). A systematic review on the effectiveness of physical and rehabilitation interventions for chronic non-specific low back pain. *European Spine Journal, 20*, 19–39.

Van Tulder, M. (2008). Non-pharmacological treatment for chronic low back pain. *British Medical Journal, 337*(417), 418.

Van Tulder, M. W., Goossens, M., Waddell, G., & Nachemson, A. (2000a). Conservative treatment of chronic low back pain. In A. Nachemson & E. Jonsson (Eds.), *Neck and back pain. The scientific evidence of causes, diagnosis, and treatment* (pp. 271–304). Philadelphia: Lippincott Williams & Wilkins.

Van Tulder, M. W., Ostelo, R., Vlaeyen, J. W. S., Linton, S. J., Morley, S. J., & Assendelft, W. J. J. (2000b). Behavioural treatment for chronic low back pain. A systematic review within the framework of the Cochrane Back review Group. *Spine, 25*, 2688–2699.

Verbeek, J., Sengers, M. J., Riemens, L., & Haafkens, J. A. (2004). Patient expectations of treatment for back pain. A systematic review of qualitative and quantitative studies. *Spine, 29*, 2309–2318.

Von Korff, M., Barlow, W., Cherkin, D., & Deyo, R. A. (1994). Effects of practice style in managing back pain. *Annals of Internal Medicine, 121*, 187–195.

Von Korff, M., Ormel, J., Keefe, F. J., & Dworkin, S. F. (1992). Grading the severity of chronic pain. *Pain, 50*, 133–149.

Waddell, G. (1987). A new clinical model for the treatment of low back pain. *Spine, 12*, 632–644.

Waddell, G. (1994). *Epidemiology review. Annex to CSAG report on back pain.* London: HMSO.

Waddell, G., & Main, C. J. (1998). A new clinical model of low back pain and disability. In G. Waddell (Ed.), *The back pain revolution* (pp. 223–240). Edinburgh: Churchill Livingstone.

Walker, B. F., Muller, R., & Grant, W. D. (2004). Low back pain in Australian adults. Prevalence and associated disability. *Journal of Manipulative and Physiological Therapeutics, 27*, 238–244.

Walsh, K., Cruddas, M., & Coggon, D. (1992). Low back pain in eight areas of Britain. *Journal of Epidemiology & Community Health, 46*, 227–230.

Waxman, R., Tennant, A., & Helliwell, P. (2000). A prospective follow-up study of low back pain in the community. *Spine, 25*, 2085–2090.

Webster, B. S., & Snook, S. H. (1994). The cost of 1989 workers' compensation low back pain claims. *Spine, 19*, 1111–1116.

Wenig, C. M., Schmidt, C. O., Kohlmann, T., & Schweikert, B. (2009). Costs of back pain in Germany. *European Journal of Pain, 13*, 280–286.

Williams, D. A., Feuerstein, M., Durbin, D., & Pezzullo, J. (1998). Health care and indemnity costs across the natural history of disability in occupational low back pain. *Spine, 23*, 2329–2336.

Wilson, P. M., Kendall, S., & Brooks, F. (2006). Nurses' responses to expert patients: The rhetoric and reality of self-management in long-term conditions: A grounded theory study. *International Journal of Nursing Studies, 43*, 803–8818.

Woolf, A. D., Zeidler, H., Haglund, U., Carr, A. J., Chaussade, S., & Cucinotta, D., et al. (2004). Musculoskeletal pain in Europe: Its impact and a comparison of population and medical perceptions of treatment in eight European countries. *Annals of the Rheumatic Diseases, 63*, 342–347.

Chapter 17
Adult Cancer-Related Pain

Sean Ransom, Timothy P. Pearman, Errol Philip, and Dominique Anwar

For people with cancer, pain can be one of the most feared and debilitating consequences of the disease, sapping quality of life and sometimes leading to wishes for hastened death. Estimations of the prevalence of cancer-related pain vary widely, but findings suggest that a majority of patients in both curative and palliative treatment experience pain (Van den Beuken-van Everdingen et al. 2007), with more than one-third of such patients classifying their pain as severe. Although the development of pain guidelines by the World Health Organization (WHO) and other groups appears to have led to a reduction in the burden of pain among those with cancer in recent decades (Hiraga et al. 1991), there is a widespread consensus that cancer-related pain continues to be a major quality of life problem for many with cancer. Recent literature reviews also suggest that for more than 40% of patients with cancer, pain continues to be significantly undertreated (Deandrea et al. 2008).

Compounding these difficulties are the challenges that healthcare personnel face in accurately treating pain. Factors as diverse as poor assessment practices, patient reluctance to report pain and to take opioids, and discomfort among physicians in prescribing large doses of opioid medications can hamper the ability to create effective pain treatment plans for patients with cancer (Von Roenn et al. 1993). The continued emphasis on pain management among various national and international medical groups as well as the ongoing transformation of palliative medicine into a truly supportive approach throughout the cancer continuum are positive developments in the treatment of cancer-related pain, but more is clearly needed.

S. Ransom, PhD (✉)
Department of Psychiatry and Behavioral Sciences, Tulane University School
of Medicine, New Orleans, LA, USA

Tulane University Medical Center, Tulane Cancer Center, New Orleans, LA, USA
e-mail: sransom@tutane.edu

T.P. Pearman, PhD
Departments of Medical Social Sciences and Psychiatry, Northwestern University
Feinberg School of Medicine, Chicago, IL, USA

Department of Supportive Oncology, Robert H. Lurie Comprehensive
Cancer Center, Chicago, IL, USA

E. Philip, PhD
Department of Psychiatry and Behavioral Sciences, Memorial Sloan-Kettering
Cancer Center, New York, NY, USA

D. Anwar, MD
Department of Medicine, Section of General Internal Medicine and Geriatrics,
Tulane University School of Medicine, New Orleans, LA, USA

R.J. Moore (ed.), *Handbook of Pain and Palliative Care: Biobehavioral Approaches for the Life Course*,
DOI 10.1007/978-1-4419-1651-8_17, © Springer Science+Business Media, LLC 2012

In addition to the patient and physician factors that contribute to difficulties in pain management in cancer patients is the fact that cancer itself is an inherently exasperating disease. Cancer can be described not as one disease but as several hundred, with each cancer site and each type of cancer at a particular site having a distinctive presentation, treatment, prognosis, and set of challenges associated with its care. So it is with cancer-related pain. While some cancers, such as leukemia, have little pain associated with the disease itself, in the late stages, the treatments for such diseases can result in various pain-associated syndromes such as mucositis, peripheral neuropathy, or abdominal discomfort associated with chemotherapy-related nausea. Other cancers may more directly create pain, such as when a solid tumor grows within bones or presses on the spinal cord or peripheral nerves. Because pain can arise from a variety of sites and through diverse means, treatments for cancer-related pain are often themselves diverse, with treatment approaches varying based on the characteristics of the disease and the pain it produces. Further complicating the diagnosis and treatment of pain are the psychological, sociocultural, behavioral, and affective aspects of pain (Ahles et al. 1983). In this chapter, we review cancer-related causes of pain and pharmacologic as well as nonpharmacologic approaches to treating pain and also focus on the challenges and future directions.

Types of Cancer Pain

Pain is not a unitary construct. Although, broadly speaking, all types of pain share the characteristics of physical discomfort and distress, different types of pain may differ markedly in their experiential nature and the optimal treatment approach based on the tissues from which the pain arises. Cancer-related pain is particularly complex because such pain can arise in nearly any area of the body and because disease processes and treatments can induce sometimes debilitating pain, as illustrated by Cherney's (2007) enumeration of more than ten dozen separate acute and chronic pain syndromes commonly found in those with cancer (see also Donovan et al. 2011). In addition, cancer-related pain may arise from a variety of sites simultaneously and via multiple different mechanisms, often offering a mixed pain presentation (Pappagallo et al. 2007). In general, however, pain can be broken down into two broad categories, nociceptive and neuropathic, with nociceptive pain further divided into somatic and visceral pain.

Somatic Pain

Pain associated with damage to the skin or the musculoskeletal system is termed *somatic pain*. Often described as sharp and localized in nature, somatic pain is both commonly experienced and, in comparison to visceral and neuropathic pain, is little discussed in the medical literature as an entity unto itself. This literary neglect is possibly partly because somatic pain can often be readily associated with a precipitating cause, such as a surgical incision or a bone fracture, and because somatic pain may be treated with a variety of narcotic and nonnarcotic pain medications that present an impressive range of potency, administration routes, and duration of effectiveness. Among those with cancer, somatic pain is highly common and can derive from a tremendous number of conditions and procedures ranging from the simple blood draw to major invasive surgeries and beyond.

This is not to say that somatic pain presents fewer problems for patients. Among the most difficult pain conditions faced by those with cancer is that of bone pain, which, unfortunately, is also the most common cause of chronic malignant pain (Pappagallo et al. 2007). Those cancers with the highest prevalence – breast, prostate, lung, etc. – all metastasize easily to the bones, as do other types, such as thyroid and kidney, and lesions to the bone are also common in multiple myeloma. Cancer can cause bone fracture as well as a series of other painful effects to the bones, including inflammation, spinal instability, and hypocalcaemia.

Visceral Pain

Both somatic and visceral pains are termed *nociceptive* in that they arise from specific nerve structures, called nociceptors, that are engineered to detect tissue damage or possible tissue damage. Nevertheless, the neurobiology of visceral pain differs substantially from that of somatic pain and thus the two different types of pain are experienced quite differently. As its name suggests, visceral pain arises from the viscera, or the internal organs, and although somatic pain is the more understood type of pain, researchers have suggested that visceral pain is the most common type of pain experienced by humans during their lifespan (Cervero and Laird 1999).

Not all organs can experience pain. Many organs, such as the liver, lungs, and kidneys, do not have afferent pain pathways arising from in the parenchyma (Cervero and Laird 1999). When these organs receive damage pain is only experienced when tissues surrounding these organs become affected, such as when tumor growth causes stretching to an organ capsule. Although some organs, particularly the hollow organs of the digestive tract, do produce pain when stretched, the pain insensitivity of much of the internal viscera can unfortunately result in the undetected development of a malignancy until the tumor grows to cause pressure to other tissues (Regan and Peng 2000). The absence of symptoms such as pain also allows these cancers to spread before they produce symptoms.

The ability to detect the source of visceral pain can also be much different from that of the more well-defined somatic types. Nociceptors in areas that create somatic pain are finely distributed, allowing a precise localization of the pain, but pain pathways in the visceral tissues arise from a smaller number of nociceptors, which creates a more diffuse area of pain localization (Cervero and Laird 1999). These pathways may lead out to the body walls and result in referred pain that is distant from the location of the tissue damage. These pathways also may converge in the spinal cord, further reducing the brain's ability to hone in on the source of the pain. Further compounding difficulties for patients, severe visceral pain can often be accompanied by noxious constellation of reflexive symptoms, such as vomiting, changes in heart rate and blood pressure, sweating, and muscle tension that can themselves produce misery in the patient (Queneau et al. 2003).

Neuropathic Pain

Pain is useful when it warns the central nervous system of possible damage and moves the individual to protect itself from dangerous stimuli. When tissue damage does occur, ongoing pain in the affected area allows the individual to protect the site to occasion better healing. However, neuropathic pain, which is felt when the nervous system sends abnormal pain signals in the absence of tissue dysfunction, does not provide such benefits because the resulting pain indicates a malfunction of this warning and protection system. Among those with cancer-related pain, neuropathic pain is thought to occur in up to 40% (Bennett 2011).

As with somatic and visceral pain, neuropathic pain can arise from numerous conditions, with the nervous system involvement resulting in the unique positive (e.g., burning, shooting, pins & needles, electric) and negative (e.g., numbness, weakness) symptoms that are characteristic of such pain. In addition, allodynia arises when afferent sensory pathways that are not normally nociceptive produce pain (Jenson and Hansson 2006). In severe cases, neuropathic allodynia can make even the slightest touch unbearable. Those with severe allodynia in the feet, for example, cannot endure the sensation of footwear, even socks, and such pain can turn a brief walk into a debilitating experience. In addition to this hypersensitivity to stimuli, neuropathic pain can also be spontaneous and it is common for such pain to be constant with flare-ups that occur when the area is stimulated.

Neuropathic pain can arise from nerve injuries (as when nerves are damaged during surgery), demyelinating side effects of chemotherapy, tumor-related nerve compression, or other conditions that affect the nervous system. Unfortunately, among those with cancer many of these injuries are commingled with other, nonneuropathic pain syndromes, and it can be a challenge to determine the extent to which pain is neuropathic or nonneuropathic (Jenson and Hansson 2006). Making this distinction, however, is an important task for the treating physician because nociceptive pain is thought to respond to different treatments than does neuropathic pain. For example, it has long been thought that opioid medications useful in treating nociceptive pain may not be effective alone to treat neuropathic pain, though they do have a role (Quigley 2005). Instead, such pain is more likely to respond to combinations of opioids with adjunctive medications such as anticonvulsants and tricyclic antidepressants. Unfortunately, despite good evidence regarding these medications' effectiveness and the inclusion of these adjunctive combinations in published guidelines (Jost and Roila 2009), such adjunctive medications are rarely used for neuropathic pain in cancer patients (Berger et al. 2006). Such low use may be partly due to these drugs' adverse side effects (Bennett 2011). In recent years, newer drugs such as duloxetine and pregabalin have become available to treat neuropathic pain in patients with cancer with more favorable side effect profiles than older agents.

Temporal Variations in Cancer Pain

In temporal terms, as with most conditions, cancer pain can be divided into that of a chronic nature vs. that which is mainly acute. Acute pain syndromes vary from the planned and necessary (i.e., bone marrow biopsy) to the feared and disabling (i.e., vertebral collapse as a result of tumor infiltration), with postoperative pain related to surgical tumor removal as one of the more common acute pain issues. By definition, acute pain is time-limited and, at least when related to treatment, is often endured willingly as the fare required for more positive outcomes. However, in cases where the pain is unexpected, acute pain can be seen as an ominous harbinger of advancing disease and may be accompanied by substantial patient anxiety until the source of the pain is definitively identified, adequately assessed, and treated (see also, Short and Vetter 2011).

Chronic pain, when disabling and poorly controlled, can be one of the great fears of a cancer diagnosis. In areas where physician-assisted suicide is legal, more patients request such an end to their lives as a result of uncontrolled chronic pain than because of any other reason. Most chronic pain is related with the tumor itself (Cherney 2007), and such tumor-related chronic pain may result from the growth of unresectable tumors in the bones or visceral tissues, compression of nerve tracts, or any of a number of various means. The vertebral column is the most common site of bone metastases (Portenoy and Lesage 1999), and tumor growth in this location may cause not only the somatic pain associated with bone fracture but also painful compression of the epidural spinal cord or cauda equina.

There is no shortage of other pain syndromes that can occur in the absence of tumor growth. These include the reemergence of herpes zoster and postherpetic neuralgia, unrelenting chemotherapy-related peripheral neuropathies, postamputation phantom pain of limbs or breast, to name just a few. Despite this, research suggests that up to 90% of patients with cancer can have their pain controlled when effective pain management guidelines are followed for opioid medications (Ventafridda et al. 1990), and additional patients able to be helped by interventional pain techniques (Miguel 2000, see also Zhao and Cope 2011).

Other research has focused on chronic pain experienced by survivors of cancer, a large group that is growing as a result of more effective cancer treatments over recent decades. Today, a majority of those diagnosed with cancer will survive their disease, but chronic pain among cancer survivors is common (Burton et al. 2007). Numerous treatment-related and psychological predictors for chronic pain among cancer survivors have been identified. For example, as many as 50% of breast cancer survivors experience chronic pain, a number that research suggests is unrelated to the type of surgery the patient undergoes (breast conserving surgery vs. mastectomy). Instead, factors such as axillary lymph node dissection and radiotherapy to the affected area appear to be greater predictors of chronic pain, as are anxiety, depression, and, especially, the severity of acute pain in the postoperative period (Burton et al. 2007; see also Short and Vetter 2011; Donovan et al. 2011).

Breakthrough Pain

Even with adequate baseline pain control, it is common for patients to experience sudden flares of pain that increase suddenly. These intense, transient pain events, called breakthrough pain (BTP), can complicate what would otherwise be a successful pain management approach. Survey research has found that between 40 and 80% of patients with chronic cancer-related pain also experience BTP (Haugen et al. 2010), with BTP occurring in a variety of ways. BTP may be somatic, visceral or neuropathic in nature, paralleling the nature of the background pain it arises from. In many cases, such pain may be associated with a precipitating event, such as motor movement (e.g., sneezing, exertion) or at the end-of-dose period when one dose of medication loses efficacy immediately prior to the next scheduled dose (Lossignol and Dumitrescu 2010). In about half of all cases, however, there is no readily identifiable precipitating event, and in these cases BTP can be difficult to predict or prevent (Portenoy et al. 1999).

Although BTP is common, findings suggest that patients who have more frequent and severe BTP also tend to experience higher levels of baseline pain without adequate baseline pain relief. Such data suggest that more problematic BTP is related with an insufficient pain management plan at baseline (Portenoy et al. 1999). Often, the management of BTP necessitates a very fast-acting, quickly eliminated pain relieving medication alongside the longer-acting baseline pain medication. The development of easily administered fentanyl solutions has enhanced the possibility that BTP may be more easily treated (Lossignol and Dumitrescu 2010).

Basic Issues in Pharmacological Treatment

The WHO Cancer Pain Ladder, designed in 1986, is a step-by-step approach to the treatment of cancer related pain (World Health Organization 1987; see also, Donovan et al. 2011; Hjermstad et al. 2011; Smith et al. 2011). It serves as an algorithm for a sequential pharmacological approach to treatment according to the intensity of pain as reported by the patient. The ladder first recommends the use of nonopioids such as acetaminophen and NSAID (Step I), then "weak" opioids such as codeine or tramadol (Step II), and, finally, more potent opioids if pain is ongoing (Step III). At each step it is also possible to add a co-analgesic or adjuvant treatment for cancer pain.

This pain ladder was an important innovation that reduced under-treatment rates (Ventafridda et al. 1990; Zech et al. 1995). However, some alterations to this model may still enhance its effectiveness. When pain is severe, Step II may be skipped, a practice sometimes called the "analgesic elevator" (Eisenberg et al. 1994). Additionally, published guidelines now recommend starting with low doses of strong opioids to relieve pain more quickly at the outset when treating those with cancer-related pain (National Comprehensive Cancer Network 2010). A randomized control trial that compared the use of strong opioids for the initial treatment of terminal cancer pain with the WHO stepped approach showed that the strong opioid arm correlated with significantly less pain, higher satisfaction, and fewer changes in therapy (Marinangeli et al. 2004).

Opioid Drugs

Very strong evidence exists now regarding the effectiveness of strong opioids in cancer pain management (see Szucs-Reed and Gallagher 2011). Morphine has been the most commonly studied and most used opioid for decades and is still considered the gold standard, although all opioids are considered effective (Mercadante et al. 2008).

Clinical recommendations suggest that opioid agonists should be used only for the management of cancer pain (Trescot et al. 2006) (Table 17.1). Meperidine and propoxyphene are not recommended because of CNS toxic metabolites. Mixed agonist–antagonists (pentazocine, nalbuphine, butorphanol, dezocine) have also been shown to have limited efficacy and should not be mixed with opioid agonist drugs. It must be remembered that their antagonist properties may precipitate a withdrawal syndrome in individuals who have developed physiological tolerance to these medications. Of note these agonist–antagonists also have a ceiling effect and therefore a potentially decreased abuse potential.

The means by which one opioid is converted to another is termed the "equianalgesic ratio," and an equianalgesic dose of two opioids is defined as the dose at which they provide (at steady-state) approximately the same pain relief in opioid-naïve patients with acute pain (Berdine and Nesbit 2006). Several opioid equivalence tables are available (see Table 17.1 for an example), but various publications question them because important and potentially clinically relevant differences in published opioid equianalgesic ratios have been identified, which may be confusing for the physician and dangerous for the patient (Anderson et al. 2001; Shaheen et al. 2009). As a consequence, equianalgesic tables should be used with caution and should only represent a first step toward the clinical

Table 17.1 Substances/equivalences (adapted from National Comprehensive Cancer Network 2010)

Opioid agonist	Oral dose	IV dose	Onset (min)	Duration (h)	Half-life (h)
Codeine[a]	200 mg	130 mg	15–30	4–6	3–4
Tramadol[b]	50–100 mg	–	15–30	3–7	No data
Morphine	30 mg	10 mg	15–30	3–7	3–4
Hydrocodone[c]	30–45 mg	–	10–20	3–5	3–4
Methadone[d]	–	–	30–60	4–8	15–120
Hydromorphone	7.5 mg	1.5 mg	15–30	4–5	2–3
Oxycodone[e]	15–20 mg	–	15–30	3–5	3–4
Oxymorphone	10 mg	1 mg	5–10	3–6	3–4
Fentanyl IV[f]	–	100 μg	7–8	1–2	1.5–6

[a]Bioactivated by CYP2D6 into morphine, no expression in 1/10 Caucasian patient, overexpression in 1/10
[b]Maximum dosage 400 mg/day (!CNS toxicity)
[c]Equivalence data not substantiated. Available in combination form only (with APAP)
[d]Expert prescription suggested. Please refer to the specific chapter on methadone in the treatment of neuropathic pain
[e]Different receptors may have less adverse effects, neuropathic pain
[f]Does not apply to transdermal fentanyl

decision, although they can give a general estimate of the doses that are safe when applied to the general population.

Evidence-based best practices not only depend upon the equivalence table, but also upon the clinician's ability to effectively tailor opioid use to the individual patient characteristics and response (see also Smith et al. 2011; Szucs-Reed and Gallagher 2011; Palermo 2011). The choice of the opioid should be made after an impeccable assessment and must target individualized care to the patient. Patient opioid naivety/tolerance, severity and type of pain (nociceptive, neuropathic, acute/chronic, etc.), overall efficacy, receptors targeted, pharmacokinetics, side-effect profile, onset of action, potential drug interactions of the opioid, specific population (pediatrics, older adult), and comorbidities (renal or liver failure, respiratory disease) must also be considered (see also Smith et al. 2011; Szucs-Reed and Gallagher 2011; Palermo 2011). Also, practical issues such as cost and availability of the drug and sometimes patient's beliefs and concerns, compliance, and drug abuse potential should be integrated. At any given time, the order of choice in the decision making may vary (Cherny 2000).

In regard to opioid tolerance, clinical observation suggests that patients are more likely to become tolerant to the side effects of opioid medications (with the exception of constipation) than they are to develop progressively worse pain control as a result of the development of tolerance to the analgesic effects of opioids (Meuser et al. 2001; see also Szucs-Reed and Gallagher 2011; Palermo 2011). Indeed, patients with stable pain management who then develop increasing pain are more likely to show disease progression rather than the development of tolerance to opioid analgesia (Passick et al. 2007), and the development of opioid tolerance to the point of requiring progressive dose escalation appears rare in clinical settings.

Unfortunately, the use of opioid medications is complicated by the reality that abuse of these drugs has been increasing and both physicians and patients work under a progressively stricter regulatory environment. In a patient with verifiable cancer-related pain, a complex risk–benefit ratio must be determined when the patient also appears to be seeking out pain medications in a nonmedically appropriate manner, with a multi-faceted harm reduction approach developed to ensure patient safety as well as the continuation of optimal pain management that considers specific patient characteristics (Passick et al. 2007). For example, the use of slower-acting opioid medications may be advisable in certain high-risk patients, with the use of rapidly administered BTP medications avoided when feasible.

Combination Drugs

Codeine, hydrocodone, and oxycodone are available at various dosages in combination with acetaminophen, ibuprofen, or acetylsalicylic acid (ASA). Although these drugs have been shown to provide relief for cancer pain, the nonopioid components of these combination drugs are not standardized and may vary with each formulation. As a consequence, care should be taken when prescribing these drugs to patients with cancer. In the case of ASA-containing formulations, it is important to balance the potential ASA component-related benefit and the risk of major adverse renal, gastrointestinal (GI), or cardiovascular effects. Regarding acetaminophen, there is a controversy which emerged in June, 2009, after the release of the recommendations of a Food and Drug Administration advisory panel of a strong caution against combination drugs and a maximum daily dosage of 2.6 g acetaminophen owing to concerns of acute liver failure (Lee 2010). Some authors will emphasize the potential benefit of combination analgesics in terms of improve efficacy and decreased side effects in the treatment of moderate pain (Raffa 2001; O'Connor and Dworkin 2009; Markman 2010). In contrast, other publications suggest that there is no benefit to adding acetaminophen to a strong opioid treatment (Axelsson et al. 2008; Israel et al. 2010).

In either case, it is important to carefully consider the patient's specific situation, and to not use these combined forms of drugs if the opioid dosage must be increased. Also, specific attention must be given to the patients' compliance and education regarding their medications, especially regarding the addition of acetaminophen-containing OTC medications, including cold medications, to the combination drug.

Initiation of Treatment and Titration

There is limited clinical guidance regarding the initiation of opioid treatment for cancer-related pain. As reported in a recent publication, there may be no direct evidence regarding the superiority of one opioid over another, whether one should begin treatment with a short- or a long-acting form of medication, or whether patients should start with an around-the-clock dose vs. doses taken on an as-needed basis (Chou et al. 2009). However, as a rule-of-thumb, pain physicians use the maxim, "start low, go slow," with initial treatment using immediate release forms of medication at a low dose to assess efficacy and tolerability. Also, despite the lack of sufficient evidence to support a specific titration protocol, certain evidence-based guidelines do suggest that dosage increases of 20–30% are indicated when the initial opioid dose does not give adequate pain control (Davis et al. 2004).

Titration must be done progressively, with assessments every 24–48 h. Once the pain score is decreased to three or below on a patient-reported 0–10 Likert pain scale, it is possible to switch to long-acting forms of opioids. These long-acting opioid formulations typically last 12 h and replace the initial short-acting forms; however, short-acting breakthrough opioids should be available when using long-acting drugs, and are usually prescribed at 10–20% of the 24-h total opioid dose.

Fentanyl

Fentanyl is a synthetic opioid whose high lipid solubility facilitates the absorption through the skin and oral membranes. The transdermal delivery system (e.g., transdermal fentanyl patch) provides a consistent rate of fentanyl to the microcirculation of the skin tissue and the steady-state rate is achieved at 72 h. Patches are replaced every 3 days. The potency of fentanyl is about 100 times that of morphine (Table 17.1), and the development of fentanyl has been a major addition to the pain-control armamentarium, but the drug also has limitations. For example, due to the limitations of patch size, dosing in small increments is not possible. In addition, the long half-life of fentanyl does not allow a rapid change of dose for patients with unstable or BTP.

Targeted education must be provided to the patient regarding the use of these patches, especially given the fact that heat can cause dangerous increases to the amount of drug released and also because the drug *must be* disposed of in a safe manner. According to recommendations made by the European Association for Palliative Care (Hanks et al. 2001), transdermal fentanyl should be reserved for patients who require stable opioid doses or for patients unable to take oral morphine as an alternative to the subcutaneous route. An Italian survey shows, however, that fentanyl may be the first-line drug of choice for chronic pain in some situations (Ripamonti et al. 2006).

In addition to transdermal formulations, three transmucosal formulations offering various dosages have been approved for the treatment of BTP: "lozenge on the stick" (lollipops) (Actiq™), buccal effervescent tablets (Fentora™) and buccal soluble films (Onsolis™). Due to their potency and cost, these formulations must be used with caution and only in opioid-tolerant patients who receive more than the equivalent dosage of 60 mg of morphine per day and in those patients who do not respond to the usual short-acting forms of opioids (Trescot et al. 2006).

Specific Situations

Impaired Renal Function

When prescribing opioids with active metabolites (especially codeine, morphine, hydromorphone), a specific attention must be paid to impaired renal function owing to the increased risk of side effects, especially opioid-related neurotoxicity (Bush and Bruera 2009). If these medications are prescribed, the dosage must either be decreased or the interval between doses increased and the patient should be carefully monitored. Oxycodone may be a better alternative choice because less than 15% of a dose is excreted in the kidneys (Davis et al. 2005). Methadone and fentanyl may also be safer options, as they do not have active metabolites.

Chemotherapy-Related Pain

A study found that 17% of patients' pain was due to adverse effects of cancer treatment (Goudas 2005). Chemotherapy-induced peripheral neuropathy (CIPN) is a common adverse effect of many agents and may be challenging to treat. Randomized controlled trials of prophylactic agents (minerals, vitamins, anticonvulsants) have shown limited efficacy in CIPN (Kottschade et al. 2011). A randomized controlled trial of tricyclic antidepressants and anticonvulsants also failed to show real benefit in the treatment of this condition (Kaley and Deangelis 2009).

Neuropathic Pain

Neuropathic pain tends to exhibit a relatively poor response to traditional opioid analgesics. In this context, additional adjuvant analgesic drugs may be required alongside the standard opioid therapy. In recent years, methadone has also been utilized in the treatment of neuropathic pain because of its additional mechanism of action as an NMDA receptor antagonist (Mannino et al. 2006).

Co-Analgesics

Co-analgesics (or adjuvant analgesics) are defined as medications whose primary indication is for a purpose other than the pain relief, but that also demonstrate some analgesic effects. Antidepressants and antiepileptics are first-line co-analgesics for the treatment of cancer-related neuropathic pain, as they target specific mechanisms commonly involved in this specific type of pain (Hempenstall and Rice 2002). Tricyclic antidepressants have long been the first choice therapy for neuropathic pain, and the analgesic efficacy of gabapentin has been shown in several types of nonmalignant neuropathic pain (Morello et al. 1999; Backonja et al. 1998; Rowbotham et al. 1998; Dallocchio et al. 2000; Rice et al. 2001; Backonja and Glanzman 2003). However, only a few studies assessed the efficacy of these drugs in cancer-related neuropathic pain (Oneschuk and al-Shari 2003) and often only anecdotal experience may guide the specific choice of a co-analgesic. A recent systematic review showed that a decrease in pain intensity of more than 1 point on a 0–10 numerical rating scale is unlikely with the usage of co-analgesics, while the increase in adverse events is likely (Bennett 2011).

Biphosphonates are effective in improving pain outcomes due to bone metastasis in multiple myeloma (Mhaskar et al. 2010) and in breast cancer (Pavlakis et al. 2005), though no specific biphosphonate has shown clear superiority in treating pain. Evidence for effectiveness in other cancers is limited. The use of biphosphonates may also be limited given the risk of significant adverse effects, including painful osteonecrosis of the jaw (Kahn et al. 2008).

Methadone

Methadone is a μ-opioid agonist, approved for oral and intramuscular use in cancer patient. It has also been used rectally, intravenously, subcutaneously, epidurally, and intrathecally (Mandalà et al. 2006). Methadone has a number of potential advantages compared with other opioids:

- In a study of cancer patients with uncontrolled pain or significant side effects from opioids, 80% of patients reported improvement in pain control and reduction of adverse effects following transition to methadone (Mercadante et al. 2001). Other studies suggest that methadone's potential efficacy in neuropathic pain is due to its action as antagonist of NMDA receptors, which are activated in chronic and neuropathic pain. However, the results of a randomized clinical trial failed to support the relatively more effective role for methadone in patients with neuropathic pain syndromes as compared with morphine (Bruera et al. 2004). A Cochrane review (Nicholson 2007) also showed no trial evidence that methadone has a particular role in neuropathic pain of malignant origin.
- Methadone may be a safer option for patients with impaired renal function as it does not have any known active metabolites and does not undergo significant renal elimination (Bruera and Sweeney 2002). Unlike morphine, it is also usually not necessary to adjust the dosage of methadone in patients with renal insufficiency.
- Methadone may be used in patients with morphine allergy because methadone is synthetic and offers no cross-allogenicity.
- Due to its low cost and efficacy, it may also be a good choice as a first-line cancer pain treatment in the global context of oncology care and cancer pain management. This also includes low-income populations or in developing countries.

Despite these substantial advantages, methadone has a long and unpredictable half-life, which makes titration difficult to achieve (Ripamonti et al. 1997, 1998) as well as large individual variations in the equianalgesic ratio of methadone to other opioids. The equianalgesic dose also varies depending on the extent of previous exposure to opioids. Caution must be exercised with methadone because of the various interactions and the potential risk of cardiac arrhythmia (Krantz et al. 2009). However, several recent studies in the palliative care cancer population have highlighted the probable safety of this potentially very useful drug (Parson et al. 2010; Reddy et al. 2010). However, more studies are warranted. Meanwhile, benefits and potential side effects of methadone must be weighed depending on the specific patient's situation and the other options available.

Managing Opioid Side Effects

The most common adverse event related to opioids is constipation, which occurs in 25–50% of patients. All patients initiating an opioid treatment should receive a laxative regimen and be provided with information on nonpharmacological approaches to constipation management such as the effects of diet and hydration on constipation.

Nausea and vomiting occur in up to 30% of patients at the initiation of an opioid treatment and antiemetics should be used as needed. Other side effects are less frequent but can be troublesome, such as pruritus and urinary retention. One of the more frightening adverse events is opioid-related toxicity, which may be caused by the effects of opioids and their metabolites in the central nervous system. Opioid-related toxicity may appear with a large variety of manifestations, such as nightmares, delirium, myoclonia, and allodynia (Mitra 2008). Careful titration and monitoring, as well as a dose reduction or opioid switch, ideally to a form without active metabolites such as methadone or fentanyl, may help avoid the development of opioid-related toxicity.

Radiation Therapy and Interventional Pain Management Strategies

Radiation therapy can be effective in reducing cancer pain, particularly when patients' pain derives from tumor growth. In randomized controlled trials of appropriate patients, 90% of patients received some relief and 25% a complete relief from radiation therapy, even if pain may worsen temporarily, or pain relief be delayed to up to 1 month. Several studies compared single- and multiple-fraction radiotherapy without finding differences in the effectiveness of pain relief (Foro Arnalot et al. 2008).

In terms of interventional strategies, including the use of nerve blocks, spinal (epidural and subarachnoid) administration of local anesthetics, opioids or alpha-2 agonists, spinal cord stimulation, and surgical interventions (see Zhao and Cope 2011; see also Adler et al. 2011), as dictated by patient condition, can be considered as a fourth step of the WHO Cancer Pain Ladder in patients in whom the pharmacological approach fails to achieve adequate pain relief or cause undesirable/intolerable side effects (Miguel 2000). Numerous interventional options are readily accessible and the majority can be performed on an outpatient basis. They can be used as the sole agents for the control of cancer pain or as useful adjuvants to supplement analgesia provided by opioids while decreasing opioid dose requirements and side effects. A careful risk–benefit ratio should also be considered prior to implementing invasive analgesic methods (Myers et al. 2010).

Psychological Influences on Cancer Pain

The conceptualization of pain within a biopsychosocial framework has prompted significant empirical enquiry into the potential role of psychological factors in explaining individual variability in pain response, along with pain assessment and treatment (see also Gatchel et al. 2011; Morris 2011; Hjermstad et al. 2011; Donovan et al. 2011). This has been particularly true within the domain of chronic noncancer pain, with an extensive literature now dedicated to detailing adaptive and maladaptive psychologically based factors that have been associated with this chronic condition (Keefe et al. 2004; Turk and Okifuji 2002; see also Donovan et al. 2011).

The role of psychological influences in the development and experience of cancer pain has received significantly less attention. However, this is changing, most notably in regard to chronic pain in cancer survivorship. As the number of cancer survivors in the USA increases (ACS 2010; Jemal et al. 2007; CDC 2004), there has been growing recognition of the potential long-term physical and psychological impact that treatment can exert, including ongoing pain conditions, and the need for comprehensive cancer care to be able to address such issues (Adler and Page 2007; Hewitt et al. 2005; see also Donovan et al. 2011). Psychological factors can exert an important influence across a range of pain-related behavior and treatment outcomes in cancer care. An individual's coping style or psychological state can influence not only one's experience of pain, but also one's ability or willingness to report pain and accept biomedical or psychological interventions for cancer pain. The assessment and treatment of cancer pain can be particularly complex, as a patient may associate pain with disease progression, and therefore may be unwilling to report their condition accurately to their healthcare provider (Lenhard et al. 2001; see also Hjermstad et al. 2011; Dy and Seow 2011).

In both noncancer- and cancer-related pain, empirical endeavors have focused on the role of three primary psychological factors: catastrophizing, coping, and emotional distress. Although the current section examines each of these factors in turn, it is important to note that their association with pain and patient behavior remains intertwined. For example, an intervention targeting the development of adaptive coping styles may enhance a patient's feeling of confidence in managing his/her pain, which in turn may be associated with a reduction in pain intensity or severity, along with a reduction in emotional distress. It is therefore important to recognize the complex and multidimensional nature of not only a patient's experience of cancer-related pain but also his/her response to this pain (see also Donovan et al. 2011).

Catastrophizing

Catastrophizing in the context of the pain experience is most frequently defined as an "exaggerated negative 'mental set' brought to bear during actual or anticipated pain" (Sullivan et al. 2001). Catastrophizing has been associated with heightened pain severity, intensity, and increased pain behaviors across a number of clinical populations (Sullivan et al. 2001), including healthy volunteers (Weissman-Fogel et al. 2008) and postoperative patients (Khan et al. 2011). This tendency to respond to pain in a reactive, exaggerated fashion is differentiated from an active coping response by its nongoal directed nature and distinction in past psychometric analyses in noncancer populations (Sullivan et al. 2001; Lawson et al. 1990). Catastrophizing has been identified as a primary factor in the Cancer Pain Inventory that was developed to assess individuals' beliefs and concerns regarding pain (Deshields et al. 2010). Khan and colleagues found that across a number of patient populations undergoing surgery, catastrophizing was associated with heightened pain severity, increased incidence of chronic pain and impaired quality of life when followed postoperatively.

One review identified catastrophizing as one of the most consistently studied psychological constructs associated with cancer pain (Zaza and Baine 2002), with high levels of catastrophizing consistently associated with negative outcomes. In the study of cancer, catastrophizing is associated with higher levels of pain and use of analgesic following breast cancer surgery (Jacobsen and Butler 1996). More recently, it was shown that oncology patients who reported moderate-to-high levels of pain also reported higher levels of catastrophizing as compared to those who reported mild pain (Utne et al. 2009). Catastrophizing has also been associated with heightened symptoms of depression and anxiety across a range of cancer sites (Fischer et al. 2010; Wilkie and Keefe 1991), as well as the over prediction of pain and less perceived control (Wilkie and Keefe 1991; Buck and Morley 2006).

Coping

The diagnosis of cancer, its treatment, and long-term management can present a myriad of challenges for patients to navigate. An individual's coping response has been conceptualized as the "constantly changing cognitive and behavioral efforts to manage specific external and/or internal demands that are appraised as taxing or exceeding the resources of the person" (Lazarus and Folkman 1984). This intentional, active, and effortful process can comprise a range of skills, techniques, and approaches. Those that have received the most empirical attention include self-efficacy for coping, and the more broad domains of active and passive coping. An extensive review of the literature concluded that the relationship between various coping mechanisms and cancer-related pain has not yet been fully defined (Zaza and Baine 2002); however, empirical pursuits in this area of research are ongoing.

In the current context, self-efficacy for coping represents an individual's perceived ability or confidence to manage stressors associated with their condition (Bandura 1989) and has been consistently associated with enhanced quality of life and disease adjustment (Bandura 1989, 1997; Linde et al. 2006; Meredith et al. 2006; Merluzzi and Martinez Sanchez 1997; Merluzzi et al. 2001). Further, it has been established that individuals who possess higher levels of self-efficacy also report lower levels of pain, both in the studies of cancer (Wilkie and Keefe 1991; Bishop and Warr 2003; Porter et al. 2008) and noncancer populations (Turk and Okifuji 2002). Active coping processes are defined as those they promote control of pain or the ability to function in spite of it, whereas passive coping processes represent those that relinquish control of pain to another person or professional. In general, active coping has been associated with more positive outcomes when compared to passive coping. In the studies of individuals diagnosed with cancer, passive coping strategies have been associated with greater self-reported disability (Bishop and Warr 2003) and increased pain (Utne et al. 2009), while more adaptive coping techniques have been associated with less anxiety, depression, and fatigue (Reddick et al. 2005).

Emotional Distress

Emotional distress is most often defined in terms of symptoms of depression and anxiety. A significant number of cancer patients will experience clinical elevations of distress at some stage of the illness trajectory (Stanton et al. 2005; Zabora et al. 2001), a statistic that has led to increased awareness regarding the identification of patients in need and the provision of effective support services. Pain and depression are the two of most frequently reported symptoms associated with cancer treatment and survivorship, and yet remain under-recognized and under-treated, with few patients receiving care from mental health professionals or pain experts. Cancer-related pain and distress frequently co-occur and can exert an additive impact on an individual's quality of life (Keefe et al. 2005; Kroenke et al. 2010). Although longitudinal studies are yet to fully elucidate a causal relationship between these factors (Laird et al. 2009), their prevalence, consistent empirical association, and frequent clinical co-morbidity provide the foundation for the ongoing pursuit to better understand and treat these conditions in cancer care.

Extensive empirical reviews have identified a strong and consistent association between emotional distress and pain (Zaza and Baine 2002; Keefe et al. 2005), with the majority of studies reviewed reporting a significant association between these two factors. In those diagnosed with cancer, patients reporting pain also report higher levels of anxiety and depression (Ahles et al. 1983; Chen et al. 2000; Spiegel et al. 1994; Velikova et al. 1995). In a study of patients diagnosed with pancreatic cancer, Kelsen et al. (1995) reported that higher levels of pain were associated with not only higher rates of depression, but also impaired functioning and quality of life. The bidirectional nature of distress and pain must once again be acknowledged, with interventions that target pain likely to lessen distress (O'Mahony et al. 2010), whereas reducing distress may also reduce the severity or intensity of experienced pain.

Psychological and Behavioral Treatments

A recent report (Green et al. 2010) of evidence-based recommendations on cancer-related pain management noted that pharmacologic and nonpharmacologic interventions, including psychological and behavioral treatments, should be combined to achieve effective pain management. Likewise, guidelines state that access to and understanding of psychosocial oncology support services should be the standard of care. Although NSAIDs and opioids are generally a first-line treatment for somatic and visceral pain, currently there are no agents approved by the US Food and Drug Administration (FDA) for the treatment of neuropathic pain in cancer patients, nor have available pharmacologic treatments proven effective (Jensen et al. 2009). Further, a recent review of opioid therapies for cancer survivors noted that cognitive behavioral and physical therapies are "extremely important aspects of pain management" (Moryl et al. 2010).

Cognitive behavioral therapy (CBT) is a useful adjunctive treatment for cancer pain (see also Donovan et al. 2011). The overall goal of treatment is to provide some behavioral control over pain. Some techniques focus more on perceptual and thought processes, and some are directed at modifying behavior patterns (Breitbart et al. 2010). All approaches incorporate two basic components, (1) education regarding how thoughts, feelings, and behaviors can influence and be influenced by pain, and (2) structured training in one or more cognitive or behavioral coping skills (Cassileth and Keefe 2010). Cognitive techniques include imagery, hypnosis, restructuring of overly negative thoughts, and distraction techniques. Behavioral techniques include activity pacing, behavioral goal setting, and progressive relaxation training.

Specific techniques include relaxation, which can decrease autonomic arousal and muscular tension to decrease pain, as well as hypnosis and self-hypnosis, which can be used to manipulate perception of pain. Self-hypnosis involves using an induction (invitation to focus awareness) and one or more specific suggestions (relaxation, changing thoughts, increasing acceptance, etc.) to modify pain.

Cognitive restructuring has also been shown to decrease pain. The keys to this technique are recognizing negative cognitions (i.e., "I can't cope with the pain") and challenging those negative cognitions. Ultimately, patients are also taught to modify their expectations of pain (i.e., "I may not be pain-free, but I can manage the pain that I have"). This has been shown to be more effective than an education-only control condition (Ehde and Jensen 2004). Other techniques include engaging in activity pacing and distraction. Biofeedback has also been used to heighten relaxation training.

Overall, CBT has been found to be effective in individual and in group settings (Andersen et al. 2008) and has been found to have biobehavioral and immune benefits, some of which could be helpful in remediating cancer pain (Andersen et al. 2010). In addition, novel uses of CBT (i.e., MP3s of patient-controlled cognitive behavioral techniques) have been investigated and found to be feasible and well-tolerated by patients (Kwekkeboom et al. 2010).

Goals of group therapy include sharing experiences and identifying successful coping strategies. Limitations of this approach are primarily practical, in that many cancer patients experiencing significant pain and with advanced disease may not be capable of traveling to group sessions and sitting in group activities for extended periods of time. However, these interventions have been found to be quite powerful and meaningful to patients (Spiegel and Bloom 1983).

Complementary Treatments

Complementary treatments are those that lie outside conventional medical treatments but are used as adjuncts to traditional medicine (National Center for Complementary and Alternative Medicine 2010; see also Kutner and Smith 2011). Complementary treatments for cancer pain include acupuncture and massage. Acupuncture stimulates the release of endogenous opioids to control pain (Carlsson and Sjölund 2001). Modern acupuncture derives from an ancient form of Oriental medicine that involves the needling and stimulation of specific anatomical points on the body. The use of acupuncture has been somewhat conflictual, with some studies finding positive results, and others concluding that the data are inconclusive. A large, randomized clinical trial found that acupuncture successfully induced analgesia in cancer patients compared to a placebo (Alimi et al. 2003).

Although a recent review of the literature suggested that the evidence base continues to lack well-designed randomized clinical trials (Hopkins Hollis 2010), experimental research suggests that acupuncture analgesia is attenuated upon the administration of naloxone (Cassileth et al. 2007), which indicates an opioid-like mechanism and suggests that future research approaches should be fruitful in both clinical applications and in elucidating previously unknown mechanisms for pain control.

Massage is the practice of applying pressure, rubbing, or stroking soft tissue and skin to promote relaxation, well-being, and circulation. Reflexology massage focuses on the feet or hands, and Reiki or light touch therapies involve the gentle brushing of hands over the body. The light touch therapies are particularly helpful for patients who cannot tolerate traditional massage therapy, as is sometimes seen in cancer patients. The National Comprehensive Cancer Network (NCCN) recommends massage therapy for treatment of refractory cancer pain (National Comprehensive Cancer Network 2009). There have been concerns raised that perhaps stimulating circulation or manipulating tissue could spread metastases. Fortunately, these concerns have been disproved (Corbin 2005).

Although there are few large-scale studies in cancer, the largest study to date, involving 1,284 cancer patients, showed that massage improved pain scores for both inpatients and outpatients by 40% (Cassileth and Vickers 2004). Other, smaller studies have suggested that massage therapy increases serotonin and dopamine, as well as natural killer cells and lymphocytes, though the clinical significance of this is unknown (Cassileth et al. 2007).

Other notable interventions which have been used in a supportive role for the treatment of cancer pain include music therapy (Nilsson et al. 2005) and exercise interventions (Penedo and Dahn 2005). Exercise has been found to favorably impact mood and provide muscular, pulmonary, and cardiovascular benefits, as well as have positive effects on bodily pain reported in cancer survivors, as well as those undergoing chemotherapy treatment.

Barriers to Effective Pain Treatment

Several issues appear critical in the care of cancer-related pain as they may lead to undertreatment of pain. Specific populations at risk of undertreatment include cultural minorities, patients with earlier stage disease, those cared for at home, those with high-school education or less, (Fairchild 2010) or the elderly population, particularly women over age 65 (Cleeland 1998; see also Green 2011).

Numerous barriers for optimal pain management have been detected. These include barriers related with the patient or the patient's support network (Morss 2010), the physician, and the healthcare system.

In regard to the patient and the patient's support network, pain management may be hampered by poor compliance, fear of addiction or side effects (Pargeon and Hailey 1999), fear of exhausting one's pain control options if opioids are taken too early in the disease course, fear of precipitating the disease when taking opioids, as well as drug abuse and drug diversion in the patient and the patient's social circle. Maladaptive beliefs of all types can contribute to patient reluctance to address their pain, further suggesting a role for cognitive therapy as an adjunctive approach.

In regard to the physician, nonspecialist physicians may be reluctant to engage in cancer pain management, especially while facing complex situations, out of concern not to be able to offer the best updated medical knowledge regarding the pain control, a reluctance to prescribe Schedule II medications, the cost-effectiveness in managing a complex pain situation, and questions regarding whether patients are truly in pain or engaging in drug-seeking behavior.

In addition, physicians may lack some of the skills necessary for an adequate pain assessment. Assessment flaws often lead to inappropriate treatment regimens. For physicians who doubt their ability to manage a complex pain problem, it is important to seek the advice of a pain care specialist, especially regarding chronic pain situations and in case of suspicion of drug diversion/abuse (see also Chang 2011; Hjermstad et al. 2011; Dy and Seow 2011; Kovach 2011).

In regard to the healthcare system, patients often lack access to drugs necessary to treat their pain, access to pain specialists who understand state-of-the-art pain management techniques, and access to interdisciplinary treatment teams to manage the multiple dimensions of their pain (see also Palermo 2011; Green 2011; Hallenbeck 2011). Often, pain management is hampered by communication difficulties between the healthcare provider and the patient or patient's family, and miscommunications may also happen among healthcare providers, themselves (Hallenbeck 2011; Brown et al. 2011; Ngo Su-mien et al. 2011; Schapira and Steensma 2011; Kreps 2011). Difficulties with access to pain management are widespread, but are particular problems among disadvantaged communities, including ethnic and linguistic minorities and the poor (see also Green 2011).

Ethnic Differences in Cancer Pain Management

In the USA, ethnic minorities are more likely to be burdened by undertreated cancer-related pain than are Caucasians (Haynes et al. 1999; see also Green 2011) and pain management programs are less likely to be implemented in cancer centers that treat primarily ethnic minorities (Todd et al. 2000). As mentioned previously, undertreatment for cancer-related pain is unfortunately common for all who have cancer, but this is even more particularly the case for African-American and Hispanic individuals with cancer. In a now-classic study, for example, Cleeland et al. (1994) found that nearly 40% of Caucasian patients with metastatic cancer failed to receive adequate pain management, whereas nearly 60% of minority patients were treated similarly poorly.

The causes of these disparities are likely to be multifaceted and complex, rooted both in discrimination and in cultural factors that present barriers to successful pain management. Research in non-cancer populations has shown unequivocally that minority patients are significantly less likely than non-Hispanic Whites to be offered appropriate pain management in situations that such medications are both clearly indicated and available, such as in an emergency room following a long bone fracture (Todd et al. 2000) or in a maternity ward during childbirth (Rust et al. 2004). When pain prescriptions are obtained, those living in predominately minority neighborhoods may find that their pharmacies are less likely to supply opioid medications (Morrison et al. 2000). Finally, cultural variables play a role in how individuals approach their own pain (Kagawa-Singer et al. 2010). Such cultural factors may lead individuals from some minority groups to be more likely to attempt to deal with pain through stoicism rather than treatment (Im et al. 2007, 2008a, b), to have greater concern over the possibility of opioid addiction (Anderson et al. 2002), to be more likely to be deferential to physicians and family members (Maly et al. 2006), be more resistant to the idea of hospice care (Mazanec et al. 2010), or hold any other number of specific behaviors that may affect the pain management they receive.

The Role of Palliative and Supportive Medicine in Cancer-Related Pain

The prevalence of cancer-related pain increases as the disease progresses, with meta-analysis suggesting nearly two-thirds of patients with advanced disease experience pain (Van den Beuken-van Everdingen et al. 2007). The goal of palliative care as supportive care is to increase patients' quality of life by reducing the burdens of symptoms such as pain. As such, medical professionals specializing in palliative care often make pain management a particular focus of their approach. Although sometimes misconstrued as end-of-life care, palliative care is increasingly provided across the spectrum of treatment, with recent findings showing that the initiation of palliative care early in treatment provides both longer survival and greater quality of life (Bakitas et al. 2009; Connor et al. 2007; Temel et al. 2010). Such treatment is also less costly as a result of reduced number of hospital stays.

In addition to assessment and treatment of symptoms, palliative care teams provide a number of other services for patients, including decision-making support, ensuring patient and family wishes are understood and addressed, and ensuring that patient care is consistent between different care settings, such as hospitals, the patient's home, and the hospice setting (Kelley and Meier 2010). Such teams have a strongly interdisciplinary focus and typically include social workers, chaplains, nutritionists, rehabilitation specialists, and others, as well as the palliative care physician. Findings show that referrals to palliative care services are among the most effective ways of addressing the persistent undertreatment of pain among those with cancer (Higginson and Evans 2010 see also Rich 2011; Fine 2011; Jones and Meier 2011).

Despite this, medical professionals appear to hold a stigma against palliative care, with surveys suggesting that many physicians see palliative services as useful only when their patients are without medical hope (Fadul et al. 2009). Fortunately, such attitudes may begin to change as research makes increasingly clear that reducing suffering is beneficial to all patients and that reducing misery is an appropriate goal for all those with cancer, regardless of whether or not their disease can be cured. Perhaps most surprising is the fact that research is only recently been developed to show the tremendous benefits of palliative care. Accordingly, the research literature continues to have weaknesses, for example, it is unclear what aspects of a multifaceted palliative care approach are most beneficial to patients, but what is already known is enough to cause many to endorse palliative care as routine and essential in the management of diseases such as cancer (Kelley and Meier 2010; see also Rich 2011; Fine 2011; Jones and Meier 2011).

Future Directions

Although pain management in oncology settings continues to improve, the improvement is neither fast enough nor widespread enough to comprehensively address the needs of an ever-expanding cancer patient population. Fortunately, positive developments in pain management approaches and the growing acceptance of palliative care provide promise that these issues may become less burdensome to patients in the future; this improvement – as well as the general improvement in cancer care, generally – highlights the need for closer multispecialty and multidisciplinary cooperation in managing pain in patients. Transitions between various treating physicians are a particularly important time when palliative issues such as pain management may lose focus. Integrating an awareness of pain management and other issues among the growing legions of cancer patient navigators, for example, could allow patients to continue receiving optimal pain control when transitions are made (citation needed).

Similarly, pain management issues should be considered as part of evidence-based routine follow-up care among cancer survivors. Although the research base continues to be lacking, a number of cancer centers now have survivorship programs to provide care summaries and individualized follow-up plans once patients complete their treatment. Pain is one such symptom that deserves attention in the short and long term, as we begin to learn more about the long-term risk of pain associated with various treatment protocols. Patient education programs should also involve information regarding pain as patients transition to long-term survivorship, including the type of pain patients should they report and whether possible pain symptoms are normal long-term sequelae of their particular cancer treatment or whether such pain may represent a change in health status.

The promise that patients may be spared from the unrelenting agony of needless cancer-related pain is one that everyone concerned with oncology should be committed to fulfilling. Although the field has made important steps, too many individuals and families, particularly those with poorer access to high-quality medical treatment, continue to suffer in ways that could be prevented. Ultimately, the field should not stand still until all those who experience suffering are provided needed care, and such efforts should form the core ethic of any future direction in this area of medicine.

References

ACS. (2010). *Cancer facts and figures 2010*. Atlanta: American Cancer Society.

Adler, B., Yarchoan, M., & Adler, J. R. (2011). Neurosurgical interventions for the control of chronic pain conditions. In R. J. Moore (Ed.), *Handbook of pain and palliative care: Biobehavioral approaches for the life course*. New York: Springer.

Adler, N. E., & Page, A. E. (Eds.). (2007). *Cancer care for the whole patient: Meeting psychosocial health needs*. Washington: National Academies Press.

Ahles, T. A., Blanchard, E. B., & Ruckdeschel, J. C. (1983). The multidimensional nature of cancer-related pain. *Pain, 17*(3), 277–288.

Alimi, D., Rubino, C., Pichard-Léandri, E., Fermand-Brule, S., Dubremit-Lemaire, M. L. & Hill, C. (2003). Analgesic effect of auricular acupuncture for cancer pain: A randomized, blinded, controlled trial. *Journal of Clinical Oncology, 21*(22), 4120–4126.

Andersen, B. L., Thornton, L. M., Shapiro, C. L., Farrar, W. B., Mundy, B. L., Yang, H. C., et al. (2010). Biobehavioral, immune, and health benefits following recurrence for psychological intervention participants. *Clinical Cancer Research, 16*(12), 3270–3278.

Andersen, B. L., Yang, H. C., Farrar, W. B., Golden-Kreutz, D. M., Emery, C. F., Thornton, L. M., et al. (2008). Psychologic intervention improves survival for breast cancer patients: A randomized clinical trial. *Cancer, 113*(12), 3450–3458.

Anderson, K. O., Richman, S. P., Hurley, J., Palos, G., Valero, V., Mendoz, T. R., et al. (2002). Cancer pain management among underserved minority outpatients: Perceived needs and barriers to optimal control. *Cancer, 94*(8), 2295–2304.

Anderson, R., Saiers, J. H., Abram, S., & Schlicht, C. (2001). Accuracy in equianalgesic dosing: Conversion dilemmas. *Journal of Pain and Symptom Management, 21*(5), 397–406.

Axelsson, B., Stellborn, P., & Ström, G. (2008). Analgesic effect of paracetamol on cancer related pain in concurrent strong opioid therapy. A prospective clinical study. *Acta Oncologica, 47*(5), 891–895.

Backonja, M., Beydoun, A., Edwards, K. R., Schwartz, S. L., Fonseca, V., Hes, M., et al. (1998). Gabapentin for the symptomatic treatment of painful neuropathy in patients with diabetes mellitus: A randomized controlled trial. *Journal of the American Medical Association, 280*, 1831–1836.

Backonja, M., & Glanzman, R. L. (2003). Gabapentin dosing for neuropathic pain: Evidence from randomized, placebo-controlled clinical trials. *Clinical Therapeutics, 25*, 81–104.

Bakitas, M., Lyons, K. D., Hegel, M. T., Balan, S., Brokan, F. C., Sevill, J., et al. (2009). Effects of a palliative care intervention on clinical outcomes in patients with advanced cancer: The Project ENABLE II randomized controlled trial. *Journal of the American Medical Association, 302*(7), 741–749.

Bandura, A. (1989). Human agency in social cognitive theory. *The American Psychologist, 44*, 1175–1184.

Bandura, A. (1997). *Self-efficacy: The exercise of control*. New York: Freeman.

Bennett, M. (2011). Effectiveness of antiepileptic or antidepressant drugs when added to opioids for cancer pain: A systematic review. *Palliative Medicine, 25*(5), 553–559.

Berdine, H. J., & Nesbit, S. A. (2006). Equianalgesic dosing of opioids. *Journal of Pain & Palliative Care Pharmacotherapy, 20*(4), 79–84.

Berger, A., Dukes, E., Mercadante, S., & Oster, G. (2006). Use of antiepileptics and tricyclic antidepressants in cancer patients with neuropathic pain. *European Journal of Cancer Care, 15*(2), 138–145.

Bishop, S. R., & Warr, D. (2003). Coping, catastrophizing and chronic pain in breast cancer. *Journal of Behavioral Medicine, 26*(3), 265–281.

Breitbart, W. S., Park, J., & Katz, A. M. (2010). Pain. In J. Holland (Ed.), *Psycho-oncology* (2nd ed., pp. 215–228). New York: Oxford University Press.

Brown, M., Crowe, A., & Cousins, S. (2011). Educating patients and caregivers about pain management: What clinicians need to know. In R. J. Moore (Ed.), *Handbook of pain and palliative care: Biobehavioral approaches for the life course*. New York: Springer.

Bruera, E., Palmer, J. L., Bosnjak, S., Rico, M. A., Moyano, J., Sweaney, C., et al. (2004). Methadone versus morphine as a first-line strong opioid for cancer pain: A randomized, double blind study. *Journal of Clinical Oncology, 1*, 185–192.

Bruera, E., & Sweeney, C. (2002). Methadone use in cancer patients with pain: A review. *Journal of Palliative Medicine, 5*, 127–138.

Buck, R., & Morley, S. A. (2006). Daily process design study of attentional pain control strategies in the self-management of cancer pain. *European Journal of Pain, 10*(5), 385–398.

Burton, A. W., Fanciullo, G. J., Beasley, R. D., & Fisch, M. J. (2007). Chronic pain in the cancer survivor: A new frontier. *Pain Medicine, 8*(2), 189–198.

Bush, S., & Bruera, E. (2009). The assessment and management of delirium in cancer patients. *The Oncologist, 14*(10), 1039–1049.

Carlsson, C. P., & Sjölund, B. H. (2001). Acupuncture for chronic low back pain: A randomized placebo-controlled study with long-term follow-up. *The Clinical Journal of Pain, 17*(4), 296–305.

Cassileth, B., Trevisan, C., & Gubili, J. (2007). Complementary therapies for cancer pain. *Current Pain and Headache Reports, 11*(4), 265–269.

Cassileth, B. R., & Keefe, F. J. (2010). Integrative and behavioral approaches to the treatment of cancer-related neuropathic pain. *The Oncologist, 15*(Suppl 2), 19–23.

Cassileth, B. R., & Vickers, A. J. (2004). Massage therapy for symptom control: Outcome study at a major cancer center. *Journal of Pain and Symptom Management, 28*(3), 244–249.

CDC. (2004). Cancer survivorship-United States, 1971–2001. *Morbidity and Mortality Weekly Report, 53*(24), 526–529.

Cervero, F., & Laird, J. M. (1999). Visceral pain. *Lancet, 353*(9170), 2145–2148.

Chang, C.-H. (2011). Dynamic pain assessment: An application of clinical infometrics to personalized pain treatment and management. In R. J. Moore (Ed.), *Handbook of pain and palliative care: Biobehavioral approaches for the life course*. New York: Springer.

Chen, M. L., Chang, H. K., & Yeh, C. H. (2000). Anxiety and depression in Taiwanese cancer patients with and without pain. *Journal of Advanced Nursing, 32*(4), 944–951.

Cherney, N. I. (2007). Cancer pain: Principles of assessment and syndromes. In A. M. Berger, J. L. Shuster Jr., & J. H. Von Roenn (Eds.), *Principles and practice of palliative care and supportive oncology* (3rd ed., pp. 3–26). Philadelphia: Lippincott, Williams & Wilkins.

Cherny, N. (2000). New strategies in opioid therapy for cancer pain. *The Journal of Oncology Management, 9*(1), 8–15.

Chou, R., Fanciullor, G. J., & Fine, P. G. (2009). Clinical guidelines for the use of chronic opioid therapy in chronic noncancer pain. *The Journal of Pain, 10*(2), 113–130.

Cleeland, C. (1998). Undertreatment of cancer pain in elderly patients. *Journal of the American Medical Association, 279*, 1914–1915.

Cleeland, C. S., Gonin, R., Hatfield, A. K., Edmonson, J. H., Blum, R. H., Stewart, J. A., et al. (1994). Pain and its treatment in outpatients with metastatic cancer. *The New England Journal of Medicine, 330*(9), 592–596.

Connor, S. R., Pyenson, B., Fitch, K., Spence, C., & Iwasaki, K. (2007). Comparing hospice and nonhospice patient survival among patients who die within a three-year window. *Journal of Pain and Symptom Management, 33*, 238–246.

Corbin, L. (2005). Safety and efficacy of massage therapy for patients with cancer. *Cancer Control, 12*(3), 158–164.

Dallocchio, C., Buffa, C., Mazzarello, P., & Chiroli, S. (2000). Gabapentin vs. amitriptyline in painful diabetic neuropathy: An open-label pilot study. *Journal of Pain and Symptom Management, 20*, 280–285.

Davis, M., Glare, P., & Hardy, J. (2005). *Opioids in cancer pain*. Oxford: Oxford University Press.

Davis, M. P., Weissman, D. E., & Arnold, R. M. (2004). Opioid dose titration for severe cancer pain: A systematic evidence-based review. *Journal of Palliative Medicine, 7*, 462–468.

Deandrea, S., Montanari, M., Moja, L., & Apolone, G. (2008). Prevalence of undertreatment in cancer pain. A review of published literature. *Annals of Oncology, 19*(12), 1985–1991.

Deshields, T. L., Tait, R. C., Manwaring, J., Trinkaus, K. M., Naughton, M., Hawkins, J., et al. (2010). The Cancer Pain Inventory: Preliminary development and validation. *Psycho-Oncology, 19*(7), 684–692.

Donovan, K. A., Thompson, L. M. A., & Jacobsen, P. B. (2011). Pain, depression and anxiety in cancer. In R. J. Moore (Ed.), *Handbook of pain and palliative care: Biobehavioral approaches for the life course*. New York: Springer.

Dy, S., & Seow, H. (2011). Quality indicators for pain in palliative care. In R. J. Moore (Ed.), *Handbook of pain and palliative care: Biobehavioral approaches for the life course*. New York: Springer.

Ehde, D. M., & Jensen, M. P. (2004). Feasibility of a cognitive restructuring intervention for treatment of chronic pain in persons with disabilities. *Rehabilitation Psychology, 49*, 254–258.

Eisenberg, E., Berkey, C. S., Carr, D. B., Mosteller, F., & Chalmers, T. C. (1994). Efficacy and safety of nonsteroidal anti inflammatory drugs for cancer pain: A meta-analysis. *Journal of Clinical Oncology, 12*(12), 2756–2765.

Fadul, N., Elsayem, A., Palmer, J. L., Del Fabbco, E., Swint, K., Li, E., et al. (2009). Supportive versus palliative care: What's in a name? A survey of medical oncologists and midlevel providers at a comprehensive cancer center. *Cancer, 115*(9), 2013–2021.

Fairchild, A. (2010). Under-treatment of cancer pain. *Current Opinion in Supportive and Palliative Care, 4*(1), 11–15.

Fine, P. (2011). Recognition and resolution of ethical barriers to palliative care research. In R. J. Moore (Ed.), *Handbook of pain and palliative care: Biobehavioral approaches for the life course.* New York: Springer.

Fischer, D. J., Villines, D., Kim, Y. O., Epstein, J. B., & Wilkie, D. J. (2010). Anxiety, depression, and pain: Differences by primary cancer. *Supportive Care in Cancer, 18*(7), 801–810.

Foro Arnalot, P., Fontanals, A. V., Galcerán, J. C., Lynd, F., Latiesas, Xs., de Dios, N. R., et al. (2008). Randomized clinical trial with two palliative radiotherapy regimens in painful bone metastases: 30 Gy in 10 fractions compared with 8 Gy in single fraction. *Radiotherapy and Oncology, 89*, 150–155.

Gatchel, R. J., Haggard, R., Thomas, C., & Howard, K. J. (2011). A biopsychosocial approach to understanding chronic pain and disability. In R. J. Moore (Ed.), *Handbook of pain and palliative care: Biobehavioral approaches for the life course.* New York: Springer.

Goudas, L. C. (2005). The epidemiology of cancer pain. *Cancer Investigation, 23*, 182–190.

Green, C. (2011). Disparities in pain management and palliative care. In R. J. Moore (Ed.), *Handbook of pain and palliative care: Biobehavioral approaches for the life course.* New York: Springer.

Green, E., Zwaal, C., Beals, C., Fitzgerald, B., Harle, I., Jores, J., et al. (2010). Cancer-related pain management: A report of evidence-based recommendations to guide practice. *The Clinical Journal of Pain, 26*(6), 449–462.

Hallenbeck, J. (2011). Pain and intercultural communication. In R. J. Moore (Ed.), *Handbook of pain and palliative care: Biobehavioral approaches for the life course.* New York: Springer.

Hanks, G. W., Conno, F., Cherny, N., Hanna, M., Kalso, E., McQuay, H. J., et al. (2001). Morphine and alternative opioids in cancer pain: The EAPC recommendations. *British Journal of Cancer, 84*(5), 587–593.

Haugen, D. F., Hjermstad, M. J., Hagen, N., Caraceni, A., Kaasa, S., & European Palliative Care Research Collaborative (EPCRC). (2010). Assessment and classification of cancer breakthrough pain: A systematic literature review. *Pain, 149*(3), 476–482.

Haynes, M. A., Smedley, B. D., & Institute of Medicine, Committee on Cancer Research among Minorities and the Medically Underserved. (1999). *The unequal burden of cancer: An assessment of NIH research and programs for ethnic minorities and the medically underserved.* Washington: National Academy Press.

Hempenstall, K., & Rice, A. S. (2002). Current treatment options in neuropathic pain. *Current Opinion in Investigational Drugs, 3*(3), 441–448.

Hewitt, M., Greenfield, S., & Stovall, E. (Eds.). (2005). *From cancer patient to cancer survivor: Lost in transition: An Institute of Medicine and National Research Council Symposium.* Washington: National Academies Press.

Higginson, I. J., & Evans, C. J. (2010). What is the evidence that palliative care teams improve outcomes for cancer patients and their families? *Cancer Journal, 16*(5), 423–435.

Hiraga, K., Mizuguchi, T., & Takeda, F. (1991). The incidence of cancer pain and improvement of pain management in Japan. *Postgraduate Medical Journal, 67*(Suppl 2), S14–S25.

Hjermstad, M., Haugen, D. F., Bennett, M. I., & Kaasa, S. (2011). Pain assessment tools in palliative care and cancer. In R. J. Moore (Ed.), *Handbook of pain and palliative care: Biobehavioral approaches for the life course.* New York: Springer.

Hopkins Hollis, A. S. (2010). Acupuncture as a treatment modality for the management of cancer pain: The state of the science. *Oncology Nursing Forum, 37*(5), E344–E348.

Im, E. O., Guevara, E., & Chee, W. (2007). The pain experience of Hispanic patients with cancer in the United States. *Oncology Nursing Forum, 34*(4), 861–868.

Im, E. O., Lim, H. J., Clark, M., & Chee, W. (2008a). African American cancer patients' pain experience. *Cancer Nursing, 31*(1), 38–46.

Im, E. O., Liu, Y., Kim, Y. H., & Chee, W. (2008b). Asian American cancer patients' pain experience. *Cancer Nursing, 31*(3), E17–E23.

Israel, F. J., Parker, G., Charles, M., & Reymond, L. (2010). Lack of benefit from paracetamol (acetaminophen) for palliative cancer patients requiring high-dose strong opioids: A randomized, double-blind, placebo-controlled, crossover trial. *Journal of Pain and Symptom Management, 39*(3), 548–554.

Jacobsen, P. B., & Butler, R. W. (1996). Relation of cognitive coping and catastrophizing to acute pain and analgesic use following breast cancer surgery. *Journal of Behavioral Medicine, 19*(1), 17–29.

Jemal, A., Siegel, R., Ward, E., Murray, T., Xu, J., Thun, J., et al. (2007). Cancer statistics, 2007. *CA: A Cancer Journal for Clinicians, 57*, 43–66.

Jensen, T. S., Madsen, C. S., & Finnerup, N. B. (2009). Pharmacology and treatment of neuropathic pains. *Current Opinion in Neurology, 22*(5), 467–474.

Jenson, T. S., & Hansson, P. T. (2006). Classification of neuropathic pain syndromes based on symptoms and signs. *Handbook of Clinical Neurology, 81,* 517–526.

Jones, A. B., & Meier, D. E. (2011). How health care reform can improve access to quality pain and palliative care services. In R. J. Moore (Ed.), *Handbook of pain and palliative care: Biobehavioral approaches for the life course.* New York: Springer.

Jost, L., & Roila, F. (2009). On behalf of the ESMO Guidelines Working Group. Management of cancer pain: ESMO clinical recommendations. *Annals of Oncology, 20*(Suppl 4), 170–173.

Kagawa-Singer, M., Dadia, A. V., Yu, M. C., & Surbone, A. (2010). Cancer, culture, and health disparities: Time to chart a new course? *CA: A Cancer Journal for Clinicians, 60*(1), 12–39.

Kaley, T. J., & Deangelis, L. M. (2009). Therapy of chemotherapy-induced peripheral neuropathy. *British Journal of Haematology, 145,* 3–14.

Keefe, F. J., Abernethy, A. P., & Campbell, L. C. (2005). Psychological approaches to understanding and treating disease-related pain. *Annual Review of Psychology, 56,* 601–630.

Keefe, F. J., Rumble, M. E., Scipio, C. D., Giordano, L. A., & Perri, L. M. (2004). Psychological aspects of persistent pain: Current state of the science. *The Journal of Pain, 5*(4), 195–211.

Kelley, A. S., & Meier, D. E. (2010). Palliative care – A shifting paradigm. *The New England Journal of Medicine, 363,* 781–782.

Kelsen, D. P., Portenoy, R. K., Thaler, H. T., Niedzwiecki, D., Passik, S. D., Tao, Y., Banks, W., Brennan, M. F., & Foley, K. M. (1995). Pain and depression in patients with newly diagnosed pancreas cancer. *Journal of Clinical Oncology, 13*(3), 748–755.

Khan, A. A., Sándor, G. K., Dore, E., et al. (2008). Canadian consensus practice guidelines for biphosphonate associated osteonecrosis of the jaw. *The Journal of Rheumatology, 35,* 1391–1397.

Khan, R. S., Ahmed, K., Blakeway, E., et al. (2011). Catastrophizing: A predictive factor of postoperative pain. *The American Journal of Surgery, 201*(1), 122–131.

Kottschade, L. A., Sloan, J. A., Mazurczak, M. A., Johnson, D. B., Murphy, E. P., et al. (2011). The use of vitamin E for the prevention of chemotherapy-induced peripheral neuropathy: Results of a randomized phase III clinical trial. *Support Care Cancer, 19*(11), 1769–1777.

Kovach, C. R. (2011). Assessing pain and unmet needs in patients with advanced dementia: The role of the serial trial intervention (STI). In R. J. Moore (Ed.), *Handbook of pain and palliative care: Biobehavioral approaches for the life course.* New York: Springer.

Krantz, M. J., Martin, J., Stimmel, B., Mehta, D., & Haigney, M. C. (2009). QTc interval screening in methadone treatment. *Annals of Internal Medicine, 150*(6), 387–395.

Kreps, G. (2011). Communication and palliative care: E-health interventions and pain management. In R. J. Moore (Ed.), *Handbook of pain and palliative care: Biobehavioral approaches for the life course.* New York: Springer.

Kroenke, K., Theobald, D., Wu, J., Norton, K., Morrison, G., Carpenter, J., & Tu, W. (2010). Effect of telecare management on pain and depression in patients with cancer: A randomized trial. *Journal of the American Medical Association, 304*(2), 163–171.

Kutner, J. S., & Smith, M. C. (2011). CAM in chronic pain and palliative care. In R. J. Moore (Ed.), *Handbook of pain and palliative care: Biobehavioral approaches for the life course.* New York: Springer.

Kwekkeboom, K. L., Abbott-Anderson, K., & Wanta, B. (2010). Feasibility of a patient-controlled cognitive-behavioral intervention for pain, fatigue, and sleep disturbance in cancer. *Oncology Nursing Forum, 37*(3), E151–E159.

Laird, B. J., Boyd, A. C., Colvin, L. A., & Fallon, M. T. (2009). Are cancer pain and depression interdependent? A systematic review. *Psycho-Oncology, 18*(5), 459–464.

Lawson, K., Reesor, K. A., Keefe, F. J., & Turner, J. A. (1990). Dimensions of pain-related cognitive coping: Cross validation of the factor structure of the Coping Strategies Questionnaire. *Pain, 42,* 195–204.

Lazarus, A., & Folkman, S. (1984). *Stress, appraisal and coping.* New York: Springer.

Lee, W. M. (2010). The case for limiting acetaminophen-related deaths: Smaller doses and unbundling the opioid-acetaminophen compounds. *Clinical Pharmacology and Therapeutics, 88*(3), 289–292.

Lenhard, R. E., Osteen, R. T., & Gansler, T. S. (2001). *Clinical oncology.* Atlanta: Wiley-Blackwell.

Linde, J. A., Rothman, A. J., Baldwin, A. S., & Jeffery, R. W. (2006). The impact of self-efficacy on behavior change and weight change among overweight participants in a weight loss trial. *Health Psychology, 25*(3), 282–291.

Lossignol, D. A., & Dumitrescu, C. (2010). Breakthrough pain: Progress in management. *Current Opinion in Oncology, 22*(4), 302–306.

Maly, R. C., Umezawa, Y., Ratliff, C. T., & Leake, B. (2006). Racial/ethnic group differences in treatment decision-making and treatment received among older breast carcinoma patients. *Cancer, 106*(4), 957–965.

Mandalà, M., Moro, C., Labianca, R., Cremonesi, M., & Barni, S. (2006). Optimizing use of opiates in the management of cancer pain. *Therapeutics and Clinical Risk Management, 2*(4), 447–453.

Mannino, R., Coyne, P., Swainey, C., Hansen, L. A., & Lyckholm, L. (2006). Methadone for cancer-related neuropathic pain: A review of the literature. *Journal of Opioid Management, 2*(5), 269–276.

Marinangeli, F., Ciccozzi, A., Leonardis, M., Aloisio, L., Mazzer, A., Paladin, A., et al. (2004). Use of strong opioids in advanced cancer pain: A randomized trial. *Journal of Pain and Symptom Management, 27*(5), 409–416.

Markman, J. D. (2010). Bundle up: It's painful out there – The case for opioid–acetaminophen combinations. *Clinical Pharmacology & Therapeutics, 88*(3), 292–294.

Mazanec, P. M., Daly, B. J., & Townsend, A. (2010). Hospice utilization and end-of-life care decision making of African Americans. *The American Journal of Hospice & Palliative Care, 27*(8), 560–566.

Mercadante, S., Casnccio, A., Fulfaro, F., Groff, L., Boff, R., Viltari, P., et al. (2001). Switching from morphine to methadone to improve analgesia and tolerability in cancer patients: A prospective study. *Journal of Clinical Oncology, 19*, 2898–2904.

Mercadante, S., Porzio, G., Ferrera, P., Fulfaro, F., Aielli, F., Verna, L., et al. (2008). Sustained-release oral morphine versus transdermal fentanyl and oral methadone in cancer pain management. *European Journal of Pain, 12*(8), 1040–1046.

Meredith, P. J., Strong, J., & Feeney, A. (2006). Adult attachment, anxiety, and pain self-efficacy as predictors of pain intensity and disability. *Pain, 123*(1–2), 146–154.

Merluzzi, T. V., & Martinez Sanchez, M. A. (1997). Perceptions of coping behaviors by persons with cancer and health providers. *Psycho-Oncology, 6*(3), 197–203.

Merluzzi, T. V., Nairn, R. C., Hedge, K., Martinez Sanchez, M. A., & Dunn, L. (2001). Self-efficacy for coping with cancer: Revision of the Cancer Behavior Inventory (version 2.0). *Psycho-Oncology, 10*(3), 206–217.

Meuser, T., Pietruck, C., Radbruch, L., Stute, P., Lehmann, K. A., Grond, S., et al. (2001). Symptoms during cancer pain treatment following WHO-guidelines: A longitudinal follow-up study of symptom prevalence, severity and etiology. *Pain, 93*(3), 247–257.

Mhaskar, R., Redzepovic, J., Wheatley, K., Clark, O. A., Miladinovic, B., Glasmaches, A., et al. (2010). Biphosphonates in multiple myeloma. *Cochrane Database of Systematic Reviews, 3*, CD003188.

Miguel, R. (2000). Interventional treatment of cancer pain: The fourth step in the World Health Organization analgesic ladder? *Cancer Control, 7*, 149–156.

Mitra, S. (2008). Opioid-induced hyperalgesia: Pathophysiology and clinical implications. *Journal of Opioid Management, 4*(3), 123–130.

Morello, C. M., Leckband, S. G., Stoner, C. P., Moorhouse, D. F., & Saragian, G. A. (1999). Randomized double-blind study comparing the efficacy of gabapentin with amitriptyline on diabetic peripheral neuropathy pain. *Archives of Internal Medicine, 159*, 1931–1937.

Morris, D. B. (2011). Narrative and pain: Towards an integrative model. In R. J. Moore (Ed.), *Handbook of pain and palliative care: Biobehavioral approaches for the life course*. New York: Springer.

Morrison, R. S., Wallenstein, S., Natale, D. K., Senzel, R. S., Huavg, L. L. (2000). "We don't carry that" – failure of pharmacies in predominantly nonwhite neighborhoods to stock opioid analgesics. *The New England Journal of Medicine, 342*, 1023–1026.

Morss, S. (2010). Evidence-based approaches to pain in advanced cancer. *Cancer Journal, 16*, 500–506.

Moryl, N., Coyle, N., Essandoh, S., & Glare, P. (2010). Chronic pain management in cancer survivors. *Journal of the National Comprehensive Cancer Network, 8*(9), 1104–1110.

Myers, J., Chan, V., Jarvis, V., & Walter-Dilks, C. (2010). Intraspinal techniques for pain management in cancer patients: A systematic review. *Supportive Care in Cancer, 18*, 137–149.

National Center for Complementary and Alternative Medicine. (2010). CAM basics. http://nccam.nih.gov/health/whatiscam/D347.pdf. Accessed on Oct 14, 2010.

National Comprehensive Cancer Network. (2009). NCCN clinical practice guidelines in oncology-adult cancer pain. http://www.nccn.org/professionals/physician_gls/f_guidelines.asp. Accessed on Oct 14, 2010.

National Comprehensive Cancer Network. (2010). *Adult Cancer Pain*, v.1.2010. www.nccn.org. Accessed on Oct 14, 2010.

Ngo Su-mien, L., Gillianne, L., Yi, G., & Penson, R. T. (2011). Hope in the context of pain and palliative care. In R. J. Moore (Ed.), *Handbook of pain and palliative care: Biobehavioral approaches for the life course*. New York: Springer.

Nicholson, A. B. (2007). Methadone for cancer pain. *Cochrane Database of Systematic Reviews*, (4), CD003971.

Nilsson, U., Unosson, M., & Rawal, N. (2005). Stress reduction and analgesia in patients exposed to calming music postoperatively: A randomized controlled trial. *European Journal of Anaesthesiology, 22*(2), 96–102.

O'Connor, A. B., & Dworkin, R. H. (2009). Treatment of neuropathic pain: An overview of recent guidelines. *The American Journal of Medicine, 122*, S22–S32.

O'Mahony, S., Goulet, J. L., & Payne, R. (2010). Psychosocial distress in patients treated for cancer pain: A prospective observational study. *Journal of Opioid Management, 6*(3), 211–222.

Oneschuk, D., & al-Shari, M. Z. (2003). The pattern of gabapentin use in a tertiary palliative care unit. *Journal of Palliative Care, 19*, 185–187.

Palermo, Y. (2011). The art of pain: The patient's perspective of chronic pain. In R. J. Moore (Ed.), *Handbook of pain and palliative care: Biobehavioral approaches for the life course*. New York: Springer.

Pappagallo, M., Shaiova, L., Perlov, E., & Knotkova, H. (2007). Difficult pain syndromes: Bone pain, visceral pain, neuropathic pain. In A. M. Berger, J. L. Shuster Jr., & J. H. Von Roenn (Eds.), *Principles and practice of palliative care and supportive oncology* (3rd ed., pp. 27–43). Philadelphia: Lippincott, Williams & Wilkins.

Pargeon, K. L., & Hailey, B. J. (1999). Barriers to effective cancer pain management: A review of the literature. *Journal of Pain and Symptom Management, 18*, 358–368.

Parson, H. A., de la Cruz, M., El Osta, B., Li, Z., Caldecon, B., Paliner, J. L., et al. (2010). Methadone initiation and rotation in the outpatient setting for patients with cancer pain. *Cancer, 116*(2), 520–528.

Passick, S. D., Olden, M., Kirsh, K. L., & Portenoy, R. K. (2007). Substance abuse issues in palliative care. In A. M. Berger, J. L. Shuster Jr., & J. H. Von Roenn (Eds.), *Principles and practice of palliative care and supportive oncology* (pp. 457–466). Philadelphia: Lippincott, Williams & Wilkins.

Pavlakis, N., Schmidt, R. L., Stockler, M. R. (2005). Biphosphonates for breast cancer. *Cochrane Database of Systematic Reviews, 3*, CD003474.

Penedo, F. J., & Dahn, J. R. (2005). Exercise and well-being: A review of mental and physical health benefits associated with physical activity. *Current Opinion in Psychiatry, 18*(2), 189–193.

Portenoy, R. K., & Lesage, P. (1999). Management of cancer pain. *Lancet, 353*(9165), 1695–1700.

Portenoy, R. K., Payne, D., & Jacobsen, P. (1999). Breakthrough pain: Characteristics and impact in patients with cancer pain. *Pain, 81*(1–2), 129–134.

Porter, L. S., Keefe, F. J., Garst, J., McBride, C. M., & Baucom, D. (2008). Self-efficacy for managing pain, symptoms, and function in patients with lung cancer and their informal caregivers: Associations with symptoms and distress. *Pain, 137*, 306–315.

Queneau, P., Navez, M., Peyron, R., & Laurent, B. (2003). Introduction à la physiopathologie de la douleur. Applications aux douleurs viscérales. *Gastroenterology & Clinical Biology, 27*(3 Suppl), S59–S67.

Quigley, C. (2005). The role of opioids in cancer pain. *Journal of the American Medical Association, 331*(7520), 825–829.

Raffa, R. B. (2001). Pharmacology of oral combination analgesics: Rational therapy for pain. *Journal of Clinical Pharmacy and Therapeutics, 26*(4), 257–264.

Reddick, B. K., Nanda, J. P., Campbell, L., Ryman, D. G., & Gaston-Johansson, F. (2005). Examining the influence of coping with pain on depression, anxiety and fatigue among women with breast cancer. *Journal of Psychosocial Oncology, 23*(2), 137–157.

Reddy, S., Hui, D., El Osta, B., de la Cruz, M., Walker, P., Palmer, J. L., et al. (2010). The effect of oral methadone on the QTc interval in advanced cancer patients: A prospective pilot study. *Journal of Palliative Medicine, 13*, 33–38.

Regan, J. M., & Peng, P. (2000). Neurophysiology of cancer pain. *Cancer Control, 7*(2), 111–119.

Rice, A. S., Maton, S., & Postherpetic Neuralgia Study Group. (2001). Gabapentin in postherpetic neuralgia: A randomised, double blind, placebo controlled study. *Pain, 94*, 215–224.

Rich, B. A. (2011). The delineation and explication of palliative options of last resort. In R. J. Moore (Ed.), *Handbook of pain and palliative care: Biobehavioral approaches for the life course*. New York: Springer.

Ripamonti, C., Fagnoni, E., Campa, T., Brunelli, C., & DeConno, F. (2006). Is the use of transdermal fentanyl inappropriate according to the WHO guidelines and the EAPC recommendations? A study of cancer patients in Italy. *Supportive Care in Cancer, 14*, 400–407.

Ripamonti, C., Groff, L., Brunelli, C., Polastri, D., Stavrakis, A., de Conno, F., et al. (1998). Switching from morphine to oral methadone in treating cancer pain: What is the equianalgesic dose ratio? *Journal of Clinical Oncology, 16*, 3216–3221.

Ripamonti, C., Zecca, E., & Bruera, E. (1997). An update on the clinical use of methadone for cancer pain. *Pain, 70*, 109–115.

Rowbotham, M., Harden, N., Stacey, B., Bernstein, P., & Magnus-Miller, L. (1998). Gabapentin for the treatment of postherpetic neuralgia: A randomized controlled trial. *Journal of the American Medical Association, 280*, 1837–1842.

Rust, G., Nembhard, W. N., Nichols, M., Omole, F., Minor, P., Barosso, G., & Mayberry, R. (2004). Racial and ethnic disparities in the provision of epidural analgesia to Georgia Medicaid beneficiaries during labor and delivery. *American Journal of Obstetrics and Gynecology, 191*, 456–462.

Schapira, L., & Steensma, D. (2011). Truth telling and palliative care. In R. J. Moore (Ed.), *Handbook of pain and palliative care: Biobehavioral approaches for the life course*. New York: Springer.

Shaheen, P. E., Walsh, D., Lasheen, W., Davis, M. P., & Lagman, R. L. (2009). Opioid equianalgesic tables: Are they all equally dangerous? *Journal of Pain and Symptom Management, 38*(3), 409–417.

Short, R., III, & Vetter, T. R. (2011). Acute to chronic pain: Transitions in the post surgical patient. In R. J. Moore (Ed.), *Handbook of pain and palliative care: Biobehavioral approaches for the life course*. New York: Springer.

Smith, H. S., Datta, S., & Manchikanti, L. (2011). Evidence-based pharmacotherapy of chronic pain. In R. J. Moore (Ed.), *Handbook of pain and palliative care: Biobehavioral approaches for the life course*. New York: Springer.

Spiegel, D., & Bloom, J. R. (1983). Pain in metastatic breast cancer. *Cancer, 52*(2), 341–345.

Spiegel, D., Sands, S., & Koopman, C. (1994). Pain and depression in patients with cancer. *Cancer, 74*(9), 2570–2578.

Stanton, A. L., Ganz, P. A., Rowland, J. H., Meyerowitz, B. E., Kruinick, J. L., Sears, S. R., et al. (2005). Promoting adjustment after treatment for cancer. *Cancer, 104*(11 Suppl), 2608–2613.

Sullivan, M. J., Thorn, B., Haythornthwaite, J. A., Gallagher, E. R., Admine, S., Jackson, V. A., et al. (2001). Theoretical perspectives on the relation of between catastrophizing and pain. *The Clinical Journal of Pain, 17*(1), 52–64.

Szucs-Reed, R. P., & Gallagher, R. M. (2011). Chronic pain and opioids. In R. J. Moore (Ed.), *Handbook of pain and palliative care: Biobehavioral approaches for the life course*. New York: Springer.

Temel, J. S., Greer, J. A., Muzikansky, A., Gallagher, E. R., Admine, S., Jackson, V. A., et al. (2010). Early palliative care for patients with metastatic non-small-cell lung cancer. *The New England Journal of Medicine, 363*(8), 733–742.

Todd, K. H., Deaton, C., D'Adamo, A. P., & Goe, L. (2000). Ethnicity and analgesic practice. *Annals of Emergency Medicine, 35*(1), 11–16.

Trescot, A. M., Boswell, M. V., Atluri, S. L., et al. (2006). Opioid guidelines in the management of chronic non-cancer pain. *Pain Physician, 9*(1), 1–39.

Turk, D. C., & Okifuji, A. (2002). Psychological factors in chronic pain: Evolution and revolution. *Journal of Consulting and Clinical Psychology, 70*(3), 678–690.

Utne, I., Miaskowski, C., Bjordal, K., Paul, S. M., Jakobsen, G., & Rustøen, T. (2009). Differences in the use of pain coping strategies between oncology inpatients with mild vs. moderate to severe pain. *Journal of Pain and Symptom Management, 38*(5), 717–726.

Van den Beuken-van Everdingen, M. H., de Rijke, J. M., Kessels, A. G., Schoten, H. C., Van Kleef, M., Patijn, J., et al. (2007). Prevalence of pain in patients with cancer: A systematic review of the past 40 years. *Annals of Oncology, 18*(9), 1437–1449.

Velikova, G., Selby, P. J., Snaith, P. R., & Kirby, P. G. (1995). The relationship of cancer pain to anxiety. *Psychotherapy and Psychosomatics, 63*(3–4), 181–184.

Ventafridda, V., Caraceni, A., Gamba, A. (1990). Field-testing of the WHO guidelines for cancer pain relief: Summary report of demonstration projects. In K. M. Foley, J. J. Bonica, V. Ventafridda (Eds.), *Advances in pain research and therapy. Proceedings of the second international congress on pain* (Vol. 16, pp. 451–464). New York: Raven Press.

Von Roenn, J. H., Cleeland, C. S., Gonin, R., Hatfield, A. K., & Pandya, K. (1993). Physician attitudes and practice in cancer pain management: A survey from the Eastern Cooperative Oncology Group. *Annals of Internal Medicine, 119*(2), 121–126.

Weissman-Fogel, I., Sprecher, E., & Pud, D. (2008). Effects of catastrophizing on pain perception and pain modulation. *Experimental Brain Research, 186*(1), 79–85.

Wilkie, D. J., & Keefe, F. J. (1991). Coping strategies of patients with lung cancer-related pain. *The Clinical Journal of Pain, 7*(4), 292–299.

World Health Organization. (1987). *Traitement de la douleur cancéreuse*. Geneva: World Health Organization.

Zabora, J., BrintzenhofeSzoc, K., Curbow, B., Hooker, C., & Piantadosi, S. (2001). The prevalence of psychological distress by cancer site. *Psycho-Oncology, 10*(1), 19–28.

Zaza, C., & Baine, N. (2002). Cancer pain and psychosocial factors: A critical review of the literature. *Journal of Pain and Symptom Management, 24*(5), 526–542.

Zech, D. F., Gron, S., Lynch, J., Hertel, D., & Lehmann, K. A. (1995). Validation of World Health Organization guidelines for cancer pain relief: A 10-year prospective study. *Pain, 63*(1), 65–76.

Zhao, Z., & Cope, D. K. (2011). Nerve blocks, trigger points, and intrathecal therapy for chronic pain. In R. J. Moore (Ed.), *Handbook of pain and palliative care: Biobehavioral approaches for the life course*. New York: Springer.

Part IV
Mechanisms

Chapter 18
Neuroanatomy of Pain and Pain Pathways

Elie D. Al-Chaer

Introduction

It may not be quite clear when the study of pain pathways began, but it is almost certain that it gained focus with the reflex theory advanced by Descartes (1664) and was rejuvenated time and again by a number of subsequent theories, such as the specificity theory (Schiff 1858), the sensory interaction theory (Noordenbos 1959) and the gate control theory (Melzack and Wall 1965). More recently, pattern and neuromatrix theories have discounted the specific function assigned to anatomic components of the nervous system (e.g., Berkley and Hubscher 1995a; Melzack 1999; Nafe 1934), particularly when it comes to pain processing; but they have been faced with challenges of their own, not the least of which is translating their theoretical framework into clinical applications. One thing we know for sure is that the perception of pain arises when neural signals originating from the terminals of nociceptors are propagated to second-order neurons in the spinal cord or brainstem, whereupon they are transmitted to specific higher-order brain areas (Price 2000). This chapter highlights recent advances in our knowledge of the pain system including our understanding of nociceptors, of the processing of nociceptive information in the spinal cord, brainstem, thalamus, and cerebral cortex and of descending pathways that modulate nociceptive activity. Some of this information might potentially lead to improvements in patient care.

Peripheral Pathways

The peripheral sensory nerves are made up of the axons of somatic and visceral sensory neurons and the connective tissue sheaths that enfold them (epineurium, perineurium, and endoneurium; Ross et al. 1995). These axons may be myelinated or unmyelinated. Large myelinated sensory axons belong to the Aβ class and are predominantly somatic, whereas small myelinated axons belong to the Aδ group and along with the unmyelinated fibers (often referred to as C fibers), they innervate

Revised and updated from "The neuroanatomy of pain pathways." In R. J. Moore PhD (Ed.), *Biobehavioral approaches to pain.* New York: Springer, 2009.

E.D. Al-Chaer, MS, PhD, JD (✉)
Center for Pain Research, Departments of Pediatrics, Internal Medicine (Gastroenterology), Neurobiology and Developmental Sciences, College of Medicine, University of Arkansas for Medical Sciences, Biomedical Research Center, Bldg. II, Suite 406-2, 4301 West Markham, Slot 842, Little Rock, AR 72205, USA
e-mail: ealchaer@uams.edu

both somatic and visceral tissues (Al-Chaer and Willis 2007). In general, only small myelinated and unmyelinated fibers are involved in pain processing; however, in some cases of peripheral neuropathy, large myelinated fibers have also been implicated (e.g., see Kajander and Bennett 1992).

Nociceptors

Sherrington defined nociceptors as sensory receptors activated by stimuli that threaten to damage or actually damage a tissue (Sherrington 1906). Nociceptors have been described in most of the structures of the body that give rise to pain sensation, including the skin, muscle, joints, and viscera (Willis and Coggeshall 2004). Some nociceptors are unresponsive to mechanical stimuli unless they are sensitized by tissue injury or inflammation. These are referred to as "silent nociceptors" (Häbler et al. 1990; Lynn and Carpenter 1982; Schaible and Schmidt 1983) and have been described in joint, cutaneous, and visceral nerves. Human studies involving microneurography and microstimulation in peripheral nerves have demonstrated that activation of nociceptors results in pain (Ochoa and Torebjörk 1989). The quality of the pain sensation depends on the tissue innervated; e.g., stimulation of cutaneous Aδ nociceptors leads to pricking pain (Konietzny et al. 1981), whereas stimulation of cutaneous C nociceptors results in burning or dull pain (Ochoa and Torebjörk 1989). However, it is important to keep in mind that pain does not always result from activation of nociceptors. Examples include cases of central pain following damage to the central nervous system (Boivie et al. 1989), functional pain residual to neonatal injury (Al-Chaer et al. 2000; Wang et al. 2008; Christianson et al. 2010) or activation of motivational-affective circuits that can also mimic pain states, particularly in patients with anxiety, neurotic depression, or hysteria (Chaturvedi 1987; Merskey 1989).

Peripheral Sensitization and Primary Hypersensitivity

Sensitization of nociceptors is commonly defined as an increase in the firing rate and a reduction in threshold of the nociceptor. In silent nociceptors, sensitization causes an "awakening" by effecting the development of spontaneous discharges and causing the receptors to become more sensitive to peripheral stimulation (Schaible and Schmidt 1985, 1988). Sensitization depends on the activation of second-messenger systems by the action of inflammatory mediators released in the damaged tissue, such as bradykinin, prostaglandins, serotonin, and histamine (Birrell et al. 1993; Davis et al. 1993; Dray et al. 1988; Schepelmann et al. 1992). A hallmark of the sensitization of peripheral nociceptors is sensory hypersensitivity classified as primary hyperalgesia or allodynia (Gold and Gebhart 2010).

Hyperalgesia is defined as an increase in the painfulness of a noxious stimulus and a reduced threshold for pain (LaMotte et al. 1983; Meyer and Campbell 1981; see Bonica 2001). Primary hyperalgesia is felt at the site of injury and is believed to be a consequence of the sensitization of nociceptors during the process of inflammation (LaMotte et al. 1982, 1983; Meyer and Campbell 1981). Allodynia is a related phenomenon in which non-noxious stimuli produce painful responses. One of the most common examples of allodynia is pain produced by lightly touching burned skin.

Primary Afferents: Somatic and Visceral

Nociceptors run in peripheral nerves as they extend toward the skin surface or other target organs in the periphery (muscles or viscera). They represent peripheral processes of dorsal root ganglion

(DRG) cells, or in the case of the head and neck, trigeminal ganglion cells. These cells are organized as groups of neurons in the peripheral nervous system and form two longitudinal chains along either side of the spinal cord (see Willis and Coggeshall 2004).

Somatic innervations of peripheral tissues follow a dermatomal distribution; however, visceral afferents innervating internal organs are broadly subdivided into splanchnic and pelvic afferents that follow the path of sympathetic and parasympathetic efferents, which project to the gut wall (see Al-Chaer and Traub 2002). Somatic afferents that innervate the striated musculature of the pelvic floor project to the sacral spinal cord via the pudendal nerve (Grundy et al. 2006). Visceral afferents have multiple receptive fields extending over a relatively wide area. Those in the serosa and mesenteric attachments respond to distortion of the viscera during distension and contraction. Other endings detect changes in the submucosal chemical milieu following injury, ischemia, or infection and may play a role in generating hypersensitivity. Intramural spinal afferent fibers have collateral branches that innervate blood vessels and enteric ganglia. These contain and release neurotransmitters during local axon reflexes that influence blood flow, motility, and secretory reflexes in the gastrointestinal tract (Maggi and Meli 1988; for a review of the neurochemistry of visceral afferents, see Al-Chaer and Traub 2002). Spinal afferents on route to the spinal cord also give off collaterals that innervate prevertebral sympathetic ganglia neurons. The same sensory information is thereby transmitted to information processing circuits in the spinal cord, enteric nervous system (ENS) and prevertebral ganglia. The main transmitters are calcitonin gene-related peptide (CGRP) and substance P, and both peptides are implicated in the induction of neurogenic inflammation (Grundy et al. 2006).

Central Pathways

Primary afferents carry sensory information from the periphery and converge onto the CNS via the dorsal roots. Their first synapse in the transmission of peripheral noxious information to the brain is in the superficial dorsal horn of the spinal cord, composed of laminae I and II (the marginal zone and substantia gelatinosa, respectively) (Sorkin and Carlton 1997). Lamina I of the spinal cord is believed to play a key role in the modulation of pain transmission; its neurons exhibit distinct response properties compared to neurons deeper in the dorsal horn (e.g., lamina V). The majority of these lamina I neurons are nociceptive-specific in their responses, a smaller number are polymodal nociceptive with an additional response to noxious cold, and a very few neurons are wide dynamic range (WDR). In lamina V the large majority are WDR, so that information transmitted from dorsal horn neurons is almost entirely nociceptive in lamina I but spans the innocuous through the noxious range in lamina V. Lamina I neurons exhibit higher thresholds for excitation and generally have smaller mechanical and heat-evoked responses and receptive fields when compared to deeper dorsal horn neurons. By contrast to lamina II, which is composed mainly of small intrinsic neurons terminating locally (Woolf and Fitzgerald 1983), lamina I neurons typically have long axons thus allowing projection to higher CNS centers (Todd 2002). The predominant ascending output from lamina I neurons appears to be the spino-parabrachial pathway in the rat (Hylden et al. 1989; Light et al. 1993; Todd 2002); however, a small proportion of lamina I neurons appears to project contralaterally via the lateral spinothalamic tract (STT), a key pathway for pain, itch, and temperature (Craig and Dostrovsky 2001; Marshall et al. 1996; Wall et al. 1988). Neurons in the deep dorsal horn (laminae V–VI), however, have predominant projections in the STT. In recent years, lamina X neurons located around the central canal have been shown to respond to somatic and visceral stimulation in the innocuous and noxious ranges (Al-Chaer et al. 1996b). Despite their morphological diversity, some of these neurons have long axons projecting in the dorsal column (DC) to the caudal medulla, specifically to the DC nuclei.

Pathways in the Ventral (Anterior) Quadrant

The Spinothalamic Tract

The STT is a major ascending pathway in primates and humans. It is classically associated with pain and temperature sensations and generally believed to mediate the sensations of pain, cold, warmth, and touch (Gybels and Sweet 1989; Willis 1985; Willis and Coggeshall 2004). This belief is based largely on the results of anterolateral cordotomies performed to relieve pain (Foerster and Gagel 1932; Spiller and Martin 1912; White and Sweet 1969) or deficits due to selective damage to the spinal cord by disease or trauma (Gowers 1878; Head and Thompson 1906; Noordenbos and Wall 1976; Spiller 1905). It is further reinforced by results of experimental studies of primates in which behavioral responses to noxious stimuli measured before and after spinal lesions were consistent with the clinical evidence (Vierck and Luck 1979; Vierck et al. 1990; Yoss 1953).

The STT arises largely from neurons in the dorsal horn of the spinal cord and projects to various areas in the thalamus (see Willis and Coggeshall 2004). The locations of the cells of origin of the STT have been mapped in the rat, cat, and monkey using retrograde tracing (Apkarian and Hodge 1989a, b; Carstens and Trevino 1978; Craig et al. 1989; Giesler et al. 1979; Kevetter and Willis 1982; Willis et al. 1979) and antidromic activation methods (Albe-Fessard et al. 1974a, b; Giesler et al. 1976; Trevino et al. 1972, 1973). In monkeys, a large fraction of STT cells is located in the lumbar and sacral enlargements, and these cells are concentrated in the marginal zone and neck of the dorsal horn in laminae I and IV–VI (Apkarian and Hodge 1989a; Willis et al. 1979). However, some spinothalamic cells are located in other laminae, including lamina X, which is around the central canal, and in the ventral horn. Tracing studies demonstrate that the STT distributes projections to several thalamic nuclei and that each have different anatomical and functional associations and, conversely, that the STT originates in several different cell groups that each have different anatomical and functional characteristics (Albe-Fessard et al. 1985; Apkarian and Hodge 1989a–c; Boivie 1979; Burton and Craig 1983; Craig et al. 1989; Le Gros Clark 1936; Mantyh 1983; Mehler et al. 1960; Willis et al. 1979). Comparison of the populations of STT cells projecting to the lateral thalamus, including the ventral posterior lateral (VPL) nucleus, and those projecting to the medial thalamus, including the central lateral (CL) nucleus, show clear differences between the two (Craig and Zhang 2006; Willis et al. 1979). Laterally projecting STT neurons are more likely to be situated in laminae I and V, whereas medially projecting cells are more likely to be situated in the deep dorsal horn and in the ventral horn. Most of the cells project to the contralateral thalamus, although a small fraction project ipsilaterally.

As a general rule, the axons of STT neurons decussate through the ventral white commissure at a very short distance from the cell body (Willis et al. 1979). They initially enter the ventral funiculus and then shift into the lateral funiculus as they ascend. Axons from STT cells of lamina I ascend more dorsally in the lateral funiculus than do the axons of STT cells in deeper layers of the dorsal horn (Apkarian and Hodge 1989b). Clinical evidence from anterolateral cordotomies indicates that spinothalamic axons in the anterolateral quadrant of the spinal cord are arranged somatotopically. At cervical levels, spinothalamic axons representing the lower extremity and caudal body are placed more laterally and those representing the upper extremity and rostral body more anteromedially (Hyndman and Van Epps 1939; Walker 1940). Recordings from spinothalamic axons in monkeys are consistent with this scheme (Applebaum et al. 1975).

In primates, STT axon terminals exist in the following nuclei: the caudal and oral parts of the VPL nucleus (VPLc and VPLo) (Olszewski 1952), the ventral posterior inferior (VPI) nucleus, the medial part of the posterior complex (POm), the CL nucleus, the ventral medial nucleus, and other intralaminar and medial thalamic nuclei (Apkarian and Hodge 1989c; Apkarian and Shi 1994;

Berkley 1980; Boivie 1979; Craig et al. 1994; Gingold et al. 1991; Kerr 1975; Mantyh 1983; Mehler et al. 1960; Mehler 1962).

Primate STT cells that project to the lateral thalamus generally have receptive fields on a restricted area of the contralateral skin (Willis et al. 1974). Cells that project to the region of the CL nucleus in the medial thalamus may also collateralize to the lateral thalamus; these cells have response properties identical to those of STT cells that project just to the lateral thalamus (Giesler et al. 1981), except for their larger receptive fields. Most of the neurons show their best responses when the skin is stimulated mechanically at a noxious intensity. However, many STT cells also respond to innocuous mechanical stimuli or noxious heating of the skin (Chung et al. 1979; Craig et al. 1994; Ferrington et al. 1987; Kenshalo et al. 1979; Price and Mayer 1975; Price et al. 1978; Surmeier et al. 1986a, b; Willis et al. 1974). Some spinothalamic neurons respond to stimulation of receptors in muscle (Foreman et al. 1979), joints (Dougherty et al. 1992), or viscera (Al-Chaer et al. 1999; Ammons et al. 1985; Ammons 1989a, b; Blair et al. 1982, 1984; Milne et al. 1981).

These observations clearly suggest that the STT comprises several distinct components that each convey ascending activity selectively associated with different spinal functions (Craig and Zhang 2006; Craig et al. 1989; Klop et al. 2005; Stepniewska et al. 2003; Truitt et al. 2003). Whether these distinct components imply segregated functions vis-à-vis the processing of pain information within the STT remains uncertain.

Several other pathways accompany the STT in the white matter of the ventrolateral quadrant of the spinal cord. These include the spinomesencephalic tract, the spinoreticular tracts, and several spino-limbic tracts. For a detailed review of these pathways, see Willis and Coggeshall (2004) and Willis and Westlund (1997).

Pathways in the Dorsal (Posterior) Quadrant

A number of pathways believed to be involved in pain processing originate in the dorsal horn and have axons that project in the dorsolateral and dorsal white matter of the spinal cord; these include the spinocervical pathway and the postsynaptic DC.

Spinocervical Pathway

The spinocervical pathway originates from neurons in the spinal cord dorsal horn and relays in the lateral cervical nucleus in segments C1 and C2 (reviewed in Willis 1985; Willis and Coggeshall 2004). The axons of neurons of the lateral cervical nucleus decussate and then ascend with the medial lemniscus to the thalamus (Ha 1971). A lateral cervical nucleus has been identified in several species, including rat, cat, and monkey (see Mizuno et al. 1967). A comparable nucleus has been observed in at least some human spinal cords (Truex et al. 1965).

In cats, the cells of origin are situated mostly in lamina IV, although some are situated in adjacent laminae of the dorsal horn and in deeper layers (Brown et al. 1980; Craig 1978). The axons of spinocervical tract neurons ascend in the dorsal part of the lateral funiculus to the upper cervical level (Nijensohn and Kerr 1975) and terminate in the lateral cervical nucleus. Cervicothalamic neurons project to the contralateral VPL nucleus and the medial part of the posterior complex (Berkley 1980; Boivie 1979; Smith and Apkarian 1991). Many of the cells also give off collaterals to the midbrain (Willis and Coggeshall 2004). Some spinocervical tract cells respond to noxious stimuli, both in cats (Brown and Franz 1969; Cervero et al. 1977) and in monkeys (Bryan et al. 1974; Downie et al. 1988); therefore, the spinocervical is considered a potential pathway through which nociceptive signals can reach the lateral thalamus.

The Dorsal Column

The dorsal funiculus, also referred to as the DC in animals or the posterior column in man, contains collateral branches of primary afferent fibers that ascend from the dorsal root entry level all the way to the medulla (Willis and Coggeshall 2004). In addition, it contains the ascending axons of tract cells of the dorsal horn (Angaut-Petit 1975a, b; Petit 1972; Rustioni 1973; Uddenburg 1966, 1968). These tract cells form the postsynaptic dorsal column (PSDC) pathway, which along with primary afferent axons, travel in the DC and synapse in the DC nuclei. The dorsal funiculus is subdivided into two components known as the fasciculus gracilis, containing the ascending afferents from levels caudal to the mid-thoracic region, and the fasciculus cuneatus, containing the ascending afferents that originate from mid-thoracic to upper cervical levels. The gracilis and cuneatus fasciculi terminate at the level of the lower medulla in the nucleus gracilis and the nucleus cuneatus respectively, collectively known as the DC nuclei.

Classical teaching holds that the DC subserves graphesthesia, two-point discrimination, and kinesthesia. This concept was adopted at the turn of the twentieth century (Brown-Sequard 1868; Head and Thompson 1906; Stanley 1840; see also Davidoff 1989) and was based on the pathologic alterations observed in certain disease states associated with DC lesions and on the skimpy knowledge of spinal tracts available at that time. On the other hand, the evidence for the importance of the DC pathway in the transmission of visceral nociceptive information is compelling. It rests on studies which highlight the great effectiveness of limited midline myelotomy in reducing intractable pelvic cancer pain in humans (Gildenberg and Hirshberg 1984; Hirshberg et al. 1996; Hitchcock 1970, 1974; Schwarcz 1976, 1978) and on a number of ground-breaking experimental observations (Al-Chaer et al. 1996a, b, 1998a, b, 1999; see also Willis et al. 1999).

In an early report on visceral nociceptive fibers in the DC, awaken human subjects experienced unbearable, excruciating pain when the DC or medial aspect of the nucleus gracilis was probed mechanically (Foerster and Gagel 1932). The pain was referred to the sacral region and perineum. Subsequent studies observed that the sensation of visceral distension was retained following extensive anterolateral cordotomy (White 1943) and that the sensation of duodenal distension was unaffected by a differential spinal block which abolished the sensation of cutaneous pinprick (Sarnoff et al. 1948) suggesting that these sensations were mediated by a posterior column pathway.

More direct clinical evidence comes from successful neurosurgical procedures aimed at treating intractable visceral pain. These procedures have often accidentally severed DC axons in and around the midline. Commissural myelotomy was introduced as a technique to produce bilateral analgesia by interrupting the decussating axons of the spinothalamic and spinoreticular tracts by means of a longitudinal midline incision extending over several segments (Armour 1927). The rostro-caudal extent of commissural myelotomy was later reduced to a localized lesion made stereotaxically by inserting a metal electrode into the midline at the C1 level with the patient awake (Hitchcock 1970, 1974; Schwarcz 1976, 1978). The clinical result was an unexpectedly widespread distribution of pain relief, similar to that found with open commissural myelotomy, despite the small extent of the lesion and its location well rostral to the decussation of most of the STT. Similar successes were reported later using limited midline myelotomy to treat pelvic visceral cancer pain (Gildenberg and Hirshberg 1984). This result compelled a major revision in thinking regarding pain pathways in the spinal cord (Gybels and Sweet 1989). Hirshberg et al. (1996) reported eight clinical cases where pelvic visceral cancer pain was successfully treated using a limited posterior midline myelotomy. The lesion was placed in the midline at the T10 level of the spinal cord and extended a few mm rostrocaudally. Following surgery the pelvic pain was found to be markedly reduced or eliminated without any demonstrable postoperative neurological deficit. The extent of the lesion in one of the patients was examined histologically postmortem and was found to interrupt axons of the posterior columns at and adjacent to the midline and anteriorly to the level of the posterior gray commissure. More recent studies have lent further support for the concept that neurosurgical interruption of a midline posterior column pathway provides significant pain relief without causing adverse neurological sequelae in cancer patients with visceral pain refractory to other therapies (Kim and Kwon 2000; Nauta et al. 1997, 2000).

Early experimental evidence that described the DC as the pathway of splanchnic afferents was obtained in rabbits, cats, and dogs (Amassian 1951) and led to the conclusion that the sense of visceral distension may be dependent on the integrity of this afferent projection system. Responses to splanchnic nerve stimulation were recorded "in logical time relationships," in the ipsilateral fasciculus gracilis of the spinal cord, in the ipsilateral nucleus gracilis, in the region of decussation of the medial lemniscus, in the medial lemniscus at various levels in the medulla, pons, and caudal thalamus, and in the VPL nucleus of the thalamus, suggesting a continuous pathway for splanchnic input that "parallels that for proprioception from the limbs and trunk" (Aidar et al. 1952). Nociceptive activity, including responses to uterine and vaginal distension, has also been demonstrated in neurons of the DC nuclei (Angaut-Petit 1975a, b; Berkley and Hubscher 1995a, b; Cliffer et al. 1992; Ferrington et al. 1988). These nociceptive responses could be triggered by unmyelinated primary afferent fibers that have been shown to ascend in the dorsal column directly to the DC nuclei (Conti et al. 1990; Patterson et al. 1989, 1990). Alternatively, they could be mediated through the PSDC pathway (Bennett et al. 1983, 1984; Noble and Riddell 1988; Uddenburg 1968). More recent studies in primates and rodents have shown that a lesion of the DC can dramatically reduce the responses of neurons in the VPL nucleus of the thalamus (Al-Chaer et al. 1996a, 1998a; Feng et al. 1998; Ness 2000) and in the DC nuclei (Al-Chaer et al. 1996b, 1999; Berkley and Hubscher 1995a) to mechanical distension of normal and acutely inflamed colons. These studies have identified the DC as being more important in visceral nociceptive transmission than the spinothalamic and spinoreticular tracts. In rats and monkeys, colorectal distension stimulates the firing of viscerosensitive VPL thalamic neurons. After a DC lesion at T10 level, the responses are reduced despite ongoing stimulation. A similar lesion of the STT at T10 does not achieve the same effect (Al-Chaer et al. 1996a, 1998a). The DC also has a role in signaling epigastric nociception (Feng et al. 1998; see Willis et al. 1999).

The correspondence between these functional studies in experimental animals and the findings from human neurosurgical studies is consistent with accumulating evidence that strongly supports the concept that the DC projection system is critical for visceral pain sensation.

Postsynaptic Dorsal Column Pathway

The PSDC pathway arises from cells distributed medial to laterally in lamina III in the dorsal horn, as well as from a few cells just lateral to lamina X (Bennett et al. 1983; Giesler et al. 1984; Rustioni 1973, 1974, 1979). The trajectories of PSDC fibers are somatotopically organized in the DC (Cliffer and Giesler 1989; Hirshberg et al. 1996; Wang et al. 1999).

Although the PSDC pathway may not have a role in cutaneous pain (Al-Chaer et al. 1996b, 1999; Giesler and Cliffer 1985), the PSDC cells in rats and monkeys were shown to respond to both mechanical and chemical irritation of viscera (Al-Chaer et al. 1996b, 1999). They receive inputs from the colon, the ureter, the pancreas, and epigastric structures (see Willis et al. 1999). Presumably, the visceral information is relayed together with cutaneous epicritic information in the medial lemniscus to the thalamus (Willis and Westlund 1997). An illustration of the STT and the PSDC trajectories in the spinal cord to the thalamus can be seen in Fig. 18.1.

Representation of Nociceptive Sensation in the Brain

In contrast to most other sensory modalities, the neuroanatomical substrates in the brain for pain sensation in general and visceral pain in particular, have only recently begun to be elucidated. Major advances in this field have come through functional anatomical and physiological studies in

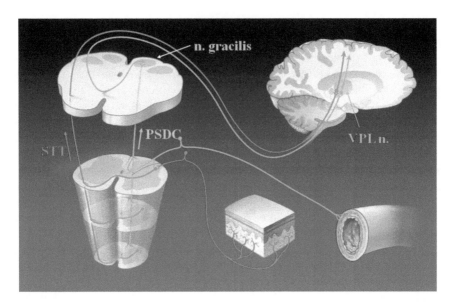

Fig. 18.1 Pain pathways. Illustration of the postsynaptic dorsal column (PSDC) and the spinothalamic tract (STT) as they arise in the dorsal horn of the spinal cord and ascend towards the brainstem and eventually the thalamus. The PSDC pathway synapses on neurons in the dorsal column nuclei (DCN; the nucleus gracilis is labeled); axons of DCN neurons subsequently cross the midline and ascend in the medial lemniscus to converge onto thalamic neurons. The axons of STT neurons cross the midline at the dorsal horn level and ascend to the VPL nucleus of the thalamus in the anterolateral quadrant of the cord. Peripheral input is shown from the colon mainly onto the PSDC pathway and from the skin mainly onto the STT to illustrate the relative importance of these pathways in the nociception arising from these tissues respectively

nonhuman primates and rats, which have identified substrates that underlie findings from functional imaging and microelectrode studies in humans.

Thalamic Representation of Pain

Electrophysiological recordings made of nociceptive responses in the VPL and ventral posteromedial (VPM) nuclei of the thalamus in rats and monkeys by many investigators showed that neurons in these thalamic nuclei can be activated by nociceptive stimulation of the periphery (Al-Chaer et al. 1996a; Apkarian and Shi 1994; Brüggemann et al. 1994; Bushnell and Duncan 1987; Bushnell et al. 1993; Casey and Morrow 1983, 1987; Chandler et al. 1992; Chung et al. 1986; Duncan et al. 1993; Gaze and Gordon 1954; Kenshalo et al. 1980; Pollin and Albe-Fessard 1979; Yokota et al. 1988).

In general, responses of nociceptive neurons in the VPL nucleus to innocuous cutaneous mechanical stimuli are weak, in contrast to their responses to noxious mechanical stimuli (Casey and Morrow 1983, 1987; Chung et al. 1986; Kenshalo et al. 1980). The location of the neurons in the VPL nucleus is somatotopic but their receptive fields are relatively small and situated on the contralateral side. Almost all of the VPL neurons tested were shown by antidromic activation to project to the primary somatosensory cortex (SI) (Kenshalo et al. 1980). Surprisingly, most neurons (85%) in the VPL nucleus respond to both cutaneous and visceral stimuli (Al-Chaer et al. 1996a, 1998b; Brüggemann et al. 1994; Chandler et al. 1992). Although the cutaneous input is somatotopic, the visceral input is not viscerotopic (Brüggemann et al. 1994).

Investigations of visceral inputs into the thalamus were made using electrical stimulation of visceral nerves (Aidar et al. 1952; Dell and Olson 1951; McLeod 1958; Patton and Amassian 1951) or natural stimulation of visceral organs (Chandler et al. 1992; Davis and Dostrovsky 1988; Emmers 1966; Rogers et al. 1979). In monkeys, the medial thalamus receives viscerosomatic input via thoracic STT neurons (Ammons et al. 1985), whereas neurons in the lateral thalamus are activated by input through the STT and the DC (Al-Chaer et al. 1998a). Lateral thalamic neurons can also be excited by colorectal distension or urinary bladder distension and by convergent input elicited by noxious stimulation of somatic receptive fields in proximal lower body regions (Chandler et al. 1992). In fact, the majority of lateral thalamic somatosensory neurons in squirrel monkeys receive somatovisceral and viscero-visceral inputs from naturally stimulated visceral organs (Brüggemann et al. 1994). In the rat, neurons in and near the thalamic ventrobasal complex respond to stimulation of different visceral organs, including the uterus, the cervix, the vagina, and the colon (Al-Chaer et al. 1996a; Berkley et al. 1993). Colorectal distension or colon inflammation excites neurons in the ventral posterolateral nucleus of thalamus (Al-Chaer et al. 1996a; Berkley et al. 1993; Brüggemann et al. 1994) and in the medial thalamus at the level of the nucleus submedius (Kawakita et al. 1997).

Microstimulation in the region of the thalamic principal sensory nucleus (the ventrocaudal nucleus) – a nucleus that corresponds to the ventral posterior nucleus in the cat and the monkey (Hirai and Jones 1989; Jones 1985) – can evoke a sensation of angina in humans (Lenz et al. 1994) and trigger in some cases pain "memories" (Davis et al. 1995). Electrical stimulation of the thalamic ventrobasal complex in animals inhibits viscerosensory processing in normal rats but facilitates visceral hypersensitivity in rats with neonatal colon pain (Saab et al. 2004). These observations coupled with an extensive repertoire of experimental data suggest that the thalamus, particularly the posterolateral nucleus, is involved in the processing of visceral information, including both noxious and innocuous visceral inputs.

Nociceptive neurons also exist in the VPI and POm nuclei (Casey and Morrow 1987; Apkarian and Shi 1994; Pollin and Albe-Fessard 1979). The cutaneous receptive fields of neurons in the VPI nucleus are somatotopically organized but tend to be larger than those of the VPL nociceptive neurons and presumably project to the secondary somatosensory cortex (SII) (Friedman et al. 1986). The cells studied in the monkey POm nucleus had small, contralateral nociceptive receptive fields. The POm nucleus projects to the retroinsular cortex in monkeys (Burton and Jones 1976).

Cortical Pain Processing

Anatomical, physiological, and lesion data implicate multiple cortical regions in the complex experience of pain (Kenshalo et al. 1988; White and Sweet 1969). These regions include primary and secondary somatosensory cortices, anterior cingulate cortex, insular cortex, and regions of the frontal cortex. Nevertheless, the role of different cortical areas in pain processing remains controversial. Studies of cortical lesions and cortical stimulation in humans did not uncover a clear role of various cortical areas in the pain experience and more recent human brain-imaging studies are not always consistent in revealing pain-related activation of somatosensory areas (see Bushnell et al. 1999). Despite this controversy, the application of functional magnetic resonance imaging (fMRI) and positron emission tomography (PET) has identified a network of brain areas that process painful sensation from a number of somatic regions including chronic pain states (see Apkarian et al. 2005; Matre and Tran 2009; Peyron et al. 2000; Veldhuijzen et al. 2007) and from a number of visceral organs such as the esophagus (Aziz et al. 1997), stomach (Ladabaum et al. 2001), and the anorectum (Hobday et al. 2001). Results of these studies show activation of the primary somatosensory cortex (SI) by a range of noxious stimuli. These studies also confirm the somatotopic organization of SI pain responses, thus supporting the role of SI in pain localization. Other imaging data that implicate SI in the sensory aspect of pain perception note that S1 activation is modulated by cognitive manipulations that alter perceived pain intensity but not by manipulations that alter unpleasantness, independent of pain intensity (Baliki et al. 2006).

Visceral sensation, on the other hand, is primarily represented in the secondary somatosensory cortex (SII). Unlike somatic sensation, which has a strong homuncular representation in SI, visceral representations in the primary somatosensory cortex are vague and diffuse (Aziz et al. 1997). This might account for visceral sensation being poorly localized in comparison with somatic sensation. Nevertheless, visceral sensation is represented in paralimbic and limbic structures (e.g., anterior insular cortex, amygdala, anterior and posterior cingulate cortex), and prefrontal and orbitofrontal cortices (Mertz et al. 2000; Silverman et al. 1997), areas that purportedly process the affective and cognitive components of visceral sensation (Derbyshire 2003).

Differential cortical activation is also seen when comparing sensation from the visceral and somatic regions of the gastrointestinal tract, for example, sensations from the esophagus vs. the anterior chest wall (Strigo et al. 2003) or the rectum vs. the anal canal (Hobday et al. 2001). Brain processing for esophageal and anterior chest wall sensations occurs in a common brain network consisting of secondary somatosensory and parietal cortices, thalamus, basal ganglia, and cerebellum (Strigo et al. 2003). Yet, differential processing of sensory information from these two areas occurred within the insular, primary sensory, motor, anterior cingulate, and prefrontal cortices. These findings are consistent with other studies which highlight similarities in the visceral and somatic pain experience and might also explain the individual's ability to distinguish between the two modalities and generate differential emotional, autonomic, and motor responses when each modality is individually stimulated.

Descending Modulatory Pathways

In addition to the afferent pathways that process nociceptive signals at different levels of the neuraxis, pain processing involves a number of modulatory controls that exist throughout the nervous system and function to enhance or dampen the intensity of the original signal or to modify its quality. At the level of the spinal cord input from non-nociceptive and nociceptive afferent pathways can interact to modulate transmission of nociceptive information to higher brain centers. In addition, the brain contains modulatory systems that affect the conscious perception of sensory stimuli. Spinal nociceptive transmission is subject to descending modulatory influences from supraspinal structures e.g., periaqueductal gray, nucleus raphe magnus, locus coeruleus, nuclei reticularis gigantocellularis, and the ventrobasal complex of the thalamus (see Besson and Chaouch 1987; Hodge et al. 1986; Light 1992; Peng et al. 1996b; Willis 1982). Descending modulation can be inhibitory, facilitatory or both depending on the context of the stimulus or the intensity of the descending signal (Saab et al. 2004; Zhuo and Gebhart 2002). The descending influence from the ventromedial medulla is mediated mainly by pathways traveling in the dorsolateral spinal cord (Zhuo and Gebhart 2002) and can be inhibitory or facilitatory based on stimulus intensity. In contrast, descending control from the thalamus is context-specific in that it may facilitate or inhibit spinal nociceptive processing depending upon the presence or absence of central sensitization (Saab et al. 2004). For instance, serotonergic (Peng et al. 1995), noradrenergic (Peng et al. 1996a; Proudfit 1992), and to a lesser extent dopaminergic projections are major components of descending modulatory pathways (Dahlström and Fuxe 1964, 1965), in addition to a major role played by opiates and enkephalins (Duggan and North 1984; Duggan et al. 1977).

Molecular Pathways

The activity of nociceptors can be affected by adequate stimuli, such as strong mechanical, thermal, or chemical stimuli (see Willis 1985; Willis and Coggeshall 2004), and also by chemical actions on surface membrane receptors of their axons. A battery of chemical mediators, including biogenic amines (such as glutamate, [gamma]-aminobutyric acid (GABA), histamine, serotonin, norepinephrine) (Dray et al. 1994; McRoberts et al. 2001), opiates (Joshi et al. 2000; Su et al. 1997), purines, prostanoids, proteases, cytokines, and other peptides (such as bradykinin, substance P, and CGRP) act in a promiscuous manner on a range of receptors expressed upon any one sensory ending (Kirkup et al. 2001).

Three distinct processes are involved in the actions of these substances on afferent nerves. First, by direct activation of receptors coupled to the opening of ion channels present on nerve terminals, the terminals are depolarized and firing of impulses is initiated. Second, by sensitization that develops in the absence of direct stimulation and results in hyperexcitability to both chemical and mechanical modalities, e.g., opiate receptors are ineffective in modulating the normal activity of joint nociceptors, but they were shown to become effective after the development of inflammation (Stein 1994). Sensitization may also involve postreceptor signal transduction that includes G-protein coupled alterations in second-messenger systems which in turn lead to phosphorylation of membrane receptors and ion channels that control excitability of the afferent endings. Third, by genetic changes in the phenotype of mediators, channels, and receptors expressed by the afferent nerve, for example after peripheral nerve injury, many afferent fibers express newly formed adrenoreceptors (Bossut and Perl 1995; Campbell et al. 1992; Sato and Perl 1991; Xie et al. 1995). A change in the ligand-binding characteristics or coupling efficiency of these newly expressed receptors could alter the sensitivity of the afferent terminals. Neurotrophins, in particular nerve growth factor and glial-derived neurotropic factor, influence different populations of visceral afferents and play an important role in adaptive responses to nerve injury and inflammation (McMahon 2004; Bielefeldt et al. 2006).

Ion channels on nociceptors act as molecular transducers that depolarize these neurons, thereby setting off nociceptive impulses along the pain pathways (Price 2000; Costigan and Woolf 2000). Among these ion channels are the members of the transient receptor potential (TRP) family, activated by changes in temperature and extracellular pH and the presence of vanilloid ligands, such as capsaicin and mustard oil (Woolf and Ma 2007). The thermosensitive TRP family constitutes an interface with the environment and includes a number of diverse channels, each with a distinct thermal threshold and a different set of chemical activators. To date, the most studied member of the TRP family is the TRPV1 receptor (Di Marzo et al. 2002; Cortright and Szallasi 2004). Activation of primary afferents can also be brought about by other types of ion channels, including the degenerin epithelial sodium channel (ENaC) family (Kellenberger and Schild 2002; Price et al. 2001) and the acid-sensing ion channel (ASIC) family, of which ASIC3 has been implicated in the perception of noxious mechanical stimulation in mammals (Mogil et al. 2005). Tissue damage also results in the release of high concentrations of ATP, which can act on ligand-gated purinergic P2X channels and P2Y receptors to activate nociceptors (Khakh and North 2006).

Voltage-gated sodium channels (VGSCs) are also critical for the initiation of action potentials in the peripheral terminals of nociceptors and conduction along axons in peripheral nerves to the spinal cord. VGSCs allow sodium ion influx in response to local membrane depolarization, such as the potential generated in the peripheral terminals of nociceptors (Cummins et al. 2007). Different roles have been attributed to each sodium channel in influencing neuronal excitability, often associated with expression in specific subclasses of DRG neurons.

In the CNS, the central axon terminals of primary afferent neurons release neurotransmitters in the dorsal horn of the spinal cord. Like most neurons in the CNS, $A\delta$ and C fiber nociceptors use glutamate as their fast neurotransmitter. Glutamate binds to ionotropic α-amino-3-hydroxy-5-methyl-4-isoxazolepropionic acid (AMPA) and N-methyl-D-aspartic acid (NMDA) receptors, as well as to metabotropic glutamate receptors expressed in the dorsal horn. AMPA receptors produce fast excitatory postsynaptic potentials that signal the onset, intensity, duration, and location of peripheral noxious stimulation. More-intense or sustained activation of C fiber nociceptors also results in the release of neuropeptide neuromodulators, such as substance P and the calcitonin-gene-related peptide (CGRP), which produce slow synaptic potentials via the neurokinin 1 receptor (NK1R) and the CGRP-1 and CGRP-2 receptors, respectively. The presence of these peptides enables considerable use-dependent functional plasticity in the control of pain transmission, since their release typically follows high-intensity stimulation (Schaible 2004; for a review, see Bingham et al. 2009).

Presynaptic voltage-gated calcium channels, such as CaV2.2, contribute substantially to controlling neurotransmitter release from synaptic vesicles in the dorsal horn. Neurotransmitter release is also regulated by presynaptic inhibition produced by the neurotransmitter γ-aminobutyric acid (GABA) acting on $GABA_A$ ion channels and $GABA_B$ receptors. Other presynaptic inhibitory receptors include the cannabinoid receptor 1 (CB1) and the three opioid receptors μ, δ, and κ. GABA also induces postsynaptic inhibition in dorsal horn neurons comparable to that caused by the neurotransmitter glycine (Woolf and Salter 2000). Each of the elements involved in the regulation of spinal neurotransmitter release constitutes potential targets for pain pharmacotherapy.

Multiple molecular mechanisms have been associated with producing the sensation of pain many of which have been largely developed through the use of genetic manipulations. These signaling pathways involve many molecular components that could potentially be targets for pharmacotherapeutic intervention, but the complexity of these systems might also mean that multiple sites must be affected simultaneously to disrupt propagation of pain signals or restore homeostatic conditions. This makes the idea of a "silver bullet" for the treatment of pain all the more challenging.

Gender Differences in Pain Processing

Gender differences are a hallmark of pain perception, particularly visceral pain; however, little is known about the biological causes of these differences (Fillingim 2000; Keogh 2009, see also Keogh 2011). Recent studies have shown that estrogen receptors located on nociceptive neurons in the spinal cord play an important role in the sexually differentiated responses of these neurons to nociceptive visceral stimuli (Al-Chaer, unpublished observations). Similarly gender differences have been reported in the cortical representation of pain. Activation in the sensory–motor and parieto-occipital areas is common in both males and females following rectal distension; however, greater activation in the anterior cingulate/prefrontal cortices has been found in women (Kern et al. 2001). These actual gender differences in the processing of sensory input substantiate reports that perceptual responses are exaggerated in female patients with chronic pain.

Conclusion

It is important to keep in mind that these pathways, while seemingly anatomically segregated and traditionally perceived as conveying specific perceptions of pain, are in fact functionally dynamic, interactive polymodal channels for visceral, cutaneous, muscular and proprioceptive sensations, in addition to possible motor, autonomic and not as yet defined functions. As such, the STT as well as the DC can be regarded as interactive polymodal channels for visceral, somatic, and autonomic events with sorted priorities for the sake of immediate, reliable, and simple readings of acute and transient but complex situations. These breakthroughs in defining pain mechanisms and pathways have advanced the field of pain research and management particularly in the areas of drug development. However, despite these extraordinarily impressive scientific advances in our understanding of the mechanisms of pain and describing some of its pathways, the field is beset by similarly and equally impressive stalemates and retreats in the actual management and cure of pain. After all, knowledge about pain and its mechanisms is only useful to the extent it helps the sufferer.

For pain relief, we naturally use anything that works; historically we used trephination, opiates, and willow bark. Today, regardless of their site of action, we continue to use some of the same techniques that worked albeit in different pharmaceutical formulae and more controlled environments… but the nervous system seems to be extremely resistant to switching off pain!

Future Directions

Translational research in the immediate and extended future can be expected to maintain ongoing progress in each of the following areas:

1. Continued mechanistic focus on the basic science of pain that includes the molecular basis for peripheral sensitization of sensory receptors by inflammatory mediators, selectivity of central pain-related transmission pathways, and higher-order central processing of nociceptive information from the periphery.
2. Integration of imaging technology and classic neurophysiological and neuropharmacological approaches for improved understanding of the neurobiology of pain.
3. Expanded investigation of the psychoneuroendocrine pathways, which are not only responsible for alteration of function during psychogenic stress and the exacerbation of chronic pain states, but which also may be partly responsible for gender differences in pain.
4. Enhanced focus on the identification of drug targets on neuronal elements of the nervous system and on non-neuronal cell types, such as glia, which release substances that alter the activity of neurons.
5. More attention to individual differences in pain reporting and efficacy of management in addition to novel phenotype-directed approaches to pain study and treatment.

However, given the immediate need for pain relief in severe conditions refractory to conventional treatment and the reported success, albeit anecdotal, of many alternative and complementary therapies, focused research on the mechanisms of these therapies is likely to yield beneficial results in the immediate future.

Acknowledgments The author would like to thank Ms. Kirsten Garner for assistance with editing the manuscript. This work was supported by NIH Grants DK077733, DK081628.

References

Aidar, O., Geohegan, W. A., & Ungewitter, L. H. (1952). Splanchnic afferent pathways in the central nervous system. *Journal of Neurophysiology, 15*, 131–138.
Albe-Fessard, D., Berkley, K. J., Kruger, L., Ralston, H. J., & Willis, W. D. (1985). Diencephalic mechanisms of pain sensation. *Brain Research Reviews, 9*, 217–296.
Albe-Fessard, D., Levante, A., & Lamour, Y. (1974a). Origin of spinothalamic and spinoreticular pathways in cats and monkeys. *Advances in Neurology, 4*, 157–166.
Albe-Fessard, D., Levante, A., & Lamour, Y. (1974b). Origin of spino-thalamic tract in monkeys. *Brain Research, 65*, 503–509.

Al-Chaer, E. D., Feng, Y., & Willis, W. D. (1998a). A role for the dorsal column in nociceptive visceral input into the thalamus of primates. *Journal of Neurophysiology, 79*, 3143–3150.

Al-Chaer, E. D., Feng, Y., & Willis, W. D. (1998b). Visceral pain: A disturbance in the sensorimotor continuum? *Pain Forum, 7*(3), 117–125.

Al-Chaer, E. D., Feng, Y., & Willis, W. D. (1999). A comparative study of viscerosomatic input onto postsynaptic dorsal column and spinothalamic tract neurons in the primate. *Journal of Neurophysiology, 82*(4), 1876–1882.

Al-Chaer, E. D., Kawasaki, M., & Pasricha, P. J. (2000). A new model of chronic visceral hypersensitivity in adult rats induced by colon irritation during postnatal development. *Gastroenterology, 119*(5), 1276–1285.

Al-Chaer, E. D., Lawand, N. B., Westlund, K. N., & Willis, W. D. (1996a). Visceral nociceptive input into the ventral posterolateral nucleus of the thalamus: A new function for the dorsal column pathway. *Journal of Neurophysiology, 76*, 2661–2674.

Al-Chaer, E. D., Lawand, N. B., Westlund, K. N., & Willis, W. D. (1996b). Pelvic visceral input into the nucleus gracilis is largely mediated by the postsynaptic dorsal column pathway. *Journal of Neurophysiology, 76*, 2675–2690.

Al-Chaer, E. D., & Traub, R. J. (2002). Biological basis of visceral pain: Recent developments. *Pain, 96*(3), 221–225.

Al-Chaer, E. D., & Willis, W. D. (2007). Neuroanatomy of visceral pain: Pathways and processes. In P. J. Pasricha, W. D. Willis, & G. F. Gebhart (Eds.), *Chronic abdominal and visceral pain: Theory and practice*. New York: Informa Health Care Inc.

Amassian, V. E. (1951). Fiber groups and spinal pathways of cortically represented visceral afferents. *Journal of Neurophysiology, 14*, 445–460.

Ammons, W. S. (1989a). Primate spinothalamic cell responses to ureteral occlusion. *Brain Research, 496*, 124–130.

Ammons, W. S. (1989b). Electrophysiological characteristics of primate spinothalamic neurons with renal and somatic inputs. *Journal of Neurophysiology, 60*, 1121–1130.

Ammons, W. S., Girardot, M. N., & Foreman, R. D. (1985). T2-T5 spinothalamic neurons projecting to medial thalamus with viscerosomatic input. *Journal of Neurophysiology, 54*, 73–89.

Angaut-Petit, D. (1975a). The dorsal column system: I. Existence of long ascending postsynaptic fibres in the cat's fasciculus gracilis. *Experimental Brain Research, 22*, 457–470.

Angaut-Petit, D. (1975b). The dorsal column system: II. Functional properties and bulbar relay of the postsynaptic fibres of the cat's fasciculus gracilis. *Experimental Brain Research, 22*, 471–493.

Apkarian, A. V., Bushnell, M. C., Treede, R. D., et al. (2005). Human brain mechanisms of pain perception and regulation in health and disease. *European Journal of Pain, 9*(4), 463–484.

Apkarian, A. V., & Hodge, C. J. J. (1989a). The primate spinothalamic pathways: I. A quantitative study of the cells of origin of the spinothalamic pathway. *The Journal of Comparative Neurology, 288*, 447–473.

Apkarian, A. V., & Hodge, C. J. J. (1989b). The primate spinothalamic pathways: II. The cells of origin of the dorsolateral and ventral spinothalamic pathways. *The Journal of Comparative Neurology, 288*, 474–492.

Apkarian, A. V., & Hodge, C. J. J. (1989c). Primate spinothalamic pathways: III. Thalamic terminations of the dorsolateral and ventral spinothalamic pathways. *The Journal of Comparative Neurology, 288*, 493–511.

Apkarian, A. V., & Shi, T. (1994). Squirrel monkey lateral thalamus. I. Somatic nociresponsive neurons and their relation to spinothalamic terminals. *The Journal of Neuroscience, 14*, 6779–6795.

Applebaum, A. E., Beall, J. E., Foreman, R. D., & Willis, W. D. (1975). Organization and receptive fields of primate spinothalamic tract neurons. *Journal of Neurophysiology, 38*, 572–586.

Armour, D. (1927). On the surgery of the spinal cord and its membranes. *The Lancet, 2*, 691–697.

Aziz, Q., Andersson, J. L., Valind, S., Sundin, A., Hamdy, S., Jones, A. K., et al. (1997). Identification of human brain loci processing esophageal sensation using positron emission tomography. *Gastroenterology, 113*, 50–59.

Baliki, M. N., Chialvo, D. R., Geha, P. Y., Levy, R. M., Harden, R. M., Parrish, T. B., & Apkarian, A. V. (2006). Chronic pain and the emotional brain: Specific brain activity associated with spontaneous fluctuations of intensity of chronic back pain. *The Journal of Neuroscience, 26*(47), 12165–12173.

Bennett, G. J., Nishikawa, N., Lu, G. W., Hoffert, M. J., & Dubner, R. (1984). The morphology of dorsal column postsynaptic (DCPS) spino-medullary neurons in the cat. *The Journal of Comparative Neurology, 224*, 568–578.

Bennett, G. J., Seltzer, Z., Lu, G. W., Nishikawa, N., & Dubner, R. (1983). The cells of origin of the dorsal column postsynaptic projection in the lumbosacral enlargements of cats and monkeys. *Somatosensory Research, 1*, 131–149.

Berkley, K. J. (1980). Spatial relationships between the terminations of somatic sensory and motor pathways in the rostral brainstem of cats and monkeys. I. Ascending somatic sensory inputs to lateral diencephalon. *The Journal of Comparative Neurology, 193*, 283–317.

Berkley, K. J., Guilbaud, G., Benoist, J., & Gautron, M. (1993). Responses of neurons in and near the thalamic ventrobasal complex of the rat to stimulation of uterus, cervix, vagina, colon, and skin. *Journal of Neurophysiology, 69*, 557–568.

Berkley, K. J., & Hubscher, C. H. (1995a). Are there separate central nervous system pathways for touch and pain? *Nature Medicine, 1*(8), 766–773.

Berkley, K. J., & Hubscher, C. H. (1995b). Visceral and somatic sensory tracks through the neuraxis and their relation to pain: Lessons from the rat female reproductive system. In G. F. Gebhart (Ed.), *Visceral pain*. Seattle: IASP Press.

Besson, J. M., & Chaouch, A. (1987). Peripheral and spinal mechanisms of nociception. *Physiological Reviews, 67*, 67–186.

Bielefeldt, K., Lamb, K., & Gebhart, G. F. (2006). Convergence of sensory pathways in the development of somatic and visceral hypersensitivity. *American Journal of Physiology. Gastrointestinal and Liver Physiology, 291*(4), G658–G665.

Bingham, B., Ajit, S. K., Blake, D. R., & Samad, T. A. (2009). The molecular basis of pain and its clinical implications in rheumatology. *Nature Clinical Practice Rheumatology, 5*(1), 28–37.

Birrell, G. J., McQueen, D. S., Iggo, A., & Grubb, B. D. (1993). Prostanoid-induced potentiation of the excitatory and sensitizing effects of bradykinin on articular mechanonociceptors in the rat ankle joint. *Neurosciences, 54*, 537–544.

Blair, R. W., Ammons, W. S., & Foreman, R. D. (1984). Responses of thoracic spinothalamic and spinoreticular cells to coronary artery occlusion. *Journal of Neurophysiology, 51*, 636–648.

Blair, R. W., Wenster, R. N., & Foreman, R. D. (1982). Responses of thoracic spinothalamic neurons to intracardiac injection of bradykinin in the monkey. *Circulation Research, 51*, 83–94.

Boivie, J. (1979). An anatomical reinvestigation of the termination of the spinothalamic tract in the monkey. *The Journal of Comparative Neurology, 186*, 343–370.

Boivie, J., Leijon, G., & Johansson, I. (1989). Central post-stroke pain – A study of the mechanisms through analyses of the sensory abnormalities. *Pain, 37*, 173–185.

Bonica, J. J. (2001). Bonica's management of pain (3rd ed). J. D. Loeser (Ed.). Philadelphia: Lippincott Williams and Wilkins.

Bossut, D. F., & Perl, E. R. (1995). Effects of nerve injury on sympathetic excitation of A[delta] mechanical nociceptors. *Journal of Neurophysiology, 73*, 1721–1723.

Brown, A. G., & Franz, D. N. (1969). Responses of spinocervical tract neurons to natural stimulation of identified cutaneous receptors. *Experimental Brain Research, 7*, 231–249.

Brown, A. G., Fyffe, R. E. W., Noble, R., Rose, P. K., & Snow, P. J. (1980). The density, distribution and topographical organization of spinocervical tract neurons in the cat. *The Journal of Physiology, 300*, 409–428.

Brown-Sequard, E. (1868). Lectures on the physiology and pathology of the central nervous system and on the treatment of organic nervous affections. *The Lancet, 2*, 593–823.

Brüggemann, J., Shi, T., & Apkarian, A. V. (1994). Squirrel monkey lateral thalamus. II. Viscerosomatic convergent representation of urinary bladder, colon, and esophagus. *The Journal of Neuroscience, 14*, 6796–6814.

Bryan, R. N., Coulter, J. D., & Willis, W. D. (1974). Cells of origin of the spinocervical tract in the monkey. *Experimental Neurology, 42*, 574–586.

Burton, H., & Craig, A. D. (1983). Spinothalamic projections in cat, raccoon and monkey: A study based on anterograde transport of horseradish peroxidase. In G. Macchi, A. Rustioni, & R. Spreafico (Eds.), *Somatosensory integration in the thalamus*. New York: Elsevier.

Burton, H., & Jones, E. G. (1976). The posterior thalamic region and its cortical projection in New World and Old World monkeys. *The Journal of Comparative Neurology, 168*, 249–302.

Bushnell, M. C., & Duncan, G. H. (1987). Mechanical response properties of ventroposterior medial thalamic neurons in the alert monkey. *Experimental Brain Research, 67*, 603–614.

Bushnell, M. C., Duncan, G. H., Hofbauer, R. K., Ha, B., Chen, J. I., & Carrier, B. (1999). Pain perception: Is there a role for primary somatosensory cortex? *Proceedings of the National Academy of Sciences of the United States of America, 96*(14), 7705–7709.

Bushnell, M. C., Duncan, G. H., & Tremblay, N. (1993). Thalamic VPM nucleus in the behaving monkey. I. Multimodal and discriminative properties of thermosensitive neurons. *Journal of Neurophysiology, 69*, 739–752.

Campbell, J. N., Meyer, R. A., & Raja, S. N. (1992). Is nociceptor activation by alpha-1 adrenoreceptors the culprit in sympathetically maintained pain? *American Society for Pain Journal, 1*, 3–11.

Carstens, E., & Trevino, D. L. (1978). Laminar origins of spinothalamic projections in the cat as determined by the retrograde transport of horseradish peroxidase. *The Journal of Comparative Neurology, 182*, 151–166.

Casey, K. L., & Morrow, T. J. (1983). Ventral posterior thalamic neurons differentially responsive to noxious stimulation of the awake monkey. *Science, 221*, 675–677.

Casey, K. L., & Morrow, T. J. (1987). Nociceptive neurons in the ventral posterior thalamus of the awake squirrel monkey: Observations on identification, modulation, and drug effects. In J. M. Besson, G. Guilbaud, & M. Peschanski (Eds.), *Thalamus and pain*. Amsterdam: Excerpta Medica.

Cervero, F., Iggo, A., & Molony, V. (1977). Responses of spinocervical tract neurons to noxious stimulation of the skin. *The Journal of Physiology, 267*, 537–558.

Chandler, M. J., Hobbs, S. F., Fu, Q.-G., Kenshalo, D. R. Jr., Blair R. W., & Foreman, R. D. (1992). Responses of neurons in ventroposterolateral nucleus of primate thalamus to urinary bladder distension. *Brain Research, 571*, 26–34.

Chaturvedi, S. K. (1987). Prevalence of chronic pain in psychiatric patients. *Pain, 29*, 231–237.

Christianson, J. A., Bielefeldt, K., Malin, S. A., & Davis, B. M. (2010). Neonatal colon insult alters growth factor expression and TRPA1 responses in adult mice. *Pain, 151*(2), 540–549.

Chung, J. M., Kenshalo, D. R., Gerhart, K. D., & Willis, W. D. (1979). Excitation of primate spinothalamic neurons by cutaneous C-fiber volleys. *Journal of Neurophysiology, 42*, 1354–1369.

Chung, J. M., Surmeier, D. J., Lee, K. H., Sorkin, L. S., Honda, C. N., Tsong, Y., et al. (1986). Classification of primate spinothalamic and somatosensory thalamic neurons based on cluster analysis. *Journal of Neurophysiology, 56*, 308–327.

Cliffer, K. D., & Giesler, G. J., Jr. (1989). Postsynaptic dorsal column pathway of the rat. III. Distribution of ascending afferent fibers. *The Journal of Neuroscience, 9*, 3146–3168.

Cliffer, K. D., Hasegawa, T., & Willis, W. D. (1992). Responses of neurons in the gracile nucleus of cats to innocuous and noxious stimuli: Basic characterization and antidromic activation from the thalamus. *Journal of Neurophysiology, 68*, 818–832.

Conti, F., De Biasi, S., Giuffrida, R., & Rustioni, A. (1990). Substance P-containing projections in the dorsal columns of rats and cats. *Neurosciences, 34*, 607–621.

Cortright, D. N., & Szallasi, A. (2004). Biochemical pharmacology of the vanilloid receptor TRPV1. An update. *European Journal of Biochemistry, 271*(10), 1814–1819.

Costigan, M., & Woolf, C. J. (2000). Pain: Molecular mechanisms. *The Journal of Pain, 1*(3 Suppl), 35–44.

Craig, A. D. (1978). Spinal and medullary input to the lateral cervical nucleus. *The Journal of Comparative Neurology, 181*, 729–744.

Craig, A. D., Bushnell, M. C., Zhang, E. T., & Blomqvist, A. (1994). A thalamic nucleus specific for pain and temperature sensation. *Nature, 372*, 770–773.

Craig, A. D., & Dostrovsky, J. (2001). Differential projections of thermoreceptive and nociceptive lamina I trigeminothalamic and spinothalamic neurons in the cat. *Journal of Neurophysiology, 86*, 856–870.

Craig, A. D., Linington, A. J., & Kniffki, K. D. (1989). Cells of origin of spinothalamic projections to medial and/or lateral thalamus in the cat. *The Journal of Comparative Neurology, 289*, 568–585.

Craig, A. D., & Zhang, E. T. (2006). Retrograde analyses of spinothalamic projections in the macaque monkey: Input to posterolateral thalamus. *The Journal of Comparative Neurology, 499*(6), 953–964.

Cummins, T. R., Sheets, P. L., & Waxman, S. G. (2007). The roles of sodium channels in nociception: Implications for mechanisms of pain. *Pain, 131*(3), 243–257.

Dahlström, A., & Fuxe, K. (1964). Evidence for the existence of monoamine-containing neurons in the central nervous system. I. Demonstration of monoamines in the cell bodies of brain stem neurons. *Acta Physiologica Scandinavica, 62*(Suppl 232), 1–55.

Dahlström, A., & Fuxe, K. (1965). Evidence for the existence of monoamine neurons in the central nervous system. II. Experimentally induced changes in the intraneuronal amine levels of bulbospinal neurons systems. *Acta Physiologica Scandinavica, 64*(Suppl 247), 1–36.

Davidoff, R. A. (1989). The dorsal columns. *Neurology, 39*, 1377–1385.

Davis, K. D., & Dostrovsky, J. O. (1988). Properties of feline thalamic neurons activated by stimulation of the middle meningeal artery and sagittal sinus. *Brain Research, 454*, 89–100.

Davis, K. D., Meyer, R. A., & Campbell, J. N. (1993). Chemosensitivity and sensitization of nociceptive afferents that innervate the hairy skin of monkey. *Journal of Neurophysiology, 69*, 1071–1081.

Davis, K. D., Tasker, R. R., Kiss, Z. H. T., Hutchison, W. D., & Dostrovsky, J. O. (1995). Visceral pain evoked by thalamic microstimulation in humans. *NeuroReport, 6*, 369–374.

Dell, P., & Olson, R. (1951). Projections thalamiques, corticales et cerebelleuses des afferences viscerales vagales. *Comptes Rendus Seances Society of Biology Forum, 145*, 1084–1088.

Derbyshire, S. W. (2003). A systematic review of neuroimaging data during visceral stimulation. *The American Journal of Gastroenterology, 98*, 12–20.

Descartes, R. (1664). *L'Homme. e.* Paris: Angot.

Di Marzo, V., Blumberg, P. M., & Szallasi, A. (2002). Endovanilloid signaling in pain. *Current Opinion in Neurobiology, 12*(4), 372–379.

Dougherty, P. M., Sluka, K. A., Sorkin, L. S., Westlund, K. N., & Willis, W. D. (1992). Neural changes in acute arthritis in monkeys. I. Parallel enhancement of responses of spinothalamic tract neurons to mechanical stimulation and excitatory amino acids. *Brain Research Reviews, 17*, 1–13.

Downie, J. W., Ferrington, D. G., Sorkin, L. S., & Willis, W. D. (1988). The primate spinocervicothalamic pathway: Responses of cells of the lateral cervical nucleus and spinocervical tract to innocuous and noxious stimuli. *Journal of Neurophysiology, 59*, 861–885.

Dray, A., Bettaney, J., Forster, P., & Perkins, N. M. (1988). Bradykinin-induced stimulation of afferent fibres is mediated through protein kinase C. *Neuroscience Letters, 91*, 301–307.

Dray, A., Urban, L., & Dickenson, A. (1994). Pharmacology of chronic pain. *Trends in Pharmacological Sciences, 15*(6), 190–197.

Duggan, A. W., Hall, J. G., & Headley, P. M. (1977). Enkephalins and dorsal horn neurons of the cat: Effects on responses to noxious and innocuous skin stimuli. *British Journal of Pharmacology, 61*, 399–408.

Duggan, A. W., & North, R. A. (1984). Electrophysiology of opioids. *Pharmacological Reviews, 35*, 219–281.

Duncan, G. H., Bushnell, M. C., Oliveras, J. L., Bastrash, N., & Tremblay, N. (1993). Thalamic VPM nucleus in the behaving monkey. III. Effects of reversible inactivation by lidocaine on thermal and mechanical discrimination. *Journal of Neurophysiology, 70*, 2086–2096.

Emmers, R. (1966). Separate relays of tactile, pressure, thermal, and gustatory modalities in the cat thalamus. *Proceedings of the Society for Experimental Biology and Medicine, 121*, 527–531.

Feng, Y., Cui, M., Al-Chaer, E. D., & Willis, W. D. (1998). Epigastric antinociception by cervical dorsal column lesions in rats. *Anesthesiology, 89*(2), 411–420.

Ferrington, D. G., Downie, J. W., & Willis, W. D. (1988). Primate nucleus gracilis neurons: Responses to innocuous and noxious stimuli. *Journal of Neurophysiology, 59*, 886–907.

Ferrington, D. G., Sorkin, L. S., & Willis, W. D. (1987). Responses of spinothalamic tract cells in the superficial dorsal horn of the primate lumbar spinal cord. *The Journal of Physiology, 388*, 681–703.

Fillingim, R. B. (Ed.). (2000). Sex, gender, and pain. Progress in pain research and management (Vol. 17). Seattle: IASP Press.

Foerster, O., & Gagel, O. (1932). Die Vorderseitenstrangdurchschneidung beim Menschen. Eine klinisch-pathophysiologisch-anatomische Studie. *Zeitschrift für die Gesamte Neurology und Psychiatry, 138*, 1–92.

Foreman, R. D., Schmidt, R. F., & Willis, W. D. (1979). Effects of mechanical and chemical stimulation of fine muscle afferents upon primate spinothalamic tract cells. *The Journal of Physiology, 286*, 215–231.

Friedman, D. R., Murray, E. A., O'Neill, J. B., & Mishkin, M. (1986). Cortical connections of the somatosensory fields of the lateral sulcus of macaques: Evidence for a corticolimbic pathway for touch. *The Journal of Comparative Neurology, 252*, 323–347.

Gaze, R. M., & Gordon, G. (1954). The representation of cutaneous sense in the thalamus of the cat and monkey. *Journal of Experiment Physiology, 39*, 279–304.

Giesler, G. J., Jr., & Cliffer, K. D. (1985). Postsynaptic dorsal column pathway of the rat. II. Evidence against an important role in nociception. *Brain Research, 326*(2), 347–356.

Giesler, G. J., Jr., Menétrey, D., & Basbaum, A. I. (1979). Differential origins of spinothalamic tract projections to medial and lateral thalamus in the rat. *The Journal of Comparative Neurology, 184*, 107–126.

Giesler, G. J., Jr., Menétrey, D., Guilbaud, G., & Besson, J. M. (1976). Lumbar cord neurons at the origin of the spinothalamic tract in the rat. *Brain Research, 118*, 320–324.

Giesler, G. J., Nahin, R. L., & Madsen, A. M. (1984). Postsynaptic dorsal column pathway of the rat. I. Anatomical studies. *Journal of Neurophysiology, 51*, 260–275.

Giesler, G. J., Yezierski, R. P., Gerhart, K. D., & Willis, W. D. (1981). Spinothalamic tract neurons that project to medial and/or lateral thalamic nuclei: Evidence for a physiologically novel population of spinal cord neurons. *Journal of Neurophysiology, 46*, 1285–1308.

Gildenberg, P. L., & Hirshberg, R. M. (1984). Limited myelotomy for the treatment of intractable cancer pain. *Journal of Neurology, Neurosurgery, and Psychiatry, 47*, 94–96.

Gingold, S. I., Greenspan, J. D., & Apkarian, A. V. (1991). Anatomic evidence of nociceptive inputs to primary somatosensory cortex: Relationship between spinothalamic terminals and thalamocortical cells in squirrel monkeys. *The Journal of Comparative Neurology, 308*, 467–490.

Gold, M. S., & Gebhart, G. F. (2010). Nociceptor sensitization in pain pathogenesis. *Nature Medicine, 16*(11), 1248–1257.

Gowers, W. R. (1878). A case of unilateral gunshot injury to the spinal cord. *Transactions of the Clinical Society of London, 11*, 24–32.

Grundy, D., Al-Chaer, E. D., Aziz, Q., Collins, S. M., Ke, M., Taché, Y., et al. (2006). Fundamentals of neurogastroenterology: Basic science. *Gastroenterology, 130*(5), 1391–1411.

Gybels, J. M., & Sweet, W. H. (Eds.). (1989). *Neurosurgical treatment of persistent pain*. Basel: Karger.

Ha, H. (1971). Cervicothalamic tract in the Rhesus monkey. *Experimental Neurology, 33*, 205–212.

Häbler, H. J., Jänig, W., & Koltzenburg, M. (1990). Activation of unmyelinated afferent fibres by mechanical stimuli and inflammation of the urinary bladder in the cat. *The Journal of Physiology, 425*, 545–562.

Head, H., & Thompson, T. (1906). The grouping of afferent impulses within the spinal cord. *Brain, 29*, 537–741.

Hirai, T., & Jones, E. G. (1989). A new parcellation of the human thalamus on the basis of histochemical staining. *Brain Research Reviews, 14*, 1–34.

Hirshberg, R. M., Al-Chaer, E. D., Lawand, N. B., Westlund, K. N., & Willis, W. D. (1996). Is there a pathway in the posterior funiculus that signals visceral pain? *Pain, 67*, 291–305.

Hitchcock, E. R. (1970). Stereotactic cervical myelotomy. *Journal of Neurology, Neurosurgery, and Psychiatry, 33*, 224–230.

Hitchcock, E. R. (1974). Stereotactic myelotomy. *Proceedings of the Royal Society of Medicine, 67*, 771–772.

Hobday, D. I., Aziz, Q., Thacker, N., Hollander, I., Jackson, A., & Thompson, D. G. (2001). A study of the cortical processing of ano-rectal sensation using functional MRI. *Brain, 124*, 361–368.

Hodge, C. J., Apkarian, A. V., & Stevens, R. T. (1986). Inhibition of dorsal-horn cell responses by stimulation of the Kölliker-Fuse nucleus. *Journal of Neurosurgery, 65*, 825–833.

Hylden, J. L., Anton, F., & Nahin, R. L. (1989). Spinal lamina I projection neurons in the rat: Collateral innervation of parabrachial area and thalamus. *Neurosciences, 28*, 27–37.

Hyndman, O. R., & Van Epps, C. (1939). Possibility of differential section of the spinothalamic tract. *Archives of Surgery, 38*, 1036–1053.

Jones, E. G. (1985). *The thalamus.* New York: Plenum.

Joshi, S. K., Su, X., Porreca, F., & Gebhart, G. F. (2000). Kappa-Opioid receptor agonists modulate visceral nociception at a novel, peripheral site of action. *The Journal of Neuroscience, 20*, 5874–5879.

Kajander, K. C., & Bennett, G. J. (1992). Onset of a painful peripheral neuropathy in rat: A partial and differential deafferentation and spontaneous discharge in A beta and A delta primary afferent neurons. *Journal of Neurophysiology, 68*(3), 734–744.

Kawakita, K., Sumiya, E., Murase, K., & Okada, K. (1997). Response characteristics of nucleus submedius neurons to colo-rectal distension in the rat. *Neuroscience Research, 28*(1), 59–66.

Kellenberger, S., & Schild, L. (2002). Epithelial sodium channel/degenerin family of ion channels: A variety of functions for a shared structure. *Physiological Reviews, 82*(3), 735–767.

Kenshalo, D. R., Chudler, E. H., Anton, F., & Dubner, R. (1988). SI nociceptive neurons participate in the encoding process by which monkeys perceive the intensity of noxious thermal stimulation. *Brain Research, 454*, 378–382.

Kenshalo, D. R., Giesler, G. J., Leonard, R. B., & Willis, W. D. (1980). Responses of neurons in primate ventral posterior lateral nucleus to noxious stimuli. *Journal of Neurophysiology, 43*, 1594–1614.

Kenshalo, D. R., Leonard, R. B., Chung, J. M., & Willis, W. D. (1979). Responses of primate spinothalamic neurons to graded and to repeated noxious heat stimuli. *Journal of Neurophysiology, 42*, 1370–1389.

Keogh, E. (2009). Sex differences in pain. In R. J. Moore (Ed.), *Biobehavioural approaches to pain.* New York: Springer.

Keogh, E. (2011). Sex differences in pain across the life course. In R. J. Moore (Ed.), *Handbook of pain and palliative care: Biobehavioral approaches for the life course.* New York: Springer.

Kern, M. K., Jaradeh, S., Arndorfer, R. C., Jesmanowicz, A., Hyde, J., & Shaker, R. (2001). Gender differences in cortical representation of rectal distension in healthy humans. *American Journal of Physiology. Gastrointestinal and Liver Physiology, 281*, G1512–G1523.

Kerr, F. W. L. (1975). The ventral spinothalamic tract and other ascending systems of the ventral funiculus of the spinal cord. *The Journal of Comparative Neurology, 159*, 335–356.

Kevetter, G. A., & Willis, W. D. (1982). Spinothalamic cells in the rat lumbar cord with collaterals to the medullary reticular formation. *Brain Research, 238*, 181–185.

Khakh, B. S., & North, R. A. (2006). P2X receptors as cell-surface ATP sensors in health and disease. *Nature, 442*(7102), 527–532.

Kim, Y. S., & Kwon, S. J. (2000). High thoracic midline dorsal column myelotomy for severe visceral pain due to advanced stomach cancer. *Neurosurgery, 46*(1), 85–92.

Kirkup, A. J., Brunsden, A. M., & Grundy, D. (2001). Receptors and transmission in the brain-gut axis: Potential for novel therapies. I. Receptors on visceral afferents. *American Journal of Physiology. Gastrointestinal and Liver Physiology, 280*, G787–G794.

Klop, E. M., Mouton, L. J., Kuipers, R., & Holstege, G. (2005). Neurons in the lateral sacral cord of the cat project to periaqueductal grey, but not to thalamus. *The European Journal of Neuroscience, 21*, 2159–2166.

Konietzny, F., Perl, E. R., Trevino, D., Light, A. & Hensel, H. (1981). Sensory experiences in man evoked by intraneural electrical stimulation of intact cutaneous afferent fibers. *Experimental Brain Research, 42*, 219–222.

Ladabaum, U., Minoshima, S., Hasler, W. L., Cross, D., Chey, W. D., & Owyang, C. (2001). Gastric distention correlates with activation of multiple cortical and subcortical regions. *Gastroenterology, 120*, 369–376.

LaMotte, R. H., Thalhammer, J. G., & Robinson, C. J. (1983). Peripheral neural correlates of magnitude of cutaneous pain and hyperalgesia: A comparison of neural events in monkey with sensory judgments in human. *Journal of Neurophysiology, 50*, 1–26.

LaMotte, R. H., Thalhammer, J. G., Torebjörk, H. E., & Robinson, C. J. (1982). Peripheral neural mechanisms of cutaneous hyperalgesia following mild injury by heat. *The Journal of Neuroscience, 2*, 765–781.

Le Gros Clark, W. E. (1936). The termination of ascending tracts in the thalamus of the macaque monkey. *Journal of Anatomy, 71*, 7–40.

Lenz, F. A., Gracely, R. H., Hope, E. J., Baker, F. H., Rowland, L. H., Dougherty, P. M., et al. (1994). The sensation of angina can be evoked by stimulation of the human thalamus. *Pain, 59*, 119–125.

Light, A. R. (1992). *The initial processing of pain and its descending control: Spinal and trigeminal systems.* Basel: Karger.

Light, A. R., Sedivec, M., Casale, E., & Jones S. L. (1993). Physiological and morphological characteristics of spinal neurons projecting to the parabrachial region of the cat. *Somatosensory & Motor Research, 10*, 309–325.

Lynn, B., & Carpenter, S. E. (1982). Primary afferent units from the hairy skin of the rat hind limb. *Brain Research, 238*(1), 29–43.

Maggi, C. A., & Meli, A. (1988). The sensory-efferent function of capsaicin-sensitive sensory neurons. *General Pharmacology, 19*, 1–43.

Mantyh, P. W. (1983). The spinothalamic tract in the primate: A re-examination using wheatgerm agglutinin conjugated to horseradish peroxidase. *Neurosciences, 9*, 847–862.

Marshall, G. E., Shehab, S. A., Spike, R. C., & Todd, A. J. (1996). Neurokinin-1 receptors on lumbar spinothalamic neurons in the rat. *Neurosciences, 72*, 255–263.

Matre, D., & Tran, T. D. (2009). Imaging modalities for pain. In R. J. Moore (Ed.), *Biobehavioural approaches to pain*. New York: Springer.

McLeod, J. G. (1958). The representation of the splanchnic afferent pathways in the thalamus of the cat. *The Journal of Physiology, 94*, 439–452.

McMahon, S. B. (2004). Sensitisation of gastrointestinal tract afferents. *Gut, 53*, ii13–ii15.

McRoberts, J. A., Coutinho, S. V., Marvizon, J. C., Grady, E. F., Tognetto, M., Sengupta, J. N., et al. (2001). Role of peripheral N-methyl-D-aspartate (NMDA) receptors in visceral nociception in rats. *Gastroenterology, 120*, 1737–1748.

Mehler, W. R. (1962). The anatomy of the so-called "pain tract" in man: An analysis of the course and distribution of the ascending fibers of the fasciculus anterolateralis. In J. D. French & R. W. Porter (Eds.), *Basic research in paraplegia*. Springfield: Charles C. Thomas.

Mehler, W. R., Feferman, M. E., & Nauta, W. J. H. (1960). Ascending axon degeneration following anterolateral cordotomy. An experimental study in the monkey. *Brain, 83*, 718–750.

Melzack, R. (1999). From the gate to the neuromatrix. *Pain, 6*, S121–S126.

Melzack, R., & Wall, P. D. (1965). Pain mechanisms: A new theory. *Science, 150*(699), 971–979.

Merskey, H. (1989). Pain and psychological medicine. In P. D. Wall & R. Melzack (Eds.), *Textbook of pain* (2nd ed.). Edinburgh: Churchill-Livingstone.

Mertz, H., Morgan, V., Tanner, G., Pickens, D., Price, R., Shyr, Y., et al. (2000). Regional cerebral activation in irritable bowel syndrome and control subjects with painful and nonpainful rectal distention. *Gastroenterology, 18*, 842–848.

Meyer, R. A., & Campbell, J. N. (1981). Myelinated nociceptive afferents account for the hyperalgesia that follows a burn to the hand. *Science, 213*, 1527–1529.

Milne, R. J., Foreman, R. D., Giesler, G. J., & Willis, W. D. (1981). Convergence of cutaneous and pelvic visceral nociceptive inputs onto primate spinothalamic neurons. *Pain, 11*, 163–183.

Mizuno, N., Nakano, K., Imaizumi, M., & Okamoto, M. (1967). The lateral cervical nucleus of the Japanese monkey (Macaca fuscata). *The Journal of Comparative Neurology, 129*, 375–384.

Mogil, J. S., Breese, N. M., Witty, M. F., Ritchie, J., Rainville, M. L., Ase, A., et al. (2005). Transgenic expression of a dominant-negative ASIC3 subunit leads to increased sensitivity to mechanical and inflammatory stimuli. *The Journal of Neuroscience, 25*(43), 9893–9901.

Nafe, J. P. (1934). The pressure, pain and temperature senses. In C. A. Murchison (Ed.), *Handbook of general experimental psychology*. Worcester: Clark University Press.

Nauta, H. J., Hewitt, E., Westlund, K. N., & Willis, W. D. (1997). Surgical interruption of a midline dorsal column visceral pain pathway. Case report and review of the literature. *Journal of Neurosurgery, 86*(3), 538–542.

Nauta, H. J., Soukup, V. M., Fabian, R. H., Lin, J. T., Grady, J. J., Williams, C. G., et al. (2000). Punctate midline myelotomy for the relief of visceral cancer pain. *Journal of Neurosurgery, 92*(2 Suppl), 125–130.

Ness, T. J. (2000). Evidence for ascending visceral nociceptive information in the dorsal midline and lateral spinal cord. *Pain, 87*(1), 83–88.

Nijensohn, D. E., & Kerr, F. W. L. (1975). The ascending projections of the dorsolateral funiculus of the spinal cord in the primate. *The Journal of Comparative Neurology, 161*, 459–470.

Noble, R., & Riddell, J. S. (1988). Cutaneous excitatory and inhibitory input to neurons of the postsynaptic dorsal column system in the cat. *The Journal of Physiology, 396*, 497–513.

Noordenbos, W. (1959). *Pain*. Amsterdam: Elsevier.

Noordenbos, W., & Wall, P. D. (1976). Diverse sensory functions with an almost totally divided spinal cord. A case of spinal cord transection with preservation of part of one anterolateral quadrant. *Pain, 2*, 185–195.

Ochoa, J., & Torebjörk, E. (1989). Sensations evoked by intraneural microstimulation of C nociceptor fibres in human skin nerves. *The Journal of Physiology, 415*, 583–599.

Olszewski, J. (1952). *The thalamus of Macaca mulatta*. New York: Karger.

Patterson, J. T., Coggeshall, R. E., Lee, W. T., & Chung, K. (1990). Long ascending unmyelinated primary afferent axons in the rat dorsal column: Immunohistochemical localizations. *Neuroscience Letters, 10*, 6–10.

Patterson, J. T., Head, P. A., McNeill, D. L., Chung, K., & Coggeshall, R. E. (1989). Ascending unmyelinated primary afferent fibers in the dorsal funiculus. *The Journal of Comparative Neurology, 290*, 384–390.

Patton, H. D., & Amassian, V. E. (1951). Thalamic relay of splanchnic afferent fibers. *The American Journal of Physiology, 167,* 815–816.

Peng, Y. B., Lin, Q., & Willis, W. D. (1995). The role of 5HT3 receptors in periaqueductal gray-induced inhibition of nociceptive dorsal horn neurons in rats. *The Journal of Pharmacology and Experimental Therapeutics, 276,* 116–124.

Peng, Y. B., Lin, Q., & Willis, W. D. (1996a). Involvement of [alpha]2-adrenoreceptors in the periaqueductal gray-induced inhibition of dorsal horn cell activity in rats. *The Journal of Pharmacology and Experimental Therapeutics, 278*(1), 125–135.

Peng, Y. B., Lin, Q., & Willis, W. D. (1996b). Effects of GABA and glycine receptor antagonists on the activity and PAG-induced inhibition of rat dorsal horn neurons. *Brain Research, 736*(1–2), 189–201.

Petit, D. (1972). Postsynaptic fibres in the dorsal columns and their relay in the nucleus gracilis. *Brain Research, 48,* 380–384.

Peyron, R., Garcia-Larrea, L., Gregoire, M. C., Convers, P., Richard, A., Lavenne, F., et al. (2000). Parietal and cingulate processes in central pain. A combined positron emission tomography (PET) and functional magnetic resonance imaging (fMRI) study of an unusual case. *Pain, 84*(1), 77–87.

Pollin, B., & Albe-Fessard, D. (1979). Organization of somatic thalamus in monkeys with and without section of dorsal spinal tracts. *Brain Research, 173,* 431–449.

Price, D. D. (2000). Psychological and neural mechanisms of the affective dimension of pain. *Science, 288*(5472), 1769–1772.

Price, D. D., Hayes, R. L., Ruda, M. A., & Dubner, R. (1978). Spatial and temporal transformations of input to spinothalamic tract neurons and their relation to somatic sensation. *Journal of Neurophysiology, 41,* 933–947.

Price, D. D., & Mayer, D. J. (1975). Neurophysiological characterization of the anterolateral quadrant neurons subserving pain in *M. mulatta. Pain, 1,* 59–72.

Price, M. P., McIlwrath, S. L., Xie, J., Cheng, C., Qiao, J., Tarr, D. E., et al. (2001). The DRASIC cation channel contributes to the detection of cutaneous touch and acid stimuli in mice. *Neuron, 32*(6), 1071–1083. Erratum in: *Neuron, 35*(2), 407, 2002.

Proudfit, H. K. (1992). The behavioral pharmacology of the noradrenergic descending system. In J.-M. Besson & G. Guilbaud (Eds.), *Towards the use of noradrenergic agonists for the treatment of pain.* New York: Elsevier.

Rogers, R. C., Novin, D., & Butcher, L. L. (1979). Hepatic sodium and osmoreceptors activate neurons in the ventrobasal thalamus. *Brain Research, 168,* 398–403.

Ross, M. H., Romrell, L. J., & Kaye, G. I. (1995). *Histology: A text and atlas* (3rd ed.). Baltimore: Williams & Wilkins.

Rustioni, A. (1973). Non-primary afferents to the nucleus gracilis from the lumbar cord of the cat. *Brain Research, 51,* 81–95.

Rustioni, A. (1974). Non-primary afferents to the cuneate nucleus in the brachial dorsal funiculus of the cat. *Brain Research, 75,* 247–259.

Rustioni, A., Hayes, N. L., & O'Neill, S. (1979). Dorsal column nuclei and ascending spinal afferents in macaques. *Brain, 102,* 95–125.

Saab, C. Y., Park, Y. C., & Al-Chaer, E. D. (2004). Thalamic modulation of visceral nociceptive processing in adult rats with neonatal colon irritation. *Brain Research, 1008*(2), 186–192.

Saab, C. Y., Wang, J., Gu, C., Garner, K. N., Al-Chaer, E. D. (2007). Microglia: a newly discovered role in visceral hypersensitivity? *Neuron Glia Biology, 2,* 271–277.

Sarnoff, S. J., Arrowood, J. G., & Chapman, W. P. (1948). Differential spinal block. IV. The investigation of intestinal dyskinesia, colonic atony, and visceral afferent fibers. *Surgery, Gynecology & Obstetrics, 86,* 571–581.

Sato, J., & Perl, E. R. (1991). Adrenergic excitation of cutaneous pain receptors induced by peripheral nerve injury. *Science, 251,* 1608–1610.

Schaible, H. G. (2004). Spinal mechanisms contributing to joint pain. *Novartis Foundation Symposium, 260,* 4–22; discussion 22–27, 100–104, 277–279, review.

Schaible, H. G., & Schmidt, R. F. (1983). Activation of groups III and IV sensory units in medial articular nerve by local mechanical stimulation of knee joint. *Journal of Neurophysiology, 49,* 35–44.

Schaible, H. G., & Schmidt, R. F. (1985). Effects of an experimental arthritis on the sensory properties of fine articular afferent units. *Journal of Neurophysiology, 54,* 1109–1122.

Schaible, H. G., & Schmidt, R. F. (1988). Time course of mechanosensitivity changes in articular afferents during a developing experimental arthritis. *Journal of Neurophysiology, 60,* 2180–2195.

Schepelmann, K., Messlinger, K., Schaible, H. G., & Schmidt, R. F. (1992). Inflammatory mediators and nociception in the joint: Excitation and sensitization of slowly conducting afferent fibers of cat's knee by prostaglandin I2. *Neurosciences, 50,* 237–247.

Schiff, J. M. (1858). *Lehrbuch der physiologie des menschen I: Muskel und nervenphysiologie.* Lahr: Nabu Press.

Schwarcz, J. R. (1976). Stereotactic extralemniscal myelotomy. *Journal of Neurology, Neurosurgery, and Psychiatry, 39,* 53–57.

Schwarcz, J. R. (1978). Spinal cord stereotactic techniques, trigeminal nucleotomy and extralemniscal myelotomy. *Applied Neurophysiology, 41*, 99–112.

Sherrington, C. S. (1906). *The integrative action of the nervous system* (2nd ed.). Newhaven: Yale University Press.

Silverman, D. H., Munakata, J. A., Ennes, H., Mandelkern, M. A., Hoh, C. K., & Mayer, E. A. (1997). Regional cerebral activity in normal and pathological perception of visceral pain. *Gastroenterology, 112*, 64–72.

Smith, M. V., & Apkarian, A. V. (1991). Thalamically projecting cells of the lateral cervical nucleus in monkey. *Brain Research, 555*, 10–18.

Sorkin, L., & Carlton, S. (1997). Spinal anatomy and pharmacology of afferent processing. In T. Yaksh, C. Lynch, W. Zapol, et al. (Eds.), *Anesthesia. Biologic foundations*. Philadelphia: Lippincott-Raven.

Spiller, W. G. (1905). The occasional clinical resemblance between caries of the vertebrae and lumbothoracic syringomyelia, and the location within the spinal cord of the fibres for the sensations of pain and temperature. *University of Pennsylvania Medical Bulletin, 18*, 147–154.

Spiller, W. G., & Martin, E. (1912). The treatment of persistent pain of organic origin in the lower part of the body by division of the anterolateral column of the spinal cord. *Journal of the American Medical Association, 58*, 1489–1490.

Stanley, E. (1840). A case of disease of the posterior columns of the spinal cord. *Medico-Chirurgical Transactions, 23*, 80–84.

Stein, C. (1994). Peripheral opioid analgesia: Mechanisms and therapeutic applications. In J. M. Besson, G. Guilbaud, & H. Ollat (Eds.), *Peripheral neurons in nociception: Physio-pharmacological aspects*. Paris: John Libbey Eurotext.

Stepniewska, I., Sakai, S. T., Qi, H. X., & Kaas, J. H. (2003). Somatosensory input to the ventrolateral thalamic region in the macaque monkey: Potential substrate for Parkinsonian tremor. *The Journal of Comparative Neurology, 455*, 378–395.

Strigo, I. A., Duncan, G. H., Boivin, M., & Bushnell, M. C. (2003). Differentiation of visceral and cutaneous pain in the human brain. *Journal of Neurophysiology, 89*, 3294–3303.

Su, X., Sengupta, J. N., & Gebhart, G. F. (1997). Effects of kappa opioid receptor-selective agonists on responses of pelvic nerve afferents to noxious colorectal distension. *Journal of Neurophysiology, 78*, 1003–1012.

Surmeier, D. J., Honda, C. N., & Willis, W. D. (1986a). Responses of primate spinothalamic neurons to noxious thermal stimulation of glabrous and hairy skin. *Journal of Neurophysiology, 56*, 328–350.

Surmeier, D. J., Honda, C. N., & Willis, W. D. (1986b). Temporal features of the responses of primate spinothalamic neurons to noxious thermal stimulation of hairy and glabrous skin. *Journal of Neurophysiology, 56*, 351–368.

Todd, A. (2002). Anatomy of primary afferents and projection neurons in the rat spinal dorsal horn with particular emphasis on substance P and the neurokinin 1 receptor. *Experimental Physiology, 87*, 245–249.

Trevino, D. L., Coulter, J. D., & Willis, W. D. (1973). Locations of cells of origin of spinothalamic tract in lumbar enlargement of the monkey. *Journal of Neurophysiology, 36*, 750–761.

Trevino, D. L., Maunz, R. A., Bryan, R. N., & Willis, W. D. (1972). Location of cells of origin of the spinothalamic tract in the lumbar enlargement of cat. *Experimental Neurology, 34*, 64–77.

Truex, R. C., Taylor, M. J., Smythe, M. Q., & Gildenberg, P. L. (1965). The lateral cervical nucleus of cat, dog and man. *The Journal of Comparative Neurology, 139*, 93–104.

Truitt, W. A., Shipley, M. T., Veening, J. G., & Coolen, L. M. (2003). Activation of a subset of lumbar spinothalamic neurons after copulatory behavior in male but not female rats. *The Journal of Neuroscience, 23*, 325–331.

Uddenburg, N. (1966). Studies on modality segregation and second-order neurons in the dorsal funiculus. *Experientia, 15*, 441–442.

Uddenburg, N. (1968). Functional organization of long, second-order afferents in the dorsal funiculus. *Experimental Brain Research, 4*, 377–382.

Veldhuijzen, D. S., Greenspan, J. D., Kim, J. H., Coghill, R. C., Treede, R. D., Ohara, S., et al. (2007). Imaging central pain syndromes. *Current Pain and Headache Reports, 11*(3), 183–189.

Vierck, C. J., Greenspan, J. D., & Ritz, L. A. (1990). Long-term changes in purposive and reflexive responses to nociceptive stimulation following anterolateral cordotomy. *The Journal of Neuroscience, 10*, 2077–2095.

Vierck, C. J., & Luck, M. M. (1979). Loss and recovery of reactivity to noxious stimuli in monkeys with primary spinothalamic cordotomies, followed by secondary and tertiary lesions of other cord sectors. *Brain, 102*, 233–248.

Walker, A. E. (1940). The spinothalamic tract in man. *Archives of Neurology and Psychiatry, 43*, 284–298.

Wall, P., Bery, J., & Saade, N. (1988). Effects of lesions to rat spinal cord lamina I cell projection pathways on reactions to acute and chronic noxious stimuli. *Pain, 35*, 327–339.

Wang, C. C., Willis, W. D., & Westlund, K. N. (1999). Ascending projections from the area around the spinal cord central canal: A *Phaseolus vulgaris* leucoagglutinin study in rats. *The Journal of Comparative Neurology, 415*(3), 341–367.

Wang, J., Gu, C., & Al-Chaer, E. D. (2008). Altered behavior and digestive outcomes in adult male rats primed with minimal colon pain as neonates. *Behavioral and Brain Functions, 4*, 28.

White, J. C. (1943). Sensory innervation of the viscera: Studies on visceral afferent neurons in man based on neurosurgical procedures for the relief of intractable pain. *Research Publications – Association for Research in Nervous and Mental Disease, 23*, 373–390.

White, J. C., & Sweet, W. H. (1969). *Pain and the neurosurgeon*. Springfield: Charles C. Thomas.

Willis, W. D. (1982). Control of nociceptive transmission in the spinal cord. In D. Ottoson (Ed.), *Progress in sensory physiology 3*. Berlin: Springer.

Willis, W. D. (1985). *The pain system*. Basel: Karger.

Willis, W. D., Al-Chaer, E. D., Quast, M. J., & Westlund, K. N. (1999). A visceral pain pathway in the dorsal column of the spinal cord. *Proceedings of the National Academy of Sciences of the United States of America, 96*(14), 7675–7679.

Willis, W. D., & Coggeshall, R. E. (2004). *Sensory mechanisms of the spinal cord* (3rd ed.). New York: Plenum Press.

Willis, W. D., Kenshalo, D. R. J., & Leonard, R. B. (1979). The cells of origin of the primate spinothalamic tract. *The Journal of Comparative Neurology, 188*, 543–574.

Willis, W. D., Trevino, D. L., Coulter, J. D., & Maunz, R. A. (1974). Responses of primate spinothalamic tract neurons to natural stimulation of hindlimb. *Journal of Neurophysiology, 37*, 358–372.

Willis, W. D., & Westlund, K. N. (1997). Neuroanatomy of the pain system and of the pathways that modulate pain. *Journal of Clinical Neurophysiology, 14*(1), 2–31.

Woolf, C., & Fitzgerald, M. (1983). The properties of neurons recorded in the superficial dorsal horn of the rat spinal cord. *The Journal of Comparative Neurology, 221*, 313–328.

Woolf, C. J., & Ma, Q. (2007). Nociceptors–noxious stimulus detectors. *Neuron, 55*(3), 353–364.

Woolf, C. J., & Salter, M. W. (2000). Neuronal plasticity: Increasing the gain in pain. *Science, 288*(5472), 1765–1769.

Xie, J., Yoon, Y. W., Yom, S. S., et al. (1995). Norepinephrine rekindles mechanical allodynia in sympathectomized neuropathic rat. *Analgesia, 1*, 107–113.

Yokota, T., Nishikawa, Y., & Koyama, N. (1988). Distribution of trigeminal nociceptive neurons in nucleus ventralis posteromedialis of primates. In R. Dubner, G. F. Gebhart, & M. R. Bond (Eds.), *Pain research and clinical management* (Vol. 3). Amsterdam: Elsevier.

Yoss, R. E. (1953). Studies of the spinal cord. Part 3. Pathways for deep pain within the spinal cord and brain. *Neurology, 3*, 163–175.

Zhuo, M., & Gebhart, G. F. (2002). Facilitation and attenuation of a visceral nociceptive reflex from the rostroventral medulla in the rat. *Gastroenterology, 122*, 1007–1019.

Chapter 19
Acute to Chronic Pain: Transition in the Post-Surgical Patient

Roland T. Short III and Thomas R. Vetter

Introduction

Pain has always been an accepted consequence of surgery, and the conventional wisdom has been that it should resolve as the patient heals. However, such symptom resolution does not always occur, leaving some patients with pain continuing well beyond the normal healing period. The fact that certain surgical procedures are more likely than others to result in chronic pain initially led to a procedure-specific approach to investigating and solving the problem, and the ability for surgery as a whole to contribute to chronic pain went under recognized. It was not until the late 1990s that the broader concept of chronic post-surgical pain (CPSP) was proposed. This represents an important shift in thinking because it suggests that there may be more similarities than differences among patients with CPSP despite their varying surgical insults. This paradigm shift began with a survey of pain medicine clinic patients throughout Great Britain, which revealed that 22.5% of patients' presenting pains were the result of a surgical procedure. The only reason for pain that was cited more often was degenerative joint disease (34.2%) (Crombie et al. 1998). Subsequently, multiple studies have evaluated the epidemiology, pathophysiology, and neuropsychology of CPSP in an attempt to better identify at-risk patient populations, implement preventative strategies, and treat those already suffering from CPSP.

The palliative care physician is in a unique position and is well suited to care for CPSP patients. The specialty cares for a group of patients with a wide variety of chronic conditions that are often associated with chronic pain. In fact, chronic pain is present in more than 50% of patients with end-stage cancer, AIDS, heart disease, COPD, and renal disease (Solano et al. 2006). As various types of surgical procedures are associated with all of these disease states, a significant portion of this chronic pain is post-surgical in nature. Furthermore, there is currently a drive to involve palliative care earlier in the management of patients with a variety of chronic conditions, many of which may be associated

R.T. Short III, MD (✉)
Department of Anesthesiology, University of Alabama School of Medicine,
619 South 19th Street, JT-862, Birmingham, AL 35249-6810, USA
e-mail: rtshort151@gmail.com

T.R. Vetter, MD, MPH
Division of Pain Medicine, Department of Anesthesiology, University of Alabama
at Birmingham School of Public Health, 619 South 19th Street, JT-862,
Birmingham, AL 35249-6810, USA

R.J. Moore (ed.), *Handbook of Pain and Palliative Care: Biobehavioral Approaches for the Life Course*,   295
DOI 10.1007/978-1-4419-1651-8_19, © Springer Science+Business Media, LLC 2012

with a normal life expectancy. While some of the more invasive pain treatment options may be deferred until end-of-life management, most of the treatment options for CPSP are applicable to patients at any point in their lifespan. Earlier involvement leads to increased opportunities for the palliative care specialist to intervene in CPSP. In the case of patients already suffering from CPSP, an adequate understanding of the pathophysiological and psychological changes that take place in the transition from acute to chronic pain also allows for design of an appropriate treatment regimen. In the case of patients for whom surgery is planned, knowledge of CPSP can help to identify those patients at greatest risk and form a plan that attempts to minimize chronic pain as an outcome (Sepulveda et al. 2002).

This chapter will provide the following overview of CPSP:

- Definition
- Epidemiology
- Pathophysiology
- Risk factors
- Management
- Overview of specific post-surgical pain syndromes

Definition

When assigned the task of finding a solution, the first step is to define the problem. However, when the problem is broad and multifactorial, this first step can be difficult. Such is the case with CPSP.

To begin, there is no agreed upon definition regarding the time required for the transition from acute to chronic pain. Bonica, in 1953, described chronic pain as that which persisted "beyond the normal time of healing." However, healing time varies depending on the type of tissue injury. For example, skin heals at a faster rate than peripheral nerves. In the case of surgical pain, a range of expected recovery times exist for different surgical procedures. The general consensus among most authorities is that a time period of 3–6 months is needed before post-surgical pain is considered chronic (Apkarian et al. 2009).

How CPSP presents varies depending on the surgery in question. Furthermore, even for the same procedure, different forms of CPSP can exist, sometimes simultaneously. For example, postamputees may suffer from stump pain, phantom limb pain, or both (see also Foell and Flor 2011). The nature of the pain complaint should be consistent with a known presentation of CPSP. Pain may develop that, although temporally related to the surgery, is new and independent of the procedure itself. It is the clinician and the caretaker's responsibility to be familiar with the types of pain that classically follow a particular surgery. It should also always be remembered that CPSP is a diagnosis of exclusion. Any other organic causes of pain such as metastases or infection should first be ruled-out.

Finally, the presence of pain prior to surgery may further confuse the picture. In patients with pre-existing pain who undergo a procedure, an attempt to differentiate procedurally induced pain from former pain must be made prior to establishing the clinical diagnosis of CPSP.

The current working definition for CPSP is as follows (Macrae and Davies 1999):

- The pain develops after a surgical procedure
- The pain is of at least 2 months duration
- Other causes of the pain have been excluded (e.g., malignancy, infection)
- The possibility that the pain is caused from a pre-existing condition should be explored and, if possible, excluded

Epidemiology

Any surgery can potentially result in chronic pain; however, certain surgeries are more likely than others to do so. Table 19.1 lists seven commonly performed surgical procedures with their respective estimated incidence of CPSP. Of note, for several reasons, the incidence range for each of these procedures is quite wide.

For reasons discussed above, establishing an appropriately inclusive definition has been challenging. However, many studies reporting on the epidemiology of certain CPSP syndromes failed to utilize any type of definition. When definitions have been used, they have often been inconsistent (Poobalan et al. 2003 #780).

Epidemiological studies of CPSP have also lacked uniformity in many ways other than definition as well. Clinical variables including the duration of follow-up, surgical technique, patient population, and what, if any, preventative therapeutic measures were undertaken have also differed from study to study. Such discrepancies likely contribute to the wide range of reported incident values (Bruce et al. 2003, 2004).

Further affecting the quality of these epidemiological studies is the fact that most are retrospective. Therefore, they rely on a patient's ability to accurately remember the amount of pre-surgical, acute post-surgical, and CPSP experienced. Such patient recall has been demonstrated to be unreliable (Tasmuth et al. 1996).

Another interesting phenomenon is that those studies in which CPSP is the primary focus tend to report a higher incidence of post-surgical pain. A striking example of this occurrence involves the reported incidence of phantom limb pain following amputation. Even though the currently accepted rate of chronic phantom limb pain is thought to range between 60 and 80%, some early literature reported incidence rates as low as 2%. This discrepancy seems most likely a result of early studies that based their incidence rates on patients' requests for pain treatment following surgery, a practice that significantly underestimates the true frequency of CPSP (Nikolajsen and Jensen 2001). It is has been historically demonstrated that patients are often unwilling to complain of phantom limb pain before being prompted due to fear of being labeled as mentally unstable (Sherman and Sherman 1983). While the rate of underreporting may vary depending on the type of post-surgical pain in question, it still begs the question of whether an unrecognized, and possibly undertreated, population of CPSP patients exists.

To date, epidemiological studies have been procedure specific, and thus the overall incidence of CPSP is not known. However, to illustrate the possible overall societal impact of CPSP, it is helpful to consider the estimated number of annual surgeries. According to the CDC National Center for Health Statistics (NCHS), in 2006, there were an estimated 46 million surgical procedures performed in the United States alone. Taking into consideration only the seven procedure types listed in

Table 19.1 Surgeries commonly resulting in CPSP, the respective estimated rates of CPSP and the estimated number of operations performed annually in the United States

Type of operation	Incidence of chronic post-surgical pain	Number of operations performed in USA in 2006 (DeFrances et al. 2008)
Coronary artery bypass graft	28% (Meyerson et al. 2001) to 56% (Eisenberg et al. 2001)	444,000
Hysterectomy	4.7–31.9% (Brandsborg et al. 2008)	560,000
Mastectomy	25–60% (Gartner et al. 2009)	60,000
Thoracotomy	21–61% (Gottschalk and Ochroch 2008)	699,000
Amputation (lower limb)	60–80% (Nikolajsen and Jensen 2001)	65,000
Cesarean section	6–18% (Vermelis et al. 2010)	1,269,000
Cholecystectomy (open+lap)	5–50% (Macrae 2008; Ure et al. 2004)	721,000

Table 19.1 and applying the lowest incidence rate for each, suggests that as many as 460,000 new patients can potentially experience CPSP each year. If one accepts the highest incidence rate for each procedure, the number of new patients suffering from CPSP each year may be as high as 1.5 million.

Pathophysiology

Pain is an evolved phenomenon comprised of both sensory-discriminative and affective-motivational components that serves the role of protecting an organism from harm. As such, it changes to adapt to the various circumstances and environments encountered. These changes can be either in the form of amplification or attenuation of sensory input, and when operating appropriately, function to promote and enhance survival. The process by which the nervous system alters how it responds to both external and internal stimuli is termed *neuronal plasticity*. A commonly cited example of extreme attenuation is that of soldiers who continued to function in battle despite sustaining severe injuries, including loss of limb, and later reported that at the time they felt little or no pain (Beecher 1946 #730, 1959 #733). More often recognized is the ability of the nervous system to increase its sensitivity following an injury so that even non-noxious stimuli begin to cause pain, a process termed *sensitization*. Such a response is appropriate to prevent further injury during the time of healing. Typically, once an injury heals, the sensitivity of the nervous system returns to baseline and pain resolves. However, in some cases the nervous system fails to reset and instead pain continues to be experienced, even long after tissue healing has finished. When this occurs, pain itself becomes the disease.

The mechanisms responsible for neuronal plasticity are multiple, and all levels of the pain signaling pathways are involved. The degree to which sensitization occurs depends on factors such as the intensity and duration of the nociceptive input, degree of inflammatory response from the tissue injury, and magnitude of any direct peripheral nerve injury that may have occurred. There is also growing evidence that genetic, environmental and developmental patterns also play a role in predisposing certain individuals to chronic pain (Papp and Sobel 2009 #777; Al-Chaer and Weaver 2009 #778). The myriad of neuroplastic changes that occur can be broadly categorized into three types based on the mechanism of action. *Activation-dependent* plasticity is attributed primarily to conformational receptor changes and/or a temporary loss of inhibition and is typically short-lasting. *Modulation* occurs via post-translational changes to receptor and ion channels and produces longer lasting but reversible increases in the sensitivity of the nervous system. *Modification* is an increase in the sensitivity of the nervous system that results from transcriptional changes in gene expression. The effects of modification tend to be more permanent (Woolf and Salter 2000).

CPSP is a syndrome based entirely on the fact that sometimes acute pain becomes chronic. Therefore, it is an ideal pain state for questioning how the transition from acute to chronic pain occurs. In fact, many investigators who use animal models to study chronic pain have incorporated surgical procedures into their methodologies for this very reason. This section attempts to provide an overview of neuroplastic changes that contribute to the development of chronic pain. While this chapter focuses on CPSP, the pathophysiology discussed below is applicable to the generalized field of chronic pain.

Basic concepts of pain signaling: Primary afferent fibers can broadly be classified based on their conduction velocity (which is dependent on size and the presence or absence of myelination) and the stimuli by which they are activated. A-beta ($A\beta$) fibers are large, myelinated fibers that conduct the fastest (35–75 m/s). A-delta ($A\delta$) fibers are smaller but also myelinated and have slower conduction speeds (>2 m/s). C fibers consist of small, unmyelinated fibers with the slowest conduction speeds (<2 m/s). $A\beta$ fibers typically respond to light touch, pressure, or vibration. $A\delta$ and C-fibers respond to the sensations of pain or temperature, and those fibers that respond specifically to pain are termed *nociceptive* nerve fibers. Most nociceptive nerve fibers are *polymodal*, meaning that they respond to all types of stimuli, including mechanical, thermal, and chemical. Nociceptive Aδ and C fibers appear to work in concert by, respectively, providing the early (sharp, intense) and late (burning, throbbing) sensations of acute pain (Meyer and Campbell 1981 #784) (see also Al-Chaer 2011).

When a nociceptive receptor is exposed to a noxious stimulus, its ion channel opens partially depolarizing the nerve ending, a process termed *transduction*. When a sufficient number of ion channels are opened, an action potential is generated that transmits an afferent signal to the dorsal horn of the spinal cord. All primary afferents use glutamate as their principle neurotransmitter and, therefore, induce excitatory postsynaptic potentials (EPSP). Many activated nociceptors also play an efferent role in pain signal transduction by peripherally releasing neuropeptides like substance P and calcitonin gene-related peptide (CGRP). These neuropeptides induce an inflammatory reaction (vasodilation, plasma extravasation, attraction of macrophages, mast cell degranulation, etc.) termed *neurogenic inflammation* (Schaible and Richter 2004).

The amount of external stimulation (e.g., heat, pressure, or chemical) that is required to generate an action potential is termed the *activation threshold*. The role of nociceptive neurons is to identify actual or potential injury, and so their activation thresholds are usually high. However, as will be discussed, the activation threshold of a neuron is not static. In fact, the ability of the nervous system to adjust its neuronal responses to external stimuli is a central concept of neuronal plasticity.

All peripheral afferent fibers direct their action potentials to the dorsal horn, which is the main hub connecting the peripheral nervous system (PNS) and the central nervous system (CNS). At the level of the dorsal horn, a confluence of ascending and descending spinal tracts interact with the central terminals of peripheral afferents. Such bidirectional signaling allows for the nervous system to both process and adjust to somatosensory input almost instantaneously.

The dorsal horn is anatomically divided into six layers or *laminae* based on the size and packing density of its neurons as identified by Rexed (1952 #782). Peripheral afferent fibers terminate within the laminae of the dorsal horn in an organized fashion according to diameter and type. Most Aδ and C-fiber central terminals are found in the superficial laminae I and II (respectively, called the *marginal layer* and the *substantia gelatinosa*) while the larger Aβ-fibers tend to arborize in the deeper laminae III–V. Ascending projection neurons relay sensory input from the dorsal horn to various supraspinal targets where processing of information continues. Descending neurons travel in the opposite direction and allow for various supraspinal regions to influence how easily sensory input flows through the dorsal horn (discussed further below). Interneurons are also found within the dorsal horn. These neurons do not travel outside of the spinal cord and tend to arborize locally. While incompletely understood, at least part of their known role is to modulate sensory throughput at the dorsal horn in response to signaling received from both peripheral afferent fibers and central descending axons.

Ascending projection neurons can be classified as either nociceptor specific (NS) or wide dynamic range (WDR) based on the type of sensory input they receive. NS neurons are predominantly found in lamina I and the outer part of lamina II of the dorsal horn where they receive input from Aδ and C-fiber nociceptive afferents. Most often NS neurons interact with their afferent inputs indirectly via interneurons; however, some direct synapses between Aδ fibers and NS projection neurons in lamina I have been identified (Grudt and Perl 2002 #785). WDR neurons are located deeper in the dorsal horn in lamina III–V. These neurons directly synapse with both low-threshold Aβ and nociceptive Aδ and C-fibers.

WDR neurons have graded responses to the sensory input that they receive so that non-noxious stimuli induce lower impulse firing rates than noxious stimuli. In contrast, NS neurons do not respond at all to non-noxious stimuli, but respond fully to noxious stimuli. While both WDR and NS neurons have spontaneous discharge rates, WDR neurons have faster basal rates (11 Hz) than NS neurons (3–5 Hz).

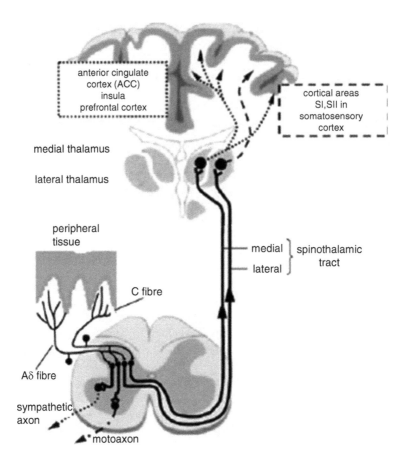

Fig. 19.1 Scheme of the nociceptive system with nociceptive. Free nerve endings in the peripheral tissue, afferent nerve fibers, and their synapses in the dorsal horn of the spinal cord. From the dorsal horn, the ascending tracts including the medial and lateral spinothalamic tracts project to the thalamus. Relay nuclei in the thalamus then project rostrally to the anterior cingulate cortex, insula, prefrontal cortex, and somatosensory cortex. Interneurons also exist in the dorsal horn that serve to modulate secondary synaptic propagation thereby attenuating or facilitating nociceptive signaling. Interneurons have also been found to interact with sympathetic and motor nerves as well (Schaible and Richter 2004)

Although WDR neurons are located primarily in the deeper laminae, they have been found to send dendritic connections to the more superficial laminae of the dorsal horn (Naim et al. 1997 #786). Such neuronal organization supports the gate control theory of pain originally proposed by Melzack and Wall (1965 #787). This theory posits that intrinsic Aβ activity inhibits nociceptive signaling by Aδ and C-fibers. In fact, the ability of such low-threshold non-noxious receptor activity to partially inhibit the conduction of nociceptive signaling at the level of the dorsal horn has been demonstrated (Bini et al. 1984). Furthermore, an established connection between non-noxious and noxious signaling pathways provides a mechanism for how certain chronic pain conditions such as allodynia (pain experienced from non-noxious stimuli) may exist.

Numerous ascending projection tracts extend from the dorsal horn to various targets in the brainstem and higher cortical regions. The destinations of these tracts provide clues into what regions of the brain are involved in pain processing and how other psychological phenomena, such as emotion or attention, may influence pain perception.

The largest and most studied of the ascending projection systems is the spinothalamic tract (Fig. 19.1). Axons of the spinothalamic tract are concentrated in two locations of the spinal cord.

The lateral spinothalamic tract travels in the middle of the lateral funiculus, and the medial spinothalamic tract travels in the middle of the anterior funiculus. The lateral spinothalamic tract projects to the somatosensory region of the brain and the medial spinothalamic tract projects to prefrontal targets including the anterior cingulate. Based on these respective destinations, historically these tracts have been associated with the sensory-discriminative and the cognitive-emotional components of pain sensation. However, emerging research continues to blur these lines, especially in the situation of chronic pain (Apkarian et al. 2009).

Other ascending tracts also exist that appear to be as vital, if not even more important, than the spinothalamic tracts regarding the development of chronic pain. Projections to the catecholamine cell groups (A1–7) are thought to be involved with the autonomic responses (Ex. tachycardia, vasoconstriction) associated with pain. The parabrachial nucleus also receives sensory input from the spinal cord that may allow it to play a role in integrating visceral and peripheral nociceptive sensation. The fact that the parabrachial nucleus projects to both the hypothalamus and reticular formation suggests that it may be involved with the neuroendocrine and arousal responses to pain. The parabrachial nucleus' interactions with the amygdala provide a potential pathway connecting pain and emotion (Price et al. 2006).

As will be discussed in greater detail (see also, Naylor et al. 2011) a variety of cortical regions appear to be involved in the higher processing of pain. For acute pain, the major contributing brain regions are the primary and secondary somatosensory, insular, anterior cingulate, and prefrontal cortices. Many of these structures have been found to receive projections both directly from the spinal cord and indirectly via the spinothalamic pathways (Price et al. 2006 #801). There is also growing recognition that in chronic pain states the relative contributions of each of these regions and the timing of their interactions with each other changes. Furthermore, patients with chronic pain engage regions of the brain that usually remain silent in healthy patients experiencing acute pain. Many of these newly engaged regions are heavily involved in cognitive and emotional functioning, providing a mechanism for the strong affective component of chronic pain that is so often seen in clinical pain population (Apkarian et al. 2005 #798, 2009 #794).

Electrophysiological Concepts of Neuroplasticity

Exposure to noxious stimuli promotes neuroplastic changes that clinically result in *hyperesthesia*. Hyperesthesia is an increased sensitivity to stimulation, both painful and nonpainful. Hyperesthesia is a broad term that includes several different types of painful sensations (Merskey and Bogduk 1994):

- *Hyperalgesia* is an increased response to a stimulus that is normally painful.
- *Allodynia* is a painful response to a stimulus that is normally not painful.
- *Dysesthesia* is an unpleasant abnormal sensation that may be either spontaneous or evoked.

While pain is a subjective phenomenon, the process of *nociception* (the encoding and processing of noxious stimuli) is an objective phenomenon that can be measured via electrophysiological testing. Electrophysiologically, hyperesthesia is observed as increased nerve fiber activity following a noxious stimulus and is termed *sensitization*. Sensitization occurs when receptors display a decreased activation threshold for stimulation, an increased response to suprathreshold stimuli, and spontaneous electrophysiological activity (Meyer et al. 2006). The relationship between the electrophysiological findings observed with sensitization and patients' subjective experiences with hyperesthesia is detailed in Table 19.2.

An individual nociceptor innervates a specific area on the skin that can be measured objectively. This area of nociceptive coverage is termed the *receptor field*. When a nociceptor is activated by a

Table 19.2 Comparison of characteristics of hyperesthesia and sensitization

Hyperesthesia (subjective response)	Sensitization (electrophysiologically recorded nerve fiber response)
Increased pain to suprathreshold stimuli (hyperalgesia)	Increased electrical response to suprathreshold stimuli
Decreased pain threshold (allodynia)	Decreased activation threshold for electrical response
Spontaneous pain (dysesthesia)	Spontaneous electrical activity

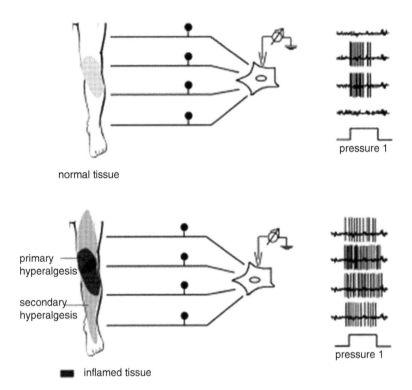

Fig. 19.2 When a noxious stimulus is applied to tissue, peripheral sensitization results in the zone of primary hyperalgesia. As result of central sensitization, the expanded zone of secondary hyperalgesia is formed (Schaible and Richter 2004)

noxious stimulus, the receptor field of that nociceptor becomes hyperalgesic, thus forming the zone *of primary hyperalgesia.* Neuroplastic changes primarily occurring in the PNS, or *peripheral sensitization,* form the zone of primary hyperalgesia. However, after a noxious stimulus, the area outside of the original receptor field can also become hyperalgesic. This surrounding area is termed the *zone of secondary hyperalgesia,* and it develops as a result of neuroplastic changes occurring in the CNS, or *central sensitization* (Fig. 19.2) (Joshi and Ogunnaike 2005).

That different mechanisms are involved in the development of the primary and secondary zones of hyperalgesia were elegantly demonstrated in an experiment by LaMotte et al. (1991). Capsaicin (a substance found in hot peppers that directly activates nociceptors producing both zones of primary and secondary hyperalgesia) was injected subcutaneously into an upper extremity that had already received a proximal nerve block, sparing the CNS of nociceptive input. By creating this interruption between the peripheral and CNS, formation of the zone of secondary hyperalgesia was entirely inhibited supporting the CNS's integral involvement in this process (LaMotte et al. 1991).

However, during surgery, nerves not only relay nociceptive input resulting from surrounding tissue injury but also suffer injury themselves. Such injury to nervous tissue results in a specific type of pain called *neuropathic pain*. Characteristics of neuropathic pain can be divided into negative and positive symptoms. Negative symptoms include the sensory and motor deficits that result from the injury. Positive symptoms include any allodynia, hyperalgesia, dysesthesia, or hyperpathia at the site of the nerve injury. *Hyperpathia* refers to a combination of dulled sensation with increased stimulus threshold and poor localization; extreme pain with repeated stimulation that persists after the stimulation has ended; and spread of the pain from the site of stimulation. Hyperpathia appears to be unique to neuropathic pain (Devor 2006).

Peripheral sensitization and the neuropathic pain resulting from nerve injury work in conjunction to send a barrage of nociceptive signaling to the dorsal horn. This massive influx of nociceptive input, in turn, causes central sensitization to occur which further amplifies what is relayed to the brain. Higher processing then incorporates behavioral and historical components such as emotion, past memories, and psychopathological conditions into received sensory information allowing these elements to also modify how pain is perceived. Furthermore, the brain utilizes the descending tracts to exert its influence over pain processing at the level of the dorsal horn as well. Some of the mechanisms thought to be responsible for the above processes will be discussed below.

Peripheral Sensitization

The sensitivity of the peripheral nociceptors increases with repeated stimulation. Heat sensitivity and thermal hyperalgesia are at least partly mediated by the capsaicin-sensitive vanilloid 1 receptor/ion channel complex (TRPV1). Increased intracellular calcium levels that occur as a result of repeated activation are believed to cause conformational changes increasing sensitivity of the receptor (Guenther et al. 1999). Mechanoreceptors are thought to open their associated ion channels in response to external pressure allowing cations to depolarize the nerve terminal, achieve activation threshold, and initiate an action potential. Swelling secondary to inflammation may allow these channels to more effectively open, thereby, increasing their sensitivity (Belmonte and Cervero 1996). Furthermore, some nociceptive fibers increase their receptive fields after activation, resulting in a greater response to stimulus ratio, which can produce more pain (Reeh et al. 1987; Thalhammer and LaMotte 1982).

Numerous inflammatory mediators are released upon exposure to a noxious stimulus or tissue injury including bradykinin, histamine, serotonin, adenosine derivatives, arachidonic acid metabolites, and various cytokines (Fig. 19.3). Some of these substances directly activate nociceptors further increasing their sensitivity by means of repeated stimulation. However, other mediators initiate modulatory changes to the PNS by initiating intracellular cascades leading to increased nociceptor sensitivity (Bhave and Gereau 2004; McMahon et al. 2006). Bradykinin both directly activates nociceptors as well as sensitizes the capsaicin receptor (TRPV1) via a protein kinase C pathway (Okuse 2007). Adenosine triphosphate (ATP) released from injured tissue appears to bind to its associated ion channel, $P2X_3$, increasing calcium influx into nociceptive nerve fibers. Pro-inflammatory cytokines such as tumor necrosis factor alpha (TNF-α), interleukin-1 (IL-1), IL-6, and the chemokine IL-8 have been shown to produce mechanical and thermal hyperalgesia following injection. However, the cytokines also appear to induce peripheral sensitization via phosphorylation of nociceptive receptors by means of various intracellular kinase pathways. The prostaglandins phosphorylate the tetrodotoxin-resistant sensory neuron specific (TTX-SNS) sodium ion channel, an ion channel

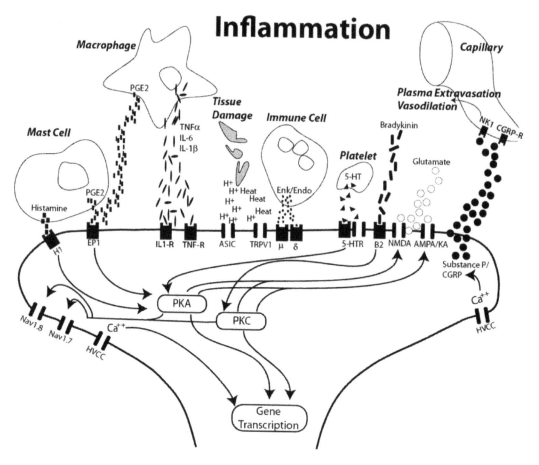

Fig. 19.3 Inflammatory mediators released in response to a noxious stimulus both directly activate some receptors as well as initiate a series of intracellular cascades that result in both post-translational receptor modulation and gene transcription modification, all of which result in peripheral sensitization (Sluka 2009)

specific to Aδ and C-fiber nerves, via a protein kinase A (PKA) or C pathway reducing its activation threshold (Cesare et al. 1999; Khasar et al. 1999).

Additionally, several pro-inflammatory mediators have been shown to recruit a special group of nociceptive nerve fibers, termed mechanically insensitive afferents (MIAs). These fibers, as their name suggests, are normally unresponsive to mechanical stimuli and not involved in nociceptive transmission. However, upon activation, they become profoundly sensitive even to subthreshold stimuli that would normally not be noxious. This finding correlates with the hypersensitivity noted immediately following an injury (Davis et al. 1993). A cyclic AMP/PKA second messenger cascade has been implicated as the mechanism by which recruitment of MIA receptors occurs (Levy and Strassman 2002).

Inflammation also releases neurotrophins such as nerve growth factor (NGF) into the involved tissue. Neurotrophins are a family of proteins that normally act to induce survival, development, and function of neurons; however, when their concentration levels are increased they function to produce a hyperalgesic response. NGF directly causes degranulation of mast cells, and as a result provides a positive feedback loop further increasing the amount of inflammatory mediators available to induce sensitization of the peripheral nociceptors. NGF also modifies gene expression by binding to receptor tyrosine kinase A (trkA). This interaction upregulates synthesis of SNS, TRPV1 channels, substance P, calcitonin-gene-related peptide (CGRP), and bradykinin receptors further contributing to peripheral sensitization (Michael and Priestley 1999; Okuse 2007; Schaible and Richter 2004; Tate et al. 1998).

Peripheral Nerve Injury

Injury to a peripheral nerve results in neuropathic pain. While healthy nerves tend to only fire after being stimulated, injured nerves often exhibit abnormal, spontaneous electrical activity termed *ectopy* (Fukuoka et al. 2000; Wu et al. 2001). These ectopic discharges involve not only the smaller Aδ and C-fiber nerves, but also the larger myelinated Aβ-fibers that typically encode innocuous mechanosensory information.

Ectopy develops because nerve injury induces internal changes that lead to a hyperexcitable state. As injured nerves undergo Wallerian degeneration, an inflammatory milieu develops causing increased levels of NGF to be expressed. NGF, in turn, induces changes in membrane ion channel expression resulting in both increased channel density as well as altered channel kinetics. A higher density of ion channels promotes ectopy by increasing the likelihood that depolarization occurs (Aurilio et al. 2008).

The specific role of ion channels in the development of ectopy is worth addressing. Nine subtypes of sodium ion channels have been identified and classified by their respective sensitivity or resistance to the neurotoxin, tetrodotoxin (TTX). The TTX-sensitive sodium channels become inactive quickly, resulting in burst-like signal transmissions that are most consistent with the electrical activity of ectopy. The TTX-resistant sodium channels which have slower inactivation and activation kinetics are most concentrated on the smaller Aδ and C-fiber neurons. Following a nerve injury, both TTX-sensitive and resistant channels are upregulated at the damaged site as well as along the neuron. These changes are thought to alter the membrane properties of the neuron, so that rapid firing rates (bursting ectopic discharges) are produced (Woolf and Mannion 1999). The ability of the intrinsically slower TTX-resistant channels to produce ectopic activity is believed to be a result of cascade mediated conformational changes that increase channel conductivity (Aurilio et al. 2008). In addition to the abnormal accumulation of sodium channels, there is evidence that nerve injury also promotes an increased number of calcium channels to be expressed that may contribute to ectopic activity (Xie et al. 1993). These specific phenotypic changes are important to understand as they may offer routes for targeted pharmocotherapy in the future. As will be discussed later, many of the medications used to treat neuropathic pain are nonspecific and, therefore, have many side effects. Developing agents with high affinities specific to these ion channels is a high priority in the pharmaceutical industry.

Normally, the sympathetic nervous system is not involved in nociception. However, some axons begin to express α-adrenoceptors following nerve injury, causing them to become sensitive to circulating catecholamines and norepinephrine released by postganglionic sympathetic terminals. In such a manner, the sympathetic nervous system may also become a source of nociceptive transduction, termed *sympathetically maintained pain* (Woolf and Mannion 1999).

Central Sensitization

Central sensitization can be viewed as having two major components. First, it serves to amplify any sensory input received at the dorsal horn. Second, it converts innocuous sensory input from non-nociceptive afferents into nociceptive transmission. In addition to CPSP, central sensitization is also involved in the development of neuropathic pain (diabetic neuropathy, postherpetic neuralgia), inflammatory pain (rheumatoid arthritis, lupus), migraine, irritable bowel syndrome (IBS), and fibromyalgia. Neurons in the dorsal horn that have been affected by central sensitization exhibit some or all of the following (Latremoliere and Woolf 2009):

- Development of or increases in spontaneous activity
- A reduction in the threshold for activation by peripheral stimuli
- Increase in the responsiveness to any suprathreshold input
- Expansion of the extent of the receptive fields of dorsal horn neurons

When inflammatory and neuropathic pain in the periphery conduct a barrage of nociceptive signaling to the spinal cord, neuroplastic changes resulting in central sensitization begin to occur. Normal nociceptive signal conduction involves the primary afferent neuron releasing the excitatory neurotransmitters, glutamate, and aspartate into the synaptic cleft. These neurotransmitters then activate the alpha-amino-3-hydroxy-5-methyl-isoxazole-4-propionic acid (AMPA) receptors on the postsynaptic membrane allowing for signal propagation to continue rostrally. However, when AMPA receptors are continuously activated, prolonged depolarization of the postsynaptic membrane occurs allowing for a normally quiescent N-methyl-D-aspartate (NMDA) channel to become activated through a loss of static inhibition by magnesium ions (Mayer et al. 1984). Activation of the NMDA receptor creates a surge in intracellular calcium which, in turn, activates numerous intracellular pathways that contribute to the maintenance of central sensitization. Together, the AMPA and NMDA receptors amplify the incoming nociceptive signal throughput in a process termed *windup*.

Additionally, depolarization triggers the release of neuropeptides, including substance P (SP) and CGRP, into the dorsal horn synapse. These neuropeptides activate G-protein coupled receptors, which slow postsynaptic depolarization, further allowing temporal summation and amplification of the nociceptive signal to occur. SP binds to its neurokinin 1 (NK-1) receptor activating a PKC pathway that phosphorylates the NMDA receptor. Phosphorylation of the NMDA receptor also stabilizes the receptor in its active state (Woolf and Salter 2006). These neuropeptides reside in vesicles located in the presynaptic terminal. When depolarization occurs, voltage sensitive calcium channels (VSCC) open increasing intracellular calcium concentrations, thereby allowing the vesicles to fuse with the presynaptic membrane and release their contents. Of the various types of calcium channels expressed in the nervous system, evidence suggests that the high-threshold N-type channels located in the superficial Rexed laminae (discussed further below) are most important to the development of central sensitization (Fig. 19.4) (Aurilio et al. 2008).

Synaptic connections at the dorsal horn are not permanent, and their rearrangement may explain how normally innocuous input from mechanosensory Aβ-fibers is perceived as painful after central sensitization has occurred. Typically, nociceptive fibers synapse superficially in the dorsal horn at Rexed laminae I and II while mechanosensitive fibers synapse at the deeper Rexed laminae. Aβ-fibers do have dendritic extensions to nociceptors in the more superficial laminae. Normally signals via these extensions are thought to be inhibited by interneurons. One theory of allodynia is that a loss of this inhibition occurs allowing for non-noxious stimuli to be miscoded as a nociceptive signal (Todd 2010 #817). Furthermore, following central sensitization the synaptic locations of the Aβ-fibers migrate superficially so that they activate secondary neurons of the nociceptive pathway (Schaible and Richter 2004). Such rearrangement of synaptic connections at the dorsal horn may extend rostrally or caudally one or more levels contiguously.

Other factors may also have roles in the development of secondary hyperalgesia. For example, tissue damage itself, particularly to low-threshold non-noxious peripheral receptors, may also facilitate this process. The normal activity of these innocuous receptors partially inhibits the conduction of pain signals upon activation of nociceptors (Bini et al. 1984). Therefore, loss of this innocuous transmission may result in a central disinhibition of nociceptor input (Meyer et al. 2006). As will be discussed in the next section, supraspinal influence at the level of the dorsal horn is also very much involved in the development of central sensitization.

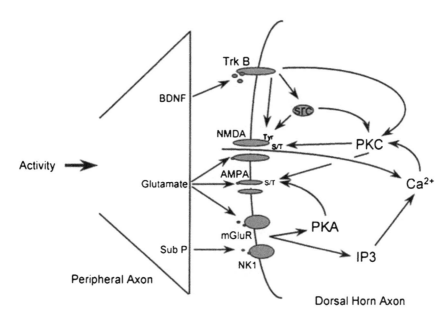

Fig. 19.4 Repeated barrage of nociceptive signaling at the dorsal horn results in activation of the NMDA receptor as well as initiation of multiple intracellular cascade pathways leading to post-translational and transcriptional changes (Woolf and Costigan 1999)

Descending Tracts

The ability of the brain to modulate nociceptive signaling at the level of the dorsal horn is dependent on two structures: the PAG and the rostral ventromedial medulla (RVM). The PAG is located in the midbrain and receives direct inputs from numerous higher structures including the anterior cingulate, insular cortex, and amygdala. Indirectly, structures such as the nucleus accumbens and lateral hypothalamus project to the PAG. The PAG also interacts with its neighboring regions, the nucleus cuneiformis, the reticular formation, the locus coeruleus, and other brainstem catecholaminergic nuclei. Finally, the PAG receives direct projections from lamina I nociceptive neurons.

The PAG exerts its influence over nociceptive processing at the dorsal horn via its interaction with the RVM. The RVM is located in the medulla and includes the midline nucleus raphe magnus and the adjacent reticular formation that lies ventral to the nucleus reticularis gigantocellularis. The major descending tracts to the dorsal horn of the spinal cord initiate from the RVM. Three classes of neurons that travel from the RVM to the dorsal horn have been identified: on-cells, off-cells, and neutral cells. These neurons are found throughout the RVM and are not anatomically separable; they have instead been classified based on their activity responses to a noxious stimulus. Off-cells display an abrupt pause in ongoing activity immediately following a noxious stimulus and are believed to contribute to the inhibitory influences of the RVM on the dorsal horn. On-cells display a burst of activity immediately following a noxious stimulus and are believed to contribute to the facilitatory influences of the RVM on the dorsal horn. Neutral cells show no change in activity related to noxious stimuli (Fields et al. 2006 #810).

While the PAG-RVM descending modulatory system is most known for the attenuating effects it has on pain, more recently there has been growing evidence that it may have significant roles in facilitating chronic pain states as well. Low-intensity electrical stimulation of the RVM or direct injection of the neurotransmitter glutamate has been shown to increase spinal nociception.

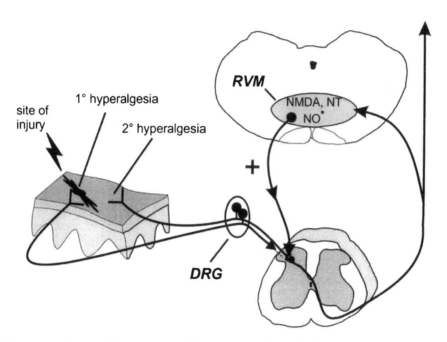

Fig. 19.5 Summary diagram illustrating a significant supraspinal contribution to secondary, but not primary, hyperalgesia. As will be discussed further, peripheral injury results in activation and sensitization of peripheral noci-ceptors and subsequent enhanced excitability of dorsal horn neurons (central sensitization) that contributes to primary hyperalgesia (at the site of injury) and secondary hyperalgesia (adjacent/distant from the site of injury). Additionally, it has been proposed that stimulation of nociceptors activates a spinobulbospinal loop, engaging centrifugal descending nociceptive facilitatory influence from the RVM. Facilitatory influences are activated by NMDA, NO⁻, and NT receptors in the RVM and descend to multiple spinal segments to contribute significantly to secondary hyperalgesia. In contrast, primary hyperalgesia does not involve descending facilitatory influences from supraspinal sites and is likely the direct result of peripheral nociceptor sensitization and neuroplasticity intrinsic to the spinal cord. For clarity, the afferent input to the spinal dorsal horn from the site of injury is illustrated as not entering the spinal cord (which it certainly does) (Urban 1999 #814)

These facilitatory influences appear to involve an anatomically separate descending projection system in the ventrolateral funiculi and to be mediated by spinal serotonin and cholecystokinin receptors. Furthermore, secondary hyperalgesia following certain pain states such as mustard oil-induced sensitization and neuropathic pain after spinal nerve ligation can be attenuated by inactivation of the RVM. NMDA, neurontensin (NT), and nitric oxide (NO⁻) receptors in the RVM appear to be involved in these processes. An illustration of this proposed spinobulbospinal pathway and its role in secondary hyperalgesia is presented in Fig. 19.5 (Urban 1999 #814).

In its healthy state, the basal tone of this processing appears to be mostly inhibitory to prevent spontaneous nociceptive signals from occurring in the absence of actual noxious stimuli or tissue injury. This inhibitory state does not appear to opioid driven given the fact that intrathecal injection of the opioid inhibitor naloxone does not cause hyperalgesia. Serotonin has been proposed as partially responsible for the tonic inhibitory state. Supporting this hypothesis are the facts that the RVM is the exclusive source of serotonin in the dorsal horn, serotonergic RVM neurons continuously slowly release serotonin into the dorsal horn, and intrathecal administration of serotonin antagonists has been found to reduce the effectiveness of the RVM to produce analgesia. However, as mentioned above at least one serotonin receptor (5-HT$_3$) appears to also be involved in facilitating certain pain states, suggesting that serotonin probably plays a more complex role in modulating pain (Fields et al. 2006 #810).

Behavioral Factors in Neuroplasticity

Certain behavioral states have consistently been shown to alter pain perception. Studies evaluating the relationship of attention and pain have reliably demonstrated that when subjects are distracted they report less pain (Levine et al. 1982 #824; Miron et al. 1989 #826). This is obviously a difficult association to unravel because pain itself is an attention-demanding phenomenon. In fact, a decreased ability to distract attention away from pain may be a feature common to chronic pain patients (Grisart and Plaghki 1999 #827).

The pathways and mechanisms behind how attention modifies pain perception are still incompletely understood. Neurophysiological studies have shown that modulation from attentional changes occurs even at the level of the dorsal horn (Villemure and Bushnell 2002 #822). The aid of functional MRI (fMRI) has also demonstrated that attention influences many of the same brain regions involved with pain processing. Tracey et al. observed that PAG activity was significantly increased when subjects were distracted from pain (Tracey et al. 2002 #829). Other areas of the brain involved in attention and pain appear to be the secondary somatosensory cortex (S2), anterior cingulate cortex, and insula (Sawamoto et al. 2000 #836).

The inability of chronic pain patients to distract themselves from the experience of pain has been proposed as one driving maladaptive behavior. Normally, the pain associated with repeated exposure to a noxious stimulus diminishes over time in a process termed *habituation* or a time-dependent decline of vigilance. The same areas of the brain thought to be crucial for maintaining vigilance are also involved in focusing attention to pain. Therefore, patients with chronic pain may exhibit a "hypervigilant" state in which they fail to return to their basal sensory states and disengage pain (Lorenz and Tracey 2009 #838).

Another central concept to understanding the relationship between behavior and pain is that of placebo and nocebo behavior (see also Pollo and Benedetti 2011). A *placebo effect* is the concept that the expectation of pain relief is able to independently provide analgesia. Mechanistically, this process is thought to be driven by the prefrontal cortex via the PAG-RVM descending modulatory system. In contrast to a placebo effect, a *nocebo effect* is that of increased pain secondary to a negative expectation of pain. fMRI has associated the S2 and posterior insula with the nocebo effect, and there is evidence that the hyperalgesia is mediated by spinal cholecystokinin. Such maladaptive behaviors such as anxiety, catastrophizing, and excessive fear of injury are believed to evoke nocebo phenomenon. Key brain regions and how they are thought to relate to behavior and pain can be seen in Fig. 19.6 (Lorenz and Tracey 2009 #838).

Risk Factors and Preventative Therapies

The pathophysiologic changes underlying CPSP are complex, and treatment after it has developed is often underwhelming. Hence, there has been a greater focus on preventative therapy. The most obvious way to prevent the development of CPSP is to not undergo the surgery. Yet, a reduction in the number of surgeries would still only partially solve the problem. No matter how selective one is, many patients ultimately require surgery, especially in the field of palliative care. Therefore, a better understanding of the predisposing risk factors, both procedurally as well as biopsychosocially, is required in order to help design a successful preventative therapeutic strategy.

Procedural

Ample evidence exists demonstrating that a given surgical approach can influence the development of CPSP. The major cause of CPSP is thought to be nerve injury, either directly from the surgical

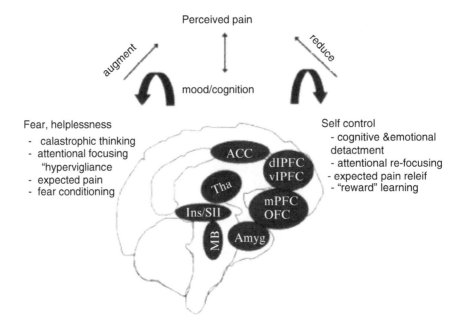

Fig. 19.6 Summary figure of main brain regions determined to be relevant in the psychological amplification and reduction of the pain experience based on bodily or psychological context. *ACC* anterior cingulate cortex; *Amyg* amygdala; *dlPFC* dorsolateral prefrontal cortex; *Ins* insular cortex; *MB* midbrain; *mPFC* medial prefrontal cortex; *OFC* orbitofrontal cortex; *SII* secondary somatosensory cortex; *Tha* thalamus; *vlPFC* ventrolateral prefrontal cortex (Lorenz and Tracey 2009 #838)

insult or from other consequences such as inflammation or scar tissue. Thus, new surgical techniques have been designed to reduce the overall amount of tissue and nerve injury, and in doing so, to help prevent CPSP. Laparoscopically assisted surgery has been shown to result in decreased long-term post-surgical pain for both hernia repair and cholecystectomy (Grant et al. 2004; Stiff et al. 1994). Nerve sparing approaches for both mastectomy and thoracotomy have also reduced post-surgical morbidity (Cerfolio et al. 2003; Jung et al. 2003). Surgical techniques such as sentinel lymph node biopsy, which were developed to reduce the number of axillary radical dissections performed, have also decreased the incidence of chronic postmastectomy pain (Sclafani and Baron 2008).

An increased risk of CPSP has been associated with a surgical duration of greater than 3 h (Peters et al. 2007). This is probably because a longer, more complicated procedure is likely to involve greater amounts of tissue injury and nerve damage. Furthermore, the incidence of CPSP has been observed to be decreased when the surgery is performed at a high vs. low volume surgical unit (Tasmuth et al. 1999). This finding is commensurate with several studies reporting a favorable association between high procedural volume centers and reduced surgical morbidity (Battaglia et al. 2006; Rectenwald and Upchurch 2007; Wilt et al. 2008).

Concomitant treatments may also increase the incidence of CPSP. Chronic pain has been reported to be increased following amputation and mastectomy when performed in close conjunction with radiation or chemotherapy (Gulluoglu et al. 2006; Smith and Thompson 1995). Whether such therapeutic regimens contribute to pain following other types of surgery is still uncertain; however, the potential for radiation or chemotherapy alone to cause neuropathic pain is also well documented (Argyriou et al. 2008; Forman 1990).

Biopsychosocial

Acute pain appears to correlate with the development of chronic pain. This relationship exists for acute pain in both the preoperative and postoperative settings. Amputees with severe preoperative pain are more likely to develop intense phantom limb pain than those who report no or only mild preoperative pain (Jensen et al. 1985; Nikolajsen et al. 1997). Similarly, severe postoperative pain has been shown to be an independent risk factor for the development of CPSP after thoracotomy (Katz et al. 1996), mastectomy (Poleshuck et al. 2006), herniorrhaphy (Aasvang and Kehlet 2005), and Cesarean section (Nikolajsen et al. 2004). These findings are consistent with the idea that neuroplastic changes begin in the acute setting.

While the true gender prevalence of chronic pain remains debated, women report more severe pain, more frequent bouts of pain, and more anatomically diffuse pain compared to men (Hurley and Adams 2008, see also Keogh 2011). This tendency for the female population to report greater pain has been observed with postthoracotomy pain (Gotoda et al. 2001). Younger age may also predispose the development of CPSP. Poleshuck et al. reported that the probability of developing chronic pain after breast surgery decreased 5% for each additional year of age (Poleshuck et al. 2006). This relationship may be partly explained by younger patients tending to have more aggressive and advanced disease, therefore, requiring more extensive surgery (Kroman et al. 2000).

Conflicting evidence exists regarding psychological predictors for CPSP. Harden et al. found that preoperative anxiety was related to the development of complex regional pain syndrome (CRPS) following total knee arthroplasty (Harden et al. 2003). However, in another study by Katz et al., no relationship was found between depression and anxiety and postthoracotomy pain (Katz et al. 1996). It should be noted, however, that Katz's study questioned patients 1 day prior to surgery, and this timing may have falsely elevated the number of patients expressing symptoms of both depression and anxiety. Traits of neuroticism and an introverted personality have been found to be related to postcholecystectomy pain (Borly et al. 1999). A recent review of the literature by Hinrichs-Rocker et al. (2009) observed that depression, psychological vulnerability, and stress to be the most reliable psychological predictors of CPSP currently known.

Pain catastrophizing may also be related to the development of CPSP. Pain catastrophizing is defined as an exaggerated negative orientation to aversive stimuli that involves rumination about painful sensations, magnification of the threat value of the painful stimulus, and perceived inability to control pain (Granot and Ferber 2005). These inappropriate pain behaviors are generally considered maladaptive coping strategies, and as such, often result in increased anxiety levels. Pain catastrophizing has been demonstrated to be a risk factor for increased chronic pain in rheumatoid arthritis patients (Keefe et al. 1989). Currently available studies evaluating the role of catastrophizing in CPSP, however, are conflicting. While catastrophizing has been shown to predict acute post-surgical pain intensity (Pavlin et al. 2005), other studies have been unable to establish such a correlation with CPSP, despite the fact that severe acute post-surgical pain is itself a risk factor for CPSP (Hanley et al. 2004; Peters et al. 2007). In fact, more frequent catastrophizing 1 month postoperatively was found to be associated with greater improvement in the pain score at 2 years postoperatively. This finding may be due to this study having only evaluated the absolute change in pain scores as opposed to actual pain scores. Therefore, a patient with frequent catastrophizing at 1 month may have a higher overall pain score, thereby giving that patient more room to improve. However, one alternative explanation provided by the authors was that early catastrophizing has a paradoxically beneficial role by prompting earlier recognition and treatment.

A patient's social environment as a predictor of CPSP has also been assessed. One study investigating the risk factors for phantom limb pain found lack of social support to be a major predictor (Jensen et al. 2002). This finding was supported in a subsequent study evaluating the incidence of postamputation pain (Hanley et al. 2004). Solicitous behavior, in which family members (often unknowingly) reinforce a patient's pain behaviors, may also be a risk factor for developing CPSP (Katz and Seltzer 2009).

Finally, there may be genetic predisposition to the development of chronic neuropathic pain that increases the likelihood of CPSP. The link has been demonstrated in animal studies, in which specific strains of mice are more likely to develop neuropathic pain after nerve injury (Seltzer et al. 2001). There is also evidence that patients with CPSP are more likely to have other functional pain syndromes such as IBS, temporomandibular joint disorder (TMJD), migraine, and fibromyalgia (Macrae 2008). Yarnitsky et al. tested patients' diffuse noxious inhibitor control (DNIC), a marker of one's overall endogenous analgesia system, prior to undergoing thoracotomy. Although the level of DNIC did not correlate with acute post-surgical pain, it was directly related to the development of chronic postthoracotomy pain. This finding suggests that not only is there likely a genetic predisposition to developing CPSP, but also that the mechanisms of acute and CPSP are most likely distinct (Yarnitsky et al. 2008).

Preventative Therapies

The nociceptive barrage that is thought to trigger the peripheral and central sensitization that ultimately causes CPSP may occur at any time point in the perioperative period – preoperative, intraoperative, and postoperative. However, CPSP is different than other forms of chronic pain in that the timing of the noxious stimulus (the surgery insult) is usually known prior to its occurrence; therefore, an opportunity may exist to proactively disrupt the chain of events that leads to CPSP in the face of severe preoperative pain. The concept of preemptive analgesia holds that the application of analgesic techniques prior to the surgical insult will block the central transmission of pain signals, thereby preventing or reducing the neuroplastic changes thought most responsible for the development of CPSP. While several animal studies have supported the role of preemptive analgesia, the ability to reliably reproduce these results in clinical situations has not been achieved (Dougherty et al. 1992; Haley et al. 1990; Yamamoto and Yaksh 1991).

Multiple reasons have been posited to explain this lack of translation from animal to human studies. As mentioned above, the presence of presurgical pain may be sufficient to independently trigger CPSP, despite adequate nociceptive suppression during the intraoperative and postoperative periods. While such preoperative pain is absent in animal studies, it is often present in human clinical settings. Additionally, animal studies typically choose a surgical procedure involving well-defined nociceptive afferents such as the tail or an extremity so that adequate nociceptive suppression can be easily achieved. However, in human studies, the nociceptive inputs are often diffuse, and complete blockade of algesic signaling is much more difficult. Surgeries in animal studies are often shorter than in comparative human study. Such brevity better ensures adequate nociceptive blockade throughout the duration of the procedure. Animal models also lack the psychological factors that have been found to greatly influence the occurrence of CPSP in humans (Aida 2005).

There may also be an intrinsic flaw in the idea of preemptive analgesia that may account for its lack of success in human trials. Studies evaluating preemptive analgesia require two groups of patients to receive an identical treatment before or after the same type of surgery. However, if the theory that CPSP may be triggered at any point in the perioperative period is accurate, then a preemptive treatment at only one time point may not be adequate to prevent the development of CPSP. Furthermore, preemptive analgesia relies on the idea that acute pain and chronic pain are causal in relationship, and therefore the latter cannot occur without the former. However, if acute pain and chronic pain are only associative in relationship, then while the factors that cause each may be interrelated, blockade of acute pain may not assure blockade of chronic pain (Katz and Seltzer 2009).

In contrast to preemptive analgesia which only provides an analgesic agent at a specific time point, the focus of preventive analgesia is attenuation of the nociceptive barrage throughout the entire perioperative period. Preventive analgesia attempts to select a synergistic combination of analgesic agents (e.g., a local anesthetic and opioid), which when given across the preoperative, intraoperative, and postoperative periods work to reduce the neuroplastic changes thought to underlie CPSP. The therapeutic benefit of preventive analgesia exists when postoperative pain and/analgesic requirements are decreased significantly beyond the duration of action (defined as more than 5.5 half-lives) of the selected preventive analgesic agents A systematic review of available preventive analgesia studies has found the benefits of preventive analgesia to be statistically significant (Katz and Clarke 2008).

Management

Pharmacology is the mainstay of treatment for CPSP today, and this chapter will focus primarily on medication management for this reason. However, other treatment modalities may also include psychological, rehabilitative, and surgical approaches, which can be vital in achieving a successful result. CPSP is a biopsychosocial phenomenon and should be treated as such. This chapter will include a short overview of some of these other therapeutic modalities as well. Regarding pharmacological management, a mechanistic approach to treating CPSP is the most rational as illustrated in Fig. 19.7 (Beydoun and Backonja 2003).

Pharmacological

Antidepressants

The antidepressant group of medications can be divided into the tricyclic antidepressants (TCAs), the selective serotonin re-uptake inhibitors (SSRIs), and the serotonin/norepinephrine re-uptake

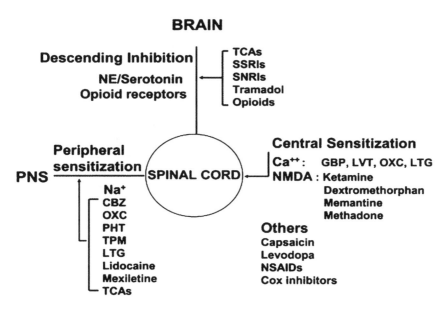

Fig. 19.7 Mechanistic stratification of antineuralgic agents that may be utilized in the treatment of chronic post-surgical pain (CPSP) (Beydoun and Backonja 2003)

inhibitors (SNRIs). The antidepressants are believed to provide analgesia by modulating the descending central inhibitory pathway through their inhibition of norepinephrine and serotonin re-uptake (Beydoun and Backonja 2003).

The TCAs have been most rigorously studied in regard to treatment of neuropathic pain. The TCAs are divided according to their structure into tertiary and secondary amines. The tertiary amines, such as amitriptyline and clomipramine, inhibit re-uptake of the biogenic amines, serotonin, and norepinephrine, compared to the secondary amines, such as nortriptyline and desipramine, which are fairly selective norepinephrine re-uptake inhibitors (Sanchez and Hyttel 1999). TCAs reduce neuropathic pain compared to placebo in patients with denervation syndromes such as postherpetic neuralgia and diabetic neuropathy (Getto et al. 1987). They are first line agents in the treatment of trigeminal neuralgia, and there is also some evidence supporting their use in the treatment of CRPS (Harden 2005; Kingery 1997).

TCAs may influence analgesic activity in other ways including alpha adrenergic blockade; anticholinergic effects; antihistaminic effects; reuptake inhibition of dopamine; effects on gamma-aminobutyric acid (GABA)-B and adenosine receptors; potassium, calcium, and sodium channel blockade; and NMDA-receptor antagonism (Jackson 2006). In particular, amitriptyline has been observed to reversibly block TTX-resistant sodium channels suggesting its potential efficacy in the role of peripheral sensitization as well (Brau et al. 2001).

Side effects of TCAs are mostly anticholinergic driven (e.g., constipation, urinary retention, blurred vision, sedation, impaired memory, etc.). Because of the common complaint of sedation, they are usually dosed at bedtime. The side effect profile of the more norepinephrine-specific secondary amines is milder than that of the tertiary amines. Furthermore, studies comparing the efficacy of these medications have found no differences between the two (Rowbotham et al. 2005). Therefore, the IASP recommends the use of secondary over tertiary amines as first line treatments of neuropathic pain.

The TCAs have also been associated with cardiovascular side effects including prolongation of QT interval, conduction blockade, and dysrhythmias such as Torsade's de pointes. Hence, it is prudent to check an EKG on patient older than 40 years of age. TCAs are contraindicated in patients who are recovering from a recent MI (particularly if a new heart block is present) and in patients already taking MAOIs (Haanpaa et al. 2010).

The SNRIs may also be viable options for the treatment of neuropathic pain associated with CPSP. Duloxetine is FDA approved for the treatment of fibromyalgia, a condition involving widespread pain that, in some ways, may be mechanistically similar to CPSP (Arnold et al. 2005). Both venlafaxine and duloxetine improve the pain of diabetic peripheral neuropathy when compared to placebo (Goldstein et al. 2005; Rowbotham et al. 2004). Milnacipran, a relatively new SNRI with greater norepinephrine re-uptake activity, also appears to be effective in the treatment of fibromyalgia (Pae et al. 2009).

It is well established that SSRIs are more often tolerated by patients. However, their analgesic effectiveness is greatly reduced in the treatment of diabetic peripheral neuropathy, postherpetic neuralgia, and CRPS when compared to medications with norepinephrine re-uptake inhibitor properties (Harden 2005; Max et al. 1992; Stacey 2005). Therefore, SSRI's should be regarded as second-line agents for patients with neuropathic pain who are unable to tolerate or unresponsive to a TCA or SNRI (Jung et al. 1997).

Anticonvulsants

Anticonvulsants have been used in the management of pain since the 1960s (Wiffen et al. 2005). These medications are generally believed to relieve neuropathic pain by stabilizing ectopic activity of injured or dysfunctioning neurons. Anticonvulsants may affect either peripheral sensitization, central sensitization, or both depending on which specific medication is chosen. As these medications are fairly nonspecific, side effects including sedation, dizziness, clouded thinking, and water retention often occur and often limit therapeutic efficacy.

Carbamazepine, oxcarbazepine, phenytoin, topiramate, and lamotrigine all act as sodium channel blockers by inhibiting high-frequency repetitive firing and/or stabilizing the slow inactivated conformation of sodium channels. As discussed above, when a peripheral nerve injury occurs, sodium channel density increases and is believed to facilitate the development of ectopy that accompanies neuropathic pain. Anticonvulsants are thought to be therapeutically effective because they are able to prevent ectopic activity of the injured nerve at concentrations lower than those required to block normal impulse generation and conduction. In addition to the common side effects associated with this class, several drug-specific side effects are also worth noting. All of these medications may cause a rash; however, severe rashes have only been reported with carbamazepine, phenytoin, and lamotrigine. For both carbamazepine and oxcarbazepine, one should monitor for hyponatremia. Phenytoin may cause gengival hyperplasia. Cases of aplastic anemia have been reported with carbamazepine (Beydoun and Backonja 2003; Porter and Meldrum 2001).

Gabapentin, pregabalin, oxcarbazepine, and lamotrigine all block the alpha2-delta subunit of the high-threshold N-type calcium channel which is thought to play a large role in central sensitization. Because the safety profiles of gabapentin and pregabalin are benign except for the generalized side effects common to all of the medications in this family, these are the two most prescribed medications for neuropathic pain. However, it is worthwhile noting that both oxcarbazepine and lamotrigine have pharmocodynamic features consistent with the ability to affect sensitization both peripherally and centrally. While evidence does not yet exist to clinically support or oppose this observation, it does present opportunities for further exploration (Beydoun and Backonja 2003; Porter and Meldrum 2001).

Many gaps in the available literature make evidence-based approaches to the use of these medications difficult. In fact, 71% of the patients treated with anticonvulsants in the US are receiving off-label prescriptions, and between 19 and 57% of the use of the six most frequently prescribed anticonvulsants is not supported by evidence from controlled trials (Chen et al. 2005; Goodyear-Smith and Halliwell 2009). There are several reasons for this lack of evidence-based practice. Most studies evaluating anticonvulsants for pain have focused on patients with either diabetic peripheral neuropathy, postherpetic neuralgia, or trigeminal neuralgis; however, neuropathic pain is a broad diagnosis that may be present in many more than just these few disease states. Furthermore, most studies have focused on more recently developed anticonvulsants, resulting in older drugs often being excluded from the literature. Finally, comparison trials of one anticonvulsant against another are lacking (Goodyear-Smith and Halliwell 2009).

Local Anesthetics

Local anesthetics interfere with signal conduction through their blockade of sodium channels. In this way, they are believed to potentially reduce neuronal excitability and ectopy following peripheral sensitization and peripheral nerve injury. In one systematic review, perioperative lidocaine infusions were found to significantly reduce pain and opioid consumption following abdominal surgical procedures (McCarthy et al. 2010). Another systematic review by Cohen et al. found intravenous lidocaine infusions to be predictive of a patient's successful response to mexiletine, an oral medication with properties similar to lidocaine, in regard to neuropathic pain (Cohen et al. 2009). Side effects are a common problem with this class of medications and include gastrointestinal symptoms (diarrhea, nausea) as well as dysrhythmias. Mexiletine is contraindicated in patients who have second or third degree conduction heart blocks (Knotkova and Pappagallo 2007).

Opioids

Opioids are one of the oldest classes of medications used to treat pain and are still heavily relied upon for the treatment of many conditions. Opioids work primarily in the CNS via activation of the μ, κ, and δ receptors in the substantia gelatinosa region of the dorsal horn. Presynaptically, opioids induce closure of VGCCs, reducing the amount of neuropeptides (Ex. glutamate, substance P) released into the synapse. Postsynaptically, opioids open potassium channels causing hyperpolarization of the cell, thereby reducing the likelihood of activation (Way et al. 2001).

While the efficacy of opioids in the treatment of acute nociceptive and inflammatory pain is universally accepted, their role in the treatment of chronic pain has classically been questioned, especially regarding neuropathic pain (Arner and Meyerson 1988). Neuropathic pain's resistance to opioid therapy is thought to be due at least in part to the fact that a downregulation of presynaptic opioid receptors occurs in this patient population. Furthermore, many of the suspected pathways thought responsible for the production of neuropathic pain, such as the NMDA-receptor mediated pathways, do not involve the opioid receptor system. Nevertheless, more recent evidence suggests there still may be a role for opioids in the management of chronic neuropathic pain (Dickenson and Kieffer 2006; Furlan et al. 2006). In fact, a recent meta-analysis found that intermediate-term trials of opioids demonstrated consistent analgesic efficacy in reducing spontaneous neuropathic pain (Eisenberg et al. 2006). When deciding which opioid medication to use, it may be worthwhile considering one with multiple receptor properties. For example, methadone also exerts NMDA-receptor antagonist activity. Tramadol, in addition to being a weak μ-opioid receptors agonist, partially antagonizes NMDA-receptors and is a weak inhibitor of norepinephrine and serotonin re-uptake (Martin et al. 2008).

Opioids are regularly associated with the stigma of abusive and addictive behaviors that can make both patients and physicians hesitant to use them. When used appropriately, however, they may substantially help to reduce a patient's overall pain. This is even more true for patients involved with a palliative care service who are often at a point in their lives where quality is difficult to achieve because of severe pain. A frank and open discussion regarding the use of these medications for the treatment of pain may help to uncover any hesitations or concerns. Furthermore, a narcotics contract with any patient started on opioids helps resolve any confusion that may exist regarding the use and expectations of this treatment modality (Manchikanti et al. 2008).

Opioid usage is associated with a myriad of side effects including sedation, nausea, itching, constipation, and potentially even life-threatening respiratory depression. These problems should be considered and addressed before initiating use of an opioid analgesic, and the patient should be monitored regularly throughout for development of any intolerances. Often side effects can be conservatively managed; however, for those patients who would otherwise benefit from opioid therapy but are side effect limited, one may consider intrathecal administration as an alternative route (Way et al. 2001).

N-Methyl-D-Aspartate Receptor Antagonists

The NMDA glutamate receptor channel is thought to be involved in the development of neuropathic pain, central sensitization, and opioid-induced hyperalgesia (Okon 2007; Silverman 2009). Because of this relationship, drugs antagonistic to the NMDA receptor have been evaluated for use in the treatment of these painful symptoms. In addition to methadone, clinically available drugs with NMDA receptor blocking properties include ketamine, dextromethorphan, memantine, and amantidine. Ketamine has been used parenterally as an adjuvant for intractable malignant pain in two palliative care studies and found to increase pain relief by 20–30% and reduce opioid consumption by 25–50% (Fitzgibbon and Viola 2005; Lossignol et al. 2005). These drugs are not licensed for use as analgesics in most countries and should be prescribed with caution. Their use is typically limited by side effects which include sedation, nausea, and cognitive deficits. Psychological disturbances involving alterations in mood or body image, floating sensations, vivid dreams, hallucinations, and delirium are also common (Knotkova and Pappagallo 2007).

Alpha-2 Receptor Agonists

Alpha-2 receptor agonists offer a potential treatment strategy for both peripheral and central sensitization. Peripherally, alpha-2 receptor agonists work presynaptically to inhibit norepinephrine release, thereby, potentially reducing sympathetically maintained pain. They may also possess anti-inflammatory properties that could reduce peripheral sensitization (Lavand'homme and Eisenach 2003). Centrally, alpha-2 receptors agonists are thought to work at both the spinal and supraspinal levels. Although still not fully understood, proposed mechanisms include central reduction of sympathetic outflow and stimulation of cholinergic interneurons in the spinal cord (Giovannoni et al. 2009).

Clonidine has been used successfully as an adjunct in regional and neuroaxial anesthesia to reduce opioid and local anesthetic requirements. However, its oral use is limited secondary to the hypotension that often accompanies its use. Tizanidine is a short-acting oral alpha-2 agonist with a much lesser hypotensive effect. It has traditionally been used for the management of spasticity. However, animal and clinical evidence exists supporting its potential role in other neuropathic-type pain states (Knotkova and Pappagallo 2007).

Nonsteroidal Anti-Inflammatory Drugs

Nonsteroidal anti-inflammatory drugs (NSAIDs) inhibit the enzyme cyclo-oxygenase (COX), thereby, reducing the production of pro-inflammatory prostaglandins formed from arachidonic acid. All NSAIDs possess anti-inflammatory, analgesic, and antipyretic properties. Two subclasses of COX enzymes have been identified. COX-1 is the most ubiquitous, being found in platelets, the gastrointestinal tract, kidneys, and most other human tissues. COX-2 is predominantly found in the kidneys and CNS; however, its expression is also increased in tissues following injury. It is via inhibition of the COX-2 enzymes that NSAIDs are believed to exert most of their peripheral anti-inflammatory and analgesic effects (Munir et al. 2007). A third subclass, COX-3 enzyme, is found primarily in the CNS and heart and has been postulated in the literature as the potential substrate by which NSAIDs exert their central analgesic effects. However, further investigation has found that COX-3 is merely a minor genetic variant of COX-1, and so this mechanism of action is unlikely (Mattia and Coluzzi 2009).

Prostaglandins are involved in processes that initiate and amplify peripheral sensitization and central sensitization (Schaible and Richter 2004). In cases of CPSP, low levels of inflammation may exist long after the initial insult, further propagating peripheral and central sensitization (De Kock 2009). NSAIDs offer blockade of this potential pain pathway and should be considered when evaluating a patient with CPSP.

NSAIDs are traditionally grouped according to their COX-2/COX-1 binding affinities as being either nonspecific or COX-2 selective. However, it should be noted that all NSAIDs developed so far have at least some affinity for both enzymes. Table 19.3 lists some of the available NSAIDs and their relative selectivity for the COX-2 enzyme (Mattia and Coluzzi 2005).

While NSAIDs lack many of the adverse effects associated with opioids such as constipation, respiratory depression, and development of physical dependence, they have less analgesic potency and several important side effects of their own. Nonselective NSAIDs have the potential to increase bleeding risks by inhibiting the formation of platelet COX-1-dependent thromboxane. This side

Table 19.3 COX-2/COX-1 ratios of various nonsteroidal anti-inflammatory drugs (NSAIDs)

NSAID	COX-2/COX-1 ratio
Naproxen	0.6
Diclofenac	7
Celecoxib	30

Table 19.4 Side effects of NSAID therapy (Munir et al. 2007 #675)

Gastrointestinal	Nausea, anorexia, abdominal pain, ulcers, anemia, gastrointestinal hemorrhage, perforation, diarrhea
Cardiovascular	Hypertension, decreased effectiveness of anti-hypertensive medications, myocardial infarction, stroke, and thromboembolic events (last three with selective COX-2 inhibitors); inhibit platelet activation, propensity for bruising and hemorrhage
Renal	Salt and water retention, edema, deterioration of kidney function, decreased effectiveness of diuretic medication, decreased urate excretion, hyperkalemia, analgesic nephropathy
Central nervous system	Headache, dizziness, vertigo, confusion, depression, lowering of seizure threshold, hyperventilation (salicylates)
Hypersensitivity	Vasomotor rhinitis, asthma, urticaria, flushing, hypotension, shock

effect is most significant with aspirin because it covalently binds to COX-1, and so its impact on platelet function is irreversible. Both traditional and COX-2 selective NSAIDs have the potential to worsen renal function in patients with already compromised renal blood flow states such as congestive heart failure, hepatic cirrhosis, chronic kidney disease, and hypovolemia. Although more prevalent with NSAIDs that have significant COX-1 activity, all NSAIDs may also cause gastrointestinal disturbances including nausea, abdominal pain, and ulcer formation that may sometimes lead to severe gastrointestinal bleeding. In fact, this relationship between COX-1 inhibition and gastrointestinal side effects was one of the major driving forces behind the development of COX-2 selective NSAIDs. So far, three COX-2 selective NSAIDs (rofecoxib, valdecoxib, and celecoxib) have been approved for use in the United States. However, rofecoxib and valdecoxib were both withdrawn from the market due to their potential cardiovascular adverse event profile. Strongly selective COX-2 inhibitors have since been found to increase the risk of cardiothrombotic events, especially in patients who already have risk factors for cardiovascular events. Certain patients also exhibit a hypersensitivity to aspirin and NSAIDs that can range from vasomotor rhinitis to profuse watery excretions, angioedema, generalized urticaria, and bronchial asthma. Therefore, aspirin intolerance is considered a contraindication to treatment with any other NSAID because of possible cross-sensitivity. A complete list of side effects associated with NSAIDs can be found in Table 19.4 (Munir et al. 2007).

Acetaminophen is a nonsalicylate that produces similar analgesic and antipyretic effects to aspirin. However, it lacks peripheral anti-inflammatory action as well as gastrointestinal, renal, and cardiovascular side effects. While its mechanism of action is unclear at this time, it seems to possess central analgesic properties. Acetaminophen may be used in combination with other medications including NSAIDs and opioids in a synergistic fashion to produce greater pain relief. Because of the potential to cause liver damage, dosage should not exceed 4 g/day, and in patients who chronically use acetaminophen daily, the dosage should probably be closer to 3 g/day. It should also be avoided in patients who are chronically alcoholic or who are experiencing worsening liver disease (Munir et al. 2007).

Topical Agents

Topical agents offer the advantage of allowing medications to exert their peripheral action while avoiding many of the systemic side effects that accompany them. Commonly used topical agents include NSAIDs, local anesthetics, and capsaicin. The mechanisms of the first two have previously been discussed. Capsaicin, with repeated application, leads to the depletion of substance P from the primary afferent neurons resulting in the relief of neuropathic pain. It has been shown to be useful in the relief of painful diabetic neuropathy, postherpetic neuralgia, chronic distal painful polyneuropathy, oral neuropathic pain, and CPSP. While adverse side effects are minimal, a disadvantage of this agent is that application is associated with a temporary but often painful burning sensation. This sensation typically decreases with time, however, and preapplication of topical lidocaine helps to reduce this pain also (McCleane 2007).

Nonpharmacologic Treatments

Physical Medicine and Rehabilitation

Numerous modalities utilized by physical and occupational therapists have the potential to aid patients suffering from CPSP. Following surgery, many patients experience a degree of deconditioning that decreases their level of physical activity and their ability to perform necessary activities of daily living. When a patient's post-surgical pain does not resolve, the severity of deconditioning can increase dramatically, even to the point that independent living is no longer sustainable. With the aid of a trained physical or occupational therapist, appropriate exercise and stretching techniques can help to regain muscle conditioning allowing for reintegration into life and society (see also, May 2011). For patients whose pain is prohibitive to any type of traditional rehabilitation therapy, aquatic therapy offers many advantages. The viscosity of water provides resistance for aerobic and strengthening exercises, compressive forces help to decrease edema, and buoyancy decreases the need for weight bearing helping to make the exercise less uncomfortable. Pool therapy is also often a group experience that may provide additional social benefit for the patient (Stanos et al. 2007).

Passive modalities include cryotherapy, heat, and electrical stimulation. Some patients' pains are responsive to the use of hot or cold therapy for providing relief. Electrical stimulation involves transmission of electrical energy to the PNS via an external stimulator and conductive gel pads on the skin. This modality is believed to stimulate non-nociceptive large afferent A-β fibers, thereby preventing the constant signaling of small fiber peripherally sensitized nociceptors from reaching the dorsal horn. This proposed mechanism of action is based on the original "Gate Theory of Pain" introduced by Melzack and Wall in the 1960s (Melzack and Wall 1965). Electrical stimulation has also been shown to release endogenous opioids and activate peripheral α_2-adrenoceptors as other potential mechanisms of action (King et al. 2005). Two forms of electrical stimulation exist. Transcutaneous electrical nerve stimulation (TENS) provides superficial electrical stimulation. Interferential current therapy (ICT) is a variant of TENS that mixes frequencies to provide stimulation of deeper tissues with decreased discomfort (Stanos et al. 2007).

Other modalities include graded exposure and mirror therapies. Graded exposure, or desensitization, therapy is based on the concept that gradually reexposing a patient to a feared setting or experience helps to reduce associated discomfort. CPSP often experience neuropathic pain in the form of allodynia. Desensitization exercises utilize gradually increasing tactile sensation with the aim of improving the patient's tolerance to external stimuli (de Jong et al. 2005). Mirror therapy is directed toward postamputee patients with phantom limb pain and involves using a mirror to create the illusion that the patient is moving the missing extremity when they actually move the existing one.

The mechanism of action of this modality is not completely understood but is believed to involve reorganization of the sensorimotor cortex (Chan et al. 2007; Diers et al. 2010) (see also Foell and Flor 2011).

Interventional Procedures

Interventional measures used to treat CPSP specifically and more broadly neuropathic pain may best be divided into those that are neuromodulatory and those that are neuroablative. Neuromodulation attempts to alter the way the nervous system responds to sensory input in order to reduce the overall perception of pain. Both chemical and electrical techniques have been utilized. Stellate or lumbar sympathetic ganglion blocks using local anesthetic may be considered for pain that is believed to be sympathetically mediated. Nerve blocks involving the brachial plexus, femoral, or sciatic nerves may be performed for extremity pain; a catheter tunneled underneath the skin may provide an infusion of local anesthetic for longer term relief. While these blocks may only provide temporary relief, they may be used to facilitate beneficial physical therapy modalities that would otherwise not be tolerated. For patients who obtain relief from opioids but are limited by side effects, one may consider an intrathecal (IT) pump. This method involves placing an intrathecal catheter that is tunneled underneath the skin to where it connects with a pump reservoir. Because the treatment solution is delivered directly to the site at which its primary mechanism of action is believed to occur, much lesser total amount of drug is needed and side effects are often greatly reduced as well (Nocom et al. 2009). Neuromodulation electrically attempts to alter nociception through the use of spinal cord stimulators (SCS). This procedure involves placing an electrical generator near the dorsal columns of the spinal cord at a level corresponding to where the patient is experiencing neuropathic pain peripherally. While SCSs are often compared to TENS units to describe how they work, their mechanism of action, although not yet understood, is probably much more complex than the "gate-theory" of pain and involves modulation of rostral nociceptive transmission via stimulation of the large diameter fibers (Chong and Bajwa 2003).

Neuroablative procedures attempt to interrupt the pain signal transmission via a lesion in the nociceptive pathway. Procedures of this type include nerve avulsion or section, dorsal rhizotomy, spinal dorsal root entry zone lesions, spinothalamic tractotomies, cingulotomy, frontal lobotomy, and destruction of the primary sensory cortex. These treatments are generally considered last-resort measures because they involve further damage to the nervous system. Furthermore, nerve injury itself is a primary cause of the neuroplastic changes that can lead to neuropathic pain. Therefore, these types of procedures have a very high risk of worsening the pain for which they are intended to relieve (Chong and Bajwa 2003).

Behavioral Medicine

Behavioral medicine is based on the concept that psychological and behavioral factors reciprocally and dynamically interact with physical health. This treatment philosophy, which began in the 1970s, was a radical swing away from the more traditional biomedical approaches to pain therapy that focused solely on the anatomical, physiological, and neurochemical processes of nociception. Today several different behavioral approaches are utilized to help patients suffering from chronic pain reduce their pain perceptions and begin to reintegrate themselves into society.

One of the most commonly used approaches is cognitive-behavioral therapy (CBT) (see also, Donovan et al. 2011). Patients with chronic pain often have misconceptions regarding how they relate to their environment that may actually lead to activities and beliefs that make their pain worse.

For instance, these patients often perceive themselves as being helpless to the world around them and unable to influence their outcome for the better. CBT attempts to reconstruct how they interpret their surroundings as well as show them how their actions can affect both themselves and their environment. Patients are first educated about how physiological processes such as sleep, activity level, and mood are able to affect their overall pain. Then they are taught behavioral skills such as breathing exercises or distraction techniques to help redirect their focus away from pain. Finally, they are taught cognitive skills to help identify activities or situations that often result in increased pain. Coping strategies are utilized to help improve functioning despite the presence of pain, and patients are taught self-efficacy or the idea that they can effectively change a situation by executing a specific course of action (Okifuji and Ackerlind 2007).

Clinical Presentation of Several CPSP Syndromes

Classically, pain is categorized as being acute, inflammatory, or neuropathic. These categorizations of pain are mostly heuristic, and in reality the lines separating the types of pain and their adaptive or maladaptive properties often become blurred. It is important to remember that a continuum of pain exists when assessing the clinical picture. Just because the pain characteristics more classically describe neuropathic pain does not mean that a component of inflammatory pain does not also exist and vice versa. Inflammatory pain often elicits symptoms of allodynia, hyperalgesia, and dysesthesia. Neuropathic pain may occur as a result of an inflammatory process (Ex. inflammation of a major nerve trunk or neuritis) (Fig. 19.7) (Devor 2006).

CPSP, at some point in time, involves all three components of pain, and it may consist of all three types of pain simultaneously. For example, a recent amputee may experience both acute and inflammatory pain at the surgical site in addition to the neuropathic condition of phantom limb pain. The clinical presentation of the more common CPSP syndromes will be discussed below (Fig. 19.8).

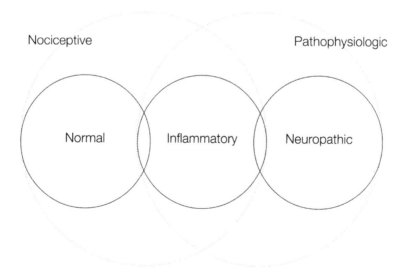

Fig. 19.8 The continuum of nociceptive, inflammatory, and neuropathic pain and their adaptive and maladaptive roles (Devor 2006)

Postamputation Pain

The two most commonly described types of pain following amputation are phantom pain and stump pain (see also Foell and Flor 2011). Phantom pain is the pain felt to be originating from the amputated limb. For most patients, phantom pain is more typically located in the distal parts (e.g., fingers and toes) of the previous extremity. Initially, pain may be more evenly distributed throughout the missing limb; however, it tends to migrate further distally over time (Jensen et al. 1985; Nikolajsen et al. 1997). Pain is usually intermittent with symptoms occurring on daily to weekly intervals, and extremes of frequency such as rare or constant pain are uncommon. Episodes of pain typically last from seconds to hours (Kooijman et al. 2000; Nikolajsen et al. 1997; Wartan et al. 1997). The pain is usually described as burning, aching, or cramping; however, a myriad of other descriptors including crushing, twisting, grinding, tingling, drawing, needlelike, knifelike, sticking, squeezing and shock-like have been used by patients (Jensen et al. 1983, 1985; Katz and Melzack 1990).

Stump pain, as the name suggests, is located at the remaining distal site of the amputated limb. Patients will often describe this type of pain as pressing, throbbing, burning, or squeezing, and the quality of the pain may be beneficial in finding an underlying cause. Many experience allodynia and hyperpathia at the stump site. Patients complaining of stump pain should be evaluated for infection, bone spurs, neuromas, excess scar tissue, and if the amputation was for cancer, recurrence of tumor (Jensen et al. 1983, 1985). It is also worthwhile to assess the temperature of the residual limb as it may exhibit features of CRPS and thereby be potentially amenable to the treatment of sympathetically maintained pain (Wilsey et al. 2001).

Postmastectomy Pain

Postmastectomy pain is often a result of injury to the intercostobrachial nerve. This nerve provides sensation to the posteromedial arm, axilla, and anterior chest well, and so pain also typically falls in this distribution. Pain descriptors often include tightness, constriction, and burning. Exacerbating factors include any type of ipsilateral arm movement, and the patients will often immobilize their arm to avoid further pain. Such immobilization may result in a frozen shoulder that further contributes to the overall pain experience and loss of function. Injury to the intercostobrachial nerve is more common following radical mastectomy with axillary node dissection and concurrent treatment with radiation. Presence of a neuroma at the surgical scar site, arm, or axilla may also be a source of discomfort. Breast reconstruction can result in damage to other nerves including the medial pectoral, lateral pectoral, thoracodorsal, and long thoracic nerves (Couceiro et al. 2009).

Postmastectomy patients may also suffer from phantom breast pain. Akin to phantom limb pain, phantom breast pain is perception of pain in the amputated breast. It usually begins within the first 3 postoperative months. A wide range of descriptors exist including sharp, burning, shooting, stabbing, lancinating, aching, crushing, and pressing. It typically begins in the nipple area and becomes more diffuse with time. Exacerbating factors include movement and tactile stimulation but may also often have affective components such as emotional distress (Hsu and Sliwa 2004).

Postthoracotomy Pain

Postthoractomy pain has been defined as "chronic dysesthetic burning and aching in the general area of the incision that persists at least 2 months after thoracotomy" (Rogers and Duffy 2000). Its etiology is generally considered to be neuropathic pain resulting from damage to one or more of the intercostal nerves (Baumrucker 2002). Sensory loss over the distribution of the involved intercostal nerve is also typically evident. Patients often experience extreme point tenderness over the edges of the incision following surgery that generally resolves with time; however, tenderness over the scar site may become chronic (Thompson 2007).

Conclusion

CPSP is a common problem possibly affecting millions in the present United States alone. The prevalence of CPSP can only be expected to grow in light of the aging population and the increased incidence of surgery among the elderly. We have discussed the pathophysiological mechanisms, predisposing risk factors, preventative strategies, and therapeutic modalities as we understand them today. For now, conservative patient selection for surgery is the key in reducing the incidence of CPSP as success with ex post facto treatment is difficult to achieve. As our basic knowledge regarding the transition from acute to chronic pain grows, our ability to prevent and treat CPSP will no doubt improve.

However, a couple of logistical problems need to first be addressed before scientific advancement can lead to change. The first is education. CPSP has been recognized among those in the field of pain medicine as a prevalent syndrome for 20 years, and yet it is still mostly under recognized in the general medical community. Health care providers need to be cognizant of the fact that CPSP exists and that their patients may not discuss the problem unless prompted. Preoperative clinics should provide patient risk stratification as well as intraoperative preventative plans and make themselves widely accessible in the health care community. Additionally, chronic pain and palliative care clinics need to be prepared to care for this patient population in a timely and effective manner. It has even been suggested that a new CPSP service be developed to "more accurately determine the true incidence of this phenomenon, to uncover the populations at risk, and to provide early treatment strategies" (De Kock 2009 #7).

The second issue is translational science. The basic sciences have outpaced the clinical practices. Numerous biochemical targets have already been identified that might offer more successful treatments with fewer side effects. However, clinicians do not rush to incorporate the new discoveries into clinical care often because they are unaware they even exist. This gap between the basic and clinical sciences has created the opportunity for an entirely new profession of translational science to serve as a bridge. The future will need willing pain and palliative care practitioners to be more involved in this field in order to improve upon our treatment strategies.

References

Aasvang, E., & Kehlet, H. (2005). Chronic postoperative pain: The case of inguinal herniorrhaphy. *British Journal of Anaesthesia, 95*(1), 69–76.

Aida, S. (2005). The challenge of preemptive analgesia. *Pain Clinical Updates, XIII*, 1–4.

Al-Chaer, E. (2011). Neuroanatomy of pain and pain pathways. In R. J. Moore (Ed.), *Handbook of pain and palliative care: Biobehavioral approaches for the life course*. New York: Springer.

Al-Chaer, E. D., & Weaver, S. A. (2009). Early Life Trauma and Chronic Pain. In E. A. Mayer & M. C. Bushnell (Eds.), *Functional pain syndromes: Presentation and pathophysiology* (pp. 423–452). Seattle: IASP Press.

Apkarian, A. V., Baliki, M. N., & Geha, P. Y. (2009). Towards a theory of chronic pain. *Progress in Neurobiology, 87*(2), 81–97.

Apkarian, A. V., Bushnell, M. C., Treede, R. D., & Zubieta, J. K. (2005). Human brain mechanisms of pain perception and regulation in health and disease. *Eur J Pain, 9*(4), 463–484.

Argyriou, A. A., Koltzenburg, M., Polychronopoulos, P., Papapetropoulos, S., & Kalofonos, H. P. (2008). Peripheral nerve damage associated with administration of taxanes in patients with cancer. *Critical Reviews in Oncology/Hematology, 66*(3), 218–228.

Arner, S., & Meyerson, B. A. (1988). Lack of analgesic effect of opioids on neuropathic and idiopathic forms of pain. *Pain, 33*(1), 11–23.

Arnold, L. M., Rosen, A., Pritchett, Y. L., D'Souza, D. N., Goldstein, D. J., Iyengar, S., et al. (2005). A randomized, double-blind, placebo-controlled trial of duloxetine in the treatment of women with fibromyalgia with or without major depressive disorder. *Pain, 119*(1–3), 5–15.

Aurilio, C., Pota, V., Pace, M. C., Passavanti, M. B., & Barbarisi, M. (2008). Ionic channels and neuropathic pain: Physiopathology and applications. *Journal of Cellular Physiology, 215*(1), 8–14.

Battaglia, T. C., Mulhall, K. J., Brown, T. E., & Saleh, K. J. (2006). Increased surgical volume is associated with lower THA dislocation rates. *Clinical Orthopaedics and Related Research, 447*, 28–33.

Baumrucker, S. J. (2002). Post-thoracotomy pain syndrome: An opportunity for palliative care. *The American Journal of Hospice & Palliative Care, 19*(2), 83–84.

Beecher, H. K. (1946). Pain in Men Wounded in Battle. *Ann Surg, 123*(1), 96–105.

Beecher, H. K. (1959). Measurement of subjective responses; quantitative effects of drugs. New York: Oxford University Press.

Belmonte, C., & Cervero, E. (1996). *Neurobiology of nociceptors*. Oxford: Oxford University Press.

Beydoun, A., & Backonja, M. M. (2003). Mechanistic stratification of antineuralgic agents. *Journal of Pain and Symptom Management, 25*(5 Suppl), S18–S30.

Bhave, G., & Gereau, R. W. T. (2004). Posttranslational mechanisms of peripheral sensitization. *Journal of Neurobiology, 61*(1), 88–106.

Bini, G., Cruccu, G., Hagbarth, K. E., Schady, W., & Torebjork, E. (1984). Analgesic effect of vibration and cooling on pain induced by intraneural electrical stimulation. *Pain, 18*(3), 239–248.

Borly, L., Anderson, I. B., Bardram, L., Christensen, E., Sehested, A., Kehlet, H., et al. (1999). Preoperative prediction model of outcome after cholecystectomy for symptomatic gallstones. *Scandinavian Journal of Gastroenterology, 34*(11), 1144–1152.

Brandsborg, B., Nikolajsen, L., Kehlet, H., & Jensen, T. S. (2008). Chronic pain after hysterectomy. *Acta Anaesthesiologica Scandinavica, 52*(3), 327–331.

Brau, M. E., Dreimann, M., Olschewski, A., Vogel, W., & Hempelmann, G. (2001). Effect of drugs used for neuropathic pain management on tetrodotoxin-resistant Na(+) currents in rat sensory neurons. *Anesthesiology, 94*(1), 137–144.

Bruce, J., Drury, N., Poobalan, A. S., Jeffrey, R. R., Smith, W. C., & Chambers, W. A. (2003). The prevalence of chronic chest and leg pain following cardiac surgery: A historical cohort study. *Pain, 104*(1–2), 265–273.

Bruce, J., Poobalan, A. S., Smith, W. C., & Chambers, W. A. (2004). Quantitative assessment of chronic postsurgical pain using the McGill Pain Questionnaire. *The Clinical Journal of Pain, 20*(2), 70–75.

Cerfolio, R. J., Price, T. N., Bryant, A. S., Sale Bass, C., & Bartolucci, A. A. (2003). Intracostal sutures decrease the pain of thoracotomy. *The Annals of Thoracic Surgery, 76*(2), 407–411; discussion 411–402.

Cesare, P., Dekker, L. V., Sardini, A., Parker, P. J., & McNaughton, P. A. (1999). Specific involvement of PKC-epsilon in sensitization of the neuronal response to painful heat. *Neuron, 23*(3), 617–624.

Chan, B. L., Witt, R., Charrow, A. P., Magee, A., Howard, R., Pasquina, P. F., et al. (2007). Mirror therapy for phantom limb pain. *The New England Journal of Medicine, 357*(21), 2206–2207.

Chen, H., Deshpande, A. D., Jiang, R., & Martin, B. C. (2005). An epidemiological investigation of off-label anticonvulsant drug use in the Georgia Medicaid population. *Pharmacoepidemiology and Drug Safety, 14*(9), 629–638.

Chong, M. S., & Bajwa, Z. H. (2003). Diagnosis and treatment of neuropathic pain. *Journal of Pain and Symptom Management, 25*(5 Suppl), S4–S11.

Cohen, S. P., Kapoor, S. G., & Rathmell, J. P. (2009). Intravenous infusion tests have limited utility for selecting long-term drug therapy in patients with chronic pain: A systematic review. *Anesthesiology, 111*(2), 416–431.

Couceiro, T. C., Menezes, T. C., & Valenca, M. M. (2009). Post-mastectomy pain syndrome: The magnitude of the problem. *Revista Brasileira de Anestesiologia, 59*(3), 358–365.

Crombie, I. K., Davies, H. T., & Macrae, W. A. (1998). Cut and thrust: Antecedent surgery and trauma among patients attending a chronic pain clinic. *Pain, 76*(1–2), 167–171.

Davis, K. D., Meyer, R. A., & Campbell, J. N. (1993). Chemosensitivity and sensitization of nociceptive afferents that innervate the hairy skin of monkey. *Journal of Neurophysiology, 69*(4), 1071–1081.

de Jong, J. R., Vlaeyen, J. W., Onghena, P., Cuypers, C., den Hollander, M., & Ruijgrok, J. (2005). Reduction of pain-related fear in complex regional pain syndrome type I: The application of graded exposure in vivo. *Pain, 116*(3), 264–275.

De Kock, M. (2009). Expanding our horizons: Transition of acute postoperative pain to persistent pain and establishment of chronic postsurgical pain services. *Anesthesiology, 111*(3), 461–463.

DeFrances, C. J., Lucas, C. A., Buie, V. C., & Golosinskiy, A. (2008). National hospital discharge survey. *National Health Statistics Report, 5*, 1–20.

Devor, M. (2006). Response of nerves to injury in relation to neuropathic pain. In S. B. McMahon & M. Koltzenburg (Eds.), *Textbook of pain* (5th ed., pp. 905–927). New York: Elsevier Churchill Stone.

Dickenson, A. H., & Kieffer, B. (2006). Opiates: Basic mechanisms. In S. B. McMahon & M. Koltzenburg (Eds.), *Textbook of pain* (5th ed., pp. 427–442). New York: Churchill-Livingstone.

Diers, M., Christmann, C., Koeppe, C., Ruf, M., & Flor, H. (2010). Mirrored, imagined and executed movements differentially activate sensorimotor cortex in amputees with and without phantom limb pain. *Pain, 149*(2), 296–304.

Donovan, K. A., Thompson, L. M. A., & Jacobsen, P. B. (2011). Pain, depression and anxiety in cancer. In R. J. Moore (Ed.), *Handbook of pain and palliative care: Biobehavioral approaches for the life course*. New York: Springer.

Dougherty, P. M., Garrison, C. J., & Carlton, S. M. (1992). Differential influence of local anesthetic upon two models of experimentally induced peripheral mononeuropathy in the rat. *Brain Research, 570*(1–2), 109–115.

Eisenberg, E., McNicol, E., & Carr, D. B. (2006). Opioids for neuropathic pain. *Cochrane Database Syst Rev, 3*, CD006146.

Eisenberg, E., Pultorak, Y., Pud, D., & Bar-El, Y. (2001). Prevalence and characteristics of post coronary artery bypass graft surgery pain (PCP). *Pain, 92*(1–2), 11–17.

Fields, H. L., Basbaum, A. I., & Heinricher, M. M. (2006). Central nervous system mechanisms of pain modulation. In P. D. Wall, S. B. McMahon & M. Koltzenburg (Eds.), *Wall and Melzack's textbook of pain* (5th ed., pp. 125–142). Philadelphia: Elsevier/Churchill Livingstone.

Fitzgibbon, E. J., & Viola, R. (2005). Parenteral ketamine as an analgesic adjuvant for severe pain: Development and retrospective audit of a protocol for a palliative care unit. *Journal of Palliative Medicine, 8*(1), 49–57.

Foell, J., & Flor, H. (2011). Phantom limb pain. In R. J. Moore (Ed.), *Handbook of pain and palliative care: Biobehavioral approaches for the life course*. New York: Springer.

Forman, A. (1990). Peripheral neuropathy in cancer patients: Clinical types, etiology, and presentation. Part 2. *Oncology (Williston Park), 4*(2), 85–89.

Fukuoka, T., Tokunaga, A., & Kondo, E. (2000). The role of neighboring intact dorsal root ganglion neurons in a rat neuropathic pain model. In M. Devor, M. Rowbotham, & Z. Wiesenfeld-Helm (Eds.), *Progress in pain research and management* (Vol. 16, pp. 137–146). Seattle: IASP Press.

Furlan, A. D., Sandoval, J. A., Mailis-Gagnon, A., & Tunks, E. (2006). Opioids for chronic noncancer pain: A meta-analysis of effectiveness and side effects. *Canadian Medical Association Journal, 174*(11), 1589–1594.

Gartner, R., Jensen, M. B., Nielsen, J., Ewertz, M., Kroman, N., & Kehlet, H. (2009). Prevalence of and factors associated with persistent pain following breast cancer surgery. *JAMA, 302*(18), 1985–1992.

Getto, C. J., Sorkness, C. A., & Howell, T. (1987). Issues in drug management. Part I. Antidepressants and chronic nonmalignant pain: A review. *Journal of Pain and Symptom Management, 2*(1), 9–18.

Giovannoni, M. P., Ghelardini, C., Vergelli, C., & Dal Piaz, V. (2009). Alpha2-agonists as analgesic agents. *Medicinal Research Reviews, 29*(2), 339–368.

Goldstein, D. J., Lu, Y., Detke, M. J., Lee, T. C., & Iyengar, S. (2005). Duloxetine vs. placebo in patients with painful diabetic neuropathy. *Pain, 116*(1–2), 109–118.

Goodyear-Smith, F., & Halliwell, J. (2009). Anticonvulsants for neuropathic pain: Gaps in the evidence. *The Clinical Journal of Pain, 25*(6), 528–536.

Gotoda, Y., Kambara, N., Sakai, T., Kishi, Y., Kodama, K., & Koyama, T. (2001). The morbidity, time course and predictive factors for persistent post-thoracotomy pain. *European Journal of Pain, 5*(1), 89–96.

Gottschalk, A., & Ochroch, E. A. (2008). Clinical and demographic characteristics of patients with chronic pain after major thoracotomy. *The Clinical Journal of Pain, 24*(8), 708–716.

Granot, M., & Ferber, S. G. (2005). The roles of pain catastrophizing and anxiety in the prediction of postoperative pain intensity: A prospective study. *The Clinical Journal of Pain, 21*(5), 439–445.

Grant, A. M., Scott, N. W., & O'Dwyer, P. J. (2004). Five-year follow-up of a randomized trial to assess pain and numbness after laparoscopic or open repair of groin hernia. *The British Journal of Surgery, 91*(12), 1570–1574.

Grisart, J. M., & Plaghki, L. H. (1999). Impaired selective attention in chronic pain patients. *Eur J Pain, 3*(4), 325–333.

Grudt, T. J., & Perl, E. R. (2002). Correlations between neuronal morphology and electrophysiological features in the rodent superficial dorsal horn. *J Physiol, 540*(Pt 1), 189–207.

Guenther, S., Reeh, P. W., & Kress, M. (1999). Rises in [Ca2+]i mediate capsaicin- and proton-induced heat sensitization of rat primary nociceptive neurons. *The European Journal of Neuroscience, 11*(9), 3143–3150.

Gulluoglu, B. M., Cingi, A., Cakir, T., Gercek, A., Barlas, A., & Eti, Z. (2006). Factors related to post-treatment chronic pain in breast cancer survivors: The interference of pain with life functions. *International Journal of Fertility and Women's Medicine, 51*(2), 75–82.

Haanpaa, M. L., Gourlay, G. K., Kent, J. L., Miaskowski, C., Raja, S. N., Schmader, K. E., et al. (2010). Treatment considerations for patients with neuropathic pain and other medical comorbidities. *Mayo Clinic Proceedings, 85*(3 Suppl), S15–S25.

Haley, J. E., Sullivan, A. F., & Dickenson, A. H. (1990). Evidence for spinal N-methyl-D-aspartate receptor involvement in prolonged chemical nociception in the rat. *Brain Research, 518*(1–2), 218–226.

Hanley, M. A., Jensen, M. P., Ehde, D. M., Hoffman, A. J., Patterson, D. R., & Robinson, L. R. (2004). Psychosocial predictors of long-term adjustment to lower-limb amputation and phantom limb pain. *Disability and Rehabilitation, 26*(14–15), 882–893.

Harden, R. N. (2005). Pharmacotherapy of complex regional pain syndrome. *American Journal of Physical Medicine & Rehabilitation, 84*(3 Suppl), S17–S28.

Harden, R. N., Bruehl, S., Stanos, S., Brander, V., Chung, O. Y., Saltz, S., et al. (2003). Prospective examination of pain-related and psychological predictors of CRPS-like phenomena following total knee arthroplasty: A preliminary study. *Pain, 106*(3), 393–400.

Hinrichs-Rocker, A., Schulz, K., Jarvinen, I., Lefering, R., Simanski, C., & Neugebauer, E. A. (2009). Psychosocial predictors and correlates for chronic post-surgical pain (CPSP) – A systematic review. *European Journal of Pain, 13*(7), 719–730.

Hsu, C., & Sliwa, J. A. (2004). Phantom breast pain as a source of functional loss. *American Journal of Physical Medicine & Rehabilitation, 83*(8), 659–662.

Hurley, R. W., & Adams, M. C. (2008). Sex, gender, and pain: An overview of a complex field. *Anesthesia and Analgesia, 107*(1), 309–317.

Jackson, K. C., II. (2006). Pharmacotherapy for neuropathic pain. *Pain Practice, 6*(1), 27–33.

Jensen, M. P., Ehde, D. M., Hoffman, A. J., Patterson, D. R., Czerniecki, J. M., & Robinson, L. R. (2002). Cognitions, coping and social environment predict adjustment to phantom limb pain. *Pain, 95*(1–2), 133–142.

Jensen, T. S., Krebs, B., Nielsen, J., & Rasmussen, P. (1983). Phantom limb, phantom pain and stump pain in amputees during the first 6 months following limb amputation. *Pain, 17*(3), 243–256.

Jensen, T. S., Krebs, B., Nielsen, J., & Rasmussen, P. (1985). Immediate and long-term phantom limb pain in amputees: Incidence, clinical characteristics and relationship to pre-amputation limb pain. *Pain, 21*(3), 267–278.

Joshi, G. P., & Ogunnaike, B. O. (2005). Consequences of inadequate postoperative pain relief and chronic persistent postoperative pain. *Anesthesiology Clinics of North America, 23*(1), 21–36.

Jung, A. C., Staiger, T., & Sullivan, M. (1997). The efficacy of selective serotonin reuptake inhibitors for the management of chronic pain. *Journal of General Internal Medicine, 12*(6), 384–389.

Jung, B. F., Ahrendt, G. M., Oaklander, A. L., & Dworkin, R. H. (2003). Neuropathic pain following breast cancer surgery: Proposed classification and research update. *Pain, 104*(1–2), 1–13.

Katz, J., & Clarke, H. (2008). Preventive analgesia and beyond: Current status, evidence, and future directions. In P. Macintyre, D. Rowbotham, & R. Howard (Eds.), *Clinical pain management: Acute pain* (pp. 154–198). London: Hodder Arnold Ltd.

Katz, J., Jackson, M., Kavanagh, B. P., & Sandler, A. N. (1996). Acute pain after thoracic surgery predicts long-term post-thoracotomy pain. *The Clinical Journal of Pain, 12*(1), 50–55.

Katz, J., & Melzack, R. (1990). Pain "memories" in phantom limbs: Review and clinical observations. *Pain, 43*(3), 319–336.

Katz, J., & Seltzer, Z. (2009). Transition from acute to chronic postsurgical pain: Risk factors and protective factors. *Expert Review of Neurotherapeutics, 9*(5), 723–744.

Keefe, F. J., Brown, G. K., Wallston, K. A., & Caldwell, D. S. (1989). Coping with rheumatoid arthritis pain: Catastrophizing as a maladaptive strategy. *Pain, 37*(1), 51–56.

Keogh, E. (2011). Sex differences in pain across the life course. In R. J. Moore (Ed.), *Handbook of pain and palliative care: Biobehavioral approaches for the life course*. New York: Springer.

Khasar, S. G., McCarter, G., & Levine, J. D. (1999). Epinephrine produces a beta-adrenergic receptor-mediated mechanical hyperalgesia and in vitro sensitization of rat nociceptors. *Journal of Neurophysiology, 81*(3), 1104–1112.

King, E. W., Audette, K., Athman, G. A., Nguyen, H. O., Sluka, K. A., & Fairbanks, C. A. (2005). Transcutaneous electrical nerve stimulation activates peripherally located alpha-2A adrenergic receptors. *Pain, 115*(3), 364–373.

Kingery, W. S. (1997). A critical review of controlled clinical trials for peripheral neuropathic pain and complex regional pain syndromes. *Pain, 73*(2), 123–139.

Knotkova, H., & Pappagallo, M. (2007). Adjuvant analgesics. *The Medical Clinics of North America, 91*(1), 113–124.

Kooijman, C. M., Dijkstra, P. U., Geertzen, J. H., Elzinga, A., & van der Schans, C. P. (2000). Phantom pain and phantom sensations in upper limb amputees: An epidemiological study. *Pain, 87*(1), 33–41.

Kroman, N., Jensen, M. B., Wohlfahrt, J., Mouridsen, H. T., Andersen, P. K., & Melbye, M. (2000). Factors influencing the effect of age on prognosis in breast cancer: Population based study. *BMJ, 320*(7233), 474–478.

LaMotte, R. H., Shain, C. N., Simone, D. A., & Tsai, E. F. (1991). Neurogenic hyperalgesia: Psychophysical studies of underlying mechanisms. *Journal of Neurophysiology, 66*(1), 190–211.

Latremoliere, A., & Woolf, C. J. (2009). Central sensitization: A generator of pain hypersensitivity by central neural plasticity. *The Journal of Pain, 10*(9), 895–926.

Lavand'homme, P. M., & Eisenach, J. C. (2003). Perioperative administration of the alpha2-adrenoceptor agonist clonidine at the site of nerve injury reduces the development of mechanical hypersensitivity and modulates local cytokine expression. *Pain, 105*(1–2), 247–254.

Levine, J. D., Gordon, N. C., Smith, R., & Fields, H. L. (1982). Post-operative pain: Effect of extent of injury and attention. *Brain Res, 234*(2), 500–504.

Levy, D., & Strassman, A. M. (2002). Distinct sensitizing effects of the cAMP-PKA second messenger cascade on rat dural mechanonociceptors. *The Journal of Physiology, 538*(Pt 2), 483–493.

Lorenz, J., & Tracey, I. (2009). Brain Correlates of Psychological Amplification of Pain. In E. A. Mayer & M. C. Bushnell (Eds.), *Functional pain syndromes: Presentation and pathophysiology* (pp. 385–401). Seattle: IASP Press.

Lossignol, D. A., Obiols-Portis, M., & Body, J. J. (2005). Successful use of ketamine for intractable cancer pain. *Supportive Care in Cancer, 13*(3), 188–193.

Macrae, W. A. (2008). Chronic post-surgical pain: 10 years on. *British Journal of Anaesthesia, 101*(1), 77–86.

Macrae, W. A., & Davies, H. (1999). Chronic postsurgical pain. In I. K. Crombie (Ed.), *Epidemiology of pain* (pp. 125–142). Seattle: IASP Press.

Manchikanti, L., Atluri, S., Trescot, A. M., & Giordano, J. (2008). Monitoring opioid adherence in chronic pain patients: Tools, techniques, and utility. *Pain Physician, 11*(2 Suppl), S155–S180.

Martin, M. O., Gomez Sancho, M., Morlion, B., & Simpson, K. (2008). The management of pain due to amputation. *Journal of Pain & Palliative Care Pharmacotherapy, 22*(1), 57–60.

Mattia, A., & Coluzzi, F. (2009). What anesthesiologists should know about paracetamol (acetaminophen). *Minerva Anestesiologica, 75*(11), 644–653.

Mattia, C., & Coluzzi, F. (2005). COX-2 inhibitors: Pharmacological data and adverse effects. *Minerva Anestesiologica, 71*(7–8), 461–470.

Max, M. B., Lynch, S. A., Muir, J., Shoaf, S. E., Smoller, B., & Dubner, R. (1992). Effects of desipramine, amitriptyline, and fluoxetine on pain in diabetic neuropathy. *The New England Journal of Medicine, 326*(19), 1250–1256.

May, S. (2011). Chronic low back pain. In R. J. Moore (Ed.), *Handbook of pain and palliative care: Biobehavioral approaches for the life course*. New York: Springer.

Mayer, M. L., Westbrook, G. L., & Guthrie, P. B. (1984). Voltage-dependent block by Mg^{2+} of NMDA responses in spinal cord neurones. *Nature, 309*(5965), 261–263.

McCarthy, G. C., Megalla, S. A., & Habib, A. S. (2010). Impact of intravenous lidocaine infusion on postoperative analgesia and recovery from surgery: A systematic review of randomized controlled trials. *Drugs, 70*(9), 1149–1163.

McCleane, G. (2007). Topical analgesics. *The Medical Clinics of North America, 91*(1), 125–139.

McMahon, S. B., Bennett, D. L. H., & Bevan, S. (2006). Inflammatory mediators and modulators of pain. In S. B. McMahon & M. Koltzenburg (Eds.), *Textbook of pain* (5th ed., pp. 49–72). New York: Churchill Livingstone.

Melzack, R., & Wall, P. D. (1965). Pain mechanisms: A new theory. *Science, 150*(699), 971–979.

Merskey, H., & Bogduk, N. (1994). *Classification of chronic pain*. Seattle: IASP Press.

Meyer, R. A., & Campbell, J. N. (1981). Myelinated nociceptive afferents account for the hyperalgesia that follows a burn to the hand. *Science, 213*(4515), 1527–1529.

Meyer, R. A., Ringkamp, M., Campbell, J. N., & Raja, S. N. (2006). Peripheral mechanisms of cutaneous nociception. In S. B. McMahon & M. Koltzenburg (Eds.), *Textbook of pain* (5th ed., pp. 3–34). New York: Churchill Livingstone.

Meyerson, J., Thelin, S., Gordh, T., & Karlsten, R. (2001). The incidence of chronic post-sternotomy pain after cardiac surgery – A prospective study. *Acta Anaesthesiologica Scandinavica, 45*(8), 940–944.

Michael, G. J., & Priestley, J. V. (1999). Differential expression of the mRNA for the vanilloid receptor subtype 1 in cells of the adult rat dorsal root and nodose ganglia and its downregulation by axotomy. *The Journal of Neuroscience, 19*(5), 1844–1854.

Miron, D., Duncan, G. H., & Bushnell, M. C. (1989). Effects of attention on the intensity and unpleasantness of thermal pain. *Pain, 39*(3), 345–352.

Munir, M. A., Enany, N., & Zhang, J. M. (2007). Nonopioid analgesics. *Anesthesiol Clin, 25*(4), 761–774, vi.

Naim, M., Spike, R. C., Watt, C., Shehab, S. A., & Todd, A. J. (1997). Cells in laminae III and IV of the rat spinal cord that possess the neurokinin-1 receptor and have dorsally directed dendrites receive a major synaptic input from tachykinin-containing primary afferents. *J Neurosci, 17*(14), 5536–5548.

Naylor, M. R., Seminowicz, D. A., Somers, T. J., & Keefe, F. J. (2011). Pain imaging. In R. J. Moore (Ed.), *Handbook of pain and palliative care: Biobehavioral approaches for the life course*. New York: Springer.

Nikolajsen, L., Ilkjaer, S., Kroner, K., Christensen, J. H., & Jensen, T. S. (1997). The influence of preamputation pain on postamputation stump and phantom pain. *Pain, 72*(3), 393–405.

Nikolajsen, L., & Jensen, T. S. (2001). Phantom limb pain. *British Journal of Anaesthesia, 87*(1), 107–116.

Nikolajsen, L., Sorensen, H. C., Jensen, T. S., & Kehlet, H. (2004). Chronic pain following Caesarean section. *Acta Anaesthesiologica Scandinavica, 48*(1), 111–116.

Nocom, G., Ho, K. Y., & Perumal, M. (2009). Interventional management of chronic pain. *Annals of the Academy of Medicine, Singapore, 38*(2), 150–155.

Okifuji, A., & Ackerlind, S. (2007). Behavioral medicine approaches to pain. *The Medical Clinics of North America, 91*(1), 45–55.

Okon, T. (2007). Ketamine: An introduction for the pain and palliative medicine physician. *Pain Physician, 10*(3), 493–500.

Okuse, K. (2007). Pain signalling pathways: From cytokines to ion channels. *The International Journal of Biochemistry & Cell Biology, 39*(3), 490–496.

Pae, C. U., Marks, D. M., Shah, M., Han, C., Ham, B. J., Patkar, A. A., et al. (2009). Milnacipran: Beyond a role of antidepressant. *Clinical Neuropharmacology, 32*(6), 355–363.

Papp, J., & Sobel, E. (2009). The Genetics of Pain. In E. A. Mayer & M. C. Bushnell (Eds.), *Functional pain syndromes: Presentation and pathophysiology* (pp. 405–422). Seattle: IASP Press.

Pavlin, D. J., Sullivan, M. J., Freund, P. R., & Roesen, K. (2005). Catastrophizing: A risk factor for postsurgical pain. *The Clinical Journal of Pain, 21*(1), 83–90.

Peters, M. L., Sommer, M., de Rijke, J. M., Kessels, F., Heineman, E., Patijn, J., et al. (2007). Somatic and psychologic predictors of long-term unfavorable outcome after surgical intervention. *Annals of Surgery, 245*(3), 487–494.

Poleshuck, E. L., Katz, J., Andrus, C. H., Hogan, L. A., Jung, B. F., Kulick, D. I., et al. (2006). Risk factors for chronic pain following breast cancer surgery: A prospective study. *The Journal of Pain, 7*(9), 626–634.

Pollo, A., & Benedetti, F. (2011). Pain and the placebo/nocebo effect. In R. J. Moore (Ed.), *Handbook of pain and palliative care: Biobehavioral approaches for the life course*. New York: Springer.

Poobalan, A. S., Bruce, J., Smith, W. C., King, P. M., Krukowski, Z. H., & Chambers, W. A. (2003). A review of chronic pain after inguinal herniorrhaphy. *Clin J Pain, 19*(1), 48–54.

Porter, R. J., & Meldrum, B. S. (2001). Antiseizure drugs. In B. G. Katzung (Ed.), *Basic and clinical pharmacology* (8th ed., pp. 395–418). New York: Lange Medical Books/McGraw-Hill.

Price, D. D., Verne, G. N., & Schwartz, J. M. (2006). Plasticity in brain processing and modulation of pain. *Prog Brain Res, 157*, 333–352.

Rectenwald, J. E., & Upchurch, G. R., Jr. (2007). Impact of outcomes research on the management of vascular surgery patients. *Journal of Vascular Surgery, 45*(Suppl A), A131–A140.

Reeh, P. W., Bayer, J., Kocher, L., & Handwerker, H. O. (1987). Sensitization of nociceptive cutaneous nerve fibers from the rat's tail by noxious mechanical stimulation. *Experimental Brain Research, 65*(3), 505–512.

Rexed, B. (1952). The cytoarchitectonic organization of the spinal cord in the cat. *J Comp Neurol, 96*(3), 414–495.

Rogers, M. L., & Duffy, J. P. (2000). Surgical aspects of chronic post-thoracotomy pain. *European Journal of Cardio-Thoracic Surgery, 18*(6), 711–716.

Rowbotham, M. C., Goli, V., Kunz, N. R., & Lei, D. (2004). Venlafaxine extended release in the treatment of painful diabetic neuropathy: A double-blind, placebo-controlled study. *Pain, 110*(3), 697–706.

Rowbotham, M. C., Reisner, L. A., Davies, P. S., & Fields, H. L. (2005). Treatment response in antidepressant-naive postherpetic neuralgia patients: Double-blind, randomized trial. *The Journal of Pain, 6*(11), 741–746.

Sanchez, C., & Hyttel, J. (1999). Comparison of the effects of antidepressants and their metabolites on reuptake of biogenic amines and on receptor binding. *Cellular and Molecular Neurobiology, 19*(4), 467–489.

Sawamoto, N., Honda, M., Okada, T., Hanakawa, T., Kanda, M., Fukuyama, H., et al. (2000). Expectation of pain enhances responses to nonpainful somatosensory stimulation in the anterior cingulate cortex and parietal operculum/posterior insula: an event-related functional magnetic resonance imaging study. *J Neurosci, 20*(19), 7438–7445.

Schaible, H. G., & Richter, F. (2004). Pathophysiology of pain. *Langenbeck's Archives of Surgery, 389*(4), 237–243.

Sclafani, L. M., & Baron, R. H. (2008). Sentinel lymph node biopsy and axillary dissection: Added morbidity of the arm, shoulder and chest wall after mastectomy and reconstruction. *Cancer Journal, 14*(4), 216–222.

Seltzer, Z., Wu, T., Max, M. B., & Diehl, S. R. (2001). Mapping a gene for neuropathic pain-related behavior following peripheral neurectomy in the mouse. *Pain, 93*(2), 101–106.

Sepulveda, C., Marlin, A., Yoshida, T., & Ullrich, A. (2002). Palliative care: The World Health Organization's global perspective. *Journal of Pain and Symptom Management, 24*(2), 91–96.

Sherman, R. A., & Sherman, C. J. (1983). Prevalence and characteristics of chronic phantom limb pain among American veterans. Results of a trial survey. *American Journal of Physical Medicine, 62*(5), 227–238.

Silverman, S. M. (2009). Opioid induced hyperalgesia: Clinical implications for the pain practitioner. *Pain Physician, 12*(3), 679–684.

Sluka, K. A. (2009). Peripheral mechanisms involved in pain processing. In K. A. Sluka (Ed.), *Mechanisms and management of pain for the physical therapist* (pp. 19–40). Seattle: IASP Press.

Smith, J., & Thompson, J. M. (1995). Phantom limb pain and chemotherapy in pediatric amputees. *Mayo Clinic Proceedings, 70*(4), 357–364.

Solano, J. P., Gomes, B., & Higginson, I. J. (2006). A comparison of symptom prevalence in far advanced cancer, AIDS, heart disease, chronic obstructive pulmonary disease and renal disease. *Journal of Pain and Symptom Management, 31*(1), 58–69.

Stacey, B. R. (2005). Management of peripheral neuropathic pain. *American Journal of Physical Medicine & Rehabilitation, 84*(3 Suppl), S4–S16.

Stanos, S. P., McLean, J., & Rader, L. (2007). Physical medicine rehabilitation approach to pain. *The Medical Clinics of North America, 91*(1), 57–95.

Stiff, G., Rhodes, M., Kelly, A., Telford, K., Armstrong, C. P., & Rees, B. I. (1994). Long-term pain: Less common after laparoscopic than open cholecystectomy. *The British Journal of Surgery, 81*(9), 1368–1370.

Tasmuth, T., Blomqvist, C., & Kalso, E. (1999). Chronic post-treatment symptoms in patients with breast cancer operated in different surgical units. *European Journal of Surgical Oncology, 25*(1), 38–43.

Tasmuth, T., Estlanderb, A. M., & Kalso, E. (1996). Effect of present pain and mood on the memory of past postoperative pain in women treated surgically for breast cancer. *Pain, 68*(2–3), 343–347.

Tate, S., Benn, S., Hick, C., Trezise, D., John, V., Mannion, R. J., et al. (1998). Two sodium channels contribute to the TTX-R sodium current in primary sensory neurons. *Nature Neuroscience, 1*(8), 653–655.

Thalhammer, J. G., & LaMotte, R. H. (1982). Spatial properties of nociceptor sensitization following heat injury of the skin. *Brain Research, 231*(2), 257–265.

Thompson, A. R. (2007). Recognizing chronic postsurgical pain syndromes at the end of life. *American Journal of Hospice Palliative Care, 24*(4), 319–322; discussion 322–314.

Todd, A. J. (2010). Neuronal circuitry for pain processing in the dorsal horn. *Nat Rev Neurosci, 11*(12), 823–836.

Tracey, I., Ploghaus, A., Gati, J. S., Clare, S., Smith, S., Menon, R. S., et al. (2002). Imaging attentional modulation of pain in the periaqueductal gray in humans. *J Neurosci, 22*(7), 2748–2752.

Ure, B. M., Jesch, N. K., & Nustede, R. (2004). Postcholecystectomy syndrome with special regard to children – A review. *European Journal of Pediatric Surgery, 14*(4), 221–225.

Vermelis, J. M., Wassen, M. M., Fiddelers, A. A., Nijhuis, J. G., & Marcus, M. A. (2010). Prevalence and predictors of chronic pain after labor and delivery. *Current Opinion in Anaesthesiology, 23*(3), 295–299.

Villemure, C., & Bushnell, M. C. (2002). Cognitive modulation of pain: How do attention and emotion influence pain processing? *Pain, 95*(3), 195–199.

Wartan, S. W., Hamann, W., Wedley, J. R., & McColl, I. (1997). Phantom pain and sensation among British veteran amputees. *British Journal of Anaesthesia, 78*(6), 652–659.

Way, W. L., Fields, H. L., & Schumacher, M. A. (2001). Opioid analgesics and antagonists. In B. G. Katzung (Ed.), *Basic and clinical pharmacology* (8th ed., pp. 512–531). New York: Lange Medical Books/McGraw-Hill.

Wiffen, P., Collins, S., McQuay, H., Carroll, D., Jadad, A., & Moore, A. (2005). Anticonvulsant drugs for acute and chronic pain. *Cochrane Database Syst Rev,* (3), CD001133.

Wilsey, B., Teicheira, D., Caneris, O. A., & Fishman, S. M. (2001). A review of sympathetically maintained pain syndromes in the cancer pain population: The spectrum of ambiguous entities of RSD, CRPS, SMP and other pain states related to the sympathetic nervous system. *Pain Practice, 1*(4), 307–323.

Wilt, T. J., Shamliyan, T. A., Taylor, B. C., MacDonald, R., & Kane, R. L. (2008). Association between hospital and surgeon radical prostatectomy volume and patient outcomes: A systematic review. *Journal of Urology, 180*(3), 820–828; discussion 828–829.

Woolf, C. J., & Costigan, M. (1999). Transcriptional and posttranslational plasticity and the generation of inflammatory pain. *Proceedings of the National Academy of Sciences of the United States of America, 96*(14), 7723–7730.

Woolf, C. J., & Mannion, R. J. (1999). Neuropathic pain: Aetiology, symptoms, mechanisms, and management. *Lancet, 353*(9168), 1959–1964.

Woolf, C. J., & Salter, M. W. (2000). Neuronal plasticity: Increasing the gain in pain. *Science, 288*(5472), 1765–1769.

Woolf, C. J., & Salter, M. W. (2006). Plasticity and pain: Role of the dorsal horn. In S. B. McMahon & M. Koltzenburg (Eds.), *Textbook of pain* (5th ed., pp. 91–105). New York: Churchill-Livingstone.

Wu, G., Ringkamp, M., Hartke, T. V., Murinson, B. B., Campbell, J. N., Griffin, J. W., et al. (2001). Early onset of spontaneous activity in uninjured C-fiber nociceptors after injury to neighboring nerve fibers. *The Journal of Neuroscience, 21*(8), RC140.

Xie, Y. K., Xiao, W. H., & Li, H. Q. (1993). The relationship between new ion channels and ectopic discharges from a region of nerve injury. *Science in China, Series B, 36*(1), 68–74.

Yamamoto, T., & Yaksh, T. L. (1991). Stereospecific effects of a nonpeptidic NK1 selective antagonist, CP-96,345: Antinociception in the absence of motor dysfunction. *Life Sciences, 49*(26), 1955–1963.

Yarnitsky, D., Crispel, Y., Eisenberg, E., Granovsky, Y., Ben-Nun, A., Sprecher, E., et al. (2008). Prediction of chronic post-operative pain: Pre-operative DNIC testing identifies patients at risk. *Pain, 138*(1), 22–28.

Chapter 20
Pain and the Placebo/Nocebo Effect

Antonella Pollo and Fabrizio Benedetti

Introduction

In order to focus on the importance of placebo mechanisms in humans, let us examine the following two pictures. *Picture 1*: 2000 B.C.; a wounded warrior is carried to the shaman tent. The respected shaman takes a look at the wound and assures the warrior that he will be healed with the proper prayers and ritual dances. He then prepares a strong-smelling mixture of herbs and seeds, and as the whole tribe chants rhythmically around the campfire, he carefully applies it to the wound, all the while uttering incomprehensible sentences passed on to him by a venerable line of ancestral shamans. *Picture 2*: 2010 A.D.; a wounded soldier is carried to the military hospital. The medical staff completes a physical examination, a CT scan to rule out internal lesions is carried out to the reassuring buzz of the most recent technology, and a respected clinician wearing a spotless white coat reassures the soldier that he will be healed with the proper drugs and physiotherapy.

One of the main aims of placebo research is to outline what these two pictures have in common. Shamans of the past and clinicians of today share instinctual knowledge that the context surrounding a therapy is an important part of the therapy itself. Rituals have changed and adapted to contemporary world, but they are still here. Across the divide of centuries, they help the two depicted patients develop hope, belief and expectation that they will eventually regain their health. Giving a placebo (i.e. a drug or a treatment devoid of specific activity for the condition being treated) consists of essentially delivering a context without the substance. It is a wrapping devoid of content. Yet, the empty box itself acts subtly on the patient's mind, just as an active drug would do, activating or silencing synapses, altering neurotransmitter content in specific brain areas and modifying brain activity in ways that are today amenable to scientific enquiry. Thus, a placebo is not only the archetypal sugar pill given to please the patient, but anything with the power to impact on the patient's expectations, be it a chemical, a physical treatment or a verbal instruction suggesting a positive outcome.

A. Pollo, MD (✉)
Department of Neuroscience, University of Turin Faculty of Pharmacy, Turin, Italy

National Institute of Neuroscience, Turin, Italy
e-mail: antonella.pollo@unito.it

F. Benedetti, MD
Department of Neuroscience, University of Turin Medical School, Turin, Italy

National Institute of Neuroscience, Turin, Italy

R.J. Moore (ed.), *Handbook of Pain and Palliative Care: Biobehavioral Approaches for the Life Course*,
DOI 10.1007/978-1-4419-1651-8_20, © Springer Science+Business Media, LLC 2012

In fact, what is important is not really the tool used, but the changes it triggers in neural activity, and how these changes ultimately affect psychological and bodily functions.

Contrary to shamans, today clinicians have the technical means to begin to exploit the placebo/context effect in a more rational and scientific way. Basic research in the fields of psychology, physiology, pharmacology and neurobiology has in the last couple of decades enlightened how in different systems and medical conditions different mechanisms are at play. With the largest number of studies, placebo analgesia probably represents the best understood placebo response. It is therefore also the best candidate to pioneer the transfer to the ward of the acquired theoretical knowledge.

The nocebo effect is the negative counterpart of the placebo effect. It is the negative consequence (e.g. symptom worsening) which follows the administration of an inert substance or treatment believed by the receiver to be harmful. As for placebos, the whole context surrounding the therapeutic act impacts on different psychological aspects to produce the end result. Knowledge of nocebo mechanisms can best be applied in clinical practice to minimize the negative aspects of the patient–provider interaction and avoid unhelpful characteristics of the therapeutic context.

The aim of this chapter is to provide the reader with an understanding of how the pain experience can be affected by a placebo or nocebo treatment, either in the form of a drug or a physical manipulation, extending the concept of placebo/nocebo to include all aspects of the context surrounding the care of the patient. Specific in-depth discussion of these issues can also be found in a number of recent books and reviews (Benedetti 2007, 2008a, b, 2010; Benedetti et al. 2011a; Enck et al. 2008; Price et al. 2008; Zubieta and Stohler 2009).

Defining Placebo and Nocebo Effects

Two terms are commonly encountered in placebo literature: placebo effect and placebo response. Although they are often used as synonymous, technically they refer to different concepts. The placebo effect is that observed in the placebo arm of a clinical trial, and is produced by the placebo biological phenomenon in addition to other potential factors contributing to symptom amelioration, such as natural history (the time course of a symptom or disease in the absence of any external intervention), regression to the mean (a statistical phenomenon whereby the second measurement of a symptom is likely to yield a value nearer to the average, i.e. an improvement), biases, judgement errors. The placebo response, on the other hand, designates the biological phenomenon in isolation, as can best be studied in specifically designed experimental protocols (Colloca et al. 2008a).

The definition of nocebo effect also needs to be stated precisely. The term nocebo (latin "I shall harm") was originally introduced to designate noxious effects produced by a placebo, e.g. side-effects of the drug the placebo is substituting for (Pogge 1963). In this instance, however, the negative outcome is produced in spite of an expectation of benefit. True nocebo effects, on the other hand, are always the result of negative expectations, specific or generic (e.g. a pessimistic attitude).

The word placebo (or nocebo) calls attention to the sham drug, but what really matters is not the drug but the changes it elicits in the patient's brain. Moerman (2002) proposed to substitute the term *placebo response* with *meaning response*, to underscore the importance of the patient's beliefs about the treatment and to also stress what is present (something inducing the expectation of a benefit) rather than what is absent (a chemical or manipulation of proven specific efficacy). At the limit, a physical substance or treatment does not need to be administered. Put differently, a placebo/nocebo effect can also be induced by raising expectations in the complete absence of a treatment, just by inducing expectations. These effects are sometimes called "placebo/nocebo-related" effects (Benedetti et al. 2007). They are often the only nocebo effects amenable to human experimental studies, because ethical constraints strongly limit the use of noxious agents.

Four Proposed Mechanisms to Explain Placebo/Nocebo Effects

Different explanatory mechanisms have been proposed for both placebo and nocebo effects, each supported by experimental evidence. They need not be mutually exclusive and can actually be at work simultaneously.

The first theory considers the placebo effect as an example of classical conditioning. As described in the studies on conditioned reflexes by the Russian physiologist Ivan Pavlov, the repeated co-occurrence of an unconditioned response to an unconditioned stimulus (e.g. salivation after the sight of food) with a conditioned stimulus (e.g. a bell ringing) induces a conditioned response (i.e. salivation that is induced by bell ringing alone). Likewise, aspects of the clinical setting (e.g. colour, taste, shape of a pill, as well as concurrent aspects of the therapeutic environment, such as white coats or the peculiar hospital smell) can also act as conditioned stimuli, eliciting a therapeutic response in the absence of an active principle, just because they have been paired with it in the past (Wikramasekera 1985; Siegel 2002; Ader 1997).

Similarly, a conditioned response can also occur for a nocebo effect. For example, nausea can be elicited by the sight of the environment where chemotherapy has been administered in the past. Conditioning has been exploited in the development of a protocol widely used in placebo studies to strengthen the ability of a sham treatment to induce a placebo response. Voudouris and colleagues paired a placebo analgesic cream with a painful stimulation, which was surreptitiously reduced with respect to a baseline condition to mislead the subject regarding the analgesic effect. Direct comparison between a conditioned and an unconditioned group showed that pain reduction following conditioning was invariably larger, indicating the effectiveness of conditioning in mediating a placebo response (Voudouris et al. 1990). Classical conditioning seems to work best where unconscious processes are at play, as in placebo/nocebo effects involving endocrine or immune systems, but it has also been documented in clinical and experimental placebo analgesia and nocebo hyperalgesia.

The second explanation centres on expectations, generated as the product of cognitive engagement, when the patient consciously foresees a positive/negative outcome, based on factors such as verbal instructions, environmental clues, emotional arousal, previous experience and the interaction with care-providers. This anticipation of the future outcome in turn triggers internal changes resulting in specific experiences (e.g. analgesia/hyperalgesia). By grading the degree of expectation, graded responses can be obtained: the same placebo cream applied onto three contiguous skin areas induces a progressively stronger analgesia, according to the strength of the accompanying words ("it is a powerful/weak analgesic cream") (Price et al. 1999). This is true also in the clinical setting, where changing the symbolic meaning of a basal physiological infusion in postoperative patients resulted in different additional painkiller request. In spite of all patients receiving a physiological solution, those who believed that they would receive an analgesic drug demanded significantly less pain reliever than those who believed that they would receive no analgesic at all. An intermediate level of certainty in those believing to have a 50% chance to receive the drug resulted in an intermediate request (Pollo et al. 2001). The expectation of forthcoming pain can further be modulated by a number of emotional and cognitive factors, like desire, self-efficacy and self-reinforcing feedback. Desire is the experiential dimension of wanting something to happen or wanting to avoid something happening (Price et al. 2008), while self-efficacy is the belief to be able to manage the disease, performing the right actions to induce positive changes, for example to withstand and lessen pain. Self-reinforcing feedback is a positive loop whereby the subject selectively attends to signs of improvement, taking them as evidence that the placebo treatment has been successful. This has sometimes been termed the "somatic focus". It is the degree to which individuals focus on their symptoms (Price et al. 2008). A related proposed mechanism posits that anxiety reduction also plays a role in placebo responses, because the subject interpretation of ambiguous sensations is turned from harmful and threatening to benign and unworthy of attention. Accordingly, Vase et al. (2005) showed decreased anxiety levels in patients with irritable bowel syndrome who received a placebo treatment.

A particular type of expectation that contributes to the genesis of placebo effects is the expectation of reward. Our brain is endowed with a so-called reward system, which through the activation of the mesolimbic and mesocortical pathways and the release of dopamine fulfils its natural task to provide pleasurable feelings in response to life-sustaining functions, such as eating, drinking or sex, in order to encourage the repetition of those functions. It has been argued that placebos also have reward properties, associated with the beneficial outcome they provide. In other words, the expected clinical benefit is a form of reward, which triggers the placebo response (Lidstone and Stoessl 2007). Along the history of humankind, when only few active treatments were available and the history of medicine largely matched that of placebo effects, individuals displaying placebo responses certainly had an evolutionary advantage (de la Fuente-Fernández 2010).

Recently, medical anthropologists have proposed a constructionist view of the placebo experience which has at its core the concept of embodiment. According to this idea, the human mind is strongly influenced and shaped by aspects of the body, such as the sensory systems and interactions with the environment and the society. Thus, our experiences can not only be consciously stored as memories, but also imprinted straight onto our body, without involvement of any cognitive process. An example of how sociocultural experiences and processes can impact on the individual's physiology is offered by studies of trauma or stress, as in post-traumatic stress disorder (PTSD), where symptoms like frightening thoughts or sleep disorders are the result of an implicit perception, the literal "incorporation" of a terrifying event from the external world, which has bypassed conscious awareness. According to this theory, the placebo effect is a positive effect of embodiment and the nocebo effect a negative one. Lived positive experiences can be channelled into objects or places, which then acquire the potential to trigger healing responses. Importantly, this process need not involve conscious expectation or conscious attribution of symbolic meaning to the object or place (Thompson et al. 2009). When a symbolic meaning is indeed attributed to an object or place, we enter the domain of the performative efficacy theory. Therapeutic performances may have per se a convincing, persuading effect. A change in the body or mind can be achieved just by the *ritual* of the therapeutic act. The performance inducing a placebo effect may be social, as in sham surgery in clinical trials producing positive outcomes in the placebo arm, or in the case of a mother's kiss on a child wound; or it may be internal, as for athletes mentally rehearsing before a competition. In this framework, a placebo effect could result from the internal act of imagining a specific change of state of the body. Central to the performative efficacy of the ritual is the patient–provider relationship, with factors such as empathy, prestige of the healer, gesture and recitation all contributing to the treatment success (Thompson et al. 2009).

All the above described mechanisms may contribute to a given placebo or nocebo effect, with varying weight and reciprocal influence in different contexts. For example, both conditioning and expectation can be triggered independently in the same experimental protocol, testing pain tolerance in arm ischemic pain, and their effects are additive (Amanzio and Benedetti 1999). In addition, it has been shown in healthy volunteers in a pain conditioning/expectation protocol that conditioning was more important than verbal instructions (inducing expectation) for placebo effects, while the opposite was true for nocebo effects (Colloca and Benedetti 2006; Colloca et al. 2008b). As both conditioning and expectation are forms of learning, it can be inferred that, in the case of placebo, learning from others is not as effective as learning by personally experimenting the association between two situations (e.g. the presence of a specific context and pain relief). On the other hand, learning from others without first-hand experience becomes very powerful in the event of noxious outcomes.

Conditioning seems to be the sole mechanisms involved in the generation of the placebo response in the case of those physiological functions which are only subconsciously controlled, like those involving the immune or the endocrine systems. Thus, placebo modulation of growth hormone (GH) and cortisol secretion could be obtained after conditioning with sumatriptan (a selective $5\text{-HT}_{1B/1D}$ receptor agonist stimulating GH and inhibiting cortisol secretion). However, it was impossible to induce the same modulation by suggestion alone, in the absence of conditioning. It was also not possible to reverse the modulation achieved by conditioning by inducing in the subjects the opposite expectation by verbal instruction. Notably, it was indeed possible to exert this counteracting effect with the induction of opposite expectations in the case of placebo analgesia/hyperalgesia, where cognitive conscious processes play an important role (Benedetti et al. 2003). Immune functions have also been repeatedly conditioned, both in animals and in humans. For instance, in multiple sclerosis patients, decrements in peripheral leucocyte counts induced by cyclophosphamide could be conditioned by pairing the drug with a strongly flavoured beverage (Giang et al. 1996), and more recently, in healthy subjects, a similar conditioning with cyclosporine A produced immunosuppression after placebo, as assessed by depressed mRNA expression of IL-2 and interferon-gamma, and lymphocyte proliferation (Goebel et al. 2002), mediated (at least in rodents) by calcineurin inhibition (Pacheco-López et al. 2008). Recently, much work has been devoted to the identification of the neural structures involved centrally (amygdala, insular cortex, hypothalamus) and peripherally (cholinergic and catecholaminergic output in the autonomic nervous system) in conditioned immunosuppression (Pacheco-López et al. 2005). Reflex control of immunity (Tracey 2009) has been proposed to be part of a neocortical-immune axis (Tuohy 2005), raising the interesting possibility of a role for cognitive factors such as expectations and beliefs in placebo immunological responses (Pacheco-López et al. 2006; Schedlowski and Pacheco-López 2010).

The Neurobiology of Placebo Analgesia

Placebo Molecules: Opioids, Cholecystokinin and Dopamine

The discovery that endogenous opioids are released following a sham treatment in the nervous system of the ailing patient hoping for pain relief can be regarded as a landmark achievement in understanding the pathway leading to the modern definition of placebo therapeutically. Until the late 1970s, when Levine and colleagues first showed that the opiate antagonist naloxone was able to reduce the placebo response in dental postoperative pain (Levine et al. 1978), the placebo effect was held as little more than a nuisance that had to be taken into account in order to properly assess the effects of medicaments in clinical trials. But Levine's and subsequent work in the 1980s and 1990s left little doubts that specific biochemical events were taking place in the pain matrix, giving the placebo effect the dignity of a scientific phenomenon worth of inquiry in its own right. Among the relevant findings, placebo responders were found to have levels of β-endorphin in the cerebrospinal fluid which were more than double those of non-responders (Lipman et al. 1990); opioids released by a placebo procedure displayed the same side-effects as exogenous opiates (Benedetti et al. 1999); naloxone-sensitive cardiac effects could be observed during placebo-induced expectation of analgesia (Pollo et al. 2003). Indirect support also came from the placebo-potentiating role of the colecystokinin (CCK) antagonist proglumide. In fact, the CCK system effects counteract those of opioids, delineating a picture where the placebo effect seems to be under the opposing influence of facilitating opioids and inhibiting CCK (Benedetti et al. 1995, 2011b), in analogy with observations in other sensory domains (Gospic et al. 2008). The endogenous opioids that are released are part of the descending antinociceptive pathway, a top-down regulatory system extending from cognitive and affective cortical brain regions to the brainstem and spinal cord dorsal horns. This system is called into action in life-threatening situations, which call for the organism to attend to more urgent needs than pain (stress-induced analgesia). In such cases, a sort of feedback loop depressing incoming nociceptive signals is activated (Millan 2002).

The opioid antinociceptive system is certainly the best studied, but not the only one implicated. Knowledge of other systems is scarce, but their existence emerges from the fact that, in some situations, a placebo effect can still occur after blockade of opioid mechanisms by naloxone (Gracely et al. 1983; Grevert et al. 1983; Vase et al. 2005). It seems that different agents can bring about different placebo effects. For example, with a morphine conditioning and/or expectation-inducing protocol, Amanzio and Benedetti could, with naloxone, completely reverse placebo analgesia induced in experimental ischemic arm pain. With the use of ketorolac, a non-opioid analgesic, in the same protocol, however, only a partial blockade was observed (Amanzio and Benedetti 1999).

Along a different line of research, dopamine has also been suggested as a putative substance involved in placebo analgesia. The placebo response was first linked to this neurotransmitter after observations in Parkinson's disease, where it usually takes the form of motor improvement following the administration of an inert substance which the patient believes to be an effective antiparkinsonian drug. Here, it is mediated by dopamine release in the *dorsal* striatum, a key structure in the motor circuit affected by the disease (de la Fuente-Fernández et al. 2001). However, it must be noted that dopamine is also released in the *ventral* striatum, notably in the nucleus accumbens, involved in the reward circuit. Contrary to the dorsal striatum, release in ventral striatum was not correlated with the experienced clinical benefit, leading the authors to suggest that this release might be related to the expectation of reward, rather than to reward itself (de la Fuente-Fernández et al. 2002; de la Fuente-Fernández and Stoessl 2002). As such, this dopamine mechanism might not be limited to effects in Parkinson's disease, but could be a generalized process underlying all placebo responses. Although at present strictly neuropharmacological evidence has not been presented for the role of dopamine in shaping the placebo response, additional support from neuroimaging studies points to a possible function of dopamine in placebo analgesia. In a study combining placebo analgesia and a monetary reward task, it was demonstrated that the subjects with stronger nucleus accumbens synaptic activation (as measured by functional magnetic resonance imaging, fMRI) during the monetary reward anticipation also showed more profound placebo responses and greater dopamine activity in the same nucleus (as measured with dopamine-agonist [^{11}C] raclopride positron emission tomography, PET) (Scott et al. 2007). Moreover, in a subsequent PET study using the μ-opioid receptor-selective radiotracer [^{11}C]carfentanil and [^{11}C]raclopride, both opioid and dopamine neurotransmission were assessed with a pain placebo procedure. It was found that they were both coupled with the placebo response, with changes of activity induced in several brain regions associated with the opioid and dopamine networks (Scott et al. 2008).

Placebo Images

Support from neuroimaging techniques is by no means limited to the role of dopamine. PET, fMRI, magneto-electroencephalography (MEG) and electro-encephalography (EEG) have all been usefully employed to characterize the spatial and temporal domains of placebo analgesia (Rainville and Duncan 2006; Kong et al. 2007; Colloca et al. 2009).

Reduced pain-related brain activation during placebo analgesia has been repeatedly and independently reported in many studies, often with strict correlation with psychophysical pain measures, supporting the view that during placebo analgesia what is altered is not the evaluation of an unchanged incoming pain information, but rather a direct modulation of nociceptive afferent signals (Wager et al. 2004; Lieberman et al. 2004; Koyama et al. 2005; Bingel et al. 2006; Kong et al. 2006; Watson et al. 2009). Areas of the pain matrix showing decreased activation include thalamus, insula, rostral anterior cingulate cortex (rACC), primary somatosensory cortex, supramarginal gyrus and left inferior parietal lobule. For example, using thermal stimuli Koyama et al. (2005) observed pain-intensity-related activation after decreased expectations of pain (expected 48°C/received 50°C) which qualitatively resembled that evoked by correctly signalled lower stimuli (expected 48°C/received 48°C). Similarly, significant differences in the ipsilateral caudal anterior cingulate cortex, the head of the caudate, cerebellum and the contralateral nucleus cuneiformis (nCF) were recorded when comparing activations after the same noxious thermal stimulus preceded by visual cues conditioned to two different pain intensities (Keltner et al. 2006). In irritable bowel syndrome patients, by long-duration rectal distension with a balloon barostat, Price et al. (2007) also showed that placebo analgesia was accompanied by reductions in brain activity similar to those resulting from lowering the strength of stimulation (in the thalamus, somatosensory cortex, insula and ACC). Notably, this study was conducted on a clinically relevant model of placebo analgesia and showed large placebo effects, consistent with the described discrepancy in magnitude between placebo responses in the experimental and clinical settings (Charron et al. 2006). Scalp laser-evoked potentials (LEPs) amplitude was also found to be reduced during the placebo analgesic response, namely in the N2-P2 components, thought to be originated in the bilateral insula and in the cingulate gyrus (Wager et al. 2006; Watson et al. 2007; Colloca et al. 2009).

Modulation of pain-related neural activity by placebo has been shown to extend down to the spinal cord level. Skin areas of heat-induced mechanical hyperalgesia (thought to derive from central sensitization) were smaller in placebo conditions relative to control (Matre et al. 2006), while expectations of reduced pain resulted in dampened spinal (withdrawal) reflexes and brain-evoked potentials after sural nerve stimulation (Goffaux et al. 2007). Recently, an elegant study demonstrated the direct involvement of the spinal cord in placebo analgesia, by showing with fMRI that the responses to painful heat stimulation are reduced under placebo analgesia in the ipsilateral dorsal horn (Eippert et al. 2009a).

Data from imaging studies neatly converge with the neuropharmacological evidence described above to support the model of the recruitment of the descending pain inhibitory system to negatively modulate pain processing during the placebo response. The first indication came from a PET study measuring regional cerebral blood flow (rCBF) in healthy volunteers, which showed overlapping of opioid-induced (by the μ-agonist remifentanil) and placebo-induced analgesia, with similar activation of the rACC and the orbital cortex by a pharmacological or a psychological means (Petrovic et al. 2002). Direct demonstration of endogenous opioid release was obtained 3 years later in another PET study, using molecular imaging with a μ-opioid receptor-selective radiotracer, a sensitive technique shown to effectively reveal the activation of opioid neurotransmission as a reduction of the in vivo availability of μ-opioid receptors to bind the radiolabelled tracer (Bencherif et al. 2002). In this study, [^{11}C]carfentanil was displaced by the activation of opioid neurotransmission, showing significant binding decrease after placebo in pregenual rACC, insula, nucleus accumbens and dorsolateral prefrontal cortex (DLPFC); in all areas except DLPFC, this decrease was correlated with placebo reduction of pain intensity reports (Zubieta et al. 2005).

Focusing strictly on the pain anticipatory phase, i.e. on the time lag between the display of a cue signalling the impending pain stimulus and the delivery of the stimulus, Wager et al. (2004) observed an increase in DLPFC activity, negatively correlated with the signal reduction in thalamus, ACC and insula and with reported pain intensity, but positively correlated with increase in a midbrain region containing the PAG. Further support for a link between limbic areas and the PAG came from a connectivity analysis showing correlation between the activation of rACC and that of PAG and bilateral amygdalae (Bingel et al. 2006). In a recent paper, the same authors also showed strict opioid-specificity of this coupling, which was abolished by naloxone administration (Eippert et al. 2009b). Observations along the same line were also made by Wager et al. (2007) in a PET study with in vivo receptor binding, where they reported potentiation of endogenous opioid responses during placebo analgesia. Similarly, a comparison between real and sham acupuncture again showed activation of right DLPFC, rACC and PAG (Pariente et al. 2005).

By piecing together all these data, a central role for cognitive and evaluative processes seems to emerge, whereby the prefrontal cortex (namely, the DLPFC) could drive the activation of the descending antinociceptive system just before the onset of placebo analgesia. Watson et al. (2009) further elaborated on the specific role of the prefrontal cortex in the anticipation phase. By fMRI, they specifically analysed anticipatory brain activity before a painful stimulus, during placebo conditioning (with stimulus intensity surreptitiously reduced) and during placebo analgesia (with stimulus intensity restored to the initial level). They found that the same areas were modulated during placebo conditioning and placebo analgesia: DLPFC, medial frontal cortex and the anterior mid-cingulate cortex (aMCC), with the addition of the OFC in placebo analgesia. They speculated that the main effect of placebo arises from the reduction of anticipation of pain during placebo conditioning that is subsequently maintained during placebo analgesia. In other words, in the conditioning block the altered activity in the cingulate cortex during anticipation leads to learning of the association via activation of the PFC; during the anticipation phase of the post-conditioning block (placebo analgesia), activation of PFC may represent retrieval from memory of the effectiveness of the sham treatment. Comparable findings were recently obtained by Lui et al. (2010), who described an overlap of anticipation of analgesia-related activity in the frontal cortex, during the conditioning and post-conditioning sessions, but detected in addition a build-up over time of fMRI signal changes related to anticipation of analgesia during conditioning.

It can be hypothesized that if prefrontal cognitive functions are impaired, placebo analgesia would also be disrupted. In Alzheimer patients loss of placebo responses on one hand and reduction of connectivity between the prefrontal lobes and the rest of the brain on the other progressed in parallel (Benedetti et al. 2006a). Transitory inhibition of excitability in the prefrontal cortex, as can be obtained by repetitive transcranial magnetic stimulation (rTMS), has also been shown to be equally effective in producing abolition of placebo analgesia (Krummenacher et al. 2010).

The Neurobiology of Nocebo Hyperalgesia

Nocebo Molecules: Cholecystokinin

To design experiments aimed at gathering information on the negative outcome of sham treatments is not an easy task, all the more so when pain is involved. Ethical constraints forbid inflicting deliberate harm, and many studies are carried out on healthy volunteers (rather than patients), in whom only expectations about incoming pain are negatively modulated, without actual administration of any drug. In this context, it is not surprising that our knowledge on nocebo hyperalgesia still lags behind the more detailed understanding of placebo analgesia (Benedetti et al. 2007; Colloca and Benedetti 2007).

In an early study, Benedetti et al. (1997) showed that nocebo pain responses induced in postoperative patients by negative expectation regarding a saline infusion could be prevented by the CCK antagonist proglumide, a non-specific CCK-1 and CCK-2 antagonist, in a dose-dependent manner. This blockade was not mediated by endogenous opioids, as it was unaffected by naloxone. As the expectation of pain increase is a highly anxiogenic process, and both anxiety and anxiety-induced hyperalgesia have been shown to be enhanced by CCK and attenuated by CCK antagonists in animal models (Lydiard 1994; Hebb et al. 2005; Andre et al. 2005), it is rational to assume that anxiolytic drugs can interfere with nocebo hyperalgesia. In a study on healthy volunteers employing a protocol of experimental ischemic arm pain, Benedetti et al. (2006b) showed that nocebo hyperalgesia can indeed be regarded as a stress response as it is accompanied by increased levels of adrenocorticotropic hormone (ACTH) and cortisol, which indicates hyperactivity of the hypothalamic–pituitary–adrenal (HPA) axis. After administration of a benzodiazepine anxiolytic drug (diazepam), both HPA hyperactivity and nocebo hyperalgesia were blocked. When proglumide was given together with nocebo suggestion, only hyperalgesia was completely prevented. There was no effect on the HPA axis. This suggests that CCK does not act on the general process of nocebo-induced anxiety, but rather specifically on nocebo/anxiety-induced hyperalgesia. Put differently, nocebo suggestions induce anxiety, which in turn separately induces both HPA and pain enhancement. While diazepam acts on anxiety, thus blocking both effects, proglumide acts only on the pain pathway, downstream of the nocebo-induced anxiety. Neither diazepam nor proglumide showed analgesic properties on baseline pain, since they act only on the increase in anxiety-induced pain.

Nocebo Images

As for placebo analgesia, neuroimaging techniques have also brought important contributions to our knowledge of nocebo hyperalgesia. Inducing negative expectations results in both amplified unpleasantness of innocuous thermal stimuli as assessed by psychophysical pain measures (verbal subject report) and increased fMRI responses in the ACC and in a region including parietal operculum and posterior insula (Sawamoto et al. 2000). Together with the hippocampus and the prefrontal cortex, these are regions also involved in pain anticipation (Koyama et al. 1998; Chua et al. 1999; Hsieh et al. 1999; Ploghaus et al. 1999, 2001; Porro et al. 2002, 2003; Koyama et al. 2005; Lorenz et al. 2005; Keltner et al. 2006). In some cases, the same study has addressed both positive (placebo) and negative (nocebo) expectations, with opposite modulation of pain-related brain areas. Thus, in the fMRI study by Koyama et al. (2005), as the magnitude of expected pain increased, activation increased in the thalamus, insula, prefrontal cortex and anterior cingulate cortex. By contrast, expectations of decreased pain reduced activation of pain-related brain regions, like the primary somatosensory cortex, the insular cortex and anterior cingulate cortex. With a different technique, by using MEG and EEG, it was demonstrated that SII-localized pain-evoked potentials were increased, in parallel with pain reporting, by cues announcing strong pain (Lorenz et al. 2005). Similarly, in the fMRI study by Keltner et al. (2006) it was found that the level of expected pain intensity altered perceived pain intensity along with the activation of different brain regions. By using two visual cues, each conditioned to one of two noxious thermal stimuli (high and low), they showed that subjects reported higher pain when the noxious stimulus was preceded by the high-intensity visual cue. By comparing the brain activations produced by the two visual cues, they found significant differences in the ipsilateral caudal anterior cingulate cortex, the head of the caudate, the cerebellum and the contralateral nucleus cuneiformis.

Recently, Kong et al. (2008) emphasized the effect of negative expectations about pain perception following sham acupuncture, and compared fMRI responses following thermal stimuli of equal intensity delivered at control sites or at sites along the suggested course of an acupuncture meridian (nocebo). Increased pain reports for the nocebo sites paralleled increased activity in several areas of the medial pain matrix (including bilateral dorsal anterior cingulate cortex, insula, left frontal and parietal operculum, orbital prefrontal cortex and hippocampus). Of particular interest is the involvement of the hippocampus (never shown so far to be involved in placebo analgesia), as its activity is also anxiety-driven (Ploghaus et al. 2001).

Negative expectations can impact clinically relevant pain. Irritable bowel syndrome, a gastrointestinal disorder often accompanied by hyperalgesia, visceral and somatic hypersensitivity, is highly modifiable by placebo and nocebo factors with synergistic interaction. This suggests that negative emotional regulation can enhance hyperalgesia, likely through the facilitation of nociceptive input (Price et al. 2009).

From all these studies it appears that the circuitry underlying nocebo hyperalgesia largely involves, with opposite modulation, the same areas engaged by placebo analgesia. The current model suggests that the DLPFC here too might exert active control on pain perception, by modulating corticosubcortical and corticocortical pathways.

Two Phenomena Along a Continuum

Placebo and nocebo effects are not two "all or none", or opposite phenomena; rather, they can be represented along a straight line going from bad to good, from worsening to improving. All experimental evidence supports this idea. Behaviourally, it is possible to turn an analgesic placebo response into a hyperalgesic nocebo one. An example is shown in the study by Benedetti et al. (2003), where pain lessening induced by pharmacological pre-conditioning with ketorolac, together with placebo suggestions, could be turned into pain exacerbation just by reversing the verbal instructions. From neurochemical studies, we have learned how the opioid and CCK-ergic systems, respectively, induce or prevent placebo effects, and how on the contrary nocebo effects can be mediated by the CCK system (Benedetti et al. 2007, 2011b). Although evidence for a role of opioids in nocebo effects is still missing, animal studies indicate that an anatomical substrate could underlie interaction between the two systems. In rats, rostroventromedial medulla neurons have been found, expressing both μ-opioid and CCK-2 receptors. Selective lesions of these cells do not alter the basal sensory thresholds but abolish the hyperalgesia induced by microinjection of CCK into the rostroventromedial medulla, suggesting that these CCK-2/μ-opioid co-expressing rostroventromedial neurons facilitate pain (Zhang et al. 2009). Finally, we know from imaging studies that often the same pain-related brain areas are modulated bidirectionally by positive or negative pain expectations. Thus, it can be speculated that the placebo–nocebo phenomenon exists on a continuum, representing a sensitive target which can be influenced and shaped in the experimental and clinical setting.

Clinical Implications

Clinical Practice

The most obvious way of clinically exploiting the potential for therapeutic benefit of a placebo procedure is of course via the administration of placebos. However, this is also a most controversial issue on ethical grounds, conflicting with the patient's right to be thoroughly informed. Although medicine has been based for centuries on remedies acting mainly by suggestion, modern accessibility to chemicals provided with biological activity warrants that the best available treatment be used. Nevertheless, even today placebo practice is widespread, as demonstrated by the high percentage of physicians surveyed who reported the use of placebo, usually to calm patients, avert requests for unnecessary medication, or as a supplemental treatment (Sherman and Hickner 2007; Nitzan and Lichtenberg 2008). It can be argued that deception is not necessarily involved in the use of a placebo, or that it can represent an effective treatment which it would be unethical to withdraw (Lichtenberg et al. 2004; Miller and Colloca 2009a). While it might be too soon to draw conclusions on ethical justifiability, there is ample space for placebo use in less direct ways in clinical medicine.

The therapeutic environment is a complex context, where the active principle contained in a drug is not the sole agent acting on the patient body. In fact, any treatment administered in routine health care can be regarded as having two components: one pharmacodynamic and the other psychosocial. As described throughout this chapter, expectations have a central role in determining this second component (placebo or nocebo), and as they can be elicited by any aspect of the therapeutic context, it is in its optimization that the knowledge on placebo/nocebo mechanisms can both fruitfully and ethically be applied. To the extreme, total elimination of context-induced expectations can be achieved with hidden drug administration carried out by a machine unbeknown to the patient. In this case, dose requirement for the achievement of a given level of analgesia are invariably higher than in the open condition (Amanzio et al. 2001).

The first and foremost aspect of the psychosocial context is the patient–provider interaction. Indeed, the placebo effect has recently been defined as a form of interpersonal healing (Miller and Colloca 2009b). A list of eight specific clinical actions has been proposed: speak positively about treatments, provide encouragement, develop trust, provide reassurance, support relationships, respect uniqueness, explore values and create ceremony (Barrett et al. 2006).

Also non-verbal clues intentionally or unintentionally conveyed by the clinician are important. It has been shown that deceiving clinicians as to the substance (placebo or drug) being administered to two groups of patients, when in fact both groups received a placebo, has resulted in a bigger effect in the group believed by the clinicians to receive a drug (Gracely et al. 1985). Equal attention should be paid to avoid nocebo suggestions. Even a seemingly innocuous act like communicating to the patient that a therapy is going to be interrupted can have a negative impact, as shown by the faster and of larger intensity relapse of pain after open, rather than hidden, interruption of morphine analgesic therapy (Colloca et al. 2004). By using a nocebo procedure, where verbal suggestions of painful stimulation were given to healthy volunteers before administration of either tactile or low-intensity painful electrical stimuli, Colloca et al. (2008b) showed that these anxiogenic verbal suggestions were capable of turning tactile stimuli into pain, as well as low-intensity painful stimuli into high-intensity pain. Therefore, by defining hyperalgesia as an increase in pain sensitivity and allodynia as the perception of pain in response to innocuous stimulation, nocebo suggestions of a negative outcome can produce both hyperalgesic and allodynic effects. Language incorporating negative suggestions should be changed to offer positive hints (e.g. from "here's your pain medicine" to "Here's some medicine to help you get better"), in order to minimize stress (Schenk 2008). Warning patients of painful or undesirable experiences can also result in greater pain and anxiety than not doing so (Lang et al. 2005).

Another important aspect is what can be learned from the context about other patient's experiences. Just by watching others, it is possible to obtain useful information (so-called social observational learning). Just like other forms of learning (prior experience, conditioning, expectation induced by verbal communication), social observational learning can induce placebo/nocebo responses. For example, healthy volunteers observing the beneficial effect of a placebo in a demonstrator showing analgesic effects also displayed placebo responses which were comparable to those induced by directly experiencing the benefit through a conditioning procedure, while verbal suggestions alone produced significantly smaller effects (Colloca and Benedetti 2009).

Clinical Trials

In clinical trials, the desired goal is just the opposite as in clinical practice, namely, to limit and reduce placebo effects as much as possible, in order to isolate the specific effect of the active principle under scrutiny. Research on placebo mechanisms has at least two important implications for clinical trials: (1) the design of protocols that circumvent the need of a placebo arm. An example is the "open/hidden" protocol, where the placebo component stands out as the difference between overt or covert drug administration, with no patients receiving sham treatment. (2) The reevaluation of clinical trial methodology. In fact, patient expectations are not usually among the controlled variables but they do have the potential to differentially influence improvement in both control (placebo) and drug arms, thus invalidating attempts to separate the pharmacodynamic effect. For example, a study on acupuncture has showed that results could be drastically reversed by redistributing the subjects according to what they believed was their group of assignment. In other words, no differences were found with the standard grouping, but the subjects expecting real acupuncture reported significant less pain than those who believed that they were in the sham group, regardless of the real assignment (Bausell et al. 2005). Similar results were obtained in another study (Linde et al. 2007).

Of great theoretical and practical importance is the notion that any drug has the potential of interacting with patient expectation mechanisms, thus the ascription of its effect to the pharmacodynamic or the psychosocial component can be difficult, if not impossible. In other words, a secondary effect of any drug can be to interfere with one or more expectation-activated biochemical mechanisms (e.g. through the opioid, CCK or dopamine systems), with no possibility for the experimenter to know if the observed effect derives from the activation of nonspecific placebo pathways or from the specific action of the drug (uncertainty principle, Colloca and Benedetti 2005).

Conclusions and Future Directions

Research on placebo/nocebo mechanisms over the last 20 years has advanced us from definitions dominated by purely theoretical entities like "suggestibility" and "power of the mind" to descriptions characterized by biological accuracy and molecular certainty, with rituals and contexts interpreted in terms of specific brain regions and biochemical pathways activated. Thus, the placebo/nocebo response represents a visible example of the capacity of the mind to affect the body. This capacity is not limited to the modulation of pain. The endocrine and immune systems, symptoms of diseases like Parkinson's disease and depression, even behaviours outside the medical domain, like athletic motor performance, respond equally well.

Many questions remain open, however. Placebo responses vary widely among individuals, and very little is known today as to why some subjects respond while others do not. Genetic, ethnic and gender differences are only now beginning to be investigated, as well as consistency of the response across different situations in the same individual. Much has still to be learned on the interaction between the different mechanisms involved, and it is to be hoped that advances in imaging techniques will allow more detailed analysis of anatomical and temporal aspects of the underlying brain processes.

References

Ader, R. (1997). The role of conditioning in pharmacotherapy. In A. Harrington (Ed.), *The placebo effect: An interdisciplinary exploration*. Cambridge: Harvard University Press.

Amanzio, M., & Benedetti, F. (1999). Neuropharmacological dissection of placebo analgesia: expectation-activated opioid systems versus conditioning-activated specific sub-systems. *Journal of Neuroscience, 19*, 484–494.

Amanzio, M., Pollo, A., Maggi, G., & Benedetti, F. (2001). Response variability to analgesics: A role for non-specific activation of endogenous opioids. *Pain, 90*, 205–215.

Andre, J., Zeau, B., Pohl, M., Cesselin, F., Benoliel, J-J., & Becker, C. (2005). Involvement of cholecystokininergic systems in anxiety-induced hyperalgesia in male rats: Behavioural and biochemical studies. *Journal of Neuroscience, 25*, 7896–7904.

Barrett, B., Muller, D., Rakel, D., Rabago, D., Marchand, L., & Scheder, J. (2006). Placebo, meaning and health. *Perspectives in Biology and Medicine, 49*, 178–198.

Bausell, R. B., Lao, L., Bergman, S., Lee, W-L., & Berman, B. M. (2005). Is acupuncture analgesia an expectancy effect? *Evaluation & the Health Professions, 28*, 9–26.

Bencherif, B., Fuchs, P. N., Sheth, R., Dannals, R. F., Campbell, J. N., & Frost, J. J. (2002). Pain activation of human supraspinal opioid pathways as demonstrated by [11C]-carfentanil and positron emission tomography (PET). *Pain, 99*, 589–598.

Benedetti, F. (2007). Placebo and endogenous mechanisms of analgesia. *Handbook of Experimental Pharmacology, 177*, 393–413.

Benedetti, F. (2008a). Mechanisms of placebo and placebo-related effects across diseases and treatments. *Annual Review of Pharmacology and Toxicology, 48*, 33–60.

Benedetti, F. (2008b). *Placebo effects: Understanding the mechanisms in health and disease*. Oxford: Oxford University Press.

Benedetti, F. (2010). *The patient's brain: The neuroscience behind the doctor-patient relationship.* Oxford: Oxford University Press.

Benedetti, F., Amanzio, M., & Maggi, G. (1995). Potentiation of placebo analgesia by proglumide. *The Lancet, 346,* 1231.

Benedetti, F., Amanzio, M., Casadio, C., Oliaro, A., & Maggi, G. (1997). Blockade of nocebo hyperalgesia by the cholecystokinin antagonist proglumide. *Pain, 71,* 135–140.

Benedetti, F., Amanzio, M., Baldi, S., Casadio, C., & Maggi, G. (1999). Inducing placebo respiratory depressant responses in humans via opioid receptors. *European Journal of Neuroscience, 11,* 625–631.

Benedetti, F., Pollo, A., Lopiano, L., Lanotte, M., Vighetti, S., & Rainero, I. (2003). Conscious expectation and unconscious conditioning in analgesic, motor and hormonal placebo/nocebo responses. *Journal of Neuroscience, 23,* 4315–4323.

Benedetti, F., Arduino, C., Costa, S., Vighetti, S., Tarenzi, L., Rainero, I., et al. (2006a). Loss of expectation-related mechanisms in Alzheimer's disease makes analgesic therapies less effective. *Pain, 121,* 133–144.

Benedetti, F., Amanzio, M., Vighetti, S., Asteggiano, G. (2006b). The biochemical and neuroendocrine bases of the hyperalgesic nocebo effect. *Journal of Neuroscience, 26,* 12014–12022.

Benedetti, F., Lanotte, M., Lopiano, L., Colloca, L. (2007). When words are painful: Unraveling the mechanisms of the nocebo effect. *Neuroscience, 147,* 260–271.

Benedetti, F., Carlino, E., & Pollo, A. (2011a). How placebos change the patient's brain. *Neuropsychopharmacology, 36,* 339–354. doi:10.1038/npp 2010.81.

Benedetti, F., Amanzio, M., & Thoen, W. (2011b). Disruption of opioid-induced placebo responses by activation of cholecystokinin type-2 receptors. *Psychopharmacology, 213,* 791–797. doi:10.1007/s00213-010-2037-y.

Bingel, U., Lorenz, J., Schoell, E., Weiller, C., & Büchel, C. (2006). Mechanisms of placebo analgesia: rACC recruitment of a subcortical antinociceptive network. *Pain, 120,* 8–15.

Charron, J., Rainville, P., & Marchand, S. (2006). Direct comparison of placebo effects on clinical and experimental pain. *The Clinical Journal of Pain, 22,* 204–211.

Chua, P., Krams, M., Toni, I., Passingham, R. & Dolan, R. (1999). A functional anatomy of anticipatory anxiety. *NeuroImage, 9,* 563–571.

Colloca, L., & Benedetti, F. (2005). Placebos and painkillers: Is mind as real as matter? *Nature Reviews. Neuroscience, 6,* 545–552.

Colloca, L., & Benedetti, F. (2006). How prior experience shapes placebo analgesia. *Pain, 124,* 126–133.

Colloca, L., & Benedetti, F. (2007). Nocebo hyperalgesia: How anxiety is turned into pain. *Current Opinion in Anaesthesiology, 20,* 435–439.

Colloca, L., & Benedetti, F. (2009). Placebo analgesia induced by social observational learning. *Pain, 144,* 28–34.

Colloca, L., Lopiano, L., Lanotte, M., & Benedetti, F. (2004). Overt versus covert treatment for pain, anxiety, and Parkinson's disease. *Lancet Neurology, 3,* 679–684.

Colloca, L., Benedetti, F., & Porro, C. A. (2008a). Experimental designs and brain mapping approaches for studying the placebo analgesic effect. *European Journal of Applied Physiology, 102,* 371–380.

Colloca, L., Sigaudo, M., & Benedetti, F. (2008b). The role of learning in nocebo and placebo effects. *Pain, 136,* 211–218.

Colloca, L., Tinazzi, M., Recchia, S., Le Pera, D., Fiaschi, A., Benedetti, F., et al. (2009). Learning potentiates neurophysiological and behavioral placebo analgesic responses. *Pain, 139,* 306–314.

de la Fuente-Fernández, R. (2010). The placebo-reward hypothesis: Dopamine and the placebo effect. *Parkinsonism & Related Disorders, 15*(S3), S72–S74.

de la Fuente-Fernández, R., & Stoessl, A. J. (2002). The placebo effect in Parkinson's disease. *Trends in Neurosciences, 6,* 302–306.

de la Fuente-Fernández, R., Ruth, T. J., Sossi, V., Schulzer, M., Calne, D. B., & Stoessl, A. J. (2001). Expectation and dopamine release: Mechanism of the placebo effect in Parkinson's disease. *Science, 293,* 1164–1166.

de la Fuente-Fernández, R., Phillips, A. G., Zamburlini, M., Sossi, V., Calne, D. B., Ruth, T. J. et al. (2002). Dopamine release in human ventral striatum and expectation of reward. *Behavioural Brain Research, 136,* 359–363.

Eippert, F., Finsterbusch, J., Bingel, U., & Büchel, C. (2009a). Direct evidence for spinal cord involvement in placebo analgesia. *Science, 326,* 404.

Eippert, F., Bingel, U., Schoell, E. D., Yacubian, J., Klinger, R., Lorenz, J., et al. (2009b). Activation of the opioidergic descending pain control system underlies placebo analgesia. *Neuron, 63,* 533–543.

Enck, P., Benedetti, F., & Schedlowski, M. (2008). New insights into the placebo and nocebo responses. *Neuron, 59,* 195–206.

Giang, D. W., Goodman, A. D., Schiffer, R. B., Mattson, D. H., Petrie, M., Cohen, N., et al. (1996). Conditioning of cyclophosphamide-induced leukopenia in humans. *The Journal of Neuropsychiatry and Clinical Neurosciences, 8,* 194–201.

Goebel, M. U., Trebst, A. E., Steiner, J., Xie, Y. F., Exton, M. S., Frede, S., et al. (2002). Behavioral conditioning of immunosuppression is possible in humans. *The FASEB Journal, 16,* 1869–1873.

Goffaux, P., Redmond, W. J., Rainville, P., & Marchand, S. (2007). Descending analgesia – When the spine echoes what the brain expects. *Pain, 130*, 137–143.

Gospic, K., Gunnarsson, T., Fransson, P., Ingvar, M., Lindefors, N., & Petrovic, P. (2008). Emotional perception modulated by an opioid and a cholecystokinin agonist. *Psychopharmacology, 197*, 295–307.

Gracely, R. H., Dubner, R., Wolskee, P. J., & Deeter, W. R. (1983). Placebo and naloxone can alter post-surgical pain by separate mechanisms. *Nature, 306*, 264–265.

Gracely, R. H., Dubner, R., Deeter, W. D., & Wolskee, P. J. (1985). Clinician's expectations influence placebo analgesia. *The Lancet, 5*, 43.

Grevert, P., Albert, L. H., & Goldstein, A. (1983). Partial antagonism of placebo analgesia by naloxone. *Pain, 16*, 129–143.

Hebb, A. L. O., Poulin, J. F., Roach, S. P., Zacharko, R. M., & Drolet, G. (2005). Cholecystokinin and endogenous opioid peptides: interactive influence on pain, cognition and emotion. *Progress in Neuro-Psychopharmacology & Biological Psychiatry, 29*, 1225–1238.

Hsieh, J. C., Stone-Elander, S., & Ingvar, M. (1999). Anticipatory coping of pain expressed in the human anterior cingulate cortex: A positron emission tomography study. *Neuroscience Letters, 262*, 61–64.

Keltner, J. R., Furst, A., Fan, C., Redfern, R., Inglis, B., & Fields, H. L. (2006). Isolating the modulatory effect of expectation on pain transmission: A functional magnetic imaging study. *Journal of Neuroscience, 26*, 4437–4443.

Kong, J., Gollub, R. L., Rosman, I. S., Webb, J. M., Vangel, M. G., Kirsch, I., et al. (2006). Brain activity associated with expectancy-enhanced placebo analgesia as measured by functional magnetic resonance imaging. *Journal of Neuroscience, 26*, 381–388.

Kong, J., Kaptchuk, T. J., Polich, G., Kirsch, I., & Gollub, R. L. (2007). Placebo analgesia: Findings from brain imaging studies and emerging hypothesis. *Reviews in the Neurosciences, 18*, 173–190.

Kong, J., Gollub, R. L., Polich, G., Kirsch, I., LaViolette, P., Vangel, M., et al. (2008). A functional magnetic resonance imaging study on the neural mechanisms of hyperalgesic nocebo effect. *Journal of Neuroscience, 28*, 13354–13362.

Koyama, T., Tanaka, Y. Z., & Mikami, A. (1998). Nociceptive neurons in the macaque anterior cingulated activate during anticipation of pain. *NeuroReport, 9*, 2663–2667.

Koyama, T., McHaffie, J. G., Laurienti, P. J., & Coghill, R. C. (2005). The subjective experience of pain: Where expectations become reality. *Proceedings of National Academy of Sciences, 102*, 12950–12955.

Krummenacher, P., Candia, V., Folkers, G., Schedlowsky, M., & Schönbächler, G. (2010). Prefrontal cortex modulates placebo analgesia. *Pain, 148*, 368–374.

Lang, E. V., Hatsiopoulou, O., Koch, T., Berbaum, K., Lutgendorf, S., Kettenmann, E., et al. (2005). Can words hurt? Patient-provider interactions during invasive procedures. *Pain, 114*, 303–309.

Levine, J. D., Gordon, N. C., & Fields, H. L. (1978). The mechanisms of placebo analgesia. *The Lancet, 2*, 654–657.

Lichtenberg, P., Heresco-Levy, U., & Nitzan, U. (2004). The ethics of the placebo in clinical practice. *Journal of Medical Ethics, 30*, 551–554.

Lidstone, S. C., & Stoessl, A. J. (2007). Understanding the placebo effect: Contributions from neuroimaging. *Molecular Imaging and Biology, 9*, 176–185.

Lieberman, M. D., Jarcho, J. M., Berman, S., Naliboff, B. D., Suyenobu, B. J., Mandelkern, M., et al. (2004). The neural correlates of placebo effects: A disruption account. *NeuroImage, 22*, 447–455.

Linde, K., Witt, C. M., Streng, A., Weidenhammer, W., Wagenpfeil, S., Brinkhaus, B., et al. (2007). The impact of patient expectations on outcomes in four randomized controlled trials of acupuncture in patients with chronic pain. *Pain, 128*, 264–271.

Lipman, J. J., Miller, B. E., Mays, K. S., Miller, M. N., North, W. C., & Birne W. L. (1990). Peak B endorphin concentration in cerebrospinal fluid: Reduced in chronic pain patients and increased during the placebo response. *Psychopharmacology, 102*, 112–116.

Lorenz, J., Hauch, M., Paur, R. C., Nakamura, Y., Zimmermann, R., Bromm, B., et al. (2005). Cortical correlates of false expectations during pain intensity judgments – A possible manifestation of placebo/nocebo cognitions. *Brain, Behavior, and Immunity, 19*, 283–295.

Lui, C., Colloca, L., Duzzi, D., Anchisi, D., Benedetti, F., & Porro., C. A. (2010). Neural bases of conditioned placebo analgesia. *Pain, 151*, 816–824. doi:10.1016/j.pain.2010.09.021.

Lydiard, R. B. (1994). Neuropeptides and anxiety: Focus on cholecystokinin. *Clinical Chemistry, 40*, 315–318.

Matre, D., Casey, K. L., & Knardahl, S. (2006). Placebo-induced changes in spinal cord pain processing. *Journal of Neuroscience, 26*, 559–563.

Millan, M. J. (2002). Descending control of pain. *Progress in Neurobiology, 66*, 355–474.

Miller, F. G., & Colloca, L. (2009a). The legitimacy of placebo treatments in clinical practice: Evidence and ethics. *American Journal of Bioethics, 9*, 39–47.

Miller, F. G., & Colloca, L. (2009b). The placebo effect. Illness and interpersonal healing. *Perspectives in Biology and Medicine, 52*, 518–539.

Moerman, D. E. (2002). *Meaning, medicine and the placebo effect*. Cambridge: Cambridge University Press.

Nitzan, U., & Lichtenberg, P. (2008). Questionnaire survey on use of placebo. *British Medical Journal, 329*, 944–946.

Pacheco-López, G., Niemi, M. B., Kou, W., Harting, M., Fandrey, J., & Schedlowski, M. (2005). Neural substrates for behaviourally conditioned immunosuppression in the rat. *Journal of Neuroscience, 25*, 2330–2337.

Pacheco-López, G., Engler, H., Niemi, M. B., & Schedlowski, M. (2006). Expectations and associations that heal: Immunomodulatory placebo effects and its neurobiology. *Brain, Behavior, and Immunity, 20*, 430–446.

Pacheco-López, G., Riether, C., Doenlen, R., Engler, H., Niemi, M. B., Engler, A., et al. (2008). Calcineurin inhibition in splenocytes induced by Pavlovian conditioning. *The FASEB Journal, 23*, 1161–1167.

Pariente, J., White, P., Frackowiak, R. S. J., & Lewith, G. (2005). Expectancy and belief modulate the neuronal substrates of pain treated by acupuncture. *NeuroImage, 25*, 1161–1167.

Petrovic, P., Kalso, E., Petersson, K. M., & Ingvar, M. (2002). Placebo and opioid analgesia-Imaging a shared neuronal network. *Science, 295*, 1737–1740.

Ploghaus, A., Tracey, I., Gati, J. S., Clare, S., Menon, R. S., Matthews, P. M., et al. (1999). Dissociating pain from its anticipation in the human brain. *Science, 64*, 1979–1981.

Ploghaus, A., Narain, C., Beckmann, C. F., Clare, S., Bantick, S., Wise, R., et al. Exacerbation of pain by anxiety is associated with activity in a hippocampal network. *Journal of Neuroscience, 21*, 9896–9903.

Pogge, R. C. (1963). The toxic placebo. Part I. Side and toxic effects reported during the administration of placebo medicine. *Medical Times, 91*, 773–778.

Pollo, A., Amanzio, M., Arslanian, A., Casadio, C., Maggi, G., & Benedetti, F. (2001). Response expectancies in placebo analgesia and their clinical relevance. *Pain, 93*, 77–83.

Pollo, A., Vighetti, S., Rainero, I., & Benedetti, F. (2003). Placebo analgesia and the heart. *Pain, 102*, 125–133.

Porro, C. A., Baraldi, P., Pagnoni, G., Serafini, M., Facchin, P., Maieron, M., et al. (2002). Does anticipation of pain affect cortical nociceptive systems? *Journal of Neuroscience, 22*, 3206–3214.

Porro, C. A., Cettolo, V., Francescato, M. P., & Baraldi, P. (2003). Functional activity mapping of the mesial hemispheric wall during anticipation of pain. *NeuroImage, 19*, 1738–1747.

Price, D. D., Milling, L. S., Kirsch, I., Duff, A., Montgomery, G. H., & Nicholls, S. (1999). An analysis of factors that contribute to the magnitude of placebo analgesia in an experimental paradigm. *Pain, 83*, 147–156.

Price, D. D., Craggs, J., Verne, G. N., Perlstein, W. M., & Robinson, M. E. (2007). Placebo analgesia is accompanied by large reductions in pain-related brain activity in irritable bowel syndrome patients. *Pain, 127*, 63–72.

Price, D. D., Finniss, D. G., & Benedetti, F. (2008). A comprehensive review of the placebo effects: Recent advances and current thought. *Annual Review of Psychology, 59*, 565–590.

Price, D. D., Craggs, J. G., Zhou, Q. Q., Verne, G. N., Perlstein, W. M., & Robinson, M. E. (2009). Widespread hyperalgesia in irritable Bowel syndrome is dynamically maintained by tonic visceral impulse input and placebo/nocebo factors: Evidence from human psychophysics, animal models, and neuroimaging. *NeuroImage, 47*, 995–1001.

Rainville, P., & Duncan, G. H. (2006). Functional brain imaging of placebo analgesia: Methodological challenges and recommendations. *Pain, 121*, 177–180.

Sawamoto, N., Honda, M., Okada, T., Hanakawa, T., Kanda, M., Fukuyama, H., et al. (2000). Expectation of pain enhances responses to non-painful somatosensory stimulation in the anterior cingulate cortex and parietal operculum/posterior insula: An event-related functional magnetic resonance imaging study. *Journal of Neuroscience, 20*, 7438–7445.

Schedlowski, M., & Pacheco-López, G. (2010). The learned immune response: Pavlov and beyond. *Brain, Behavior, and Immunity, 24*, 176–185.

Schenk, P. W. (2008). "Just breathe normally": Word choices that trigger nocebo responses in patients. *American Journal of Nursing, 108*, 52–57.

Scott, D. J., Stoher, C. S., Egnatuk, C. M., Wang, H., Koeppe, R. A., & Zubieta J. K. (2007). Individual differences in reward responding explains placebo-induced expectations and effects. *Neuron, 55*, 325–336.

Scott, D. J., Stoher, C. S., Egnatuk, C. M., Wang, H., Koeppe, R. A., & Zubieta J. K. (2008). Placebo and nocebo effects are defined by opposite opioid and dopaminergic responses. *Archives of General Psychiatry, 65*, 220–231.

Sherman, R., & Hickner, J. (2007). Academic physicians use placebos in clinical practice and believe in the mind-body connection. *Journal of General Internal Medicine, 23*, 7–10.

Siegel, S. (2002). Explanatory mechanisms for placebo effects: Pavlovian conditioning. In H. A. Guess, A. Kleinman, J. W. Kusek, & L. W. Engel (Eds.), *The science of the placebo: Toward an interdisciplinary research agenda*. London: BMJ Books.

Thompson, J. J., Ritenbaugh, C., & Nichter, M. (2009). Reconsidering the placebo response from a broad anthropological perspective. *Culture, Medicine and Psychiatry, 33*, 112–152.

Tracey, K. J. (2009). Reflex control of immunity. *Nature Reviews. Immunology, 9*, 419–428.

Tuohy, V. K. (2005). The neocortical-immune axis. *Journal of Neuroimmunology, 158*, 1–2.

Vase, L., Robinson, M. E., Verne, G. N., & Price D. D. (2005). Increased placebo analgesia over time in irritable bowel syndrome (IBS) patients is associated with desire and expectation but not endogenous opioid mechanisms. *Pain, 115*, 338–347.

Voudouris, N. J., Peck, C. L., & Coleman, G. (1990). The role of conditioning and verbal expectancy in the placebo response. *Pain, 43*, 121–128.

Wager, T. D., Rilling, J. K., Smith, E. E., Sokolik, A., Casey, K. L., Davidson, R. J. et al. (2004). Placebo-induced changes in fMRI in the anticipation and experience of pain. *Science, 303*, 1162–1166.

Wager, T. D., Matre, D., & Casey, K. L. (2006). Placebo effects in laser-evoked pain potentials. *Brain, Behavior, and Immunity, 20*, 219–230.

Wager, T. D., Scott, D. J., & Zubieta, J. K. (2007). Placebo effects on human μ-opioid activity during pain. *PNAS, 104*, 11056–11061.

Watson, A., El-Dereby, W., Vogt, B. A., & Jones, A. K. P. (2007). Placebo analgesia is not due to compliance or habituation: EEG and behavioural evidence. *NeuroReport, 18*, 771–775.

Watson, A., El-Deredy, W., Iannetti, G. D., Lloyd, D., Tracey, I., Vogt, B. A., et al. (2009). Placebo conditioning and placebo analgesia modulate a common brain network during pain anticipation and perception. *Pain, 145*, 24–30.

Wikramasekera, I. (1985). A conditioned response model of the placebo effect: Predictions of the model. In L. White, B. Tursky, & G. E. Schwartz (Eds.), *Placebo: Theory, research and mechanisms.* New York: Guilford Press.

Zhang, W., Gardell, S., Zhang, D., Xie, J. Y., Agnes, R. S., Badghisi, H., et al. (2009). Neuropathic pain is maintained by brainstem neurons co-expressing opioid and cholecystokinin receptors. *Brain, 132*, 778–787.

Zubieta, J. K., Bueller, J. A., Jackson, L. R., Scott, D. J., Xu, Y., Koeppe, R. A., et al. (2005). Placebo effects mediated by endogenous opioid activity on μ-opioid receptors. *Journal of Neuroscience, 25*, 7754–7762.

Zubieta, J. K., & Stohler, C. S. (2009). Neurobiological mechanisms of placebo responses. *Annals of the New York Academy of Sciences, 1156*, 198–210.

Chapter 21
Sex Differences in Pain Across the Life Course

Edmund Keogh

Introduction

The past 20 years have seen an increased interest in the role that sex and gender have on the perception and experience of pain (Berkley 1997; Berkley et al. 2002; Bernardes et al. 2008; Dao and LeResche 2000; Fillingim 2000b; Fillingim et al. 2009; Holdcroft and Berkley 2005; Keogh 2008; Paller et al. 2009; Unruh 1996). Such is this interest in the disparity between men's and women's pain experiences that a special interest group (SIG) of the International Association for the Study of Pain (IASP) was formed in 1999, with the specific goal of bringing basic scientists and clinicians together in order to better understand this phenomenon. In 2007–2008, IASP dedicated its annual global campaign to the topic of pain in women, and a consensus report from the SIG published (Greenspan et al. 2007), both of which highlighted the importance and interest in sex differences in pain.

The primary aim of this chapter is to provide readers with a brief overview of the various developments that have occurred over the past 2 decades and summarize what we currently know and understand about sex differences in pain. Given the focus of this volume is on pain across the life course, a secondary aim of this chapter will be to highlight research that has considered sex differences across different age groups, i.e., child, adult, and older adult groups. It will also cover epidemiological, laboratory, and clinical studies, as well as consider some of the reasons why there may be sex differences in the experience of pain across the life span. Given that sex differences in pain are likely to reflect a range of different influences, the mechanisms that underpin men's and women's pain will stem from biological, psychological, and social origins (Fillingim 2000a; Fillingim et al. 2009; Gatchel et al. 2007). However, and as will become apparent, the focus within this chapter will be more on psychosocial influences. This choice should not be taken to mean that biological factors are considered unimportant, but was instead taken because there are already some excellent reviews that cover this material in detail (Aloisi 2003; Aloisi and Bonifazi 2006; Berkley et al. 2002; Fillingim 2000a; Holdcroft 2002a; Holdcroft and Berkley 2005). In contrast, there are fewer reviews that focus on psychosocial factors (Bernardes et al. 2008), hence the decision to focus on these issues here.

E. Keogh, PhD (✉)
Department of Psychology and Centre for Pain Research, University of Bath,
Claverton Down, Bath, BA2 7AY, UK
e-mail: e.m.keogh@bath.ac.uk

R.J. Moore (ed.), *Handbook of Pain and Palliative Care: Biobehavioral Approaches for the Life Course*, 347
DOI 10.1007/978-1-4419-1651-8_21, © Springer Science+Business Media, LLC 2012

Epidemiology of Sex Differences in Pain

Perhaps the first place to start when considering sex differences in pain is epidemiology, and whether there are sex-related differences in the prevalence of painful conditions. The general pattern that emerges for a range of pain-related conditions is that sex differences exist, with women showing a greater susceptibility to pain than men (Berkley 1997; Bingefors and Isacson 2004; Blyth et al. 2001; Fillingim et al. 2009; Johannes et al. 2010; Rustoen et al. 2004a, b; Unruh 1996). In two, now classic and often cited papers, Unruh (1996) and Berkley (1997) reviewed the available evidence from a range of different sources and concluded that women are generally more vulnerable to pain than men. Unruh (1996) observed that women exhibited more frequent pain symptoms, as well as more intense and recurrent painful episodes, whereas Berkley (1997) noted that when looking at painful conditions that show a sex-related bias there are more female-prevalent than male-prevalent conditions. This pattern has continued to be reported, much of which has recently been summarized by Fillingim et al. (2009), who note women are more vulnerable to a range of common pain-related conditions including musculoskeletal pain, headache, rheumatoid arthritis, fibromyalgia, abdominal pain, lower back pain, cancer-related pain, and postoperative pain (Johannes et al. 2010; Logan and Rose 2004; Mayer et al. 2004; Rollman and Lautenbacher 2001; Shinal and Fillingim 2007; Taenzer et al. 2000; Theis et al. 2007; Wijnhoven et al. 2006).

Given that women are more likely to develop painful conditions than men, the question now turns to whether these sex differences occur across the life course or whether they are more likely to occur at certain stages. The general pattern that emerges is that this female-related bias is stronger during the reproductive years, i.e., puberty to menopause (Fillingim et al. 2009; LeResche 1999). For example, LeResche (1999) notes that conditions such as migraine headache and temporomandibular disorder show greater sex-related differences during adult working years, with fewer differences during early childhood and later life. A similar conclusion has recently been made by Fillingim et al. (2009) in their comprehensive review of sex differences in various painful conditions. However, this peak around the reproductive years is not the case for all conditions, and there are reports that not only suggest strong sex differences in older adult groups, but that some painful events may peak in older age as well (Blyth et al. 2001; Cain et al. 2009; Elliott et al. 1999; Portenoy et al. 2004; Sjogren et al. 2009). For example, Blyth et al. (2001) report a large telephone based survey of 17,543 adult Australians, in which they confirmed that females (20%) were more likely to report suffering from a pain condition compared to men (17.1%). However, they also found that the peak age prevalence was different between the sexes, with peak age being aged 65–69 for men and 80–85 for women. Interestingly, they also found that interference caused by pain was higher in women (84.3%) than men (75.9%) within the younger age groups (20–24 years), suggesting age-related differences in the effects pain has on men and women. More recently, a survey found that for some common chronic pain conditions the differences between the sexes are more apparent in older aged adults (Tsang et al. 2008), whereas a separate internet-based survey not only found that women report more chronic pain than men, but that these differences seem to occur in all age groups for most conditions (Johannes et al. 2010).

Although sex differences in pain are most often reported in adulthood, this does not preclude sex differences in painful conditions occurring in children and adolescents (Hakala et al. 2002; Krekmanova et al. 2009; Merlijn et al. 2003; Perquin et al. 2000; Stovner et al. 2007) (see also Vetter 2011). Indeed, epidemiological evidence also suggests sex differences occur in both acute and chronic childhood pain, with a greater incidence of pain in girls than boys (Perquin et al. 2000). There is also clinical evidence to suggest that there are sex differences in how children and adolescents respond to medical procedures, including postoperative pain (Fowler-Kerry and Lander 1991; Goodenough et al. 1997, 1999; Hodgins and Lander 1997; Logan and Rose 2004). For example, Logan and Rose (2004) report a study on postoperative pain and analgesia within a group of 104 adolescents (47 males, 57 females). They found sex differences in postoperative pain, although it did depend on the type of measure of pain used. Females reported more average and lowest pain levels, but were similar in terms of the amount of highest pain reported. However, there are contradictions, with some studies showing a male pain bias for some conditions. For example, one study reports finding an earlier age of onset for migraine headache in boys than girls (Stewart et al. 1991). An additional problem is that considerable developmental changes occur in children and adolescents, and because participants are often grouped together it can be difficult to determine at what point sex differences in childhood pain emerge. There is evidence to suggest that when a finer investigation of sex differences across childhood is made differences in pain report seem to emerge around 8 years (Goodenough et al. 1999).

Given that the reproductive years seem to be particularly important when it comes to sex difference in pain, and that they are marked by important changes in hormonal profiles, this has led to the suggestion that sex hormones play an important role in explaining why there are sex differences in pain, and possibility why some painful conditions show greater female prevalence at certain life stages. This hormonal explanation is further supported by evidence that some clinical pain symptoms not only vary across the menstrual cycle, but also seem to change around key changes in hormonal status, such as during menses, pregnancy, and menopause (Heitkemper and Chang 2009; LeResche et al. 2003; Martin 2009; Martin and Behbehani 2006; Sherman et al. 2005). For example, migraine headache and gastrointestinal disorders seem to peak around menses and menopause (Heitkemper and Chang 2009; Martin and Behbehani 2006), and some clinical pain conditions show temporary remission during pregnancy (Drossaers-Bakker et al. 2002; Hazes 1991; Hazes et al. 1990).

Thus, it seems that although sex differences in pain occur at all stages of life, generally it seems that the reproductive years show the strongest differences. However, peak prevalence does depend on the condition.

Experimental Laboratory-Based Studies

An alternative approach used to examine for sex differences in pain has been to use experimental laboratory-based methods (Fillingim 2002, 2003; Fillingim et al. 2009; Fillingim and Ness 2000; Rollman et al. 2000). These studies are valuable as they allow for the careful administration and measurement of pain in a highly controlled manner, which is not possible in clinical pain. There are a range of different methods for inducing pain in an objective manner, including pressure pain, thermal heat/cold, electrical stimulation, and ischemic pain. Common outcome measures include pain threshold and pain tolerance, which respectively refer to first point that pain is detected, and the point at which a painful stimulus can no longer be tolerated and so elicits withdrawal. These methods have been used to examine pain sensitivity in men and women across a large number of studies (Fillingim et al. 2009; Riley et al. 1998, 1999). The general pattern that emerges is that there are indeed reliable sex differences in pain sensitivity, with females exhibiting lower pain thresholds and pain tolerance levels when compared to males. However, it has also been shown that this female sensitivity may vary in terms of the strength of effect, and depends on the type of pain induction method used. For example, in a meta-analysis of experimental pain induction studies, Riley et al. (1999) found the strongest sex differences were for pressure pain and electrical stimulation, with comparatively weaker effects for thermal pain. This conclusion is reiterated in a more recent review by Fillingim et al. (2009), which also indicates a relatively weak effect for ischemic pain. Interestingly, Fillingim et al. (2009) also highlight recent developments in the use of experimental methods to examine sex differences in pain, including temporal and spatial summation, as well as the use of techniques to isolate potential central mechanisms that may be involved, e.g., diffuse noxious inhibitory control (Popescu et al. 2010). Unfortunately, it is still too early to draw any conclusions about many of these new methods, but this position is likely to change with additional research and more focused summaries of core findings.

Most experimental studies that look at sex differences have been conducted on adult samples, with few focusing on either children or older adults. This means that it is difficult to determine whether these sex differences occur consistently across the life course or whether these differences change as a product of age. Few studies have examined for sex differences in experimental pain within older adult samples or compared across different age groups. There are, however, some studies on child groups, but they tend to provide mixed evidence for sex differences (Chambers et al. 2002; Fanurik et al. 1993; Myers et al. 2006; Piira et al. 2002). As with other child pain studies, age-related developmental changes may be important. For example, when Piira et al. (2002) looked at different age groups of children, they found that sex differences were more apparent in the older child group, suggesting that sex differences in experimental pain sensitivity develop with age.

Reasons for such developmental changes in pain are wide ranging, and may reflect changing biology, as well as psychosocial influences. For example, gender roles have been used to help explain why there are sex differences in experimental (and other) pain reports (Bernardes et al. 2008). Socially learnt gender roles develop during childhood by modeling behaviors observed at both individual (e.g., parents, peers) and wider sociocultural (e.g., schooling, media) levels (Bussey and Bandura 1999; Tobin et al. 2010). Interestingly, although prototypical gender roles may be acquired during childhood, they are by no means fixed and are thought to be continually shaped by experience, e.g., workplace (Bussey and Bandura 1999). From this we might expect variation in how gender roles related to pain affect experimental pain sensitivity across the life course. Unfortunately, this possibility has yet to be examined.

As well as demonstrating that there are differences between the sexes, experimental methods have also been used to explore the sex hormone hypothesis. For example, studies have examined whether experimental pain sensitivity varies across the menstrual cycle (Fillingim et al. 2009; Riley et al. 1999; Sherman and LeResche 2006). Indeed, if sex hormones do help account for some of the differences in pain sensitivity, then we might expect to see changes in experimental pain reports across the menstrual cycle. In a meta-analysis of these studies, Riley et al. (1999) found that pain sensitivity was greatest during the luteal phase of the cycle for most pain induction methods, with electrical stimulation being a notable exception. At least one study has also shown that the effects of opioid analgesics on experimental pain responses vary across the menstrual cycle (Ribeiro-Dasilva et al. 2011). However, reviews since 1999 suggest that the picture is less clear than perhaps first thought (Fillingim et al. 2009; Sherman and LeResche 2006), with some studies reporting phase-related differences, whereas others do not (Klatzkin et al. 2010; Kowalczyk et al. 2006, 2010; Teepker et al. 2010). Part of the problem is the variation in methods employed, such as phase and method of testing (Fillingim et al. 2009; Sherman and LeResche 2006). However, it does also seem as if under some conditions, hormonal factors may indeed play a role in explaining some of the variation in pain sensitivity that occurs in women during reproductive ages.

Thus, it seems that although sex differences in experimental pain exist, with females showing a greater general sensitivity, there is a paucity of research that examines these differences across different ages. It is difficult to say whether similar sex differences exist across the life span.

Sex Differences in Pain Intervention Responses

As well as examining for sex differences in pain sensitivity, there have also been investigations into whether or not men and women differ in their responses to pain treatments. This section will focus on sex differences in analgesia across the life span.

Sex differences in responses to pharmacological pain interventions have been examined in both the laboratory and the clinic, although with fairly mixed results. For example, some studies reported that females exhibit stronger analgesic effects than males, while others have failed to find such effects, or in fact report the opposite (Fillingim et al. 2004, 2005a, b; Ip et al. 2009; Olofsen et al. 2005; Sarton et al. 2000). From this it has been suggested that if there are sex differences in analgesia, then effects may be fairly restricted, and certainly not consistent. Part of the problem is the variability in methods and approaches used, such as type of analgesic and type of pain (Fillingim 2002). For example, Fillingim (2002) found that methodological parameters associated with the type of pain induction approach adopted can affect the strength of the sex difference found. There are also suggestions that men and women differ in terms of side effects associated with a range of drugs, including analgesics (Ciccone and Holdcroft 1999; Fillingim et al. 2005b; Holdcroft 2002b; Light et al. 2006; Pleym et al. 2003; Wu et al. 2006). Thus, one reason why females may consume less analgesics could be to avoid unwanted side effects, rather than because of better analgesia.

In light of such inconsistencies and an associated need to determine whether there are sex differences in analgesia, there have been attempts to summarize this work, but with mixed conclusions (Ip et al. 2009; Niesters et al. 2010). For example, a study by Ip et al. (2009) on postoperative analgesic consumption failed to find supporting evidence for sex differences, whereas Niesters et al. (2010) reported differences under certain conditions. In their systematic review and meta-analysis of 25 clinical and 25 experimental studies in opioid analgesia, Niesters et al. (2010) found evidence that females gained greater analgesia, although it was dependent on the type of pain and opioid under investigation. Specifically, greater opioid analgesia in females was found in studies that examined morphine in experimental pain settings, or if in clinical studies, when the focus was on patient controlled analgesia (PCA). Interestingly, there was also a suggestion that the sex differences in PCA analgesia increased over testing time, indicating that study protocols are important.

There are few studies that directly examine whether there are age-related effects when considering sex differences in analgesia. Of those that have considered this, results are also mixed (Aubrun et al. 2005; Logan and Rose 2004). For example, Logan and Rose (2004) examined postoperative analgesia consumption in adolescents (aged 12–18). Although girls reported more postoperative pain (e.g., average pain), they failed to find any evidence for sex differences in analgesia consumption. It is also unclear whether sex differences in analgesia exist within older groups. For example, Aubrun et al. (2005) examined for age- and sex-related effects in the postoperative morphine consumption of 4,317 adult patients (54% male). While women required a higher dose, this sex effect seemed to be reduced in older age groups (those aged 75 or above). However, in their systematic review, Niesters et al. (2010) failed to find evidence for sex differences in opioid analgesia within younger groups, although differences were found in older adult samples.

Alongside pharmacological studies, there have also been attempts to see whether men and women differ in terms of other types of interventions for pain (Lofgren and Norrbrink 2009; Lund et al. 2005). For example, Lund et al. (2005) found that women were more likely to show TENS-related increases in experimental pain thresholds when compared to men. A number of these studies highlight the psychological component and include experimental studies with healthy individuals, as well as clinically based pain treatments. Experimental approaches include studies that have examined whether men and women differ in experimental pain responses when using various coping instructions (Keogh and Birkby 1999; Keogh et al. 2000, 2005a; Keogh and Herdenfeldt 2002). For example, Keogh et al. (2000) found that men benefited from the use of pain focusing instructions, compared to when instructed to avoid such sensations; coping instruction did not seem to affect women's pain scores. In a second study, Keogh and Herdenfedlt (2002) not only showed that men benefited from sensory focusing, but that women reported worse pain when focusing on emotional qualities. Another approach has been to compare coping instructions designed to reflect two different cognitive-behavioral approaches used in clinical pain management. Keogh et al. (2005a) found that instructions designed to reflect acceptance-type approaches were of greater benefit to women than more traditional cognitive-control type instructions. However, there has been a failure to replicate this finding (Keogh et al. 2006b).

There are also a few studies that have examined whether men and women with clinical pain differ in terms of responses to nonpharmacological treatments. Again findings are mixed, in that some report differences, whereas others do not. Such discrepancies are possibility due to the wide range of methods and types of treatment used (Burns 1997; Edwards et al. 2003; Hampel et al. 2009; Hansen et al. 1993; Hechler et al. 2010; Hooten et al. 2009; Jensen et al. 2001; Keogh et al. 2005b; Krogstad et al. 1996; McGeary et al. 2003). Such measurement variation is important, as it can affect when differences are found, even within studies. For example, Keogh et al. (2005a, b) examined sex differences in patients who attended an intensive chronic pain management intervention. Although men and women initially showed benefits in a range of outcomes directly following the intervention, there was evidence that at a 3-month follow-up point women reported pain and catastrophizing levels that were similar to those expressed prior to treatment. However, it should be noted that for certain key outcome variables, such as disability, both men and women maintained posttreatment improvements. This indicates that although there may be sex differences in responses to treatment, great care needs to be paid to the outcome measures under investigations, as well as the goal of the treatment (e.g., reduce pain or improve disability).

In terms of age-related effects, there are very few studies that have compared across different age groups. In one of the few that has looked at treatment outcomes in adolescents, Hechler et al. (2010) examined the pain and coping responses of 141 adolescents (aged 11–18) before and after (3-month) multimodal pain treatment. Overall no sex differences were found in the degree of change in pain at 3 months. However, changes in coping were related to changes in pain in a sex-specific manner. Specifically, a greater reduction in the tendency to make use of social support was related to a reduction in pain intensity in females, but not males. There are few studies that examine age-related differences or focus on sex differences in the treatment responses of older adults.

Sex Differences in Pain Behavior

When considering sex differences in pain, we can also think about what men and women do when they are in pain. There is evidence that there are general sex differences in healthcare utilization, with women engaging and using much more healthcare at all levels (Green and Pope 1999; Koopmans and Lamers 2007). For example, women are more likely to seek healthcare support from physicians and to consult with healthcare professionals. This could of course be due to men under-utilizing healthcare; we know that men tend to underreport healthcare concerns, are much less likely to approach and consult with their physician. However, at least one study has shown that when controlling for health needs, women (above 65 years) may actually underutilize healthcare services (Cameron et al. 2010). Health behavior is complex, but it remains possible that there are sex differences across various age groups in the behaviors people engage in when in pain.

In terms of healthcare utilization for pain, the pattern that emerges with respect to sex differences is that women are more likely to seek out support (Eriksen et al. 2004; Kaur et al. 2007; Weir et al. 1996). For example, Weir et al. (1996) showed that women made greater use of chronic pain services when compared to men. Pain-related healthcare utilization can also be seen in the use of both prescribed and over-the-counter analgesics (Antonov and Isacson 1996, 1998; Isacson and Bingefors 2002; Paulose-Ram et al. 2003; Turunen et al. 2005). For example, a study conducted by Paulose-Ram et al. (2003) in a sample of over 20,000 US adults found that women were more likely to report using both prescribed and over-the-counter analgesics.

Interestingly, such surveys usually report medication use in working age adults, and do not tend to examine whether there are sex differences in the pain medications used by infants (or at least their parent's usage) and/or older adults. There have been suggestions that the female bias in analgesic usage also occurs in adolescents (Boyd et al. 2006; McCabe et al. 2007; Wu et al. 2008), although their usage in younger children is less well known. In terms of older adults, again it is not as clear whether there are sex differences in pain mediation use. There have been suggestions that women and older adults are, individually, more likely to make use and claim for opioids (Williams et al. 2008). There is also some evidence that older women may be particularly more likely to make use of medical services, including those associated with pain (Pokela et al. 2010; Williams et al. 2008). However, others raise concerns about older adults not receiving adequate pain relief (Wilder-Smith 2005).

Alongside pharmacological behaviors associated with managing pain, there have also been investigations into the coping strategies that men and women report using. There seem to be general sex differences in coping behavior, with women reporting greater use of social support and emotion-focused approaches, and men greater use of problem-focused coping (Tamres et al. 2002). In terms of pain coping strategies, there also seem to be sex differences (Unruh 1996; Unruh et al. 1999). For example, Unruh et al. (1999) found that women were more likely to use a greater range of strategies for alleviating pain when compared to men. This includes alternative and complimentary approaches to dealing with pain, a finding which has been reported elsewhere to varying degrees (Bishop and Lewith 2010; Fouladbakhsh and Stommel 2010; Ndao-Brumblay and Green 2010). There are also suggestions that women are more likely to make use of social support as a coping strategy for pain when compared to men (Unruh et al. 1999).

This female bias for social and/or emotional support has also been reported within adolescent pain groups as well (Keogh and Eccleston 2006; Lu et al. 2007; Lynch et al. 2007). For example, Keogh and Eccleston (2006) report a study on adolescents with chronic pain, in which females reported making a greater use of social support, whereas males tended to report a greater use of distraction. Lynch et al. (2007) also found that social support was more likely in females, and distraction in males. Interestingly, in this study, younger (aged 8–12 years) and older (aged 13–18 years) children were compared, but this did not seem to affect any of the sex differences in coping strategy that were found. There may also be sex differences in the way in which interventions promote change in coping, and the effect this may have on adolescent pain. As mentioned in the previous section, Hechler et al. (2010) found a greater reduction in the use of social support following a pain intervention was related to a reduction in pain intensity within female, but not male, adolescents. While this may suggest that younger males and females differ, others have failed to find sex differences in pain coping behaviors (Kaczynski et al. 2009).

Emotions and Pain

Pain is more than just a sensory experience, in that it also includes emotional and cognitive components. If there are differences in the way in which emotions affect men and women, then it is possible that this may be relevant to our understanding of sex differences in pain. Generally, there seem to be sex differences in emotional expressions and responses (Vigil 2009), in that women are generally more emotionally expressive than men (Hall 1978, 2006; LaFrance et al. 2003) and are more likely to suffer from common emotional conditions, such as anxiety or depression (Bekker and van Mens-Verhulst 2007; Gater et al. 1998; Marcus et al. 2008; McLean and Anderson 2009; Ustun 2000). Given that anxiety and depression are common in chronic pain groups, the possibility that these two emotions have a differential effect on men's and women's pain has been considered (Rhudy and Williams 2005).

Depression is a commonly experienced mood state associated chronic pain, and there is evidence to suggest that the relationship between depression and pain is stronger in women than in men (Bingefors and Isacson 2004; Keogh et al. 2006b; Tsang et al. 2008). For example, Bingefors and

Isacson (2004) report an epidemiological study in which they not only confirmed that females reported more pain than males, but that there was a higher likelihood of comorbid anxiety and depression in women. Tsang et al. (2008) reported a large cross-cultural study that incorporated the responses of over 42,000 individuals from 17 countries, which showed not only higher chronic pain prevalence in females, but also a greater likelihood of comorbid anxiety/depression, when compared to men. Depression has also been related to pain-related disability in a sex-specific way. For example, Keogh et al. (2006b) found that depression was more strongly related to pain-related disability in women than men. However, there are examples where this has not been found, as well as examples where men show a stronger relationship for some outcomes (Keogh et al. 2006b). Even so, the general picture that seems to emerge is that depression seems to be a particular issue when considering pain in women.

As well as depression there has been interest in anxiety, which is also commonly reported by those in pain (Rhudy and Williams 2005). Like depression, anxiety also seems to show a female-related prevalence bias and has also been examined within the context of sex differences in pain. Unlike depression, however, anxiety seems to generally show a stronger relationship in men than women, in both healthy experimental studies as well as those that focus on clinical pain (Edwards et al. 2000; Elklit and Jones 2006; Jones et al. 2002, 2003; Jones and Zachariae 2002; McCracken and Houle 2000). For example, in a laboratory-based study, Jones et al. (2003) found that low anxious men exhibited greater cold pressor tolerance than high anxious men, but no such effect of anxiety was found in women. Similarly, in clinical pain studies, both Edwards et al. (2000) and McCracken and Houle (2000) found that pain-related anxiety had a stronger relationship with pain outcomes in men than women. While it may seem as if there is a male-related vulnerability to the effects of anxiety, there is a noticeable exception to this. Specifically, there is a type of anxiety, called anxiety sensitivity, which is a panic-like construct associated with the fear of anxiety-related sensations, and seems to show a stronger relationship with pain in women than men (Keogh and Asmundson 2004; Keogh et al. 2004, 2006a; Keogh and Birkby 1999; Thompson et al. 2008). For example, both Keogh and Birkby (1999) and Thompson et al. (2008) have shown this female-related susceptibility to experimental pain, whereas Keogh et al. (2004) found this in a group of chest pain patients. Why pain anxiety and anxiety sensitivity would have different sex-related effects is unclear at present, and this is not helped by the relatively few studies that consider the moderating effect of sex on the relationship between anxiety sensitivity and pain (Ocanez et al. 2010).

Given the current focus on life span, the question now turns to whether similar sex-specific emotion–pain relationships are found in different age groups. There have been investigations in child groups, but with mixed results (Egger et al. 1999; Kaczynski et al. 2009; Logan and Rose 2004). For example, Egger et al. (1999) found that depression was related to musculoskeletal pain in both male and female children, and that anxiety was related to range of different somatic complaints (as well as headaches and stomach pains) in girls, but not boys. Similarly, Logan and Rose (2004) found that among female adolescents undergoing a surgical intervention, anticipatory distress was found to predict postoperative pain. This was not the case for males. More recently, Kaczynski et al. (2009) report a study on children with chronic pain, and the role that depression and anxiety has with various pain outcomes. No sex differences were found in levels of pain, although a relationship was found between pain-related disability and a tendency to internalizing symptoms (which is common to both anxiety and depression) in females, but not in males. In terms of older groups, there are few studies that look for sex differences in emotion and pain. However, there is an interesting developmental change associated with emotional experiences that has recently emerged, which would be interesting to consider in the context of pain. Specially, it seems that despite an increase in health-related conditions in older age, this group generally report greater emotional stability (Scheibe and Carstensen 2010). It has yet to be shown whether these changes in emotional well-being during older age impacts in a sex-specific way on the experience of pain and pain-related disability.

Role of Cognition: Thoughts, Beliefs, and Expectations

Closely linked to the emotions we feel in pain, there is also interest in the thoughts and beliefs we have about pain. Such thoughts are considered important to the current discussion, as it is possible that if there are sex differences in health cognitions, then this might influence pain behaviors, including coping and healthcare utilization (Galdas et al. 2005; Moller-Leimkuhler 2002). One health belief that has been considered within the context of sex differences is pain-related catastrophizing, which is defined as a tendency to engage in negative rumination and worry about pain, with an exaggerated focus on the negative consequences it may have. What has been shown in a range of different studies is that women report engaging in more pain-related catastrophizing than men, in laboratory based studies with healthy volunteers, as well as in a range of different pain conditions (Dixon et al. 2004; Jensen et al. 1994; Osman et al. 2000; Sullivan et al. 1995). Although there are some examples where such sex differences have not been found (Unruh et al. 1999), on the whole there seems to be a fairly consistent sex difference (Geisser et al. 2003). Of particular interest are findings that indicate that pain-related catastrophizing may actually explain why there are sex differences in some types of experimental and clinical pain (Edwards et al. 2004; Keefe et al. 2000; Keogh and Eccleston 2006; Keogh et al. 2005b; Khan et al. 2011; Sullivan et al. 2000, 2001). Furthermore, sex differences in responses to some interdisciplinary pain interventions may be mediated by changes in pain catastrophizing (Keogh et al. 2005b). Unfortunately, there are few studies that have considered sex differences in catastrophizing within younger or older adults, or examined for age-related changes in pain. In one of the few studies that have looked at this, Keogh and Eccleston (2006) found that sex differences in adolescent pain were also explained by levels of catastrophizing. It therefore seems that while pain-related catastrophizing has been identified as an important cognitive factor that helps explain why there are sex differences in pain, it is not clear whether this is consistently found across different age groups or whether it changes with age.

A second set of cognitive beliefs and expectations that have been examined within the context of sex differences in pain are those associated with gender role identity (Defrin et al. 2009; Keogh and Denford 2009; Myers et al. 2006; Pool et al. 2007; Robinson et al. 2001, 2003a, b, 2004a, b; Robinson and Wise 2003, 2004; Wise et al. 2002). Stemming from Bandura's social learning model of cognitive development (Bussey and Bandura 1999), it has been argued that we acquire a gender role identity through various learning models, such as parents, siblings, as well as society (e.g., media). It is argued that we possess expectations and beliefs associated with our male and female gender roles that affect the way we behave, which includes how we report and respond to pain (Bernardes et al. 2008). For example, it has been shown that both sexes hold the general belief that men are less willing to report pain, whereas women are more pain sensitive (Robinson et al. 2001). It has also been shown that such gender-role expectations exist for pain behaviors as well, such as coping. For example, Keogh and Denford (2009) found that both male and female participants viewed the typical women as much more likely to engage in pain-related catastrophizing. Research has also shown that these beliefs may explain some of the sex differences in pain behavior. For example, gender role expectations have been found to mediate sex differences in experimental pain (Robinson et al. 2004b), and it has been shown that by manipulating gender role expectations it is also possible to influence sex differences in pain (Robinson and Wise 2003). Unfortunately, we are not aware of any research that has examined whether there are age-related differences in such gender role expectations, or when they might develop, and if once acquired are maintained over time.

There are other examples of cognitive beliefs and expectations that may be important in helping us to understand why there are sex differences in pain. For example, there is evidence that there may be sex differences in pain self-efficacy, which refers to the belief that one has in one's own ability to deal with situations (Jackson et al. 2002; Lackner and Carosella 1999; Tait et al. 1982). For example, Jackson et al. (2002), in a study on the cold pressor pain responses of healthy adults, reported that sex differences in pain were mediated by levels of self-efficacy. However, others have failed to find similar sex differences (Beckham et al. 1994; Chong et al. 2001; Strong et al. 1992). Interestingly, although Chong et al. (2001) failed to find sex-related differences in self-efficacy reports of chronic pain patients, they found that younger adult males and females (aged 17–35 years) reported lower self-efficacy than those in their middle aged group (aged 36–55 years). An additional area of potential interest is the possibility that there may be sex differences in placebo expectation (Fillingim et al. 2009) (see also Pollo and Benedetti 2011). However, there are too few studies to draw any definite conclusions, especially given the mixed results found (Aslaksen and Flaten 2008; Averbuch and Katzper 2001; Bruehl et al. 2010; Compton et al. 2003; Flaten et al. 1999; Gear et al. 1999; Lyby et al. 2010; Pud et al. 2006). What these studies do, however, is suggest the potentially interesting role that pain cognitions may have in understanding why there are sex differences in pain across the life span.

Social Context and Communication

This final section will consider some of the wider social issues associated with the experience of pain and analgesia. What is becoming more and more apparent is that social context is an important factor when considering men's and women's pain (Bernardes et al. 2008; Craig 2009). Given that a person's pain can be influenced by others, such as spouse, parents, other family members, as well as healthcare professionals and the healthcare context, it is also possible that the sex of the person observing a patient in pain may play a role. One way this has been examined has been through laboratory-based studies, which examine whether the sex of the experimenter (observer) has an effect on the pain reports of men and women (Aslaksen et al. 2007; Kallai et al. 2004; Levine and Desimone 1991; Weisse et al. 2005). For example, Levine and DeSimone (1991) found that male participants exhibited less pain if the experimenter was female. This finding has not only been replicated, but it has also been shown that similar effects might also occur in females when the experimenter is male (Kallai et al. 2004).

Considering how the sex of the observer affects pain reports, there have also been studies that examine whether the sex of the person in pain affects the behaviors of those observing them. Much of this work has examined whether treatment decisions differ according to the sex of the person in pain (Calderone 1990; Chen et al. 2008; Cicero et al. 2009; Lord et al. 2009; Michael et al. 2007; Roger et al. 2000; Weisse et al. 2001). For example, some studies have looked at whether there are biases in the administration of analgesics to patients prior to entering hospital. In a study on 953 prehospital cases of individuals with an isolated extremity injury, Michael et al. (2007) found that men (32.8%) were more likely to receive analgesia than women (26.7%). Although Lord et al. (2009) failed to find sex differences in prehospital analgesics administration, they did find that of those that received analgesics, women were less likely to receive morphine than men, even when controlling for age and pain severity. Interestingly, there were no sex differences in analgesic refusal rates.

There are also potential sex-related prescription/treatment biases in hospital settings (Calderone 1990; Chen et al. 2008; Roger et al. 2000; Weisse et al. 2001). For example, Calderone (1990) found that men were more likely to receive analgesics, whereas women seemed more likely to receive sedatives following surgery. More recently, Hirsh et al. (2008) created virtual reality (VR) patients to help medical students in pain assessment training. The VR patients were varied in terms of the age and sex, in order to see whether this would affect observer impressions. Female VR patients were viewed as having more pain, and in need of treatment, than male VR patients. There were also some age-related effects, with older VR patients being viewed as worse than younger ones. In terms of potential age-related sex differences, few studies have examined these variables together. However, when Cicero et al. (2009) examined a medical insurance claims database for any differences in analgesic use, they not only showed more females in the chronic pain category and a greater level of healthcare utilization, but that this pattern increased with age. They also found that older females were much more likely to receive a weak opioid than a strong one, which the authors suggest could at least partially reflect a bias in physician prescription decision-making.

Another set of studies have considered sex differences in the social communication and interactions that occur between family members, such between parent and child, patient and spouse (Chambers et al. 2002; Evans et al. 2008a, b, 2009; Jackson et al. 2002; Keefe et al. 1990; Smith et al. 2004). For example, Evans et al. conducted an interesting series of studies in which they consider the relationships between parent and child, and how this affects a child's responses to experimentally induced pain (see also Vetter 2011). In one study, Evans et al. (2009) found that mother's level of self-reported negative life events was positively related to experimental pain levels in girls, whereas it was negatively related in boys. In adult dyads, the relationship between patient and spouse has also been examined (Romano et al. 1995, 2000; Smith et al. 2004). For example, Smith et al. (2004) report a study in which they examined spousal support of patients with osteoarthritis who were completing a painful household task. They found that wives were more likely to engage in facilitative behaviors when compared to husbands. Again it is very difficult to examine these studies for potential changes or differences in communication across the life span, especially considering the already complex nature of these studies and the variety of methods used.

Finally, there is interest in the nonverbal behaviors associated with pain, which involves investigating both the encoding (presentation) and decoding (recognition) of cues in various channels (e.g., face, voice, and movement). Unfortunately, few studies have directly examined for sex differences in pain behaviors, although some have looked at biases in the facial domain. However, limited evidence has emerged from these studies, in that there are few consistent examples of sex differences in the encoding of pain expression within adults (Kunz et al. 2009; Prkachin 1992; Prkachin and Solomon 2009; Simon et al. 2008). In terms of age-related effects, like adult studies, there are some examples in groups of children, in both facial and vocal domains, but again outcomes are generally inconsistent (Ginsburg and Drake 2002; Grunau et al. 1990; Grunau and Craig 1987; Guinsburg et al. 2000; Kunz et al. 2009; Moon et al. 2008; Piira et al. 2007). This lack of consistency is puzzling, especially given the evidence that there are sex differences in the encoding and decoding of emotional expressions (Hall 1978, 2006; Vigil 2009). It is, therefore, not currently possible to make any definite conclusions as to whether there are sex differences in the encoding and decoding of nonverbal pain expressions, or whether they change across the life span.

Summary and Conclusions

What emerges from a range of different sources is that, when compared to men, women experience more pain, are more susceptible to pain-related conditions, and may even respond in different ways to pain-related interventions when compared to men. There also seem to be differences in how men and women behave when in pain, as well as differences in the roles that cognitive and emotional factors play. There is emerging recognition that pain does not occur in a vacuum, and that context, and social interactions and communication between men and women also plays a role. However, more research is required that considers the wider role that social influences have on sex differences in pain, especially in terms of how assumptions related to a patient's gender may affect how observers respond to those in pain.

Although there may be sex differences in pain and pain behaviors, this may depend on age (LeResche 1999). Indeed, it has been suggested that male–female differences in pain are most apparent during the reproductive years, with weaker differences observed prior to puberty and following menopause. However, recent evidence has questioned some of these assumptions. Part of the problem is that the vast majority of research that considers sex differences focuses on adults of working age and so there is relatively little research that examines these differences across the life span. Whereas it may be the case that more consistent evidence exists for sex differences across the reproductive years, the lack of research that has focused on both younger and older groups means that it is difficult to draw conclusions. However, the relatively recent emergence of research that focuses on pediatric or elderly populations, developing new approaches and tools that are focused on the needs of these groups, means that we might soon be in a better position to reconsider the impact that sex and gender have on the pain experienced at different life stages. Future research, therefore, needs to consider the potential for sex differences at all life phases. In doing so, this will hopefully help us understand the developmental trajectory of sex differences in pain, ascertain when and in what way differences are likely to occur across the life course, as well as consider the impact they may have on treatment.

Answers to these questions are more likely if there is a general change in the way future research is conducted, with the reporting of sex differences made more routine. Indeed, many studies still do not actively analyze for and report possible sex differences, despite calls for such changes to be made (Greenspan et al. 2007). With more research that routinely considers these differences we should, in time, be able to better explain why being male or female impacts on the perception and experience of pain. This in turn should help us develop more appropriate and effective approaches to pain management.

Acknowledgments This writing of this book chapter was partly made possible by a research sabbatical awarded to the author during 2009–2010 by the University of Bath.

References

Aloisi, A. M. (2003). Gonadal hormones and sex differences in pain reactivity. *The Clinical Journal of Pain, 19,* 168–174.

Aloisi, A. M., & Bonifazi, M. (2006). Sex hormones, central nervous system and pain. *Hormones and Behavior, 50,* 1–7.

Antonov, K. I., & Isacson, D. (1996). Use of analgesics in Sweden-the importance of sociodemographic factors, physical fitness, health and health-related factors, and working conditions. *Social Science & Medicine, 42,* 1473–1481.

Antonov, K. I., & Isacson, D. G. (1998). Prescription and nonprescription analgesic use in Sweden. *The Annals of Pharmacotherapy, 32,* 485–494.

Aslaksen, P. M., & Flaten, M. A. (2008). The roles of physiological and subjective stress in the effectiveness of a placebo on experimentally induced pain. *Psychosomatic Medicine, 70,* 811–818.

Aslaksen, P. M., Myrbakk, I. N., Hoifodt, R. S., & Flaten, M. A. (2007). The effect of experimenter gender on autonomic and subjective responses to pain stimuli. *Pain, 129,* 260–268.

Aubrun, F., Salvi, N., Coriat, P., & Riou, B. (2005). Sex- and age-related differences in morphine requirements for postoperative pain relief. *Anesthesiology, 103,* 156–160.

Averbuch, M., & Katzper, M. (2001). Gender and the placebo analgesic effect in acute pain. *Clinical Pharmacology and Therapeutics, 70,* 287–291.

Beckham, J. C., Rice, J. R., Talton, S. L., Helms, M. J., & Young, L. D. (1994). Relationship of cognitive constructs to adjustment in rheumatoid arthritis patients. *Cognitive Therapy and Research, 18,* 479–496.

Bekker, M. H., & van Mens-Verhulst, J. (2007). Anxiety disorders: Sex differences in prevalence, degree, and background, but gender-neutral treatment. *Gender Medicine, 4,* S178–S193.

Berkley, K. J. (1997). Sex differences in pain. *The Behavioral and Brain Sciences, 20,* 371–380.

Berkley, K. J., Hoffman, G. E., Murphy, A. Z., & Holdcroft, A. (2002). Pain: Sex/gender differences. In D. Pfaff, A. Arnold, A. Etgen, S. Fahrbach, & R. Rubin (Eds.), *Hormones, brain and behavior* (Vol. 5, pp. 409–442). London: Academic.

Bernardes, S. F., Keogh, E., & Lima, M. L. (2008). Bridging the gap between pain and gender research: A selective literature review. *European Journal of Pain, 12,* 427–440.

Bingefors, K., & Isacson, D. (2004). Epidemiology, co-morbidity, and impact on health-related quality of life of self-reported headache and musculoskeletal pain – a gender perspective. *European Journal of Pain, 8*(5), 435–450.

Bishop, F. L., & Lewith, G. T. (2010). Who uses CAM? A narrative review of demographic characteristics and health factors associated with CAM use. *Evidence-Based Complementary and Alternative Medicine, 7,* 11–28.

Blyth, F. M., March, L. M., Brnabic, A. J., Jorm, L. R., Williamson, M., & Cousins, M. J. (2001). Chronic pain in Australia: A prevalence study. *Pain, 89*, 127–134.

Boyd, C. J., Esteban McCabe, S., & Teter, C. J. (2006). Medical and nonmedical use of prescription pain medication by youth in a Detroit-area public school district. *Drug and Alcohol Dependence, 81*, 37–45.

Bruehl, S., Burns, J. W., Chung, O. Y., Magid, E., Chont, M., Gilliam, W., et al. (2010). Hypoalgesia associated with elevated resting blood pressure: Evidence for endogenous opioid involvement. *Journal of Behavioral Medicine, 33*, 168–176.

Burns, J. W. (1997). Anger management style and hostility: Predicting symptom-specific physiological reactivity among chronic low back pain patients. *Journal of Behavioral Medicine, 20*, 505–522.

Bussey, K., & Bandura, A. (1999). Social cognitive theory of gender development and differentiation. *Psychological Review, 106*, 676–713.

Cain, K. C., Jarrett, M. E., Burr, R. L., Rosen, S., Hertig, V. L., & Heitkemper, M. M. (2009). Gender differences in gastrointestinal, psychological, and somatic symptoms in irritable bowel syndrome. *Digestive Diseases and Sciences, 54*, 1542–1549.

Calderone, K. L. (1990). The influence of gender on the frequency of pain and sedative medication administered to postoperative patients. *Sex Roles, 23*, 713–725.

Cameron, K. A., Song, J., Manheim, L. M., & Dunlop. D. D. (2010). Gender disparities in health and healthcare use among older adults. *Journal of Women's Health, 19*, 1643–1650.

Chambers, C. T., Craig, K. D., & Bennett, S. M. (2002). The impact of maternal behavior on children's pain experiences: An experimental analysis. *Journal of Pediatric Psychology, 27*, 293–301.

Chen, E. H., Shofer, F. S., Dean, A. J., Hollander, J. E., Baxt, W. G., Robey, J. L., et al. (2008). Gender disparity in analgesic treatment of emergency department patients with acute abdominal pain. *Academic Emergency Medicine, 15*, 414–418.

Chong, G. S., Cogan, D., Randolph, P., & Racz, G. (2001). Chronic pain and self-efficacy: The effects of age, sex, and chronicity. *Pain Practice, 1*, 338–343.

Ciccone, G. K., & Holdcroft, A. (1999). Drugs and sex differences: A review of drugs relating to anaesthesia. *British Journal of Anaesthesia, 82*, 255–265.

Cicero, T. J., Aylward, S. C., & Meyer, E. R. (2003). Gender differences in the intravenous self-administration of mu opiate agonists. *Pharmacology Biochemistry & Behavior, 74*, 541–549.

Cicero, T. J., Wong, G., Tian, Y., Lynskey, M., Todorov, A., & Isenberg, K. (2009). Co-morbidity and utilization of medical services by pain patients receiving opioid medications: Data from an insurance claims database. *Pain, 144*, 20–27.

Compton, P., Charuvastra, V. C., & Ling, W. (2003). Effect of oral ketorolac and gender on human cold pressor pain tolerance. *Clinical and Experimental Pharmacology & Physiology, 30*, 759–763.

Craig, K. D. (2009). The social communication model of pain. *Canadian Psychology, 50*, 22–32.

Dao, T. T., & LeResche, L. (2000). Gender differences in pain. *Journal of Orofacial Pain, 14*, 169–184.

Defrin, R., Shramm, L., & Eli, I. (2009). Gender role expectations of pain is associated with pain tolerance limit but not with pain threshold. *Pain, 145*, 230–236.

Dixon, K. E., Thorn, B. E., & Ward, L. C. (2004). An evaluation of sex differences in psychological and physiological responses to experimentally-induced pain: A path analytic description. *Pain, 112*, 188–196.

Drossaers-Bakker, K. W., Zwinderman, A. H., van Zeben, D., Breedveld, F. C., & Hazes, J. M. (2002). Pregnancy and oral contraceptive use do not significantly influence outcome in long term rheumatoid arthritis. *Annals of the Rheumatic Diseases, 61*, 405–408.

Edwards, R. R., Augustson, E. M., & Fillingim, R. B. (2000). Sex-specific effects of pain-related anxiety on adjustment to chronic pain. *The Clinical Journal of Pain, 16*, 46–53.

Edwards, R. R., Doleys, D. M., Lowery, D., & Fillingim, R. B. (2003). Pain tolerance as a predictor of outcome following multidisciplinary treatment for chronic pain: Differential effects as a function of sex. *Pain, 106*, 419–426.

Edwards, R. R., Haythornthwaite, J. A., Sullivan, M. J., & Fillingim, R. B. (2004). Catastrophizing as a mediator of sex differences in pain: Differential effects for daily pain versus laboratory-induced pain. *Pain, 111*, 335–341.

Egger, H. L., Costello, E. J., Erkanli, A., & Angold, A. (1999). Somatic complaints and psychopathology in children and adolescents: Stomach aches, musculoskeletal pains, and headaches. *Journal of the American Academy of Child and Adolescent Psychiatry, 38*, 852–860.

Elklit, A., & Jones, A. (2006). The association between anxiety and chronic pain after whiplash injury: Gender-specific effects. *The Clinical Journal of Pain, 22*, 487–490.

Elliott, A. M., Smith, B. H., Penny, K. I., Smith, W. C., & Chambers, W. A. (1999). The epidemiology of chronic pain in the community. *The Lancet, 354*, 1248–1252.

Eriksen, J., Sjogren, P., Ekholm, O., & Rasmussen, N. K. (2004). Health care utilization among individuals reporting long-term pain: An epidemiological study based on Danish National Health Surveys. *European Journal of Pain, 8*, 517–523.

Evans, S., Tsao, J. C., Lu, Q., Kim, S. C., Turk, N., Myers, C. D., et al. (2009). Sex differences in the relationship between maternal negative life events and children's laboratory pain responsivity. *Journal of Developmental and Behavioral Pediatrics, 30*, 279–288.

Evans, S., Tsao, J. C., Lu, Q., Myers, C., Suresh, J., & Zeltzer, L. K. (2008a). Parent-child pain relationships from a psychosocial perspective: A review of the literature. *Journal of Pain Management, 1*, 237–246.

Evans, S., Tsao, J. C., & Zeltzer, L. K. (2008b). Relationship of child perceptions of maternal pain to children's laboratory and non-laboratory pain. *Pain Research & Management, 13*, 211–218.

Fanurik, D., Zeltzer, L. K., Roberts, M. C., & Blount, R. L. (1993). The relationship between children's coping styles and psychological interventions for cold pressor pain. *Pain, 53*, 213–222.

Fillingim, R. B. (2000a). Sex, gender and pain: A biopsychosocial framework. In R. B. Fillingim (Ed.), *Sex, gender and pain* (pp. 1–6). Seattle: IASP Press.

Fillingim, R. B. (Ed.). (2000b). *Sex, gender, and pain* (Vol. 17). Seattle: IASP Press.

Fillingim, R. B. (2002). Sex differences in analgesic responses: Evidence from experimental pain models. *European Journal of Anaesthesiology, 19*, 16–24.

Fillingim, R. B. (2003). Sex-related influences on pain: A review of mechanisms and clinical implications. *Rehabilitation Psychology, 48*, 165–174.

Fillingim, R. B., Hastie, B. A., Ness, T. J., Glover, T. L., Campbell, C. M., & Staud, R. (2005a). Sex-related psychological predictors of baseline pain perception and analgesic responses to pentazocine. *Biological Psychology, 69*, 97–112.

Fillingim, R. B., King, C. D., Ribeiro-Dasilva, M. C., Rahim-Williams, B., & Riley, J. L., III. (2009). Sex, gender, and pain: A review of recent clinical and experimental findings. *The Journal of Pain, 10*, 447–485.

Fillingim, R. B., & Ness, T. J. (2000). Sex-related hormonal influences on pain and analgesic responses. *Neuroscience & Biobehavioural Reviews, 24*, 485–501.

Fillingim, R. B., Ness, T. J., Glover, T. L., Campbell, C. M., Hastie, B. A., Price, D. D., et al. (2005b). Morphine responses and experimental pain: Sex differences in side effects and cardiovascular responses but not analgesia. *The Journal of Pain, 6*, 116–124.

Fillingim, R. B., Ness, T. J., Glover, T. L., Campbell, C. M., Price, D. D., & Staud, R. (2004). Experimental pain models reveal no sex differences in pentazocine analgesia in humans. *Anesthesiology, 100*, 1263–1270.

Flaten, M. A., Simonsen, T., & Olsen, H. (1999). Drug-related information generates placebo and nocebo responses that modify the drug response. *Psychosomatic Medicine, 61*, 250–255.

Fouladbakhsh, J. M., & Stommel, M. (2010). Gender, symptom experience, and use of complementary and alternative medicine practices among cancer survivors in the U.S. cancer population. *Oncology Nursing Forum, 37*, E7–E15.

Fowler-Kerry, S., & Lander, J. (1991). Assessment of sex differences in children's and adolescents' self-reported pain from venipuncture. *Journal of Pediatric Psychology, 16*, 783–793.

Galdas, P. M., Cheater, F., & Marshall, P. (2005). Men and health help-seeking behaviour: Literature review. *Journal of Advanced Nursing, 49*(6), 616–623.

Gatchel, R. J., Peng, Y. B., Peters, M. L., Fuchs, P. N., & Turk, D. C. (2007). The biopsychosocial approach to chronic pain: Scientific advances and future directions. *Psychological Bulletin, 133*, 581–624.

Gater, R., Tansella, M., Korten, A., Tiemens, B. G., Mavreas, V. G., & Olatawura, M. O. (1998). Sex differences in the prevalence and detection of depressive and anxiety disorders in general health care settings: Report from the World Health Organization Collaborative Study on Psychological Problems in General Health Care. *Archives of General Psychiatry, 55*, 405–413.

Gear, R. W., Miaskowski, C., Gordon, N. C., Paul, S. M., Heller, P. H., & Levine, J. D. (1999). The kappa opioid nalbuphine produces gender- and dose-dependent analgesia and antianalgesia in patients with postoperative pain. *Pain, 83*, 339–345.

Geisser, M. E., Robinson, M. E., Miller, Q. L., & Bade, S. M. (2003). Psychosocial factors and functional capacity evaluation among persons with chronic pain. *Journal of Occupational Rehabilitation, 13*, 259–276.

Ginsburg, G. S., & Drake, K. L. (2002). Anxiety sensitivity and panic attack symptomatology among low-income African-American adolescents. *Journal of Anxiety Disorders, 16*, 83–96.

Goodenough, B., Kampel, L., Champion, G. D., Laubreaux, L., Nicholas, M. K., Ziegler, J. B., et al. (1997). An investigation of the placebo effect and age-related factors in the report of needle pain from venipuncture in children. *Pain, 72*, 383–391.

Goodenough, B., Thomas, W., Champion, G. D., Perrott, D., Taplin, J. E., von Baeyer, C. L., et al. (1999). Unraveling age effects and sex differences in needle pain: Ratings of sensory intensity and unpleasantness of venipuncture pain by children and their parents. *Pain, 80*, 179–190.

Green, C. A., & Pope, C. R. (1999). Gender, psychosocial factors and the use of medical services: A longitudinal analysis. *Social Science & Medicine, 48*, 1363–1372.

Greenspan, J. D., Craft, R. M., LeResche, L., Arendt-Nielsen, L., Berkley, K. J., Fillingim, R., et al. (2007). Studying sex and gender differences in pain and analgesia: A consensus report. *Pain, 132*(Suppl 1), S26–S45.

Grunau, R. V., Johnston, C. C., & Craig, K. D. (1990). Neonatal facial and cry responses to invasive and non-invasive procedures. *Pain, 42*, 295–305.

Grunau, R. V. E., & Craig, K. D. (1987). Pain expression in neonates – Facial action and cry. *Pain, 28*, 395–410.

Guinsburg, R., de Araujo Peres, C., Branco de Almeida, M. F., de Cassia Xavier Balda, R., Cassia Berenguel, R., Tonelotto, J., et al. (2000). Differences in pain expression between male and female newborn infants. *Pain, 85*, 127–133.

Hakala, P., Rimpela, A., Salminen, J. J., Virtanen, S. M., & Rimpela, M. (2002). Back, neck, and shoulder pain in Finnish adolescents: National cross sectional surveys. *British Medical Journal, 325*, 743.

Hall, J. A. (1978). Gender effects in decoding nonverbal cues. *Psychological Bulletin, 85*, 845–857.

Hall, J. A. (2006). Women's and men's nonverbal communication: Similarities, differences, stereotypes, and origins. In V. Manusov & M. L. Patterson (Eds.), *The SAGE handbook of nonverbal communication* (pp. 208–218). London: Sage Publishers.

Hampel, P., Graef, T., Krohn-Grimberghe, B., & Tlach, L. (2009). Effects of gender and cognitive-behavioral management of depressive symptoms on rehabilitation outcome among inpatient orthopedic patients with chronic low back pain: A 1 year longitudinal study. *European Spine Journal, 18*, 1867–1880.

Hansen, F. R., Bendix, T., Skov, P., Jensen, C. V., Kristensen, J. H., Krohn, L., et al. (1993). Intensive, dynamic back-muscle exercises, conventional physiotherapy, or placebo-control treatment of low-back pain. A randomized, observer-blind trial. *Spine, 18*, 98–108.

Hazes, J. M. (1991). Pregnancy and its effect on the risk of developing rheumatoid arthritis. *Annals of the Rheumatic Diseases, 50*, 71–72.

Hazes, J. M., Dijkmans, B. A., Vandenbroucke, J. P., de Vries, R. R., & Cats, A. (1990). Pregnancy and the risk of developing rheumatoid arthritis. *Arthritis and Rheumatism, 33*, 1770–1775.

Hechler, T., Kosfelder, J., Vocks, S., Monninger, T., Blankenburg, M., Dobe, M., et al. (2010). Changes in pain-related coping strategies and their importance for treatment outcome following multimodal inpatient treatment: Does sex matter? *The Journal of Pain, 11*, 472–483.

Heitkemper, M. M., & Chang, L. (2009). Do fluctuations in ovarian hormones affect gastrointestinal symptoms in women with irritable bowel syndrome? *Gender Medicine, 6*, 152–167.

Hirsh, A. T., Alqudah, A. F., Stutts, L. A., & Robinson, M. E. (2008). Virtual human technology: Capturing sex, race, and age influences in individual pain decision policies. *Pain, 140*, 231–238.

Hodgins, M. J., & Lander, J. (1997). Children's coping with venipuncture. *Journal of Pain and Symptom Management, 13*, 274–285.

Holdcroft, A. (2002a). Pharmacological differences between men and women. *Acta Anaesthesiologica Belgica, 53*, 299–303.

Holdcroft, A. (2002b). Sex differences and analgesics. *European Journal of Anaesthesiology Supplement, 26*, 1–2.

Holdcroft, A., & Berkley, K. J. (2005). Sex and gender differences in pain and its relief. In S. B. McMahon, M. Koltzenburg, P. D. Wall, & R. Melzack (Eds.), *Wall and Melzack's textbook of pain* (5th ed., pp. 1181–1197). Edinburgh: Elsevier Churchill Livingstone.

Hooten, W. M., Townsend, C. O., Bruce, B. K., Shi, Y., & Warner, D. O. (2009). Sex differences in characteristics of smokers with chronic pain undergoing multidisciplinary pain rehabilitation. *Pain Medicine, 10*, 1416–1425.

Ip, H. Y., Abrishami, A., Peng, P. W., Wong, J., & Chung, F. (2009). Predictors of postoperative pain and analgesic consumption: A qualitative systematic review. *Anesthesiology, 111*, 657–677.

Isacson, D., & Bingefors, K. (2002). Epidemiology of analgesic use: A gender perspective. *European Journal of Anaesthesiology, 19*, 5–15.

Jackson, T., Iezzi, T., Gunderson, J., Nagasaka, T., & Fritch, A. (2002). Gender differences in pain perception: The mediating role of self-efficacy beliefs. *Sex Roles, 47*, 561–568.

Jensen, I., Nygren, A., Gamberale, F., Goldie, I., & Westerholm, P. (1994). Coping with long-term musculoskeletal pain and its consequences: Is gender a factor? *Pain, 57*, 167–172.

Jensen, I. B., Bergstrom, G., Ljungquist, T., Bodin, L., & Nygren, A. L. (2001). A randomized controlled component analysis of a behavioral medicine rehabilitation program for chronic spinal pain: Are the effects dependent on gender? *Pain, 91*, 65–78.

Johannes, C. B., Le, T. K., Zhou, X., Johnston, J. A., & Dworkin, R. H. (2010). The prevalence of chronic pain in United States adults: Results of an internet-based survey. *The Journal of Pain, 11*, 1230–1239.

Jones, A., Spindler, H., Jorgensen, M. M., & Zachariae, R. (2002). The effect of situation-evoked anxiety and gender on pain report using the cold pressor test. *Scandinavian Journal of Psychology, 43*, 307–313.

Jones, A., & Zachariae, R. (2002). Gender, anxiety, and experimental pain sensitivity: An overview. *Journal of the American Medical Women's Association, 57*, 91–94.

Jones, A., Zachariae, R., & Arendt-Nielsen, L. (2003). Dispositional anxiety and the experience of pain: Gender-specific effects. *European Journal of Pain, 7*, 387–395.

Kaczynski, K. J., Claar, R. L., & Logan, D. E. (2009). Testing gender as a moderator of associations between psychosocial variables and functional disability in children and adolescents with chronic pain. *Journal of Pediatric Psychology, 34*, 738–748.

Kallai, I., Barke, A., & Voss, U. (2004). The effects of experimenter characteristics on pain reports in women and men. *Pain, 112*, 142–147.

Kaur, S., Stechuchak, K. M., Coffman, C. J., Allen, K. D., & Bastian, L. A. (2007). Gender differences in health care utilization among veterans with chronic pain. *Journal of General Internal Medicine, 22*, 228–233.

Keefe, F. J., Crisson, J., Urban, B. J., & Williams, D. A. (1990). Analyzing chronic low back pain: The relative contribution of pain coping strategies. *Pain, 40*, 293–301.

Keefe, F. J., Lefebvre, J. C., Egert, J. R., Affleck, G., Sullivan, M. J., & Caldwell, D. S. (2000). The relationship of gender to pain, pain behavior, and disability in osteoarthritis patients: The role of catastrophizing. *Pain, 87*, 325–334.

Keogh, E. (2008). Sex differences in pain. In J. M. Moore (Ed.), *Biobehavioral approaches to pain*. New York: Springer.

Keogh, E., & Asmundson, G. J. G. (2004). Negative affectivity, catastrophizing and anxiety sensitivity. In G. J. G. Asmundson, J. W. Vlaeyen, & G. Crombez (Eds.), *Understanding and treating fear of pain* (pp. 91–115). Oxford: Oxford University Press.

Keogh, E., Barlow, C., Mounce, C., & Bond, F. W. (2006a). Assessing the relationship between cold pressor pain responses and dimensions of the anxiety sensitivity profile in healthy men and women. *Cognitive Behavior Therapy, 35*, 198–206.

Keogh, E., & Birkby, J. (1999). The effect of anxiety sensitivity and gender on the experience of pain. *Cognition & Emotion, 13*, 813–829.

Keogh, E., Bond, F. W., Hanmer, R., & Tilston, J. (2005a). Comparing acceptance- and control-based coping instructions on the cold-pressor pain experiences of healthy men and women. *European Journal of Pain, 9*, 591–598.

Keogh, E., & Denford, S. (2009). Sex differences in perceptions of pain coping strategy usage. *European Journal of Pain, 13*, 629–634.

Keogh, E., & Eccleston, C. (2006). Sex differences in adolescent chronic pain and pain-related coping. *Pain, 123*, 275–284.

Keogh, E., Hamid, R., Hamid, S., & Ellery, D. (2004). Investigating the effect of anxiety sensitivity, gender and negative interpretative bias on the perception of chest pain. *Pain, 111*, 209–217.

Keogh, E., Hatton, K., & Ellery, D. (2000). Avoidance versus focused attention and the perception of pain: Differential effects for men and women. *Pain, 85*, 225–230.

Keogh, E., & Herdenfeldt, M. (2002). Gender, coping and the perception of pain. *Pain, 97*, 195–201.

Keogh, E., McCracken, L. M., & Eccleston, C. (2005b). Do men and women differ in their response to interdisciplinary chronic pain management? *Pain, 114*, 37–46.

Keogh, E., McCracken, L. M., & Eccleston, C. (2006b). Gender moderates the association between depression and disability in chronic pain patients. *European Journal of Pain, 10*, 413–422.

Khan, R. S., Ahmed, K., Blakeway, E., Skapinakis, P., Nihoyannopoulos, L., Macleod, K., et al. (2011). Catastrophizing: A predictive factor for postoperative pain. *American Journal of Surgery, 201*(1), 122–131.

Klatzkin, R. R., Mechlin, B., & Girdler, S. S. (2010). Menstrual cycle phase does not influence gender differences in experimental pain sensitivity. *European Journal of Pain, 14*, 77–82.

Koopmans, G. T., & Lamers, L. M. (2007). Gender and health care utilization: The role of mental distress and help-seeking propensity. *Social Science & Medicine, 64*, 1216–1230.

Kowalczyk, W. J., Evans, S. M., Bisaga, A. M., Sullivan, M. A., & Comer, S. D. (2006). Sex differences and hormonal influences on response to cold pressor pain in humans. *The Journal of Pain, 7*, 151–160.

Kowalczyk, W. J., Sullivan, M. A., Evans, S. M., Bisaga, A. M., Vosburg, S. K., & Comer, S. D. (2010). Sex differences and hormonal influences on response to mechanical pressure pain in humans. *The Journal of Pain, 11*, 330–342.

Krekmanova, L., Bergius, M., Robertson, A., Sabel, N., Hafstrom, C., Klingberg, G., et al. (2009). Everyday- and dental-pain experiences in healthy Swedish 8–19 year olds: An epidemiological study. *International Journal of Paediatric Dentistry, 19*, 438–447.

Krogstad, B. S., Jokstad, A., Dahl, B. L., & Vassend, O. (1996). The reporting of pain, somatic complaints, and anxiety in a group of patients with TMD before and 2 years after treatment: Sex differences. *Journal of Orofacial Pain, 10*, 263–269.

Kunz, M., Prkachin, K., & Lautenbacher, S. (2009). The smile of pain. *Pain, 145*, 273–275.

Lackner, J. M., & Carosella, A. M. (1999). The relative influence of perceived pain control, anxiety, and functional self efficacy on spinal function among patients with chronic low back pain. *Spine, 24*, 2254–2260.

LaFrance, M., Hecht, M. A., & Paluck, E. L. (2003). The contingent smile: A meta-analysis of sex differences in smiling. *Psychological Bulletin, 129*, 305–334.

LeResche, L. (1999). Gender considerations in the epidemiology of chronic pain. In I. K. Crombie, P. R. Croft, S. J. Linton, L. LeResche, & M. Von Korff (Eds.), *Epidemiology of pain* (pp. 43–52). Seattle: IASP Press.

LeResche, L., Mancl, L., Sherman, J. J., Gandara, B., & Dworkin, S. F. (2003). Changes in temporomandibular pain and other symptoms across the menstrual cycle. *Pain, 106*, 253–261.

Levine, F. M., & Desimone, L. L. (1991). The effects of experimenter gender on pain report in male and female subjects. *Pain, 44*, 69–72.

Light, K. P., Lovell, A. T., Butt, H., Fauvel, N. J., & Holdcroft, A. (2006). Adverse effects of neuromuscular blocking agents based on yellow card reporting in the U.K.: Are there differences between males and females? *Pharmacoepidemiology and Drug Safety, 15*, 151–160.

Lofgren, M., & Norrbrink, C. (2009). Pain relief in women with fibromyalgia: A cross-over study of superficial warmth stimulation and transcutaneous electrical nerve stimulation. *Journal of Rehabilitation Medicine, 41*, 557–562.

Logan, D. E., & Rose, J. B. (2004). Gender differences in post-operative pain and patient controlled analgesia use among adolescent surgical patients. *Pain, 109*, 481–487.

Lord, B., Cui, J., & Kelly, A. M. (2009). The impact of patient sex on paramedic pain management in the prehospital setting. *The American Journal of Emergency Medicine, 27*, 525–529.

Lu, Q., Tsao, J. C., Myers, C. D., Kim, S. C., & Zeltzer, L. K. (2007). Coping predictors of children's laboratory-induced pain tolerance, intensity, and unpleasantness. *The Journal of Pain, 8*, 708–717.

Lund, I., Lundeberg, T., Kowalski, J., & Svensson, E. (2005). Gender differences in electrical pain threshold responses to transcutaneous electrical nerve stimulation (TENS). *Neuroscience Letters, 375*, 75–80.

Lyby, P. S., Aslaksen, P. M., & Flaten, M. A. (2010). Is fear of pain related to placebo analgesia? *Journal of Psychosomatic Research, 68*, 369–377.

Lynch, A. M., Kashikar-Zuck, S., Goldschneider, K. R., & Jones, B. A. (2007). Sex and age differences in coping styles among children with chronic pain. *Journal of Pain and Symptom Management, 33*, 208–216.

Marcus, S. M., Kerber, K. B., Rush, A. J., Wisniewski, S. R., Nierenberg, A., Balasubramani, G. K., et al. (2008). Sex differences in depression symptoms in treatment-seeking adults: Confirmatory analyses from the Sequenced Treatment Alternatives to Relieve Depression study. *Comprehensive Psychiatry, 49*, 238–246.

Martin, V. T. (2009). Ovarian hormones and pain response: A review of clinical and basic science studies. *Gender Medicine, 6*, 168–192.

Martin, V. T., & Behbehani, M. (2006). Ovarian hormones and migraine headache: Understanding mechanisms and pathogenesis – part I. *Headache, 46*, 3–23.

Mayer, E. A., Berman, S., Lin, C., & Naliboff, B. D. (2004). Sex-based differences in gastrointestinal pain. *European Journal of Pain, 8*, 451–463.

McCabe, S. E., Boyd, C. J., & Young, A. (2007). Medical and nonmedical use of prescription drugs among secondary school students. *Journal of Adolescent Health, 40*, 76–83.

McCracken, L. M., & Houle, T. (2000). Sex-specific and general roles of pain-related anxiety in adjustment to chronic pain: A reply to Edwards et al. *The Clinical Journal of Pain, 16*, 275–276.

McGeary, D. D., Mayer, T. G., Gatchel, R. J., Anagnostis, C., & Proctor, T. J. (2003). Gender-related differences in treatment outcomes for patients with musculoskeletal disorders. *The Spine Journal, 3*, 197–203.

McLean, C. P., & Anderson, E. R. (2009). Brave men and timid women? A review of the gender differences in fear and anxiety. *Clinical Psychology Review, 29*, 496–505.

Merlijn, V. P., Hunfeld, J. A., van der Wouden, J. C., Hazebroek-Kampschreur, A. A., Koes, B. W., & Passchier, J. (2003). Psychosocial factors associated with chronic pain in adolescents. *Pain, 101*, 33–43.

Michael, G. E., Sporer, K. A., & Youngblood, G. M. (2007). Women are less likely than men to receive prehospital analgesia for isolated extremity injuries. *American Journal of Emergency Medicine, 25*, 901–906.

Moller-Leimkuhler, A. M. (2002). Barriers to help-seeking by men: A review of sociocultural and clinical literature with particular reference to depression. *Journal of Affective Disorders, 71*, 1–9.

Moon, E. C., Chambers, C. T., Larochette, A. C., Hayton, K., Craig, K. D., & McGrath, P. J. (2008). Sex differences in parent and child pain ratings during an experimental child pain task. *Pain Research & Management, 13*, 225–230.

Myers, C. D., Tsao, J. C., Glover, D. A., Kim, S. C., Turk, N., & Zeltzer, L. K. (2006). Sex, gender, and age: Contributions to laboratory pain responding in children and adolescents. *The Journal of Pain, 7*, 556–564.

Ndao-Brumblay, S. K., & Green, C. R. (2010). Predictors of complementary and alternative medicine use in chronic pain patients. *Pain Medicine, 11*, 16–24.

Niesters, M., Dahan, A., Kest, B., Zacny, J., Stijnen, T., Aarts, L., et al. (2010). Do sex differences exist in opioid analgesia? A systematic review and meta-analysis of human experimental and clinical studies. *Pain, 151*, 61–68.

Ocanez, K. L., Kathryn McHugh, R., & Otto, M. W. (2010). A meta-analytic review of the association between anxiety sensitivity and pain. *Depression and Anxiety, 27*, 760–767.

Olofsen, E., Romberg, R., Bijl, H., Mooren, R., Engbers, F., Kest, B., et al. (2005). Alfentanil and placebo analgesia – No sex differences detected in models of experimental pain. *Anesthesiology, 103*, 130–139.

Osman, A., Barrios, F. X., Gutierrez, P. M., Kopper, B. A., Merrifield, T., & Grittmann, L. (2000). The Pain Catastrophizing Scale: Further psychometric evaluation with adult samples. *Journal of Behavioral Medicine, 23*, 351–365.

Paller, C. J., Campbell, C. M., Edwards, R. R., & Dobs, A. S. (2009). Sex-based differences in pain perception and treatment. *Pain Medicine, 10*, 289–299.

Paulose-Ram, R., Hirsh, R., Dillon, C., Losonczy, K., Cooper, M., & Ostchega, Y. (2003). Prescription and non-prescription analgesic use among the US adult population: Results from the third National Health and Nutrition Examination Survey (NHANES III). *Pharmacoepidemiology and Drug Safety, 12*, 315–326.

Perquin, C. W., Hazebroek-Kampschreur, A. A., Hunfeld, J. A., Bohnen, A. M., van Suijlekom-Smit, L. W., Passchier, J., et al. (2000). Pain in children and adolescents: A common experience. *Pain, 87*, 51–58.

Piira, T., Champion, G. D., Bustos, T., Donnelly, N., & Lui, K. (2007). Factors associated with infant pain response following an immunization injection. *Early Human Development, 83*, 319–326.

Piira, T., Taplin, J. E., Goodenough, B., & von Baeyer, C. L. (2002). Cognitive-behavioural predictors of children's tolerance of laboratory-induced pain: Implications for clinical assessment and future directions. *Behavior Research & Therapy, 40*, 571–584.

Pleym, H., Spigset, O., Kharasch, E. D., & Dale, O. (2003). Gender differences in drug effects: Implications for anesthesiologists. *Acta Anaesthesiologica Scandinavica, 47*, 241–259.

Pokela, N., Bell, J. S., Lihavainen, K., Sulkava, R., & Hartikainen, S. (2010). Analgesic use among community dwelling people aged 75 years and older: A population based interview study. *The American Journal of Geriatric Pharmacotherapy, 8*, 233–244.

Pollo, A., & Benedetti, F. (2011). Pain and the placebo/nocebo effect. In R. J. Moore (Ed.), *Handbook of pain and palliative care: Biobehavioral approaches for the life course*. New York: Springer.

Pool, G. J., Schwegler, A. F., Theodore, B. R., & Fuchs, P. N. (2007). Role of gender norms and group identification on hypothetical and experimental pain tolerance. *Pain, 129*, 122–129.

Popescu, A., LeResche, L., Truelove, E. L., & Drangsholt, M. T. (2010). Gender differences in pain modulation by diffuse noxious inhibitory controls: A systematic review. *Pain, 150*(2), 309–318.

Portenoy, R. K., Ugarte, C., Fuller, I., & Haas, G. (2004). Population-based survey of pain in the United States: Differences among white, African American, and Hispanic subjects. *The Journal of Pain, 5*, 317–328.

Prkachin, K. M. (1992). The consistency of facial expressions of pain: A comparison across modalities. *Pain, 51*, 297–306.

Prkachin, K. M., & Solomon, P. E. (2009). The structure, reliability and validity of pain expression: Evidence from patients with shoulder pain. *Pain, 139*, 267–274.

Pud, D., Yarnitsky, D., Sprecher, E., Rogowski, Z., Adler, R., & Eisenberg, E. (2006). Can personality traits and gender predict the response to morphine? An experimental cold pain study. *European Journal of Pain, 10*, 103–112.

Rhudy, J. L., & Williams, A. E. (2005). Gender differences in pain: Do emotions play a role? *Gender Medicine, 2*, 208–226.

Ribeiro-Dasilva, M. C., Shinal, R. M., Glover, T., Williams, R. S., Staud, R., Riley, J. L., & Fillingim, R. B. (2011). Evaluation of menstrual cycle effects on morphine and pentazocine analgesia. *Pain, 152*, 614–622.

Riley, J. L., Robinson, M. E., Wise, E. A., Myers, C. D., & Fillingim, R. B. (1998). Sex differences in the perception of noxious experimental stimuli: A meta-analysis. *Pain, 74*, 181–187.

Riley, J. L., Robinson, M. E., Wise, E. A., & Price, D. D. (1999). A meta-analytic review of pain perception across the menstrual cycle. *Pain, 81*, 225–235.

Robinson, M. E., Gagnon, C. M., Dannecker, E. A., Brown, J. L., Jump, R. L., & Price, D. D. (2003a). Sex differences in common pain events: Expectations and anchors. *The Journal of Pain, 4*, 40–45.

Robinson, M. E., Gagnon, C. M., Riley, J. L., & Price, D. D. (2003b). Altering gender role expectations: Effects on pain tolerance, pain threshold, and pain ratings. *The Journal of Pain, 4*, 284–288.

Robinson, M. E., George, S. Z., Dannecker, E. A., Jump, R. L., Hirsh, A. T., Gagnon, C. M., et al. (2004a). Sex differences in pain anchors revisited: Further investigation of "most intense" and common pain events. *European Journal of Pain, 8*, 299–305.

Robinson, M. E., Riley, J. L., Myers, C. D., Papas, R. K., Wise, E. A., Waxenberg, L. B., et al. (2001). Gender role expectations of pain: Relationship to sex differences in pain. *The Journal of Pain, 2*, 251–257.

Robinson, M. E., & Wise, E. A. (2003). Gender bias in the observation of experimental pain. *Pain, 104*, 259–264.

Robinson, M. E., & Wise, E. A. (2004). Prior pain experience: Influence on the observation of experimental pain in men and women. *The Journal of Pain, 5*, 264–269.

Robinson, M. E., Wise, E. A., Gagnon, C., Fillingim, R. B., & Price, D. D. (2004b). Influences of gender role and anxiety on sex differences in temporal summation of pain. *The Journal of Pain, 5*, 77–82.

Roger, V. L., Farkouh, M. E., Weston, S. A., Reeder, G. S., Jacobsen, S. J., Zinsmeister, A. R., et al. (2000). Sex differences in evaluation and outcome of unstable angina. *Journal of the American Medical Association, 283*, 646–652.

Rollman, G. B., & Lautenbacher, S. (2001). Sex differences in musculoskeletal pain. *The Clinical Journal of Pain, 17*, 20–24.

Rollman, G. B., Lautenbacher, S., & Jones, K. S. (2000). Sex and gender differences in response to experimentally induced pain in humans. In R. B. Fillingim (Ed.), *Sex, gender, and pain* (pp. 165–190). Seattle: IASP Press.

Romano, J. M., Jensen, M. P., Turner, J. A., Good, A. B., & Hops, H. (2000). Chronic pain patient-partner interactions: Further support for a behavioral model of chronic pain. *Behavior Therapy, 31*, 415–450.

Romano, J. M., Turner, J. A., Jensen, M. P., Friedman, L. S., Bulcroft, R. A., Hops, H., et al. (1995). Chronic pain patient-spouse behavioral interactions predict patient disability. *Pain, 63*, 353–360.

Rustoen, T., Wahl, A. K., Hanestad, B. R., Lerdal, A., Paul, S., & Miaskowski, C. (2004a). Gender differences in chronic pain-findings from a population-based study of Norwegian adults. *Pain Management Nursing, 5*, 105–117.

Rustoen, T., Wahl, A. K., Hanestad, B. R., Lerdal, A., Paul, S., & Miaskowski, C. (2004b). Prevalence and characteristics of chronic pain in the general Norwegian population. *European Journal of Pain, 8*, 555–565.

Sarton, E., Olofsen, E., Romberg, R., den Hartigh, J., Kest, B., Nieuwenhuijs, D., et al. (2000). Sex differences in morphine analgesia – An experimental study in healthy volunteers. *Anesthesiology, 93*, 1245–1254.

Scheibe, S., & Carstensen, L. L. (2010). Emotional aging: Recent findings and future trends. *The Journals of Gerontology Series B, 65B*, 135–144.

Sherman, J. J., & LeResche, L. (2006). Does experimental pain response vary across the menstrual cycle? A methodological review. *American Journal of Physiology – Regulatory, Integrative and Comparative Physiology, 291*(2), R245–R256.

Sherman, J. J., LeResche, L., Mancl, L. A., Huggins, K., Sage, J. C., & Dworkin, S. F. (2005). Cyclic effects on experimental pain response in women with temporomandibular disorders. *Journal of Orofacial Pain, 19*, 133–143.

Shinal, R. M., & Fillingim, R. B. (2007). Overview of orofacial pain: Epidemiology and gender differences in orofacial pain. *Dental Clinics of North America, 51*, 1–18, v.

Simon, D., Craig, K. D., Gosselin, F., Belin, P., & Rainville, P. (2008). Recognition and discrimination of prototypical dynamic expressions of pain and emotions. *Pain, 135*, 55–64.

Sjogren, P., Ekholm, O., Peuckmann, V., & Gronbaek, M. (2009). Epidemiology of chronic pain in Denmark: An update. *European Journal of Pain, 13*, 287–292.

Smith, S. J., Keefe, F. J., Caldwell, D. S., Romano, J., & Baucom, D. (2004). Gender differences in patient-spouse interactions: A sequential analysis of behavioral interactions in patients having osteoarthritic knee pain. *Pain, 112*, 183–187.

Stewart, W. F., Linet, M. S., Celentano, D. D., Van Natta, M., & Ziegler, D. (1991). Age- and sex-specific incidence rates of migraine with and without visual aura. *American Journal of Epidemiology, 134*, 1111–1120.

Stovner, L., Hagen, K., Jensen, R., Katsarava, Z., Lipton, R., Scher, A., et al. (2007). The global burden of headache: A documentation of headache prevalence and disability worldwide. *Cephalalgia, 27*, 193–210.

Strong, J., Ashton, R., & Chant, D. (1992). The measurement of attitudes towards and beliefs about pain. *Pain, 48*, 227–236.

Sullivan, M. J., Thorn, B., Haythornthwaite, J. A., Keefe, F., Martin, M., Bradley, L. A., et al. (2001). Theoretical perspectives on the relation between catastrophizing and pain. *The Clinical Journal of Pain, 17*, 52–64.

Sullivan, M. J. L., Bishop, S. R., & Pivik, J. (1995). The Pain Catastrophizing Scale: Development and validation. *Psychological Assessment, 7*, 524–532.

Sullivan, M. J. L., Tripp, D. A., & Santor, D. (2000). Gender differences in pain and pain behavior: The role of catastrophizing. *Cognitive Therapy and Research, 24*, 121–134.

Taenzer, A. H., Clark, C., & Curry, C. S. (2000). Gender affects report of pain and function after arthroscopic anterior cruciate ligament reconstruction. *Anesthesiology, 93*, 670–675.

Tait, R., DeGood, D., & Carron, H. (1982). A comparison of health locus of control beliefs in low-back patients from the U.S. and New Zealand. *Pain, 14*, 53–61.

Tamres, L. K., Janicki, D., & Helgeson, V. S. (2002). Sex differences in coping behavior: A meta-analytic review and an examination of relative coping. *Personality and Social Psychology Review, 6*, 2–30.

Teepker, M., Peters, M., Vedder, H., Schepelmann, K., & Lautenbacher, S. (2010). Menstrual variation in experimental pain: Correlation with gonadal hormones. *Neuropsychobiology, 61*, 131–140.

Theis, K. A., Helmick, C. G., & Hootman, J. M. (2007). Arthritis burden and impact are greater among U.S. women than men: Intervention opportunities. *Journal of Women's Health, 16*, 441–453.

Thompson, T., Keogh, E., French, C. C., & Davis, R. (2008). Anxiety sensitivity and pain: Generalisability across noxious stimuli. *Pain, 134*, 187–196.

Tobin, D. D., Menon, M., Menon, M., Spatta, B. C., Hodges, E. V. E., & Perry, D. G. (2010). The intrapsychics of gender: A model of self-socialization. *Psychological Review, 117*, 601–622.

Tsang, A., Von Korff, M., Lee, S., Alonso, J., Karam, E., Angermeyer, M. C., et al. (2008). Common chronic pain conditions in developed and developing countries: Gender and age differences and co-morbidity with depression-anxiety disorders. *The Journal of Pain, 9*, 883–891.

Turunen, J. H., Mantyselka, P. T., Kumpusalo, E. A., & Ahonen, R. S. (2005). Frequent analgesic use at population level: Prevalence and patterns of use. *Pain, 115*, 374–381.

Unruh, A. M. (1996). Gender variations in clinical pain experience. *Pain, 65*, 123–167.

Unruh, A. M., Ritchie, J., & Merskey, H. (1999). Does gender affect appraisal of pain and pain coping strategies? *The Clinical Journal of Pain, 15*, 31–40.

Ustun, T. B. (2000). Cross-national epidemiology of depression and gender. *The Journal of Gender-Specific Medicine, 3*, 54–58.

Vetter, T. R. (2011). Pediatric chronic pain. In R. J. Moore (Ed.), *Handbook of pain and palliative care: Biobehavioral approaches for the life course*. New York: Springer.

Vigil, J. M. (2009). A socio-relational framework of sex differences in the expression of emotion. *The Behavioral and Brain Sciences, 32*, 375–390.

Weir, R., Browne, G., Tunks, E., Gafni, A., & Roberts, J. (1996). Gender differences in psychosocial adjustment to chronic pain and expenditures for health care services used. *The Clinical Journal of Pain, 12*, 277–290.

Weisse, C. S., Foster, K. K., & Fisher, E. A. (2005). The influence of experimenter gender and race on pain reporting: Does racial or gender concordance matter? *Pain Medicine, 6*, 80–87.

Weisse, C. S., Sorum, P. C., Sanders, K. N., & Syat, B. L. (2001). Do gender and race affect decisions about pain management? *Journal of General Internal Medicine, 16*, 211–217.

Wijnhoven, H. A. H., de Vet, H. C. W., & Picavet, H. S. J. (2006). Prevalence of musculoskeletal disorders is systematically higher in women than in men. *The Clinical Journal of Pain, 22*, 717–724.

Wilder-Smith, O. H. (2005). Opioid use in the elderly. *European Journal of Pain, 9*, 137–140.

Williams, R. E., Sampson, T. J., Kalilani, L., Wurzelmann, J. I., & Janning, S. W. (2008). Epidemiology of opioid pharmacy claims in the United States. *Journal of Opioid Management, 4*, 145–152.

Wise, E. A., Price, D. D., Myers, C. D., Heft, M. W., & Robinson, M. E. (2002). Gender role expectations of pain: Relationship to experimental pain perception. *Pain, 96*, 335–342.

Wu, C. L., Rowlingson, A. J., Cohen, S. R., Michaels, R. K., Courpas, G. E., Joe, E. M., et al. (2006). Gender and post-dural puncture headache. *Anesthesiology, 105*, 613–618.

Wu, L. T., Pilowsky, D. J., & Patkar, A. A. (2008). Non-prescribed use of pain relievers among adolescents in the United States. *Drug and Alcohol Dependence, 94*, 1–11.

Chapter 22
Stress and Pain

Catherine M. Stoney

Abbreviations

CBT	Cognitive behavioral therapy
DHEA	Dehydroepiandrosterone
fMRI	Functional magnetic resonance imaging
HPA	Hypothalamic-pituitary-adrenal
MRI	Magnetic resonance imaging
OTC	Over-the-counter
PSP	Perceived Stress Scale
PTSD	Posttraumatic stress disorder
SES	Socioeconomic status

Defining Psychosocial Stress

While the definition of both acute and chronic pain will be covered in other chapters, the purpose of this chapter is to focus on psychological stress and its relationship to pain, in terms of both the nature and causes of that relationship, as well as how that relationship might suggest possibilities for treatment. Thus, a discussion of how stress is conceptualized and measured is both an appropriate and necessary first step in understanding how stress and pain are sometimes linked.

Unless otherwise stated, this chapter will focus primarily on psychosocial stress, rather than on environmental (cold stress), physical (starvation stress), or other types of extreme circumstances and burden on the body that is sometimes referred to as a stressor. In some cases, these burdens may result in the subsequent experience of psychosocial stress – for example, some environmental stressors (extreme crowding) may result in the experience of psychological stress, but for the most part the literature studying the relationship between psychosocial stressors and health outcomes comes from studying phenomenon that have direct impact on psychological functioning and social interactions.

There are several definitions of psychosocial stress in the literature, and there is little consensus across the field about which is most appropriate under which conditions. Particularly in clinical

C.M. Stoney, PhD (✉)
The National Institutes of Health, National Heart, Lung, and Blood Diseases,
6701 Rockledge Drive, Bethesda, MD 20892, USA
e-mail: stoneyc@mail.nih.gov

R.J. Moore (ed.), *Handbook of Pain and Palliative Care: Biobehavioral Approaches for the Life Course*,
DOI 10.1007/978-1-4419-1651-8_22, © Springer Science+Business Media, LLC 2012

situations and the lay public, psychosocial stress is most commonly referred to as the impact of an environmental or "external" event, such as work burden, family burden, and certain traumas. In these examples, stress is considered to occur to an individual and is thought of as being an invariant consequence of that event. References to stress exposure, trauma exposure, and exposure to a natural or man-made disaster are in line with this way of conceptualizing stress. Although often labeled as stress, these might best be considered stressors, since they are precipitants or potential precipitants of a cascade of events. While many external events or exposures might universally be considered to be stressors (the trauma of being held hostage, for example), there is actually considerable individual variation in response to such events and exposures, both in terms of perceptions of the events, as well as health outcomes. Thus, it is useful to consider alternative views of stress to account for such individual differences.

A more cognitive conceptualization of stress considers stress to be the perception of not having sufficient resources to adequately cope with perceived demands. Here, stress is considered to be quite individualized and based on perceptions of one's own abilities and resources, as well as one's own notions of what it means to cope or meet the perceived demands appropriately or adequately. An example might be the stress experienced by students when confronted with a very difficult school curriculum. With this conceptualization, some researchers still consider the demands to be primarily external or environmental ones (work, school, stress, etc.), although more cognitively focused views of this type of stress would include perceptions of demands, such as individual notions of what demands are required to be met. Thus, this latter conceptualization allows for individual differences in perceiving the same environmental demand (school curriculum) as being either stressful or not. In this example, a difficult school curriculum might be perceived as being a stressor for those students for whom the perceived demand is the necessity to excel at the curriculum at all times regardless of the difficulty, with the perception that adequately meeting the demands would be indicated by the highest possible grades. For those students for whom the difficult curriculum is perceived as a challenge to do ones best regardless of grades, a very challenging academic curriculum may not be perceived as a stressor. Environmental demands then, under this conceptualization, are quite broad and include not only external demands, but internally focused ones as well.

Still other conceptualizations of psychosocial stress view stress as the consequence of an interaction between perceived demands (which could be cognitive and environmental and which might include, for example, expectations of others or perceived expectations of others) with an individual's perceived ability to meet those demands. In this model, stress would be considered to be present when one has the perception of an inability to meet those perceived demands. With this broad conceptualization of stress, it is important to note that the perception of an inability to meet perceived demands may or may not be accurate, and may vary over time. In fact, in this conceptualization, the assessment or appraisal of one's perceptions is an ongoing experience which allows for feedback to alter the experience and perception of stress. This explains why, for example, an initial challenging experience may be perceived as stressful, but once the challenge is experienced and perceived as no longer threatening, subsequent appraisals would likely consider the same experience as nonstressful. This explains why the same or similar circumstances for different individuals may be perceived as either stressful or not, depending on how our initial and ongoing appraisals alter those perceptions.

Finally, stress is sometimes considered to be a physiological response of an individual, such as an elevation in blood pressure or increased secretion of cortisol. While this very nonspecific notion of stress can be useful when undertaking stress research using animal models and can be used in human research to verify the "stressfulness" of an experience, it is more helpful to view these factors as consequences of stressful experiences, especially when trying to understand the link between psychosocial stress and disease.

The Measurement of Stress and Stressors

Patient-Reported Measures of Stress

The most common way of measuring psychosocial stress in humans is by self-report, and a large number of instruments have been developed and validated for this purpose. These vary according to how stress is conceptualized. For example, one of the most common self-report measures is the Perceived Stress Scale (PSS), which as the name suggests, queries individuals with regard to the type and amount of stress they have perceived in their lives over the previous few weeks. Several versions of the PSS are available (Cohen et al. 1983; Cohen and Williamson 1988), and all have demonstrated good reliability and validity. This measure is easy to use when the clinician or researcher wishes to have a meaningful index of how a particular individual perceives his or her experiences. Other common self-report measures focus on external events to index the magnitude of stress (Holmes and Rahe 1967; Sarason et al. 1978), and query individuals about discrete experiences (change in job, marriage, relocation, death of a loved one) that have occurred over some discrete period of time. The events are weighted and numerically tabulated for a "stress index." These events, which can have both positive and negative valence, have the common element of requiring significant change and adjustment. Still other self-report measures query individuals about common and often daily annoyances. Such "hassles" measures are thought to be useful because they include experiences that are quite common and may give a more accurate picture of how individuals cope with common and mild stressors (Lazarus and Folkman 1989).

Event-Driven Measures of Stress

Life events measures index the number and, in some cases, the impact of certain life events, and make the assumption that a larger number of changes in ones' life – whether positive or negative – will necessarily increase the perception of stress. Some life events scales, which are primarily based on self-reports, incorporate the meaning or valence of the event in determining the amount of stress that may accumulate as a result of the events. An example of the same event resulting in different perceptions of stress is the birth of a child. Although a significant life event in nearly any situation, it can have different meaning under different circumstances. In the first and more typical case, it is viewed as a positive event. Although it will necessitate changes in the lives of the parents, these are typically anticipated and desired. However, sometimes the birth of a child is not anticipated or planned, and can place significant economic, physical, and psychological burden on the mother and/ or family, in which case the event may result in perceptions of an inability to cope with the situation and resultant perceptions of stress. Thus, the valence of the event can be a salient factor to take into consideration when measuring life events as potential stressors. Similarly, the extent to which the event is perceived as one with which one is able to cope effectively can have an impact on whether the event is perceived as a stressor. Finally, regardless of the valence or perceptions of coping, the absolute impact of life events can be a significant factor in whether the event is perceived as a stressor. For example, moving to a different city can be both positive and can be effectively coped with, but when moving has a significant impact on one's social integration, the impact of such a move can be perceived as a stressor.

Biological Markers of Stress

A number of putative biomarkers of stressors and stress have been suggested in both the animal and human literature, and these generally focus on functioning of the autonomic nervous system, the hypothalamic-pituitary-adrenal (HPA) axis, and the sympathetic neural axis. Both acute and chronic psychosocial stressors frequently are associated with transient increases in blood pressure and heart rate, and decreases with parasympathetic tone (heart rate variability, for example). Such changes are often cited as the potential biological mechanisms linking stressors with certain health and physiological outcomes such as hypertension and flare-ups of underlying autoimmune disorders. However, they are also sometimes considered as biomarkers of psychosocial stress; for example, cortisol, dehydroepiandrosterone (DHEA), and alpha-amyloid are typically increased during psychosocial stressors. Although each can have significant biological impact, they also are sensitive to changes in self-reports of psychological stress or external (apparently) stressors. Thus, they are sometimes considered to be markers of stress, and sometimes considered to be biological outcomes of stress. Work is continuing to determine the value of adding one or a panel of biomarkers of psychosocial stress to the self-report and other-report measures of stress, in the service of a reliable, comprehensive, and valid metric that can be applied across humans and model systems.

Behavioral and Other-Report Measures of Stress

Behavioral indices of stress are employed most frequently in studies of young children and in animal studies. Among children, reports from parents and teachers are commonly used because children may be less able to provide accurate self-reports of psychosocial stress. For some behaviors and in certain situations, behavioral indications of stress in children can be monitored by unrelated observers, who can sometimes be less biased in their observations. Examples of behavioral indices that are closely monitored as indicators of childhood stress include hostile and aggressive behaviors and conduct disorders, impulsivity, behavioral regression, sleep disorders, withdrawal, sleep disruption, and expressions of persistent worries. Animal models use other behaviors as indications of stress, including altered posturing, decreased grooming, and alternations in activity, depending on the specific animals being observed.

Psychosocial Explanations for the Comorbidity Between Stress and Pain

Psychosocial stress and pain are frequently comorbid and this relationship has led to several hypotheses and studies regarding why this is the case and how it can inform treatment strategies. Traumatic stressors and development of posttraumatic stress disorder (PTSD) in childhood is strongly associated with subsequent development of chronic pain disorders (Arguelles et al. 2006). Even mild stressors such as sleep deprivation have been linked with pain (McBeth et al. 2007). There are several psychosocial mechanisms by which stress and pain can become comorbid.

Acute pain, in particular, can sometimes lead to a certain level of acute stress because of fear regarding the origins and meaning of the pain (what could the pain be due to?), discomfort, short-term use of pain medication which in certain individuals can cause distress, and a temporary condition of having to alter one's lifestyle because of functional restrictions due to the pain. Acute pain also often requires questions regarding when and if to seek healthcare services, which can be stressful, particularly when access to such services is restricted. When the immediate cause of the acute pain is clear, stress is lessened, both because of the clarity regarding the meaning of the pain, understanding regarding treatment and time course, and the knowledge that the acute pain will dissipate.

If the pain is or becomes chronic in nature, the level of distress typically rises. In fact, psychological sequela is typically more prevalent and likely during chronic pain conditions, relative to acute pain experiences. This is because of continuing questions on the factors regarding the nature and understanding of the pain condition, increasing use of narcotic and other medications, and difficulty in interacting with healthcare providers who are often at a loss of how to manage, understand, or diagnosis the pain condition. Over time, chronic pain can lead to social isolation, a complete change of lifestyle and, sometimes, livelihood, and perseverance with the pain. The average chronic pain patient has experienced pain for 7 years by the time they arrive at a chronic pain treatment center (Flor et al. 1992). Living with chronic pain for this length of time without treatment is disruptive to nearly all aspects of these patients' social lives and well-being, so that often by the time treatment at such a facility is initiated, their lives have been profoundly disrupted. For some individuals, an inability to understand where the pain comes from can lead to depression, helplessness, and poor family and social relationships. In cases where the chronic pain results from a known and pervasive or terminal condition, such as pain related to cancer or rheumatologic conditions, fear frequently accompanies the stress, not only because of the dire diagnosis, but also because such a diagnosis often suggests the pain will remain chronic. The incidence of a psychiatric disorder among chronic pain patients is at least twice that of the general population (Turk et al. 2010).

However, there are significant individual differences in the magnitude of psychological distress reported by chronic pain patients, as well as differences in reports of overall health-related quality of life, regardless of disease and pain severity and disability (Bazzichi et al. 2005). For some chronic pain patients, personality factors such as hostility (positive prediction) and a high sense of coherence (negative prediction) are reasonably good predictors of the level of stress reported by chronic pain patients (Bai et al. 2009). The implications of this direction of research are primarily treatment related; this might involve, for example, such personality factors to be considered within the context of a psychological coping treatment plan. In addition, findings such as these, if maintained, could provide additional information regarding the mechanisms relating to pain and stress.

In any case, it is clear that the experience of stress can exacerbate pain conditions and, in some cases, take a minor acute pain condition and alter it to a more severe state. In fact, in both chronic and even acute pain conditions, it is frequently the case that the experience of stress exacerbates the pain and makes it less likely that patients will be able to be successful in developing and maintaining coping strategies to manage the pain (Gill et al. 2004). For example, among patients with sickle-cell disease, stress and negative affect are associated with increased pain. In addition, pain-related functional impairment reduces the ability to effectively cope in some situations, such as seeking out social networks and family support, adhering to medical advice, and increasing functional status.

Strongly related to the comorbidity between pain and stress is that between pain and depression, because depression and stress are so strongly related. The depression that can arise with increasing levels of pain-related distress can be especially debilitating. Pain is in fact a common complaint among those with major depressive disorders, in addition to the experience of depression as a consequence of pain. Along with the increased difficulty in coping with comorbid pain and depression, it becomes more difficult to recognize, diagnose, and treat the pain condition when depression is present. The link between depression and pain is so common that the term depression-pain dyad has been coined, to emphasize the possibility of underlying similar biological pathways involved in both (Bair et al. 2003). Anxiety is the other common psychiatric diagnosis that is comorbid with chronic pain; however, there are significant individual differences in the occurrence of comorbid psychiatric disorders among chronic pain patients, some of which is due to coping strategies used when living with chronic pain (Clauw 2009).

Biological Relationships Between Stress and Pain

Because of the relationships between trauma and psychological stressors on the one hand and pain on the other, there has been significant interest in understanding the biological and neural underpinnings of this relationship, which could potentially inform clinical interventions and treatments. For example, it is well known that both pain and stress are associated with the increased release of circulating cortisol, although there are clearly individual differences in the magnitude of the responses (Kanegane et al. 2009). As indicated previously, cortisol is a typical consequence and indication of the experience of stress, and can similarly involve exaggerated or abnormal HPA axis responses and autonomic function. Interestingly, many functional pain disorders such as fibromyalgia, irritable bowel syndrome, and interstitial cystitis are associated with autonomic dysfunction (Demitrack and Crofford 1998). One study has found that women with major depressive disorder had higher circulating levels of Substance P and calcitonin-gene-related peptide than did nondepressed women. Both of these neuropeptides play a mediating role in pain symptoms (Hartman et al. 2006), albeit in different ways. The elevation in Substance P among women with major depressive disorder is particularly interesting because it is involved in both the serotonergic and norepinephrine systems by which pain and depression are influenced (Bondy et al. 2003).

Stress in the Absence of a Diagnosed Underlying Pain Condition

It is certainly the case that stress can actually cause pain in the absence of a specific pain condition. Common examples include headache, backache, and neck ache, similar to the other physiological consequences of stress, such as increased blood pressure, heart rate, and gastrointestinal distress. These latter stress-related physiological changes – caused by increases in cortisol, proinflammatory cytokines, and muscular changes – may also be responsible for the pain associated with stress (Mayer 2000). This phenomenon is especially the case for severe, trauma-related stress. In such cases, pain often emerges after a significant period of time has elapsed, and has been hypothesized to reflect a dysregulation of the HPA axis (Heim et al. 2001), activation of the autonomic nervous system (Nilsen et al. 2007), and may be moderated by the activity of the amygdala (Staud et al. 2007). This phenomenon is prevalent with traumatic stressors in particular; traumatic events and in some cases even more moderate stressors are thought to trigger the initiation of certain pain disorders, such as fibromyalgia and other functional pain disorders, among individuals with a genetic predisposition to these conditions (Clauw 2009).

The Neuromatrix Theory of Pain

The gate control theory of pain, developed by Melzack and Wall (1965), integrates physiological and psychological aspects of pain perception and incorporates sensory-discriminative, motivational-affective, and cognitive-evaluative domains. The theory describes how cortical factors (stress, memory, attention) interact with the peripheral gating system in the spine to affect pain perception. Melzack (1999, 2001) has developed these ideas further, in an attempt to understand how pain might occur in the absence of peripheral afferent stimulation. A key example is phantom limb pain, which is often severe and cannot be explained without understanding the vital and sometimes initial role of central processes in pain perceptions. Melzack provides a theoretical framework to understand the neurological underpinnings of how chronic pain and stress may be closely linked, emphasizing the multiple levels involved. The model is particularly useful in postulating how stress can be the starting point that leads to chronic pain syndromes and experiences. Termed the neural matrix, the theory outlines the complexities of neural connections that integrate somatosensory, cognitive, and perceptual information and interpretations, behaviors and emotions, and homeostatic processes. Melzack proposes that particular patterns of neural firing in particular configurations, both temporal and spatial, produce a neural signature. These neural firing patterns, which evolve over time to become neural signatures, can also become the basis for certain chronic pain experiences which can then be activated by either sensory or central triggers. For example, as the network processes impulses, neurosignature patterns are produced which trigger perceptions and emotions. Interestingly, the neural firing patterns in stress experiences are also part of the neural matrix and may be part of the neural signatures associated with pain, because both pain and stress share common pathways. Thus, the theory may provide not only a framework in which to better understand conditions such as phantom limb pain, but also why stress can precipitate bouts of pain among patients with functional pain disorders or precipitate the disorder itself among susceptible individuals.

Psychosocial and Emotional Aspects of Pain

In addition to stress, a number of other psychological and social precipitants and sequela of pain can be identified, and are important because they share many characteristics with pain syndromes themselves and are often comorbid with pain. Such factors include sleep disorders, social isolation, fatigue, socioeconomic status (SES) and cognitive dysfunction, and depression, among others. Although psychological problems and pain do have some common characteristics, these psychological phenomena are distinct both in terms of their interactions with pain, as well as being psychologically distinct experiences, and understanding the contributions of each is important in identifying appropriate assessment and treatment.

One of the most common comorbid conditions with pain is depression, with the comorbidity between depression and pain is so frequent that some clinicians and researchers refer to a depression-pain syndrome. Clinically depressed patients often present with a number of somatic complaints (Croft et al. 1995), and in fact somatic symptoms are part of the diagnostic criteria for major depressive disorder. Not infrequently, such somatic complaints include pain from undetermined causes. For example, those with diagnoses of major depressive disorder have a significantly increased likelihood of reporting pain symptoms; between 50 and 70% of such patients report having pain (Ohayon and Schatzberg 2010), and pain intensity has been shown to be positively correlated with the severity of depression (Hartman et al. 2006). Interestingly, symptoms of depressed mood also predict subsequent pain symptoms, suggesting that there may be some common neural pathways linking persistent depressed mood with pain symptoms. One piece of evidence in this regard is that antidepressant medications are sometimes effective for relieving both pain and depression.

From the opposite perspective, it is not difficult to understand how pain – and in particular chronic pain – can lead to depression and depressive symptoms because of loss of functionality, fear and frustration regarding inadequate treatment strategies, and disrupted family and social relationships. Interestingly, however, the two conditions are not only comorbid but also appear to have some common biological pathways and may be similarly responsive to a single treatment strategy. Thus, the connection between either clinical depression or depressed mood on the one hand, and pain symptoms on the other may have important implications for a mechanistic understanding of both phenomena, as well as for treatment strategies.

Other aspects of negative affect related to pain but somewhat distinct from stress include fear and anger. When either or both are present during the experience of pain, they can have influences not only on behavioral responses to pain, but also on subsequent experiences of stress.

Anxiety disorders, closely related to stress but diagnosable as distinct disorders, are particularly interesting when comorbid with pain because anxiety (as well as high levels of stress if detected by healthcare providers) can prevent the identification and subsequent treatment of pain, particularly chronic pain. This is a diagnostic issue which can occur when the overwhelming presenting symptoms are those of anxiety. Interestingly, the opposite is also true – pain can mask the identification of both clinical anxiety and depression, and lead to a failure to appropriately and fully treat the patient presenting with these comorbid conditions (Bair et al. 2003). As with depression, which is frequently comorbid with anxiety, anxiety intensity is positively correlated with pain intensity (Hartman et al. 2006). In acute situations, simply the anticipation of pain increases anxiety and stress (Kanegane et al. 2009), regardless of whether stress was measured by self-report or by increased levels of salivary cortisol.

Learning and cognition also interact with pain through both behavioral responses and complex neural networks. Responses of caregivers, family members, healthcare providers, and even coworkers to symptom reports or pain behaviors (grimacing, sighing, and other behaviors indicating the presence of pain) have feed-forward and feedback consequences on future behaviors, reports, and perceptions. Pain behaviors also include visits to healthcare providers, use of pain medications, expressions of stress, and time off from work. All of these can be absolutely appropriate responses to pain, but in some cases and in particularly with chronic pain, have the potential to reinforce the pain behaviors. It is possible that these behaviors may become so conditioned that they actually reinforce the perception of pain.

Economic disparities occur in pain, as they do across many mental and physical health conditions (Adler and Ostrove 1999). Stress is reported more frequently among those at lower SES, in part because there are a larger number of stressful life events and fewer resources to cope with those events among individuals at lower socioeconomic levels (Gallo and Matthews 2003). Among patients with rheumatoid arthritis, for example, financial worry and stress were positively related to reports of pain (Skinner et al. 2004). A recent report verifies this finding and supports the notion that stress and pain are especially linked among those with financial stress and is generalized to a broad range of patients and pain conditions (Rios and Zautra 2011).

Finally, pain can alter the social environment significantly, which can have downstream effects on how likely the pain is to cause stress, and how well individuals cope with that stress. As chronic pain persists without effective treatment or relief, patients become more stressed and anxious, pain behaviors tend to increase as a sign to others that "something needs to be done," mobility and daily functions can often diminish, and patients gradually become more socially isolated.

It is important to note that the relationships noted between stress and pain occur over a broad range of clinical conditions and patient populations, and does not appear to depend on whether the pain is associated with a terminal or life-shortening illness or not. Thus, it appears that the pain itself, along with the sequela of the pain, is most important with regard to the association with stress than is the disease (when identifiable) itself (Crosbie et al. 2009).

Ways in Which Stress Affects the Experience of Pain

One of the curious aspects of the relationship between stress and pain involves the many and sometimes contradictory ways that the two impact each other. These differences are likely related to the type, severity, and chronicity of the pain, individual differences in coping and in the meaning of the pain, and the type, severity, and chronicity of the particular stressor(s) involved. Two specific examples of how psychosocial stress and pain interact in seemingly opposite ways follow.

Stress-Induced Analgesia

The first documented demonstration of the strong relationship between stress and pain came from medics in World War II working in battleground areas. They noticed that seriously wounded soldiers would frequently fail to report pain shortly after being wounded; after a day or two, as the shock of their wounds wore off, reports of pain increased significantly. This phenomenon of stress-induced analgesia has been subsequently tested in both humans and animals and has been clearly demonstrated in individuals experiencing both mild and severe pain. In some cases, generally less severe pain, the analgesia is mediated by the activation of the opioidergic neural mid-brain system as well as by peripheral opioid release from the adrenal and pituitary gland. In more severe pain and under different stressor conditions, stress-induced analgesia appears to be mediated by nonopioid mechanisms, although some of the same neural networks appear to be similarly activated. In addition, however, other peripheral systems operate during nonopioid stress-induced analgesia such as release of vasopressin, activation of the HPA axis, and other systems that vary according to the specific stressor and conditions (Amit and Galina 1986). Overall, the biological mechanisms explaining stress-induced analgesia are not fully developed, but the phenomenon does clearly indicate that psychological factors such as stress play an important role in the perception of pain. Stress-induced analgesia may serve as a short-term, biologically adaptive response when temporary pain suppression is necessary in order to move oneself to safety or to cope with extreme pain; thus, when stress is strongly coupled with pain, the consequent analgesia might be considered initially adaptive. However, longer term analgesia may not be adaptive, such as when some action is needed to decrease the bodily damage and subsequent pain. In such cases, stress-induced analgesia may be frankly damaging. In such cases, other phenomenon may come into play, such as the opposite condition of stress-induced hyperalgesia.

Stress-Induced Hyperalgesia

In contrast to stress-induced analgesia, the phenomenon of stress-induced hyperalgesia also occurs. In this case, exposure to stressors leads to an exaggerated perception of pain (Simone 1992). This phenomenon has been less well studied than has stress-induced analgesia, and most experimental evidence has been dedicated to animal studies. However, among humans, evidence for the phenomenon includes the demonstration that stress can enhance the perception of pain in some individuals; that stress can decrease the ability of pain-relieving medications to be optimally effective; and that stressed patients tend to be hypersensitive to pain than less stressed patients. Although it is difficult to reconcile stress-induced analgesia and stress-induced hyperalgesia, a better understanding of the biological and psychological underpinnings of both will clarify the conditions under which either occurs. Interestingly, both phenomena can be classically conditioned, underscoring the importance of how illness behavior and the responses of family and friends toward those experiencing pain can influence the experience of pain.

The Role of Stress in the Transition from Acute to Chronic Pain

In general, the mechanisms by which acute pain or injury leads to chronic pain conditions are not well delineated, but psychosocial mechanisms have been proposed as playing a significant role. When the initial experiences of injury and pain are accompanied by significant fear regarding the pain, the consequence can be to engage in a variety of maladaptive behaviors to decrease the experience of even small amounts of pain. These might include such behaviors as inactivity and illness behaviors, and a strong desire to avoid any behaviors that will increase the experience of the pain itself (Vlaeyen and Linton 2000). Disability can then ensue, leading to a chronic pain condition.

On the other hand, when the pain is not accompanied by fear, the avoidance of adaptive and healthy behaviors does not occur and the acute pain is alleviated.

Physiological events that accompany stress may also play a significant role in whether or not there is a transition from acute to chronic pain. Acute injury engages the physiological stress responses of increased cortisol, activation of the sympathetic nervous system, and activation of central neurobiological pain pathways, which can be exaggerated to result in the above dysregulated pattern (McLean et al. 2005).

Related to this is the phenomenon of phantom limb pain or the experience of pain which is perceived to be associated with an amputated limb. Early studies identified blood flow near the amputated limb and muscle spasms were associated with phantom limb pain (Arena et al. 1990), but more current data using fMRI suggests that maladaptive cortical reorganization is more likely to be operating (Flor 2008). In all of these cases, however, the suggestion is that the pain is due to physiological causes. However, there is also a body of literature showing a relationship between the periodic onset of phantom limb pain and psychological stress (Arena et al. 1990). The direction of the association has been shown to be bidirectional in certain individuals under certain conditions – that is, phantom limb pain leads ultimately to increased reporting of stress, and the experience of psychological stress (independent of pain) predisposes to the onset of phantom limb pain. Such a relationship has been demonstrated with other periodic pain conditions as well, such as headache (Arena et al. 1984).

Many chronic pain patients truly live their pain – it becomes a pervasive albeit unwanted part of their lives and much of their time is spent within the healthcare system seeking diagnosis, treatment, and, often, simply acknowledgment of the pain. By the time patients are seen by healthcare systems focused specifically on the management of chronic pain, they have been living with pain for a mean duration of 7 years (Flor et al. 1992). Because of the pervasive and long-term nature of chronic pain, and because of obstacles often encountered not only within family and work environments, but also within the healthcare system, it is virtually impossible for individuals with chronic pain to not develop some type of psychological sequela, with perceptions of stress topping the list. Up to 50% of chronic pain patients report psychological stress (Cairns et al. 2003).

Some of the distress experienced by the chronic pain patient is due directly or indirectly to interactions with the healthcare system. Pain, by its nature, is patient reported and therefore a subjective experience. As such, it is difficult to understand comparisons that are made across individuals. Because pain is typically viewed as a consequence of disease or injury, and pain and disease or injury are linearly and positively correlated (with greater tissue damage typically associated with greater pain), pain patients seeking treatment who do not have a diagnosable disease or apparent injury that can be related to their pain, pain can be difficult for healthcare providers to treat, and frustrating for the patients. This tends to lead to a protracted process of patients seeking health care from one practitioner to another, seeking alleviation or even acknowledgement of pain that is difficult or impossible to "see" and healthcare providers seeing these as difficult patients to treat. As the stress and frustration of the patient mount, hope and self-efficacy decrease, making it more likely that the ability to engage in nonpharmacologic self-management strategies for the pain decreases.

Whether experiencing chronic or acute stress, the stress of living with the pain is frequently compounded by the additional stress associated with secondary consequences of the pain, such as necessary changes in lifestyle, mobility, functional status, economic conditions, and social engagement. The psychological impact of these stressors may be the same, whether the pain is acute or chronic. However, it is generally acknowledged that psychosocial factors are likely to play a larger role in pain and pain perception when pain is chronic rather than acute.

While there are both pharmacologic and nonpharmacologic approaches to the treatment of pain, it is difficult to know a priori which treatment, dosage, and regimen will be effective for any particular pain in a patient. The medical system tends to err on the side of underutilization of narcotics for pain management, yet is generally not well trained in nonpharmacologic pain management.

Treatment Strategies

Because of the relationships between psychosocial stress and pain, stress-reduction interventions may serve as appropriate treatment approaches for certain pain conditions and may be appropriate to consider, particularly for chronic pain conditions. A discussion of the methodology involved in obtaining accurate assessment of pain is not the purpose of this chapter, but assessment of pain and its sequela can be critical in determining appropriate treatment strategies. It is important to evaluate not only the various dimensions of pain (severity, location, chronicity, quality of the pain) and functional impairments, but also the psychosocial consequences of the pain in order to target an appropriate treatment approach. This includes evaluating stress related to the experience of pain, assessing pain behaviors, and the impact on quality of life and related factors such as employment, social and family relationships, substance use and abuse, functional capacity, current coping strategies, environmental barriers that may make coping with pain more difficult, control and self-efficacy, and expectations regarding pain management and treatment.

Although there are a number of treatment strategies that focus on alleviating the stress and associated psychosocial consequences associated with pain, for some conditions, populations, and types of pain, these strategies are not fully satisfactory for reducing either the stress nor the pain or pain condition. Treatments that focus on the stress associated with acute pain are generally different than those that focus on treatments of stress associated with chronic pain conditions. In most cases, the main goal is to ameliorate the stress associated with pain in order to either decrease the perception of pain or to increase quality of life and functional status. Of course, pain reduction in most cases will serve to reduce the stress related to pain; these pain-reduction strategies are the focus of other chapters.

Patient-Based Psychosocial Management Strategies

A variety of patient-based strategies can be taught and used to manage pain, and in particular to manage the stress associated with pain which often increases the experience of pain. Adaptive strategies that patients can employ themselves include distraction; support from friends, family, and other support networks; lifestyle strategies that enhance self-efficacy and help individuals find meaning in life; and altering cognitive appraisals of the pain and the meaning and consequences of the pain. Many of these require training and practice to learn. Each decreases the stress associated with pain, and each has been shown to have positive effects on the perception of pain as well. One example is the use of distraction during anticipated acute stress with children. A systematic review of the literature on strategies for reducing both pain and stress associated with immunizations in children concluded that distraction and breathing exercises (using party blowers or bubbles) are particularly effective in reducing reports of the stress that children report, but also reduce child reports of pain associated with immunization (Chambers et al. 2009).

In addition to adaptive patient-based strategies that manage both pain and stress, there are also a variety of strategies that pain patients use which are maladaptive – that is, they increase pain, increase stress, or both. There are clinically important reasons to identify these maladaptive strategies because they shed light on how patients themselves cope with stress. For example, even among individuals without pain, over-the-counter (OTC) use of analgesics is influenced by psychosocial factors and has been thought to be used as a way of coping with stressors often in the absence of pain (Stasio et al. 2008), especially because of the association between OTC analgesic use and psychiatric morbidity (Abbott and Fraser 1998). One cross-sectional study using data from 4,739 individuals from the Danish Health Interview Survey showed an association between self-reported stress and OTC analgesic use, even after adjusting for symptoms of pain and discomfort (Koushede et al. 2010). Thus, self-medication with OTC analgesic preparations may be one of many poor coping strategies, even among pain patients.

Another maladaptive strategy is pain catastrophizing. Patients who catastrophize their pain – that is, they experience and describe their pain as being unbearable – tend to elicit greater responses from those around them than individuals who are less likely to catastrophize their pain. The increased attention and concern from others who mean well may in fact reinforce the catastrophizing behaviors, as well as the pain experience itself. Such patients are less likely to use distraction as an effective pain coping strategy (Campbell et al. 2010) and may be less able to use other psychological coping strategies as well. Pain catastrophizing is related to depression and may likely also be related to high perceptions of stress, in part because of the distorted view of pain. For example, magnetic resonance imaging (MRI) studies of fibromyalgia patients have examined brain activation areas in high and low pain catastrophizers. Data indicate that brain structures related to the anticipation of pain (the medial frontal cortex and cerebellum), attention to pain (the dorsal anterior cingulate gyrus and dorsolateral prefrontal cortex), and the emotional aspects of pain (amygdale and claustrum) are activated more in those who are pain catastrophizers than those who were not classified as pain catastrophizers (Gracely et al. 2003). These important data suggest that pain catastrophizing has an important influence on pain perception and can enhance the emotional response to pain, including the stress response.

Beliefs about pain can both increase and decrease perceptions of stress and also alter perceptions of pain. When chronic pain patients become helpless with regard to their pain, they feel they are no longer able to manage or cope with the pain. The result is a cascade of negative effects, ranging from increased stress and depression, to decreased adaptive health behaviors such as seeking appropriate medical care and adhering to medical advice, to becoming socially isolated.

Provider-Based Psychosocial Management Strategies

The role of the healthcare provider can be pivotal in helping to diagnose the source and cause of pain, the existence of comorbid psychosocial stress, and to develop an effective treatment strategy that incorporates treatment of both the pain and stress.

One of the most common psychological strategies for alleviating chronic pain is cognitive behavioral therapy (CBT), which incorporates behavioral techniques to cope with the pain (such as distraction, enhancing social support, appropriate self-care) and cognitive techniques such as finding positive meaning with the pain, decreasing catastrophizing thoughts about the pain, enhancing self-efficacy in managing the pain, and stress management. Most elements of CBT are most effective for chronic pain conditions; simple behavioral strategies such as distraction can be most useful for acute pain conditions. Distraction is used frequently and effectively especially in children undergoing painful medical procedures, as well as other acute pain experiences.

Other strategies that can be effective in alleviating both pain and stress include biofeedback, which can be useful for muscle-related pain in particular, relaxation techniques, and hypnosis (Hoffman et al. 2007). In general, such interventions are modestly useful for both pain and the stress associated with the pain, and are most effective when used in conjunction with a nonpsychological intervention.

Predictors of Outcomes

Reports of relatively low levels of psychosocial stress and articulation of specific strategies for coping with stress are likely the best predictors of which patients will cope well with chronic pain, as well as which may respond well to treatment interventions focused as much on stress as on other pain management techniques (Jensen et al. 1991). One study found that stress at work in patients with acute radicular pain and a lumbar disk prolapsed or protrusion was the best predictor of early retirement, and that persistent pain was more likely to be present in patients with not only highly levels of pain symptoms, but also fewer psychological and social resources to draw from and poorer pain coping strategies (Hasenbring et al. 1994). Resilience, a trait-like factor that refers to the ability to recover quickly and which is generally thought of as nearly opposite to the concept of stress, has been shown to be part of an adaptive strategy after severe injury, and is increased by social support and lessened by pain (Quale and Schanke 2010). Mastery or the perception of control over pain is an important predictor of those who cope well with chronic pain, as well as an important component of perceived stress. As mentioned previously, increasing evidence suggests that selected other personality traits such as hostility and a sense of coherence can impact the degree to which stress impacts coping and quality of life in some chronic pain patients (Bai et al. 2009). All of these factors may provide information regarding other pathways by which stress management treatment techniques are able to improve outcomes for chronic pain patients.

Conclusions

Pain and psychological stress are frequently comorbid. This chapter outlined the notion that while pain can and does lead to the experience of stress, it is also the case that psychosocial stress can lead to pain. Several theoretical frameworks have proposed how such connections occur, with the neural matrix theory proposed by Melzack (1999, 2001) describing a compelling and comprehensive picture of how consistent neural firing patterns can lead to neural signatures, which can then be triggered by both peripheral and central (cognitive) stimuli. Ultimately, the goal of developing more effective treatment strategies for pain patients clearly must acknowledge the role of psychological stress and incorporate strategies for stress management in treating pain. The development of future treatments will benefit from a more comprehensive and systems-based approach to understanding how and under what conditions central and peripheral processes interact during pain, and the potentially critical role that psychological stress plays in that interaction.

References

Abbott, F. V., & Fraser, M. I. (1998). Use and abuse of over-the-counter analgesic agents. *Journal of Psychiatry & Neuroscience, 23*, 13–34.

Adler, N. E., & Ostrove, J. M. (1999). Socioeconomic status and health: What we know and what we don't. *Annals of the New York Academy of Science, 896*, 3–15.

Amit, Z., & Galina, Z. H. (1986). Stress-induced analgesia: Adaptive pain suppression. *Physiological Reviews, 66*, 1091–1120.

Arena, J. G., Blanchard, E. B., & Andrasik, F. (1984). The role of affect in the etiology of chronic headache. *Journal of Psychosomatic Research, 28*, 79–86.

Arena, J. G., Sherman, R. A., Bruno, G. M., & Smith, J. D. (1990). The relationship between situational stress and phantom limb pain: Cross-lagged correlational data from six month pain logs. *Journal of Psychosomatic Research, 34*, 71–77.

Arguelles, L. M., Afrai, N., Buchwald, D. S., Clauw, D. J., Ferner, S., & Soldbert, J. (2006). A twin study of posttraumatic stress disorder symptoms and chronic widespread pain. *Pain, 124*, 150–157.

Bai, M., Tomenson, B., Creed, F., Mantis, D., Tsifetaki, N., Voulgari, P. V., Drosos, A. A., & Hyphantis, T. N. (2009). The role of psychological distress and personality variables in the disablement process in rheumatoid arthritis. *Scandanavian Journal of Rheumatology, 38*, 419–430.

Bair, M. J., Robinson, R. L., Katon, W., & Kroenke, K. (2003). Depression and pain comorbidity: A literature review. *Archives of Internal Medicine, 163*, 2433–2445.

Bazzichi, L., Maser, J., Piccinni, A., Rucci, P., Del Debbio, A., Vivarelli, L., et al. (2005). Quality of life in rheumatoid arthritis: Impact of disability and lifetime depressive spectrum symptomatology. *Clinical and Experimental Rheumatology, 23*, 783–788.

Bondy, B., Baghal, T. C., Minov, C., Schule, C., Schwarz, M. J., Zwanzger, P., Rupprecht, R., & Moller, J. J. (2003). Substance P serum levels are increase in major depression: Preliminary results. *Biological Psychology, 53*, 538–542.

Cairns, M. C., Foster, N. E., Wright, C. C., & Pennington, D. (2003). Level of distress in a recurrent low back pain population referred for physical therapy. *Spine, 28*, 952–959.

Campbell, C. M., Witmer, K., Simango, M., Carteret, A., Loggia, M. L., Campbell, J. N., Haythornthwaite, J. A., & Edwards, R. R. (2010). Catastrophizing delays the analgesic effect of distraction. *Pain, 149*, 202–207.

Chambers, C. T., Taddio, A., Uman, L. S., McMurtry, C. M.; for the HELPinKIDS Team. (2009). Psychological interventions for reducing pain and distress during routine childhood immunizations: A systematic review. *Clinical Therapeutics. 31*(Suppl B), S77–S103.

Clauw, D. J. (2009). Fibromyalgia: An overview. *The American Journal of Medicine, 122*, S3–S13.

Cohen, S., Kamarck, T., & Mermelstein, R. (1983). A global measure of perceived stress. *Journal of Health and Social Behavior, 24*, 385–396.

Cohen, S., & Williamson, G. (1988). Perceived stress in a probability sample of the United States. In S. Spacapam & S. Oskamp (Eds.), *The social psychology of health: Claremont Symposium on applied social psychology*. Newbury Park: Sage.

Croft, P. R., Papageorgiou, A. C., Ferry, S., Thomas, E., Jayson, M. I., & Silman, A. J. (1995). Psychological distress and low back pain: Evidence from a prospective study in the general population. *Spine, 20*, 2731–2737.

Crosbie, T. W., Packman, W., & Packman, S. (2009). Psychological aspects of patients with Fabry disease. *Journal of Inherited Metabolic Diseases, 32*, 745–753.

Demitrack, M. A., & Crofford, L. J. (1998). Evidence for and pathophysiologic implications of hypothalamic-pituitary-adrenal axis dysregulation in fibromyalgia and chronic fatigue syndrome. *Annals of the New York Academy of Science, 840*, 684–697.

Flor, H. (2008). Maladaptive plasticity, memory for pain and phantom limb pain: Review and suggestions for new therapies. *Expert Review of Neurotherapeutics, 8*, 809–818.

Flor, H., Fydrich, T., & Turk, D. C. (1992). Efficacy of multidisciplinary pain treatment centers: A meta-analytic review. *Pain, 49*, 221–230.

Gallo, L. C., & Matthews, K. A. (2003). Understanding the association between socioeconomic status and physical health: Do negative emotions play a role? *Psychological Bulletin, 129*, 10–51.

Gill, K. M., Carson, J. W., Porter, L. S., Scipio, C., Bediako, S. M., & Orringer, E. (2004). Daily mood and stress predict pain, health care use, and work activity in African American adults with sickle-cell disease. *Health Psychology, 23*, 267–274.

Gracely, R. H., Feisser, M. E., Fiesecke, T., Grant, M. A. B., Petzke, F., Williams, D. A., & Clauw, D. J. (2003). Pain catastrophizing and neural responses to pain among persons with fibromyalgia. *Brain, 127*, 835–843.

Hartman, J. M., Berger, A., Baker, K., Bolle, J., Handel, D., Mannes, A., Pereira, D., St. Germain, D., et al. (2006). Quality of life and pain in premenopausal women with major depressive disorder: The POWER Study. *Health and Quality of Life Outcomes, 4*, 2–6.

Hasenbring, M., Marienfeld, G., Kuhlendahl, D., & Soyka, D. (1994). Risk factors of cronicity in lumbar disc patients: A prospective investigation of biologic, psychologic, and social predictors of therapy outcome. *Spine, 19*, 2759–2765.

Heim, C., Newport, D. J., Bonsall, R., Miller, A. H., & Nemeroff, C. B. (2001). Altered pituitary-adrenal axis responses to provocative challenge tests in adult survivors of childhood abuse. *The American Journal of Psychiatry, 158*, 575–581.

Hoffman, B. M., Papas, R. K., Chatkoff, D. K., et al. (2007). Meta-analysis of psychological interventions for chronic low back pain. *Health Psychology, 26*, 1–9.

Holmes, T. H., & Rahe, R. H. (1967). The social readjustment rating scale. *Journal of Psychosomatic Research, 11*, 213–218.

Jensen, M. P., Turner, J. A., Romano, J. M., & Karoly, P. (1991). Coping with chronic pain: A critical review of the literature. *Pain, 47*, 249–283.

Kanegane, K., Penha, S. S., Munhoz, C. D., & Rocha, R. G. (2009). Dental anxiety and salivary cortisol levels before urgent dental care. *Journal of Oral Science, 51*, 515–520.

Koushede, V., Holstein, B., Andersen, A., Ekholm, L., & Hansen, E. H. (2010). Use of over-the-counter analgesics and perceived stress among 25–44 year olds. *Pharmacopeidemiology and Drug Safety, 19*, 351–357.

Lazarus, R. S., & Folkman, S. (1989). *Hassles and uplifts scales*. Palo Alto: Consulting Psychologists Press.

Mayer, E. A. (2000). The neurobiology of stress and gastrointestinal disease. *Gut, 47*, 861–869.

McBeth, J., Siolman, A. J., Gupta, A., et al. (2007). Moderation of psychosocial risk factors through dysfunction of the hypothalamic-pituitary-adrenal stress axis in the onset of chronic widespread musculoskeletal pain: Findings of a population-based prospective cohort study. *Arthritis and Rheumatology, 56*, 360–371.

McLean, S. A., Clauw, D. J., Abelson, J. L., & Liberzon, I. (2005). The development of persistent pain and psychological morbidity after motor vehicle collision: Integrating the potential role of stress response systems into a biopsychosocial model. *Psychosomatic Medicine, 67,* 783–790.

Melzack, R. (1999). Pain and stress: A new perspective. In R. J. Gatchel & D. C. Turk (Eds.), *Psychosocial factors in pain* (pp. 89–106). New York: Guilford Press.

Melzack, R. (2001). Pain and the neuromatrix in the brain. *Journal of Dental Education, 65,* 1378–1382.

Melzack, R., & Wall, P. D. (1965). Pain mechanisms: A new theory. *Science, 150,* 971–979.

Nilsen, K. B., Sand, T., Westgaard, R. H., et al. (2007). Autonomic activation and pain in response to low-grade mental stress in fibromyalgia and shoulder/neck pain patients. *European Journal of Pain, 11,* 743–755.

Ohayon, M. M., & Schatzberg, A. F. (2010). Chronic pain and major depressive disorder in the general population. *Journal of Psychiatric Research, 44,* 454–461.

Quale, A. J., & Schanke, A. K. (2010). Resilience in the face of coping with a severe physical injury: A study of trajectories of adjustment in a rehabilitation setting. *Rehabilitation Psychology, 55,* 12–22.

Rios, R., & Zautra, A. J. (2011). Socioeconomic disparities in pain: The role of economic hardship and daily financial worry. *Health Psychology, 30,* 58–66.

Sarason, I., Johnson, J., & Siegel, J. (1978). Assessing the impact of life changes: Development of the life experiences survey. *Journal of Consulting and Clinical Psychology, 46*(5), 932–946.

Simone, D. A. (1992). Neural mechanisms of hyperalgesia. *Current Opinions in Neurobiology, 2,* 479–483.

Skinner, M. A., Zautra, A. J., & Reich, J. W. (2004). Financial stress predictors and the emotional and physical health of chronic pain patients. *Cognitive Therapy and Research, 28,* 695–713.

Stasio, M. J., Curry, K., Sutton-Skinner, K. M., & Glassman, D. M. (2008). Over-the-counter medication and herbal or dietary supplement use in college: Dose frequency and relationship to self-reported distress. *Journal of American College Health, 56,* 535–547.

Staud, R., Craggs, J. G., Robinson, M. E., et al. (2007). Brain activity related to temporal summation of C-fiber evoked pain. *Pain, 129,* 130–142.

Turk, D. C., Audette, J., Lecy, R. M., Mackey, S. C., & Stanos, S. (2010). Assessment and treatment of psychosocial comorbidities in patients with neuropathic pain. *Mayo Clinic Proceedings, 85*(Suppl), S42–S50.

Vlaeyen, J. W. S., & Linton, S. J. (2000). Fear-avoidance and its consequences in chronic musculoskeletal pain: A state of the art. *Pain, 85,* 317–332.

Chapter 23
Hope in the Context of Pain and Palliative Care

Richard T. Penson, Lynette Su-Mien Ngo, and Gillianne Lai

Hope is a good thing, maybe the best thing, and no good thing ever dies.

Andy Dufresne, The Shawshank Redemption (1994 film)

Hope has been defined as "an inner power that facilitates the transcendence of the present situation and movement toward new awareness and enrichment of being" (Herth 1990). It is the belief in a positive outcome related to events and circumstances in one's life (Pickett et al. 2000). Qualitative studies including phenomenological, grounded theory, and ethnography suggest that hope is a complex, multidimensional, and dynamic set of biobehavioral factors that affect resilience, healing, coping, and quality of life in both healthy individuals and in medically ill and vulnerable patients (Cutcliffe 1998; Herth 1992; Miller and Powers 1988). Those confronted with life-threatening situations describe hope as a "positive expectation that goes beyond visible facts" (Fitzgerald 1979), a positive psychological and biophysical energy in situations of adversity (Frankl 1963; Korner 1970; McGee 1984). In this chapter, we primarily emphasize the biobehavioral understandings of hope in patients with cancer and related pain, with implications for pain in patients with other chronic illnesses.

Cancer and Pain: One Context for Understanding Hope

A universal and fundamental part of living, hope is recognized as a valuable human response (Dufault and Martocchio 1985) and an important coping mechanism (Herth 1989). Yet, from its diagnosis through the course of illness to progression to an incurable illness, cancer threatens hope and places patients in a very vulnerable position. Patients have to negotiate through feelings of anger, grief, despair, fear, anxiety, loss, and loneliness. The presence of pain in the context of cancer can also potentially threaten hope since patients are forced to face the threat of an uncertain future, including death. These are some of the barriers to hopefulness. Indeed, several studies have demonstrated that

R.T. Penson, MD, MRCP (✉)
Massachusetts General Hospital, Harvard Medical School, Boston, MA, USA
e-mail: rpenson@partners.org

L.S.-M. Ngo, MBBS, MRCP
National Cancer Centre Singapore, Singapore

G. Lai
National University of Singapore, Singapore

R.J. Moore (ed.), *Handbook of Pain and Palliative Care: Biobehavioral Approaches for the Life Course,*   383
DOI 10.1007/978-1-4419-1651-8_23, © Springer Science+Business Media, LLC 2012

pain and uncertainty separately influence the levels of hope in patients with cancer. A patient and survivor's ability to cope with new physical symptoms, increased disability, and the possibility of death also very much depends on their ability to re-define meaning in life, and to positively reframe hope and hopelessness in the context of living with a chronic illness (Park and Folkman 1997; Davis et al. 1998; Evans et al. 2006).

The Psychology of Hope: Factors Associated with Hope and Hopelessness

Studies have long sought to elucidate the meaning of hope in patients with cancer. Variations across age and stage of illness have also been described. Adolescents with cancer may see hope as a belief that a personal tomorrow exists (Hinds and Martin 1988). Elderly patients with advanced illness have described hope as an inner resource and spirituality as a coping mechanism essential for their quality of life (Duggleby and Wright 2005). In Benzein et al.'s narrative interview with 11 elderly patients, tension between hoping for a cure and living in the hope that encompassed reconciliation, comfort with life and death was noted to be a recurring theme (Benzein et al. 2001).

Other research suggests that levels of hope are not necessarily related to an individual's stage of cancer. Rather, potential threats to hope include a decline in physical well-being (McGill and Paul 1993), low socioeconomic status (McGill and Paul 1993) educational level (Rustoen and Wiklund 2000), as well as physical or psychological fatigue (Lee 2001). Put differently, hope and pain influence one another in a vicious cycle, with pain diminishing hope, and hopelessness in turn worsening pain. Christman examined the relationship between uncertainty, hope, symptom severity, control preference, and psychosocial adjustment in patients receiving radiotherapy for cancer (Christman 1990). At the end of treatment, an increase in severity of symptoms was associated with a significant increase in uncertainty and feeling less hopeful. Greater uncertainty and less hope were also associated with problems with adjustment across culturally diverse cancer patient populations. Raleigh interviewed 90 patients who reported that their levels of hope had an immediate influence on their experience of symptoms relating to their illness (Raleigh 1992). Coping strategies for pain management thus included utilization of family, friends, and religious beliefs to help support hope. In a study of Taiwanese lung cancer patients (Hsu et al. 2003), pain severity and interference with daily activities of living were found to be negatively correlated to hope. Brandt (1987) and Hwang et al. (1996) also reported similar outcomes in their studies, while Herth (1995) found that the engendering of hope was hampered by unrelieved cancer pain. It is clear that identifying and treating pain early while at the same time nurturing hope can prevent the downward spiral of uncontrolled pain and hopelessness.

One might also expect a difference in levels of hope between patients who are curatively and palliatively treated, yet no association was found between treatment intent and levels of hope in a survey done by Sanatani et al. on 50 patients, which showed that overall hope was maintained over time (Sanatani et al. 2008). There was, however, a trend towards fewer patients hoping for cure as time progressed. Similarly, Ballard et al. (1997) found no difference in the levels of hope between 20 patients with newly diagnosed cancer and 18 patients with recurrent cancer. Of note, married patients were found to have more hope, suggesting the importance of social support as a factor in fostering hope.

There have also been few well-controlled studies of interventions at the end of life, with the majority of observational studies focusing on overtreatment fuelled by the collusion of patient and clinician (Ho et al. 2011). However, a hugely important study published in the New England Journal of Medicine in 2010 documented an unexpected survival advantage in metastatic lung cancer patients anticipated to be in their last year of life who received early palliative care (Temel et al. 2010).

Although not in the primary analysis, the authors subsequently wrote that treatment of symptoms, particularly depression, may have been the major factor improving survival, and strongly suggested that hope is fueled by more than just chemotherapy.

Not many studies have examined the differences in hope by gender or ethnicity in cancer patients with adequate controls. Three themes appear in the literature: (1) young men cope relatively poorly with psychological interventions, even with negative counter-intuitive (Moynihan et al. 1999); (2) older and more isolated patients are more vulnerable to poorer quality of life and depression (Kornblith et al. 2010); (3) social, cultural, and ethnic discrimination as well as educational disadvantages have profound impacts on healthcare outcomes that likely cross all medical fields and all medical conditions (Diez Roux et al. 2001). These associations are currently not well understood and are certainly important hypotheses for future study (see also Green 2011).

The importance for adequate pain relief and attention to symptom control in cancer care cannot be further emphasized. The World Health Organization's (WHO) Cancer Unit has worked tirelessly from 1982 to implement global public health programs aimed at improving cancer pain relief, roll out cancer pain management protocols, and improve training and educational programs for healthcare workers. Since the publication of the interim guidelines (World Health Organization 1982) and the official handbook, *Cancer Pain Relief* (World Health Organization 1986) that followed in 1986, major advances have been made in the understanding, identification, and pharmaceutical management of cancer pain. Yet, more needs to be done. Today, two-thirds of adults with advanced malignant disease still experience pain despite advances in medical pain management. Perhaps a deeper understanding of the experience and meaning of pain, as well as the psychosocial and spiritual aspects of pain is still lacking.

Impact of Hope on Behavior

Hope can positively impact an individual's behavior and choices. Snyder conceptualized hope as a cognitive set that influenced behavior and affective functioning, and validated his theory in both healthy and medically ill patients (Snyder 1994, 2000, 2002; Snyder et al. 1991). He illustrated his theory with studies showing that higher dispositional hopeful thinking was associated with better social functioning (Kwon 2002; Barnum et al. 1998; Snyder et al. 1997), more adaptive physical health outcomes such as the acquisition of health knowledge (Irving et al. 1998) and ease of adjustment to chronic illnesses (Jackson et al. 1998; Elliott et al. 1991; Tennen and Affleck 1999). In healthy individuals, higher levels of hope were also found to be associated with superior performance in the academic (Chang 1998) and athletic arenas (Curry et al. 1997). Hence, facilitating hope in patients with terminal illnesses enables many to pursue attainable and meaningful goals, and better cope with dying.

Gum and Snyder (2002) proposed three strategies for health care providers to increase or maintain hope in patients. This can be done by assisting patients in developing alternative, important but achievable goals, actively identifying pathways for patients to reach these goals and enhancing patients' ability to overcome obstacles and pursue their goals. Current group or individual psychosocial interventions to increase hope include components of these suggested strategies (Klausner et al. 1998). At present, results from studies examining the benefits of cognitive behavioral therapy focusing on facilitating hope and successful goal pursuit in patients are divided, with many suffering methodological flaws such as small patient numbers or presence of other confounding factors. A literature review of psychosocial interventions for couples living with cancer cited heterogeneity in intervention programs and the instruments for measuring hope as the main reason for the widely varying outcomes and difficulty in drawing any conclusions (Busch et al. 2009). Even so, the results of the review found that psychosocial interventions generally decreased the levels of depression and hopelessness in both partners. These psychosocial interventions also highlight how with hope, patients are better able to identify meaningful and realistic desired outcomes, and harness the resources for pursuing those outcomes.

The Biology of Hope

In an attempt to better understand and appreciate the complexities of patients' coping responses through the progression of their illness, researchers have begun to study biobehavioral changes that occur at the molecular level in medically ill populations and have found mounting scientific evidence pointing to the involvement of the neuroendocrine system as well as inflammatory pathways in the regulation of behavior (Miller et al. 2008; Miller 1998). Clinical studies in cancer patients have revealed associations between immune cytokines, such as interleukin (IL)-6 (Musselman et al. 2001; Jehn et al. 2006; Meyers et al. 2005; Costanzo et al. 2005; Greenberg et al. 1993; Wratten et al. 2004; Mills et al. 2005; Geinitz et al. 2001; Ahlberg et al. 2004; Pusztai et al. 2004; Shafqat et al. 2005; Bower et al. 2002, 2003, 2007; Collado-Hidalgo et al. 2006; Knobel et al. 2000; Dimeo et al. 2004; Morant et al. 1993; Rich et al. 2005) as well as markers of systemic inflammation such as C-reactive protein (CRP) (Wratten et al. 2004; Morant et al. 1993; Brown et al. 2005) with depression, fatigue, sleep disturbances, and cognitive dysfunction.

Cytokines have been shown to alter the metabolism of neurotransmitters such as serotonin, norepinephrine, and dopamine, all of which play major roles in regulating behavior (Capuron et al. 2003; Bonaccorso et al. 2002; Zhu et al. 2005, 2006; Evans et al. 1986; Carlson et al. 2003), including the development and maintenance of depression, anxiety, and chronic pain states. There is also evidence that shows that cancer patients with major depression exhibit neuroendocrine changes that predispose to activation of inflammatory responses (Meyers et al. 2005; Costanzo et al. 2005; Andersen et al. 2007).

Biobehavioral Interventions

Given the relationship between inflammatory processes and depression, fatigue, sleep disturbance, and cognitive dysfunction, behavioral scientists began studying the significance of cognitive-behavioral, supportive, and psychoeducational interventions in relation to immune responses.

Several studies have shown that psychological interventions alleviate psychological distress in cancer patients, as well as normalize diurnal cortisol secretion and increase lymphocyte proliferative responses (Carlson et al. 2003; Andersen et al. 2004, 2007; Antoni et al. 2006; Cruess et al. 2000; McGregor et al. 2004; Kiecolt-Glaser et al. 1985). In a randomized controlled study by Fawzy et al. (1990, 1993), postsurgical patients with early stage malignant melanoma who received a 6-week structured group intervention consisting of health education, stress management techniques such as relaxation and psychological support not only demonstrated reduced psychological distress, they were also found to have significant increases in the percentage of large granular lymphocytes (defined as CD57 with Leu-7) and natural killer (NK) cells (defined as CD16 with Leu-11 and CD56 with NKH1) when compared with the control group of patients who received standard treatment. There were also indications of increased NK cytotoxic activity and a small decrease in the percentage of helper/inducer (CD4) T cells. Similarly, Anderson et al. (2004) who randomly assigned 227 women with surgically treated regional breast cancer to psychoeducational intervention, which included strategies to reduce stress, improve mood, and alter health behaviors or to regular assessment only, found stable or increased T-cell proliferation in response to stimulation with phytohemagglutinin and concanavalin A, in addition to significant lowering of anxiety, improvement in perceived social support, dietary habits, and reduction in smoking in the intervention group compared to the control group.

While there are no studies directly linking programs primarily aimed at fostering hope to changes in the neuroendocrine or immune pathways, this research does suggest that interventions which nurture, inspire, and maintain hope (Yancey et al. 1994; Koopmeiners et al. 1997; Rustoen et al. 1998; Herth 2000, 2001) can not only play an important role in helping patients cope effectively and improving their emotional well-being but may also enhance the biologic regulation of behavioral responses.

Additionally, exercise has been shown to change levels of cytokines and to decrease anxiety in cancer patients and survivors (Ligibel 2011). Exercise modulates behavior by increasing the white count by adrenergic effects on demargination of circulating leucocytes and steroidal effects on the bone marrow (Weight et al. 1991).

A number of studies have also been conducted on acupuncture and have demonstrated that this treatment is associated with higher white cell counts which fall less with chemotherapy (Lu et al. 2009). However, there is substantial controversy about studies that claim a link to more important outcomes like survival.

Hope and Patient Outcomes

Hope and Length of Survival

It is increasingly clear that hope can enhance quality of life in cancer patients. Can embracing hope extend the length of cancer survival? This question was addressed by two seminal randomized controlled trials in the USA. In 1989, Spiegel's group at Stanford showed survival benefit among 50 women with metastatic breast cancer receiving weekly supportive-expressive group therapy compared with standard medical therapy (Spiegel et al. 1989). Fawzy et al. (1993) evaluated long-term survival in 68 patients with malignant melanoma who participated in a 6-week psychiatric group intervention. He reported a statistically significant greater rate of death for patients in the control group compared with patients who participated in the 1.5-h weekly structured group meetings consisting of education, stress management, enhancement of coping skills, and psychological support. Multivariate analysis revealed that only two factors – having melanoma with a Breslow depth of 1.5 mm or greater and psychoeducational group intervention – were predictive of survival.

More than 20 psychoeducational intervention studies have since been conducted, amidst conflicting results and much heated debate and controversy. These include small sample sizes with their inherent sampling biases and survival not being a primary endpoint were these studies' main weaknesses. Fox (1995, 1999); Fox et al. (1989) examined the long-term survival of patients in Spiegel et al.'s study (1989) and compared them with a similar group of patients using the National Cancer Institute's Surveillance, Epidemiology and End Results (SEER) data. He found that the survival curves of the control sample of Spiegel's study and the regional population differed strikingly after 20 months, with only 2.8% of the control patients surviving beyond 5 years in contrast to 32% of patients from the SEER data who were alive at 5 years, suggesting that randomization failed to equalize baseline characteristics with a small control group. Similarly, critics (Coyne et al. 2007; Relman and Angell 2002) pointed out that survival was not a primary endpoint in Fawzy's study (1993), analyses were not intent to treat, and the sample was so small that the results lost statistical significance when one patient was reclassified.

Replication studies of psychoeducational intervention employing larger cohort sizes, specifying survival as the primary endpoint, and applying CONSORT guidelines (Altman et al. 2001) and intention-to-treat analyses have reported no survival benefit (Boesen et al. 2007; Goodwin et al. 2001; Kissane et al. 2004, 2007; Spiegel et al. 2007; Kissane and Li 2008). Three meta-analyses have also failed to find an overall effect of psychotherapy on survival (Chow et al. 2004; Edwards et al. 2004; Smedslund and Ringdal 2004).

Hope and Quality of Survival

Psychoeducational interventions do play a role in improving the quality of life for patients coping with cancer and its treatment (Kissane 2007). A systematic review reported positive effects of cognitive-behavioral interventions in women with gynecological cancer, with counseling appearing to be the most promising intervention strategy for addressing quality of life concerns (Hersch et al. 2009), while another meta-analysis of 37 published, controlled studies supported the effectiveness of psychosocial interventions for improving quality of life in adult cancer patients (Rehse and Pukrop 2003).

Hope in Social Networks: Coping with Cancer

A positive social well-being would intuitively contribute to a patient's inherent ability to cope with cancer. While the efficacy of psychotherapy and other related interventions in prolonging survival may be debatable, the impact of a strong social support network is being increasingly established. A prospective study by Epplein et al. (2010) evaluated the effects of various measures of quality of life on mortality and recurrence, and demonstrated that social well-being remained a good prognostic factor even after adjusting for known clinical predictors. Social networks conceivably improve emotion processing by increasing acceptance and decreasing distress, and this has been demonstrated to be distinctively protective against mortality in a study by Weihs et al. (2008). Though critics have cited statistical concerns about this study (Coyne and Thombs 2008), this is congruent with findings from a recent meta-analysis that showed an association between better social support and a 12–25% risk reduction in cancer mortality (Pinquart and Duberstein 2009).

An association between social well-being and improved disease outcomes would suggest that interventions to improve this factor would lead to prolonged survival and reduced recurrence. However, interventional studies to modify social well-being have generally not been able to demonstrate improved outcomes (Smedslund and Ringdal 2004; Falagas et al. 2007), suggesting that social networks reflect inherent socioeconomic, educational and access to care advantages more than a resilient ability to adjust, but there is enormous interest in the field (Christakis and Fowler 2011).

Hope in Palliative Care: When Hopelessness Hurts

A common fear is that when the patient gives up, the disease takes over, and relatives often plead for a loved one to not give up. How much this reflects subtle signals of disease progression as opposed to treatable problems like depression is often hard to discern. Accepting the inevitable is an important dignity and how this interfaces with hopelessness hurting is poorly studied.

A recent study seeking to identify the specific needs of patients with advanced, incurable cancer (Rainbird et al. 2009) revealed that areas of unmet need were in the psychological and the medical communication domains. Up to 40% of the patients reported a moderate to high level of need in the area of informational and psychological support.

Patients also consistently stated in studies on patient preferences for oncologist communication that they wanted to hear biomedical information about their disease and treatment (Innes and Payne 2009; Hagerty et al. 2004; Wright et al. 2004). Although the majority of patients wanted their oncologist to be honest and realistic, they also want truth-telling to be balanced with hope (Innes and Payne 2009; Parker et al. 2001; Clayton et al. 2005a; Ptacek and Eberhardt 1996) (see also Schapira and Steensma 2011).

In a study by Kutner et al. (1999), all of the 56 patients interviewed wanted the doctor to be honest, yet 91% wanted the approach to be optimistic. Similarly, in a systematic narrative review of 13 studies identified (Innes and Payne 2009), four studies found that while almost all patients wanted qualitative information (i.e., that their illness was life limiting), fewer wanted quantitative information like statistics and timeframes. Hope was a recurring theme; while for some patients, hope was the possibility of recovery, for others it was engendered by honesty, knowledge, and feeling in control. A good death inventory, developed from a bereaved family member's perspective, included maintaining hope as one of the ten key domains (Miyashita et al. 2008).

Hope in Complementary and Alternative Medicine

The use of alternative and complementary therapies (CAM) is becoming increasingly popular, especially among cancer patients (Eisenberg et al. 1998; Ernst and Cassileth 1998; Navo et al. 2004; Shen et al. 2002) (see also Kutner and Smith 2011). From 1990 to 1997, the use of CAM had increased by 65% to an estimated 42.1% of the US adult population (83 million people) (Eisenberg et al. 1998). A 1998 systematic review of studies assessing the prevalence of CAM in 13 countries concluded that about 31% of cancer patients use some form of CAM, with rates ranging up to 64% (Ernst and Cassileth 1998).

Verhoef et al. (2005) conducted a systematic review of 500 published studies on the motivations for cancer patients to use CAM and identified perceived beneficial response, desire for control, and a strong belief in CAM as prominent motivators for the use of CAM.

The benefit of CAM therapies in cancer is highly controversial. Several published systematic reviews of clinical trials on CAM in cancer patients suggest a role for acupuncture, therapeutic touch, hypnosis, and music therapy in the palliation of cancer-related pain, dyspnea, and anxiety (Pan et al. 2000; Rajasekaran et al. 2005; Spence and Olson 1997; Hilliard 2005). Unfortunately, while seemingly promising, evidence supporting the use of CAM has been plagued by a lack of rigorously conducted systematic reviews or well-designed, multi-institutional randomized controlled trials (Lee et al. 2005; Bardia et al. 2006; Sood et al. 2005). Numerous flaws in research design, such as insufficient statistical power or duration of study, poor controls or lack of sham controls, and treatment variation within and between subjects, have been the subject of criticism (Nahin and Straus 2001). Some therapies have been noted to be no more effective than placebo (Shang et al. 2005), while others have been found to have harmful, adverse effects (Pinn 2001; Saper et al. 2004; Ko 1998; Angell and Kassirer 1998; Izzo and Ernst 2001). Moreover, studies have shown that patients frequently do not discuss CAM therapies with their treating physicians (Eisenberg et al. 1998; Adler and Fosket 1999; Kaye et al. 2000) and that many oncologists have limited knowledge of CAM (Newell and Sanson-Fisher 2000).

Yet, the popularity of CAM therapies among cancer patients continues to rise. This has been attributed to the underlying theme of harnessing hope with CAM (Penson et al. 2001). In the face of cancer, with its impending threat of death, deteriorating physical well-being, and associated psychological distress, CAM provides a positive source of hope in enhancing quality of life. In a UK survey of cancer patients, patients report to being less anxious, emotionally stronger, and more hopeful about the future, even if the cancer remained. Strong practitioner–patient relationships, clarity of explanations, and the treatment environment were cited as reasons for the high satisfaction that they experienced (Back et al. 2003). While these reasons may serve to augment the therapeutic outcome of treatment, thus serving as potential contributory factors to the "placebo effect," it may arguably be reasonable to employ CAM solely for maintaining hope and improving patients' quality of life (Penson et al. 2007).

Though the role of CAM in cancer treatment is still highly contentious, it is widely agreed that all cancer patients should be managed by multidisciplinary teams, including doctors, nurses, and practitioners in professions complementary to medicine for the best chance of cure or prolonging life, palliation, and psychosocial and spiritual support.

Hope That Disappoints: The Ethics of Honesty and Hope

Providing and sustaining hope for patients with cancer has been increasingly recognized by physicians as an important element in helping patients cope with their illness. Similarly, many patients seek physicians who are strong advocates of prolonging life, positive about treatment outcomes, and who will search every avenue of hope (Back et al. 2003). Yet, this expectation can place the physician in a dilemma of being unrealistic and encouraging false hope.

Focusing exclusively on hope can leave patients unaware of their limited life expectancy (Lamont and Christakis 2001). It can also deny them the opportunity to adequately manage pain and other symptoms, address fears and uncertainties, clarify priorities, or make financial, psychosocial, and spiritual preparations, factors identified as important components of a good death (Steinhauser et al. 2000; Singer et al. 1999).

Back et al. believes that truth-telling and maintaining hope need not be mutually exclusive (Back et al. 2003) (see also Schapira and Steensma 2011). He also provides a framework for physicians to help patients "hope for the best and prepare for the worst" by (1) giving equal air time to hoping and preparing, (2) aligning patient and physician hopes, (3) encouraging but not imposing the dual agenda of hoping and preparing, (4) supporting the evolution of hope and preparation over time, and (5) respecting hopes and fears and responding to emotions. Moreover, holding a frank and honest discussion about the patient's illness and prognosis engenders trust and strengthens the doctor–patient relationship (Butow et al. 2002; Sapir et al. 2000; Friedrichsen et al. 2000). Helft suggested a "metered" way of communicating prognosis with patients, dosing information like a drug depending on their clinical situation (Helft 2006).

Communication skills and appropriateness of time and environment plays an important role in maintaining hope in prognostic communication with cancer patients. Recent systematic reviews of published studies exploring cancer patients' preferences towards information provision and prognosis communication suggested that the majority of patients desired detailed prognostic information (Innes and Payne 2009; Hagerty et al. 2005a; Parker et al. 2007; Clayton et al. 2008), presented in an open and honest manner (Kutner et al. 1999; Wenrich et al. 2001; Kirk et al. 2004; Clayton et al. 2005b), while at the same time conveying a sense of hope (Clayton et al. 2005a; Ptacek and Eberhardt 1996; Wenrich et al. 2001; Hagerty et al. 2005b). Not knowing one's clinical reality is often associated with uncertainty and unrealistic fears. Being well informed enables patients to maintain hope by freeing them from anxiety and fear (Wenrich et al. 2001). Recognizing the importance of providing hope and sensitivity while at the same time delivering prognostic information with honesty and realism, a national initiative in Australia was undertaken in the form of the Australian Psychosocial Clinical Practice Guidelines (Initiative NBCCaNCC 2003) to make recommendations addressing appropriate communication techniques.

When All Hope Is Gone: A "Good Death,", a "Good Life"

Patients often feel that they must choose between hoping for a cure and preparing for death when they are faced with a life-threatening illness (Delvecchio Good et al. 1990). Yet, in a systematic review of 27 studies, patients seem to be able to maintain a sense of hope despite acknowledging the terminal nature of their illness (Clayton et al. 2008). When cure of the disease is out of reach, patients with high levels of hope may redefine priorities to be more realistic and to have more meaningful goals.

The concept of a good death was examined by Kehl with an analysis of 42 published papers (Kehl 2006). A good death was found to be highly individual, changeable over time, and based on perspective and experience. Common attributes of a good death included being in control, being comfortable, having a sense of closure, honoring beliefs and values, minimizing burdens, and leaving a legacy.

In his seminal text, *How we die: Reflections of Life's Final* Chapters (Nuland 1994), Nuland stresses that doctors should instill in patients the hope not for a miraculous cure, but for dignity and a high quality of life. As Nuland states eloquently, "the greatest dignity to be found in death is the dignity of the life that precedes it. This is a form of hope we can all achieve."

Palliative care physician and past president of the American Academy of Hospice and Palliative Medicine, Ira Byock, provides further guidance and empowers people with life-threatening illnesses to die well by living well. Cautioning against the use of the phrase "A Good Death" which evokes images of preparing for the final terminal event, Byock urges one to strive for an experiential personal journey encompassing meaning, purpose, emotional healing, and a sense of completion. In his book, *Dying Well: The prospect for growth at the end of life* (Byock 1997), he lists the key to living well and thus dying well, as an expression of the five Things of Relationship Completion: "I forgive you"; "Forgive me"; "Thank you"; "I love you," and "Goodbye."

The value of improving the level of palliative care and palliative care education has also been emphasized by journalist Bill Moyers in his recent television program *Dying in America*. In an intimate glimpse of the final days of several patients and the challenges faced in living with dying, the importance of the contribution by palliative care providers is poignantly captured.

Hope and Spirituality: How Spirituality Sustains Hope

Spirituality is an important component of holistic palliative care (*see also* Wachholtz and Makowski 2011). Despite the endless debate on the definition of spirituality, there is general consensus that spiritual care is an essential component of end-of-life care. Spiritual well-being is identified by the Institute of Medicine as one of the six domains of quality end-of-life care (Field and Cassel 1997). The WHO describes effective palliative care as one which encompasses the integration of the psychological and spiritual aspects of care in the supportive care of the dying (WHO 2011). After convening an end-of-life consensus panel, The American College of Physicians published guidelines stating that physicians should extend their care for those with serious medical illness by attentiveness to psychosocial, existential, or spiritual suffering (Lo et al. 1999).

Spirituality can mean different things to different people. A review of publications by Unruh et al. in the occupational therapy literature alone yielded a staggering 92 definitions of spirituality (Unruh et al. 2002). However, common themes have emerged whereby spiritual peace is thought to encompass a sense of transcendence, where meaning in life, suffering, and death is grasped and experienced, be it in the context of religious values and beliefs or in relationships with loved ones, nature, or other forms of expression such as art or music. In a recent qualitative analysis of published medical literature on spirituality in the past 10 years (Vachon et al. 2009), 11 dimensions for the concept of end-of-life spirituality were identified: meaning and purpose in life, self-transcendence, transcendence with a higher being, feelings of communion and mutuality, belief and faith, hope, attitude toward death, appreciation of life, reflection upon fundamental values, the developmental nature of spirituality, and its conscious aspect. Hope emerged as a significant component of spirituality, ranging from hoping for life after death to hoping for a painless death or to conclude unfinished business. Kissane et al. advocated the use of the term Demoralization syndrome as a relevant diagnostic tool for spiritual distress in palliative care. He defined Demoralization syndrome as "a psychiatric state in which hopelessness, helplessness, meaninglessness, and existential distress are the core phenomena" (Kissane et al. 2001).

Spiritual distress exacerbates symptoms of pain, anxiety, and depression (Chochinov et al. 1995; Breitbart et al. 2000; McClain et al. 2003; Kaczorowski 1989). Conversely, patients with increased spiritual well-being have improved quality of life and coping skills (Cotton et al. 1999; Fehring et al. 1997). Moadel et al. 1999 investigated the spiritual and existential needs of 248 ethnically diverse urban sample of cancer patients in New York, USA and identified areas of unmet spiritual or existential needs to include needing help in overcoming fears, finding hope and meaning in life, finding spiritual resources and having someone to talk with about the meaning of life and death and finding peace of mind.

Acknowledging spiritual distress can in itself be therapeutic. Helping patients find meaning and facilitating hope reduces existential or spiritual suffering. More importantly, making ourselves available and walking with patients in their journey comforts and contributes to spiritual healing.

The strength of spirituality is beautifully summed up by Rabbi Harold Kushner in his book, *The Lord is My Shepherd*, based on the twenty-third psalm of the Bible. He states: "…and somehow they found the strength to go on. They found a sense of purpose to their lives, refusing to let tragedy define them. Let God take you by the hand as he did for them and lead you through the valley of darkness" (Kushner 2003).

Conclusion

Hope can exist, even when the challenge is impossible, the odds long, and the time short. There is a privilege and responsibility in patient–caregiver relationships to nurture realistic hopefulness and to not abandon patients to fear and despair in their last days. The best care demands the science of medicine and the art of compassion. Then we can all speak the language of hope, trust, and respect.

References

Adler, S. R., & Fosket, J. R. (1999). Disclosing complementary and alternative medicine use in the medical encounter: A qualitative study in women with breast cancer. *Journal of Family Practice, 48*, 453–458.

Ahlberg, K., Ekman, T., & Gaston-Johansson, F. (2004). Levels of fatigue compared to levels of cytokines and hemoglobin during pelvic radiotherapy: A pilot study. *Biological Research for Nursing, 5*, 203–210.

Altman, D. G., Schulz, K. F., Moher, D., et al. (2001). The revised CONSORT statement for reporting randomized trials: Explanation and elaboration. *Annals of Internal Medicine, 134*, 663–694.

Andersen, B. L., Farrar, W. B., Golden-Kreutz, D. M., et al. (2004). Psychological, behavioral, and immune changes after a psychological intervention: A clinical trial. *Journal of Clinical Oncology, 22*, 3570–3580.

Andersen, B. L., Farrar, W. B., Golden-Kreutz, D., et al. (2007). Distress reduction from a psychological intervention contributes to improved health for cancer patients. *Brain, Behavior, and Immunity, 21*, 953–961.

Angell, M., & Kassirer, J. P. (1998). Alternative medicine–the risks of untested and unregulated remedies. *The New England Journal of Medicine, 339*, 839–841.

Antoni, M. H., Wimberly, S. R., Lechner, S. C., et al. (2006). Reduction of cancer-specific thought intrusions and anxiety symptoms with a stress management intervention among women undergoing treatment for breast cancer. *The American Journal of Psychiatry, 163*, 1791–1797.

Back, A. L., Arnold, R. M., & Quill, T. E. (2003). Hope for the best, and prepare for the worst. *Annals of Internal Medicine, 138*, 439–443.

Ballard, A., Green, T., McCaa, A., et al. (1997). A comparison of the level of hope in patients with newly diagnosed and recurrent cancer. *Oncology Nursing Forum, 24*, 899–904.

Bardia, A., Barton, D. L., Prokop, L. J., et al. (2006). Efficacy of complementary and alternative medicine therapies in relieving cancer pain: A systematic review. *Journal of Clinical Oncology, 24*, 5457–5464.

Barnum, D. D., Snyder, C. R., Rapoff, M. A., et al. (1998). Hope and social support in the psychological adjustment of children who have survived burns and their matched controls. *Children's Health Care, 27*, 15–30.

Benzein, E., Norberg, A., & Saveman, B. I. (2001). The meaning of the lived experience of hope in patients with cancer in palliative home care. *Palliative Medicine, 15*, 117–126.

Boesen, E. H., Boesen, S. H., Frederiksen, K., et al. (2007). Survival after a psychoeducational intervention for patients with cutaneous malignant melanoma: A replication study. *Journal of Clinical Oncology, 25*, 5698–5703.

Bonaccorso, S., Marino, V., Puzella, A., et al. (2002). Increased depressive ratings in patients with hepatitis C receiving interferon-alpha-based immunotherapy are related to interferon-alpha-induced changes in the serotonergic system. *Journal of Clinical Psychopharmacology, 22*, 86–90.

Bower, J. E., Ganz, P. A., Aziz, N., et al. (2002). Fatigue and proinflammatory cytokine activity in breast cancer survivors. *Psychosomatic Medicine, 64*, 604–611.

Bower, J. E., Ganz, P. A., Aziz, N., et al. (2003). T-cell homeostasis in breast cancer survivors with persistent fatigue. *Journal of the National Cancer Institute, 95*, 1165–1168.

Bower, J. E., Ganz, P. A., Aziz, N., et al. (2007). Inflammatory responses to psychological stress in fatigued breast cancer survivors: Relationship to glucocorticoids. *Brain, Behavior, and Immunity, 21*, 251–258.

Brandt, B. T. (1987). The relationship between hopelessness and selected variables in women receiving chemotherapy for breast cancer. *Oncology Nursing Forum, 14*, 35–39.

Breitbart, W., Rosenfeld, B., Pessin, H., et al. (2000). Depression, hopelessness, and desire for hastened death in terminally ill patients with cancer. *JAMA, 284*, 2907–2911.

Brown, D. J., McMillan, D. C., & Milroy, R. (2005). The correlation between fatigue, physical function, the systemic inflammatory response, and psychological distress in patients with advanced lung cancer. *Cancer, 103*, 377–382.

Busch, A. K., Schnepp, W., & Spirig, R. (2009). Psychosocial interventions for couples living with cancer. A literature review. *Pflege, 22*, 254–265.

Butow, P. N., Dowsett, S., Hagerty, R., et al. (2002). Communicating prognosis to patients with metastatic disease: What do they really want to know? *Supportive Care in Cancer, 10*, 161–168.

Byock, I. (1997). *Dying well: The prospect for growth at the end of life.* Riverhead Books: New York.

Capuron, L., Neurauter, G., Musselman, D. L., et al. (2003). Interferon-alpha-induced changes in tryptophan metabolism. Relationship to depression and paroxetine treatment. *Biological Psychiatry, 54*, 906–914.

Carlson, L. E., Speca, M., Patel, K. D., et al. (2003). Mindfulness-based stress reduction in relation to quality of life, mood, symptoms of stress, and immune parameters in breast and prostate cancer outpatients. *Psychosomatic Medicine, 65*, 571–581.

Chang, E. C. (1998). Hope, problem-solving ability, and coping in a college student population: Some implications for theory and practice. *Journal of Clinical Psychology, 54*, 953–962.

Chochinov, H. M., Wilson, K. G., Enns, M., et al. (1995). Desire for death in the terminally ill. *The American Journal of Psychiatry, 152*, 1185–1191.

Chow, E., Tsao, M. N., & Harth, T. (2004). Does psychosocial intervention improve survival in cancer? A meta-analysis. *Palliative Medicine, 18*, 25–31.

Christakis, N. A., & Fowler, J. H. (2011). Connected: The surprising power of our social networks and how they shape our lives. 352 pages. Little, Brown and Company (September 28, 2009). Boston, MA.

Christman, N. J. (1990). Uncertainty and adjustment during radiotherapy. *Nursing Research, 39*, 17–20. 47.

Clayton, J. M., Butow, P. N., Arnold, R. M., et al. (2005a). Fostering coping and nurturing hope when discussing the future with terminally ill cancer patients and their caregivers. *Cancer, 103*, 1965–1975.

Clayton, J. M., Butow, P. N., Arnold, R. M., et al. (2005b). Discussing life expectancy with terminally ill cancer patients and their carers: A qualitative study. *Supportive Care in Cancer, 13*, 733–742.

Clayton, J. M., Hancock, K., Parker, S., et al. (2008). Sustaining hope when communicating with terminally ill patients and their families: A systematic review. *Psycho-Oncology, 17*, 641–659.

Collado-Hidalgo, A., Bower, J. E., Ganz, P. A., et al. (2006). Inflammatory biomarkers for persistent fatigue in breast cancer survivors. *Clinical Cancer Research, 12*, 2759–2766.

Costanzo, E. S., Lutgendorf, S. K., Sood, A. K., et al. (2005). Psychosocial factors and interleukin-6 among women with advanced ovarian cancer. *Cancer, 104*, 305–313.

Cotton, S. P., Levine, E. G., Fitzpatrick, C. M., et al. (1999). Exploring the relationships among spiritual well-being, quality of life, and psychological adjustment in women with breast cancer. *Psycho-Oncology, 8*, 429–438.

Coyne, J. C., Stefanek, M., & Palmer, S. C. (2007). Psychotherapy and survival in cancer: The conflict between hope and evidence. *Psychological Bulletin, 133*, 367–394.

Coyne, J. C., & Thombs, B. D. (2008). Was it shown that "Close relationships and emotional processing predict decreased mortality in women with breast cancer?" a critique of Weihs et al. (2008). *Psychosomatic Medicine. 70*, 737–738; author reply 738–739.

Cruess, D. G., Antoni, M. H., McGregor, B. A., et al. (2000). Cognitive-behavioral stress management reduces serum cortisol by enhancing benefit finding among women being treated for early stage breast cancer. *Psychosomatic Medicine, 62*, 304–308.

Curry, L. A., Snyder, C. R., Cook, D. L., et al. (1997). Role of hope in academic and sport achievement. *Journal of Personality and Social Psychology, 73*, 1257–1267.

Cutcliffe, J. R. (1998). Hope, counselling and complicated bereavement reactions. *Journal of Advanced Nursing, 28*, 754–761.

Davis, C. G., Nolen-Hoeksema, S., & Larson, J. (1998). Making sense of loss and benefiting from the experience: Two construals of meaning. *Journal of Personality and Social Psychology, 75*, 561–574.

Delvecchio Good, M. J., Good, B. J., Schaffer, C., et al. (1990). American oncology and the discourse on hope. *Culture, Medicine and Psychiatry, 14*, 59–79.

Diez Roux, A. V., Merkin, S. S., Arnett, D., et al. (2001). Neighborhood of residence and incidence of coronary heart disease. *The New England Journal of Medicine, 345*, 99–106.

Dimeo, F., Schmittel, A., Fietz, T., et al. (2004). Physical performance, depression, immune status and fatigue in patients with hematological malignancies after treatment. *Annals of Oncology, 15*, 1237–1242.

Dufault, K., & Martocchio, B. C. (1985). Symposium on compassionate care and the dying experience. Hope: Its spheres and dimensions. *Nursing Clinics of North America, 20*, 379–391.

Duggleby, W., & Wright, K. (2005). Transforming hope: How elderly palliative patients live with hope. *Canadian Journal of Nursing Research, 37*, 70–84.

Edwards, A. G., Hailey, S., & Maxwell, M. (2004). Psychological interventions for women with metastatic breast cancer. *Cochrane Database of Systematic Reviews*. (2), CD004253.

Eisenberg, D. M., Davis, R. B., Ettner, S. L., et al. (1998). Trends in alternative medicine use in the United States, 1990–1997: Results of a follow-up national survey. *JAMA, 280*, 1569–1575.

Elliott, T. R., Witty, T. E., Herrick, S., et al. (1991). Negotiating reality after physical loss: Hope, depression, and disability. *Journal of Personality and Social Psychology, 61*, 608–613.

Epplein, M., Zheng, Y., Zheng, W., et al. (2010). Quality of life after breast cancer diagnosis and survival. *Journal of Clinical Oncology, 29*, 406–412.

Ernst, E., & Cassileth, B. R. (1998). The prevalence of complementary/alternative medicine in cancer: A systematic review. *Cancer, 83*, 777–782.

Evans, D. L., McCartney, C. F., Nemeroff, C. B., et al. (1986). Depression in women treated for gynecological cancer: Clinical and neuroendocrine assessment. *The American Journal of Psychiatry, 143*, 447–452.

Evans, W. G., Tulsky, J. A., Back, A. L., et al. (2006). Communication at times of transitions: How to help patients cope with loss and re-define hope. *Cancer Journal, 12*, 417–424.

Falagas, M. E., Zarkadoulia, E. A., Ioannidou, E. N., et al. (2007). The effect of psychosocial factors on breast cancer outcome: A systematic review. *Breast Cancer Research, 9*, R44.

Fawzy, F. I., Fawzy, N. W., Hyun, C. S., et al. (1993). Malignant melanoma. Effects of an early structured psychiatric intervention, coping, and affective state on recurrence and survival 6 years later. *Archives of General Psychiatry, 50*, 681–689.

Fawzy, F. I., Kemeny, M. E., Fawzy, N. W., et al. (1990). A structured psychiatric intervention for cancer patients. II. Changes over time in immunological measures. *Archives of General Psychiatry, 47*, 729–735.

Fehring, R. J., Miller, J. F., & Shaw, C. (1997). Spiritual well-being, religiosity, hope, depression, and other mood states in elderly people coping with cancer. *Oncology Nursing Forum, 24*, 663–671.

Field, M. J., & Cassel, C. K. (1997). Institute of Medicine (U.S.) Committee on Care at the End of Life. Approaching death: Improving care at the end of life. Washington: National Academy Press.

Fitzgerald, R. (1979). *The sources of hope*. Rushcutters Bay: Pergamon Press.

Fox, B. H. (1995). Some problems and some solutions in research on psychotherapeutic intervention in cancer. *Supportive Care in Cancer, 3*, 257–263.

Fox, B. H. (1999). Clarification regarding comments about a hypothesis. *Psycho-Oncology, 8*, 366–367.

Fox, B. H., et al. (1989). A hypothesis about Spiegel et al.'s,1989 paper on Psychosocial intervention and breast cancer survival. *Psycho-Oncology, 7*(361–70), 1998.

Frankl, V. E. (1963). *Man's search for meaning; an introduction to logotherapy*. Boston: Beacon Press.

Friedrichsen, M. J., Strang, P. M., & Carlsson, M. E. (2000). Breaking bad news in the transition from curative to palliative cancer care–patient's view of the doctor giving the information. *Supportive Care in Cancer, 8*, 472–478.

Geinitz, H., Zimmermann, F. B., Stoll, P., et al. (2001). Fatigue, serum cytokine levels, and blood cell counts during radiotherapy of patients with breast cancer. *International Journal of Radiation Oncology, Biology, and Physics, 51*, 691–698.

Goodwin, P. J., Leszcz, M., Ennis, M., et al. (2001). The effect of group psychosocial support on survival in metastatic breast cancer. *The New England Journal of Medicine, 345*, 1719–1726.

Green, C. (2011). Disparities in pain management and palliative care. In R. J. Moore (Ed.), *Handbook of pain and palliative care: Biobehavioral approaches for the life course*. New York: Springer.

Greenberg, D. B., Gray, J. L., Mannix, C. M., et al. (1993). Treatment-related fatigue and serum interleukin-1 levels in patients during external beam irradiation for prostate cancer. *Journal of Pain and Symptom Management, 8*, 196–200.

Gum, A., & Snyder, C. R. (2002). Coping with terminal illness: The role of hopeful thinking. *Journal of Palliative Medicine, 5*, 883–894.

Hagerty, R. G., Butow, P. N., Ellis, P. A., et al. (2004). Cancer patient preferences for communication of prognosis in the metastatic setting. *Journal of Clinical Oncology, 22*, 1721–1730.

Hagerty, R. G., Butow, P. N., Ellis, P. M., et al. (2005a). Communicating prognosis in cancer care: A systematic review of the literature. *Annals of Oncology, 16*, 1005–1053.

Hagerty, R. G., Butow, P. N., Ellis, P. M., et al. (2005b). Communicating with realism and hope: Incurable cancer patients' views on the disclosure of prognosis. *Journal of Clinical Oncology, 23*, 1278–1288.

Helft, P. R. (2006). An intimate collaboration: Prognostic communication with advanced cancer patients. *The Journal of Clinical Ethics, 17*, 110–121.

Hersch, J., Juraskova, I., Price, M., et al. (2009). Psychosocial interventions and quality of life in gynaecological cancer patients: A systematic review. *Psycho-Oncology, 18*, 795–810.

Herth, K. A. (1989). The relationship between level of hope and level of coping response and other variables in patients with cancer. *Oncology Nursing Forum, 16*, 67–72.

Herth, K. (1990). Fostering hope in terminally-ill people. *Journal of Advanced Nursing, 15*, 1250–1259.

Herth, K. (1992). Abbreviated instrument to measure hope: Development and psychometric evaluation. *Journal of Advanced Nursing, 17*, 1251–1259.

Herth, K. (1995). Engendering hope in the chronically and terminally ill: Nursing interventions. *The American Journal of Hospice & Palliative Care, 12*, 31–39.

Herth, K. (2000). Enhancing hope in people with a first recurrence of cancer. *Journal of Advanced Nursing, 32*, 1431–1441.

Herth, K. A. (2001). Development and implementation of a Hope Intervention Program. *Oncology Nursing Forum, 28*, 1009–1016.

Hilliard, R. E. (2005). Music therapy in hospice and palliative care: A review of the empirical data. *Evidence Based Complementary and Alternative Medicine, 2*, 173–178.

Hinds, P. S., & Martin, J. (1988). Hopefulness and the self-sustaining process in adolescents with cancer. *Nursing Research, 37*, 336–340.

Ho, T. H., Barbera, L., Saskin, R., et al. (2011). Trends in the aggressiveness of end-of-life cancer care in the Universal Health Care System of Ontario, Canada. *Journal of Clinical Oncology, 29*, 1587–1591.

Hsu, T. H., Lu, M. S., Tsou, T. S., et al. (2003). The relationship of pain, uncertainty, and hope in Taiwanese lung cancer patients. *Journal of Pain and Symptom Management, 26*, 835–842.

Hwang, R., Ku, N., Mao, H., et al. (1996). Hope and related factors of breast cancer women. *Nursing Research, 4*, 35–45.

Initiative NBCCaNCC. (2003). *Clinical practice guidelines for the psychosocial care of adults with cancer*. Camperdown: National Breast Cancer Centre.

Innes, S., & Payne, S. (2009). Advanced cancer patients' prognostic information preferences: A review. *Palliative Medicine, 23*, 29–39.

Irving, L. M., Snyder, C. R., & Crowson, J. J., Jr. (1998). Hope and coping with cancer by college women. *Journal of Personality, 66*, 195–214.

Izzo, A. A., & Ernst, E. (2001). Interactions between herbal medicines and prescribed drugs: A systematic review. *Drugs, 61*, 2163–2175.

Jackson, W. T., Taylor, R. E., Palmatier, A. D., et al. (1998). Negotiating the reality of visual impairment: Hope, coping and functional ability. *Journal of Clinical Psychology in Medical Settings, 5*, 173–185.

Jehn, C. F., Kuehnhardt, D., Bartholomae, A., et al. (2006). Biomarkers of depression in cancer patients. *Cancer, 107*, 2723–2729.

Kaczorowski, J. M. (1989). Spiritual well-being and anxiety in adults diagnosed with cancer. *The Hospice Journal, 5*, 105–116.

Kaye, A. D., Clarke, R. C., Sabar, R., et al. (2000). Herbal medicines: Current trends in anesthesiology practice– a hospital survey. *Journal of Clinical Anesthesia, 12*, 468–471.

Kehl, K. A. (2006). Moving toward peace: An analysis of the concept of a good death. *The American Journal of Hospice & Palliative Care, 23*, 277–286.

Kiecolt-Glaser, J. K., Glaser, R., Williger, D., et al. (1985). Psychosocial enhancement of immunocompetence in a geriatric population. *Health Psychology, 4*, 25–41.

Kirk, P., Kirk, I., & Kristjanson, L. J. (2004). What do patients receiving palliative care for cancer and their families want to be told? A Canadian and Australian qualitative study. *British Medical Journal, 328*, 1343.

Kissane, D. W. (2007). Letting go of the hope that psychotherapy prolongs cancer survival. *Journal of Clinical Oncology, 25*, 5689–5690.

Kissane, D. W., Clarke, D. M., & Street, A. F. (2001). Demoralization syndrome–a relevant psychiatric diagnosis for palliative care. *Journal of Palliative Care, 17,* 12–21.

Kissane, D. W., Grabsch, B., Clarke, D. M., et al. (2007). Supportive-expressive group therapy for women with metastatic breast cancer: Survival and psychosocial outcome from a randomized controlled trial. *Psycho-Oncology, 16,* 277–286.

Kissane, D., & Li, Y. (2008). Effects of supportive-expressive group therapy on survival of patients with metastatic breast cancer: A randomized prospective trial. *Cancer. 112,* 443–444; author reply 444.

Kissane, D. W., Love, A., Hatton, A., et al. (2004). Effect of cognitive-existential group therapy on survival in early-stage breast cancer. *Journal of Clinical Oncology, 22,* 4255–4260.

Klausner, E. J., Clarkin, J. F., Spielman, L., et al. (1998). Late-life depression and functional disability: The role of goal-focused group psychotherapy. *International Journal of Geriatric Psychiatry, 13,* 707–716.

Knobel, H., Loge, J. H., Nordoy, T., et al. (2000). High level of fatigue in lymphoma patients treated with high dose therapy. *Journal of Pain and Symptom Management, 19,* 446–456.

Ko, R. J. (1998). Adulterants in Asian patent medicines. *The New England Journal of Medicine, 339,* 847.

Koopmeiners, L., Post-White, J., Gutknecht, S., et al. (1997). How healthcare professionals contribute to hope in patients with cancer. *Oncology Nursing Forum, 24,* 1507–1513.

Kornblith, A. B., Mirabeau-Beale, K., Lee, H., et al. (2010). Long-term adjustment of survivors of ovarian cancer treated for advanced-stage disease. *Journal of Psychosocial Oncology, 28,* 451–469.

Korner, I. N. (1970). Hope as a method of coping. *Journal of Consulting and Clinical Psychology, 34,* 134–139.

Kushner, H. S. (2003). *The Lord is my shepherd: Healing wisdom of the twenty-third Psalm* (1st ed.). New York: Alfred A. Knopf.

Kutner, J. S., & Smith, M. C. (2011). CAM in chronic pain and palliative care. In R. J. Moore (Ed.), *Handbook of pain and palliative care: Biobehavioral approaches for the life course.* New York: Springer.

Kutner, J. S., Steiner, J. F., Corbett, K. K., et al. (1999). Information needs in terminal illness. *Social Science & Medicine, 48,* 1341–1352.

Kwon, P. (2002). Hope, defense mechanisms, and adjustment: Implications for false hope and defensive hopelessness. *Journal of Personality, 70,* 207–231.

Lamont, E. B., & Christakis, N. A. (2001). Prognostic disclosure to patients with cancer near the end of life. *Annals of Internal Medicine, 134,* 1096–1105.

Lee, E. H. (2001). Fatigue and hope: Relationships to psychosocial adjustment in Korean women with breast cancer. *Applied Nursing Research, 14,* 87–93.

Lee, H., Schmidt, K., & Ernst, E. (2005). Acupuncture for the relief of cancer-related pain–a systematic review. *European Journal of Pain, 9,* 437–444.

Ligibel, J. A. (2011). Role of adjuvant and posttreatment exercise programs in breast health. *Journal of the National Comprehensive Cancer Network, 9,* 251–256.

Lo, B., Quill, T., & Tulsky, J. (1999). Discussing palliative care with patients. ACP-ASIM End-of-Life Care Consensus Panel. American College of Physicians-American Society of Internal Medicine. *Annals of Internal Medicine, 130,* 744–749.

Lu, W., Matulonis, U. A., Doherty-Gilman, A., et al. (2009). Acupuncture for chemotherapy-induced neutropenia in patients with gynecologic malignancies: A pilot randomized, sham-controlled clinical trial. *Journal of Alternative and Complementary Medicine, 15,* 745–753.

McClain, C. S., Rosenfeld, B., & Breitbart, W. (2003). Effect of spiritual well-being on end-of-life despair in terminally-ill cancer patients. *The Lancet, 361,* 1603–1607.

McGee, R. F. (1984). Hope: A factor influencing crisis resolution. *ANS. Advances in Nursing Science, 6,* 34–44.

McGill, J. S., & Paul, P. B. (1993). Functional status and hope in elderly people with and without cancer. *Oncology Nursing Forum, 20,* 1207–1213.

McGregor, B. A., Antoni, M. H., Boyers, A., et al. (2004). Cognitive-behavioral stress management increases benefit finding and immune function among women with early-stage breast cancer. *Journal of Psychosomatic Research, 56,* 1–8.

Meyers, C. A., Albitar, M., & Estey, E. (2005). Cognitive impairment, fatigue, and cytokine levels in patients with acute myelogenous leukemia or myelodysplastic syndrome. *Cancer, 104,* 788–793.

Miller, A. H. (1998). Neuroendocrine and immune system interactions in stress and depression. *The Psychiatric Clinics of North America, 21,* 443–463.

Miller, A. H., Ancoli-Israel, S., Bower, J. E., et al. (2008). Neuroendocrine-immune mechanisms of behavioral comorbidities in patients with cancer. *Journal of Clinical Oncology, 26,* 971–982.

Miller, J. F., & Powers, M. J. (1988). Development of an instrument to measure hope. *Nursing Research, 37,* 6–10.

Mills, P. J., Parker, B., Dimsdale, J. E., et al. (2005). The relationship between fatigue and quality of life and inflammation during anthracycline-based chemotherapy in breast cancer. *Biological Psychology, 69,* 85–96.

Miyashita, M., Morita, T., Sato, K., et al. (2008). Good death inventory: A measure for evaluating good death from the bereaved family member's perspective. *Journal of Pain and Symptom Management, 35,* 486–498.

Moadel, A., Morgan, C., Fatone, A., et al. (1999). Seeking meaning and hope: self-reported spiritual and existential needs among an ethnically-diverse cancer patient population. *Psycho-Oncology, 8,* 378–385.

Morant, R., Stiefel, F., Berchtold, W., et al. (1993). Preliminary results of a study assessing asthenia and related psychological and biological phenomena in patients with advanced cancer. *Supportive Care in Cancer, 1,* 101–107.

Moynihan, C., Horwich, A., & Bliss, J. (1999). Counselling is not appropriate for all patients with cancer. *British Medical Journal, 318,* 128.

Musselman, D. L., Miller, A. H., Porter, M. R., et al. (2001). Higher than normal plasma interleukin-6 concentrations in cancer patients with depression: Preliminary findings. *The American Journal of Psychiatry, 158,* 1252–1257.

Nahin, R. L., & Straus, S. E. (2001). Research into complementary and alternative medicine: Problems and potential. *British Medical Journal, 322,* 161–164.

Navo, M. A., Phan, J., Vaughan, C., et al. (2004). An assessment of the utilization of complementary and alternative medication in women with gynecologic or breast malignancies. *Journal of Clinical Oncology, 22,* 671–677.

Newell, S., & Sanson-Fisher, R. W. (2000). Australian oncologists' self-reported knowledge and attitudes about non-traditional therapies used by cancer patients. *The Medical Journal of Australia, 172,* 110–113.

Nuland, S. B. (1994). How we die: Reflections on life's final chapter (1st ed). New York: A.A. Knopf (Distributed by Random House, Inc.)

Pan, C. X., Morrison, R. S., Ness, J., et al. (2000). Complementary and alternative medicine in the management of pain, dyspnea, and nausea and vomiting near the end of life. A systematic review. *Journal of Pain and Symptom Management, 20,* 374–387.

Park, C., & Folkman, S. (1997). Meaning in the context of stress and coping. *Review of General Psychology, 1,* 115–144.

Parker, P. A., Baile, W. F., de Moor, C., et al. (2001). Breaking bad news about cancer: Patients' preferences for communication. *Journal of Clinical Oncology, 19,* 2049–2056.

Parker, S. M., Clayton, J. M., Hancock, K., et al. (2007). A systematic review of prognostic/end-of-life communication with adults in the advanced stages of a life-limiting illness: Patient/caregiver preferences for the content, style, and timing of information. *Journal of Pain and Symptom Management, 34,* 81–93.

Penson, R. T., Castro, C. M., Seiden, M. V., et al. (2001). Complementary, alternative, integrative, or unconventional medicine? *The Oncologist, 6,* 463–473.

Penson, R. T., Gu, F., Harris, S., et al. (2007). Hope. *The Oncologist, 12,* 1105–1113.

Pickett, J. P., et al. (eds.) (2000). The American Heritage dictionary of the English language (4th ed). Boston: Houghton Mifflin

Pinn, G. (2001). Adverse effects associated with herbal medicine. *Australian Family Physician, 30,* 1070–1075.

Pinquart, M., & Duberstein, P. R. (2009). Associations of social networks with cancer mortality: A meta-analysis. *Critical Reviews in Oncology/Hematology, 75,* 122–137.

Ptacek, J. T., & Eberhardt, T. L. (1996). Breaking bad news. A review of the literature. *JAMA, 276,* 496–502.

Pusztai, L., Mendoza, T. R., Reuben, J. M., et al. (2004). Changes in plasma levels of inflammatory cytokines in response to paclitaxel chemotherapy. *Cytokine, 25,* 94–102.

Rainbird, K., Perkins, J., Sanson-Fisher, R., et al. (2009). The needs of patients with advanced, incurable cancer. *British Journal of Cancer, 101,* 759–764.

Rajasekaran, M., Edmonds, P. M., & Higginson, I. L. (2005). Systematic review of hypnotherapy for treating symptoms in terminally ill adult cancer patients. *Palliative Medicine, 19,* 418–426.

Raleigh, E. D. (1992). Sources of hope in chronic illness. *Oncology Nursing Forum, 19,* 443–448.

Rehse, B., & Pukrop, R. (2003). Effects of psychosocial interventions on quality of life in adult cancer patients: Meta analysis of 37 published controlled outcome studies. *Patient Education and Counseling, 50,* 179–186.

Relman, A. S., & Angell, M. (2002). Resolved: Psychosocial interventions can improve clinical outcomes in organic disease (con). *Psychosomatic Medicine, 64,* 558–563.

Rich, T., Innominato, P. F., Boerner, J., et al. (2005). Elevated serum cytokines correlated with altered behavior, serum cortisol rhythm, and dampened 24-hour rest-activity patterns in patients with metastatic colorectal cancer. *Clinical Cancer Research, 11,* 1757–1764.

Rustoen, T., & Wiklund, I. (2000). Hope in newly diagnosed patients with cancer. *Cancer Nursing, 23,* 214–219.

Rustoen, T., Wiklund, I., Hanestad, B. R., et al. (1998). Nursing intervention to increase hope and quality of life in newly diagnosed cancer patients. *Cancer Nursing, 21,* 235–245.

Sanatani, M., Schreier, G., & Stitt, L. (2008). Level and direction of hope in cancer patients: An exploratory longitudinal study. *Supportive Care in Cancer, 16,* 493–499.

Saper, R. B., Kales, S. N., Paquin, J., et al. (2004). Heavy metal content of ayurvedic herbal medicine products. *JAMA, 292,* 2868–2873.

Sapir, R., Catane, R., Kaufman, B., et al. (2000). Cancer patient expectations of and communication with oncologists and oncology nurses: The experience of an integrated oncology and palliative care service. *Supportive Care in Cancer, 8,* 458–463.

Schapira, L., & Steensma, D. (2011). Truth telling and palliative care. In R. J. Moore (Ed.), *Handbook of pain and palliative care: Biobehavioral approaches for the life course.* New York: Springer.

Shafqat, A., Einhorn, L. H., Hanna, N., et al. (2005). Screening studies for fatigue and laboratory correlates in cancer patients undergoing treatment. *Annals of Oncology, 16*, 1545–1550.

Shang, A., Huwiler-Muntener, K., Nartey, L., et al. (2005). Are the clinical effects of homoeopathy placebo effects? Comparative study of placebo-controlled trials of homoeopathy and allopathy. *The Lancet, 366*, 726–732.

Shen, J., Andersen, R., Albert, P. S., et al. (2002). Use of complementary/alternative therapies by women with advanced-stage breast cancer. *BMC Complementary and Alternative Medicine, 2*, 8.

Singer, P. A., Martin, D. K., & Kelner, M. (1999). Quality end-of-life care: Patients' perspectives. *JAMA, 281*, 163–168.

Smedslund, G., & Ringdal, G. I. (2004). Meta-analysis of the effects of psychosocial interventions on survival time in cancer patients. *Journal of Psychosomatic Research. 57*, 123–131; discussion 133–135.

Snyder, C. R. (1994). *The psychology of hope: You can get there from here.* Free Press: New York.

Snyder, C. R. (2000). *Handbook of hope: Theory, measures & applications.* San Diego: Academic.

Snyder, C. R. (2002). Hope theory: Rainbows in the mind. *Psychol Inquiry, 13*, 249–275.

Snyder, C. R., Harris, C., Anderson, J. R., et al. (1991). The will and the ways: Development and validation of an individual-differences measure of hope. *Journal of Personality and Social Psychology, 60*, 570–585.

Snyder, C. R., Hoza, B., Pelham, W. E., et al. (1997). The development and validation of the Children's Hope Scale. *Journal of Pediatric Psychology, 22*, 399–421.

Sood, A., Sood, R., Bauer, B. A., et al. (2005). Cochrane systematic reviews in acupuncture: Methodological diversity in database searching. *Journal of Alternative and Complementary Medicine, 11*, 719–722.

Spence, J. E., & Olson, M. A. (1997). Quantitative research on therapeutic touch. An integrative review of the literature 1985–1995. *Scandinavian Journal of Caring Sciences, 11*, 183–190.

Spiegel, D., Bloom, J. R., Kraemer, H. C., et al. (1989). Effect of psychosocial treatment on survival of patients with metastatic breast cancer. *The Lancet, 2*, 888–891.

Spiegel, D., Butler, L. D., Giese-Davis, J., et al. (2007). Effects of supportive-expressive group therapy on survival of patients with metastatic breast cancer: A randomized prospective trial. *Cancer, 110*, 1130–1138.

Steinhauser, K. E., Christakis, N. A., Clipp, E. C., et al. (2000). Factors considered important at the end of life by patients, family, physicians, and other care providers. *JAMA, 284*, 2476–2482.

Temel, J. S., Greer, J. A., Muzikansky, A., et al. (2010). Early palliative care for patients with metastatic non-small-cell lung cancer. *The New England Journal of Medicine, 363*, 733–742.

Tennen, H., & Affleck, G. (1999). Finding benefits in adversity. In C. R. Synder (Ed.), *Coping: The psychology of what works.* New York: Oxford University Press.

Unruh, A. M., Versnel, J., & Kerr, N. (2002). Spirituality unplugged: A review of commonalities and contentions, and a resolution. *Canadian Journal of Occupational Therapy, 69*, 5–19.

Vachon, M., Fillion, L., & Achille, M. (2009). A conceptual analysis of spirituality at the end of life. *Journal of Palliative Medicine, 12*, 53–59.

Verhoef, M. J., Balneaves, L. G., Boon, H. S., et al. (2005). Reasons for and characteristics associated with complementary and alternative medicine use among adult cancer patients: A systematic review. *Integrative Cancer Therapies, 4*, 274–286.

Wachholtz, A., & Makowski, S. (2011). Spiritual dimensions of pain and suffering. In R. J. Moore (Ed.), *Handbook of pain and palliative care: Biobehavioral approaches for the life course.* New York: Springer.

Weight, L. M., Alexander, D., & Jacobs, P. (1991). Strenuous exercise: Analogous to the acute-phase response? *Clinical Science (London, England), 81*, 677–683.

Weihs, K. L., Enright, T. M., & Simmens, S. J. (2008). Close relationships and emotional processing predict decreased mortality in women with breast cancer: Preliminary evidence. *Psychosomatic Medicine, 70*, 117–124.

Wenrich, M. D., Curtis, J. R., Shannon, S. E., et al. (2001). Communicating with dying patients within the spectrum of medical care from terminal diagnosis to death. *Archives of Internal Medicine, 161*, 868–874.

World Health Organization. WHO draft interim guidelines handbook on relief of cancer pain. *Report of a WHO Consultation, Milan*, 14–16 October, 1982.

World Health Organization. (1986). *Cancer pain relief.* Geneva: WHO.

WHO. (2011). Retrieved from http://www.who.int/cancer/palliative/definition/en/ on 10/14/11.

Wratten, C., Kilmurray, J., Nash, S., et al. (2004). Fatigue during breast radiotherapy and its relationship to biological factors. *International Journal of Radiation Oncology, Biology, and Physics, 59*, 160–167.

Wright, E. B., Holcombe, C., & Salmon, P. (2004). Doctors' communication of trust, care, and respect in breast cancer: Qualitative study. *British Medical Journal, 328*, 864.

Yancey, D., Greger, H. A., & Coburn, P. (1994). Effects of an adult cancer camp on hope, perceived social support, coping, and mood states. *Oncology Nursing Forum, 21*, 727–733.

Zhu, C. B., Blakely, R. D., & Hewlett, W. A. (2006). The proinflammatory cytokines interleukin-1beta and tumor necrosis factor-alpha activate serotonin transporters. *Neuropsychopharmacology, 31*, 2121–2131.

Zhu, C. B., Carneiro, A. M., Dostmann, W. R., et al. (2005). p38 MAPK activation elevates serotonin transport activity via a trafficking-independent, protein phosphatase 2A-dependent process. *Journal of Biological Chemistry, 280*, 15649–15658.

Chapter 24
Temporomandibular Disorders and its Relationship with Fibromyalgia

Ana Mirian Velly, Hong Chen, João R. Ferreira, and James R. Fricton

Abbreviations

ACR   American College of Rheumatology diagnostic criteria
ASICs Acid-sensing ion channels
BDNF   Brain-derived neurotrophic factor
EPI   Epinephrine
FM   Fibromyalgia
MPS   Myofascial pain
NE   Norepinephrine
NGF   Nerve growth factor
NMDA N-methyl-D-aspartate
RDC   Research Diagnostic Criteria
TeP   Tender points
TMD   Temporomandibular Disorder
TrP   Trigger points

A.M. Velly, DDS, PhD (✉)
Department of Dentistry, Centre for Clinical Epidemiology and Community Studies,
Jewish General Hospital, 3755, Chemin de la Côte Ste-Catherine, Suite H-485,
Montréal, QC H3T 1E2, Canada

Department of Diagnostic and Biological Sciences, Division of TMD
and Orofacial Pain, University of Minnesota, Minneapolis, MN, USA
e-mail: ana.velly@mcgill.ca

H. Chen, DDS, MS
Center for Neurosensory Disorders, Orofacial Pain Clinic, University
of North Carolina - Chapel Hill, School of Dentistry, Campus Box #7450,
Chapel Hill, NC 27599, USA

J.R. Ferreira, DDS, MS
NC Oral Health Institute, University of North Carolina, School of Dentistry, UNC-Chapel Hill, CB#7454,
Chapel Hill, NC 27599-7454, USA

J.R. Fricton, DDS, MS
University of Minnesota, Minneapolis, MN, USA

R.J. Moore (ed.), *Handbook of Pain and Palliative Care: Biobehavioral Approaches for the Life Course*,
DOI 10.1007/978-1-4419-1651-8_24, © Springer Science+Business Media, LLC 2012

Introduction

Temporomandibular Disorder (TMD) is the second most commonly occurring musculoskeletal condition resulting in orofacial pain and disability, after chronic low back pain (National Institute of Dental and Craniofacial Research Facial pain). Most TMD cases are mild in nature, fluctuate over time, and do not constitute a disability to the patient (Schiffman et al. 1990; Von Korff et al. 1988). However, about 10% of early TMD subjects develop more severe chronic pain (Fricton and Haley 1982). In addition, 20% of patients develop long-term (5 or more years) disability, and 50% of those seeking care still have pain 5 years later (Schiffman et al. 1990). This particular TMD group constitutes those patients who are most severely affected by the disorder, and thus require the most attention from health care providers. The treatment of TMD has been an increasing financial burden with annual U.S. costs doubling in the last decade to $4 billion annually (National Institute of Dental and Craniofacial Research Facial pain).

Several studies have suggested that specific central modulating processes associated with comorbidities such as fibromyalgia syndrome (FMS) may play a significant role in perpetuation of TMD (Balasubramaniam et al. 2007; Hoffmann et al. 2011; Lim et al. 2010; Velly et al. 2010). This chapter reviews the relationship between TMD and FMS and presents clinical implications regarding these findings.

Temporomandibular Disorders and Fibromyalgia Definitions and Prevalence

TMD is a collective used to describe musculoskeletal conditions characterized by pain in the muscle of mastication, the temporomandibular joint, or both (Laskin et al. 1983). The more common type of TMD appears to be 14 myofascial pain (MPS) and arthralgia followed by disc displacement with reduction (Truelove et al. 1992). MPS is characterized by myalgia with consistent patterns of referred pain and localized tenderness in specific points of muscle bands (Fricton 1990; Fricton et al. 1985; Fricton 2004).

Painful TMD occurs in about 5–10% of the general population (Dworkin and LeResche 1992; Isong et al. 2008; Okeson 1996), its prevalence declines after 45–50 years (LeResche 1997) and it is more common among females (2–18%) than males (0–10%) (LeResche 1997; Drangsholt and LeResche 1999). The female-to-male gender prevalence ratio ranges from 1.2 to 2.6 (Drangsholt and LeResche 1999).

The common hallmark in FMS is chronic widespread pain and tenderness, and a mosaic of cognitive, sleep, fatigue, and other somatic symptoms (Wolfe et al. 1990, 2010). The previous American College of Rheumatology (ACR) diagnostic criteria for FMS included widespread pain (in 3 of 4 quadrants) and generalized tenderness (11 of 18 tender points) (Wolfe et al. 1990). Recently, the ACR diagnostic criteria for FMS were modified. The ACR preliminary diagnostic criteria for FMS in 2010 (ACR 2010) purged the tender point examination, thus making it possible to study FMS in epidemiology surveys and clinical research. The current diagnostic criteria for FMS are satisfied if three conditions are met (1) the Widespread Pain Index (WPI) ≥ 7 and the Symptom Severity Score (SS) ≥ 5, or the WPI is 3–6 and the SS ≥ 9, (2) symptoms have been present at a similar level for at least 3 months, and (3) the patient does not have a disorder that would otherwise explain the pain (Wolfe et al. 2010).

The prevalence of FMS ranges from 2 to 4% (Lawrence et al. 2008; Wolfe et al. 1995). It is higher among females than males (Wolfe et al. 1995; Aaron et al. 2000; Clauw and Crofford 2003) and increases with age (Wolfe et al. 1995). FMS is also characterized by sleep disturbance, fatigue, and often psychological distress (Wolfe et al. 1985, 1990, 1995; Aaron and Buchwald 2001a) high level of functional disability and reduced health-related quality of life (HRQOL) (Wolfe et al. 1997b). The average yearly cost for service utilization among FMS patients is considerably high ($2,274) (Wolfe et al. 1997a).

Fibromyalgia Among Temporomandibular Disorders Subjects

Various studies and reviews reported that FMS commonly presents in patients with TMD (Aaron and Buchwald 2001a, 2003; Korszun et al. 1998; Leblebici et al. 2007; Plesh et al. 1996; Velly et al. 2002; Yunus 2008). Plesh et al. (1996) observed that among 39 patients with TMD, 18% presented also FMS. This prevalence is higher than that found in Velly et al. (2010) study of 572 TMD subjects, but similar to the widespread pain prevalence (20%) (Velly et al. 2010). In addition, Leblebici et al. (2007), based on a sample of 21 TMD patients, found that the prevalence of FMS was significantly higher for those with both arthralgia and MPS than those with MPS only.

Several studies examined the co-existence of FMS or widespread pain in TMD to determine their relationship to treatment outcomes or progression to more severe TMD problems. Raphael and Marbach (2001) found MPS TMD patients with widespread pain (possibly related to FMS) did not improve with an active splint while those patients with local pain who received the active splint did. This result may be explained by the finding that widespread pain and FMS contribute to the development of dysfunction TMD pain as well as its persistence (John et al. 2003; Velly et al. 2010).

Temporomandibular Disorders Among Fibromyalgia Subjects

Diagnosis and signs and symptoms of TMD are very common in FMS subjects (Aaron and Buchwald 2001a, 2003; Balasubramaniam et al. 2007; Eriksson et al. 1988; Hedenberg-Magnusses et al. 1999; Leblebici et al. 2007; Korszun et al. 1998; Pennacchio et al. 1998; Plesh et al. 1996; Rhodus et al. 2003; Yunus 2008). Plesh et al. (1996) reported that 75% of 60 subjects with FMS according to the American College of Rheumatology 1990 Criteria for the Classification of FMS satisfied criteria for muscular (myofascial) TMD. A significant greater prevalence of TMD (68 vs. 20%) was also found among 67 subjects diagnosed with FMS based on the American College of Rheumatology criteria compared to age and sex-matched controls (Rhodus et al. 2003). In Balasubramaniam et al. (2007) and Leblebici et al. (2007), patients with FMS also commonly present TMD (37–80%, respectively) where the diagnosis of MPS was more frequent.

Korszun et al. (1998) studied 92 patients who fulfilled the criteria for chronic fatigue syndrome or FMS (or both) and found that 42% reported TMD. The majority of the 39 TMD patients reported an onset of generalized symptoms before the onset of facial pain and 75% of them had been treated exclusively for painful TMD without consideration for the FMS. Hedenberg-Magnusson et al. (1999) studied 191 FMS patients who returned a self-report survey and found that 94% reported local pain, most commonly in the temples from the temporomandibular system with a mean duration of 12 years. General body pain had a significantly longer duration than TMD, suggesting again that FMS have been initiated in other parts of the body and later involved the temporomandibular region.

Clinical Characteristics of Temporomandibular Disorders and Fibromyalgia

Pain

The most common diagnosis of TMD among subjects with FMS is masticatory MPS (>75.0%) (Plesh et al. 1996; Balasubramaniam et al. 2007; Leblebici et al. 2007). The quality of pain found with MPS TMD and among FMS is frequently described as a *chronic dull aching pain* and is central to the diagnosis of both disorders. Typically, TMD pain localizes to the jaw, in front of the ear, or in the temple area (Dworkin et al. 1992), although TMD patients may report pain outside of orofacial region, such as in the neck, shoulder, and back (Lim et al. 2010). In a study including 39 consecutive patients with TMD seen in a TMD clinic and 60 patients with FMS examined according to Research Diagnostic Criteria (RDC) for TMD and the American College of Rheumatology 1990 Criteria for the classification of FMS, patients with FMS showed more painful body regions (Plesh et al. 1996). This higher number of painful body regions among patients with FMS is directly related to the classification criteria (ACR 1990): FMS patients need to have pain in at least two diagonally opposed quadrants plus axial skeletal pain (Wolfe et al. 1990).

Pain in FMS is considerably more severe and spread over a larger body area than the pain found in patients with TMD. It is relatively stable and consistent in contrast to MPS TMD, which can vary in intensity and location depending on which muscles are involved (Fricton 1990, 2004). Facial intensity and daily pattern, however, appears to be similar between MPS TMD and FMS patients (Dao et al. 1997). Cimino et al. (1998) also did not find a statistically significant difference on the levels of tenderness to palpation, pain during mandibular function when 23 women with MPS TMD were compared to 23 women with FMS. Furthermore, pain duration is significantly longer in FMS patients than in TMD patients (Pfau et al. 2009).

Tenderness and Thermal and Pressure Pain Thresholds

Both tender points (TeP) and trigger points (TrP) represent hypersensitivity to mechanical pressure. Fernandez-de-Las-Penas et al. (2010) demonstrated the existence of multiple active muscle TrPs in masticatory and neck-shoulder muscles of subjects with MPS TMD. Ge et al. (2010), Gerwin (2011), and Simons (1990) pointed out that the most of FMS TeP sites lie at well-known TrP sites. Furthermore, total number of active, but not latent, TrP is positively associated with FM pain intensity (Ge et al. 2010). Finally, these TrP may act as a peripheral pain generator driving central sensitization in FMS (Ge et al. 2010).

Thermal and pressure pain thresholds have been shown to be significantly lower in FMS and TMD patients compared to controls (Berglund et al. 2002; Desmeules et al. 2003; Farella et al. 2000; Granges and Littlejohn 1993; Kosek et al. 1996a; Lautenbacher et al. 1994; Maixner et al. 1995; Maixner et al. 1998; Pfau et al. 2009; Plesh et al. 1996; Rolke et al. 2006). Hedenberg-Magnusson et al. (1997) compared 23 patients with FMS, 23 patients with masticatory myalgia (i.e., muscular or myogenic TMD), and 20 controls and found that the number of tender muscles was higher, while pressure pain threshold and tolerance levels were lower, in the FMS group as compared to the masticatory myalgia group. Both groups were different than the control group.

Contributing Factors to Temporomandibular Disorders and Fibromyalgia

Environmental and Genetic Factors

Environmental triggers and genetic predisposition have been suggested to be implicated in the dysregulation of pain modulatory system (Clauw and Chrousos 1997; Aaron and Buchwald 2001a; Dadabhoy et al. 2008).

Environmental triggers may act by increasing stress and thus altering the sympathetic and parasympathetic activity of the autonomic nervous system such as decreasing heart variability. These effects have been reported among patients with FMS or TMD (Cohen et al. 2000; Dadabhoy et al. 2008; de Abreu et al. 1993; Elam et al. 1992; Giske et al. 2008; Glass et al. 2004; Hamaty et al. 1989; Jones et al. 1997; Legangneux et al. 2001; Light et al. 2009; Maekawa et al. 2002, 2003; Martinez-Lavin 2007; Perry et al. 1989; Schmidt and Carlson 2009; Solberg Nes et al. 2010).

In addition, another link between stress response and FMS or TMD is supported by studies that demonstrate alterations of the hypothalamic-pituitary-adrenal axis (Adler et al. 1999; Crofford et al. 2004; Gur et al. 2004; Korszun et al. 2002; McCain and Tilbe 1989; McLean et al. 2005). Korszun et al. (2002) measured cortisol levels in 15 women with well-defined TMD and 15 matched controls by sampling blood at 10-min intervals over 24 h in a controlled environment. TMD patients showed markedly increased daytime cortisol level of 30–50% higher than those of controls and a 1-h phase delay in the timing of maximum cortisol levels. In another study, an elevation of cortisol in the late evening quiescent period was evident in the FMS patients compared with their matched control group (Crofford et al. 2004).

Epidemiologic studies also demonstrated that psychological features such as depression, anxiety, and cognitive factors are observed among subjects with TMD or FMS (Dworkin et al. 1989; Garofalo et al. 1998; Gatchel et al. 1996, 2007; Gracely et al. 2004; Jensen and Karoly 1991; Jensen et al. 1991, 1994; LeResche et al. 2007; Litt et al. 2004, 2009; Turner and Aaron 2001; Turner et al. 2005; 2001; Velly et al. 2002, 2003; Wright et al. 2004). All these factors may share a *common mechanistic basis* for these conditions (Woolf 2010). These factors could also contribute to the development of the pain condition (LeResche et al. 2007; Slade et al. 2007), influence pain perception through alteration of attention and anticipation, heighten emotional responses to pain (Gracely et al. 2004), and modifying the stress response (Dadabhoy et al. 2008).

Polymorphisms in the catechol-*O*-methyltransferase gene have also been implicated in TMD and FMS (Diatchenko et al. 2005a, 2005b; Gursoy et al. 2003). Particularly, this polymorphism has an effect on the metabolism or transport of monoamines, compounds that have a critical role in both sensory processing (Zubieta et al. 2003; Nackley et al. 2007). COMT was also related to pathogenesis of inflammatory states (Shabalina et al. 2009) and to psychological factors such as anxiety, depression, and stress (Domschke et al. 2004; Enoch et al. 2003; Hamilton et al. 2002).

Modulatory Mechanisms of Temporomandibular Disorders and Fibromyalgia

Causes of TMD and FMS are not yet fully understood. FMS and TMD pain may coexist due to the disruption of central nervous system mechanisms that process painful or stressful stimuli. (Aaron and Buchwald 2001a, 2001b; 2003; Bradley et al. 2000; Loeser and Melzack 1999). Woolf (2010) explained that the commonality of these pain conditions resides in the presence of pain hypersensitivity,

Table 24.1 Characteristics of muscle fiber types I, IIA, and IIB in skeletal muscles. Type IIC and IIM are primarily involved in growth and development and not often seen in skeletal muscles as noted in Table 24.2. (Loeser and Melzack 1999)

	Major Fiber Types		
	Type I (red)	Type IIA (pink)	Type IIB (white)
Staining	Weak –ATPase (light pink)	Strong –ATPase (light pink)	Strong –ATPase (light pink)
	Strong NADH-TR (dark pink)	Strong NADH-TR (dark pink)	Weak NADH-TR (dark pink)
Contraction speed and fatigue	Slow twitch	Fast twitch	Slow twitch
	Without fatigue	Fatigue resistant	Fatigue resistant
	Gradual recruitment to maximal force	Higher threshold to recruitment	Developes highest muscle tension
Cellular characteristics	Low glycogen	Low glycogen	Rich in glycogen
	High # of mitochondria	Low # of mitochondria	Low # of mitochondria
	High oxidative enzymes	Low oxidative enzymes	Low oxidative enzymes
	Slow myosin	Fast myosin	Fast myosin
Morphology	Less in deep masseter with short face	More in deep masseter with short face	Hypertrophy with long face
	More with loss of teeth	Less with loss of teeth	Less with loss of teeth
Function	Posture	Long term use	Strength
	Sustained low force contraction	Sustained high force contraction	Brief high force contraction
	Increase muscle length does not alter function or morphology	Increase muscle length does not alter function or morphology	Increase muscle length does not alter function or morphology
Response to Electrical Stimulation	At 50 Hz: Type I to II	At 10 Hz: Type II to I	At 10 Hz: Type II to I
	Increase glycogen	Decrease glycogen	Decrease glycogen
	Decreased Mitochondria	Increased Mitochondria	Increased Mitochondria
Metabolism	Oxidative phophorylation	Glycolytic	Glycolytic

which might reflect a primary dysfunction of the nervous system. FMS and TMD pain are thought to result from dysregulation of pain modulatory systems involving altered interactions among the central (CNS) and peripheral nervous systems and the immune system (Buskila 2001; Clauw and Chrousos 1997; Katz et al. 2007; Maixner et al. 1995; 1998; Price et al. 2002).

Peripheral Mechanisms

The skeletal muscle has different proportions of muscle fiber types classified as type I, type IIA, and type IIB (Table 24.1) (Eriksson and Thornell 1983; Fricton 2004). Type IIC and IIM are involved in development and are not frequently seen in the adult masticatory muscles. Type I muscle fiber types are functionally associated with static muscle tone and posture. They are slow twitch, fatigue resistant fibers with a high number of mitochondria needed for oxidative phosphorylation used in energy metabolism (Fricton 2004). Type II fibers are functionally associated with increased velocity and force of contraction over brief periods. They are fast twitch fibers that fatigue easily, are rich in glycogen, and use anaerobic glycolysis for energy metabolism. These fiber types can transform from one type to another depending on the demands placed on a muscle. For example, Uhlig and colleagues found signs of fiber transformation from type I to type IIc fibers in cervical muscles associated with pain and dysfunction after spondylodesis (Uhlig 1995). This is consistent with transformation associated with prolonged inactivity due to the injury. Furthermore, Mayo and colleagues found decreases in the cross sectional diameter of muscle fiber type I and II in the masticatory system in rhesus monkeys undergoing maxillomandibular fixation (Mayo et al. 1988). Thus, transformation due to inactivity and pain can decrease both the percent and size of type I fibers available to maintain normal postural and resting muscle activity. On the other hand, an increase in demands of postural muscle activity may result in an increase in type I fibers and a decrease in type II fibers in muscle pain patients (Bengtsson et al. 1986b, 1986c). If the increased demand placed on the type I fiber types due to repetitive strain from activities such as back or shoulder tensing is beyond normal physiologic parameters, the intracellular components of these fibers may be damaged. This will result in hyperpolarization outside the muscle due to high levels of K+ from sustained motor unit activity and K+ pump damage, damage to the actin and myosin myofilaments, disruption of the sarcoplasmic reticulum and the calcium pump, and decrease in local blood flow. Specific factors that appear to be important in this process include both direct macro-trauma and indirect micro-trauma from repetitive muscle strain factors (Yunus 1992).

Metabolic Distress at the Motor End Plates

In explaining the local nature of MPS TrPs, Simons (1990, 2008) suggests that the damage to the muscle occurs primarily at the motor endplates, creating an energy crisis at the TrP. He suggests that this crisis occurs from grossly abnormal increase in acetylcholine release at the endplate and generation of numerous miniature endplate potentials, resulting in an increase in energy demand, sustained depolarizaton of the postjunction membrane, and mitochondrial changes. Other studies also support this proposed mechanism. For example, Hubbard and Berkoff (1993) found spontaneous EMG activity at the TrP (Hubbard and Berkoff 1993). EMG characteristics of the local twitch response are generated locally without input from the CNS (Hong 1994; Hong and Torigoe 1994).

Histologic studies also provide some support for this mechanism. They have shown myofibrillar lysis, moth eaten fibers, and ragged red type I fibers with deposition of glycogen and abnormal mitochondria but little evidence of cellular inflammation hypothesis (Bengtsson et al. 1986b; Yunus et al. 1986). Studies of muscle energy metabolism found a decrease in the levels of ATP, ADP, and phosphoryl creatine and abnormal tissue oxygenation in muscles with TrPs (Bengtsson et al. 1986a). El-Labban and colleagues demonstrated that TMJ ankylosis will result in degenerative changes in masseter and temporalis muscles (El-Labban et al. 1990). These studies suggest that localized progressive increases in oxidative metabolism and depleted energy supply in type I fibers may result in abnormal muscle changes that initially include reactive dysfunctional changes to muscle fiber type I and surrounding connective tissue but eventually may involve degenerative changes and increased connective tissue in the muscle.

The Activation of Muscle Nociceptors

The resulting metabolic by-products of this damage can result in peripheral sensitization of nociceptors the muscle, fatigue (Mao et al. 1993). Muscle strain may lead to localized progressive increases in oxidative metabolism, particularly in muscle fiber type I with depleted energy supply, increased metabolic by-products, and resultant muscle nociception at the periphery. This is supported by our recent findings that MPS TMD subjects present higher salivary and serum oxidative stress levels (8-hydroxydeoxyguanosine (8-OHdG), malondialdehyde (MDA), and total antioxidant status (TAS)) in comparison to controls (Rodriguez de Sotillo et al. 2011).

It is unknown what specific mediators are involved in this sensitization, but these may include high potassium concentration and hyperpolarization outside the muscle due to K+ pump damage, high calcium concentration from damage to the sarcoplasmic reticulum, or inflammatory mediators from tissue damage. Localized tenderness and pain in the muscle involve type III and IV muscle nociceptors and has shown to be activated by noxious substances including K+, bradykinin, histamine, or prostaglandins that can be released locally from the damage and trigger tenderness (Fricton 2004; Kniffki et al. 1978; Mense 1993). It is important to note the K+ activated a higher percent of type IV muscle nociceptors than other agents, providing support for the idea that localized increases in K+ at the neuromuscular junction may be responsible for sensitization of nociceptors. This peripheral sensitization is thought to play a major role in local tenderness and pain, which together with central sensitization produces hyperalgesia in patients with persistent muscle pain, particularly in TMD affecting masticatory and cervical muscles (Dubner 61; Fernandez-de-Las-Penas et al. 2010; Fricton 2004).

Central Mechanisms

The afferent inputs from type III and IV muscle nociceptors in the body are transmitted to the CNS through cells such as those of the lamina I, V, and possibly IV of the dorsal horn on the way to the cortex, resulting in perception of local pain (Dubner and Bennett 1983; Sessle 1995b, 1995a). In the trigeminal system, these afferent inputs project to the second order neurons in the brain stem regions including the superficial lamina of trigeminal subnucleus caudalis as well as its more rostral lamina such as interpolaris and oralis (Sessle 1995b). These neurons can then project to neurons in higher levels of the CNS such as the thalamus, cranial motor nuclei, or the reticular formation (Sessle 1995a). In the thalamus, the ventro basal complex, the posterior group of nuclei, and parts of the medial thalamus are involved in receiving and relaying somatosensory information. These inputs can also converge with other visceral and somatic inputs from tissues such as the joint or skin and be responsible for referred pain perception (Fricton 2004; Melzack 1981).

Both FMS and MPS TMD need to be considered as a primary disorder of central pain perception. Although nociceptive input from the periphery does occur, it has been shown to be modified by multiple factors in its transmission to the CNS. For example, low- and high-intensity electrical stimulation of sensory nerves or noxious stimulation of sites remote from the site of pain will suppress nociceptive responses of trigeminal brain stem neurons and related reflexes (Kashima et al. 1999). This provides support that afferent inputs can be inhibited by multiple peripherally or centrally initiated alterations in neural input to the brain stem through various treatment modalities such as cold, heat, analgesic medications, massage, muscular injections, and transcutaneous electrical stimulation (Melzack 1981). For example, Kashima et al. (1999) found increased pain sensitivity of the upper extremities of TMD patients with myalgia to experimentally evoked noxious stimulation, suggesting the possibility of central sensitization. Ta et al. (2002) studied 32 TMJ implant patients and found an altered sensitivity to sensory stimuli, a higher number of tender points with a diagnosis of FMS, increased self-report of chemical sensitivity, higher psychologic distress, and significantly lower functional ability (Fricton 2004).

Likewise, persistent peripheral or central nociceptive activity can result in an increase in abnormal neuroplastic changes in cutaneous and deep neurons. These neuroplastic changes may include prolonged responsiveness to afferent inputs, increased receptive field size, and spontaneous bursts of activity (Guilbaud 1991; Dubner 1992). Thus, peripheral inputs from muscles may also be facilitated or accentuated by multiple peripherally or centrally initiated alterations in neural input with further sustained neural activity such as persistent joint pain, sustained muscle activity habits or postural tension, or CNS alterations such as depression and anxiety that can support the central sensitization further perpetuating the problem. This sensitization may be subserved by a number of neuropeptides, including substance P, glutamate, serotonin, dopamine, norepinephrine, and endorphins. Reduced CSF levels of the major metabolites of serotonin, dopamine, and norepinephrine were found in FMS patients indicating a low turnover of these neurotransmitters. Conversely, elevated levels of substance P and glutamate were present in the CSF (Russell et al. 1994; Sarchielli et al. 2007). Furthermore, the combination of elevated glutamate and substance P and reduced serotonin supports a role for central amplification in the pain transmission and perception of patients with FMS (Vaeroy et al. 1988; Russell 1989). Moreover, researchers also found that CSF levels of two neurotrophins, nerve growth factor (NGF) and brain-derived neurotrophic factor (BDNF), were elevated in patients with FMS (Giovengo et al. 1999; Laske et al. 2007; Sarchielli et al. 2007). The increased levels of NGF and BDNF correlated with increased CSF glutamate levels of FMS patients. These researchers speculated that NGF acted indirectly to increase BDNF expression, which then modulated N-methyl-D-aspartate (NMDA) receptor activity (which is essential in both initiating and maintaining activity-dependent central amplification) to increase the excitatory amino acids glutamate and aspartate, supporting the involvement of a central mechanism in the pathophysiology of FMS (Fricton 2004; Laske et al. 2007).

Central pain amplification is well known to cause hyperalgesia (increased pain from normally painful stimuli), allodynia (pain from normally nonpainful stimuli), and referred pain (Meeus and Nijs 2007). Central pain amplification has also been supported by preclinical studies, where several animal models reproducing widespread, long-lasting hyperalgesia or allodynia have been developed to model FMS muscle pain (DeSantana and Sluka 2008; Nagakura et al. 2009). Increased glutamate and aspartate release in the mice spinal cord followed the injection of acidic saline to the gastrocnemius muscle, which correlated with hyperalgesia development in the paw (Skyba et al. 2005; Sluka et al. 2001). This hyperalgesic effect was reversed by NMDA and non-NMDA receptor antagonists, suggesting that elevated glutamate played a role in mechanical hyperalgesia (Skyba et al. 2002). Inhibitors of adenylate cyclase or protein kinase A have also been found to reverse the mechanical hyperalgesia and allodynia (Hoeger-Bement and Sluka 2003). In addition, acid-sensing ion channels (ASICs) located on afferent fibers, which respond to pH changes, can also be involved in the mechanical hyperalgesia induced by acidic saline injections in mice. This hyperalgesia has been prevented by pretreatment of the muscle with a nonselective ASIC antagonist, suggesting a role for ASICs in the development of central amplification (Sluka et al. 2003, 2007). Consequently, ASICs may be another therapeutic target for FMS pain therapy. ASICs are also important targets in neuropathic pain models, in which the role of central amplification has been well established (Poirot et al. 2006).

There is also evidence that patients with FMS may have abnormalities associated with the immune system that may distinguish FMS from MPS patients, and support the more systemic nature of FMS. Several studies have found that most patients with chronic fatigue and immune dysfunction syndrome (CFIDS) fulfill the criteria for FMS and that they may have several serum abnormalities of immune function (Komaroff and Goldenberg 1989; Moldofsky 2001; Russell 1989). The clinical overlap between these conditions may reflect a shared underlying pathophysiologic basis involving dysregulation of the hypothalamic-pituitary-adrenal stress hormone axis in predisposed individuals (Fricton 2004).

These biochemical changes underlie an integrated "central biasing mechanism" in the CNS that will dampen or accentuate peripheral input (Melzack 1971, 1981). This mechanism may explain many of the characteristics of MPS TMD and FMS including the broad regions of pain referral, the recruitment of additional muscles in chronic cases, the inter-relationship between muscle and joint pain, and the ability of many treatments including pharmacological approaches, spray and stretch modalities, massage therapy, and TrP injections to reduce the pain for longer than the duration of action (Fricton 2004).

Several studies indicated a deficiency of diffuse noxious inhibitory control (DNIC) in subjects with TMD and FMS. DNIC involves testing the pain threshold at baseline, followed by administering a painful stimulus that leads to an analgesic effect, presumably by activating endogenous analgesic systems (Dadabhoy et al. 2008). Deficient DNIC was found in four cross-sectional studies among TMD and FM patients (Julien et al. 2005; Kosek et al. 1996b; Lautenbacher and Rollman 1997; Maixner et al. 1995).

Treatment Implications

Treatment of TMD can range from simple cases with transient mild pain and fatigue to complex cases involving multiple pain locations and many interrelating contributing factors including the presence of FMS. The difficulty in management of both disorders lies in the critical need to match the level of complexity of the management program with the complexity of the patient. Failure to address the entire problem, including all involved muscles and joints, concomitant diagnoses including FMS, and contributing factors may lead to failure to improve the pain, improve function, and perpetuation of the problem. Many authors have found success in treatment of both TMD and FMS using a wide variety of techniques such as exercise, trigger point injections, vapocoolant spray and stretch, TENS, biofeedback, postural correction, tricyclic antidepressants, muscle relaxants, pregabulin, nonsteroidal anti-inflammatories, and other medications, as well as addressing perpetuating factors (Fricton and Dall' Arancio 1994; Fricton 2004; Goldenberg 2002; Travell 1998).

Although there are no controlled studies examining progression of chronic pain syndromes, results from clinical studies reveal that many patients with TMD and FMS have seen many clinicians and received numerous medications and multiple other singular treatments for years without receiving more than temporary improvement. In one study of 164 TMD patients, the mean duration of pain was 5.8 years for males and 6.9 years for females with a mean of 4.5 past clinicians seen for the study (Fricton and Haley 1982). Patients with TMD and FMS have a worse prognosis (only 5% sustained remission after treatment) than those without FMS.

These and other studies of chronic pain suggest that regardless of the pathogenesis of muscular pain, a major characteristic of some of these patients is the failure of traditional approaches to completely resolve the problem. Each clinician confronted with a patient with chronic TMD and FMS needs to recognize that there is no single treatment that is effective and only by addressing the whole problem can you maximize the potential for a successful outcome. Treating only those patients whose complexity matches the treatment strategy available to the clinician can improve success. Simple cases with minimal behavioral and psychosocial involvement can typically be managed by a single clinician. Complex TMD patients, particularly those who also have FMS should be managed within an interdisciplinary pain clinic setting that uses a team of clinicians to address different aspects of the problem in a concerted fashion (Fricton 2004).

Management includes exercises, direct therapy to muscles, and reduction of all contributing factors. The short-term goal is to restore normal function of muscles and joints, posture, and full joint range of motion with exercises and muscle therapy. This is followed in the long term with a regular muscle stretching, postural, conditioning, and strengthening exercise program as well as control of contributing factors. Long-term control of pain depends on patient education, self-responsibility, and development of long-term doctor–patient relationships. This often requires shifting the paradigms implicit in patient care (Table 24.2). The difficulty in long-term management often lies not in treating the muscle and joints, but rather in the complex task of changing the identified contributing factors

Table 24.2 Shifting the doctor/patient paradigms involves each member of the team following the same concepts by conveying the same messages implicit in their dialogue with the patient (Fricton and Haley 1982; Garofalo et al. 1998; Gatchel et al. 1996)

Concept	Statement
Self responsibility	You have more influence on your problem than we do
Self-care order	You will need to make daily changes in to improve your condition
Education	We can teach you how to make the changes
Long-term change	It will take at least 6 months for the changes to have an effect
Strong doctor-patient relationship	We will support you as you make the changes
Patient motivation	Do you want to make the changes

since they can be integrally related to the patient's attitudes, lifestyle, and social and physical environment. Interdisciplinary teams integrate various health professionals in a supportive environment to accomplish both long-term treatment of illness and modification of these contributing factors. Many approaches such as habit reversal techniques, biofeedback, and stress management have been used to achieve this within a team approach (Fricton 2004).

Conclusion

Although most cases of TMD are mild and self-limiting, about 15% develop severe disorders associated with chronic pain. It has been found that the widespread pain, depression, and sleep disorders associated with FMS may play a significant role in chronicity of patients with TMD.

Both TMD and FMS may have similar clinical characteristics, and peripheral and central modulatory pain mechanisms resulting from complex genetic and environmental contributions.

The poor prognosis for TMD patients with FMS (only 5% sustained remission after treatment) highlights the importance of recognizing whether perpetuation of TMD symptoms is due to the continuous FMS central pain amplification mechanisms. Understanding both TMD and FMS will lead to better recognition and management of these patients.

References

Aaron, L. A., & Buchwald, D. (2001a). Fibromyalgia and other unexplained clinical conditions. *Current Rheumatology Reports, 3*, 116–122.

Aaron, L. A., & Buchwald, D. (2001b). A review of the evidence for overlap among unexplained clinical conditions. *Annals of Internal Medicine, 134*, 868–881.

Aaron, L. A., & Buchwald, D. (2003). Chronic diffuse musculoskeletal pain, fibromyalgia and co-morbid unexplained clinical conditions. *Best Practice & Research: Clinical Rheumatology, 17*, 563–574.

Aaron, L. A., Burke, M. M., & Buchwald, D. (2000). Overlapping conditions among patients with chronic fatigue syndrome, fibromyalgia, and temporomandibular disorder. *Archives of Internal Medicine, 160*, 221–227.

Adler, G. K., Kinsley, B. T., Hurwitz, S., Mossey, C. J., & Goldenberg, D. L. (1999). Reduced hypothalamic-pituitary and sympathoadrenal responses to hypoglycemia in women with fibromyalgia syndrome. *The American Journal of Medicine, 106*, 534–543.

Balasubramaniam, R., de Leeuw, R., Zhu, H., Nickerson, R. B., Okeson, J. P., & Carlson, C. R. (2007). Prevalence of temporomandibular disorders in fibromyalgia and failed back syndrome patients: a blinded prospective comparison study. *Oral Surgery, Oral Medicine, Oral Pathology, Oral Radiology, and Endodontics, 104*, 204–216.

Bengtsson, A., Henriksson, K. G., Jorfeldt, L., Kagedal, B., Lennmarken, C., & Lindstrom, F. (1986a). Primary fibromyalgia. A clinical and laboratory study of 55 patients. *Scandinavian Journal of Rheumatology, 15*, 340–347.

Bengtsson, A., Henriksson, K. G., & Larsson, J. (1986b). Reduced high-energy phosphate levels in the painful muscles of patients with primary fibromyalgia. *Arthritis and Rheumatism, 29*, 817–821.

Berglund, B., Harju, E. L., Kosek, E., & Lindblom, U. (2002). Quantitative and qualitative perceptual analysis of cold dysesthesia and hyperalgesia in fibromyalgia. *Pain, 96*, 177–187.

Bradley, L. A., McKendree-Smith, N. L., & Alarcon, G. S. (2000). Pain complaints in patients with fibromyalgia versus chronic fatigue syndrome. *Current Review of Pain, 4*, 148–157.

Buskila, D. (2001). Fibromyalgia, chronic fatigue syndrome, and myofascial pain syndrome. *Current Opinion in Rheumatology, 13*, 117–127.

Cimino, R., Michelotti, A., Stradi, R., & Farinaro, C. (1998). Comparison of clinical and psychologic features of fibromyalgia and masticatory myofascial pain. *Journal of Orofacial Pain, 12*, 35–41.

Clauw, D. J., & Chrousos, G. P. (1997). Chronic pain and fatigue syndromes: overlapping clinical and neuroendocrine features and potential pathogenic mechanisms. *Neuroimmunomodulation, 4*, 134–153.

Clauw, D. J., & Crofford, L. J. (2003). Chronic widespread pain and fibromyalgia: what we know, and what we need to know. *Best Practice & Research. Clinical Rheumatology, 17*, 685–701.

Cohen, H., Neumann, L., Shore, M., Amir, M., Cassuto, Y., & Buskila, D. (2000). Autonomic dysfunction in patients with fibromyalgia: application of power spectral analysis of heart rate variability. *Seminars in Arthritis and Rheumatism, 29,* 217–227.

Crofford, L. J., Young, E. A., Engleberg, N. C., Korszun, A., Brucksch, C. B., McClure, L. A., Brown, M. B., & Demitrack, M. A. (2004). Basal circadian and pulsatile ACTH and cortisol secretion in patients with fibromyalgia and/or chronic fatigue syndrome. *Brain, Behavior, and Immunity, 18,* 314–325.

Dadabhoy, D., Crofford, L. J., Spaeth, M., Russell, I. J., & Clauw, D. J. (2008). Biology and therapy of fibromyalgia. Evidence-based biomarkers for fibromyalgia syndrome. *Arthritis Research & Therapy, 10,* 211.

Dao, T. T., Reynolds, W. J., & Tenenbaum, H. C. (1997). Comorbidity between myofascial pain of the masticatory muscles and fibromyalgia. *Journal of Orofacial Pain, 11,* 232–241.

de Abreu, T. C., Nilner, M., Thulin, T., & Vallon, D. (1993). Office and ambulatory blood pressure in patients with craniomandibular disorders. *Acta Odontologica Scandinavica, 51,* 161–170.

Rodriguez de Sotillo, D., Velly, A.M., Hadley, M., Fricton, J.R. (2011). Evidence of oxidative stress in temporomandibular disorders: a pilot study. *Journal of Oral Rehabilitation 38(10), 722–728.*

DeSantana, J. M., & Sluka, K. A. (2008). Central mechanisms in the maintenance of chronic widespread noninflammatory muscle pain. *Current Pain and Headache Reports, 12,* 338–343.

Desmeules, J. A., Cedraschi, C., Rapiti, E., Baumgartner, E., Finckh, A., Cohen, P., Dayer, P., & Vischer, T. L. (2003). Neurophysiologic evidence for a central sensitization in patients with fibromyalgia. *Arthritis and Rheumatism, 48,* 1420–1429.

Diatchenko, L., Slade, G., Nackley, A., Bhalang, K., Sigurdsson, A., Belfer, I., Goldman, D., Xu, K., Shabalina, S., Shagin, D., Max, M., Makarov, S., & Maixner, W. (2005). Genetic basis for individual variations in pain perception and the develoopment of a chronic pain condition. *Human Molecular Genetics, 14,* 135–143.

Domschke, K., Freitag, C. M., Kuhlenbaumer, G., Schirmacher, A., Sand, P., Nyhuis, P., Jacob, C., Fritze, J., Franke, P., Rietschel, M., Garritsen, H. S., Fimmers, R., Nothen, M. M., Lesch, K. P., Stogbauer, F., & Deckert, J. (2004). Association of the functional V158M catechol-O-methyl-transferase polymorphism with panic disorder in women. *The International Journal of Neuropsychopharmacology, 7,* 183–188.

Drangsholt, M., & LeResche, L. (1999). Temporomandibular Disorders Pain. In I. K. Crombie, P. R. Croft, S. J. Linton, L. LeResche, & M. Von Korff (Eds.), *Epidemiology of Pain.* Seattle, WA: IASP.

Dubner, R. (1992). Neuronal plasticity in the spinal dorsal horn following tissue inflammation. In R. Inoki, Y. Shigenaga, & M. Tohyama (Eds.), *Processing and Inhibition of Nociceptive Information* (pp. 35–41). Excerpta medica: Tokyo.

Dubner, R. (61). Hyperalgesia in Response to Injury to Cutaneous and Deep Tissues. In O. Pain, T. Disorders, J. Fricton, & R. Dubner (Eds.), *New* (pp. 71–1995). York: Raven Press, Ltd.

Dubner, R., & Bennett, G. J. (1983). Spinal and trigeminal mechanisms of nociception. *Annual Review of Neuroscience, 6,* 381–418.

Dworkin, S. F., & LeResche, L. (1992). Research diagnostic criteria for temporomandibular disorders: review, criteria, examinations and specifications, critique [Review]. *Journal of Craniomandibular Disorders, 6,* 301–355.

Dworkin, S. F., LeResche, L., Fricton, J. R., Mohl, N., Sommers, E., & Truelove, E. (1992). Research diagnostic criteria, Part II, Axis I: Clinical TMD Conditions[Review]. *Journal of Craniomandibular Disorders, 6,* 327–330.

Dworkin, S. F., LeResche, L., Von Korff, M., Truelove, E., & Sommers, E. (1989). Predicting Continued Presence and Level of TMD Pain: An Epidemiologic Study. *Journal of Dental Research, 68,* 194.

Elam, M., Johansson, G., & Wallin, B. G. (1992). Do patients with primary fibromyalgia have an altered muscle sympathetic nerve activity? *Pain, 48,* 371–375.

El-Labban, N. G., Harris, M., Hopper, C., & Barber, P. (1990). Degenerative changes in masseter and temporalis muscles in limited mouth opening and TMJ ankylosis. *Journal Oral Pathology Medicine, 19,* 423–425.

Enoch, M. A., Xu, K., Ferro, E., Harris, C. R., & Goldman, D. (2003). Genetic origins of anxiety in women: A role for a functional catechol-O-methyltransferase polymorphism. *Psychiatric Genetics, 13,* 33–41.

Eriksson, P. O., Lindman, R., Stal, P., & Bengtsson, A. (1988). Symptoms and signs of mandibular dysfunction in primary fibromyalgia syndrome (PSF) patients. *Swedish Dental Journal, 12,* 141–149.

Eriksson, P. O., & Thornell, L. E. (1983). Histochemical and morphological muscle-fibre characteristics of the human masseter, the medial pterygoid, and the temporal muscles. *Archives of Oral Biology, 28,* 781–795.

Farella, M., Michelotti, A., Steenks, M. H., Romeo, R., Cimino, R., & Bosman, F. (2000). The diagnostic value of pressure algometry in myofascial pain of the jaw muscles. *Journal of Oral Rehabilitation, 27,* 9–14.

Fernandez-de-Las-Penas, C., Galan-Del-Rio, F., Alonso-Blanco, C., Jimenez-Garcia, R., Arendt-Nielsen, L., & Svensson, P. (2010). Referred pain from muscle trigger points in the masticatory and neck-shoulder musculature in women with temporomandibular disorders. *The Journal of Pain, 11,* 1295–1304.

Fricton, J. (1990). Myofascial Pain syndrome: Characteristics and epidemiology. In J. Fricton & E. Awad (Eds.), *Advances in Pain Research and Therapy* (pp. 107–127). New York: Raven Press.

Fricton, J. R. (2004). The relationship of temporomandibular disorders and fibromyalgia: Implications for diagnosis and treatment. *Current Pain and Headache Reports, 8,* 355–363.

Fricton, J., & Dall' Arancio, D. (1994). Myofascial pain of the head and neck: Controlled outcome study of an inter-disciplinary pain program. *Journal of Musculoskeletal Pain, 2,* 81–99.

Fricton, J. R. K. R., & Haley, D. (1982). Myofascial pain syndrome: A review of 164 cases. *Oral Surgery, 60,* 615–623.

Fricton, J., Kroening, R., Haley, D., & Siegert, R. (1985). Myofascial pain syndrome of the head and neck: A review of clinical characteristics of 164 patients. *Oral Surgery, Oral Medicine, and Oral Pathology, 60,* 615–623.

Garofalo, J. P., Gatchel, R. J., Wesley, A. L., & Ellis, E., 3rd. (1998). Predicting chronicity in acute temporomandibular joint disorders using the research diagnostic criteria. *The Journal of the American Dental Association, 129,* 438–447.

Gatchel, R. J., Garofalo, J. P., Ellis, E., & Holt, C. (1996). Major psychological disorders in acute and chronic TMD: an initial examination. *The Journal of the American Dental Association, 127,* 1365–1374.

Gatchel, R. J., Peng, Y. B., Peters, M. L., Fuchs, P. N., & Turk, D. C. (2007). The biopsychosocial approach to chronic pain: Scientific advances and future directions. *Psychological Bulletin, 133,* 581–624.

Ge, H. Y., Wang, Y., Danneskiold-Samsoe, B., Graven-Nielsen, T., & Arendt-Nielsen, L. (2010). The predetermined sites of examination for tender points in fibromyalgia syndrome are frequently associated with myofascial trigger points. *The Journal of Pain, 11,* 644–651.

Gerwin, R. D. (2011). Fibromyalgia tender points at examination sites specified by the American College of Rheumatology criteria are almost universally myofascial trigger points. *Current Pain and Headache Reports, 15,* 1–3.

Giovengo, S. L., Russell, I. J., & Larson, A. A. (1999). Increased concentrations of nerve growth factor in cerebrospinal fluid of patients with fibromyalgia. *The Journal of Rheumatology, 26,* 1564–1569.

Giske, L., Vollestad, N. K., Mengshoel, A. M., Jensen, J., Knardahl, S., & Roe, C. (2008). Attenuated adrenergic responses to exercise in women with fibromyalgia–a controlled study. *European Journal of Pain, 12,* 351–360.

Glass, J. M., Lyden, A. K., Petzke, F., Stein, P., Whalen, G., Ambrose, K., Chrousos, G., & Clauw, D. J. (2004). The effect of brief exercise cessation on pain, fatigue, and mood symptom development in healthy, fit individuals. *Journal of Psychosomatic Research, 57,* 391–398.

Goldenberg, D. L. (2002). Office management of fibromyalgia. *Rheumatic Diseases Clinics of North America, 28,* 437–446.

Gracely, R. H., Geisser, M. E., Giesecke, T., Grant, M. A., Petzke, F., Williams, D. A., & Clauw, D. J. (2004). Pain catastrophizing and neural responses to pain among persons with fibromyalgia. *Brain, 127,* 835–843.

Granges, G., & Littlejohn, G. (1993). Pressure pain threshold in pain-free subjects, in patients with chronic regional pain syndromes, and in patients with fibromyalgia syndrome. *Arthritis and Rheumatism, 36,* 642–646.

Guilbaud, G. (1991). Central neurophysiological processing of joint pain on the basis of studies performed in normal animals and in models of experimental arthritis. *Canadian Journal of Physiology and Pharmacology, 69,* 637–646.

Gur, A., Cevik, R., Nas, K., Colpan, L., & Sarac, S. (2004). Cortisol and hypothalamic-pituitary-gonadal axis hormones in follicular-phase women with fibromyalgia and chronic fatigue syndrome and effect of depressive symptoms on these hormones. *Arthritis Research & Therapy, 6,* R232–238.

Gursoy, S., Erdal, E., Herken, H., Madenci, E., Alasehirli, B., & Erdal, N. (2003). Significance of catechol-O-methyltransferase gene polymorphism in fibromyalgia syndrome. *Rheumatology International, 23,* 104–107.

Hamaty, D., Valentine, J. L., Howard, R., Howard, C. W., Wakefield, V., & Patten, M. S. (1989). The plasma endorphin, prostaglandin and catecholamine profile of patients with fibrositis treated with cyclobenzaprine and placebo: a 5-month study. *The Journal of Rheumatology. Supplement, 19,* 164–168.

Hamilton, S. P., Slager, S. L., Heiman, G. A., Deng, Z., Haghighi, F., Klein, D. F., Hodge, S. E., Weissman, M. M., Fyer, A. J., & Knowles, J. A. (2002). Evidence for a susceptibility locus for panic disorder near the catechol-O-methyltransferase gene on chromosome 22. *Biological Psychiatry, 51,* 591–601.

Hedenberg-Magnusses, B., Ernberg, M., & Koop, S. (1999). Presence of orofacial pain and temporomandibular disorders in fibromyalgia. *Swedish Dental Journal, 23,* 185–192.

Hedenberg-Magnusson, B., Ernberg, M., & Kopp, S. (1997). Symptoms and signs of temporomandibular disorders in patients with fibromyalgia and local myalgia of the temporomandibular system. A comparative study. *Acta Odontologica Scandinavica, 55,* 344–349.

Hoeger-Bement, M. K., & Sluka, K. A. (2003). Phosphorylation of CREB and mechanical hyperalgesia is reversed by blockade of the cAMP pathway in a time-dependent manner after repeated intramuscular acid injections. *Journal of Neuroscience, 23,* 5437–5445.

Hoffmann, R. G., Kotchen, J. M., Kotchen, T. A., Cowley, T., Dasgupta, M., & Cowley, A. W., Jr. (2011). Temporomandibular disorders and associated clinical comorbidities. *The Clinical Journal of Pain, 27,* 268–274.

Hong, C.-Z. (1994). Persistence of local twitch response with loss of conduction to and from the spinal cord. *Archives of Physical Medicine and Rehabilitation, 75,* 12–16.

Hong, C.-Z., & Torigoe, Y. (1994). Electrophysiological charateristics of localized twitch responses in responsive taut bands of rabbit skeletal muscle. *Journal of Musculoskeletal Pain, 2,* 17–43.

Hubbard, D. R., & Berkoff, G. M. (1993). Myofascial trigger points show spontaneous needle EMG activity. *Spine (Philadelphia, Pa. 1976), 18*, 1803–1807.

Isong, U., Gansky, S. A., & Plesh, O. (2008). Temporomandibular joint and muscle disorder-type pain in U.S. adults: the National Health Interview Survey. *Journal of Orofacial Pain, 22*, 317–322.

Jensen, M. P., & Karoly, P. (1991). Control beliefs, coping efforts, and adjustment to chronic pain. *Journal of Consulting and Clinical Psychology, 59*, 431–438.

Jensen, M. P., Turner, J. A., & Romano, J. M. (1991). Self-efficacy and outcome expectancies: Relationship to chronic pain coping strategies and adjustment. *Pain, 44*, 263–269.

Jensen, M. P., Turner, J. A., Romano, J. M., & Lawler, B. K. (1994). Relationship of pain-specific beliefs to chronic pain adjustment. *Pain, 57*, 301–309.

John, M. T., Miglioretti, D. L., LeResche, L., Von Korff, M., & Critchlow, C. W. (2003). Widespread pain as a risk factor for dysfunctional temporomandibular disorder pain. *Pain, 102*, 257–263.

Jones, D. A., Rollman, G. B., & Brooke, R. I. (1997). The cortisol response to psychological stress in temporomandibular dysfunction. *Pain, 72*, 171–182.

Julien, N., Goffaux, P., Arsenault, P., & Marchand, S. (2005). Widespread pain in fibromyalgia is related to a deficit of endogenous pain inhibition. *Pain, 114*, 295–302.

Kashima, K., Rahman, O. I., Sakoda, S., & Shiba, R. (1999). Increased pain sensitivity of the upper extremities of TMD patients with myalgia to experimentally-evoked noxious stimulation: Possibility of worsened endogenous opioid systems. *Cranio, 17*, 241–246.

Katz, D. L., Greene, L., Ali, A., & Faridi, Z. (2007). The pain of fibromyalgia syndrome is due to muscle hypoperfusion induced by regional vasomotor dysregulation. *Medical Hypotheses, 69*, 517–525.

Kniffki, K. D., Mense, S., & Schmidt, R. F. (1978). Responses of group IV afferent units from skeletal muscle to stretch, contraction and chemical stimulation. *Experimental Brain Research, 31*, 511–522.

Komaroff, A. L., & Goldenberg, D. (1989). The chronic fatigue syndrome: Definition, current studies and lessons for fibromyalgia research. *The Journal of Rheumatology. Supplement, 19*, 23–27.

Korszun, A., Papadopoulos, E., Demitrack, M., Engleberg, C., & Crofford, L. (1998). The relationship between temporomandibular disorders and stress-associated syndromes. *Oral Surgery, Oral Medicine, Oral Pathology, Oral Radiology, and Endodontics, 86*, 416–420.

Korszun, A., Young, E. A., Singer, K., Carlson, N. E., Brown, M. B., & Crofford, L. (2002). Basal circadian cortisol secretion in women with temporomandibular disorders. *Journal of Dental Research, 81*, 279–283.

Kosek, E., Ekholm, J., & Hansson, P. (1996a). Modulation of pressure pain thresholds during and following isometric contraction in patients with fibromyalgia and in healthy controls. *Pain, 64*, 415–423.

Kosek, E., Ekholm, J., & Hansson, P. (1996b). Sensory dysfunction in fibromyalgia patients with implications for pathogenic mechanisms. *Pain, 68*, 375–383.

Laske, C., Stransky, E., Eschweiler, G. W., Klein, R., Wittorf, A., Leyhe, T., Richartz, E., Kohler, N., Bartels, M., Buchkremer, G., & Schott, K. (2007). Increased BDNF serum concentration in fibromyalgia with or without depression or antidepressants. *Journal of Psychiatric Research, 41*, 600–605.

Laskin, D., Greenfield, E., Gale, E., Ruth, J., Neff, P., Alling, C., et al. (1983). *The President's conference on the examination, diagnosis and management of temporomandibular disorders*. Chicago: American Dental Association.

Lautenbacher, S., & Rollman, G. B. (1997). Possible deficiencies of pain modulation in fibromyalgia. *The Clinical Journal of Pain, 13*, 189–196.

Lautenbacher, S., Rollman, G. B., & McCain, G. A. (1994). Multi-method assessment of experimental and clinical pain in patients with fibromyalgia. *Pain, 59*, 45–53.

Lawrence, R. C., Felson, D. T., Helmick, C. G., Arnold, L. M., Choi, H., Deyo, R. A., Gabriel, S., Hirsch, R., Hochberg, M. C., Hunder, G. G., Jordan, J. M., Katz, J. N., Kremers, H. M., & Wolfe, F. (2008). Estimates of the prevalence of arthritis and other rheumatic conditions in the United States Part II. *Arthritis and Rheumatism, 58*, 26–35.

Leblebici, B., Pektas, Z. O., Ortancil, O., Hurcan, E. C., Bagis, S., & Akman, M. N. (2007). Coexistence of fibromyalgia, temporomandibular disorder, and masticatory myofascial pain syndromes. *Rheumatology International, 27*, 541–544.

Legangneux, E., Mora, J. J., Spreux-Varoquaux, O., Thorin, I., Herrou, M., Alvado, G., & Gomeni, C. (2001). Cerebrospinal fluid biogenic amine metabolites, plasma-rich platelet serotonin and [3H]imipramine reuptake in the primary fibromyalgia syndrome. *Rheumatology (Oxford, England), 40*, 290–296.

LeResche, L. (1997). Epidemiology of temporomandibular disorders: Implications for the investigation of etiologic factors. *Critical Reviews in Oral Biology and Medicine, 8*, 291–305.

LeResche, L., Mancl, L. A., Drangsholt, M. T., Huang, G., & Von Korff, M. (2007). Predictors of onset of facial pain and temporomandibular disorders in early adolescence. *Pain, 129*, 269–278.

Light, K. C., Bragdon, E. E., Grewen, K. M., Brownley, K. A., Girdler, S. S., & Maixner, W. (2009). Adrenergic dysregulation and pain with and without acute beta-blockade in women with fibromyalgia and temporomandibular disorder. *The Journal of Pain, 10*, 542–552.

Lim, P. F., Smith, S., Bhalang, K., Slade, G. D., & Maixner, W. (2010). Development of temporomandibular disorders is associated with greater bodily pain experience. *The Clinical Journal of Pain, 26*, 116–120.

Litt, M. D., Shafer, D. M., Ibanez, C. R., Kreutzer, D. L., & Tawfik-Yonkers, Z. (2009). Momentary pain and coping in temporomandibular disorder pain: exploring mechanisms of cognitive behavioral treatment for chronic pain. *Pain, 145*, 160–168.

Litt, M. D., Shafer, D., & Napolitano, C. (2004). Momentary mood and coping processes in TMD pain. *Health Psychology, 23*, 354–362.

Loeser, J. D., & Melzack, R. (1999). Pain: An overview. *The Lancet, 353*, 1607–1609.

Maekawa, K., Clark, G. T., & Kuboki, T. (2002). Intramuscular hypoperfusion, adrenergic receptors, and chronic muscle pain. *The Journal of Pain, 3*, 251–260.

Maekawa, K., Twe, C., Lotaif, A., Chiappelli, F., & Clark, G. T. (2003). Function of beta-adrenergic receptors on mononuclear cells in female patients with fibromyalgia. *The Journal of Rheumatology, 30*, 364–368.

Maixner, W., Fillingim, R., Booker, D., & Sigurdsson, A. (1995). Sensitivity of patients with painful temporomandibular disorders to experimentally evoked pain. *Pain, 63*, 341–351.

Maixner, W., Fillingim, R., Sigurdsson, A., Kincaid, S., & Silva, S. (1998). Sensitivity of patients with painful temporomandibular disorders to experimentally evoked pain: evidence for altered temporal summation of pain. *Pain, 76*, 71–81.

Mao, J., Stein, R. B., & Osborn, J. W. (1993). Fatigue in Human Jaw Muscles: A Review. *Journal of Orofacial Pain, 7*, 135–142.

Martinez-Lavin, M. (2007). Biology and therapy of fibromyalgia. Stress, the stress response system, and fibromyalgia. *Arthritis Research & Therapy, 9*, 216.

Mayo, K. H., Ellis, E., III, & Carlson, D. S. (1988). Histochemical characteristics of masseter and temporalis muscles after 5 weeks of maxillomandibular fixation- An investigation in Macaca mulatta. *Oral Surgery, Oral Medicine, and Oral Pathology, 66*, 421–426.

McCain, G. A., & Tilbe, K. S. (1989). Diurnal hormone variation in fibromyalgia syndrome: a comparison with rheumatoid arthritis. *The Journal of Rheumatology. Supplement, 19*, 154–157.

McLean, S. A., Williams, D. A., Harris, R. E., Kop, W. J., Groner, K. H., Ambrose, K., Lyden, A. K., Gracely, R. H., Crofford, L. J., Geisser, M. E., Sen, A., Biswas, P., & Clauw, D. J. (2005). Momentary relationship between cortisol secretion and symptoms in patients with fibromyalgia. *Arthritis and Rheumatism, 52*, 3660–3669.

Meeus, M., & Nijs, J. (2007). Central sensitization: a biopsychosocial explanation for chronic widespread pain in patients with fibromyalgia and chronic fatigue syndrome. *Clinical Rheumatology, 26*, 465–473.

Melzack, R. (1971). Phantom limb pain: Concept of a central biasing mechanism. *Clinical Neurosurgery, 18*, 188–207.

Melzack, R. (1981). Myofascial trigger points: Relation to acupuncture and mechanisms of pain. *Archives of Physical Medicine and Rehabilitation, 62*, 114–117.

Mense, S. (1993). Nociception from Skeletal Muscle in Relation to Clinical Muscle Pain. *Pain, 54*, 241–289.

Moldofsky, H. K. (2001). Disordered sleep in fibromyalgia and related myofascial facial pain conditions. *Dental Clinics of North America, 45*, 701–713.

Nackley, A. G., Tan, K. S., Fecho, K., Flood, P., Diatchenko, L., & Maixner, W. (2007). Catechol-O-methyltransferase inhibition increases pain sensitivity through activation of both beta2- and beta3-adrenergic receptors. *Pain, 128*, 199–208.

Nagakura, Y., Oe, T., Aoki, T., & Matsuoka, N. (2009). Biogenic amine depletion causes chronic muscular pain and tactile allodynia accompanied by depression: A putative animal model of fibromyalgia. *Pain, 146*, 26–33.

National Institute of Dental and Craniofacial Research. (2009). Facial pain. Retrieved from: http://www.nidcr.nih.gov/DataStatistics/FindDataByTopic/FacialPain/.

Okeson, J. (1996). Differential diagnosis and management considerations of temporomandibular disorders. In J. Okeson (Ed.), *Orofacial pain* (pp. 113–184). Chicago: Quintessence.

Pennacchio, E. A., Borg-Stein, J., & Keith, D. A. (1998). The incidence of pain in the muscles of mastication in patients with fibromyalgia. *Journal of the Massachusetts Dental Society, 47*, 8–12.

Perry, F., Heller, P. H., Kamiya, J., & Levine, J. D. (1989). Altered autonomic function in patients with arthritis or with chronic myofascial pain. *Pain, 39*, 77–84.

Pfau, D. B., Rolke, R., Nickel, R., Treede, R. D., & Daublaender, M. (2009). Somatosensory profiles in subgroups of patients with myogenic temporomandibular disorders and Fibromyalgia Syndrome. *Pain, 147*, 72–83.

Plesh, O., Wolfe, F., & Lane, N. (1996). The relationship between fibromyalgia and temporomandibular disorders: Prevalence and symptom severity. *The Journal of Rheumatology, 23*, 1948–1952.

Poirot, O., Berta, T., Decosterd, I., & Kellenberger, S. (2006). Distinct ASIC currents are expressed in rat putative nociceptors and are modulated by nerve injury. *Journal of Physiology, 576*, 215–234.

Price, D. D., Staud, R., Robinson, M. E., Mauderli, A. P., Cannon, R., & Vierck, C. J. (2002). Enhanced temporal summation of second pain and its central modulation in fibromyalgia patients. *Pain, 99*, 49–59.

Raphael, K. G., & Marbach, J. J. (2001). Widespread pain and the effectiveness of oral splints in myofascial face pain. *The Journal of the American Dental Association, 132*, 305–316.

Rhodus, N. L., Fricton, J., Carlson, P., & Messner, R. (2003). Oral symptoms associated with fibromyalgia syndrome. *The Journal of Rheumatology, 30*, 1841–1845.

Rolke, R., Magerl, W., Campbell, K. A., Schalber, C., Caspari, S., Birklein, F., & Treede, R. D. (2006). Quantitative sensory testing: A comprehensive protocol for clinical trials. *European Journal of Pain, 10*, 77–88.

Russell, I. J. (1989). Neurohormonal aspects of fibromyalgia syndrome. *Rheumatic Diseases Clinics of North America, 15*, 149–168.

Russell, I. J., Orr, M. D., Littman, B., Vipraio, G. A., Alboukrek, D., Michalek, J. E., Lopez, Y., & MacKillip, F. (1994). Elevated cerebrospinal fluid levels of substance P in patients with the fibromyalgia syndrome. *Arthritis and Rheumatism, 37*, 1593–1601.

Sarchielli, P., Mancini, M. L., Floridi, A., Coppola, F., Rossi, C., Nardi, K., Acciarresi, M., Pini, L. A., & Calabresi, P. (2007). Increased levels of neurotrophins are not specific for chronic migraine: evidence from primary fibromyalgia syndrome. *The Journal of Pain, 8*, 737–745.

Schiffman, E. L., Fricton, J. R., Haley, D. P., & Shapiro, B. L. (1990). The prevalence and treatment needs of subjects with temporomandibular disorders. *The Journal of the American Dental Association, 120*, 295–303.

Schmidt, J. E., & Carlson, C. R. (2009). A controlled comparison of emotional reactivity and physiological response in masticatory muscle pain patients. *Journal of Orofacial Pain, 23*, 230–242.

Sessle, B. (1995a). Brainstem Mechanisms of Orofacial Pain. In J. Fricton & R. Dubner (Eds.), *Orofacial Pain and Temporomandibular Disorders* (pp. 43–60). New York: Raven Press.

Sessle, B. (1995b). Masticatory Muscle Disorders: Basic Science Perspectives. In B. J. Sessle, P. S. Bryant, & R. A. Dionne (Eds.), *Temporomandibular Disorders and Related Pain Conditions: Progress in Pain Research and Therapy* (pp. 47–61). IASP Press: Seatle.

Shabalina, S. A., Zaykin, D. V., Gris, P., Ogurtsov, A. Y., Gauthier, J., Shibata, K., Tchivileva, I. E., Belfer, I., Mishra, B., Kiselycznyk, C., Wallace, M. R., Staud, R., Spiridonov, N. A., Max, M. B., Goldman, D., Fillingim, R. B., Maixner, W., & Diatchenko, L. (2009). Expansion of the human mu-opioid receptor gene architecture: novel functional variants. *Human Molecular Genetics, 18*, 1037–1051.

Simons, D. (1990). Muscle pain syndromes. In J. Fricton & E. Awad (Eds.), *Myofascial Pain and Fibromyalgia* (pp. 1–41). New York: Raven Press.

Simons, D. G. (2008). New views of myofascial trigger points: etiology and diagnosis. *Archives of Physical Medicine and Rehabilitation, 89*, 157–159.

Skyba, D. A., King, E. W., & Sluka, K. A. (2002). Effects of NMDA and non-NMDA ionotropic glutamate receptor antagonists on the development and maintenance of hyperalgesia induced by repeated intramuscular injection of acidic saline. *Pain, 98*, 69–78.

Skyba, D. A., Lisi, T. L., & Sluka, K. A. (2005). Excitatory amino acid concentrations increase in the spinal cord dorsal horn after repeated intramuscular injection of acidic saline. *Pain, 119*, 142–149.

Slade, G. D., Diatchenko, L., Bhalang, K., Sigurdsson, A., Fillingim, R. B., Belfer, I., Max, M. B., Goldman, D., & Maixner, W. (2007). Influence of psychological factors on risk of temporomandibular disorders. *Journal of Dental Research, 86*, 1120–1125.

Sluka, K. A., Kalra, A., & Moore, S. A. (2001). Unilateral intramuscular injections of acidic saline produce a bilateral, long-lasting hyperalgesia. *Muscle & Nerve, 24*, 37–46.

Sluka, K. A., Price, M. P., Breese, N. M., Stucky, C. L., Wemmie, J. A., & Welsh, M. J. (2003). Chronic hyperalgesia induced by repeated acid injections in muscle is abolished by the loss of ASIC3, but not ASIC1. *Pain, 106*, 229–239.

Sluka, K. A., Radhakrishnan, R., Benson, C. J., Eshcol, J. O., Price, M. P., Babinski, K., Audette, K. M., Yeomans, D. C., & Wilson, S. P. (2007). ASIC3 in muscle mediates mechanical, but not heat, hyperalgesia associated with muscle inflammation. *Pain, 129*, 102–112.

Solberg Nes, L., Carlson, C. R., Crofford, L. J., de Leeuw, R., & Segerstrom, S. C. (2010). Self-regulatory deficits in fibromyalgia and temporomandibular disorders. *Pain, 151*, 37–44.

Ta, L., Phero, J., Pillemer, S., Hale-Donze, H., McCartney-Francis, N., Kingman, A., Max, M., Gordon, S., Wahl, S., & Dionne, R. (2002). Clinical evaluation of patients with temporomandibular joint implants. *Journal of Oral and Maxillofacial Surgery, 60*, 1389–1399.

Travell, J. S. D. (1998). *Myofascial Pain and Dysfunction: The Trigger Point Manual*. Baltimore: Williams & Wilkins Co.

Truelove, E. L., Sommers, E. E., LeResche, L., Dworkin, S. F., & Von Korff, M. (1992). Clinical diagnostic criteria for TMD. New classification permits multiple diagnoses. *The Journal of the American Dental Association, 123*, 47–54.

Turner, J. A., & Aaron, L. A. (2001). Pain-related catastrophizing: What is it? *The Clinical Journal of Pain, 17*, 65–71.

Turner, J. A., Brister, H., Huggins, K., Mancl, L., Aaron, L. A., & Truelove, E. L. (2005). Catastrophizing is associated with clinical examination findings, activity interference, and health care use among patients with temporomandibular disorders. *Journal of Orofacial Pain, 19*, 291–300.

Turner, J. A., Dworkin, S. F., Mancl, L., Huggins, K. H., & Truelove, E. L. (2001). The roles of beliefs, catastrophizing, and coping in the functioning of patients with temporomandibular disorders. *Pain, 92*, 41–51.

Uhlig, Y. (1995). Fiber composition and fiber transformation in neck muscles of patients with dysfunction of the cervical spine. *Journal of Orthopaedic Research, 13*, 240–249.

Vaeroy, H., Helle, R., Forre, O., Kass, E., & Terenius, L. (1988). Elevated CSF levels of substance P and high incidence of Raynaud phenomenon in patients with fibromyalgia: new features for diagnosis. *Pain, 32*, 21–26.

Velly, A. M., Gornitsky, M., & Philippe, P. (2002). A case-control study of temporomandibular disorders: Symptomatic disc displacement. *Journal of Oral Rehabilitation, 29*, 408–416.

Velly, A. M., Gornitsky, M., & Philippe, P. (2003). Contributing factors to chronic myofascial pain: A case-control study. *Pain, 104*, 491–499.

Velly, A. M., Look, J. O., Schiffman, E., Lenton, P. A., Kang, W., Messner, R. P., Holcroft, C. A., & Fricton, J. R. (2010). The effect of fibromyalgia and widespread pain on the clinically significant temporomandibular muscle and joint pain disorders–a prospective 18-month cohort study. *Journal of pain, 11*, 1155–1164.

Von Korff, M., Dworkin, S. F., Le Resche, L., & Kruger, A. (1988). An epidemiologic comparison of pain complaints. *Pain, 32*, 173–183.

Wolfe, F., Anderson, J., Harkness, D., Bennett, R. M., Caro, X. J., Goldenberg, D. L., Russell, I. J., & Yunus, M. B. (1997a). A prospective, longitudinal, multicenter study of service utilization and costs in fibromyalgia. *Arthritis and Rheumatism, 40*, 1560–1570.

Wolfe, F., Anderson, J., Harkness, D., Bennett, R. M., Caro, X. J., Goldenberg, D. L., Russell, I. J., & Yunus, M. B. (1997b). Work and disability status of persons with fibromyalgia. *The Journal of Rheumatology, 24*, 1171–1178.

Wolfe, F., Clauw, D. J., Fitzcharles, M. A., Goldenberg, D. L., Katz, R. S., Mease, P., Russell, A. S., Russell, I. J., Winfield, J. B., & Yunus, M. B. (2010). The American College of Rheumatology preliminary diagnostic criteria for fibromyalgia and measurement of symptom severity. *Arthritis Care Research (Hoboken), 62*, 600–610.

Wolfe, F., Hawley, D. J., Cathey, M. A., Caro, X., & Russell, I. J. (1985). Fibrositis: symptom frequency and criteria for diagnosis. An evaluation of 291 rheumatic disease patients and 58 normal individuals. *The Journal of Rheumatology, 12*, 1159–1163.

Wolfe, F., Ross, K., Anderson, J., Russell, I. J., & Hebert, L. (1995). The prevalence and characteristics of fibromyalgia in the general population. *Arthritis and Rheumatism, 38*, 19–28.

Wolfe, F., Smythe, H. A., Yunus, M. B., Bennett, R. M., Bombardier, C., Goldenberg, D. L., Tugwell, P., Campbell, S. M., Abeles, M., Clark, P., et al. (1990). The American College of Rheumatology 1990 Criteria for the Classification of Fibromyalgia. Report of the Multicenter Criteria Committee. *Arthritis and Rheumatism, 33*, 160–172.

Woolf, CJ. (2010). Central sensitization: Implications for the diagnosis and treatment of pain. *Pain.* 152(3), S2–15

Wright, A. R., Gatchel, R. J., Wildenstein, L., Riggs, R., Buschang, P., & Ellis, E., 3rd. (2004). Biopsychosocial differences between high-risk and low-risk patients with acute TMD-related pain. *Journal of American Dental Association, 135*, 474–483.

Yunus, M. B. (1992). Towards a model of pathophysiology of fibromyalgia: Aberrant central pain mechanisms with peripheral modulation. *Journal of Rheumatology, 19*, 846–850.

Yunus, M. B. (2008). Central sensitivity syndromes: a new paradigm and group nosology for fibromyalgia and overlapping conditions, and the related issue of disease versus illness. *Seminars in Arthritis Rheumatism, 37*, 339–352.

Yunus, M. B., Kalyan-Raman, U. P., Kalyan-Raman, K., & Masi, A. T. (1986). Pathologic changes in muscle in primary fibromyalgia syndrome. *American Journal of Medicine, 81*, 38–42.

Zubieta, J. K., Heitzeg, M. M., Smith, Y. R., Bueller, J. A., Xu, K., Xu, Y., Koeppe, R. A., Stohler, C. S., & Goldman, D. (2003). COMT val158met genotype affects mu-opioid neurotransmitter responses to a pain stressor. *Science, 299*, 1240–1243.

Chapter 25
Phantom Limb Pain

Jens Foell and Herta Flor

The phenomenon of phantom limb pain, the feeling of pain in a body part that has been lost in an accidental or clinical amputation, has been known to medicine for a long time. In 1552, Ambroise Paré described this seemingly strange occurrence and postulated that the causal factor of phantom limb pain might not be some type of mental illness, like it was thought before, but a pain memory or peripheral factors (Keil 1990). The phenomenon received its modern name from Mitchell in 1872.

Phantom limb pain has to be distinguished from nonpainful sensations in the lost limb (phantom sensations), including the general perception that the limb is still there (phantom awareness), and residual limb (or stump) pain or nonpainful residual limb phenomena (Hunter et al. 2008). Whereas the majority of people who have had an amputation experience the feeling that the limb is still there (Hunter et al. 2003), phantom limb pain occurs in about 50–80% of amputees (Ephraim et al. 2005). While most amputations, both medical and accidental, affect arms or legs, painful and nonpainful phantom sensations have also been reported after the loss of other body parts like the breast (Rothemund et al. 2004) or a tooth (Marbach and Raphael 2000) and can also occur after spinal cord injury (Melzack and Loeser 1978) or brachial plexus avulsion (Finnerup et al. 2010).

The development, intensity and quality of phantom limb pain, compared between individuals, tends to be very heterogeneous. Some people report occasional short bursts of pain, divided by long stretches of painlessness, while others constantly experience the pain. The intensity ranges from a slightly annoying perception of pin pricks to a severe and excruciating experience of pain. Usually felt as more intense in the distal part of the phantom, it can also be experienced in a variety of different ways, including throbbing, burning, and cramping. In keeping with the general heterogeneity of the syndrome, the onset of phantom limb pain can occur immediately after the amputation or years later. In many cases, phantom limb pain can be elicited or exacerbated by a variety of environmental factors, like a change in the weather, psychological factors, or emotional distress. Similar variations are visible in nonpainful phantom phenomena: Patients can experience a numbness or a change in temperature of the phantom limb, the feeling that the missing limb is staying in a specific position (in some cases in a position that would be physically impossible for an actual limb) as well as voluntary and involuntary movements of the phantom. Onset and intensity of these nonpainful sensations are also heterogeneous. While most of this variability remains unexplained, factors such as age and gender do not seem to have an influence on the development of phantom limb pain (Hanley et al. 2007). Both phantom limb pain and nonpainful phantom phenomena are only very rarely reported in

J. Foell, Dipl. Psych (✉) • H. Flor, PhD
Department of Cognitive and Clinical Neuroscience, Central Institute of Mental Health,
University of Heidelberg, Mannheim, Germany
e-mail: Jens.Foell@li-mannheim.de

R.J. Moore (ed.), *Handbook of Pain and Palliative Care: Biobehavioral Approaches for the Life Course*,
DOI 10.1007/978-1-4419-1651-8_25, © Springer Science+Business Media, LLC 2012

patients with congenital limb deficiency (Wilkins et al. 1998) and it is unclear how those rare cases are to be interpreted in terms of a model of phantom limb pain (Price 2006).

In the light of the described variability, it is crucial to identify causal factors for phantom limb pain in order to prevent it from developing or to determine alleviating factors as a foundation for possible therapies. While there is a correlation between preoperative pain and phantom limb pain, recent improvements in pre- and perioperative pain treatments still have not led to a decrease in the number of new phantom limb pain sufferers (Nikolajsen and Jensen 2005). Also, if preoperative pain is an important factor for whether or not phantom limb pain will develop, we would expect a higher rate of phantom limb pain among amputees in the next few years or decades, as (at least in the Western world) an ever-increasing proportion of amputations are performed due to the effects of vascular diseases. In these cases, there have usually been painful sensations in the affected limb for months or even years prior to the amputation.

The removal of a limb not only changes the peripheral nervous system by cutting nerve fibers, but it also causes changes in the central nervous system, because the brain has to adapt to a new and different situation. In order to determine whether peripheral or central factors are responsible for eliciting phantom limb pain, Birbaumer et al. (1997) anesthetized the brachial plexus of amputees suffering from phantom limb pain, thereby ensuring that for a certain amount of time no peripheral input could be processed. They found that this method eliminated pain in 50% of the participants, raising questions about the influence of central and peripheral factors in the experience of pain. The knowledge of both types of causal factors is crucial if we are to prevent as well as provide effective pain relief for patients with phantom limb pain.

Peripheral Factors

Since neurons are flexible entities, which can grow and change their shapes to some degree, the damage caused to nerve fibers during an amputation can have differing consequences in individual cases. Sometimes, the terminal swelling that is formed and the axonal sprouting that occurs after a nerve cell is cut can lead to the formation of a neuroma. These are tangled knots of nerve tissue that develop because the axons are unable to reconnect properly. The activity of such malformed neurons can be spontaneous and unpredictable (Fried et al. 1991). Ectopic signals produced by these neuromas might also be responsible for some forms of pain in amputees.

Changes in the electrical properties of cell membranes can increase the excitability of damaged nerve cells. The mechanisms responsible for these changes involve the upregulation or novel expression, as well as the trafficking, of voltage-sensitive sodium channels and decreased potassium channel expression (Devor 2006). Another factor are altered transduction molecules for the sensitivities to heat, cold, and mechanical stimulation of the neuroma (Gorodetskaya et al. 2003). These alterations in the firing behavior of injured neurons might lead to the often reported exacerbating effects of changing temperatures on phantom limb pain, as well as the elicitation of phantom limb pain by nonpainful tactile stimulation of the stump (Nikolajsen and Jensen 2005).

However, the formation of neuromas is not instantaneous. Thus, the described effects cannot account for the frequent reports of phantom limb pain immediately after the amputation. Thus, researchers have looked for other sources of ectopic activation and found such activity, which can even summate with the ectopic discharges described earlier, in the dorsal root ganglion (DRG). This is a module on a dorsal root, containing the cell bodies of afferent neurons in the spine. Interactions between neighboring neurons can amplify the overall ectopic signal and thus exacerbate the pain. Moreover, both spontaneous and triggered sympathetic activation can elicit or intensify ectopic discharges (Chen et al. 1996), which might be one reason why the experience of phantom limb pain is generally stronger during times of emotional distress. This sympathetic-sensory coupling occurs both at the level of the neuroma and at the level of the DRG. Recently, it has been shown that there might be a genetically determined disposition to develop ectopic neuroma and DRG discharge (Devor 2005a, b). The genetic influence on the development of phantom limb pain, though understudied at this point in time, could also explain some of the observed differences in the experience of pain between individuals with very similar medical histories and kinds of amputation.

Central Factors: The Spinal Cord

There have been reports of usually pain-free amputees who have experienced phantom limb pain during spinal anesthesia (Schmidt et al. 2005). This phenomenon, paired with results from animal studies on neuropathic pain, suggests that changes in the spinal cord might be an important factor in the development of phantom limb pain. Altered activity in peripheral neurons can lead to enduring changes in the behavior of nerve cells at the level of the spinal cord: Increased nociceptive input related to inflammatory pain causes long-term changes in the synaptic responsiveness of neurons in the dorsal horn of the spinal cord, in a process known as central sensitization (Woolf and Salter 2005). It is feasible that a similar process of hyperexcitability is caused by the nerve damage also occurs during amputation. Increased firing of the dorsal horn neurons, structural changes at the central endings of the primary sensory neurons, and reduced inhibitory processes can be spinal effects of injured nerves (Woolf 2004). Interneurons containing the inhibitory substance γ-aminobutyric acid (GABA) or inhibitory glycinergic interneurons in the spinal cord may actually be destroyed by rapid ectopic discharge or other effects of axotomy (Woolf 2004), or they might change from their usually inhibitory to an excitatory effect, being influenced by BDNF (brain-derived neurotrophic factor), which is released by microglia cells (Coull et al. 2005).

The described mechanisms might all contribute to the hyperexcitability of the spinal cord circuitry after major nerve damage. Joining them is the downregulation of opioid receptors, both on primary afferent endings and intrinsic spinal neurons (Wang et al. 2005), which is expected to reduce activity of the inhibitory neurotransmitters GABA and glycine, thus increasing the disinhibition in the spinal cord. The upregulation of cholecystokinin, an endogenous inhibitor of the opiate receptor, which occurs in injured neural tissue (Wiesenfeld-Hallin et al. 2002), can also add to this effect.

Long-term changes in firing behavior also occur in ascending projection neurons from the spine to supraspinal centers. For example, the response of N-methyl-D-aspartate (NMDA) receptors to the primary afferent neurotransmitter glutamate can be facilitated after nerve damage (Torsney and MacDermott 2006). Interestingly, in some instances the behavioral change of neurons after tissue damage is not confined to an altered sensitivity: After injury, the large and myelinated Aβ-fibers, which usually carry nonnociceptive information, may express substance P. This neuropeptide is attributed to the sensation of pain and is usually expressed only by Aδ-afferents and C-afferents, most of which are nociceptors. These nociceptors conduct quick, sharp pain and secondary, delayed pain, respectively. This means that the damage caused by an amputation can cause low-threshold afferents to become fractionally connected to ascending spinal projection neurons which carry nociceptive information to supraspinal centers (Ueda 2006), thus being effectively transformed into nociceptors contributing to phantom limb pain.

The physical damage caused to neurons can be exacerbated by the degeneration of central projection axons. After dorsal root injury, or their separation from the spinal cord, deafferentation occurs on a large scale. If a region of the spine is vacated because of injured afferents, the neighboring regions can invade this area, which results in a spreading of hyperexcitability in the spinal cord. In animals, it has been shown that this spinal reorganization can lead to an expansion of the receptive fields on the parts of the skin next to the deafferented area (Devor and Wall 1978). As we shall see, similar effects of reorganization play an even more important role when it comes to the brainstem and cortex.

Central Factors: Brainstem, Thalamus, and Cortex

The peripheral and spinal causes that have been discussed cannot be the only determining factors associated with the development of phantom limb pain. For example, the fact that spinal anesthesia does not always alleviate phantom limb pain (Baron and Maier 1995) suggests that supraspinal changes can also influence this phenomenon. It is, of course, possible that the spinal changes discussed earlier may also have a strong influence on the supraspinal alterations, although this "bottom-up" model of sensory processing has been challenged by Ergenzinger et al. (1998), who caused alterations in receptive field characteristics of monkeys by suppressing cortical activity. Changes contributing to the occurrence and severity of phantom limb pain can be found in the cerebral cortex, the brainstem, the thalamus, and the anterior cingulated cortex (Zhang et al. 2005). In the cortex, the process of axonal sprouting, where new nerve endings and new connections between neurons are created, can lead to reorganization, as has been shown in amputation experiments with monkeys (Merzenich et al. 1984; Florence et al. 1998). Reorganization at the level of the thalamus has been shown in human amputees as well as in monkeys (Jain et al. 2008) and seems to be connected to the development of phantom awareness and phantom limb pain: Davis et al. (1998) elicited phantom sensations via thalamic stimulation. Brainstem, thalamus, and the cerebral cortex are connected by a variety of fibers and the alterations that occur in one of these parts after tissue damage could be at least partially responsible for changes in the other structures, although the exact nature and direction of these influences are not yet clear.

In order to better understand this process of cortical reorganization, Merzenich et al. (1984) used microelectrode recordings to measure the cortical activity of adult owl monkeys before and after removal of their digits. They looked at the primary somatosensory (SI) cortex. This is the region on the surface of the brain where the perceptive input from the body is processed and ordered in a somatotopic map. They showed that the areas next to the representation zone of the fingers that had been severed invaded the area that was no longer used. This way, cortical resources that are no longer necessary may be put to a new use and the representation of different body parts in the brain can shift by several millimeters. This shift is not found in patients with congenital limb deficiency (Montoya et al. 1998). A quite large representational shift, in the order of centimeters, was reported by Pons et al. (1991) after they performed a dorsal rhizotomy of the monkey's arms. They found that the representation of the cheek, which is next to the representational zones of arm and hand in the SI cortex, invaded these adjacent areas. This phenomenon has been postulated as being responsible for certain nonpainful referred sensations (Ramachandran et al. 1992): Some amputees, for example, report sensations in their phantom limb when they touch their cheeks or lips, usually while they are shaving or applying makeup. The connection between changes in the SI cortex and these referred sensations has since been challenged (Grüsser et al. 2001) and they might actually be related to alterations in the premotor cortex and parietal areas (Grüsser et al. 2004). Referred sensations can be recreated in a laboratory setting and their sensational quality is usually maintained, so that, for example, a vibrating stimulus applied to the correct spot on the cheek elicits the feeling of vibration in the phantom limb (Flor et al. 2000).

However, the relationship between referred sensations and phantom limb pain is still unclear. The described sensations are only experienced by a small proportion of amputees (Grüsser et al. 2001), some who may suffer from phantom limb pain and some who will not. It has been shown that the cortical remapping can vary strongly over time (Halligan et al. 1994), whereas phantom limb pain seems to be much more rigid over several years. Also, the shift of the mouth representation in SI into the representational zone of the hand, which occurs in upper extremity amputees, has been shown to be tightly connected to the severity of phantom limb pain (Flor et al. 1995). This means that the intensity of phantom limb pain increases the further the hand zone in SI is invaded by the neighboring mouth representation. The varying extent of cortical reorganization between individuals might be caused by peripheral factors like loss of C-fibers, since those fibers appear to play an important role in maintaining cortical maps (Calford and Tweedale 1991).

Another important point about cortical reorganization is that it occurs in several distinct stages. The first stage is represented by the unmasking of neural connections that are normally inhibited. Mechanisms that are involved in this process are an increased release of excitatory neurotransmitters, a higher density of postsynaptic receptors (so that the same amount of released transmitters results in a stronger excitatory reaction), an altered conductance of neural membranes, decreased inhibitory inputs, and the removal of inhibition from excitatory inputs (Kaas and Florence 1997). This results in a higher cortical excitability in amputees with phantom limb pain (Karl et al. 2004). The second stage involves structural rather than biochemical changes and includes processes such as axonal sprouting and changes in synaptic strength. Another important factor is Hebbian learning, which leads to reorganization based on the usage of certain cell networks or assemblies, as well as long-term potentiation (Elbert et al. 1997). Churchill et al. (1998) propose a use-dependent third stage of cortical reorganization characterized by a refinement of receptive fields.

Perceptual Illusions Related to Phantom Limb Pain

There are several experimental paradigms to create illusory perceptions that shed some light on the workings of phantom limb pain. For example, Botvinick and Cohen (1998) established the so-called rubber hand illusion (RHI), in which one of the participant's hands is hidden from view and replaced in the visual field by a more or less lifelike artificial hand. The hidden hand and the rubber hand are then stimulated in a synchronous manner using brush strokes or cotton swabs. Thus, the visual and tactile senses report congruently and the rubber hand looks and feels like the participant's actual hand. In this situation, a feeling of ownership towards the rubber hand is reported and the perceived position of the hidden hand shifts towards the rubber hand. In measurements using functional magnetic resonance imaging (fMRI) during the application of the RHI it has been shown that not only the somatosensory cortex is involved in creating the illusion (as would be suggested by the mechanisms discussed earlier), but also frontal and parietal areas (Ehrsson et al. 2004), suggesting that bottom-up processes of visuo-tactile integration and top-down processes stemming from the representation of the participant's own body interact to create illusory perceptions such as the RHI (Tsakiris 2010). The crucial factors in creating the illusion of an artificial hand belonging to one's own body are so far only partially known: On the one hand, Armel and Ramachandran (2003) showed that the visual similarity between rubber hand and actual hand do not seem to be very important. They also noted a feeling of ownership towards a two-dimensional picture of a hand that was projected onto a table. On the other hand, if a rubber hand is used and put into a physically impossible position relative to the participant's body, the illusion does not occur (Ehrsson et al. 2005).

The effects and workings of the RHI have several implications for neuropsychological aspects of amputations: It shows under which circumstances a more or less external object, like the phantom limb or a prosthetic replacement for the lost limb, will be successfully integrated into the body image. In regard to the integration of prostheses, the results suggest congruent tactile feedback to be crucial. If, for example, a prosthesis collects tactile information (using pressure sensors in the fingertips of the artificial hand) and relays this data to the body by stimulating the stump, the patient's ability to accept this external object as a part of the body will most probably depend on the temporal and spatial congruence between the visual and tactile modalities. If there is too much discordance between the senses, this incongruence will lead the patient to reject the prosthesis as a part of their body and might even have adverse consequences, as discussed below.

Another illusion with important implications on phantom limb pain has been examined by McCabe et al. (2005): Here, a mirror was put between the arms or legs of healthy participants in such a manner that the limb seen as a mirror image was viewed at the same angle and in the same position as the limb that is hidden behind the mirror. In this setup, when participants are asked to move both limbs in a congruent manner (e.g., lifting both arms or both legs up at the same time), the mirror image behaves exactly like the hidden limb. If, however, the participants are instructed to do incongruent movements (e.g., moving the left arm or leg up while moving the other one down), the mirror image contradicts the body movement, leading to an incongruence between the sensory modalities of vision and proprioception. McCabe et al. (2005) report a variety of subjective reactions to this sensory incongruence, ranging from a general feeling of uneasiness and paresthesias like numbness or tickling to the perception of an altered number of limbs and even to pain. These perceptions only occurred in some participants and did not occur when the mirror was replaced with a whiteboard. The implication for phantom limb pain and related phenomena is that the sensorimotor incongruence caused by an amputation might induce the abnormal sensations that are part of many neuropathic pain syndromes. However, this study was not controlled and did not include measures other than verbal descriptions of subjective sensations.

Functional neuroimaging studies suggest that the activity in primary cortical areas during illusory perception experiments reflects the perceived, subjective input rather than the stimulus that was applied physically (Chen et al. 2003; Blankenburg et al. 2006). This also seems to be the case in the phenomenon of telescoping: This term refers to the feeling, reported by many amputees, that the size and length of the phantom limb change over time, sometimes shortening so far that the phantom fingers are perceived as being attached directly to the stump. In this way, telescoping might be an additional source of sensory incongruence. In the light of the aforementioned strong correlation between SI reorganization and the severity of phantom limb pain, it is not surprising that the extent of telescoping has been found to be associated with phantom limb pain (Grüsser et al. 2001). These studies also indicate that visual, somatosensory and motor feedback to the cortex might not only be an important determining factor of phantom limb pain, but also a potential gateway to effective feedback-based therapies.

Pain Memory

Prospective studies similar to the one by Nikolajsen et al. (1997) have postulated that chronic pain before amputation as a predictor for phantom limb pain, although it has to be pointed out that these studies usually include only a very limited number of traumatic amputees and many patients with long-term pain problems, since they rely on those cases of amputations that can in some way be expected and therefore be evaluated in a prospective manner. There also seems to be a similarity in pain quality between preoperative pain and phantom limb pain, although the likelihood of this similarity has a wide range and seems to depend on the type and time of assessment (Katz and Melzack 1990). The effects of pain memory in phantom limb pain patients may be similar to sufferers from chronic back pain, where the representational area of the back in the SI cortex increases with increased chronicity (Flor et al. 1997). This effect is an example for implicit pain memories: This term refers to central nervous changes regarding nociceptive input that lead to changes in the processing of somatosensory input and do not require changes in conscious processing of the pain (Flor et al. 2003). Thus, long-term noxious input can lead to long-lasting alterations in the cortex, affecting the subsequent processing of somatosensory input. The prominent role of the SI and motor cortex in the processing of phantom limb pain is supported by reports that the surgical removal of parts of this cortex abolishes phantom limb pain, while the stimulation of this area can elicit it (Head and Holmes 1911; Appenzeller and Bicknell 1969; Knotkova and Cruciani 2010). With an established pain memory in this cortex, the invasion of the cortical amputation zone by neighboring areas might preferentially activate neurons coding for pain. Because these neurons used to be assigned to the limb that has been amputated, the responding sensation is felt in this limb (Doetsch 1998).

As a result of these findings and the idea that central anesthesia might not be sufficient protection against the afferent nociceptive input during amputation, peripheral anesthesia has been added for some time before and during surgery to prevent central sensitization (Woolf and Chong 1993). The effectiveness of this approach, however, has been challenged by several studies (e.g., Nikolajsen et al. 1997). That said, NMDA receptor antagonists given during the operation and the postoperative weeks might be beneficial (Wiech et al. 2001; Schley et al. 2007). These neurotransmitters are expected to erase preexisting somatosensory pain memories and inhibit the creation of new ones.

The role of individual preexisting sensitivities including psychological and genetic susceptibility in the processing of nociceptive stimuli might also account for some of the observed interindividual variation in the proneness to develop phantom limb pain after amputation. This is also suggested by a study showing a connection between pain thresholds relating to pressure before the amputation and the occurrence of postoperative phantom limb pain (Nikolajsen et al. 2000). Since it is unclear which phases of the life course and which pain experiences have the largest influence on this sensitivity, additional data from longitudinal studies including those that highlight the role of biobehavioral factors to better understand the role of pain memory in the development of phantom limb pain are warranted.

Therapy

One can easily imagine that a phenomenon with such a wide range of diverse and complex origins and contributing factors will be quite resistant to simple therapeutic approaches (Sherman et al. 1980). Phantom limb pain has been treated by medication (including barbiturates, muscle relaxants, antidepressants, anticonvulsants, or neuroleptics) or other somatic interventions (such as local anesthesia, sympathectomy, dorsal root entry zone lesions, or neurostimulation), but the maximal beneficial effect of these strategies did not exceed about 30% and is therefore not higher than the placebo effect that has been reported in other studies (Finnerup et al. 2007). There are alternatives in the form of behavioral therapeutic approaches to chronic pain which will not be discussed in detail here since they are not specific to phantom limb pain (see also Donovan et al. 2011). They include treatments based on operant learning, cognitive-behavioral therapies, biofeedback, and relaxation as well as extinction training (Flor and Diers 2007).

Pharmacological Treatments

In animal models, cortical reorganization could be prevented and reversed using NMDA receptor antagonists or GABA agonists, both of which work by disrupting the mechanisms of cortical reorganization. In human phantom limb pain patients, short-term pain alleviation was achieved using the NMDA antagonist ketamine (Eichenberger et al. 2008). However, the NMDA receptor antagonist memantine was not effective (Maier et al. 2003). A reduction of phantom limb pain has been shown in several studies regarding the effect of opioids (see Huse et al. 2008). Certain pharmaceutical treatments seem to be effective only in patients with a specific cause of phantom limb pain: The anesthetic lidocaine improved the situation of patients with neuromas (Chabal et al. 1992), whereas patients with a strong contribution of peripheral factors seem to benefit from biofeedback treatments which aim for vasodilation of or decreased muscle tension in the residual limb (Sherman et al. 1997). A recent study noted that pain alleviation in sufferers from phantom limb pain after administering duloxetine, an antidepressant, and pregabalin, an anticonvulsant, with each drug influencing a different part of the nociceptive pathway (Spiegel et al. 2010). Gabapentin, a widely used treatment for neuropathic pain (Baillie and Power 2006), was not shown to reduce stump pain or phantom limb pain in a controlled study (Nikolajsen et al. 2006).

Treatments Based on Cortical Plasticity

The findings regarding the connection between phantom limb pain and cortical reorganization discussed earlier have led to the development of several innovative and promising treatments, all of which include the notion of providing the brain with at least part of the informational input that it would expect from a functioning limb (Flor 2008). The treatments discussed in the following have been shown to be effective in a clinical setting.

Prosthesis Use

Different types of prostheses vary in the amount and quality of feedback that they provide for the patient. While a cosmetic prosthesis only looks like an intact limb, without its sensory or functional properties, a myoelectric prosthesis can be controlled by the patient using contractions in the muscles of the residual limb: Possible actions are grasp movements, turning the wrist or flexing the elbow. The goal is to increase the potential to use the artificial limb in an effective and intuitive manner that should be able to influence and enhance cortical reorganization, thereby reducing phantom limb pain. Lotze et al. (1999) investigated the effects of using a myoelectric prosthesis and indeed found a reduction of phantom limb pain and cortical reorganization after intensive use. Unfortunately, it has been shown that many patients discard their prostheses, mostly because the prosthesis is not considered to be useful or because it can worsen residual limb pain (Raichle et al. 2008).

The important finding by Lotze et al. (1999) underlines current efforts to develop more effective artificial limbs which use sophisticated mechanical and electronic systems to achieve improved controllability. In a similar fashion, current trends in prosthesis development aim to collect tactile information via sensors in the artificial fingertips and to relay this information to the residual limb using tactile or electrical stimulation. Although the main goal behind this innovation is to help the patients manage everyday situations, there is reason to assume that such a system might also effectively alleviate phantom limb pain: Weiss et al. (1999) found a decrease of phantom limb pain in patients using a functionally effective Sauerbruch prosthesis as opposed to patients using nonfunctional cosmetic prostheses. They propose that by providing the brain with afferent input being transmitted by the same nerve fibers that were used for the limb before the amputation, the relevant cortical areas are being stimulated and thus the process of cortical reorganization is diminished. However, the capability of using a functional prosthesis depends on properties of the stump (including length, shape, muscle damage, and wound healing) and some patients are still not able to use one. For this reason, current efforts aim at creating a virtual environment in which an artificial functional limb can be simulated (e.g., Murray et al. 2007; Cole et al. 2009). Some patients might also benefit from biorobotics. Rossini et al. (2010) implanted electrodes directly into the median and ulnar nerves of upper limb amputees and were able to derive signals that can be used to control a robotic arm. Based on the concepts of cortical reorganization described earlier, such a robotic limb might be able to alleviate or even prevent phantom limb pain by providing the brain with a lifelike replica of the lost body part.

Sensory Discrimination

Flor et al. (2001) used a 2-week discrimination training, where the patients were asked to determine the location and frequency of different stimuli on the residual limb. The treatment consisted of ten sessions lasting 90 min each with an increasing level of difficulty of the task. As a result, the ability of the patients to discriminate between two distinct stimuli which are presented close together on the stump improved significantly. More importantly, patients reported a 60% reduction of phantom limb pain and a reversal of cortical reorganization that could be measured, with a shift of the area representing the mouth back to its original location on the cortex. A continuous discrimination task like this one can be induced in certain sophisticated prostheses or it can be applied as a separate therapeutic effort, where it can also be used for patients who cannot use a prosthesis (e.g., when there is no stump or when it is too sensitive or too weak).

Mirrors and Virtual Reality

Ramachandran and Rogers-Ramachandran (1996) created a mirror illusion for phantom limb pain patients: they constructed a box with a mirror which reflects the intact arm in such an angle that the patient obtains the visual impression of having two intact arms. If the patients are then asked to perform symmetrical movements with both their intact hand and their phantom hand, the mental image of the lost hand is accompanied by a visual image depicting the same movement. Ramachandran et al. reported that this setup can enable some patients to regain control over their phantom hand, thereby reducing cramps and alleviating phantom limb pain. Chan et al. (2007) compared a 4-week mirror training with mental imagery and with a whiteboard condition and found an alleviation of pain only in the mirror condition. However, they only collected the subjective pain ratings from the patients, without providing physiological or neuropsychological measures that might support the reported data. Current efforts try to determine whether some patients benefit more from this kind of therapy than others and if or how treatment effectiveness might be improved.

Imagery

MacIver et al. (2008) used functional MRI measurements before and after a mental imagery training to look for cortical changes that might be correlated with the alleviation of phantom limb pain. They found that the area representing the patients' lips in the somatosensory cortex, which had invaded the adjacent area representing the hand, had changed during the training: Before, as was expected based on the findings discussed earlier, the lip area on the affected side of the brain was spread out in comparison to the unaffected side. After the training, the lip area was more focused and the activation was similar to that known from healthy controls. It is interesting to note that a mental imagery training, which was successful on a subjective and on a cortical level in MacIver et al.'s study, was used as an ineffective control condition by Chan et al. (2007). This contradiction might suggest that the exact nature and application of the training affect its outcome, but also that a mirror training with actual visual feedback may be superior to mental imagery. As another variation of observed movements, Giraux and Sirigu (2003) used prerecorded videos of hand movements. Here, patients were instructed to watch these movements and to try to fit their phantom limb to the observed hand. This led to pain relief in some, but not all, patients, with pain alleviation accompanied by an increase in motor cortex activity. A good alternative to training programs using mirrors, mentalizations, or videos might be virtual reality setups in which the user can freely adjust a wide variety of factors, such as the appearance and responsiveness of the limb or properties of the task or the environment. Apart from its clinical applications, such a tool could also help to identify and test the training parameters that are best suited to alleviate phantom limb pain.

Central Stimulation

Behavioral treatments are not the only way to alter cortical reorganization. Since neurons react primarily to electrical pulses, their firing pattern can be influenced through the application of electricity. Nguyen et al. (2000) implanted electrodes over the motor cortex of their patients to modulate cortical excitability. They reported positive results in some patients. However, the invasive nature of this method is prone to complications and requires extreme caution. In recent years, there have been studies using similar, but less risky methods: In transcranial magnetic stimulation (TMS), a magnetic coil is placed over the patient's head in such a way that the magnetic field induces electricity in a specific area of the cortex. Transcranial direct current stimulation (tDCS) uses electric currents to stimulate the neurons directly. Both methods have been used repeatedly with minimal side effects and have been used successfully to alleviate phantom limb pain at least in some patients (Knotkova and Cruciani 2010; Fregni et al. 2006). However, the therapeutic effects are only short term and current technology does not yet allow for the patients to receive these kinds of therapy in their homes (Fregni et al. 2007).

Conclusions

Phantom limb pain is a multilayered and biobehavioral phenomenon with a variety of causal and exacerbating factors. Thus, the only feasible way to eliminate chronic phantom limb pain would be a combination of several treatments, each acting on a specific level of the phenomenon. In cases where it is possible to do so, the first step of treatment should take place prior to the amputation: Pain before the amputation should be eliminated by using analgesics as well as substances that interfere with the consolidation of pain memories. The next important part is the prevention of changes in cortical organization immediately after the amputation. The best way to achieve this might be an early training phase with a myoelectric prosthesis providing tactile feedback, in combination with virtual reality training. A combination of behavioral and pharmaceutical treatments, adapted to the specific background and needs of the individual patient, might be the best way to eliminate chronic phantom limb pain.

References

Appenzeller, O., & Bicknell, J. M. (1969). Effects of nervous system lesions on phantom experience in amputees. *Neurology, 19*, 141–146.

Armel, K. C., & Ramachandran, V. S. (2003). Projecting sensations to external objects: Evidence from skin conductance response. *Proceedings of the Royal Society of London B Biological Sciences, 270*, 1499–1506.

Baillie, J. K., & Power, I. (2006). The mechanism of action of gabapentin in neuropathic pain. *Current Opinion in Investigational Drugs, 7*, 33–39.

Baron, R., & Maier, C. (1995). Phantom limb pain: are cutaneous nociceptors and spinothalamic neurons involved in the signaling and maintenance of spontaneous and touch-evoked pain? A case report. *Pain, 60*, 223–228.

Birbaumer, N., Lutzenberger, W., Montoya, P., Larbig, W., Unertl, K., Töpfner, S., Grodd, W., Taub, E., & Flor, H. (1997). Effects of regional anesthesia on phantom limb pain are mirrored in changes in cortical reorganization. *The Journal of Neuroscience, 17*, 5503–5508.

Blankenburg, F., Ruff, C. C., Deichmann, R., Rees, G., & Driver, J. (2006). The cutaneous rabbit illusion affects human primary sensory cortex somatotopically. *PLoS Biology, 4*, e69. doi:10.1371/journal.pbio.0040069.

Botvinick, M., & Cohen, J. (1998). Rubber hands "feel" touch that eyes see. *Nature, 391*, 756.

Calford, M. B., & Tweedale, R. (1991). C-fibres provide a source of masking inhibition to primary somatosensory cortex. *Proceedings of the Biological Sciences, 243*, 269–275.

Chabal, C., Jacobson, L., Russell, L. C., & Burchiel, K. J. (1992). Pain response to peri-neuromal injection of normal saline, epinephrine, and lidocaine in humans. *Pain, 49*, 9–12.

Chan, B. L., Witt, R., Charrow, A. P., Magee, A., Howard, R., Pasquina, P. F., Heilman, K. M., & Tsao, J. W. (2007). Mirror therapy for phantom limb pain. *The New England Journal of Medicine, 357*, 2206–2207.

Chen, L. M., Friedman, R. M., & Roe, A. W. (2003). Optical imaging of a tactile illusion in area 3b of the primary somatosensory cortex. *Science, 302*, 881–885.

Chen, Y., Michaelis, M., Jänig, W., & Devor, M. (1996). Adrenoreceptor subtype mediating sympathetic sensory coupling in injured sensory neurons. *Journal of Neurophysiology, 76*, 3721–3730.

Churchill, J. D., Muja, N., Myers, W. A., Besheer, J., & Garraghty, P. E. (1998). Somatotopic consolidation: a third phase of reorganization after peripheral nerve injury in adult squirrel monkeys. *Experimental Brain Research, 118*, 189–196.

Cole, J., Crowle, S., Austwick, G., & Slater, D. H. (2009). Exploratory findings with virtual reality for phantom limb pain; from stump motion to agency and analgesia. *Disability and Rehabilitation, 31*, 846–854.

Coull, J. A., Beggs, S., Boudreau, D., Boivin, D., Tsuda, M., Inoue, K., Gravel, C., Salter, M. W., & De Koninck, Y. (2005). BDNF from microglia causes the shift in neuronal anion gradient underlying neuropathic pain. *Nature, 438*, 1017–1021.

Davis, K. D., Kiss, Z. H., Luo, L., Tasker, R. R., Lozano, A. M., & Dostrovsky, J. O. (1998). Phantom sensations generated by thalamic microstimulation. *Nature, 391*, 385–387.

Devor, M. (2005a). In M. Koltzenburg & S. B. McMahon (Eds.). Response of nerres to injury in relation to neuropathic pain. *Wall and Melzack's textbook of pain* (pp. 905–927). Amsterdam: Elsevier.

Devor, M. (2005b). Sodium channels and mechanisms of neuropathic pain. *Pain, 7*, 3–12.

Devor, M. (2006). Sodium channels and mechanisms of neuropathic pain. *J. pain, 7*, S3–S12.

Devor, M., & Wall, P. D. (1978). Reorganisation of spinal cord sensory map after peripheral nerve injury. *Nature, 276*, 75–76.

Doetsch, G. S. (1998). Perceptual significance of somatosensory cortical reorganization following peripheral denervation. *Neuroreport, 9*, 29–35.

Donovan, K. A., Thompson, L. M. A., & Jacobsen, P. B. (2011). Pain, depression and anxiety in cancer. In R. J. Moore (Ed.), *Handbook of pain and palliative care: Biobehavioral approaches for the life course.* New York: Springer.

Ehrsson, H. H., Holmes, N. P., & Passingham, R. E. (2005). Touching a rubber hand: feeling of body ownership is associated with activity in multisensory brain areas. *The Journal of Neuroscience, 25*, 10564–10573.

Ehrsson, H. H., Spence, C., & Passingham, R. E. (2004). That's my hand! Activity in premotor cortex reflects feeling of ownership of a limb. *Science, 305*, 875–877.

Eichenberger, U., Neff, F., Sveticic, G., Björgo, S., Petersen-Felix, S., Arendt-Nielsen, L., & Curatolo, M. (2008). Chronic phantom limb pain: the effects of calcitonin, ketamine, and their combination on pain and sensory thresholds. *Anesthesia and Analgesia, 106*, 1265–1273.

Elbert, T., Sterr, A., Flor, H., Rockstroh, B., Knecht, S., Pantev, C., Wienbruch, C., & Taub, E. (1997). Input-increase and input-decrease types of cortical reorganization after upper extremity amputation in humans. *Experimental Brain Research, 117*, 161–164.

Ephraim, P. L., Wegener, S. T., MacKenzie, E. J., Dillingham, T. R., & Pezzin, L. E. (2005). Phantom pain, residual limb pain, and back pain in amputees: results of a national survey. *Archives of Physical Medicine and Rehabilitation, 86*, 1910–1919.

Ergenzinger, E. R., Glasier, M. M., Hahm, J. O., & Pons, T. P. (1998). Cortically induced thalamic plasticity in the primate somatosensory system. *Nature Neuroscience, 1*, 226–229.

Finnerup, N. B., Norrbrink, C., Fuglsang-Frederiksen, A., Terkelsen, A. J., Hojlund, A. P., & Jensen, T. S. (2010). Pain, referred sensations, and involuntary muscle movements in brachial plexus injury. *Acta Neurologica Scandinavica, 121*, 320–327.

Finnerup, N. B., Otto, M., Jensen, T. S., & Sindrup, S. H. (2007). An evidence-based algorithm for the treatment of neuropathic pain. *Medscape General Medicine, 9*, 36.

Flor, H. (2008). Maladaptive plasticity, memory for pain and phantom limb pain: review and suggestions for new therapies. *Expert Review of Neurotherapeutics, 8*, 809–818.

Flor, H., Braun, C., Elbert, T., & Birbaumer, N. (1997). Extensive reorganization of primary somatosensory cortex in chronic back pain patients. *Neuroscience Letters, 224*, 5–8.

Flor, H., Denke, C., Schaefer, M., & Grüsser, S. (2001). Effect of sensory discrimination training on cortical reorganisation and phantom limb pain. *The Lancet, 357*, 1763–1764.

Flor, H., Devor, M., & Jensen, T. (2003). Phantom limb pain: Causes and cures. In J. Dostrovsky, M. Koltzenburg, & D. Carr (Eds.), *Proceedings of the 10th world congress on pain* (pp. 725–738). Seattle: IASP Press.

Flor, H., & Diers, M. (2007). Limitations of pharmacotherapy: behavioral approaches to chronic pain. *Handbook of Experimental Pharmacology, 177*, 415–427.

Flor, H., Elbert, T., Wienbruch, C., Pantev, C., Knecht, S., Birbaumer, N., Larbig, W., & Taub, E. (1995). Phantom-limb pain as a perceptual correlate of cortical reorganization following arm amputation. *Nature, 375*, 482–484.

Flor, H., Mühlnickel, W., Karl, A., Denke, C., Grüsser, S., Kurth, R., & Taub, E. (2000). A neural substrate for non-painful phantom limb phenomena. *Neuroreport, 11,* 1407–1411.

Florence, S. L., Taub, H. B., & Kaas, J. H. (1998). Large-scale sprouting of cortical connections after peripheral injury in adult macaque monkeys. *Science, 282,* 1117–1121.

Fregni, F., Boggio, P. S., Lima, M. C., Ferreira, M. J. L., Wagner, T., Rigonatti, S. P., Castro, A. W., Souza, D. R., Riberto, M., Freedman, S. D., Nitsche, M. A., & Pascual-Leone, A. (2006). A sham-controlled, phase II trial of transcranial direct current stimulation for the treatment of central pain in traumatic spinal cord injury. *Pain, 122,* 197–209.

Fregni, F., Freedman, S., & Pascual-Leone, A. (2007). Recent advances in the treatment of chronic pain with non-invasive brain stimulation techniques. *Lancet Neurology, 6,* 188–191.

Fried, K., Govrin-Lippmann, R., Rosenthal, F., Ellisman, M. H., & Devor, M. (1991). Ultrastructure of afferent axon endings in a neuroma. *Journal of Neurocytology, 20,* 682–701.

Giraux, P., & Sirigu, A. (2003). Illusory movements of the paralyzed limb restore motor cortex activity. *NeuroImage, 20,* 107–111.

Gorodetskaya, N., Constantin, C., & Jänig, W. (2003). Ectopic activity in cutaneous regenerating afferent nerve fibers following nerve lesion in the rat. *The European Journal of Neuroscience, 18,* 2487–2497.

Grüsser, S. M., Mühlnickel, W., Schaefer, M., Villringer, K., Christmann, C., Koeppe, C., & Flor, H. (2004). Remote activation of referred phantom sensation and cortical reorganization in human upper extremity amputees. *Experimental Brain Research, 154,* 97–102.

Grüsser, S. M., Winter, C., Mühlnickel, W., Denke, C., Karl, A., Villringer, K., & Flor, H. (2001). The relationship of perceptual phenomena and cortical reorganization in upper extremity amputees. *Neurosciences, 102,* 263–272.

Halligan, P. W., Marshall, J. C., & Wade, D. T. (1994). Sensory disorganization and perceptual plasticity after limb amputation: a follow-up study. *Neuroreport, 27,* 1341–1345.

Hanley, M. A., Jensen, M. P., Smith, D. G., Ehde, D. M., Edwards, W. T., & Robinson, L. R. (2007). Preamputation pain and acute pain predict chronic pain after lower extremity amputation. *The Journal of Pain, 8,* 102–109.

Head, H., & Holmes, G. (1911). Sensory disturbances from cerebral lesions. *Brain, 34,* 102–254.

Hunter, J. P., Katz, J., & Davis, K. D. (2003). The effect of tactile and visual sensory inputs on phantom limb awareness. *Brain, 126,* 579–589.

Hunter, J. P., Katz, J., & Davis, K. D. (2008). Stability of phantom limb phenomena after upper limb amputation: A longitudinal study. *Neurosciences, 156,* 939–949.

Huse, E., Larbig, W., Flor, H., & Birbaumer, N. (2008). The effects of opioids on phantom limb pain and cortical reorganization. *Pain, 90,* 47–55.

Jain, N., Qi, H., Collins, C. E., & Kaas, J. H. (2008). Large-scale reorganization in the somatosensory cortex and thalamus after sensory loss in macaque monkeys. *The Journal of Neuroscience, 28,* 11042–11060.

Kaas, J. H., & Florence, S. L. (1997). Mechanisms of reorganization in sensory systems of primates after peripheral nerve injury. *Advances in Neurology, 73,* 147–158.

Karl, A., Diers, M., & Flor, H. (2004). P300-amplitudes in upper limb amputees with and without phantom limb pain in a visual oddball paradigm. *Pain, 110,* 40–46.

Katz, J., & Melzack, R. (1990). Pain "memories" in phantom limbs: review and clinical observations. *Pain, 43,* 319–336.

Keil, G. (1990). So-called initial description of phantom pain by Ambroisé Paré. "Chose digne d'admiration et quasi incredible": the "douleur ès parties mortes et amputées". *Fortschritte der Medizin, 108,* 62–66.

Knotkova, H., & Cruciani, R. A. (2010). Non-invasive transcranial direct current stimulation for the study and treatment of neuropathic pain. *Methods in Molecular Biology, 617,* 505–515.

Lotze, M., Grodd, W., Birbaumer, N., Erb, M., Huse, E., & Flor, H. (1999). Does use of a myoelectric prosthesis reduce cortical reorganization and phantom limb pain? *Nature Neuroscience, 2,* 501–502.

MacIver, K., Lloyd, D. M., Kelly, S., Roberts, N., & Nurmikko, T. (2008). Phantom limb pain, cortical reorganization and the therapeutic effect of mental imagery. *Brain, 131,* 2181–2191.

Maier, C., Dertwinkel, R., Mansourian, N., Hosbach, I., Schwenkreis, P., Senne, I., Skipka, G., Zenz, M., & Tegenthoff, M. (2003). Efficacy of the NMDA-receptor antagonist memantine in patients with chronic phantom limb pain – results of a randomized double-blinded, placebo-controlled trial. *Pain, 103,* 277–283.

Marbach, J. J., & Raphael, K. G. (2000). Phantom tooth pain: A new look at an old dilemma. *Pain Medicine, 1,* 68–77.

McCabe, C. S., Haigh, R. C., Halligan, P. W., & Blake, D. R. (2005). Simulating sensory-motor incongruence in healthy volunteers: implications for a cortical model of pain. *Rheumatology, 44,* 509–516.

Melzack, R., & Loeser, J. D. (1978). Phantom body pain in paraplegics: evidence for a "central pattern generating mechanism" for pain. *Pain, 4,* 195–210.

Merzenich, M. M., Nelson, R. J., Stryker, M. P., Cynader, M. S., Schoppmann, A., & Zook, J. M. (1984). Somatosensory cortical map changes following digit amputation in adult monkeys. *The Journal of Comparative Neurology, 224,* 591–605.

Montoya, P., Ritter, K., Huse, E., Larbig, W., Braun, C., Töpfner, S., Lutzenberger, W., Grodd, W., Flor, H., & Birbaumer, N. (1998). The cortical somatotopic map and phantom phenomena in subjects with congenital limb atrophy and traumatic amputees with phantom limb pain. *The European Journal of Neuroscience, 10*, 1095–1102.

Murray, C. D., Pettifer, S., Howard, T., Patchick, E. L., Caillette, F., Kulkarni, J., & Bamford, C. (2007). The treatment of phantom limb pain using immersive virtual reality: three case studies. *Disability and Rehabilitation, 29*, 1465–1469.

Nguyen, J. P., Lefaucheur, J. P., Le Guerinel, C., Fontaine, D., Nakano, N., Sakka, L., Eizenbaum, J. F., Pollin, B., & Keravel, Y. (2000). Treatment of central and neuropathic facial pain by chronic stimulation of the motor cortex: value of neuronavigation guidance systems for the localization of the motor cortex. *Neurochirurgie, 46*, 483–491.

Nikolajsen, L., Ilkjaer, S., & Jensen, T. S. (2000). Relationship between mechanical sensitivity and postamputation pain: a prospective study. *European Journal of Pain, 4*, 327–334.

Nikolajsen, L., Ilkjaer, S., Kroner, K., Christensen, J. H., & Jensen, T. S. (1997). The influence of preamputation pain on postamputation stump and phantom pain. *Pain, 72*, 393–405.

Nikolajsen, L. J., Finnerup, N. B., Kramp, S., Vimtrup, A. S., Keller, J., & Jensen, T. S. (2006). A randomized study of the effects of gabapentin on postamputation pain. *Anesthesiology, 105*, 1008–1015.

Nikolajsen, L. J., & Jensen, T. S. (2005). In M. Koltzenburg & S. B. McMahon (Eds.). Phanton limb. *Wall and Melzack's textbook of pain* (pp. 961–971). Amsterdam: Elsevier.

Pons, T. P., Garraghty, P. E., Ommaya, A. K., Kaas, J. H., Taub, E., & Mishkin, M. (1991). Massive cortical reorganization after sensory deafferentation in adult macaques. *Science, 252*, 1857–1860.

Price, E. H. (2006). A critical review of congenital phantom limb cases and a developmental theory for the basis of body image. *Consciousness and Cognition, 15*, 310–322.

Raichle, K. A., Hanley, M. A., Molton, I., Kadel, N. J., Campbell, K., Phelps, E., Ehde, D., & Smith, D. G. (2008). Prosthesis use in persons with lower- and upper-limb amputation. *Journal of Rehabilitation Research and Development, 45*, 961–972.

Ramachandran, V. S., & Rogers-Ramachandran, D. (1996). Synesthesia in phantom limbs induced with mirrors. *Proceedings of the Royal Society of London B Biological Sciences, 263*, 377–386.

Ramachandran, V. S., Stewart, M., & Rogers-Ramachandran, D. C. (1992). Perceptual correlates of massive cortical reorganization. *Neuroreport, 3*, 583–586.

Rossini, P. M., Micera, S., Benvenuto, A., Carpaneto, J., Cavallo, G., Citi, L., Cipriani, C., Denaro, L., Denaro, V., Di Pino, G., Ferreri, F., Guglielmelli, E., Hoffmann, K. P., Raspopovic, S., Rigosa, J., Rossini, L., Tombini, M., & Dario, P. (2010). Double nerve intraneural interface implant on a human amputee for robotic hand control. *Clinical Neurophysiology, 121*, 777–783.

Rothemund, Y., Grüsser, S. M., Liebeskind, U., Schlag, P. M., & Flor, H. (2004). Phantom phenomena in mastectomized patients and their relation to chronic and acute pre-mastectomy pain. *Pain, 107*, 140–146.

Schley, M., Topfner, S., Wiech, K., Schaller, H. E., Konrad, C. J., Schmelz, M., & Birbaumer, N. (2007). Continuous brachial plexus blockade in combination with the NMDA receptor antagonist memantine prevents phantom pain in acute traumatic upper limb amputees. *European Journal of Pain, 11*, 299–308.

Schmidt, A. P., Takahashi, M. E., & de Paula Posso, I. (2005). Phantom limb pain induced by spinal anesthesia. *Clinics, 60*, 263–264.

Sherman, R. A., Davis, G. D., & Wong, M. F. (1997). Behavioral treatment of exercise-induced urinary incontinence among female soldiers. *Military Medicine, 162*, 690–694.

Sherman, R. A., Sherman, C. J., & Gall, N. G. (1980). A survey of current phantom limb pain treatment in the United States. *Pain, 8*, 85–99.

Spiegel, D. R., Lappinen, E., & Gottlieb, M. (2010). A presumed case of phantom limb pain treated successfully with duloxetine and pregabalin. *General Hospital Psychiatry, 32*, 228.

Torsney, C., & MacDermott, A. B. (2006). Disinhibition opens the gate to pathological pain signaling in superficial neurokinin 1 receptor-expressing neurons in rat spinal cord. *The Journal of Neuroscience, 26*, 1833–1843.

Tsakiris, M. (2010). My body in the brain: A neurocognitive model of body-ownership. *Neuropsychologia, 48*, 703–712.

Ueda, H. (2006). Molecular mechanisms of neuropathic painphenotypic switch and initiation mechanisms. *Pharmacology and Therapeutics, 109*, 57–77.

Wang, S., Lim, G., Yang, L., Zeng, Q., Sung, B., Jeevendra Martyn, J. A., & Mao, J. (2005). A rat model of unilateral hindpaw burn injury: slowly developing rightwards shift of the morphine dose-response curve. *Pain, 116*, 87–95.

Weiss, T., Miltner, W. H. R., Adler, T., Bruckner, L., & Taub, E. (1999). Decrease in phantom limb pain associated with prosthesis-induced increased use of an amputation stump in humans. *Neuroscience Letters, 272*, 131–134.

Wiech, K., Töpfner, S., Kiefer, T., Preissl, H., Braun, C., Haerle, M., et al. (2001). Prevention of phantom limb pain and cortical reorganization in the early phase after amputation in humans. *Society for Neuroscience Abstracts, 28*, 163–169.

Wiesenfeld-Hallin, Z., Xu, X. J., & Hökfelt, T. (2002). The role of spinal cholecystokinin in chronic pain states. *Pharmacology and Toxicology, 91*, 398–403.

Wilkins, K. L., McGrath, P. J., Finley, G. A., & Katz, J. (1998). Phantom limb sensations and phantom limb pain in child and adolescent amputees. *Pain, 78,* 7–12.

Woolf, C. J. (2004). Dissecting out mechanisms responsible for peripheral neuropathic pain: implications for diagnosis and therapy. *Life Sciences, 74,* 2605–2610.

Woolf, C. J., & Chong, M. S. (1993). Preemptive analgesia – treating postoperative pain by preventing the establishment of central sensitization. *Anesthesia and Analgesia, 77,* 362–379.

Woolf, C. J., & Salter, M. W. (2005). In M. Koltzenburg & S. B. McMahon (Eds.). Plasticity and pain: role of the dorsal horn. *Wall and Melzack's textbook of pain* (pp. 91–105). Amsterdam: Elsevier.

Zhang, L., Zhang, Y., & Zhao, Z. (2005). Anterior cingulate cortex contributes to the descending facilitatory modulation of pain via dorsal reticular nucleus. *The European Journal of Neuroscience, 22,* 1141–1148.

Chapter 26
Pharmacogenetics of Pain: The Future of Personalized Medicine

Lynn R. Webster

Genetics of Pain Processing

Individuals within any population exhibit common variations in DNA sequences (polymorphisms). Polymorphisms occur with molecules that involve transduction of sensory information and genes largely responsible for analgesia. Single-nucleotide polymorphisms (SNPs) are segments of the gene that are linked to a variety of responses in pain sensitivity and modulation. Most research takes place using animal models, healthy human volunteers, and postoperative patients; however, certain SNPs point to vulnerabilities for developing chronic pain diseases. The aim of this chapter is to provide the reader with an overview of the potential clinical implications of understanding the unique genetic pain processing of the individual and how pharmacogenetic therapy might inform personalized medical care.

Candidate Genes Implicated in Pain Processing

Several candidate genes have been studied extensively for their involvement in pain processing, and some have been associated with specific pain complaints (Belfer et al. 2004). However, research is inconclusive, and candidate genes associated with pain sensitivity do not necessarily coincide with the factors leading to the development of chronic widespread pain (Holliday et al. 2009).

What follows is a sample of candidate genes studied for pain processing and their associations with specific pain complaints.

Transient Receptor Potential Vanilloid 1

Transient receptor potential vanilloid (TRPV) is a family of transient receptor potential ion channels sensitive to temperature and chemical activation found throughout the body. The first member of the family discovered was the TRPV1 receptor, which is also called the capsaicin receptor. In the work by Kim et al., gender, ethnicity, and temperament were shown to contribute to individual variation in thermal and cold pain sensitivity by interactions with TRPV1 SNPs (Kim et al. 2004). TRPV1 has two SNPs in its exons that produce amino acid substitutions: One is in codon 315 (TRPV1 Met[315]Ile) and the other in 585 (TRPV1 Ile[585]Val). Female European Americans with the TRPV1 Val[585] allele showed

L.R. Webster, MD, FACPM, FASAM (✉)
Lifetree Clinical Research, Salt Lake City, UT, USA

American Academy of Pain Medicine, Glenview, IL, USA

R.J. Moore (ed.), *Handbook of Pain and Palliative Care: Biobehavioral Approaches for the Life Course*, DOI 10.1007/978-1-4419-1651-8_26, © Springer Science+Business Media, LLC 2012

longer cold withdrawal times than the other ethnic groups, including African American, Hispanic and Asian American, in the cold-pressor experimental pain model. Sex differences were also found with European males tolerating longer times of cold submersion than females. Harm avoidance and reward dependence were measures of temperament also found to be associated with the polymorphisms.

SC9NA

Extreme mutations of SCN9A are found in people with congenital insensitivity to pain and in those who exhibit extreme pain states (Reimann et al. 2010). More common SNPs of the gene are associated with altered pain perception and heightened pain sensitivity (Reimann et al. 2010). In a recent study of 1,277 patients with osteoarthritis, sciatica, phantom pain, pancreatitis, or pain after lumbar discectomy, the A allele of rs6746030 was associated with significantly increased pain as compared with the more common G allele (combined $p=0.0001$) (Reimann et al. 2010). Heightened pain sensitivity was also observed in 186 healthy women with the same variant, indicating a possible sex-specific expression with this SNP. Females have been reported to be more sensitive to pain than males (Nielsen et al. 2008; Fillingim et al. 2009); however, some findings are inconsistent, including sex differences in pain treatment response (Fillingim et al. 2009).

Interleukin-1

Research suggests an association between interleukin-1 (IL-1) gene locus polymorphisms to the pathogenesis of low back pain. In a subgroup of a Finnish cohort study, 131 middle-age men from three occupational groups (machine drivers, carpenters, and office workers) who carried the IL-1RNA(1812) allele showed increased pain frequency, more days with pain, and limitation of daily activities (Solovieva et al. 2004).

Further study suggests that inhibiting IL-1 could be therapeutic in preventing and reversing disc degeneration (Le Maitre et al. 2005) and that delivering an IL-1 antagonist directly or by gene therapy inhibits intervertebral disc matrix degradation (Le Maitre et al. 2007).

KCNK18

A recent study found that a mutation in the KCNK18 gene inhibits TRESK, a protein that helps regulate pain sensitivity (Ronald et al. 2010). The investigators linked the gene variant to migraine with the discovery that a large family of sufferers of migraine with aura carry it. TRESK is found in the trigeminal ganglia and dorsal root ganglia, areas of the brain linked to the development of pain and migraine. The hope is that increasing TRESK activity might serve to decrease neuron excitability, reducing migraine severity or frequency.

Catechol-*O*-Methyltransferase gene

Catechol-*O*-methyltransferase (COMT) is an enzyme that metabolizes catecholamines; inhibited COMT has been associated with heightened experimental pain sensitivity and risk for developing temporomandibular joint disorder (TMD) (Diatchenko et al. 2005). Reduced COMT activity has produced enhanced mechanical and thermal pain sensitivity in rats, an effect that was blocked by administering β_2- and β_3-adrenergic antagonists but not β_1-adrenergic, α-adrenergic, or dopaminergic receptor antagonists (Nackley et al. 2007).

The COMT polymorphism VA1158met introduces an amino acid variation associated with greater pain sensitivity. Research suggests that this polymorphism affected cerebral pain processing by increasing activity in the anterior cingulate cortex in 57 subjects (27 males) homozygous for the met158 allele (Mobascher et al. 2010).

The findings that COMT variations mediate pain modulation seem well supported. However, haplotype analysis has failed to confirm evidence of the association between chronic widespread pain and COMT SNPs associated with pain sensitivity (Nicholl et al. 2010).

Genetics of Drug Response

Interpersonal genetic variations impact not only how patients perceive and experience painful stimuli but how they absorb, metabolize, and excrete medications. Research shows 30–40% of subjects in clinical pain trials are non-responders (Argoff 2010), evidence of the large inter-individual variabilities in response to analgesic medications. Common variants in the genes encoding mu-receptors, transporters, and metabolizing enzymes are linked to the individual's opioid response and, thus, may largely dictate analgesic needs.

Data, however, are inconsistent. For example, a recent study using the association technique in 2,294 opioid-treated patients failed to show any association between a group of polymorphisms in candidate genes (OPRM1, OPRD1, OPRK1, ARRB2, GNAZ, HINT1, Stat6, ABCB1, COMT, HRH1, ADRA2A, MC1R, TACR1, GCH1, DRD2, DRD3, HTR3A, HTR3B, HTR2A, HTR3C, HTR3D, HTR3E, HTR1, or CNR1) with opioid efficacy (Klepstad et al. 2011). This finding may illustrate the difficulty in using the association technique in identifying potential genetic markers for analgesic sensitivity. The sample size in the study would be considered large for most studies but may have not been large enough to detect a genetic signal.

What follows is a discussion of common polymorphisms studied for their effects on opioid response

OPRM1 118G

The mu-opioid receptor allele A118G influences variations in postoperative analgesic needs (Zhang et al. 2010). Postsurgical patients who were 118G homozygotes needed more morphine to control pain after total knee arthroplasty (Chou et al. 2006, knee) and hysterectomy (Chou et al. 2006, hysterect) compared with 118A homozygotes.

Cytochrome P450, Including CYP2D6

Polymorphic cytochrome P450 enzymes are linked to differences in speed of drug metabolism (Fishbain et al. 2004), supporting the clinical observation that equal doses of opioids do not produce equal pain control for all patients. Among the drugs metabolized through CYP450 enzymes are codeine, tramadol, tricyclic antidepressants, and nonsteroidal anti-inflammatory drugs (Stamer & Stüber 2007).

Numerous polymorphisms within CYP2D6 influence opioid effectiveness, and researchers have identified four categories of opioid responders: poor metabolizers (PMs), intermediate metabolizers (IMs), extensive metabolizers (EMs), and ultra-rapid metabolizers (UMs) (Ingelman-Sundberg 2005). PMs are at risk for toxicity from drug accumulation, while UMs can fail to achieve adequate analgesia.

Methods of Analysis

Studies designed around twins using structural equation modeling have the advantage of enabling the analysis of genetic vs. environmental contribution to the development of a phenotype. Shared alleles and environmental effects are analyzed based on whether the twins are monozygotic (sharing 100% of alleles) or dizygotic (sharing on average 50% of alleles) (Nielsen et al. 2008). Twin studies, besides being purely correlational, are not randomly derived and, therefore, not generalizable to the larger population.

In contrast, association studies are performed in subjects unrelated to one another and are restricted to a limited set of candidate genes (Belfer et al. 2004). Association studies have greater power than family linkage studies to detect even slight genetic effects but must have far greater density of markers. Another limitation of association studies is that, often, SNPs have only a small predictive value for the studied effect.

Sex and Ethnic Variations of Pain and Medication Responses

Observable differences in pain and medication response between the sexes and among ethnic groups are linked to allelic variants. For example, approximately 7% of white Americans could be classified as PMs, compared with only 2% of black Americans based on polymorphisms within CYP2D6 (Evans et al. 1993). In contrast, in a study of healthy Ethiopians, 29% of the investigated population had duplicated or multiple copies of CYP2D6 genes, linked to ultrarapid metabolism (Aklillu et al. 1996). African Americans when compared to non-Hispanic whites have been associated with greater experimental pain sensitivity and clinical pain with indication that the difference is endogenous (Campbell et al. 2008).

Women have more postsurgical pain than men, requiring 30% more morphine on a per-weight basis to achieve similar analgesia (Cepeda & Carr 2003). Females have been shown to respond more to kappa-agonist opioids than males (Gear et al. 1996), yet they seem to have more sensitivity to pain than males (Nielsen et al. 2008). Research in animal studies (mice) and humans also show the sex difference could stem from the melanocortin-1 receptor (MC1R) gene (Mogil et al. 2003). Women with two nonfunctional *MC1R* alleles – a phenotype associated with red hair and pale skin – achieved significantly greater analgesia from the administration of the kappa-agonist pentazocine than did women without the gene variant or men (Mogil et al. 2003).

Sex hormones are suspected contributors to painful conditions seen primarily in women. Fluctuations in ovarian hormones associated with the menstrual cycle appear to influence pain response (Martin 2009). One study suggested that a polymorphism in the estrogen receptor increases the risk of women developing TMDs (Ribeiro-Dasilva et al. 2009). Although sex hormones have not been directly linked to the development of fibromyalgia, a connection to fibromyalgia syndrome may lie in the discovery that sex hormones influence serotonergic receptor response, which affects sleep and pain perception (Akkuş et al. 2000; Buskila and Sarzi-Puttini 2006).

The variability in gender and race response to drugs may explain why it is difficult to predict a drug effect when the drug is studied in a relatively homogenous population. Industry would be wise to consider gender and race difference in responses to pain stimuli and analgesics in drug development.

Environmental Vs. Genetic Contributions to Pain Processing

Some interpersonal variance in opioid response and pain sensitivity is explained by factors outside genetic vulnerability, including age, the severity of the pain stimulus, psychological coping mechanisms, concurrent medications, and differences among patients in the disease process.

Medical and psychiatric comorbidities may exacerbate or modulate pain perception, and lifestyle habits such as diet and exercise also contribute.

Nevertheless, evidence supports that genetic differences play a significant role in patient variability (Miller 2010).

Implications for Clinical Practice

In the future, genetic profiles may suggest the most effective pain therapy for the individual, whether opioid or nonopioid. Clearly, genotype variants influence the individual patient's required opioid dose. However, for pharmacogenetics as for other medical fields, research breakthroughs are not immediately accessible to inform most daily clinical decisions. For example, knowing, prior to initiating opioid therapy, whether a patient metabolizes opioids poorly would require genetic testing, which is not currently the standard of care. Therefore, for safety's sake, clinicians must assume every patient is a PM at risk for toxicity when instituting opioid therapy for pain. In addition to practicing conservative initiation, conversion, and titration of opioid doses, clinicians should also use caution when co-administering antidepressants and other substances that increase risk for toxicity due to inhibition of associated enzymes.

Opioid response during a trial may predict successful opioid therapy, but mu-opioid receptor agonists often lose effectiveness with continued administration. The degree of tolerance varies widely among patients as does cross-tolerance to other opioids, a phenomenon that may be partially explained by the presence of multiple receptor subtypes (Pasternak 2001). A lack of cross-tolerance can be beneficial. When a patient has lost response to the analgesic effect of one opioid, switching to another opioid can often restore analgesia at less than the expected equivalent dose (Pasternak 2001). A systematic review indicated that greater than 50% of patients with chronic pain who respond poorly to one opioid improve after being rotated to another opioid (Mercadante & Bruera 2006).

Pharmacogenetic science is not yet adequate to fully inform personalized opioid prescribing; however, certain data are available to help clinicians avoid toxicity and other adverse reactions in patients:

- For older patients or others on multi-drug regimens, the clinician should avoid CYP450 enzyme-mediated opioids to reduce drug–drug reaction risk. For instance, the clinician should consider using morphine, hydromorphone, or oxymorphone (Argoff 2010).
- Consider methadone for patients with renal failure (Argoff 2010). Initiate and titrate conservatively, e.g., 2.5 mg every 8 h, with dose increases occurring no more frequently than weekly in opioid-naïve patients; doses not to exceed 30–40 mg a day even in patients to be converted from high doses of other opioids (Chou et al. 2009).
- Avoid codeine in PMs, who are also likely to experience poor efficacy, or UMs, who may experience excessive side effects or exaggerated analgesia (Argoff 2010).
- In all patients, expect variability, monitor opioid therapy response, and adjust as needed (Argoff 2010).

To inform clinical decision making, genetic tests are commercially available to identify patients with particular polymorphisms. However, several do not have approval from the Food and Drug Administration (FDA), which is working with genetic companies to improve its oversight of these products to ensure scientific accuracy, reliability, and to ensure standards that protect the privacy of genetic information (Hamburg & Collins 2010). To facilitate the distribution of information regarding available genetic tests, the National Institutes of Health (NIH) is also providing federal oversight to the creation of a genetic testing registry (NLM 2010) where developers and manufacturers of products may voluntarily submit scientific validity data, indications for use, and other test information.

Future Considerations

In the future, genetic research could help explain the mystery of who will develop the disease of chronic pain in response to insults to the central nervous system. Chronic pain conditions may be prevented if they can be identified through genetic testing and averted or treated aggressively. Likewise, as pharmacogenetic science advances, clinicians should improve their own ability to effectively match patients and medications based on genotype, improving patient outcomes. However, the discovery process is complex and genetic scientists are moving away from the concept of single-gene diseases toward a theory of complex polygenics that interact with the environment. This evolution is likely to inform the development of pain medicine.

The need exists for online electronic health databases containing a wealth of genetic information to support informed clinical decisions (e.g., dosage amounts based on genotypes). Currently available resources include the *Online Mendelian Inheritance in Man (OMIM)*, a searchable database created by staff at Johns Hopkins University School of Medicine and hosted online by the National Center for Biotechnology Information (NCBI) (OMIM 2010). *OMIM* contains summaries of research on genes, genetic traits, and hereditary disorders and is written mainly by genetic scientists. Current plans for user friendly, clinically relevant resources include *Gene Reviews*, sponsored by the University of Washington and funded through the NIH. *Gene Reviews* provides expert-penned descriptions that pair genetic testing to diagnosis, management, and patient counseling (GeneReviews 2010). *The Pain Genes Database* offers an online browser of manuscripts detailing findings from pain-relevant knockout studies (Lacroix-Fralish et al. 2007). The consolidation of various genetic registries can be expected to evolve to support clinical practice and scientific discovery pertaining to pain medicine and all medical fields.

A question remains as to how health-related agencies, insurance carriers, and other decision makers will make informed clinical recommendations regarding new genetically based treatments based on level of evidence, clinical utility, and risk vs. benefit. The Evaluation of Genomic Applications in Practice and Prevention (EGAPP) Working Group (2009) analyzed data and issued some recommendations, including one that discourages CYP450 testing in adults to be treated for depression using selective serotonin reuptake inhibitors, citing inconsistent evidence (EGAPP WG 2009). While genomics must be held to a high evidentiary standard, yardsticks such as comparative effectiveness (which asks whether a treatment helps the majority of people) may conflict with personalized medicine, which is inherently individual. Cost and political considerations are certain to factor into the discussion as well.

At the present time, the US biotechnology industry lacks the financial incentive to explore treatments for pain linked to genetic findings, because there are many candidate genes, genomic sequencing is still costly, the genomic vs. environmental contributions to various chronic pain phenotypes are difficult to discern, and much of the evidence is still inconclusive.

Public–private partnerships are needed to fund research, update regulatory standards, and encourage development of innovative products.

Summary

Patients' genetic responses to pain stimuli and medication vary, thus so do their therapeutic needs. Although clinical testing methods are currently limited, knowledge that each patient carries an individual genetic imprint can inform current treatment decisions. Future research will further illuminate the genetics of pain management, yielding targeted therapies. Applied pharmacogenetics could well constitute the future of personalized medicine and of optimal pain therapy.

Acknowledgment Dr. Webster acknowledges the contribution of medical writer Beth Dove of Lifetree Clinical Research and Pain Clinic, Salt Lake City, Utah, in the preparation of this manuscript.

References

Akkuş, S., Delibaş, N., & Tamer, M. N. (2000). Do sex hormones play a role in fibromyalgia? *Rheumatology (Oxford, England), 39*(10), 1161–1163.

Aklillu, E., Persson, I., Bertilsson, L., et al. (1996). Frequent distribution of ultrarapid metabolizers of debrisoquine in an Ethiopian population carrying duplicated and multiduplicated functional CYP2D6 alleles. *J Pharmacol Exp Ther, 278*, 441–446.

Argoff, C. E. (2010). Clinical implications of opioid pharmacogenetics. *The Clinical Journal of Pain, 26*(Suppl 10), S16–S20.

Belfer, I., Wu, T., Kingman, A., et al. (2004). Candidate gene studies of human pain mechanisms: methods for optimizing choice of polymorphisms and sample size. *Anesthesiology, 100*(6), 1562–1572.

Buskila, D., & Sarzi-Puttini, P. (2006). Biology and therapy of fibromyalgia. Genetic aspects of fibromyalgia syndrome. *Arthritis Research & Therapy, 8*(5), 218.

Campbell, C. M., France, C. R., Robinson, M. E., Logan, H. L., Geffken, G. R., & Fillingim, R. B. (2008). Ethnic differences in diffuse noxious inhibitory controls. *The Journal of Pain, 9*(8), 759–766.

Cepeda, M. S., & Carr, D. B. (2003). Women experience more pain and require more morphine than men to achieve a similar degree of analgesia. *Anesth Analg, 97*(5), 1464–1468.

Chou, R., Fanciullo, G. J., Fine, P. G., American Pain Society-American Academy of Pain Medicine Opioids Guidelines Panel, et al. (2009). Clinical guidelines for the use of chronic opioid therapy in chronic noncancer pain. *The Journal of Pain, 10*(2), 113–130.

Chou, W. Y., Wang, C. H., Liu, P. H., et al. (2006). Human opioid receptor A118G polymorphism affects intravenous patient-controlled analgesia morphine consumption after total abdominal hysterectomy. *Anesthesiology, 105*(2), 334–337.

Chou, W. Y., Yang, L. C., Lu, H. F., et al. (2006). Association of mu-opioid receptor gene polymorphism (A118G) with variations in morphine consumption for analgesia after total knee arthroplasty. *Acta Anaesthesiologica Scandinavica, 50*(7), 787–792.

Diatchenko, L., Slade, G. D., & Nackley, A. G. (2005). Genetic basis for individual variations in pain perception and the development of a chronic pain condition. *Human Molecular Genetics, 14*(1), 135–143.

EGAPP Working Group Recommendations. CDC's Office of Public Health Genomics, Evaluation of Genomic Applications in Practice and Prevention (EGAPP). Available at: http://www.egappreviews.org/recommendations/index.htm. Accessed October 6, 2010.

Evans, W. E., Relling, M. V., Rahman, A., McLeod, H. L., Scott, E. P., & Lin, J. S. (1993). Genetic basis for a lower prevalence of deficient CYP2D6 oxidative drug metabolism phenotypes in black Americans. *The Journal of Clinical Investigation, 91*(5), 2150–2154.

Fillingim, R. B., King, C. D., Ribeiro-Dasilva, M. C., Rahim-Williams, B., & Riley, J. L., III. (2009). Sex, gender, and pain: a review of recent clinical and experimental findings. *The Journal of Pain, 10*(5), 447–485. Review.

Fishbain, D. A., Fishbain, D., Lewis, J., et al. (2004). Genetic testing for enzymes of drug metabolism: does it have clinical utility for pain medicine at the present time? A structured review. *Pain Medicine, 5*, 81–93.

Gear, R. W., Miaskowski, C., Gordon, N. C., et al. (1996). Kappa-opioids produce significantly greater analgesia in women than in men. *Nature Medicine, 2*(11), 1248–1250.

GeneReviews. Bethesda, MD: National Center for Biotechnology Information, National Library of Medicine; 2010. Available at: http://www.ncbi.nlm.nih.gov/sites/GeneTests/review?db=genetests. Accessed October 6, 2010.

Genetic Testing Registry. Bethesda, MD: Office of Science Policy, National Library of Medicine; 2010. Available at: http://www.ncbi.nlm.nih.gov/gtr. Accessed October 5, 2010.

Hamburg, M. A., & Collins, F. S. (2010). The path to personalized medicine. *The New England Journal of Medicine, 363*(4), 301–304.

Holliday, K. L., Nicholl, B. I., Macfarlane, G. J., Thomson, W., Davies, K. A., & McBeth, J. (2009). Do genetic predictors of pain sensitivity associate with persistent widespread pain? *Molecular Pain, 5*, 56.

Ingelman-Sundberg, M. (2005). Genetic polymorphisms of cytochrome P450 2D6 (CYP2D6): clinical consequences, evolutionary aspects and functional diversity. *The Pharmacogenomics Journal, 5*(1), 6–13.

Kim, H., Neubert, J. K., San Miguel, A., et al. (2004). Genetic influence on variability in human acute experimental pain sensitivity associated with gender, ethnicity and psychological temperament. *Pain, 109*(3), 488–496.

Klepstad, P., Fladvad, T., Skorpen, F., On behalf of the European Palliative Care Research Collaborative (EPCRC) and the European Association for Palliative Care Research Network, et al. (2011). Influence from genetic variability on opioid use for cancer pain: A European genetic association study of 2294 cancer pain patients. *Pain, 152*(5), 1139–1145.

Lacroix-Fralish, M. L., Ledoux, J. B., & Mogil, J. S. (2007). The Pain Genes Database: An interactive web browser of pain-related transgenic knockout studies. *Pain, 1–2*, 3.e1–4.

Le Maitre, C. L., Freemont, A. J., & Hoyland, J. A. (2005). The role of interleukin-1 in the pathogenesis of human intervertebral disc degeneration. *Arthritis Research & Therapy, 7*(4), R732–R745.

Le Maitre, C. L., Hoyland, J. A., & Freemont, A. J. (2007). Interleukin-1 receptor antagonist delivered directly and by gene therapy inhibits matrix degradation in the intact degenerate human intervertebral disc: an in situ zymographic and gene therapy study. *Arthritis Research & Therapy, 9*(4), R83.

Martin, V. T. (2009). Ovarian hormones and pain response: a review of clinical and basic science studies. *Gender Medicine, 6*(Suppl 2), 168–192.

Mercadante, S., & Bruera, E. (2006). Opioid switching: a systematic and critical review. *Cancer Treatment Reviews, 32*, 304–315.

Miller G. Genetics of opioid prescribing: many questions, few answers. Pain Medicine News 2010 Feb; 8(02). Available at: http://www.painmedicinenews.com/index.asp?section_id=82&show=dept&issue_id=600&article_id=14613. Accessed September 29, 2010.

Mobascher, A., Brinkmeyer, J., Thiele, H., et al. (2010). The val158met polymorphism of human catechol-O-methyltransferase (COMT) affects anterior cingulate cortex activation in response to painful laser stimulation. *Molecular Pain, 6*, 32.

Mogil, J. S., Wilson, S. G., Chesler, E. J., et al. (2003). The melanocortin-1 receptor gene mediates female-specific mechanisms of analgesia in mice and humans. *Proceedings of the National Academy of Sciences of the United States of America, 100*(8), 4867–4872.

Nackley, A. G., Tan, K. S., Fecho, K., Flood, P., Diatchenko, L., & Maixner, W. (2007). Catechol-O-methyltransferase inhibition increases pain sensitivity through activation of both beta2- and beta3-adrenergic receptors. *Pain, 128*(3), 199–208.

Nicholl, B. I., Holliday, K. L., Macfarlane, G. J., European Male Ageing Study Group, et al. (2010). No evidence for a role of the catechol-O-methyltransferase pain sensitivity haplotypes in chronic widespread pain. *Annals of the Rheumatic Diseases, 69*(11), 2009–2012.

Nielsen, C. S., Stubhaug, A., Price, D. D., Vassend, O., Czajkowski, N., & Harris, J. R. (2008). Individual differences in pain sensitivity: genetic and environmental contributions. *Pain, 136*(1–2), 21–29.

Online Mendelian Inheritance in man (OMIM). Bethesda, MD: National Center for Biotechnology Information, National Library of Medicine; 2010. Available at: http://www.ncbi.nlm.nih.gov/omim. Accessed October 6, 2010.

Pasternak, G. W. (2001). Incomplete cross tolerance and multiple mu opioid peptide receptors. *Trends in Pharmacological Sciences, 22*(2), 67–70. Review.

Reimann, F., Cox, J. J., Belfer, I., et al. (2010). Pain perception is altered by a nucleotide polymorphism in SCN9A. *Proceedings of the National Academy of Sciences of the United States of America, 107*(11), 5148–5153.

Ribeiro-Dasilva, M. C., Peres Line, S. R., Santos MC, Leme Godoy dos, Arthuri, M. T., Hou, W., Fillingim, R. B., et al. (2009). Estrogen receptor-alpha polymorphisms and predisposition to TMJ disorder. *The Journal of Pain, 10*(5), 527–533.

Ronald, G., Lafrenière, M. Zameel, Cader, Jean-François Poulin, et al. (2010). A dominant-negative mutation in the TRESK potassium channel is linked to familial migraine with aura. *Nature Medicine, 16*, 1157–1160.

Solovieva, S., Leino-Arjas, P., Saarela, J., Luoma, K., Raininko, R., & Riihimäki, H. (2004). Possible association of interleukin 1 gene locus polymorphisms with low back pain. *Pain, 109*(1–2), 8–19.

Stamer, U. M., & Stüber, F. (2007). Genetic factors in pain and its treatment. *Current Opinion in Anaesthesiology, 20*(5), 478–484.

Zhang, W., Chang, Y. Z., Kan, Q. C., et al. (2010). Association of human micro-opioid receptor gene polymorphism A118G with fentanyl analgesia consumption in Chinese gynaecological patients. *Anaesthesia, 65*(2), 130–135.

Chapter 27
Pain Imaging

Magdalena R. Naylor, David A. Seminowicz, Tamara J. Somers, and Francis J. Keefe

Introduction

Pain is an inseparable aspect of life experience and contains both sensory and emotional dimensions. Sensory qualities associated with pain are usually unpleasant and are accompanied by the pain-related emotional response often referred to as "suffering." However, emotions do not simply occur in parallel with pain, but rather there is an overlap between pain and emotion-related neurophysiological processes (Melzack 2001; Price and Bushnell 2004). Novel brain imaging methods combined with psychophysical methods have clearly shown that pain with its sensory, cognitive and affective dimensions can be modified by attention, emotions and environmental factors. Over the past decade, developments in brain imaging methods have enabled us not only to understand changes in brain function associated with persistent pain but also changes in brain structure. The purpose of this chapter is to provide a review of research on neuroimaging of pain. The chapter is divided into four sections: (1) an overview of imaging methods; (2) imaging studies that examine pain and its modulation by emotional and cognitive factors, (3) imaging studies of clinical pain states, and (4) future directions for research on this topic.

Imaging Methods

The major imaging techniques that can provide meaningful information about brain structure and function include PET (positron emission tomography), MEG (magnetoencephalography), EEG (electroencephalography), and MRI (magnetic resonance imaging). We will briefly review techniques using each of the above technologies and then concentrate on those relevant to the study of pain.

M.R. Naylor, MD, PhD (✉)
Department of Psychiatry, The University of Vermont, Burlington, VT, USA
e-mail: magdalena.naylor@uvm.edu

D.A. Seminowicz, PhD
Department of Neural and Pain Sciences, University of Maryland School of Dentistry,
Baltimore, MD, USA

T.J. Somers, PhD • F.J. Keefe, PhD
Department of Psychiatry and Behavioral Sciences, Duke University Medical Center,
Durham, NC, USA

R.J. Moore (ed.), *Handbook of Pain and Palliative Care: Biobehavioral Approaches for the Life Course*,
DOI 10.1007/978-1-4419-1651-8_27, © Springer Science+Business Media, LLC 2012

Positron Emission Tomography

Utilized in fields of biological research ranging from cardiology and oncology to neuroscience and psychiatry, PET is an important imaging tool for the study of pain. PET is a method by which radioactive tracers may be located and visualized within the body. Since radioactive molecules can be incorporated into almost any biological marker, the applications of PET to research are broad. The primary advantage of the method is its versatility. By radioactively labeling different markers, it is possible to quantify cellular metabolism, blood flow, ligand binding, neurotransmitter localization, and so on. In the study of pain, PET is frequently used to visualize regional cerebral blood flow (rCBF) through the labeling of $H_2^{15}O$, neuronal glucose metabolism using 2-deoxy-2-[^{18}F]fluoro-D-glucose (FDG), and by directly localizing pertinent receptors such as those sensitive to opioids, serotonin, and dopamine. Local concentrations of these ligands may also be estimated.

Radiolabeled Receptor Ligands

One of the most common uses of PET in the study of pain is the localization of specific types of receptors and the quantification of receptor availability by radioactively labeling specific receptor ligands. Because radioactively labeled ligands compete with endogenous ligands to bind to receptors, binding potentials may be calculated by comparing levels of radioactive ligand binding under different conditions. Not surprisingly, opioid receptors, serotonin receptors, and dopamine receptors are all common PET targets in pain research.

PET Analysis of Opioids and Opioid Receptors

Some of the more common radioactive opioid receptor ligands utilized include [^{11}C]-carfentanil (a highly selective μ-opioid receptor agonist), [^{11}C]-diprenorphine, and [^{18}F]-fluorodiprenorphine (nonselective opioid antagonists). These radiotracers have been effectively used to show that subjects with higher sensitivities to noxious cold stimuli exhibit lower basal opioidergic binding potentials in pain-processing-related brain regions such as the insular cortex and orbitofrontal cortex (OFC) (Mueller et al. 2010), supporting evidence for the role that opioidergic peptides play in modulating pain sensitivity. Further, administration of acute experimental pain results in reduced opioidergic radiotracer binding (and therefore an increased concentration of endogenous opioids) in the rostral anterior cingulate cortex (rACC) and the insular cortex, as well as in the thalamus (Bencherif et al. 2002; Sprenger et al. 2006b). The acute changes in opioidergic binding potential observed in the thalamus were also shown to vary directly with subject ratings of pain intensity. These findings suggest that acute pain results in an increase in opioidergic signaling within various supraspinal regions of the pain matrix.

PET is also useful for the investigation of disorders such as central neuropathic pain (CNP). Patients with CNP due to poststroke central nervous system damage demonstrate a lower degree of endogenous opioid binding in the anterior cingulate cortex (ACC), insular cortex, thalamus, and a portion of the inferior parietal cortex, a finding that may begin to explain why CNP patients typically require higher concentrations of opioid medication for effective analgesia (Jones et al. 2004).

PET is also frequently used to test the efficacy of various novel treatments for pain. For example, acupuncture has been shown to decrease the sensation of acute thermal heat pain and to alter opioidergic activity in key brain regions including elevated opioid levels in the ipsilateral medial OFC, insula, and thalamus, and in the contralateral medial prefrontal cortex (PFC); as well as decreased opioid levels in bilateral insular cortex regions, contralateral OFC, and in ipsilateral PFC, ACC, and brainstem (Dougherty et al. 2008). PET research has even opened new doors into the investigation of the placebo effect, showing that opioid activity in response to acute pain and anticipation of acute pain after administration of a nonbiologically active placebo increases within the periaqueductal gray (PAG), dorsal raphe nucleus, amygdala, OFC, insular cortex, rACC, and regions of the PFC (Wager et al. 2007). Interestingly, the PAG and dorsal raphe are both involved in the serotonergic system as well as in opioidergic pathways, another common target in the study of pain using PET.

PET Analysis of Serotonin and Serotonin Receptors

Demonstrating the role of serotonin in the modulation of pain, Kupers et al. (2009, 2010) used PET to examine the roles of radiolabeled ligands for the 5-HT2*a* receptor ($[^{18}F]$-altanserin) and the SERT serotonin transport ($[^{11}C]$-DASB). Significant positive correlations were shown between reported ratings of tonic pain and levels of $[^{18}F]$-altanserin binding within the OFC and posterior cingulate gyrus, among other regions, yet no significant correlation between binding potentials and pain threshold/tolerance levels was reported. Tonic heat pain ratings negatively correlated with SERT binding in the hypothalamus and anterior insula (aINS), while pain tolerance and SERT binding in the hypothalamus showed a positive correlation. The authors interpret these findings to suggest that serotonin may play a role in modulating the affective component of tonic pain perception.

PET Analysis of Dopamine and Dopamine Receptors

Recently, dopamine has become a neurotransmitter of interest in the field of pain research, as well. The D2 and D3 receptor ligand $[^{11}C]$-raclopride has been used to support mounting evidence that dopamine neurotransmission within the basal ganglia may play a role in the perception of pain in addition to its involvement in movement. Specifically, subject ratings of both sensory and affective pain intensity were positively associated with increased dopamine release in the dorsal and ventral basal ganglia (Scott et al. 2006). Further, fibromyalgia patients have been shown to demonstrate atypical dopaminergic responses to pain. The amount of dopamine released in the basal ganglia of healthy subjects exposed to deep muscle pain (hypertonic saline injection) correlated strongly with the reported severity of the pain, whereas no dopamine elevation was observed in the basal ganglia of fibromyalgia patients (Wood et al. 2007).

Measuring Regional Cerebral Blood Flow Using $H_2^{15}O$

Another extremely useful application of PET to the study of pain is its ability to measure rCBF, the same phenomenon that is indirectly measured by functional MRI (fMRI). By radioactively labeling the oxygen atom within a molecule of water, blood flow within the brain can be visualized using PET. This technique can be used to study rCBF changes due to actual painful stimuli, as well as to investigate potential treatments for pain. For example, clinical allodynia resulted in increased rCBF in contralateral OFC and ipsilateral insula whereas nonallodynic stimuli in the same patients resulted in increased rCBF in primary and association somatosensory cortices (SI and SII). Increased activity in ACC was also observed in a subset of clinical allodynia patients, though not significantly in a group analysis (Witting et al. 2006). Other research has used $H_2^{15}O$ PET to show the dose-dependent effects of opioid analgesia within the brain. Opioid infusion (compared to saline) during acute heat pain resulted in decreased rCBF to the thalamus, insula, anterior and posterior cingulate cortices; and increased rCBF in PAG and the perigenual ACC (Wagner et al. 2007). The authors suggest that these findings support the role of opioid transmission in the modulation of inhibitory pain circuitry.

As for testing the efficacy of potential treatments for pain, PET has been used to show that motor cortex stimulation, a treatment for CNP, has the ability to increase rCBF to the cingulate cortex and dorsolateral PFC (DLPFC), changes that correlate with patient ratings of pain relief (Peyron et al. 2007). Spinal cord stimulation for the treatment of CNP has also been shown to result in increases in rCBF, specifically within contralateral thalamus, bilateral parietal association cortices, ACC, and regions of the PFC (Kishima et al. 2010).

Indirect Measure of Neural Metabolism Using [18]FDG

PET has also been used to indirectly measure neural metabolism. FDG is an analog of the glucose that neurons utilize for energy, but one that becomes phosphorylated and trapped once transported within cells. The concentration of FDG within cells of specific brain regions may be used to model neural activity more directly than by examining rCBF. Kulkarni et al. (2007) used FDG PET to compare acute experimental pain with actual arthritic pain in patients and showed that while both conditions activate regions of the pain matrix, arthritic pain results in higher levels of neural metabolism in the cingulate cortex, thalamus, and amygdala.

This method is also a useful approach to researching the mechanisms behind treatments for pain-related disorders. For example, occipital nerve stimulation (ONS), a slow-acting but long-lasting treatment for intractable cluster headaches, has been found to increase neural metabolism in the hypothalamus, midbrain, and the lower pons. In just the patients who reported clinical improvements after ONS, FDG signaling was also increased within the perigenual ACC, supporting ONS as a potential long-term treatment for cluster headaches (Magis et al. 2011).

MRI

This section will provide an overview of common current MRI techniques used for pain research. By far, the most commonly used technique is functional MRI (fMRI), while methods like diffusion tensor imaging (DTI) and magnetic resonance spectroscopy (MRS) are being used more and more frequently, they are relatively new on the scene. Pharmacological MRI (phMRI) is an approach that has exciting potential for clinical purposes that has not yet been fully put to use. A newer fMRI technique, arterial spin labeling (ASL), has great promise for experimental designs not suitable for blood-oxygen-level-dependent (BOLD) fMRI. Structural MRI – looking at changes in gray matter density or cortical thickness – provides another way of assessing brain abnormalities in patients, and its use has grown rapidly in recent years (see section "Structural Analysis (T1, DTI)"). Each of the following subsections will provide an overview of the imaging method in pain research and a description of its first – to our knowledge – use in pain research, to give a historical perspective.

Functional MRI

fMRI is a useful tool in pain research. In the first fMRI study conducted to assess pain-related brain activity, Davis et al. (1995) applied painful electrical median nerve stimulation to healthy subjects and observed consistent activation in the cingulate and SI cortices, similar to what had been reported previously in PET studies. The advantages of fMRI over PET include longer run times, better temporal and spatial resolution, and improved within-subject statistical power. To date, approximately 250 pain fMRI studies have been published. Section "The 'Pain Matrix'" describes the typical regions activated in pain fMRI studies.

A typical pain fMRI experiment involves a subject receiving brief noxious stimuli, which could be thermal, electrical or mechanical, and innocuous control stimuli. A statistical map of the differences between noxious and innocuous activations reveals pain-related activity. Those activations common to both innocuous and noxious stimulations, on the other hand, would be considered somatosensory-related activity.

During the fMRI experiment, subjects can be asked to give ratings, either continuously, or at given intervals. In most cases, pain levels are kept constant – for example, all subjects in an experiment will receive a noxious stimulus that he or she would consistently rate as 5/10. The signal intensity of pain-related activations depends on the amount of pain an individual is experiencing; thus, an individual who is sensitive to noxious stimuli will have much higher pain-related activity than someone less sensitive to the same stimulus (Coghill et al. 2003).

Almost all pain fMRI studies have used BOLD imaging, which relies on the signal change associated with the overflow of oxygenated blood to regions of high metabolic (presumably neuronal) activity. Recently, however, ASL or perfusion-weighted imaging has been applied to pain research (Owen et al. 2008, 2010; Zeidan et al. 2011). The major advantage of ASL is that it allows for signal quantification, similarly to PET studies, but it is less invasive than PET. ASL can also be used to overcome some of the limitations of BOLD imaging, such as short stimulus durations, and it can account for physiological effects due to respiration.

fMRI studies have also revealed differences in pain-related activity between patients and healthy controls, but these are usually because the stimulus used in the study was painful for the patients, but not for the controls. In studies where the intensity of the pain is equal between controls and patients, studies have reported only subtle differences, if any, between groups (Baliki et al. 2010; Giesecke et al. 2004; Gracely et al. 2002). Furthermore, some of these regions might be explained by differences in the affective state of the patient. Giesecke et al. (2005) found that pain-related activation in areas considered to be part of the affective component of pain (i.e., amygdale and aINS), but not the areas involved in the sensory component, was explained by differences in depression in patients with fibromyalgia. Thus, it is important in studies of clinical pain neuroimaging to consider the psychological as well as the sensory aspects of pain.

Another way to examine pain mechanisms is in patients with and without pain relief (see also section "Pharmacological fMRI"). Apkarian et al. (2001) showed that patients with sympathetically maintained pain had heightened activity in frontal and limbic areas, which was reduced when the patients received an effective treatment (sympathetic block or placebo).

Structural MRI

Apkarian et al. (2004) published the first pain voxel-based morphometry (VBM) study, where they showed that people with chronic low back pain have relatively decreased cortical gray matter density in the frontal lobes and the thalamus compared to healthy controls. Since then, approximately 50 studies on T1-weighted measures of brain anatomy in pain patient populations have been published (see section "Structural Analysis (T1, DTI)" for more details).

T1-weighted structural MRI studies examine differences in global or regional volume, tissue densities (white matter, gray matter, cerebrospinal fluid), and/or cortical thickness. The most common approach is VBM, which examines gray matter density by first segmenting the brain into tissue classes, removing the CSF and white matter, smoothing the resultant gray matter image, and comparing the regional densities between groups of patients and controls. For a review of these methods, see Ashburner and Friston (2000). Cortical thickness analysis (CTA), as the name implies, involves measuring thickness at multiple points across the cortex. An example of a study that combines VBM and CTA is Davis et al. (2008).

Diffusion Tensor Imaging

DTI has quickly become a very popular technique for assessing white matter tract anatomy and functionality in the normal brain and in many neurological disorders. For a review of the technique and its applications, see Johansen-Berg and Behrens (2006) and Johansen-Berg and Rushworth (2009).

Different types of studies need to be considered in separate contexts with this method. For example, the earliest report of DTI changes related to pain was a case study of central poststroke pain which reported altered thalamo-SI connectivity (Seghier et al. 2005). Combined with fMRI, this study showed how a white matter lesion, characterized by DTI, could affect pain-related activity. Another use for DTI is tractography in healthy subjects. Aiming to show pathways that might be involved in descending modulation of pain, Hadjipavlou et al. (2006) searched for tracts from the brainstem to the PFC, thalamus, and amygdala in eight subjects. The findings indicate the existence of these tracts, but their actual function can only be speculated.

Geha et al. (2008b) reported aberrant connectivity patterns from the anterior insular cortex in a group of CRPS patients compared to healthy controls. Furthermore, they showed an interesting abnormality in the relationship between whole brain gray matter density and whole brain fractional anisotropy (the extent that a voxel contains fibers in primarily one direction, which is considered a marker of white matter integrity), where the two measures were strongly correlated in controls, but not in patients.

Magnetic Resonance Spectroscopy

In comparison to other MRI techniques, MRS has rarely been used in pain neuroimaging studies, although as the technology improves it is likely to become more common. MRS is a type of neurochemical imaging, like PET, but it is limited by its low sensitivity, the number of chemicals that can be identified (e.g., N-acetyl aspartate, glucose, glutamine/glutamate), and the number and size of regions that can be investigated in one study (generally a few, usually quite large, regions). MRS has the potential for diagnosis and treatment of chronic pain and related brain disorders. For a review, see van der Graaf (2010).

Grachev et al. (2000) reported lower than normal N-acetyl aspartate and glucose levels in dorsolateral prefrontal and cingulate cortices in chronic low back pain patients. Harris et al. (2009) demonstrated that people with fibromyalgia had increased glutamate levels in the posterior insula relative to controls, and that the level of glutamate in this region correlated with pain sensitivity. This finding suggests that the posterior insula might be more excitable in fibromyalgia patients, providing a potential mechanism for their pain hypersensitivity.

Pharmacological fMRI

Pharmacological fMRI (phMRI) is a term sometimes used to describe fMRI experiments in which the manipulation involves the use of a drug. It is a technique that has recently been applied and has great potential for understanding brain mechanisms of pain modulation. The basic experimental design in phMRI involves the comparison of brain activity associated with a noxious stimulus before and after administration of a drug or a placebo, with pain ratings in both states. The difference in activity before and after the drug administration can thus be considered a result of the pharmacological effect of that drug. Baliki et al. (2005) administered a COX-2 inhibitor (Celebrex® (Celocoxib)) in a single patient with psoriatic arthritis and showed that 1 h after administration, both pain ratings associated with joint manipulation and activity in SII and aINS were significantly decreased. A more recent study reported that administration of a TNF-alpha blocker reduced nociceptive fMRI signals in both mice and humans (Hess et al. 2011).

Electroencephalography and Magnetoencephalography

Over the past century, EEG has been widely used in clinical practice (e.g., to diagnose and monitor brain states in epilepsy or under anesthesia). More recently, it has also emerged as a powerful tool for research in pain. EEG is sensitive to the radial currents in cortical neurons, particularly those located close to the scalp. The magnetic fields produced by neuronal currents can be measured by MEG. In contrast to EEG, MEG is less sensitive to distortions introduced by the skull and the meninges, and more sensitive to the ambient electromagnetic noise, necessitating better shielding of the recording environment. EEG and MEG afford an opportunity to study the rhythmic firing of neuronal ensembles as well as the sequence and speed of neural events. Integrating information across and within individual brain regions is believed to take place by synchronization of neuronal populations (e.g., Schroeder et al. 2010). EEG and MEG measure synchronous activity of aligned neurons. The differences in such synchronous activity can be detected by analyzing the spectral properties of the ongoing electrical oscillations. Additionally, stimulus-locked EEG and MEG activity can be averaged across multiple trials and the resultant evoked responses can be analyzed to determine stages of neural processing. While these methods are largely insensitive to neuronal activations from deeper brain structures (including major parts of the pain neuromatrix, e.g., cingulate cortex and insula), high-density EEG recordings in combination with source localization algorithms can aid in visualizing neural activity stemming from these regions (Brown and Jones 2010; Kakigi et al. 2005). These methodologies are reviewed below in the context of available literature on pain.

Spectral Analyses

Spectral analyses are particularly well-suited for studying tonic pain, a more clinically meaningful pain model as compared to brief phasic pain. Theoretical considerations predict that tonic painful stimulation should produce decreased synchronization of cortical rhythms in the alpha band (8–12 Hz) over sensory regions contralateral to the stimulus, signaling reduced cortical idling. However, as discussed by Dowman et al. (2008), there is inconsistency in the direction and the topographical distribution of these tonic pain effects across studies. In addition to the findings from tonic pain studies, there is some evidence that anticipation of predictable phasic pain is reflected by alpha-band desynchronization (Babiloni et al. 2003, 2008; Del Percio et al. 2006). This elecrophysiological response is believed to be a marker of "gating" in the thalamocortical and cortico-cortical networks (Rossini et al. 1999) and can be modulated by top–down control in a task-relevant fashion (Klimesch et al. 2007). At the same time, in chronic pain populations, there is notable thalamocortical arrhythmia, as evidenced by alterations in the alpha band frequencies and a general slowing down of dominant frequency bands (e.g., Boord et al. 2007; Sarnthein et al. 2006; Stern et al. 2006; Walton et al. 2010). Interestingly, the arrhythmia of neurogenic pain can be normalized by therapeutically effective surgical lesions of the thalamus (Sarnthein et al. 2006). Intracranial sources of this therapeutic improvement localized to the cingulate and insular cortices (Stern et al. 2006). In a different treatment intervention, Ray et al. (2009) used MEG to study patients undergoing deep brain stimulation and correlated their perceptual ratings of pain with power in the theta (6–9 Hz) and beta (12–30 Hz) bands. In sum, spectral analyses are sensitive to therapeutic interventions in research and clinical practice.

Evoked Potentials

Painful somatosensory stimulation results in a well-described sequence of evoked potentials when stimulus-locked physiological activity is averaged. The major ERP components include N1 (i.e., first negative deflection), P1 (i.e., the first positive deflection), N2 and P2 (e.g., Kakigi et al. 2005).

Earlier sensory components in the primary and secondary somatosensory cortices have also been identified (Kakigi et al. 2005). However, since they represent relatively weak signals, a high number of trials are required to achieve adequate signal-to-noise ratios. EEG and MEG source localization algorithms are effective in differentiating activity stemming from the SI, SII/insula and anterior cingulate. Separating SII and insula is not always possible and bilateral anterior cingulate sources may cancel one another when they are oriented in opposite directions (Kakigi et al. 2005). Thus, care must be taken not to over-interpret results of inverse solutions. Combined EEG and MEG recordings are sometimes used for better modeling of intracranial sources (e.g., Hauck et al. 2007; Quante et al. 2008). Diers et al. (2007) examined pain-evoked potentials in chronic low back pain patients. Compared to healthy controls, an early sensory-discriminative component at 80 ms was enhanced, while a later component around 260 ms was reduced in the patient sample. These results highlight the differences in pain perception in the chronic pain population. There is mounting evidence for the cortical disinhibition of acute pain response in chronic pain populations. Buchgreitz et al. (2008) compared somatosensory-evoked potentials during induced tonic muscle pain in control subjects and patients with chronic tension-type headache. While the magnitude of the evoked potentials in control subjects was reduced under tonic pain conditions, it remained intact in patients. Quante et al. (2008) reached similar conclusions after investigating simultaneously present tonic and phasic pain in chronic osteoarthritis. The central descending "pain-inhibits-pain" perceptual effect was absent in this population, possibly due to the reduced activity in the cingulate gyrus (but not SII). Evoked potentials have also been used on an individual basis to monitor treatment-related cortical changes (e.g., McGeoch et al. 2009). However, as compared to spectral analyses, they are more methodologically advanced, require additional stimulus delivery equipment and may require longer testing times for better sensitivity to treatment effects.

Limitations to Imaging Methods

As described above, imaging methods have many uses, but they also have limitations. The constraints imposed by the experimental environment limit all types of pain neuroimaging. Subjects generally need to keep still while usually brief, repetitive pain stimuli are used. This differs from the way pain is normally experienced.

The major limitations of PET are its invasiveness (radiation exposure), relatively poor spatial and temporal resolution compared to other imaging modalities, and the logistics of producing, acquiring and preserving radioactive tracers. The temporal resolution of PET is limited by the time required for radiotracers to be transported into cells and to bind to receptors. Spatial resolution is an issue because PET is insensitive to anatomical information and location of nonradioactive structures, although this limitation may be addressed by coupling PET with CT or even MRI to acquire anatomical images upon which PET data can be mapped. While the typical levels of radiation exposure produced by PET are relatively low, exposing patients or research subjects to even a potentially small amount of harm always merits careful consideration. For patient and subject safety, it is usually advisable to utilize radioactive tracers with short half-lives in order to limit the duration of radiation exposure. The downsides of this approach are that short half-life radiotracers must be used quickly after being produced in order for them to remain detectable and dosing must sometimes be recalculated several times throughout the course of a day as a radiotracer decays. As a result, many institutions and hospitals are restricted to using only radiotracers that can be produced nearby or on-site.

While MRI offers much better spatial resolution than PET, MEG, and EEG, its temporal resolution is still on the scale of seconds. Some patients will not be able to undergo an MRI scan because of obesity, claustrophobia, or the presence of ferromagnetic implanted devices (e.g., pacemakers or infusion pumps). In addition, MRI equipment is expensive to purchase, maintain, and operate.

While MEG and EEG provide millisecond temporal resolution, they suffer in spatial resolution and cannot provide reliable information about subcortical sources of brain activity. The skull, meninges and cerebrospinal fluid interfere with the EEG signal, obscuring its intracranial source.

Imaging Pain

The "Pain Matrix"

Brain imaging research over the past 2 decades has aimed to determine (1) which brain areas are involved in experiencing pain, (2) which aspects of the pain experience the brain regions are involved in, and (3) whether the activity in these areas can be modulated. In this section, we will define pain-related activations, show the dimensionality of these activations, and discuss the strengths and limitations of the current research field.

Pain is a multidimensional experience comprised of sensory-discriminative, affective-motivational, and cognitive-evaluative components (Melzack and Casey 1968). The sensory-discriminative and affective-motivational components are intuitive parts of the pain experience, the former involving detecting, locating, and differentiating the properties of a stimulus, and the latter to do with the way the experience leaves us feeling and moves us to react. The cognitive component is likely the most difficult to distinguish and embodies the sensory and affective domains: it is generally agreed that without consciousness and thus lack of cognitive function – specifically the ability to attend to environmental features – one cannot experience pain. We thus focus here on the sensory and affective components of pain.

First, a brief note on neuroanatomy nomenclature: two brain areas commonly reported in pain neuroimaging studies are the cingulate cortex and the insula. There are generally two outstanding nomenclatures for the cingulate, but here we will use that defined by Vogt (2005) and described in detail by Palomero-Gallagher et al. (2008, 2009). The main inconsistency is the labeling of ACC in pain literature, which most often would fall under the area MCC (mid cingulate cortex), according to Vogt. The term rACC in the literature is used vaguely, and is sometimes within the Vogt's ACC and other times the MCC. Because of their vicinity and the often poor spatial resolution in brain imaging, the secondary somatosensory cortex (SII) and the posterior insula (pINS) are often difficult to discriminate from one another (Eickhoff et al. 2006a, b).

One of the first pain neuroimaging studies (using PET) reported pain-related activations in the cingulate cortex, SI, and SII (Talbot et al. 1991). Several reviews and meta-analyses have summarized the key brain structures identified in pain imaging studies (Apkarian et al. 2005; Farrell et al. 2005; Garcia-Larrea et al. 2003; Peyron et al. 2000, 2002; Treede et al. 1999). The most commonly reported pain-related activations include the SI, OP, MCC, aINS, PFC, including the dorsolateral PFC (DLPFC), anterolateral PFC (ALPFC), medial PFC (MPFC), and thalamus. Other areas, such as the amygdala, cerebellum, basal ganglia, brainstem including the periaqueductal gray (PAG), posterior parietal cortex (PPC), supplementary motor area, and primary motor cortex (MI) have also been reported in pain imaging studies. EEG and MEG studies of laser-evoked potentials have reported that the dipoles most commonly described were in the MCC/SMA/pre-SMA and OP, and sometimes SI (Garcia-Larrea et al. 2003).

Several different models for nociceptive processing in the brain have been described. One of the areas of heated debate is whether nociceptive information reaches brain structures through specific channels, or labeled lines, as described by Craig (2003), or whether it is mediated by convergence of multiple inputs. In the convergence model, nociceptive information is carried by both nociceptive-specific (NS) and wide dynamic range (WDR) (Willis et al. 2002) pathways to the thalamus and brainstem. Sensory, immediate affective, and secondary affective dimensions of pain can be dissociated based on the brain regions involved or the interactions between these regions (Price 2002). In the labeled lines theory, pain is considered a homeostatic emotion, whereby the primary role of the system is to detect a homeostatic imbalance (specifically in the posterior insula, which responds to thermal and noxious stimuli). In this model, the right aINS has a specific role in interoceptive awareness, and it is activated by all forms of subjective feelings (Craig 2009). The theories appear to be in conflict, and as Perl (2007) suggested, it is likely a combination of both theories that is closest to the truth.

Another system used to describe cerebral pain processing was proposed by Treede (2002). This model contains two parts: the lateral system, stemming from the lateral sensory thalamic nuclei to SI and SII; and the medial system, from the medial thalamic nuclei to MCC and insula. The lateral system is usually associated with the sensory-discriminative dimension, while the medial system is usually associated with the affective-motivational dimension. This model is an extension of a seminal model proposed by Melzack and Casey (1968). In many neuroimaging studies, this medial/lateral system is used to describe the findings (e.g., Kulkarni et al. 2005; Sprenger et al. 2006a).

It seems likely that regardless of the theory one selects, the processing of pain in the brain occurs in parallel, and is influenced by past, present, and future aspects of an individual's psychological makeup.

An extension of Melzack's neuromatrix, the term "pain matrix" has become common in the pain neuroimaging realm. The pain matrix is presumed to encompass the psychological domains of the pain experience in different brain regions. Thus, for example, the sensory-discriminative dimension is supplied by sensory cortices SI and OP, the affective-motivational by M/ACC and aINS, and the cognitive-evaluative by PFC. The idea that there is a pain-specific network of brain regions has recently been called into question by studies showing activation of so-called pain matrix areas by other sensory modalities (Iannetti et al. 2008; Mouraux et al. 2011), indicating that salience or the ability of a stimulus to grab one's awareness is responsible for these activations. Pain is highly salient, and certainly part of the activations seen in the "pain matrix" can be explained by the salience of the stimulus, as was described by Downar et al. (2003).

Is there an area that we can call "pain cortex" analogous to visual or auditory cortices? Only one area of cortex – the insula – can elicit pain when stimulated (Isnard et al. 2004; Mazzola et al. 2006, 2009; Ostrowsky et al. 2002). Lesions to this same area have led to losses or reductions of pain or temperature sensation (Greenspan et al. 1999; Schmahmann and Leifer 1992) or central pain condition (Garcia-Larrea et al. 2010). However, even very large lesions to the insula do not result in a loss of the ability to experience pain, although it may have some role in the experience (Starr et al. 2009). Thus, the insula appears to be a key area in pain, but the involvement of other brain areas may be sufficient and necessary to experience pain.

Sensory-Discriminative Aspects of Pain

The sensory-discriminative component of pain includes identifying the location, intensity, and quality of a painful stimulus. For location, the somatotopic organization of SI is well known and could be involved in location of noxious stimulation (Bingel et al. 2004; Ruben et al. 2001). More recently, studies have shown pain-related somatotopy in the insula (Bingel et al. 2004; Brooks et al. 2005; Henderson et al. 2007, 2011; Ruben et al. 2001) and putamen (Bingel et al. 2004).

For pain intensity encoding, SI (Bushnell et al. 1999), OP, and aINS are likely involved. While one study reported widespread activation of pain intensity-related activation in PET (Coghill et al. 1999), but others reported that only SI, OP, and anterior or mid insula encode pain intensity (Baliki et al. 2009; Bornhovd et al. 2002; Downar et al. 2003). In an MEG study, Timmermann et al. (2001) reported a pain intensity-related increase in SI as well as in OP.

Another part of the sensory-discriminative component is pain quality. Davis et al. (2002) have used percept-related fMRI, in which subjects provide real-time ratings of a given sensory quality, to show areas related to prickle (including ACC, PFC, mid insula) and paradoxical heat (right aINS) (Davis et al. 2004), which is the feeling of warmth that some subjects experience at the offset of a cool stimulus. It thus appears that the aINS has an important role in processing both pain intensity and pain quality.

Affective-Motivational Aspects of Pain

The affective-motivational component of pain is the suffering aspect of pain and involves how unpleasant, bothersome, and unbearable the pain is. While there are several ways of determining the brain regions involved in this component, in this section we will focus on one specific type of "pain" that presumably involves the affective, but not the sensory components: pain empathy. A recent meta-analysis of pain empathy studies reported that the areas activated while watching someone in pain, experiencing pain vicariously, or seeing picture of potentially painful situations (e.g., a thumb being caught in a car door), included bilateral aINS, and M/ACC (Lamm et al. 2011). These areas overlap with activations in studies in which participants received painful stimulation, but do not include sensory areas SI or OP. Thus, experiencing pain through observing others can activate an emotional pain response in the absence of sensory input. Interestingly, these brain areas can be activated even in people with congenital insensitivity to pain (Danziger et al. 2009), e.g., people who have never experienced the sensory aspect of pain.

Pain Modulation

Effect of Attention and Distraction

The effects of attention and distraction on individuals' perception of pain have been demonstrated across the lifespan. Infants have a decreased pain response when distracted by a sweet taste (e.g., sucrose) during a painful procedure (e.g., needle prick, circumcision) and children, adolescents, and adults report less pain when distraction techniques are conjunctively used with painful medical procedures (e.g., bone marrow transplant, venipuncture; Christensen and Fatchett 2002; Leibovici et al. 2009). New and exciting work has just begun to use brain imaging techniques to explore the areas of the brain that are likely involved in this phenomena of attention and distraction modulating pain (e.g., see Fig. 27.1). Past work has suggested that one of the brain regions that may be particularly important in understanding the effect of attention and distraction on pain is the ACC (Davis et al. 1997; Hsieh et al. 1995).

Immersive virtual reality (VR) distraction is one particularly intriguing application of distraction that is designed to provide multisensory input (e.g., visual, aural, tactile) while blocking visual and aural input from the immediate environment. Several studies have suggested that immersive VR is effective in reducing clinical pain reports in both experimental settings and with patients undergoing painful procedures for burn injuries (Malloy and Milling 2010). New work is just beginning to explore the neural correlates associated with the use of immersive VR for pain reduction.

In one such study, Hoffman et al. (2007) assessed the impact of immersive VR on both subjective pain ratings and fMRI pain-related brain activity in response to thermal pain stimulation in healthy volunteers. This study compared three experimental conditions to examine the analgesic effects of immersive VR: immersive VR distraction alone, opioid alone, immersive VR distraction + opioid, and no treatment. Results indicated that use of both immersive VR distraction and opioid medication

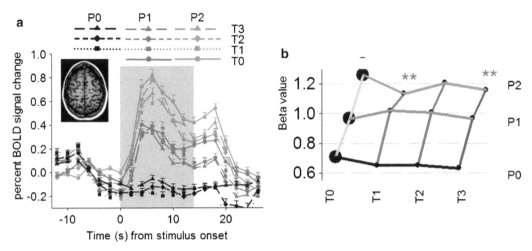

Fig. 27.1 Effects of pain and concurrent cognitive demand on SI activity. (**a**) Event-related average for primary somatosensory/motor cortex. *Shaded gray area* shows the duration of the condition. The SI/MI region whose activity is plotted is shown in axial brain image. (**b**) Modulation profile for SI/MI. This plot shows the influence of pain, cognitive load, and the interaction of pain and cognition. For example, looking only at the *cyan line* (T0, or minimal cognitive load), increasing pain (P2 (moderate pain) vs. P1 (mild pain) vs. P0 (non-painful stimulation)), activity in this region increases. This effect is significant across all task difficulty levels (T0–T3 (where T3 represents the highest cognitive demand)). However, the *asterisks* indicate that compared with P2T0, both P2T1 and P2T3 have significantly (*P*<0.01) reduced activity. In other words, SI/MI moderate pain-related activity is significantly reduced by the easy (T1) and difficult (T3) cognitive tasks. Beta values are created from the general linear model analysis and represent the estimated fit of the data to the predictive model (from Seminowicz and Davis (2007) (*Cerebral Cortex*), used with permission)

either alone or in combination generally resulted in lower subjective pain scores and lower pain-related brain activity compared to no treatment. Specifically, compared to the no treatment condition, immersive VR distraction alone significantly reduced pain-related brain activity in the insula, thalamus, and SII, while opioid alone reduced pain-related brain activity only in the insula and thalamus. When comparing the immersive VR distraction + opioid condition to other groups, the combined condition produced lower pain-related brain activity in the ACC and insula compared to the no treatment group, lower levels of pain-related brain activity in the SII compared to both the opioid alone group and the no treatment group, and lower levels of brain activity in the thalamus compared to the immersive VR distraction alone group and the no treatment group.

The study by Hoffman et al. (2007) found that participants in the immersive VR distraction + opioid group demonstrated reduced subjective (i.e., pain report) and objective (i.e., pain-related brain activity) pain markers compared to participants in the opioid alone group. The results of this study are important because they suggest that patients undergoing a painful medical procedure may receive additional pain relief from the use of distraction techniques such as immersive VR. This could be particularly important in instances where the traditional use of pain medications (i.e., opioids) for acute pain relief is not possible or desirable or is not providing adequate pain relief. The use of VR may be particularly useful because past work has shown that it has positive effects across the lifespan (i.e., both in children and adults). While this work was done in healthy volunteers in a laboratory setting, it would be interesting to understanding how this distraction technique would impact brain activity in patients with clinical pain or in patients undergoing a painful medical procedure.

In another recent study, Richter et al. (2010) employed a unique study design to examine brain activity during attention and distraction in response to pain stimuli. The aim of the study was to investigate unique brain activation in response to pain-related words compared to negative, positive, and neutral words during two attention tasks (i.e., imagination, distraction). These investigators aimed to determine if brain activity in response to pain stimuli is distinct from a general negative response and/or increased arousal. Of particular relevance to attention and distraction as pain modulators, participants' brain activity was measured in response to paying close attention to the meaning of the words and when distracted from the meaning of the words. In the attention task, participants were asked to imagine a situation or sensation associated with the particular word. In the distraction task, participants were distracted from the word itself by being instructed to count the vowels of the words and be prepared to report them after the task. When participants were asked to focus their attention on the meaning of the words, increased brain activity was found in the DLPFC, inferior parietal gyri, and precuneus when processing pain-related words compared to the other words. When participants were asked to use a distraction task (count the vowels in the words), decreased activation was demonstrated in the dorsal anterior cingulate and increased activation was demonstrated in the subgenual ventral anterior cingulate when processing pain-related words compared to the other words. The results suggest that activations of pain-related brain regions are strongly modulated by attention and distraction processes and that the processing of pain-related words is specific to pain stimuli and not simply a result of negative response or increased arousal.

These results provide additional information regarding brain activation involved in the phenomena of attention and distraction to pain. The investigators suggest that their results indicate that the perception of pain-related words changes the central nervous processing associated with the cognitive dimensions of pain. This processing may be of particular importance for the effects of distraction in individuals facing acute pain due to medical procedures and/or chronic pain due to a chronic condition. The results support the notion that the words used by an individual can impact the pain experience. For example, how patients and/or healthcare professionals talk about pain may have the potential to increase or decrease patients' levels of pain. An interesting direction for future research would be to examine how common types of pain-related language (e.g., support, reassurance, instructions, descriptions) used by health professional, caregivers, and even the patient influence pain-related brain activity in patients dealing with pain. If pain words have a clear effect on pain-related brain activity, protocols could be developed to coach individuals to alter how they talk about pain language so as to reduce negative effects.

Effect of Expectation and Hypnosis

Expectation. Heightened pain expectation, or anticipation of pain, is in and of itself adaptive in that people can remove themselves from harm's way. However, heightened pain expectation can also result in increased fear and anxiety that are not only distressing, but can lead to more distress and to more pain (Crombez et al. 1999). Patients receiving palliative care have often experienced a myriad of painful medical interventions and may be particularly vulnerable to the deleterious effects of pain expectation. Empirical work has shown that high pain expectation or anxiety before a medical procedure can lead to increased postprocedural pain (Schupp et al. 2005). High levels of pain expectation can also be problematic when they lead to behavioral avoidance of situations associated with pain (Vlaeyen et al. 1995). Investigators have begun to use innovative methods of research to examine differences in brain activity in response to expectation of pain and actual pain stimuli.

In a study using fMRI, Ziv et al. (2010) assessed brain activity before and during cued or uncued thermal pain applied to the wrist. These investigators were particularly interested in examining the differential brain activity in the amygdala and hippocampus to cued and uncued pain stimuli. They also examined the relationship between anxiety-related personality traits and differences in pain reports to cued and uncued pain stimuli (i.e., pain expectancy scores) and how these two constructs (i.e., anxiety, pain expectancy) were associated with increased brain activity. Twelve individuals (seven female, mean age = 25) received a sequence of twelve intense pain stimuli. Half of the stimuli were cued with the words "Get Ready" imaged in red on a computer screen and half of the stimuli had no cue. Participants rated the pain intensity of the thermal stimuli using a 10-point visual analog scale (VAS) after each stimulus. This study had a number of interesting findings. First, on average, when the pain stimuli were preceded by a cue, noxious stimuli were experienced as more painful relative to unexpected (i.e., no cue) noxious stimuli of the same intensity. Second, the investigators found that the amygdala was more active during trials in which a cue preceded delivery of the pain stimulus and that hippocampal activity was increased (compared to baseline) during both cued and uncued trials.

Third, participants who scored higher on the personality trait of anxiety showed increased activity in the amygdala when expecting pain (i.e., after the cue and prior to the stimulus application). Participants who had higher pain expectancy scores (i.e., the difference in pain report to cued and uncued noxious stimuli) demonstrated increased levels of hippocampal activity when expecting pain and during the pain stimuli. These findings support the notion that the amygdala plays a role in the "fight or flight" response to dangerous stimuli, in this case pain. Findings also suggest that the hippocampus is involved in both the expectancy of pain and appraisal of stimuli value.

In another study, Wise et al. (2007) examined the influence of midazolam (i.e., a short-acting anxiety medication) on brain activity associated with pain expectancy and pain. They hypothesized that brain activity associated with the anticipation of pain would be reduced when participants were administered midazolam (compared to administration of saline) but that the brain activity associated with pain stimuli would not change. To examine this, they conditioned healthy volunteers to expect either a painfully hot stimulus or a nonpainful warm stimulus on the basis of two different visual cues. As predicted, results of this work found that midazolam administration did modulate the brain activity associated with anticipation of pain. Three specific brain regions – contralateral aINS, anterior cingulate, and ipsilateral SII – associated with pain anticipation showed decreases in activity when anticipating pain under midazolam application, but not under the control condition (i.e., saline administration). Midazolam application did not have a significant effect on pain-related brain activity. Participants receiving midazolam compared to saline did, however, rate the pain stimulus as significantly lower. This suggests that midazolam produced some analgesic effect evidenced by pain report, but that it did not alter brain activity related to the stimuli. This is a very important finding because it suggests that pharmacological agents can have differential neural effects on pain and on the anticipation of pain.

Hypnosis. Hypnosis for pain has been used in both acute and chronic pain settings to produce an analgesic effect (Barber 1996; Crawford et al. 1993). It has been shown to be beneficial for managing pain due to a number of medical conditions including sickle cell disease, advanced cancer pain, osteoarthritis pain, and disability-related pain (Dinges et al. 1997; Elkins et al. 2004; Gay et al. 2002; Jensen et al. 2005). Hypnosis for pain usually includes two phases: (1) patients are led through an induction phase which includes imaging a sequence of calming statements or images (e.g., "everything is just right," or a peaceful green meadow) and (2) patients are given suggestions of experiencing less pain, less stress, more energy, and more control (Keefe et al. 2010).

In an interesting study design, Derbyshire et al. (2004) compared brain activity across three different conditions: (a) noxious stimuli application, (b) hypnotic suggestion of a painful state in the absence of noxious stimuli (i.e., hypnotically induced pain), and (c) imagined pain. Participants reported pain ratings for the noxious stimuli application and hypnotically induced pain in the absence of noxious stimuli using a verbal rating scale where 0 = no pain and 10 = maximal pain. Average pain rating following the noxious stimuli was 5.7 (range 3–10) and during the hypnotically induced pain was 2.8 (range 1–9). Brain activity in response to noxious stimulus application and hypnotically induced pain was similar – that is, the thalamus, ACC, midanterior insula, and parietal and prefrontal cortices showed similar activity in the two conditions. Imagined pain did not involve the same degree or pattern of activation as the other two conditions (i.e., noxious stimulus application, hypnotically induced pain). These results suggest that brain activation is similar in response to both actual noxious stimulation and suggestion of noxious stimuli. They are particularly important because they suggest that actual noxious stimulation is not necessary to activate pain-related brain regions.

Abrahamsen et al. (2010) explored whether hypnotically induced hypoalgesia or hyperalgesia would modulate the pain experience and associated brain responses in patients with a common chronic pain condition (i.e., temporomandibular disorder (TMD)). They investigated whether individual susceptibility to hypnosis measured by changes in perceived pain intensity and unpleasantness would correlate with brain activity during hypoalgesia and hyperalgesia. In this study, 19 patients were divided into three different experimental conditions: hypnotic hypoalgesia, hypnotic hyperalgesia, and a control condition (i.e., patients in normal alert state). In all three conditions, patients were subjected to repetitive pin-prick stimuli of identical intensity. The results of this study demonstrated that hypnotic modulation can increase or decrease patients' perception of pain and unpleasantness of painful stimuli and that these changes are associated with distinctly different brain activation patterns. Specifically, when compared to the control condition, painful stimulation during hypnotic hyperalgesia was associated with increased activity in right posterior insula and BA6 and left BA40 and hypnotic hypoalgesia was only associated with activity in right posterior insula. These findings indicate that hypnotic hypoalgesia produces significant decreases in brain activity in response to pain stimuli in patients with a chronic pain condition. An interesting feature of this study is that it was conducted in a population of persons suffering from chronic pain. This contrasts with most imaging studies of hypnosis that have relied on samples of healthy volunteers. Understanding how hypnosis is related to pain-related brain activity in patients with chronic pain conditions is particularly important as hypnosis may be a promising treatment to decrease the negative influence of pain.

Effect of Emotions

There is growing evidence that negative emotions, particularly anxiety and depression, are related to increased pain and that increased pain can lead to increased emotional distress (Fishbain et al. 1997; Fishbain 2002; Mee et al. 2006). Fully understanding the relationship between pain and emotional distress is important so that efforts can be made to interrupt a negative cycle of increased pain and emotional distress. Several common brain regions have been implicated in both pain and emotion (e.g., ACC, insula). However, the interrelationship of brain activity between pain and emotions is just beginning to be explored and explained.

Ploghaus et al. (2001) conducted one of the earliest studies using imaging to investigate the effects of anxiety on pain. In this study, participants were presented with a visual signal, which was always followed by a mild thermal nociceptive stimulus, thus making this particular visual signal induce low anxiety. A second signal was presented, which was usually followed by the same mild thermal nociceptive stimulus, but occasionally was followed by a very intense thermal noxious stimulus, resulting in a cue producing high anxiety. A manipulation check to ensure that the conditions produced the expected anxiety levels was completed in a separate group of participants; anxiety was significantly higher in the condition expected to produce higher anxiety. The investigators cited the importance of obtaining anxiety ratings in a separate group as conscious self-assessment of both processes in the same subject might lead to hypothesis-driven correlations. Imaging results found that pain-related brain activity in the entorhinal cortex was increased by expectation-induced anticipatory anxiety of pain stimuli. Increased activation in the entorhinal cortex was related to activity in the cingulate cortex and the insula (i.e., other pain-related areas). The results of this study suggest that anxiety can modulate activity in pain-responsive areas of the brain. Patients receiving painful medical treatments (e.g., bone marrow transplants, chemotherapy) may experience increased brain activity in response to environmental cues (e.g., hospital parking lot, hallways), which signal pending treatment. Future studies should focus on understanding the neural correlates of interventions, which produce anxiety responses related to impending painful events.

In a recent study, Roy et al. (2009) combined fMRI of the brain with recording of a spinal noci-ceptive reflex to explore the effects of emotion on pain. Participants underwent trials where two noxious electrical stimuli were applied as they viewed pleasant, unpleasant, or neutral images. Standardized images from the International Affective Picture System were used to evoke emotion (Lang et al. 1998). Several interesting findings were noted. First, when participants were viewing unpleasant compared to pleasant images, their report of pain during the electrical stimulation was significantly greater. Second, emotions induced by either pleasant or unpleasant images modulated patients' response to pain in the right insula, paracentral lobule, parahippocampal gyrus, thalamus, and amygdala (i.e., decreased activity in response to pleasant, increased activity in response to unpleasant). Third, when patients were viewing unpleasant compared to pleasant images, larger brain activations in the paracentral lobule, bilateral parahippocampal gyrus, and right ipsilateral insula were seen in response to the electrical stimulation. Finally, activity in the thalamus, amygdala, and several prefrontal areas was associated with the modulation of the spinal reflex responses. In sum, these results demonstrate that emotions modulate patients' pain perception, brain activity in response to pain, and spinal nociceptive processes related to pain.

Giesecke et al. (2005) examined the relationship between depressive symptoms and experimen-tally induced pain in patients with fibromyalgia. These investigators found that depressive symptoms were positively related with experimentally induced pain activation of affective brain areas. Higher levels of depressive symptoms were associated with activation of the amygdala and contralateral aINS. Interestingly, patients' rating of their fibromyalgia pain was associated with activation of the contralateral aINS, anterior cingulate cortex, and PFC. These findings provide evidence of a close relationship between pain and emotion at a cortical level.

The results of these studies are particularly important as strong emotions are likely to emerge in acute and chronic pain contexts. Future work should consider the relationships between pain-related brain activity and emotions in the context of acute pain (e.g., medical procedures) and chronic pain (e.g., diseases like arthritis and cancer). The findings from these imaging studies confer with clinical research suggesting that efforts to decrease negative emotions and increase positive emotions may have a positive impact on patients' pain and overall well-being. A better understanding of how emo-tions impact patients (vs. healthy experimental subjects) facing acute and chronic pain can help direct the application of pain interventions.

Effect of Cognition

Over the past decade there has been growing interest in the effects of cognition on pain experience. One of the strongest cognitive predictors of pain is pain catastrophizing. When faced with pain, persons who catastrophize tend to focus on pain sensations, magnify how threatening pain is, and negatively evaluate their own ability to deal with pain.

To date, three imaging studies have examined how pain catastrophizing relates neural responses to pain stimulation. Gracely et al. (2004) conducted an imaging study of pain catastrophizing in fibro-myalgia patients who were exposed to painful pressure stimulation. The fibromyalgia patients were divided into two categories (high vs. low) based on their level of catastrophizing. When compared to those in the low pain catastrophizing group, patients who scored high on pain catastrophizing showed increased activation in a number of brain regions related to pain: (1) areas related to sensory aspects of pain (SII), (2) areas involved in the anticipation of pain (cerebellum, medial frontal gyrus), (3) areas related to behavioral responses to pain (premotor cortex), and (4) brain regions related to atten-tion and emotional aspects of pain (ACC). In a study conducted in healthy volunteers, Seminowicz and Davis (2006) examined how pain catastrophizing related to brain activation in response to pain. Brain imaging data were collected under two conditions: (1) during exposure to mild, electrical pain stimulation, and (2) during exposure to more intense, electrical pain stimulation. The level of pain

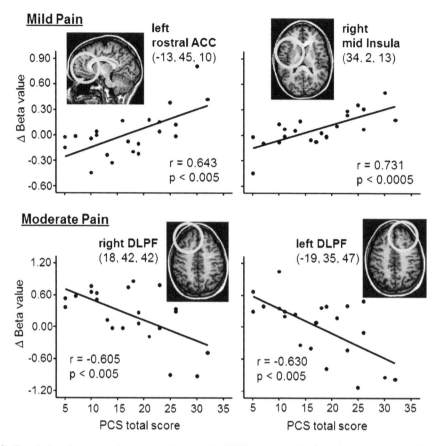

Fig. 27.2 Correlations between pain catastrophizing scale (PCS) scores and brain activity evoked by mild pain (*top*) and moderate pain (*bottom*). With mild pain, catastrophizing was associated with increased activity in rACC (a.k.a. pregenual ACC) and mid insula, areas considered to be involved in the affective component of pain, while with moderate activation catastrophizing was associated with a lack of activation of DLPF, which is thought to be involved in descending modulation of pain. *ACC* Anterior cingulate cortex; *DLPF* dorsolateral prefrontal cortex. Talairach coordinates shown (from Seminowicz and Davis (2006), used with permission)

catastrophizing was found to be correlated with brain activation patterns during both mild stimulation, with catastrophizers showing higher activity in brain regions related to vigilance and attention; and intense stimulation – where catastrophizers showed an impaired ability to activate areas of the brain responsible for descending modulation of pain (Fig. 27.2). The third and most recent study (Lu et al. 2010) used 3T-fMRI to examine the effects of pain catastrophizing on placebo analgesia in health volunteers undergoing lab-based esophageal pain stimulation. This study found no evidence of a relationship between pain catastrophizing and the activation of brain regions related to placebo effects. Taken together, the results of these studies provide some initial support for the notion that catastrophizing may be related to patterns of brain activation during pain stimulation.

Clinical observations suggest that a variety of cognitive behaviors can influence pain. For example, individuals having chronic pain often report that thinking about or imagining themselves engaged in a painful movement can increase their pain. Similarly, Gustin et al. (2008) found that persons with a complete spinal cord injury who were unable to physically move their ankle, reported increased pain when asked to imagine making movements of the ankle. More recently, these investigators (Gustin et al. 2010) conducted an fMRI study to examine the neural correlates of pain evoked by such movement imagery. A sample of 11 patients with complete thoracic level spinal cord injury and neuropathic pain experienced below the level of their injury and 19 controls were given 7 days of movement imagery training in which they were asked to imagine right ankle flexion and dorsiflexion movements 3 times daily for 8 min while listening to a recording of a car accelerator respectively accelerating and decelerating. All participants then underwent fMRI while imagining the ankle movements. Nine of the eleven patients reported increased pain with the imagined movements. During the movement imagery, both the patients and the controls showed increased activity in the supplementary motor area and cerebral cortex. However, the spinal cord injury patients showed significantly greater activity in perigenual anterior cingulate cortex and right dorsolateral frontal cortex. Interestingly, the level of activation in these areas was correlated with ratings of pain provided during the movement imagery. These findings are intriguing in that they provide evidence that a cognitive task can evoke pain and associated activation of areas of the pain neuromatrix.

Seeking social support from a loved one is one of the most common ways that people can cope with pain. Younger et al. (2010) recently used fMRI to examine the effects of viewing pictures of a new romantic partner on experimental pain. A sample of 15 undergraduates, all of whom were within the first 9 months of a romantic relationship, were exposed to moderate and high thermal pain stimulation under three different conditions: (1) while viewing pictures of their romantic partner, (2) while viewing pictures of an equally attractive friend, and (3) while engaged in a word-association task designed to distract them from pain. Results showed that viewing pictures of the romantic partner (but not the friend) decreased pain ratings. The word distraction task, which involved silently thinking of as many word associations that they could, also reduced pain ratings. Analysis of the fMRI data suggested that the mechanisms for pain relief differed for the viewing romantic partner vs. the distraction task. Specifically, viewing pictures of the romantic partner led to increased activation of areas of the brain involved in the reward system (i.e., head of the caudate, nucleus accumbens, lateral OFC, amygdala, and DLPFC) whereas the distraction task did not increase activity in these areas. These findings suggest that the pain relief that comes from viewing pictures of a new romantic partner can produce reductions in pain by activating reward systems. Future studies should examine whether thinking of a loved one or a romantic partner with whom one has been in a long-term relationship may foster pain relief through similar mechanisms, though as the authors point out more complex motivational, evaluative, emotional, and memory processes may be involved in such a case.

Pain Imaging in Patients

While pain neuroimaging over the last 2 decades has given us a general understanding of pain-related brain activity, one of the great challenges in the field is to understand how the central nervous system gets restructured as a result of suffering from chronic pain. Here, we focus on four areas of research which have addressed this issue.

Structural Analysis (T1, DTI)

Probably the most frequently reported neuroimaging studies comparing people with chronic pain and healthy controls is structural MRI, gray matter differences (VBM) or CTA. While the brain regions involved are somewhat variable, overwhelmingly, the results of these many studies indicate gray matter density loss in multiple brain areas is a common consequence of chronic pain (see reviews by May (2008) and Schweinhardt et al. (2008)); in particular, these studies implicate the cingulate and insular cortices, as well as prefrontal and parietal regions. Studies have also reported that decreased gray matter density or cortical thickness in patients is reversible with effective treatment (Gwilym et al. 2010; Rodriguez-Raecke et al. 2009; Seminowicz et al. 2010). A longitudinal study in a rat model of neuropathic pain reported prefrontal cortical volume decreases several months after the injury, and this morphometric change coincided with the onset of anxiety-like behaviors (Seminowicz et al. 2009). Thus, the evidence indicates that chronic pain causes brain atrophy, and that relief from chronic pain can restore normal brain anatomy. Furthermore, affective changes associated with chronic pain are likely partly responsible for these brain changes.

A few studies to date have examined the structural connectivity changes with DTI. Geha et al. (2008a) reported aberrant connectivity patterns from the anterior insular cortex in people with chronic regional pain syndrome compared to healthy controls, as mentioned in section "Diffusion Tensor Imaging." Other groups have shown altered white matter tracts in migraine (Moulton et al. 2011), CPSP (Seghier et al. 2005), and fibromyalgia (Lutz et al. 2008; Sundgren et al. 2007). This technique seems particularly helpful when used in combination with fMRI or VBM, where one can show a relationship between abnormal structure or function, and connections to or from that region.

Resting State fMRI

In resting state fMRI, subjects are usually asked to lie awake and relaxed in the scanner, with eyes open or closed. This technique is useful for assessing functional networks in the resting brain, i.e., without any task imposed. Several resting state networks have been identified, including a sensorimotor network (Biswal et al. 1995), a default mode network (DMN; Greicius et al. 2003; Raichle et al. 2001), which is a set of regions normally deactivated during task execution (i.e., areas that are active at rest), and several others (De Luca et al. 2005).

Two anti-correlate networks were identified by Fox et al. (2005), and called the task-positive network, which resembles the set of regions normally activated by performance of a cognitively demanding task, and a task-negative network, which resembles the DMN. Seminowicz and Davis (2007) reported that this task-positive network could be enhanced in healthy individuals when pain was evoked with electrical nerve stimulation, suggesting that pain acts as an additional cognitive load (Fig. 27.3). Patients with chronic low back pain have reduced deactivations in task-negative areas (Baliki et al. 2008), suggesting that these areas might be less active at rest, perhaps because of hyperactivity of task-positive regions. Mantini et al. (2009) supported these findings, reporting that in healthy individuals pain evoked with electrical nerve stimulation led to reduced DMN activity. Thus, chronic and experimental pain can modulate brain activity at rest, and this effect might be explained by the effects of pain on cognitive networks.

Other studies have reported altered resting state activity in chronic pain conditions, including changes in spatial networks (Cauda et al. 2009, 2010; Napadow et al. 2010; Tagliazucchi et al. 2010), and in the temporal (frequency) aspects (Malinen et al. 2010). One of the great advantages of resting state fMRI is that many different networks – cognitive, salience (Seeley et al. 2007; Taylor et al. 2009), or sensorimotor – can be interrogated from a single dataset. Data sharing projects now let researchers access tens of thousands of resting state scans from different settings, and this will allow for comparisons of resting state networks in many different disorders.

Effect of Cognitive Behavioral Therapy

Although cognitive behavioral therapy (CBT) interventions have been used in the management of persistent pain for some time (see also Donovan et al. 2011), relatively little attention has been given to the mechanisms by which CBT achieves pain relief. To our knowledge, only one published study has examined the effects of a CBT protocol on patterns of brain activation during a painful inducing task (rectal balloon distension) (Lackner et al. 2006). In this study, the responses of six irritable bowel syndrome patients who had undergone CBT were compared to that of five healthy controls.

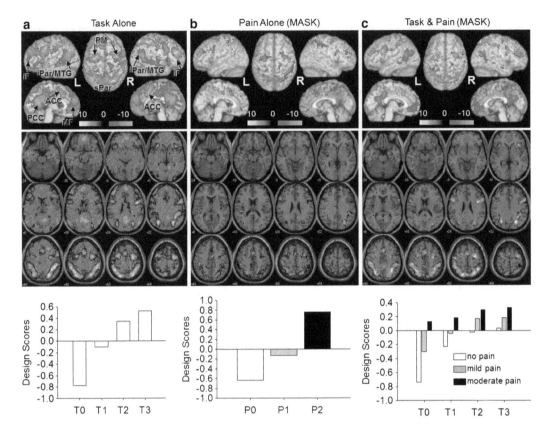

Fig. 27.3 Pain and cognitive load activate an intrinsic task-negative/task-positive network. An attention-specific network was identified in a partial least squares analysis with four levels of cognitive demand in a pain-free state and displayed as a covariance map. (**a**) Design scores (*bottom*) indicate how the covariance pattern was represented by each condition. For example, for T0 (minimal cognitive load), the design score value was negative, so *blue areas* covary positively with this task and *red areas* covary negatively with the task and with the *blue areas*; T3 (maximum cognitive load) covaried most strongly with the task-positive network (*red*) and negatively with the task-negative network (*blue*). From this spatial pattern of activity, a mask was created, including only those voxels that were significantly associated with the design. (**b**) Conditions with no, mild, and moderate pain during the control task (T0) were included in the analysis in which the mask was applied to limit the areas to the task-positive and -negative networks. The design scores (*bottom*) indicate that as pain increases, activity in the task-positive network also increases (with one difference: bilateral SII/posterior insula are included in the task-positive here, whereas those regions were part of the task-negative network identified using only task conditions). Thus pain alone activates the task-positive network. (**c**) All pain and task conditions. The results indicate that task difficulty is associated with increased activity of the task-positive network and reduced activity in the task-negative network, and pain further activates the task-positive network, and suppresses the task-negative network. *iF* Middle/inferior frontal; *iPar/MTG* inferior parietal/middle temporal gyrus; *ACC* anterior cingulate cortex; *PM* premotor cortex; *MF* medial frontal; *PCC* precuneus/posterior cingulate cortex; *sPar* superior parietal (from Seminowicz and Davis (2007) (*Journal of Neurophysiology*), Am. Physiol. Soc., used with permission)

All patients in the study underwent an imaging session before and after completing a 10-week CBT protocol which included training in several coping skills such as self-monitoring, cognitive reappraisal of pain, strategies for controlling worry, and problem solving. Data analyses showed that, after completing CBT, patients had reductions in neural activity in the parahippocampal gyrus and inferior portion of the right cingulate cortex when compared to both their pretreatment responses and the responses of healthy controls. Interestingly, the magnitude of change in these neural responses was found to be significantly correlated with reductions in a number of gastrointestinal symptoms including pain, as well as reductions in anxiety. The authors concluded that changes in the activation of brain structures, involved in attention and emotion regulation, may represent one mechanism by which CBT achieves its effects on pain and other symptoms of irritable bowel syndrome. Naylor et al. (manuscripts submitted for publication) studied the effects of CBT on brain function and structure in patients with chronic musculoskeletal pain. After 11 weeks of CBT patients showed increased activity in the insula, reduced activity in the amygdala and frontal areas associated with emotional processes of pain. This activity was correlated with subjective measures of pain and coping. In this study Naylor et al. also assessed the neuroplasticity of gray matter atrophy previously reported in patients with chronic musculoskeletal pain. CBT was associated with increased gray matter volume (GMV) in DLPFC and aACC. The post-CBT increase in gray matter volume was correlated with a decrease of pain catastrophizing (Naylor et al).

Given the interest in the neural correlates of CBT treatments for emotional disorders (e.g., panic disorder) (de Carvalho et al. 2010), the relative lack of studies of CBT for pain relief is surprising. This is clearly an important direction for future research.

Effects of Placebo

Interest in the neural correlates of placebo analgesia has been high (see also Pollo and Benedetti 2011). A number of studies support the notion that placebo analgesia is related to activation of the brain regions involved in endogenous opioid pain modulation (Bingel et al. 2006; Petrovic et al. 2010; Wager et al. 2004; Zubieta et al. 2005) – the same regions involved in opioid analgesia.

An interesting possibility is that placebo analgesia not only affects pain processing at the level of the brain but also at the level of the spinal cord. Eippert et al. (2009) used fMRI imaging of the cervical spinal cord to test this possibility. Administration of a placebo agent, which reduced ratings of thermal pain by 26%, what posterior parietal cortex, left DLPFC found to be associated with a significant reduction in BOLD responses at the ipsilateral dorsal horn of the spinal cord. These results are consistent with the notion that descending pain control systems responsible for placebo analgesia influence the gating of nociceptive input at the level of the spinal cord.

Recently, researchers have been interested in the effects of placebo conditioning trials on the effects of placebo analgesia. In placebo conditioning trials, patients are provided with repeated exposures to a placebo (e.g., a placebo cream applied to an area of pain stimulation) and this is matched with intentionally lowered level of pain stimulation to increase patients' expectations of placebo analgesia. Watson et al. (2009) studied the effects of placebo conditioning on brain activity occurring in response to a laser pain stimulus. Participants, 11 healthy individuals, underwent brain imaging before, during, and after the placebo conditioning trials as well as administration of the placebo analgesia. Data were collected during both anticipation of pain stimulation and during pain stimulation. Anticipation of pain stimulation was associated with activation of the left DLPFC, medial frontal cortex, and anterior mid-cingulate cortex for both the placebo conditioning and placebo administration conditions. Delivery of pain stimulation was associated with activation of the anterior MCC and posterior cingulate. The authors suggest that their findings support the notion that placebo conditioning produces activations in prefrontal and mid-cingulate cortices which persist during placebo analgesia.

Investigators have examined the possibility that there may be differences in the mechanisms underpinning opioid analgesia and endogenous opioid analgesia. Petrovic et al. (2010) argued that during administration of opioids, patients' expectations that they will obtain effective pain relief are met and are matched with corresponding changes in the processing of nociceptive input. This contrasts with a placebo condition during which patients' expectations for effective pain relief are not necessarily matched by corresponding changes in the processing of nociceptive input. Given prior findings that prefrontal mechanisms are involved in expectation processes and the matching of expectations with sensory input, Petrovic et al. (2010) hypothesized that these regions might be more active in placebo analgesia vs. opioid analgesia. To test this possibility, they reanalyzed data from an fMRI study contrasting opioid analgesia and placebo analgesia. Their findings indicated that, when compared to opioid analgesia, placebo analgesia was associated with substantial increases in activity in prefrontal areas (specifically, the lateral OFC and ventrolateral PFC). A connectivity analysis showed that activation of these prefrontal regions covaried with activation of the right ACC. The authors concluded that the mechanism of placebo analgesia is distinct from opioid analgesia in that it involves greater activation in prefrontal brain areas related to the processing of how expectations fit with sensory input.

Future Directions

We demonstrated in this chapter that there is considerable overlap among brain regions participating in processing of pain, cognition and emotions, including ACC, insula, amygdala, thalamus and PFC. A challenge for future research will be to unravel the mechanisms through which complex mental activities, such as cognitive behaviors (expectations, attention, distraction, catastrophizing) and emotions are able to influence brain functions and structures. As placebo analgesia is embedded in pain treatment, studying placebo effects on pain intensity and brain function would bring better understanding of how placebo analgesia can be used in clinical treatments. There is a clear need for additional studies of neural correlates of CBT treatments for pain and recent studies of the effects of CBT for emotional disorders could have implications for this research. Furthermore, more studies are needed to understand not only cortical processes but also involvement of white matter tracts in development of chronic pain and its response to psychosocial interventions and medications. Finally, we need to address long-term efficacy of psychological interventions for pain and their neural correlates.

References

Abrahamsen, R., Dietz, M., Lodahl, S., Roepstorff, A., Zachariae, R., Østergaard, L., & Svensson, P. (2010). Effect of hypnotic pain modulation on brain activity in patients with temporomandibular disorder pain. *Pain, 151*(3), 825–833.

Apkarian, A., Bushnell, M., Treede, R., & Zubieta, J. (2005). Human brain mechanisms of pain perception and regulation in health and disease. *European Journal of Pain, 9*, 463–484.

Apkarian, A., Sosa, Y., Sonty, S., Levy, R., Harden, R., Parrish, T., & Gitelman, D. (2004). Chronic back pain is associated with decreased prefrontal and thalamic gray matter density. *The Journal of Neuroscience, 24*, 10410–10415.

Apkarian, A. V., Thomas, P. S., Krauss, B. R., & Szeverenyi, N. M. (2001). Prefrontal cortical hyperactivity in patients with sympathetically mediated chronic pain. *Neuroscience Letters, 311*, 193–197.

Ashburner, J., & Friston, K. (2000). Voxel-based morphometry – The methods. *NeuroImage, 11*, 805–821.

Babiloni, C., Brancucci, A., Babiloni, F., Capotosto, P., Carducci, F., Cincotti, F., Arendt-Nielsen, L., Chen, A. C., & Rossini, P. M. (2003). Anticipatory cortical responses during the expectancy of a predictable painful stimulation. A high-resolution electroencephalography study. *The European Journal of Neuroscience, 18*, 1692–1700.

Babiloni, C., Capotosto, P., Brancucci, A., Del Percio, C., Petrini, L., Buttiglione, M., Cibelli, G., Romani, G. L., Rossini, P. M., & Arendt-Nielsen, L. (2008). Cortical alpha rhythms are related to the anticipation of sensorimotor interaction between painful stimuli and movements: A high-resolution EEG study. *The Journal of Pain, 9*, 902–911.

Baliki, M. N., Geha, P. Y., & Apkarian, A. V. (2009). Parsing pain perception between nociceptive representation and magnitude estimation. *Journal of Neurophysiology, 101*, 875–887.

Baliki, M., Geha, P., Apkarian, A., & Chialvo, D. (2008). Beyond feeling: Chronic pain hurts the brain, disrupting the default-mode network dynamics. *The Journal of Neuroscience, 28*, 1398–1403.

Baliki, M. N., Geha, P. Y., Fields, H. L., & Apkarian, A. V. (2010). Predicting value of pain and analgesia: Nucleus accumbens response to noxious stimuli changes in the presence of chronic pain. *Neuron, 66*, 149–160.

Baliki, M., Katz, J., Chialvo, D. R., & Apkarian, A. V. (2005). Single subject pharmacological-MRI (phMRI) study: Modulation of brain activity of psoriatic arthritis pain by cyclooxygenase-2 inhibitor. *Molecular Pain, 1*, 32.

Barber, J. E. (1996). *Hypnosis and suggestion in the treatment of pain: A clinical guide.* New York, NY: WW Norton.

Bencherif, B., Fuchs, P. N., Sheth, R., Dannals, R. F., Campbell, J. N., & Frost, J. J. (2002). Pain activation of human supraspinal opioid pathways as demonstrated by [11C]-carfentanil and positron emission tomography (PET). *Pain, 99*, 589–598.

Bingel, U., Glascher, J., Weiller, C., & Buchel, C. (2004). Somatotopic representation of nociceptive information in the putamen: An event-related fMRI study. *Cerebral Cortex, 14*, 1340–1345.

Bingel, U., Lorenz, J., Schoell, E., Weiller, C., & Büchel, C. (2006). Mechanisms of placebo analgesia: rACC recruitment of a subcortical antinociceptive network. *Pain, 120*, 8–15.

Biswal, B., Yetkin, F. Z., Haughton, V. M., & Hyde, J. S. (1995). Functional connectivity in the motor cortex of resting human brain using echo-planar MRI. *Magnetic Resonance in Medicine, 34*, 537–541.

Boord, P. R., Rennie, C. J., & Williams, L. M. (2007). Integrating "brain" and "body" measures: Correlations between EEG and metabolic changes over the human lifespan. *Journal of Integrative Neuroscience, 6*, 205–218.

Bornhovd, K., Quante, M., Glauche, V., Bromm, B., Weiller, C., & Buchel, C. (2002). Painful stimuli evoke different stimulus-response functions in the amygdala, prefrontal, insula and somatosensory cortex: A single-trial fMRI study. *Brain, 125*, 1326–1336.

Brooks, J., Zambeanu, L., Godinez, A., Craig, A., & Tracey, I. (2005). Somatotopic organisation of the human insula to painful heat studied with high resolution functional imaging. *NeuroImage, 27*, 201–209.

Brown, C. A., & Jones, A. K. (2010). Meditation experience predicts less negative appraisal of pain: Electrophysiological evidence for the involvement of anticipatory neural responses. *Pain, 150*, 428–438.

Buchgreitz, L., Egsgaard, L. L., Jensen, R., Arendt-Nielsen, L., & Bendtsen, L. (2008). Abnormal pain processing in chronic tension-type headache: A high-density EEG brain mapping study. *Brain, 131*, 3232–3238.

Bushnell, M., Duncan, G., Hofbauer, R., Ha, B., Chen, J.-I., & Carrier, B. (1999). Pain perception: Is there a role for primary somatosensory cortex? *Proceedings of the National Academy of Sciences of the United States of America, 96*, 7705–7709.

Cauda, F., D'Agata, F., Sacco, K., Duca, S., Cocito, D., Paolasso, I., Isoardo, G., & Geminiani, G. (2010). Altered resting state attentional networks in diabetic neuropathic pain. *Journal of Neurology, Neurosurgery, and Psychiatry, 81*, 806–811.

Cauda, F., Sacco, K., D'Agata, F., Duca, S., Cocito, D., Geminiani, G., Migliorati, F., & Isoardo, G. (2009). Low-frequency BOLD fluctuations demonstrate altered thalamocortical connectivity in diabetic neuropathic pain. *BMC Neuroscience, 10*, 138.

Christensen, J., & Fatchett, D. (2002). Promoting parental use of distraction and relaxation in pediatric oncology patients during invasive procedures. *Journal of Pediatric Oncology Nursing, 19*, 127.

Coghill, R., McHaffie, J., & Yen, Y. (2003). Neural correlates of interindividual differences in the subjective experience of pain. *Proceedings of the National Academy of Sciences of the United States of America, 100*, 8538–8542.

Coghill, R., Sang, C., Maisog, J., & Iadarola, M. (1999). Pain intensity processing within the human brain: A bilateral, distributed mechanism. *Journal of Neurophysiology, 82*, 1934–1943.

Craig, A. D. (2003). Pain mechanisms: Labeled lines versus convergence in central processing. *Annual Review of Neuroscience, 26*, 1–30.

Craig, A. D. (2009). How do you feel – Now? The anterior insula and human awareness. *Nature Reviews. Neuroscience, 10*, 59–70.

Crawford, H. J., Gur, R. C., Skolnick, B., Gur, R. E., & Benson, D. M. (1993). Effects of hypnosis on regional cerebral blood flow during ischemic pain with and without suggested hypnotic analgesia. *International Journal of Psychophysiology, 15*, 181–195.

Crombez, G., Vlaeyen, J. W. S., Heuts, P. H. T. G., & Lysens, R. (1999). Pain-related fear is more disabling than pain itself: Evidence on the role of pain-related fear in chronic back pain disability. *Pain, 80*, 329–339.

Danziger, N., Faillenot, I., & Peyron, R. (2009). Can we share a pain we never felt? Neural correlates of empathy in patients with congenital insensitivity to pain. *Neuron, 61*, 203–212.

Davis, K. D., Pope, G., Chen, J., Kwan, C. L., Crawley, A. P., & Diamant, N. E. (2008). Cortical thinning in IBS: Implications for homeostatic, attention and pain processing. *Neurology, 70*, 153–154.

Davis, K. D., Pope, G. E., Crawley, A. P., & Mikulis, D. J. (2002). Neural correlates of prickle sensation: A percept-related fMRI study. *Nature Neuroscience, 5*, 1121–1122.

Davis, K. D., Pope, G. E., Crawley, A. P., & Mikulis, D. J. (2004). Perceptual illusion of "paradoxical heat" engages the insular cortex. *Journal of Neurophysiology, 92*, 1248–1251.

Davis, K., Taylor, S., Crawley, A., Wood, M., & David, J. (1997). Functional MRI of pain- and attention-related activations in the human cingulate cortex. *Journal of Neurophysiology, 77*, 3370–3380.

Davis, K., Wood, M., Crawley, A., & Mikulis, D. (1995). fMRI of human somatosensory and cingulate cortex during painful electrical nerve stimulation. *Neuroreport, 7*, 321–325.

de Carvalho, M. R., Rozenthal, M., & Nardi, A. E. (2010). The fear circuitry in panic disorder and its modulation by cognitive-behaviour therapy interventions. *The World Journal of Biological Psychiatry, 11*, 188–198.

De Luca, M., Smith, S., De, S. N., Federico, A., & Matthews, P. M. (2005). Blood oxygenation level dependent contrast resting state networks are relevant to functional activity in the neocortical sensorimotor system. *Experimental Brain Research, 167*, 587–594.

Del Percio, C., Le Pera, D., Arendt-Nielsen, L., Babiloni, C., Brancucci, A., Chen, A. C., De Armas, L., Miliucci, R., Restuccia, D., Valeriani, M., & Rossini, P. M. (2006). Distraction affects frontal alpha rhythms related to expectancy of pain: An EEG study. *NeuroImage, 31*, 1268–1277.

Derbyshire, S. W. G., Whalley, M. G., Stenger, V. A., & Oakley, D. A. (2004). Cerebral activation during hypnotically induced and imagined pain. *NeuroImage, 23*, 392–401.

Diers, M., Koeppe, C., Diesch, E., Stolle, A. M., Holzl, R., Schiltenwolf, M., van Ackern, K., & Flor, H. (2007). Central processing of acute muscle pain in chronic low back pain patients: An EEG mapping study. *Journal of Clinical Neurophysiology, 24*, 76–83.

Dinges, D. F., Whitehouse, W. G., Orne, E. C., Bloom, P. B., Carlin, M. M., Bauer, N. K., Gillen, K. A., Shapiro, B. S., Ohene-Frempong, K., & Dampier, C. (1997). Self-hypnosis training as an adjunctive treatment in the management of pain associated with sickle cell disease. *The International Journal of Clinical and Experimental Hypnosis, 45*, 417–432.

Donovan, K. A., Thompson, L. M. A., & Jacobsen, P. B. (2011). Pain, depression and anxiety in cancer. In R. J. Moore (Ed.), *Handbook of pain and palliative care*. New York, NY: Springer.

Dougherty, D. D., Kong, J., Webb, M., Bonab, A. A., Fischman, A. J., & Gollub, R. L. (2008). A combined [11C] diprenorphine PET study and fMRI study of acupuncture analgesia. *Behavioural Brain Research, 193*, 63–68.

Dowman, R., Rissacher, D., & Schuckers, S. (2008). EEG indices of tonic pain-related activity in the somatosensory cortices. *Clinical Neurophysiology, 119*, 1201–1212.

Downar, J., Mikulis, D. J., & Davis, K. D. (2003). Neural correlates of the prolonged salience of painful stimulation. *NeuroImage, 20*, 1540–1551.

Eickhoff, S. B., Amunts, K., Mohlberg, H., & Zilles, K. (2006a). The human parietal operculum. II. Stereotaxic maps and correlation with functional imaging results. *Cerebral Cortex, 16*, 268–279.

Eickhoff, S. B., Schleicher, A., Zilles, K., & Amunts, K. (2006b). The human parietal operculum. I. Cytoarchitectonic mapping of subdivisions. *Cerebral Cortex, 16*, 254–267.

Eippert, F., Finterbusch, B., Bingel, U., & Buchel, C. (2009). Direct evidence for spinal cord involvement in placebo analgesia. *Science, 326*, 404.

Elkins, G., Marcus, J., Palamara, L., & Stearns, V. (2004). Can hypnosis reduce hot flashes in breast cancer survivors? A literature review. *The American Journal of Clinical Hypnosis, 47*, 29.

Farrell, M. J., Laird, A. R., & Egan, G. F. (2005). Brain activity associated with painfully hot stimuli applied to the upper limb: A meta-analysis. *Human Brain Mapping, 25*, 129–139.

Fishbain, D. A. (2002). The pain-depression relationship. *Psychosomatics, 43*, 341.

Fishbain, D., Cutler, R., Rosomoff, H., & Rosomoff, R. (1997). Chronic pain-associated depression: Antecedent or consequence of chronic pain? A review. *The Clinical Journal of Pain, 13*, 116–137.

Fox, M. D., Snyder, A. Z., Vincent, J. L., Corbetta, M., Van Essen, D. C., & Raichle, M. E. (2005). The human brain is intrinsically organized into dynamic, anticorrelated functional networks. *Proceedings of the National Academy of Sciences of the United States of America, 102*, 9673–9678.

Garcia-Larrea, L., Frot, M., & Valeriani, M. (2003). Brain generators of laser-evoked potentials: From dipoles to functional significance. *Neurophysiologie Clinique, 33*, 279–292.

Garcia-Larrea, L., Perchet, C., Creac'h, C., Convers, P., Peyron, R., Laurent, B., Mauguiere, F., & Magnin, M. (2010). Operculo-insular pain (parasylvian pain): A distinct central pain syndrome. *Brain, 133*, 2528–2539.

Gay, M. C., Philippot, P., & Luminet, O. (2002). Differential effectiveness of psychological interventions for reducing osteoarthritis pain: A comparison of Erickson hypnosis and Jacobson relaxation. *European Journal of Pain, 6*, 1–16.

Geha, P., Baliki, M., Harden, R., Bauer, W., Parrish, T., & Apkarian, A. (2008). The brain in chronic CRPS pain: Abnormal gray-white matter interactions in emotional and autonomic regions. *Neuron, 60*, 570–581.

Giesecke, T., Gracely, R. H., Grant, M. A., Nachemson, A., Petzke, F., Williams, D. A., & Clauw, D. J. (2004). Evidence of augmented central pain processing in idiopathic chronic low back pain. *Arthritis and Rheumatism, 50*, 613–623.

Giesecke, T., Gracely, R. H., Williams, D. A., Geisser, M. E., Petzke, F. W., & Clauw, D. J. (2005). The relationship between depression, clinical pain, and experimental pain in a chronic pain cohort. *Arthritis and Rheumatism, 52*, 1577–1584.

Gracely, R., Geisser, M., Giesecke, T., Grant, M., Petzke, F., Williams, D., & Clauw, D. (2004). Pain catastrophizing and neural responses to pain among persons with fibromyalgia. *Brain: A Journal of Neurology, 127*, 835–843.

Gracely, R., Petzke, F., Wolf, J., & Clauw, D. (2002). Functional magnetic resonance imaging evidence of augmented pain processing in fibromyalgia. *Arthritis and Rheumatism, 46*, 1333–1343.

Grachev, I. D., Fredrickson, B. E., & Apkarian, A. V. (2000). Abnormal brain chemistry in chronic back pain: An in vivo proton magnetic resonance spectroscopy study. *Pain, 89*, 7–18.

Greenspan, J. D., Lee, R. R., & Lenz, F. A. (1999). Pain sensitivity alterations as a function of lesion location in the parasylvian cortex. *Pain, 81*, 273–282.

Greicius, M. D., Krasnow, B., Reiss, A. L., & Menon, V. (2003). Functional connectivity in the resting brain: A network analysis of the default mode hypothesis. *Proceedings of the National Academy of Sciences of the United States of America, 100*, 253–258.

Gustin, S. M., Wrigley, P. J., Gandevia, S. C., Middleton, J. W., Henderson, L. A., & Siddall, P. J. (2008). Movement imagery increases pain in people with neuropathic pain following complete thoracic spinal cord injury. *Pain, 137*, 237–244.

Gustin, S. M., Wrigley, P. J., Henderson, L. A., & Siddall, P. J. (2010). Brain circuitry underlying pain in response to imagined movement in people with spinal cord injury. *Pain, 148*, 438–445.

Gwilym, S. E., Fillipini, N., Douaud, G., Carr, A. J., & Tracey, I. (2010). Thalamic atrophy associated with painful osteoarthritis of the hip is reversible after arthroplasty: A longitudinal voxel-based-morphometric study. *Arthritis and Rheumatism, 62*(10), 2930–2940.

Hadjipavlou, G., Dunckley, P., Behrens, T. E., & Tracey, I. (2006). Determining anatomical connectivities between cortical and brainstem pain processing regions in humans: A diffusion tensor imaging study in healthy controls. *Pain, 123*, 169–178.

Harris, R. E., Sundgren, P. C., Craig, A. D., Kirshenbaum, E., Sen, A., Napadow, V., & Clauw, D. J. (2009). Elevated insular glutamate in fibromyalgia is associated with experimental pain. *Arthritis and Rheumatism, 60*, 3146–3152.

Hauck, M., Lorenz, J., Zimmermann, R., Debener, S., Scharein, E., & Engel, A. K. (2007). Duration of the cue-to-pain delay increases pain intensity: A combined EEG and MEG study. *Experimental Brain Research, 180*, 205–215.

Henderson, L. A., Gandevia, S. C., & Macefield, V. G. (2007). Somatotopic organization of the processing of muscle and cutaneous pain in the left and right insula cortex: A single-trial fMRI study. *Pain, 128*, 20–30.

Henderson, L. A., Rubin, T. K., & Macefield, V. G. (2011). Within-limb somatotopic representation of acute muscle pain in the human contralateral dorsal posterior insula. *Human Brain Mapping, 32*(10), 1592–1601.

Hess, A., Axmann, R., Rech, J., Finzel, S., Heindl, C., Kreitz, S., Sergeeva, M., Saake, M., Garcia, M., Kollias, G., Straub, R. H., Sporns, O., Doerfler, A., Brune, K., & Schett, G. (2011). Blockade of TNF-alpha rapidly inhibits pain responses in the central nervous system. *Proceedings of the National Academy of Sciences of the United States of America, 108*, 3731–3736.

Hoffman, H. G., Richards, T. L., Van Oostrom, T., Coda, B. A., Jensen, M. P., Blough, D. K., & Sharar, S. R. (2007). The analgesic effects of opioids and immersive virtual reality distraction: Evidence from subjective and functional brain imaging assessments. *Anesthesia and Analgesia, 105*, 1776.

Hsieh, J. C., Belfrage, M., Stone-Elander, S., Hansson, P., & Ingvar, M. (1995). Central representation of chronic ongoing neuropathic pain studied by positron emission tomography. *Pain, 63*, 225–236.

Iannetti, G. D., Hughes, N. P., Lee, M. C., & Mouraux, A. (2008). Determinants of laser-evoked EEG responses: Pain perception or stimulus saliency? *Journal of Neurophysiology, 100*, 815–828.

Isnard, J., Guenot, M., Sindou, M., & Mauguiere, F. (2004). Clinical manifestations of insular lobe seizures: A stereo-electroencephalographic study. *Epilepsia, 45*, 1079–1090.

Jensen, M. P., Hanley, M. A., Engel, J. M., Romano, J. M., Barber, J., Cardenas, D. D., Kraft, G. H., Hoffman, A. J., & Patterson, D. R. (2005). Hypnotic analgesia for chronic pain in persons with disabilities: A case series abstract. *The International Journal of Clinical and Experimental Hypnosis, 53*, 198–228.

Johansen-Berg, H., & Behrens, T. E. (2006). Just pretty pictures? What diffusion tractography can add in clinical neuroscience. *Current Opinion in Neurology, 19*, 379–385.

Johansen-Berg, H., & Rushworth, M. F. (2009). Using diffusion imaging to study human connectional anatomy. *Annual Review of Neuroscience, 32*, 75–94.

Jones, A. K., Watabe, H., Cunningham, V. J., & Jones, T. (2004). Cerebral decreases in opioid receptor binding in patients with central neuropathic pain measured by [11C]diprenorphine binding and PET. *European Journal of Pain, 8*, 479–485.

Kakigi, R., Inui, K., & Tamura, Y. (2005). Electrophysiological studies on human pain perception. *Clinical Neurophysiology, 116*, 743–763.

Keefe, F. J., Abernethy, A. P., Wheeler, J. L., & Somers, T. J. (2010). Psychological interventions for cancer pain. In E. Bruera, R. K. Portenoy, & E. Corporation (Eds.), *Cancer pain: Assessment and management*. New York, NY: Cambridge University Press.

Kishima, H., Saitoh, Y., Oshino, S., Hosomi, K., Ali, M., Maruo, T., Hirata, M., Goto, T., Yanagisawa, T., Sumitani, M., Osaki, Y., Hatazawa, J., & Yoshimine, T. (2010). Modulation of neuronal activity after spinal cord stimulation for neuropathic pain; H(2)15O PET study. *NeuroImage, 49*, 2564–2569.

Klimesch, W., Sauseng, P., & Hanslmayr, S. (2007). EEG alpha oscillations: The inhibition-timing hypothesis. *Brain Research Reviews, 53*, 63–88.

Kulkarni, B., Bentley, D. E., Elliott, R., Julyan, P. J., Boger, E., Watson, A., Boyle, Y., El-Deredy, W., & Jones, A. K. (2007). Arthritic pain is processed in brain areas concerned with emotions and fear. *Arthritis and Rheumatism, 56*, 1345–1354.

Kulkarni, B., Bentley, D. E., Elliott, R., Youell, P., Watson, A., Derbyshire, S. W. G., Frackowiak, R. S. J., Friston, K. J., & Jones, A. K. P. (2005). Attention to pain localization and unpleasantness discriminates the functions of the medial and lateral pain systems. *The European Journal of Neuroscience, 21*, 3133–3142.

Kupers, R., Frokjaer, V. G., Erritzoe, D., Naert, A., Budtz-Joergensen, E., Nielsen, F. A., Kehlet, H., & Knudsen, G. M. (2010). Serotonin transporter binding in the hypothalamus correlates negatively with tonic heat pain ratings in healthy subjects: A [11C]DASB PET study. *NeuroImage, 54*, 1336–1343.

Kupers, R., Frokjaer, V. G., Naert, A., Christensen, R., Budtz-Joergensen, E., Kehlet, H., & Knudsen, G. M. (2009). A PET [18F]altanserin study of 5-HT2A receptor binding in the human brain and responses to painful heat stimulation. *NeuroImage, 44*, 1001–1007.

Lackner, J., Coad, M., Mertz, H., Wack, D., Katz, L., Krasner, S., Firth, R., Mahl, T., & Lockwood, A. (2006). Cognitive therapy for irritable bowel syndrome is associated with reduced limbic activity, GI symptoms, and anxiety. *Behaviour Research and Therapy, 44*, 621–638.

Lamm, C., Decety, J., & Singer, T. (2011). Meta-analytic evidence for common and distinct neural networks associated with directly experienced pain and empathy for pain. *NeuroImage, 54*(3), 2492–2502.

Lang, P., Bradley, M., & Cuthbert, B. (1998). Emotion and motivation: Measuring affective perception. *Journal of Clinical Neurophysiology, 15*, 397–408.

Leibovici, V., Magora, F., Cohen, S., & Ingber, A. (2009). Effects of virtual reality immersion and audiovisual distraction techniques for patients with pruritus. *Pain Research & Management: The Journal of the Canadian Pain Society, 14*, 283.

Lu, H. C., Hsieh, J. C., Lu, C. L., Niddam, D. M., Wu, Y. T., & Yeh, T. C. (2010). Neuronal correlates in the modulation of placebo analgesia in experimentally-induced esophageal pain: A 3T-fMRI study. *Pain, 148*, 75–83.

Lutz, J., Jager, L., de, Q. D., Krauseneck, T., Padberg, F., Wichnalek, M., Beyer, A., Stahl, R., Zirngibl, B., Morhard, D., Reiser, M., & Schelling, G. (2008). White and gray matter abnormalities in the brain of patients with fibromyalgia: A diffusion-tensor and volumetric imaging study. *Arthritis and Rheumatism, 58*, 3960–3969.

Magis, D., Bruno, M. A., Fumal, A., Gerardy, P. Y., Hustinx, R., Laureys, S., & Schoenen, J. (2011). Central modulation in cluster headache patients treated with occipital nerve stimulation: An FDG-PET study. *BMC Neurology, 11*, 25.

Malinen, S., Vartiainen, N., Hlushchuk, Y., Koskinen, M., Ramkumar, P., Forss, N., Kalso, E., & Hari, R. (2010). Aberrant temporal and spatial brain activity during rest in patients with chronic pain. *Proceedings of the National Academy of Sciences of the United States of America, 107*(14), 6493–6497.

Malloy, K. M., & Milling, L. S. (2010). The effectiveness of virtual reality distraction for pain reduction: A systematic review. *Clinical Psychology Review, 30*(8), 1011–1018.

Mantini, D., Caulo, M., Ferretti, A., Romani, G. L., & Tartaro, A. (2009). Noxious somatosensory stimulation affects the default mode of brain function: Evidence from functional MR imaging. *Radiology, 253*(3), 797–804.

May, A. (2008). Chronic pain may change the structure of the brain. *Pain, 137*, 7–15.

Mazzola, L., Isnard, J., & Mauguiere, F. (2006). Somatosensory and pain responses to stimulation of the second somatosensory area (SII) in humans. A comparison with SI and insular responses. *Cerebral Cortex, 16*, 960–968.

Mazzola, L., Isnard, J., Peyron, R., Guenot, M., & Mauguiere, F. (2009). Somatotopic organization of pain responses to direct electrical stimulation of the human insular cortex. *Pain, 146*, 99–104.

McGeoch, P. D., Williams, L. E., Song, T., Lee, R. R., Huang, M., & Ramachandran, V. S. (2009). Post-stroke tactile allodynia and its modulation by vestibular stimulation: A MEG case study. *Acta Neurologica Scandinavica, 119*, 404–409.

Mee, S., Bunney, B. G., Reist, C., Potkin, S. G., & Bunney, W. E. (2006). Psychological pain: A review of evidence. *Journal of Psychiatric Research, 40*, 680–690.

Melzack, R. (2001). Pain and the neuromatrix in the brain. *Journal of Dental Education, 65*, 1378–1382.

Melzack, R., & Casey, K. L. (1968). Sensory, motivational, and central control determinants of pain: A new conceptual model. In D. R. Kenshalo (Ed.), *The skin senses* (pp. 423–439). Springfield, IL: Chas C. Thomas.

Moulton, E. A., Becerra, L., Maleki, N., Pendse, G., Tully, S., Hargreaves, R., Burstein, R., & Borsook, D. (2011). Painful heat reveals hyperexcitability of the temporal pole in interictal and ictal migraine states. *Cerebral Cortex, 21*(2), 435–448.

Mouraux, A., Diukova, A., Lee, M. C., Wise, R. G., & Iannetti, G. D. (2011). A multisensory investigation of the functional significance of the "pain matrix". *NeuroImage, 54*(3), 2237–2249.

Mueller, C., Klega, A., Buchholz, H. G., Rolke, R., Magerl, W., Schirrmacher, R., Schirrmacher, E., Birklein, F., Treede, R. D., & Schreckenberger, M. (2010). Basal opioid receptor binding is associated with differences in sensory perception in healthy human subjects: A [18F]diprenorphine PET study. *NeuroImage, 49*, 731–737.

Napadow, V., LaCount, L., Park, K., As-Sanie, S., Clauw, D. J., & Harris, R. E. (2010). Intrinsic brain connectivity in fibromyalgia is associated with chronic pain intensity. *Arthritis and Rheumatism, 62*, 2545–2555.

Naylor, M. R., Krauthamer, G. M., Dumas, J. A., Mantegna, J., Filippi, C., Newhouse, P.A. Functional MRI treatment effects of cognitive behavioral therapy in chronic pain. Submitted for publication.

Naylor, M. R., Shpaner, M., Krauthamer, G. M., Mantegna, J., Keaser, M. L., Seminowicz, D. A. Prefrontal anatomical changes after cognitive behavioral therapy in chronic musculoskeletal pain. Submitted for publication.

Ostrowsky, K., Magnin, M., Ryvlin, P., Isnard, J., Guenot, M., & Mauguiere, F. (2002). Representation of pain and somatic sensation in the human insula: A study of responses to direct electrical cortical stimulation. *Cerebral Cortex, 12*, 376–385.

Owen, D. G., Bureau, Y., Thomas, A. W., Prato, F. S., & St Lawrence, K. S. (2008). Quantification of pain-induced changes in cerebral blood flow by perfusion MRI. *Pain, 136*, 85–96.

Owen, D. G., Clarke, C. F., Ganapathy, S., Prato, F. S., & St Lawrence, K. S. (2010). Using perfusion MRI to measure the dynamic changes in neural activation associated with tonic muscular pain. *Pain, 148*, 375–386.

Palomero-Gallagher, N., Mohlberg, H., Zilles, K., & Vogt, B. (2008). Cytology and receptor architecture of human anterior cingulate cortex. *The Journal of Comparative Neurology, 508*, 906–926.

Palomero-Gallagher, N., Vogt, B. A., Schleicher, A., Mayberg, H. S., & Zilles, K. (2009). Receptor architecture of human cingulate cortex: Evaluation of the four-region neurobiological model. *Human Brain Mapping, 30*, 2336–2355.

Perl, E. R. (2007). Ideas about pain, a historical view. *Nature Reviews. Neuroscience, 8*, 71–80.

Petrovic, P., Kalso, E., Petersson, K. M., Andersson, J., Fransson, P., & Ingvar, M. (2010). A prefrontal non-opioid mechanism in placebo analgesia. *Pain, 150*, 59–65.

Peyron, R., Faillenot, I., Mertens, P., Laurent, B., & Garcia-Larrea, L. (2007). Motor cortex stimulation in neuropathic pain. Correlations between analgesic effect and hemodynamic changes in the brain. A PET study. *NeuroImage, 34*, 310–321.

Peyron, R., Frot, M., Schneider, F., Garcia-Larrea, L., Mertens, P., Barral, F. G., Sindou, M., Laurent, B., & Mauguiere, F. (2002). Role of operculoinsular cortices in human pain processing: Converging evidence from PET, fMRI, dipole modeling, and intracerebral recordings of evoked potentials. *NeuroImage, 17*, 1336–1346.

Peyron, R., Laurent, B., & Garcia-Larrea, L. (2000). Functional imaging of brain responses to pain. A review and meta-analysis. *Clinical Neurophysiology, 30*, 263–288.

Ploghaus, A., Nairain, C., Beckmann, C., Clare, S., Bantick, S., Wise, R., Matthews, P., Rawlins, N., & Tracey, I. (2001). Exacerbation of pain by anxiety is associated with activity in a hippocampal network. *The Journal of Neuroscience, 21*, 9896–9903.

Pollo, A., & Benedetti, F. (2011). Pain and the placebo/nocebo effect. In R. J. Moore (Ed.), *Handbook of pain and palliative care*. New York, NY: Springer.

Price, D. D. (2002). Central neural mechanisms that interrelate sensory and affective dimensions of pain. *Molecular Interventions, 2*, 392–403.

Price, D., & Bushnell, M. (2004). *Psychological methods of pain control: Basic science and clinical perspectives* (308 pp). Seattle, WA: IASP Press.

Quante, M., Hille, S., Schofer, M. D., Lorenz, J., & Hauck, M. (2008). Noxious counterirritation in patients with advanced osteoarthritis of the knee reduces MCC but not SII pain generators: A combined use of MEG and EEG. *Journal of Pain Research, 1*, 1–8.

Raichle, M. E., MacLeod, A. M., Snyder, A. Z., Powers, W. J., Gusnard, D. A., & Shulman, G. L. (2001). A default mode of brain function. *Proceedings of the National Academy of Sciences of the United States of America, 98*, 676–682.

Ray, N. J., Jenkinson, N., Kringelbach, M. L., Hansen, P. C., Pereira, E. A., Brittain, J. S., Holland, P., Holliday, I. E., Owen, S., Stein, J., & Aziz, T. (2009). Abnormal thalamocortical dynamics may be altered by deep brain stimulation: Using magnetoencephalography to study phantom limb pain. *Journal of Clinical Neuroscience, 16*, 32–36.

Richter, M., Eck, J., Straube, T., Miltner, W. H. R., & Weiss, T. (2010). Do words hurt? Brain activation during the processing of pain-related words. *Pain, 148*, 198–205.

Rodriguez-Raecke, R., Niemeier, A., Ihle, K., Ruether, W., & May, A. (2009). Brain gray matter decrease in chronic pain is the consequence and not the cause of pain. *The Journal of Neuroscience, 29*, 13746–13750.

Rossini, P. M., Babiloni, C., Babiloni, F., Ambrosini, A., Onorati, P., Carducci, F., & Urbano, A. (1999). "Gating" of human short-latency somatosensory evoked cortical responses during execution of movement. A high resolution electroencephalography study. *Brain Research, 843*, 161–170.

Roy, M., Piché, M., Chen, J. I., Peretz, I., & Rainville, P. (2009). Cerebral and spinal modulation of pain by emotions. *Proceedings of the National Academy of Sciences of the United States of America, 106*, 20900.

Ruben, J., Schwiemann, J., Deuchert, M., Meyer, R., Krause, T., Curio, G., Villringer, K., Kurth, R., & Villringer, A. (2001). Somatotopic organization of human secondary somatosensory cortex. *Cerebral Cortex, 11*, 463–473.

Sarnthein, J., Stern, J., Aufenberg, C., Rousson, V., & Jeanmonod, D. (2006). Increased EEG power and slowed dominant frequency in patients with neurogenic pain. *Brain, 129*, 55–64.

Schmahmann, J. D., & Leifer, D. (1992). Parietal pseudothalamic pain syndrome. Clinical features and anatomic correlates. *Archives of Neurology, 49*, 1032–1037.

Schroeder, C. E., Wilson, D. A., Radman, T., Scharfman, H., & Lakatos, P. (2010). Dynamics of active sensing and perceptual selection. *Current Opinion in Neurobiology, 20*, 172–176.

Schupp, C. J., Berbaum, K., Berbaum, M., & Lang, E. V. (2005). Pain and anxiety during interventional radiologic procedures: Effect of patients' state anxiety at baseline and modulation by nonpharmacologic analgesia adjuncts. *Journal of Vascular and Interventional Radiology, 16*, 1585–1592.

Schweinhardt, P., Kuchinad, A., Pukall, C. F., & Bushnell, M. C. (2008). Increased gray matter density in young women with chronic vulvar pain. *Pain, 140*, 411–419.

Scott, D. J., Heitzeg, M. M., Koeppe, R. A., Stohler, C. S., & Zubieta, J. K. (2006). Variations in the human pain stress experience mediated by ventral and dorsal basal ganglia dopamine activity. *The Journal of Neuroscience, 26*, 10789–10795.

Seeley, W. W., Menon, V., Schatzberg, A. F., Keller, J., Glover, G. H., Kenna, H., Reiss, A. L., & Greicius, M. D. (2007). Dissociable intrinsic connectivity networks for salience processing and executive control. *The Journal of Neuroscience, 27*, 2349–2356.

Seghier, M. L., Lazeyras, F., Vuilleumier, P., Schnider, A., & Carota, A. (2005). Functional magnetic resonance imaging and diffusion tensor imaging in a case of central poststroke pain. *The Journal of Pain, 6*, 208–212.

Seminowicz, D., & Davis, K. (2006). Cortical responses to pain in healthy individuals depends on pain catastrophizing. *Pain, 120*, 297–306.

Seminowicz, D., & Davis, K. (2007). Pain enhances functional connectivity of a brain network evoked by performance of a cognitive task. *Journal of Neurophysiology, 97*, 3651–3659.

Seminowicz, D. A., Laferriere, A. L., Millecamps, M., Yu, J. S. C., Coderre, T. J., & Bushnell, M. C. (2009). MRI structural brain changes associated with sensory and emotional function in a rat model of long-term neuropathic pain. *NeuroImage, 47*, 1007–1014.

Seminowicz, D. A., Wideman, T. H., Naso, L., Hatami-Khoroushahi, Z., Fallatah, S., Ware, M. A., et al. (2010). *Treating chronic low back pain reverses structural brain changes*. In Montreal, Quebec, Canada.

Sprenger, T., Valet, M., Boecker, H., Henriksen, G., Spilker, M. E., Willoch, F., Wagner, K. J., Wester, H. J., & Tolle, T. R. (2006a). Opioidergic activation in the medial pain system after heat pain. *Pain, 122*, 63–67.

Sprenger, T., Willoch, F., Miederer, M., Schindler, F., Valet, M., Berthele, A., Spilker, M. E., Forderreuther, S., Straube, A., Stangier, I., Wester, H. J., & Tolle, T. R. (2006b). Opioidergic changes in the pineal gland and hypothalamus in cluster headache: A ligand PET study. *Neurology, 66*, 1108–1110.

Starr, C. J., Sawaki, L., Wittenberg, G. F., Burdette, J. H., Oshiro, Y., Quevedo, A. S., & Coghill, R. C. (2009). Roles of the insular cortex in the modulation of pain: Insights from brain lesions. *The Journal of Neuroscience, 29*, 2684–2694.

Stern, J., Jeanmonod, D., & Sarnthein, J. (2006). Persistent EEG overactivation in the cortical pain matrix of neurogenic pain patients. *NeuroImage, 31*, 721–731.

Sundgren, P. C., Petrou, M., Harris, R. E., Fan, X., Foerster, B., Mehrotra, N., Sen, A., Clauw, D. J., & Welsh, R. C. (2007). Diffusion-weighted and diffusion tensor imaging in fibromyalgia patients: A prospective study of whole brain diffusivity, apparent diffusion coefficient, and fraction anisotropy in different regions of the brain and correlation with symptom severity. *Academic Radiology, 14*, 839–846.

Tagliazucchi, E., Balenzuela, P., Fraiman, D., & Chialvo, D. R. (2010). Brain resting state is disrupted in chronic back pain patients. *Neuroscience Letters, 485*(1), 26–31.

Talbot, J., Marrett, S., Evans, A., Meyer, E., Bushnell, M., & Duncan, G. (1991). Multiple representations of pain in human cerebral cortex. *Science, 251*, 1355–1358.

Taylor, K. S., Seminowicz, D. A., & Davis, K. D. (2009). Two systems of resting state connectivity between the insula and cingulate cortex. *Human Brain Mapping, 30*, 2731–2745.

Timmermann, L., Ploner, M., Haucke, K., Schmitz, F., Baltissen, R., & Schnitzler, A. (2001). Differential coding of pain intensity in the human primary and secondary somatosensory cortex. *Journal of Neurophysiology, 86*, 1499–1503.

Treede, R. D. (2002). Spinothalamic and thalamocortical nociceptive pathways. *The Journal of Pain, 3*, 109–112.

Treede, R., Kenshalo, D., Gracely, R., & Jones, A. (1999). The cortical representation of pain. *Pain, 79*(2–3), 105–111.

van der Graaf, M. (2010). In vivo magnetic resonance spectroscopy: Basic methodology and clinical applications. *European Biophysics Journal, 39*, 527–540.

Vlaeyen, J., Haazen, I., Schuerman, J., Kole-Snijders, A., & van Eek, H. (1995). Behavioural rehabilitation of chronic low back pain: Comparison of an operant treatment, an operant-cognitive treatment and an operant-respondent treatment. *British Journal of Clinical Psychology, 34*, 95–118.

Vogt, B. A. (2005). Pain and emotion interactions in subregions of the cingulate gyrus. *Nature Reviews. Neuroscience, 6*, 533–544.

Wager, T., Rilling, J., Smith, E., Sokolik, A., Casey, K., Davidson, R., Kosslyn, S., Rose, R., & Cohen, J. (2004). Placebo-induced changes in fMRI in the anticipation and experience of pain. *Science, 303*, 1162–1167.

Wager, T. D., Scott, D. J., & Zubieta, J. K. (2007). Placebo effects on human mu-opioid activity during pain. *Proceedings of the National Academy of Sciences of the United States of America, 104*, 11056–11061.

Wagner, K. J., Sprenger, T., Kochs, E. F., Tolle, T. R., Valet, M., & Willoch, F. (2007). Imaging human cerebral pain modulation by dose-dependent opioid analgesia: A positron emission tomography activation study using remifentanil. *Anesthesiology, 106*, 548–556.

Walton, K. D., Dubois, M., & Llinas, R. R. (2010). Abnormal thalamocortical activity in patients with complex regional pain syndrome (CRPS) type I. *Pain, 150*, 41–51.

Watson, A., El-Deredy, W., Iannetti, G. D., Lloyd, D., Tracey, I., Vogt, B. A., Nadeau, V., & Jones, A. K. P. (2009). Placebo conditioning and placebo analgesia modulate a common brain network during pain anticipation and perception. *Pain, 145*, 24–30.

Willis, W. D., Jr., Zhang, X., Honda, C. N., & Giesler, G. J., Jr. (2002). A critical review of the role of the proposed VMpo nucleus in pain. *The Journal of Pain, 3*, 79–94.

Wise, R. G., Lujan, B. J., Schweinhardt, P., Peskett, G. D., Rogers, R., & Tracey, I. (2007). The anxiolytic effects of midazolam during anticipation to pain revealed using fMRI. *Magnetic Resonance Imaging, 25*, 801–810.

Witting, N., Kupers, R. C., Svensson, P., & Jensen, T. S. (2006). A PET activation study of brush-evoked allodynia in patients with nerve injury pain. *Pain, 120*, 145–154.

Wood, P. B., Schweinhardt, P., Jaeger, E., Dagher, A., Hakyemez, H., Rabiner, E. A., Bushnell, M. C., & Chizh, B. A. (2007). Fibromyalgia patients show an abnormal dopamine response to pain. *The European Journal of Neuroscience, 25*, 3576–3582.

Younger, J., Aron, A., Parke, S., Chatterjee, N., & Mackey, S. (2010). Viewing pictures of a romantic partner reduces experimental pain: Involvement of neural reward systems. *PloS One, 5*, e13309.

Zeidan, F., Martucci, K. T., Kraft, R. A., Gordon, N. S., McHaffie, J. G., & Coghill, R. C. (2011). Brain mechanisms supporting the modulation of pain by mindfulness meditation. *The Journal of Neuroscience, 31*, 5540–5548.

Ziv, M., Tomer, R., Defrin, R., & Hendler, T. (2010). Individual sensitivity to pain expectancy is related to differential activation of the hippocampus and amygdala. *Human Brain Mapping, 31*, 326–338.

Zubieta, J. K., Bueller, J. A., Jackson, L. R., Scott, D. J., Xu, Y., Koeppe, R. A., Nichols, T. E., & Stohler, C. S. (2005). Placebo effects mediated by endogenous opioid activity on {micro}-opioid receptors. *The Journal of Neuroscience, 25*, 7754.

Part V
Interventions

Chapter 28
Evidence-Based Pharmacotherapy of Chronic Pain

Howard S. Smith, Sukdeb Datta, and Laxmaiah Manchikanti

Introduction

Pharmacotherapy for chronic pain remains an art. In general, the optimal management of patients with chronic pain requires a combination of pharmacologic and nonpharmacologic therapies. Pharmacotherapy should be utilized as one component of a multimodal treatment plan for chronic pain by an interdisciplinary team. In addition to pharmacologic therapy of chronic pain, other approaches to treatment include: physical medicine, behavioral medicine, neuromodulation, interventional, surgical, and complementary and alternative approaches. Although many of the studies of chronic pain suffer from a low number of patients, one center location, suboptimal study designs, high placebo response rates and difficulties translating study findings to the average outpatient pain clinic, existing evidence from the pain literature is still superior to anecdotal stories, case reports, and expert opinion. Furthermore, most studies in the pain literature investigate the efficacy of single analgesic agents with significantly fewer studies of comparative efficacy of analgesics; and even less studies which evaluate combinations of analgesics. This is despite that it appears that the majority of patients with chronic pain are being treated with multiple analgesics.

Strength of Evidence

The major sources of information are meta-analysis, systematic reviews, and some RCTs. In some reviews, the magnitude of treatment effect as a continuous outcome was reported as an effect size (ES), calculated as the mean change in the treatment group minus mean change in the control group divided by the pooled standard deviation. By convention, an effect size of ≤ 0.2 is considered trivial; $0.2–0.5$ as small; $0.5–0.8$ as moderate; $0.8–1.2$ as important and ≥ 1.2 as very important. When comparing

H.S. Smith, MD (✉)
Department of Anesthesiology, Albany Medical College, 47 New Scotland Avenue,
MC-131, Albany, NY 12208, USA
e-mail: smithh@mail.amc.edu

S. Datta, MD
New Jersey Spine & Rehabilitation, 24 Friar Tuck Circle, Summit, NJ 07901, USA

L. Manchikanti, MD
Pain Management Center of Paducah, Anesthesiology and Perioperative Medicine,
University of Louisville, 2831 Lone Oak Road, Paducah, KY 42003, USA

R.J. Moore (ed.), *Handbook of Pain and Palliative Care: Biobehavioral Approaches for the Life Course*, 471
DOI 10.1007/978-1-4419-1651-8_28, © Springer Science+Business Media, LLC 2012

response rates on a categorical variable (e.g. "improved" or "≥50% reduction in pain"), the number needed to treat (NNT) was sometimes reported. For example, if 60% improve on analgesics vs. 35% on placebo, there is an absolute difference of 25%. The NNT is the reciprocal of this absolute difference $1/0.25 = 4$. This means that for every four patients who receive this analgesic, one additional patient would achieve a therapeutic response over and above placebo.

Nonopioid Analgesics

Nonopioid analgesics are a heterogenous group of anti-inflammatory and other agents (not grouped) with "adjuvants or co-analgesics." Nonopioid analgesics do not produce analgesia in a large part by binding to opioid receptors with subsequent G protein signaling leading to opioid receptor activation, induced analgesia but rather they lead to analgesia largely by other means. These agents generally include: acetaminophen, "traditional" – nonselective nonsteroidal anti-inflammatory drugs (NSAIDs), and cyclooxygenase 2 (COX-2) inhibitors. Some would also group specific agents which may lead to analgesia in certain circumstances/conditions such as bisphosphonates or denosumab into the nonopioid analgesic category. Nonopioid analgesics should generally be used as first-line agents or at least before opioids to treat nociceptive pain.

Acetaminophen

Para-acetylaminophenol known as acetaminophen in the United States (and paracetamol in Europe) is the most commonly over-the-counter administered oral analgesic. The FDA approved acetaminophen in 1951. Acetaminophen is available in multiple formulations including liquids, chewable tablets, coated caplets, gel caps, gel tabs, suppositories, and an intravenous formulation. The oral dose for adults is 325–650 mg every 4–6 h with a maximum daily dose of 4 g/day. The analgesic mechanisms of acetaminophen remain uncertain (Smith 2009). Theories include: inhibition of cyclooxygenases (e.g., cyclooxygenase 3), modulation of the endogenous cannabinoid system (one metabolite of acetaminophen is AM404); which may inhibit the uptake of the endogenous cannabinoid TRPV1 agonist anandamide and AM404 also inhibits sodium channels (Ottani et al. 2006).

Acetaminophen (paracetamol) is a core recommendation for use as an analgesic in 16/16 existing guidelines for the management of hip or knee OA (Zhang et al. 2007). Current European (EULAR) recommendations for the management of hip (Zhang et al. 2005) and knee (Jordan et al. 2003) OA suggest that, because of its safety and efficacy, doses of up to 4 g/day should be the oral analgesic of first choice for mild/moderate pain, and if successful, should be used as the preferred long-term oral analgesic. However, in recent years both the efficacy (Case et al. 2003) and the safety (Garcia Roderiguez and Hernandez-Diaz 2001; Rahme et al. 2002) of long-term use of acetaminophen at this dose have been questioned.

Towheed et al. (2006) performed a Cochrane Review of acetaminophen for osteoarthritis and found reasonable evidence that acetaminophen is modestly superior in efficacy compared with placebo.

Fifteen RCTs involving 5,986 participants were included in this review (Towheed et al. 2006). Seven RCTs compared acetaminophen to placebo and ten RCTs compared acetaminophen to NSAIDs. In the placebo-controlled RCTs, acetaminophen was superior to placebo in 5 of the 7 RCTs and had a similar safety profile. Compared to placebo, a pooled analysis of five trials of overall pain using multiple methods demonstrated a statistically significant reduction in pain (standardized mean differences) (SMD −0.13, 95% CI −0.22 to −0.04), which was of questionable clinical significance (Towheed et al. 2006).

The evidence to date suggests that NSAIDs are superior to acetaminophen for improving knee and hip pain in people with OA (Towheed et al. 2006).

In the United States, paracetamol is the commonest cause of acute liver failure and incidence seems to be increasing (Larson et al. 2005). The potential for concerns about possible hepatotoxicity may exist even at therapeutic doses of acetaminophen, especially in patients with chronic alcohol use (Jalan et al. 2006).

Sustained consumption of paracetamol at therapeutic doses (4 g daily) can lead to asymptomatic increases of blood hepatic aminotransferase concentrations after more than 4 days of consumption (Watkins et al. 2006; Temple et al. 2007; Heard et al. 2007). Such changes do not necessarily suggest an increased risk of progression to acute liver failure, and a systematic review found no prospective study of sustained therapeutic dosing that reported serious liver injury or death (Dart and Bailey 2007).

Traditional NSAIDs

NSAIDs (not all of which are in United States) may not be classified as: salicyclic acid derivatives (aspirin, sulfasalazine), indole and indene acetic acids (tolmentin, diclofenac, ketorolac), arylpropionic acids (ibuprofen, naproxen, fluriprofen, ketoprofen, fenoprofen, oxaprozin), anthranillic acid (fenamates) (mefeamic acid, meclofenamic acid), enolic acids – oxicams (piroxicam, tenoxicam), pyrazolidinediones (phenybutaxone, oxyphenthatrozaone), and alkanones (nabumetone). All patients taking NSAIDs should take the lowest effective dose for the shortest time necessary to control symptoms.

NSAIDs have been utilized for analgesic multiple painful conditions including: perioperative pain (Jirarattanaphochai and Jung 2008; Nauta et al. 2009; Barden et al. 2009), dysmenorrheal (Marjoribanks et al. 2010), chronic nonspecific low back pain (Kuijpers et al. 2011), and acute migraine headaches (Rabbie et al. 2010).

Roelofs et al. performed an updated Cochrane Review on NSAIDs for low back pain. In total, 65 trials (total number of patients = 11,237) were included in this review. Twenty-eight trials (42%) were considered high quality. Statistically significant effects were found in favor of NSAIDs compared with placebo, but at the cost of more statistically significant side effects (Roelofs et al. 2008). Furthermore, there does not seem to be a specific type of NSAID, which is clearly more effective than others. The selective COX-2 inhibitors showed fewer side effects compared with traditional NSAIDs in the randomized controlled trials included in their review (Roelofs et al. 2008).

NSAIDs can cause serious GI complications such as peptic ulcers, perforations and bleeds (PUBS) and this risk increases with age, concurrent use of other medications, and probably with the duration of therapy (Tramer et al. 2000). A MA of severe upper GI complications of NSAIDs showed an OR of 5.36 (95% CI 1.79, 16.1) in 16 NSAID vs. placebo trials in 4,431 patients and a pooled OR for PUBS of 3.0 (95% CI 2.5, 3.7).

In a 2006 systematic review and MA of atherothrombotic complications of COX-2 selective and nonselective NSAIDs, the incidence of serious vascular events was 1% per annum in patients treated with COX-2 selective agents compared with 0.9% in those on traditional NSAIDs (RR¼ 1.16, 95% CI 0.97, 1.38) (Kearney et al. 2006). There was, however, some heterogeneity in risk among the traditional NSAIDs with a modest increase in risk of CV events with ibuprofen (RR¼ 1.51, 95% CI 0.96, 2.37) and diclofenac (RR¼ 1.63, 95% CI 1.12, 2.37), but not with naproxen (RR¼ 0.92, 95% CI 0.67, 1.26) (Kearney et al. 2006).

COX-2 Inhibitors

Jones and Lamdin performed a systematic review and meta-analysis evaluating oral COX-2 inhibitors vs. NSAIDs, and other oral analgesics for acute soft tissue injury with nine RCTs evaluated in the meta-analysis included 3,060 patients (Jones and Lamdin 2010). Coxibs were found to be equal to NSAIDs (day 7+, $n=1,884$, 100 mm visual analogue scale [VAS]), WMD=0.18 mm (95% CI $-1.76, 2.13$), $p=0.85$ and tramadol (day 7+, $n=706$, 100 mm VAS), WMD=-6.6 mm (95% CI -9.63, -3.47) (single study, difference clinically insignificant) for treating pain after soft tissue injuries. Coxibs had fewer gastrointestinal AEs than NSAIDs, even with short-term use (RR 0.59 [95% CI 0.41, 0.85], $p=0.004$) (low quality evidence0 (Jones and Lamdin 2010).

COX-2 selective inhibitors (not all of which are available at all or in United States) include: rofecoxib, celecoxib, valdecoxib, parecoxib, etoricoxib, and lumiracoxib. Celecoxib is the only COX-2 inhibitor available in the United States. All COX-2 inhibitors should be relatively contraindicated in patients with ischemic heart disease and/or stroke, and should be avoided in patients with significant risk factors for coronary artery disease. Kearney et al. (2006) analyzed multiple trials of COX-2 inhibitors and found a "class-effect" in increasing cardiovascular risk. As noted, there was significant increase in the rate ratio for myocardial infarction with COX-2 inhibitors compared with placebo 1.86 (1.33–2.59; $p=0.0003$). Similar analyses (data not shown) include rate ratio of 1.42 (1.13–1.78; $p=0.0003$) for vascular events, 1.02 (0.71–1.47; $p=0.9$) for stroke and 1.49 (0.97–2.29; $p=0.07$) for vascular death with COX-2 inhibitors compared with placebo (Kearney et al. 2006).

Tramadol

Although the mode of action of tramadol is not completely understood, it exerts an analgesic effect to binding to the mu opioid receptor as an agonist (Opioid effect) and weakly inhibits the reuptake of serotonin and norepinephrine (nonopioid affect), similar to the effect of tricyclic antidepressants (TCAs). Tramadol has proven effective in osteoarthritis, fibromyalgia, and neuropathic pain. Because Tramadol is an unscheduled drug, clinician may not be aware of its opioid effect. However, it should be used with some caution in patients recovering from substance use disorder. A randomized trial of 11,352 participants with chronic noncancer pain compared the abuse potential of tramadol, NSAID and hydrocodone (Adams et al. 2006). Depending on the criteria used, the potential for abuse over 12 months was 0.5–2.5% for NSAIDs, 0.7–2.7% for tramadol and 1.2–4.9% for hydrocodone. While the degree of physical dependence usually appears variably mild (rarely, it can be severe), patients can report psychic dependence symptoms of tramadol craving when discontinuing the drug (McDiarmid and Mackler 2005). Seizures have been reported with tramadol as serotonin syndrome. There were patients with a history of seizures and those taking a tricyclic or SSRI antidepressant, monoamine oxidase inhibitor (MAOI), an antipsychotic drug or other opioids may be at increased risk (Sansone and Sansone 2009; Raffa and Stone 2008). Daily dose of tramadol should not exceed 400 mg. Dose reduction is recommended in all adult patients (older than 75) and in those with renal impairment or cirrhosis.

Opioids

Opioids are versatile and potent broad-spectrum analgesics which continue to have a key place among pharmacologic agents available for the treatment of chronic pain. Appropriate use of these drugs requires skills in opioid prescribing, knowledge of the principles of addiction medicine, and a commitment to performing and documenting a comprehensive assessment repeatedly over time.

Inadequate assessment can lead to undertreatment, compromise the effectiveness of therapy when implemented, and prevent an appropriate response when problematic drug-related behaviors occur (Joint Commission 1999; Max et al. 1999; Katz 2002).

Practicing in the "middle of the road" by employing the appropriate use of opioids in the context of good medical practice, as well as focusing appropriate attention on the risk assessment and management of opioid abuse (being cognizant of potential abuse, addiction, and diversion), has become known as "balance" (WHO 2000; Zacny et al. 2003; Joint 2004).

Common opioid side effects may include constipation, nausea and vomiting, sedation, and pruritus. Other adverse effects may include: cognitive disturbances, perceptual distortions, delirium, myoclonus, endocrinopathies, immunologic effects, urinary retention, headache and/or dizziness, fatigue, anorexia, dry mouth, sweating, decreased sexual desire (libido), abdominal discomfort/cramping/bloating, and infrequent respiratory depression.

Opioid Rotation

The practice of changing from one opioid to another, referred to as *opioid rotation*, is most commonly undertaken when adequate analgesia is limited by the occurrence of problematic side effects. The principle of rotation is based on the observation that a patient's response can vary from opioid to opioid, both for analgesia and adverse effects.

Mercadante and Bruera found that opioid rotation results in clinical improvement in at least 50% of patients with chronic pain presenting with a poor response to a particular opioid (Mercadante and Bruera 2006), a Cochrane review (Quigley 2004) revealed that there are no randomized controls for opioid rotation.

Key Points for Opioid Rotation

- Utilize an opioid equianalgesic table that is appropriate/relevant for your practice, and use it consistently.
- In deciding on an alternative opioid, consider all patient factors (e.g., What is the best route of drug delivery in this patient? Which drug is most convenient for the patient/treating team? Is cost going to be an issue? Is the new drug available in the community?).
- In rotating opioids, consider all medical factors that may be relevant (e.g., renal function, liver function, age, comorbidities), and adjust equianalgesic dose based on these factors.
- In rotating to an opioid other than methadone or fentanyl, decrease the equianalgesic dose by 25–50%.
- In rotating to methadone, reduce the dose by 75–90%.
- In rotating to transdermal fentanyl, maintain the equianalgesic dose.
- In rotating because of uncontrolled pain, consider a lesser dose reduction than usual.
- Ensure that appropriate rescue/breakthrough doses are available. Use 5–15% of the total daily opioid dose as a guide, and reassess and retitrate the new opioid.

Opioid Use for Clinical Analgesia

Kalso et al. (2004) reviewed data from 1,145 patients initially randomized in 15 placebo-controlled trials of potent opioids used in the treatment of severe pain; these opioids were analyzed for efficacy and safety in chronic noncancer pain. Four studies tested intravenous opioids in neuropathic pain in a crossover design, with 115 of 120 patients completing the protocols. Using either pain intensity difference or pain relief as the endpoint, all four studies reported average pain relief of 30–60% with opioids. Eleven studies (1,025 patients) compared oral opioids with placebo for 4 days to 8 weeks.

Six of the 15 trials that were included had an open-label follow-up of 6–24 months. The mean decrease in pain intensity in most studies was at least 30% with opioids and was comparable in neuropathic and musculoskeletal pain. Roughly 80% of patients noted at least one adverse effect. The most common adverse effects were constipation (41%), nausea (32%), and somnolence (29%). Only 44% of 388 patients on open-label treatments were still on opioids after therapy for between 7 and 24 months. Adverse effects and lack of efficacy were two common reasons for discontinuation.

Eisenberg et al. (2005) examined 22 studies that met inclusion criteria and were classified as short-term (<24 h; $n + 14$) or intermediate-term (median + 28 days; range of 8–56 days; $n + 8$) trials. They reported contradictory results in the short-term trials. However, all eight intermediate-term trials demonstrated opioid efficacy for spontaneous neuropathic pain. A fixed-effects model meta-analysis of six intermediate-term trials showed mean post-treatment scores of pain intensity (on a visual analog scale) after opioids to be 14 units lower on a scale from 0 to 100 than after placebo (95% confidence interval [CI] −18 to −10; $p < 0.001$). As the mean initial pain intensity recorded from four of the intermediate-term trials ranged from 46 to 69, this 14-point difference was considered to correspond to a 20–30% greater reduction with opioids than with placebo.

When the number needed to harm (NNH) is considered, the most common adverse event was nausea (NNH, 3.6; 95% CI, 2.9–4.8), followed by constipation (NNH, 4.6; 95% CI, 3.4–7.1), drowsiness (NNH, 5.3; 95% CI, 3.7–8.3), vomiting (NNH, 6.2; 95% CI, 4.6–11), and dizziness (NNH, 6.7; 95% CI, 4.8–10.0) (Eisenberg et al. 2005). Eisenberg et al. (2005) concluded that although short-term studies provide only equivocal evidence regarding the efficacy of opioids in reducing the intensity of neuropathic pain, intermediate-term studies demonstrate significant efficacy of opioids over placebo. They also concluded that further randomized, controlled trials are needed in order to establish the long-term efficacy of opioids for neuropathic pain, the safety of long-term opioids (including addiction potential), and the effects of opioids on quality of life. Rowbotham et al. (2003) demonstrated a dose-dependent analgesic effect in patients with mixed neuropathies and reported that high-dose levorphanol yielded significantly more pain relief than did lower doses of this agent.

Short-term efficacy and safety of opioid therapy for chronic low back pain (CLBP) and OA are supported by a substantial body of clinical trial data (Furlan et al. 2006; Kalso et al. 2004). Nuesch et al. performed a meta-analysis on the use of opioids in patients with OA and concluded that the moderate benefits of opioids (other than tramadol) are outweighed by the risk of AEs (Nuesch et al. 2009); therefore, Nuesch recommends that opioids not be used routinely, even for severe pain. Similarly, a meta-analysis by Deshpande et al. on the use of opioids in CLBP concluded that there are insufficient data to recommend long-term opioid therapy in this population (Deshpande et al. 2007). However, a more recent Cochrane review by Noble et al. (2010) of 26 studies of long-term opioid therapy for CNCP concluded that although many patients discontinue long-term therapy owing to inadequate analgesia or AEs, patients who are amenable to continued treatment derive clinically significant benefits.

Tapentadol Hydrochloride

Tapentadol produces analgesia toward dual mechanism of action: Mu opioid receptor activation and norepinephrine reuptake inhibition. Its efficacy has been reported in a number of animal studies, as well as in phase II–III clinical trials. Primary pain disorders in which efficacy has been reported include dental extraction pain, pain after a bunionectomy surgery, osteoarthritis pain of the knee and hip, and low back pain (Wade and Spruill 2009). Initial recommended dose of Tapentadol, immediate release (IR) which is Schedule II controlled substance is 50, 75, or 100 mg every 4–6 h with individualization according to the severity of pain (Wade and Spruill 2009). On the first day of dosing, the second dose may be administered as early as 1 h after the initial dose if satisfactory pain relief is not achieved. Daily doses exceeding 700 mg on day of therapy and 600 mg/day thereafter are not recommended as higher doses have not been studied. No dosage adjustments are necessary in patients with mild to moderate renal impairment; however, the drug has not been studied in subjects with severe renal disease and Tapentadol is not recommended in these individuals. Dosage adjustments are not necessary in patients with mild hepatic impairment, however with moderate liver disease, Tapentadol IR should be initiated at 50 mg with a dosage interval of no less than every 8 h for the first 24 h; subsequent doses may be given at longer or shorter intervals based on tolerability and analgesic needs of the patient. Use in severe hepatic impairment is not recommended. Dosage adjustments are not necessary in the elderly with normal, renal, or hepatic function. In those with liver or kidney disease, dosage adjustments are recommended, as described previously. Tapentadol is listed in pregnancy category C (Wade and Spruill 2009). Patients with significant respiratory depression, acute or severe bronchial asthma, or hypercapnia in unmonitored settings, or in the absence of resuscitative equipment should not receive Tapentadol (Wade and Spruill 2009). Administration of Tapentadol with selective serotonin reuptake inhibitors (SSRIs), serotonin and norepinephrine reuptake inhibitors (NRIs), tricyclic antidepressants, MAOIs, as well as other agents that impair serotonin metabolism and triptans may result in development of potentially life-threatening serotonin syndrome. Tapentadol may produce spasms of the sphincter of Oddi in patients with biliary tract disease, including acute pancreatitis and should be used in caution in this population. Finally, withdrawal symptoms may occur with abrupt discontinuation of Tapentadol. Gradual tapering of the dose usually reduces such symptoms.

Studies completed to date suggest that this agent has comparable or greater efficacy than morphine or oxycodone and greater efficacy than placebo in multiple acute and chronic pain syndromes. Oral absorption is rapid, with C_{max} typically reached in less than 2 h. The drug follows linear pharmacokinetics, has a $T_{1/2}$ of 4 h, and it is primarily excreted renally (Wade and Spruill 2009). Tapentadol has not been found to induce or inhibit CYP enzymes to a significant degree and is therefore thought to have a low probability of interfering with metabolism of other drugs that followed the CYP metabolic pathway.

Adverse affects associated with Tapentadol are primarily of central nervous system or gastrointestinal nature and have been reported less frequently than in patients treated with oxycodone. Efficacy has been reported for Tapentadol in patients with pain associated with dental extraction, bunionectomy surgery, arthritis of the hip and knee and low back pain. An advantage of Tapentadol compared with pure opioid agonist is efficacy in pain of neuropathic and/or inflammatory etiology.

Adverse Effects of Opioids

Common opioid side effects may include constipation, nausea and vomiting, sedation, and pruritus. Other adverse effects may include cognitive disturbances, perceptual distortions, delirium, myoclonus, urinary retention, headache and/or dizziness, fatigue, anorexia, dry mouth, sweating, decreased sexual desire (libido), opioid-induced endocrinopathy/opioid-induced androgen deficiency, abdominal discomfort/cramping/bloating, and infrequent respiratory depression. Opioid toxicity will be different between individuals. Individuals do not develop every potential adverse effect/toxicity and differ greatly as to the magnitude of various effects and how much distress is experienced. In general, tolerance develops to most side effects. There remains a dearth of high-quality evidence for the treatment of opioid side effects in populations both with and without cancer pain (McNicol et al. 2003).

General Principles of Opioid Prescribing

The Pre-Opioid Prescribing Period (POPP)

The pre-opioid prescribing period (POPP) is the period during which the physician determines whether opioids should be prescribed and, if the decision to prescribe such an agent is made, in which necessary controls are put in place prior to initiating therapy (Smith 2008).

Goal-Directed Therapy Agreements

Perhaps one of the most important principles in initiating and maintaining chronic opioid therapy (COT) for persistent noncancer pain is to "know where you are and where you are going." Goal-directed therapy agreements (GDTA) may be helpful in initiating COT for persistent noncancer pain (Smith 2006).

Ongoing assessment of these main domains not only improves pain outcomes for the patient but protects your practice for those patients on an opioid regimen. Passik and Weinreb (2000) have described a useful mnemonic for following the relevant domains of outcome in pain management. The so-called four A's (analgesia, activities of daily living, adverse events, and aberrant drug-taking behaviors) are the clinical domains that reflect progress toward the larger goal of a full and rewarding life.

The POPP is last chance to conduct a complete patient evaluation while the patient is still off opioids. The evaluation should include:

− Pain assessment and history
− Physical examination
− Review of laboratory and diagnostic studies
− Analgesic and other medication history, history of all attempted treatments
− Personal history of psychiatric issues
− Family history of substance abuse/psychiatric problems
− Assessment of comorbidities

The evaluation should also essentially "paint a picture" of the patient's life in the POPP-emotional status, occupational status, functional status and functional capacity, range of motion, recreational activities, sexual activities, social activities, activities of daily living, and status of relationships with family and friends. Accurate record keeping in the POPP is vitally important to support future decision making to increase opioid dose, continue opioid dose, or discontinue opioids.

In the POPP, when considering the risk of benefit ratio of whether or not to initiate COT, Fine and Portenoy (2007) have proposed the following questions which may be helpful to consider:

1. What is conventional practice for this patient's medical condition?
2. Are the other reasonable alternative treatments?
3. What is the risk of adverse events?
4. Is the patient likely to be a responsible drug-taker?

The Screener and Opioid Assessment for Patients with Pain-Revised (SOAPP-R) predicts aberrant medication-related behaviors in patients with chronic pain who are being considered for COT (Butler et al. 2008). It is an empirically derived, 24-item self-report questionnaire which has been shown to be reliable and valid (Butler et al. 2008). The patient scores each of the 24 items on a scale of 0–4. After summation, a total score of ≥18 identifies about 90% of high-risk patients.

Informed Consent

The prescriber must discuss the opioid treatment plan clearly with the patient and answer any questions the patient may have. The patient must be informed of the anticipated benefits of LTOT as well as the foreseeable risks, including the issues of addiction, physical dependence, and tolerance (Webster and Webster 2005). The American Academy of Pain Medicine has a sample informed consent form titled "Consent for Chronic Opioid Therapy," available in both English and Spanish on their Web site at www.painmed.org/productpub/statements.

Chronic Opioid Trial Agreements

It may also be reasonable to use an opioid contract when prescribing LTOT for patients with persistent noncancer pain. However, such a contract may not be necessary for all patients in all settings. Therefore, the use of opioid contracts is left to the clinician's judgment and/or policies. Elements of opioid contracts may include the following:

- Only one physician prescribing opioids while the patient is being treated at a pain clinic
- Use of only one pharmacy for medications
- Random drug (blood or urine) screens and/or pill counts allowed
- Refill requests must be made according to pain clinic policy and not on nights or weekends
- Selling, trading, or sharing opioids with anyone constitutes grounds for discontinuation of opioids and possible dismissal
- Forged or abused prescriptions constitute grounds for discontinuation of opioids and dismissal
- Use of any illegal controlled substances (e.g., marijuana, cocaine) constitutes grounds for discontinuation of opioids and possible dismissal
- Opioids must be safeguarded from loss or theft (lost or stolen opioids will not be replaced)
- The patient agrees to take medication exactly as prescribed
- All unused opioid medication must be brought to the pain clinic at every visit

An extension of the traditional contract is the use of a trilateral opioid contract, which is seen, agreed upon, and signed by the pain specialist, patient, and patient's primary care physician (Fishman et al. 2002). The American Academy of Pain Medicine has a sample agreement form.

Maintenance of Chronic Opioid-Therapy Documentation

Follow-up visits should also carefully document how the patient is doing and compare their current status with that of the POPP. Ongoing assessment of various domains not only improves pain outcomes for the patient but also protects your practice for those patients on an opioid regimen. Passik and Weinreb (2000) have described a useful mnemonic for following the relevant domains of outcome in pain management. The so-called four A's (analgesia, activities of daily living, adverse events, and aberrant drug-taking behaviors) are the clinical domains that reflect progress toward the larger goal of a full and rewarding life.

Current Opioid Misuse Measure

The Current Opioid Misuse Measure (COMM) was established for continued assessment of current opioid use, examining various items reflecting those patient activities that are suggestive of current, ongoing aberrant drug-related behaviors (Butler et al. 2007).

There is no single behavior that is pathognomonic of a substance use disorder, thus there is no foolproof instrument that can reliably assess the risk of opioid addiction (Gourlay and Heit 2006). As the prevalence of addiction in the general population is not insignificant, it seems prudent to utilize the ten steps of "universal precautions" in patients receiving long-term opioid therapy (COT) (Gourlay and Heit 2005). These are (1) reasonable attempts to make a diagnosis with an appropriate differential; (2) comprehensive patient assessment including risk of addictive disorders; (3) informed consent; (4) treatment agreement; (5) pre- and postintervention assessment of pain level and function; (6) appropriate trial of opioid therapy ± "adjunctive" medications; (7) reassessment of pain score and level of function; (8) regular assessment of the four "A's" of pain medicine; (9) periodic review of pain diagnosis and comorbid conditions, including addictive disorders; and (10) documentation. Application of the universal precautions is intended to help the clinician identify and interpret aberrant behavior and, where they exist, diagnose underlying substance misuse disorders.

Popular risk-management elements include obtaining informed consent for COT, using opioid contracts or agreements, performing urine drug tests, unscheduled pill counts, prescriptions with small number of pills, and implementing specific policies to manage aberrant behaviors.

Urine Drug Testing

The practice of urine drug testing (UDT) is more common in a noncancer pain setting than in an oncology or primary care setting; however, it sometimes seems to be incorrectly utilized in a punitive manner to "catch" the patient with an inappropriate positive or negative test. Unfortunately, this often results in dismissal of the patient from the practice. While drug testing can be used in a variety of ways, it is most commonly used for two quite different purposes: to identify substances that should not be present in the urine (i.e., forensic testing) and to detect the presence of prescribed medications (compliance testing).

The use of UDT in efforts to monitor patients on COT treated in a pain clinic is reasonable. This type of testing is not mandatory for all patients on COT in all settings. UDT should be utilized based on the clinical judgment of the prescribing clinician; however, some clinicians and/or clinics test all patients on COT sporadically based on policy. Katz and Fanciullo (2002) have proposed that although further research is needed, it may be easier and more uniform to conduct routine urine toxicology testing in patients with chronic pain treated with opioids. By adopting a uniform policy of testing, stigma is reduced while ensuring that those persons dually diagnosed with pain and substance use disorders may receive optimal care. With careful explanation of the purpose of testing, any patient concerns can be easily addressed (Heit and Gourlay 2004). Caveats to the use of UDT include the following:

1. Ensuring the proper collection, handling, and documentation of the urine specimen
2. Being knowledgeable regarding interpretation of UDT results
3. Knowing exactly what your patient consumed and when it was consumed prior to the urine collection
4. Knowing what you are looking for and what you will do when various results come back

The health-care professional must know which drugs to test for and by what methods, as well as the expected use of the results. It is critical that the clinician be knowledgeable regarding the limitations of the tests (i.e., low sensitivity of immunoassay for semisynthetic and synthetic opioids). Confirmatory tests should be specifically requested. If the purpose of testing is to find unprescribed or illicit drug use, combination techniques such as GC/MS or HPLC are the most specific for identifying individual drugs or their metabolites (Vandevenne et al. 2000).

Caution must be exercised in interpreting UDT results in a pain practice.

True negative urine results for prescribed medication may indicate a pattern of binging rather than drug diversion. Time of last use of the drug(s) can be helpful in interpreting the results.

In certain cases, a UDT may detect traces of unexplained opioids secondary to drug metabolism. For example, a patient taking codeine may show trace quantities of hydrocodone (up to 11%) that is unrelated to hydrocodone use (Oyler et al. 2000). Detection of minor amounts of hydrocodone in urine containing a high concentration of codeine should not be interpreted as evidence of hydrocodone misuse. In the case of a patient who is prescribed hydrocodone, quantities of hydromorphone may also be detected due to hydrocodone metabolism (Heit and Gourlay 2004). Morphine may be metabolized to produce small amounts of hydromorphone (up to 10%) through a minor metabolic pathway (Cone et al. 2006).

If UDT is utilized, it is crucial to avoid inappropriate interpretation of results, which may adversely affect clinical decision making. Health-care providers should not jump to conclusions of noncompliance or appropriate opioid use vs. opioid misuse based on positive or negative detection of opioid in the urine. Clinicians should use the results of the drug test in conjunction with other clinical information when deciding whether to alter the treatment plan.

Christo et al. (2011) have described an algorithmic approach for UDT, an approach developed based on evidence (Pesce et al. 2011). However, for UDT including accuracy, validity, and cost-effectiveness, there is a paucity of evidence. Consequently, a step-wise process for UDT may be performed as a baseline measure of risk, as well as monitoring for compliance. Figure 28.1 illustrates an algorithmic approach for UDT in chronic pain as described by Christo et al. (2011), which includes various steps for baseline UDT, monitoring for compliance, interpretation of the results, and managing patients with abnormal UDT.

Antidepressants

Tricyclic Antidepressants

Antidepressants are a heterogeneous group of drugs which have all demonstrated beneficial activity for patients with major depressive order. Additionally, these agents may have beneficial effects in patients with anxiety disorders (e.g. panic disorder, generalized anxiety disorder, social anxiety, post-traumatic stress disorder, and obsessive–compulsive disorder), eating disorders, attention deficit hyperactivity disorders, premenstrual dysphoric disorder, and chronic pain. Many antidepressants possess analgesic qualities for a broad range of pain conditions independent of their effects on mood.

Antidepressant medications may be classified as follows (Smith 2007):

1. Cyclic antidepressants, including the TCAs and tetracyclic antidepressants (e.g., maprotiline)
2. Selective serotonin reuptake inhibitors (SSRIs)
3. Serotonin norepinephrine reuptake inhibitors (SNRIs)
4. Dopamine norepinephrine reuptake inhibitors (DNRIs)
5. Norepinephrine reuptake inhibitors (NRIs)
6. Monoamine oxidase inhibitors (MAOIs)
7. The miscellaneous category of "atypical antidepressants"

Although the role of SSRIs in providing effective analgesia is uncertain, it appears limited at best (Saarto and Wiffen 2007). Two classes of antidepressants have significant analgesic properties, the TCAs, and SNRIs. Both TCAs and SNRIs (e.g., venlafaxine) have NNT roughly in the neighborhood of three (Saarto and Wiffen 2007).

Most potent effects on the noradrenergic system is desipramine [also going along with it being least sedating] (nortriptyline also exhibits preferential inhibition of NE reuptake over 5-HT reuptake). Doxepin has the most potent anti-histaminergic effects.

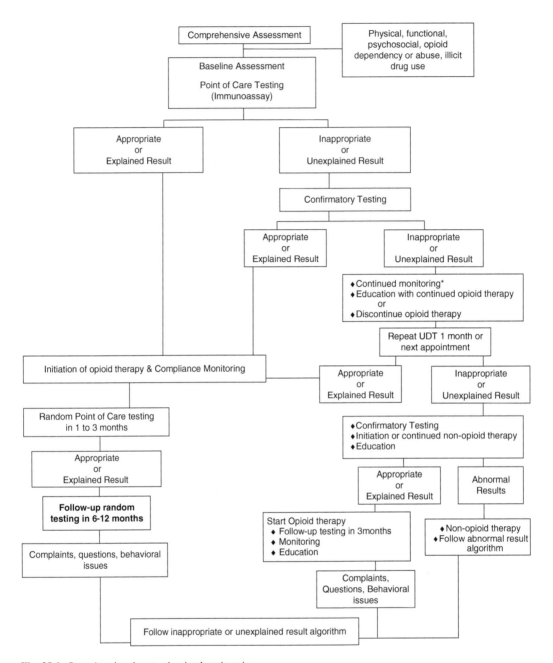

Fig. 28.1 Steps in urine drug testing in chronic pain

The TCAs can be divided into amines and their demethylated secondary amine derivatives. In addition, maprotiline (Ludiomil) is classified as a tetracyclic.

The tertiary amine TCAs include the following:

- Amitriptyline (Elavil)
- Imipramine (Tofranil)
- Trimipramine (Surmontil)

- Clomipramine (Anafranil)
- Doxepin (Sinequan)

The secondary amine TCAs include the following:

- Nortriptyline (Pamelor)
- Desipramine (Norpramin)
- Protriptyline (Vivactil)
- Amoxapine (Asendin)

TCAs, although having reasonable analgesic properties, may also possess multiple undesirable adverse effects. These adverse effects may vary depending on the individual agent. Among the TCAs, amitriptyline has the most potent anticholinergic effects and desipramine has the least, and thus is the least sedating.

Multiple placebo-controlled RCTs have found TCAs to be efficacious for several different types of neuropathic pain (Dworkin et al. 2007; Finnerup et al. 2005, 2007, 2010; Saarto and Wiffen 2007; Sindrup et al. 2005). In addition, TCAs are efficacious for the treatment of depression, a common comorbidity in patients with chronic pain, but the analgesic efficacy in neuropathic pain has been established in nondepressed patients, which establishes their beneficial effect in neuropathic pain cannot be explained simply by antidepressant effects. Anticholinergic adverse effects are common and include dry mouth, orthostatic hypotension, constipation, and urinary retention. These effects can be reduced by starting with low dosages administered at bedtime and with slow titration to higher dosage as well as by using a secondary amine TCAs (e.g., nortriptyline or desipramine).

The Neuropathic Special Interest Group (NeuPSIG) of the International Association for the Study of Pain (IASP) developed guidelines which recommend prescribing TCAs, with caution in patients with ischemic cardiac disease or ventricular conduction abnormalities, limiting the dosages to less than 100 mg/day when possible and obtaining a screening electrocardiogram for patients older than 40 years (Dworkin et al. 2007).

It can take up to 6–8 weeks, including 2 weeks at the highest dosage tolerated, for an adequate trial of treatment with TCA however, analgesia tends to be evident quicker (after about a week) and at lower does than when these agents are utilized to treat depression (Dworkin et al. 2007; Finnerup et al. 2005).

Antidepressants with Both Norepinephrine and Serotonin Reuptake Inhibition

There are four SNRIs available in the United States. Venlafaxine (Effexor) and Desvenlafaxine (Pristiq) are FDA-approved for the treatment of major depressive disorder. Milnacipran is FDA-approved for the treatment of fibromyalgia. Duloxetine and venlafaxine are selective SNRIs that have been studied in peripheral neuropathic pain (another SNRI, milnacipran has been studied only in fibromyalgia).

Venlafaxine has shown efficacy in painful diabetic peripheral neuropathy and painful polyneuropathies of different origins, but not in postherpetic neuralgia (Dworkin et al. 2007). Typically 2–4 weeks are required to titrate to an efficacious dosage (that is 150–225 mg/day); venlafaxine is available in short- and long-acting preparations. At very low doses, venlafaxine tends to "act" more like an SSRI but is clearly an SNRI as the dose is increased. Cardiac conduction abnormalities have been reported in a small number of patients, and blood pressure increases can occur; therefore venlafaxine should be prescribed with caution in patients with cardiac disease. In addition, venlafaxine should be tapered when treatment is being discontinued because of withdrawal symptoms.

The U.S. Food and Drug Administration approved duloxetine hydrochloride to treat chronic musculoskeletal pain on November 4, 2010, including discomfort from osteoarthritis and chronic lower back pain. Cymbalta was first used to treat major depressive disorder in 2004. Since its initial approval, over 30 million patients in the United States have used duloxetine. It was approved for the treatment of diabetic peripheral neuropathy in 2004; generalized anxiety disorder and maintenance treatment of major depression in 2007; and fibromyalgia in 2008. More than 29,000 patients have used duloxetine in clinical trials, and more than 600 patients were studied in the clinical trials involving osteoarthritis and CLBP. The safety evaluation for duloxetine included review of data from the clinical trials as well as postmarketing data from the previously approved patient populations. The FDA assessed the efficacy of duloxetine in CLBP and osteoarthritis in four double-blind, placebo-controlled, randomized clinical trials. At the end of the study period, patients taking duloxetine had a significantly greater pain reduction compared with placebo. The most common side effects reported with duloxetine include nausea, dry mouth, insomnia, drowsiness, constipation, fatigue, and dizziness. Other serious side effects include liver damage, allergic reactions such as hives, rashes and/or swelling of the face, pneumonia, depressed mood, suicide, suicidal thoughts and behavior.

Skljarevski et al. (2010) conducted a randomized, double-blind, placebo-controlled study; and assessed efficacy and safety of duloxetine in patients with CLBP. Adults ($n=401$) with a nonneuropathic CLBP and average pain intensity of ≥ 4 on an 11-point numerical scale (Brief Pain Inventory [BPI]) were treated with either duloxetine 60 mg once daily or placebo for 12 weeks. The primary measure was BPI average pain (Skljarevski et al. 2010). Compared with placebo-treated patients, duloxetine-treated patients reported a significantly greater reduction in BPI average pain ($p \leq 0.001$). Similarly, duloxetine-treated patients reported significantly greater improvements in PGI-I, BPI-S, BPI-I, 50% response rates, and some health outcomes. The RMDQ and 30% response rate showed numerical improvements with duloxetine treatment. Significantly more patients in the duloxetine group (15.2%) than patients in the placebo group (5.4%) discontinued because of adverse events ($p=0.002$). Nausea and dry mouth were the most common treatment-emergent adverse events with rates significantly higher in duloxetine-treated patients (Skljarevski et al. 2010).

Duloxetine has shown consistent efficacy in painful polyneuropathy (DPN) (Dworkin et al. 2007) with effectiveness sustained for 1 year in an open label trial (Raskin et al. 2006). Unfortunately, Duloxetine has not been studied in any other types of neuropathic pain and so its efficacy in such conditions is unknown. The most common adverse affect of Duloxetine is nausea, which seems to be reduced by administering 30 mg once daily for 1 week before increasing to 60 mg once daily. Duloxetine does not seem to produce clinically important electrocardiographic or blood pressure changes and our recent review concluded that aminotransferase monitoring is unnecessary.

Calcium Channel Alpha 2-Delta Ligands (Gabapentin and Pregabalin)

Gabapentin and pregabalin each bind to the voltage-gated calcium channels at the alpha 2-delta subunit and inhibit neurotransmitter release. They have shown efficacy vs. placebo in several neuropathic pain conditions (Dworkin et al. 2007; Finnerup et al. 2005; Finnerup and Jensen 2007; Finnerup 2010). Although gabapentin and pregabalin have few drug interactions, both can produce dose-dependent dizziness and sedation, which can be reduced by starting with lower dosages and titrating cautiously. Both medications also require dosage reduction in patients with renal insufficiency and dosage adjustments can be made in relation to creatinine clearance.

Gabapentin is absorbed slowly after oral administration, with maximum plasma concentrations attained within 3–4 h (Bockbrader et al. 2010). Orally administered gabapentin exhibits saturable absorption – a nonlinear (zero-order) process – making its pharmacokinetics less predictable. Plasma concentrations of gabapentin do not increase proportionally with increasing dose (Bockbrader et al. 2010). Orally administered pregabalin is absorbed more rapidly, with maximum plasma concentrations attained within 1 h. Absorption is linear (first order), with plasma concentrations increasing proportionately with increasing dose. The absolute bioavailability of gabapentin drops from 60 to 33% as the dosage increases from 900 to 3,600 mg/day, while the absolute bioavailability of pregabalin remains at ≥90% irrespective of the dosage (Bockbrader et al. 2010). Treatment should be initiated at low dosage with gradual increases until pain relief, dose-limiting adverse affects, or 3,600 mg/day in three divided doses reached. An adequate trial of treatment with gabapentin can require 2 months or more.

A systematic review of 15 trials (1,468 participants) evaluating gabapentin included 1 acute pain trial and 14 trials in neuropathic (7 in diabetic neuropathy, 2 in postherpetic neuralgia and 1 each in cancer-related neuropathy, phantom limb pain, spinal cord injury, Guillain–Barre syndrome and miscellaneous neuropathies) (Wiffen et al. 2005). In the 14 chronic neuropathic pain trials, 42% of the participants improved on gabapentin (that is pain relief of 50% or greater on gabapentin vs. 19% on placebo, and the NNT for improvement in all trials with evaluable data was 4.3 (95% CI, 3.5–5.7)). Withdrawal rates were 14% for gabapentin vs. 10% for placebo.

In an updated Cochrane Review evaluating gabapentin for chronic neuropathic pain and fibromyalgia in adults, Moore et al. (2011) found that gabapentin provides pain relief of a high level in about a third of people who take it for painful neuropathic pain. Using the Initiative on Methods, Measurement and Pain Assessment in Clinical Trials (IMMPACT) definition of at least moderate benefit, gabapentin was superior to placebo in 14 studies with 2,831 participants, 43% improving with gabapentin and 26% with placebo; the NNT was 5.8 (4.8–7.2) (Moore et al. 2011). Using the IMMPACT definition of substantial benefit, gabapentin was superior to placebo in 13 studies with 2,627 participants, 31% improving with gabapentin and 17% with placebo; the NNT was 6.8 (5.6–8.7) (Moore et al. 2011).

Pregabalin may provide analgesia more quickly then gabapentin because initial dosage of 150 mg/day has been found to be efficacious in some trials and because of the time required to titrate to a full dosage is less (Stacey et al. 2008).

Moore et al. (2009) performed a Cochrane Review of pregabalin for acute and chronic pain. For chronic pain, pregabalin at 150 mg daily was generally ineffective. Efficacy was demonstrated for dichotomous outcomes equating to moderate or substantial pain relief, alongside lower rates for lack of efficacy discontinuations with increasing dose. The best (lowest) NNT for each condition for at least 50% pain relief over baseline (substantial benefit) for 600 mg pregabalin daily compared with placebo were 3.9 (95% confidence interval 3.1–5.1) for postherpetic neuralgia, 5.0 (4.0–6.6) for painful diabetic neuropathy, 5.6 (3.5–14) for central neuropathic pain, and 11 (7.1–21) for fibromyalgia (Moore et al. 2009). The FDA has improved pregabalin for treatment of neuropathic pain associated with diabetic peripheral neuropathy and postherpetic neuralgia and for treatment of fibromyalgia; evidence from these trials is discussed under specific disorders.

Skeletal Muscle Relaxants

Most muscle relaxants are FDA-approved for either spasticity (baclofen, dantrolene, and tizanidine) or musculoskeletal conditions (carisoprodol, chlorzoxazone, cyclobenzaprine, metaxalone, methocarbamol, or orphenadrine) (Chou et al. 2004). The mechanism of action for the latter category of agents is unclear, but may be related in part to sedative effects. Cyclobenzaprine is structurally very similar to amitriptyline and may have similar mechanisms of action. Studies to date have not shown differences amongst most skeletal muscle relaxants with respect to their efficacy, adverse affects or safety. A systemic review (Chou et al. 2004) concluded that there was "insufficient data to assess comparative abuse and addiction of skeletal muscle relaxants of almost all case reports an abuse and addiction have been in patients taking carisoprodol." Most trials are focused on acute rather than chronic pain. Cyclobenzaprine is the best studied of muscle relaxant in musculoskeletal disorders overall; in 21 fair quality trials it is consistently proven superior to placebo for fibromyalgia, as well as for pain relief, muscle spasm and functional status in other disorders. Cyclobenzaprine 5 mg t.i.d. tends to be as equally effective as 10 mg t.i.d. but has fewer side effects.

Topical Analgesics

Lidocaine 5% Patch

The 5% lidocaine patch has shown efficacy and excellent tolerability in trials involving patients with postherpetic neuralgia and allodynia and in patients with allodynia due to different types of peripheral neuropathic pain (Davies and Galer 2004; Khaliq et al. 2007). As a topical treatment without substantial systemic absorption, the most common adverse effects are mild local reactions. The lack of systemic adverse affects and drug interactions can be particularly advantageous in all the patients or patients with complex neuropathic pain. Lidocaine gel (5%), which is less expensive than the lidocaine patch, has also shown efficacy in patients with postherpetic neuralgia and allodynia. Topical lidocaine is most appropriate in well-localized neuropathic pain and is likely to be of benefit in patients with central neuropathic pain. Unfortunately, attempts to predict which patients are most likely to respond to this treatment with topical lidocaine have been generally unsuccessful.

Capsaicin

Capsaicin is an alkaloid derived from chili peppers; repeated application is thought to lead to depletion of substance from primary afferent neurons (Lee et al. 1991). The main disadvantage of capsaicin is the initial burning sensation, which may persist for days. Capsaicin must be applied 3–4 times per day over the entire painful area for up to 6–8 weeks before optimal pain relief can be achieved. Mason et al. (2004a) reviewed the clinical trial evidence for capsaicin, including six trials in neuropathic pain and three trials in musculoskeletal conditions. They found that 57% of patients with neuropathic pain achieved at least 50% pain relief with capsaicin, compared with 42% of patient of placebo; for patients with musculoskeletal conditions, the capsaicin response was 38 vs. 25% for placebo (Mason et al. 2004a). Approximately one-third of the patients experienced local adverse events with capsaicin.

Derry et al. (2009) performed a Cochrane review that included six studies (389 participants in total) which compared regular application of low-dose (0.075%) capsaicin cream with placebo cream; the NNT for any pain relief over 6–8 weeks was 6.6 (4.1–17). Two studies (709 participants in total) compared a single application of high-dose (8%) capsaicin patch with placebo patch; the NNT for ≥30% pain relief over 12 weeks was 12 (6.4–70). Local skin reactions were more common with capsaicin, usually tolerable, and attenuated with time; the NNH for repeated low-dose application was 2.5 (2.1–3.1) (Derry et al. 2009).

Topical NSAIDs

Massey et al. (2010) performed a Cochrane Review of topical NSAIDs for acute pain in adults. Forty-seven studies were included; most compared topical NSAIDs in the form of a gel, spray, or cream with a similar placebo, with 3,455 participants in the overall analysis of efficacy. For all topical

NSAIDs combined, compared with placebo, the number needed to treat to benefit (NNT) for clinical success, equivalent to 50% pain relief, was 4.5 (3.9–5.3) for treatment periods of 6–14 days. Topical diclofenac, ibuprofen, ketoprofen, and piroxicam were of similar efficacy (Massey et al. 2010).

Topical Salicylate

Topical salicylate has proven superior to placebo in both acute pain (three trials, 182 patients; NNT is equal to 2.1; 95% confidence CI; 1.7–2.8) and chronic pain (six trials, 429 patients; NNT equals 5.3; 95% CI; 3.6–10.2) (Mason et al. 2004b). However, larger more rigorous trials tended to be negative.

Topical Diclofenac

Diclofenac is available in the United States in a topical formulation as: a topical diclofenac sodium 1% (DSG) gel (Voltaren Gel®), a 1.5% diclofenac solution (Pennsaid®), or as a diclofenac epolamine topical patch (DETP) 1.3% (Flector Patch®). Baraf et al. (2011) analyzed pooled data from three randomized, double-blind, parallel-group, placebo-controlled, multicenter trials which evaluated the safety and efficacy of topical diclofenac sodium gel for knee osteoarthritis in elderly and younger patients. They found that diclofenac sodium gel was effective and generally well tolerated in adults regardless of age. These data support the topical application of DSG for relief of OA knee pain in elderly and younger patients (Baraf et al. 2011).

Towheed (2006) performed a systematic review and meta-analysis of randomized controlled trials of Pennsaid® therapy for osteoarthritis of the knee. Pennsaid is an effective topical NSAID in patients with OA of the knee. Apart from minor localized skin reactions, Pennsaid was as safe as VCP (Towheed 2006). Galer et al. (2000) reported the results of a multicenter controlled clinical trial evaluating the topical diclofenac patch for minor sports injury pain. They found that the diclofenac epolamine patch is an effective and safe pain reliever for treatment of minor sports injury pain.

Kuehl (2010) analyzed eight studies utilizing the DETP (1.3%) for patients with acute pain due to soft tissue injuries. The search identified six placebo-controlled clinical studies, one active-comparator-controlled clinical study, and one open-label comparator clinical study of the efficacy and tolerability of the DETP in patients with soft tissue injuries (Kuehl 2010). Three studies reported on tolerability. Primary analyses among the eight studies reported DETP-associated reductions in spontaneous pain from baseline, assessed using a visual analog scale, ranging from 26 to 88% on day 7 and 56–61% on day 14. The use of the DETP was associated with significantly greater reductions in pain scores compared with a placebo patch (two studies) on day 7 (88 vs. 74%; $p=0.001$) and day 14 (56.5 vs. 46.8%; $p=0.001$) and compared with diclofenac diethylammonium topical gel (one study) on day 14 (60.8 vs. 40.8%; $p<0.001$) (Kuehl 2010).

High Concentration Capsaicin Patch

A high concentration (8%) capsaicin patch has been studied in multiple RCTs in patients with postherpetic neuralgia (Backonja et al. 2008, 2010; Irving et al. 2011) and reviewed (Jones et al. 2011). A single high-concentration capsaicin patch application utilized to provide analgesia for patients with painful HIV neuropathy resulted in a mean pain reduction of 22.8% during weeks 2–12 as compared to a 10.7% reduction for controls ($p=0.0026$, Simpson et al. 2008). One-third of high-concentration capsaicin patch-treated patients reported ≥30% pain decrease from baseline as compared to 18% of controls ($p = 0.0092$). Self-limited, mild-to-moderate local skin reactions were commonly observed (Simpson et al. 2008). However, in a second HIV neuropathy trial, the effects of high concentration capsaicin patches did not meet the primary endpoint of the study (Noto et al. 2009).

Application of the high-concentration capsaicin patch in patients with postherpetic neuralgia appears to be safe and well tolerated, and adverse effects were limited to transient increases in pain, as well as location reactions associated with patch application (e.g., application site reactions [pain, erythema]). After a single 1-h application (Webster et al. 2010), the high concentration capsaicin patch may be associated with some sustained reductions in pain that persist for 2–3 months. Simpson et al. (2010) concluded that repeated treatments administered over a 1-year period are generally safe and well tolerated.

Botulinum Toxin

Botulinum toxin (BTX) is a potent neurotoxin produced by the anaerobic bacterium, Clostridium botulinum. Out of the seven known serotypes, three type-A preparations, BOTOX® (onabotulinumtoxinA, product of Allergan, Inc. Irvine, CA), Xeomin® (incobotulinumtoxinA, product of Merz Pharmaceuticals, LLC, Greensboro, NC) and Dysport® (abobotulinumtoxinA, product of Medicis Pharmaceutical Inc., Scottsdale, AZ) have been developed. Currently, Type B is commercially available as Myobloc® in the United States.

Botulinum toxin Type A (BTX-A) is FDA-approved for multiple medical conditions including the treatment of cervical dystonia and more recently for chronic migraine headaches. It also appears that BTX-A may provide analgesic effect for patients with neuropathic pain (Ranoux et al. 2008).

Xiao et al. investigated the therapeutic benefits of BTX-A in subjects with PHN in a randomized, double-blind, placebo-controlled study. Sixty subjects with PHN were randomly and evenly distributed into BTX-A, lidocaine, and placebo groups (Xiao et al. 2010). Compared with pretreatment, VAS pain scores decreased at day 7 and 3 months posttreatment in all three groups ($p < 0.01$). However, the VAS pain scores of the BTX-A group decreased more significantly compared with lidocaine and placebo groups at day 7 and 3 months posttreatment ($p < 0.01$). Sleep time (hours) had improved at day 7 and at 3 months compared with pretreatment in all three groups, but the BTX-A group improved more significantly compared with lidocaine and placebo groups ($p < 0.01$). The percent of subjects using opioids posttreatment in the BTX-A group was the lowest (21.1%) compared with the lidocaine (52.6%) and placebo (66.7%) groups ($p < 0.01$) (Xiao et al. 2010). Thus, subcutaneous administration of BTX-A significantly decreased pain in PHN and reduced opioid use compared with lidocaine and placebo at day 7 and 3 months posttreatment. It also increased subjects' sleep times (Xiao et al. 2010).

Spinal Analgesics

Opioids have been and continue to be a mainstay agent for intraspinal therapy. The guidelines developed at the Polyanalgesic Consensus Conference suggest that the first-line intraspinal agent should be an opioid alone (e.g., preservative-free, sterile morphine sulfate or hydromorphone) or ziconotide, and suggest switching from one agent to another opioid agent, or adding agents if the suggested "maximum" dose is reached (e.g., 15 mg/day of morphine), if acceptable analgesia is not achieved, or if side effects occur (Deer et al. 2007).

Treatment Considerations for Neuropathic Pain

The International Association for the study of Pain Neuropathic Pain Special Interest Guidelines for the treatment of neuropathic pain recommended three classes of medications as first-line treatments: antidepressants with both norepinephrine and serotonin reuptake inhibition (TCAs and selective serotonin and norepinephrine reuptake inhibitors [SSNRIs]), calcium channel $\alpha2$-δ ligands (gabapentin and pregabalin) and topical lidocaine (lidocaine patch 5%) (Dworkin et al. 2007). Opioids and tramadol were recommended as generally second-line treatments, except in certain specific situations in which it was recommended that first-line use could be considered. A number of medications were considered as third line treatments.

The guidelines acknowledge that a combination of medication with efficacy for neuropathic pain may provide greater analgesia than use of individual medications as monotherapy, although such combination therapy may also be associated with increased side effects, inconvenience, risk of drug interaction and cost (Dworkin et al. 2007). Nevertheless, because 50% of patients in neuropathic pain trials typically achieve satisfactory pain control, many patients in clinical practice will require treatments with combinations of medications. Such combination therapy is incorporated into a stepwise management strategy for patients with partial response to treatment with first-line medications.

Treatment Considerations for Fibromyalgia

Five types of medications are effective in FM (see also Velly et al. 2011) V: (1) TCAs, (2) Cyclobenzaprine, (3) tramadol, (4) SNRIs (duloxetine, milnacipran), and (5) calcium channel $\alpha2$-δ-ligands (gabapentin and pregabalin). Although classified as a muscle relaxant, cyclobenzaprine has a chemical structure closely related to TCAs, which may partially account for its effectiveness in FM. While trials have shown the efficacy of tramadol in FM, the few studies of potent full mu agonist opioids have not shown benefit. There is no RCT evidence that NSAIDs are effective monotherapy for FM.

A meta-analysis of antidepressants published in 2000 found 13 trials with evaluable data involving three classes of antidepressants: TCAs (9 trials), SSRIs (3 trials), and s-adenosylmethionine (2 trials) (O'Malley et al. 2000). Overall, antidepressants were superior to placebo with an NNT of 4. The effect sizes for pain, fatigue, sleep and overall well-being were all moderate (ES, 0.39–0.52). In the five studies where there was adequate assessment for treatment response independent of depression, only one study found a correlation between symptom improvement and depression scores. Antidepressant class did not make a difference, although only three trials tested SSRIs (O'Malley et al. 2000).

Nishishinya et al. (2008) reported that there is some evidence to support the short-term efficacy of amitriptyline 25 mg/day in fibromyalgia. Overall, Häuser et al. (2009) in a meta-analysis concluded that antidepressant medications are associated with improvement in pain, depression, fatigue, sleep disturbances, and health-related quality of life in patients with fibromyalgia. There is no gold standard pharmacologic agent for fibromyalgia, however, it is conceivable that amitriptyline may be useful in reducing overall symptoms (e.g., pain, sleep disturbances, fatigue, and limitations of health-related quality of life); duloxetine may be useful in reducing pain, sleep disturbances, and limitations of health-related quality of life; and milnacipran may be particularly useful in reducing fatigue (Häuser et al. 2011).

A meta-analysis of four trials found that cyclobenzaprine (10–40 mg) was also superior to placebo (Arnold et al. 2000). Additionally, Tofferi et al. (2004) performed a meta-analysis on five randomized, placebo-control trials and reported that cyclobenzaprine-treated patients were three times as likely to report overall improvement and to report moderate reductions in individual symptoms, particularly sleep. Two trials involving 100 patients (Russell et al. 2000) and 313 patients (Bennett et al. 2003) showed that tramadol was superior to placebo in treating FM, although the largest trial combined tramadol with acetaminophen.

Most researches on pharmacotherapy for FM have involved use of SNRI antidepressants and the α2-δ ligand anticonvulsants. Pregabalin, milnacipran, and duloxetine have each proven effective in several phase III trials and the first effective drugs FDA-approved for the treatment of FM. Gabapentin was positive in a single trial (Arnold et al. 2007). Venlafaxine was tested in 15 patients with an open clinical low dose trial (75 mg); thus, no significant conclusion can be reached (Dwight et al. 1998).

In phase III trials, pregabalin was dosed at 300–450 mg/day (divided into b.i.d. dosing), duloxetine at 60–120 mg once a day and milnacipran at 50–100 mg twice a day. In all trials, separation of the higher dose from the lower dose of the drug was small to minimal, while side effect rates were somewhat increased at higher doses. The most bothersome side effect of duloxetine and milnacipran (as well as venlafaxine) is nausea, which may be lessened by starting at a lower dose for 1–2 weeks and taking the drug with food. The most bothersome side effect with pregabalin and gabapentin are somnolence (which often increases with treatment and may be reduced by a low starting dose and by starting with the only dose or the highest dose at bedtime), dizziness, and weight gain.

Treatment Considerations in Older Persons

Acetaminophen should be typically tried prior to NSAIDs because of slightly higher risk/benefit ratio of NSAIDs in older adults (see also McCarberg and Cole 2011). When using NSAIDs in persons 60 years and older, a proton pump inhibitor should be added as a prophylaxis against GI bleeding in those with GI symptoms (dyspepsia or gastroesophageal reflux) or who are on antiplatelet agents (e.g., aspirin, clopidogrel) or corticosteroids. Amitriptyline and cyclobenzaprine should be avoided due to highly anticholinergic effects. A TCA (e.g., nortriptyline) would only be used in a low dose early in the algorithm for low back pain and be deferred later in the algorithm for neuropathic pain and fibromyalgia which have more non-TCA evidence-based treatments. Opioids should be started at low doses and titrated slowly, with special attention paid to prevent constipation.

Summary

Pharmacologic approaches to the treatment of chronic pain are vitally important but in general should be coupled with nonpharmacologic approaches as well. Nonpharmacologic approaches include: physical medicine, behavioral medicine, neuromodulation, interventional, surgical, and complementary and alternative medicine approaches. Pharmacologic analgesic agents may include: acetaminophen, traditional NSAIDs, COX-2 selective inhibitors, tramadol, opioids (e.g., morphine, hydrocodone/acetaminophen, oxycodone, hydromorphone, fentanyl, oxymorphone, bupenorphine, methadone, tapentadol), calcium channel alpha-2 delta ligands, skeletal relaxants (baclofen, tizanidine, cyclobenzaprine, metaxalone, methocarbamol, orphenadrine), topical analgesics (lidocaine 5% patch, capsaicin/high concentration capsaicin patch, topical NSAIDs), and BTXs.

A greater appreciation of the individual patient's comorbidities/organ reserves, metabolic machinery, the pharmacokinetic/pharmacodynamic properties and adverse effects of specific analgesic agents, and the levels of evidence for the clinical use of various pharmacologic agents in various clinical painful conditions should hopefully lead to optimal patient outcomes maximizing analgesia and minimizing adverse effects.

References

Adams, E. H., Breiner, S., Cicero, T. J., et al. (2006). A comparison of abuse liability of tramadol, NSAIDs and hydrocodone in patients with chronic pain. *Journal of Pain and Symptom Management, 31*, 465–476.

Arnold, L. M., Goldenberg, D. L., Stanford, S. B., et al. (2007). Gabapentin in the treatment of fibromyalgia: A randomized, double-blind, placebo-controlled, multicenter trial. *Arthritis and Rheumatism, 56*, 1336–1344.

Arnold, L. M., Keck, P. E., Jr., & Welge, J. A. (2000). Antidepressant treatment of fibromyalgia. A metaanalysis and review. *Psychosomatics, 41*, 104–113.

Backonja, M. M., Malan, T. P., Vanhove, G. F., et al. (2010). NGX-4010, a high-concentration capsaicin patch, for the treatment of postherpetic neuralgia: A randomized, double-blind, controlled study with an open-label extension. *Pain Medicine, 11*, 600–608.

Backonja, M. M., Wallace, M. S., Blonsky, E. R., et al. (2008). NGX-4010, a high-concentration capsaicin patch, for the treatment of postherpetic neuralgia: A randomized, double-blind, controlled study. *Lancet Neurology, 7*, 1106–1112.

Baraf, H. S., Gloth, F. M., Barthel, H. R., et al. (2011). Safety and efficacy of topical diclofenac sodium gel for knee osteoarthritis in elderly and younger patients: Pooled data from three randomized, double-blind, parallel-group, placebo-controlled, multicentre trials. *Drugs & Aging, 28*, 27–40.

Barden, J., Derry, S., McQuay, H. J., et al. (2009). Single dose oral ketoprofen and dexketoprofen for acute postoperative pain in adults. *Cochrane Database Systemic Reviews,* (4), CD007355.

Bennett, R. M., Kamin, M., Karim, R., et al. (2003). Tramadol and acetaminophen combination tablets in the treatment of fibromyalgia pain: A double-blind, randomized, placebo-controlled study. *The American Journal of Medicine, 114*, 537–545.

Bockbrader, H. N., Wesche, D., Miller, R., et al. (2010). A comparison of the pharmacokinetics and pharmacodynamics of pregabalin and gabapentin. *Clinical Pharmacokinetics, 49*, 661–669.

Butler, S. F., Budman, S. H., Fernandez, K., et al. (2007). Development and validation of the Current Opioid Misuse Measure. *Pain, 130*, 114–156.

Butler, S. F., Fernandez, K., Benoit, C., et al. (2008). Validation of the revised Screener and Opioid Assessment for Patients with Pain (SOAPP-R). *The Journal of Pain, 9*(4), 360–372.

Case, J. P., Baliunas, A. J., & Black, J. A. (2003). Lack of efficacy of acetaminophen in treating symptomatic knee osteoarthritis: A randomized, double-blind, placebo controlled comparison trial with diclofenac sodium. *Archives of Internal Medicine, 163*, 169e78.

Chou, R., Peterson, K., & Helfand, M. (2004). Comparative efficacy and safety of skeletal muscle relaxants for spasticity and musculoskeletal conditions: A systematic review. *Journal of Pain and Symptom Management, 28*, 140–175.

Christo, P. J., Manchikanti, L., Ruan, X., et al. (2011). Urine drug testing in chronic pain. *Pain Physician, 14*, 123–143.

Cone, E. J., Heit, H. A., Caplan, Y. H., et al. (2006). Evidence of morphine metabolism to hydromorphone in pain patients chronically treated with morphine. *Journal of Analytical Toxicology, 30*, 1–5.

Dart, R. C., & Bailey, E. (2007). Does therapeutic use of acetaminophen cause acute liver failure? *Pharmacotherapy, 27*, 1219–1230.

Davies, P. S., & Galer, B. S. (2004). Review of lidocaine patch 5% studies in the treatment of postherpetic neuralgia. *Drugs, 64*, 937–947.

Deer, T., Krames, E. S., Hassenbusch, S. J., et al. (2007). Polyanalgesic consensus conference 2007: Recommendations for the management of pain by intrathecal (intraspinal) drug delivery: Report of an interdisciplinary expert panel. *Neuromodulation, 10*, 300–328.

Derry, S., Lloyd, R., Moore, R. A., et al. (2009). Topical capsaicin for chronic neuropathic pain in adults. *Cochrane Database Systemic Reviews,* (4), CD007393.

Deshpande, A., Furlan, A., Mailis-Gagnon, A., et al. (2007). Opioids for chronic low-back pain. *Cochrane Database Systemic Reviews,* (3), CD004959.

Dwight, M. M., Arnold, L. M., O'Brien, H., et al. (1998). An open clinical trial of venlafaxine treatment of fibromyalgia. *Psychosomatics, 39*, 14–17.

Dworkin, R. H., O'Connor, A. B., Backonja, M., et al. (2007). Pharmacologic management of neuropathic pain: Evidence based recommendation. *Pain, 132*, 237–251.

Eisenberg, E., McNicol, E. D., & Carr, D. B. (2005). Efficacy and safety of opioid agonists in the treatment of neuropathic pain of nonmalignant origin: Systematic review and meta-analysis trials. *Journal of American Medical Association, 293*, 3043–3052.

Fine, P. G., & Portenoy, R. K. (2007). Initiating and optimizing opioid therapy. In P. Fine (Ed.), *A clinical guide to opioid analgesia.* New York: Vendome Group, LLC.

Finnerup, N. B., & Jensen, T. S. (2007). Clinical use of pregabalin in the management of central neuropathic pain. *Neuropsychiatric Disease and Treatment, 3*, 885–891.

Finnerup, N. B., Otto, M., Jensen, T. S., et al. (2007). An evidence-based algorithm for the treatment of neuropathic pain. *MedGenMed, 9*, 36.

Finnerup, N. B., Otto, M., McQuay, H. J., et al. (2005). Algorithm for neuropathic pain treatment: An evidence based proposal. *Pain, 118*, 289–305.

Finnerup, N. B., Sindrup, S. H., & Jensen, T. S. (2010). The evidence for pharmacological treatment of neuropathic pain. *Pain, 150*, 573–581.

Fishman, S. M., Mahajan, G., Jung, S. W., et al. (2002). The trilateral opioid contract. Bridging the pain clinic and the primary care physician through the opioid contract. *Journal of Pain and Symptom Management, 24*, 335–344.

Furlan, A. D., Sandoval, J. A., Mailis-Gagnon, A., et al. (2006). Opioids for chronic noncancer pain: A meta-analysis of effectiveness and side effects. *Canadian Medical Association Journal, 174*, 1589–1594.

Galer, B. S., Rowbotham, M., Perander, J., et al. (2000). Topical diclofenac patch relieves minor sports injury pain: Results of a multicenter controlled clinical trial. *Journal of Pain and Symptom Management, 19*, 287–294.

Garcia Roderiguez, L. A., & Hernandez-Diaz, S. (2001). Risk of upper gastrointestinal complications among users of acetaminophen and non-steroidal anti-inflammatory drugs. *Epidemiology, 12*, 570e6.

Gourlay, D., & Heit, H. A. (2006). Universal precautions: A matter of mutual trust and responsibility. *Pain Medicine, 7*, 210–211.

Gourlay, D. L., & Heit, H. A. (2005). Universal precautions in pain medicine: A rational approach to the treatment of chronic pain. *Pain Medicine, 6*, 107–112.

Häuser, W., Bernardy, K., Uçeyler, N., et al. (2009). Treatment of fibromyalgia syndrome with antidepressants: A meta-analysis. *Journal of American Medical Association, 301*, 198–209.

Häuser, W., Petzke, F., Üçeyler, N., et al. (2011). Comparative efficacy and acceptability of amitriptyline, duloxetine and milnacipran in fibromyalgia syndrome: A systematic review with meta-analysis. *Rheumatology (Oxford, England), 50*, 532–543.

Heard, K., Green, J. L., Bailey, J. E., et al. (2007). A randomized trial to determine the change in alanine aminotransferase during 10 days of paracetamol (acetaminophen) administration in subjects who consume moderate amounts of alcohol. *Alimentary Pharmacology & Therapeutics, 26*, 283–290.

Heit, H. A., & Gourlay, D. L. (2004). Urine drug testing in pain medicine. *Journal of Pain and Symptom Management, 27*, 260–267.

Irving, G. A., Backonja, M. M., Dunteman, E., et al. (2011). A multicenter, randomized, double-blind, controlled study of NGX-4010, a high-concentration capsaicin patch, for the treatment of postherpetic neuralgia. *Pain Medicine, 12*, 99–109.

Jalan, R., Williams, R., & Bernuau, J. (2006). Paracetamol: Are therapeutic doses entirely safe? *The Lancet, 368*, 2195–2196.

Jirarattanaphochai, K., & Jung, S. (2008). Nonsteroidal antiinflammatory drugs for postoperative pain management after lumbar spine surgery: A meta-analysis of randomized controlled trials. *Journal of Neurosurgery. Spine, 9*, 22–31.

Joint Commission on the Accreditation of Healthcare Organizations. (1999). Patient rights and organization ethics. Referenced from the comprehensive accreditation manual for hospitals, update 3, 1999. Walter Reed Army Medical Center Web site. Retrieved July 5, 2007, from http://www.wramc.army.mil/JCAHO/Division.cfm?D_Id+1

Joint statement from 21 health organizations and the Drug Enforcement Administration. Promoting pain relief and preventing abuse of pain medications: A critical balancing act. Biomedical Computing Group, University of Wisconsin Medical School Web site. Retrieved August 4, 2004, from http://www.medsch.wisc.edu/painpolicy/Consensus2.pdf

Jones, P., & Lamdin, R. (2010). Oral cyclo-oxygenase 2 inhibitors versus other oral analgesics for acute soft tissue injury: Systematic review and meta-analysis. *Clinical Drug Investigation, 30*, 419–437.

Jones, V. W., Moore, K. A., & Peterson, D. M. (2011). Capsaicin 8% topical patch (qutenza) – a review of the evidence. *Journal of Pain & Palliative Care Pharmacotherapy, 25*, 32–41.

Jordan, K. M., Arden, N. K., Doherty, M., et al. (2003). EULAR recommendations 2003: An evidence based approach to the management of knee osteoarthritis: Report of a Task Force of the Standing Committee for International Clinical Studies Including Therapeutic Trials (ESCISIT). *Annals of the Rheumatic Diseases, 62*, 1145e55.

Kalso, E., Edwards, J. E., Moore, R. A., et al. (2004). Opioids in chronic non-cancer pain: A systematic review of efficacy and safety. *Pain, 112*, 372–380.

Katz, N. (2002). The impact of pain management on quality of life. *Journal of Pain and Symptom Management, 24*, S38–S47.

Katz, N., & Fanciullo, G. (2002). Role of urine toxicology testing in the management of chronic opioid therapy. *The Clinical Journal of Pain, 18*, 576–582.

Kearney, P. M., Baigent, C., Godwin, J., et al. (2006). Do selective cyclo-oxygenase inhibitors and traditional non-steroidal anti-inflammatory drugs increase the risk of atherothrombosis? Meta-analysis of randomised trials. *British Medical Journal, 332*, 1302e8.

Khaliq, W., Alam, S., Puri, N. (2007). Topical lidocaine for the treatment of postherpetic neuralgia. *Cochrane Database Systemic Reviews, 18*(2), CD004846.

Kuehl, K. S. (2010). Review of the efficacy and tolerability of the diclofenac epolamine topical patch 1.3% in patients with acute pain due to soft tissue injuries. *Clinical Therapeutics, 32*, 1001–1014.

Kuijpers, T., van Middelkoop, M., Rubinstein, S. M., et al. (2011). A systematic review on the effectiveness of pharmacological interventions for chronic non-specific low-back pain. *European Spine Journal, 20*, 40–50.

Larson, A. M., Polson, J., Fontana, R. J., et al. (2005). Acetaminophen-induced acute liver failure: Results of a United States multicenter, prospective study. *Hepatology, 42*, 1364–1372.

Lee, S. S., Sphn, Y. W., Yoo, E. S., et al. (1991). Neurotoxicity and long lasting analgesia induced by capsaicinoids. *The Journal of Toxicological Sciences, 16*, 3–20.

Marjoribanks, J., Proctor, M., Farquhar, C., et al. (2010). Nonsteroidal anti-inflammatory drugs for dysmenorrhoea. *Cochrane Database Systemic Reviews, 20*(1), CD001751.

Mason, L., Moore, R. A., Derry, S., et al. (2004a). Systematic review of topical capsaicin for the treatment of chronic pain. *British Medical Journal, 328*, 991–994.

Mason, L., Moore, R. A., Edwards, J. E., et al. (2004b). Systematic review of efficacy of topical rubefacients containing salicylates for the treatment of acute and chronic pain. *British Medical Journal, 328*, 995–997.

Massey, T., Derry, S., Moore, R. A., et al. (2010). Topical NSAIDs for acute pain in adults. *Cochrane Database Systemic Reviews, 16*(6), CD007402.

Max, M. B., Payne, R., Edwards, W. T., et al. (1999). *Principles of analgesic use in the treatment of acute pain and cancer pain* (4th ed.). Glenview: American Pain Society.

McCarberg, B., & Cole, B. (2011). Pain in the older person. In R. J. Moore (Ed.), *Handbook of pain and palliative care: Biobehavioral approaches for the life course*. New York: Springer.

McDiarmid, T., & Mackler, L. (2005). What is the addiction risk associated with tramadol? *The Journal of Family Practice, 54*, 72–73.

McNicol, E., Horowicz-Mehler, N., Risk, R., et al. (2003). Management of opioid side effects in cancer related and chronic noncancer pain: A systematic review. *The Journal of Pain, 4*, 231–256.

Mercadante, S., & Bruera, E. (2006). Opioid switching: A systematic and critical review. *Cancer Treatment Reviews, 32*, 304–315.

Moore, R. A., Straube, S., Wiffen, P. J., et al. (2009). Pregabalin for acute and chronic pain in adults. *Cochrane Database Systemic Reviews, 8*(3), CD007076.

Moore, R. A., Wiffen, P. J., Derry, S., et al. (2011). Gabapentin for chronic neuropathic pain and fibromyalgia in adults. *Cochrane Database Systemic Reviews, 16*(3), CD007938.

Nauta, M., Landsmeer, M. L., & Koren, G. (2009). Codeine-acetaminophen versus nonsteroidal anti-inflammatory drugs in the treatment of post-abdominal surgery pain: A systematic review of randomized trials. *The American Journal of Surgery, 198*, 256–261.

Nishishinya, B., Urrútia, G., Walitt, B., et al. (2008). Amitriptyline in the treatment of fibromyalgia: A systematic review of its efficacy. *Rheumatology (Oxford, England), 47*, 1741–1746.

Noble, M., Treadwell, J. R., Tregear, S. J., et al. (2010). Long-term opioid management for chronic noncancer pain. *Cochrane Database Systemic Reviews*, (1), CD006605.

Noto, C., Pappagallo, M., & Szallasi, A. (2009). NGX-4010, a high-concentration capsaicin dermal patch for lasting relief of peripheral neuropathic pain. *Current Opinion in Investigational Drugs, 10*, 702–710.

Nuesch, E., Rutjes, A. W., Husni, E., et al. (2009). Oral or transdermal opioids for osteoarthritis of the knee or hip. *Cochrane Database Systemic Reviews*, (4), CD003115.

O'Malley, P. G., Balden, E., Tomkins, G., Santoro, J., Kroenke, K., & Jackson, J. L. (2000). Treatment of fibromyalgia with antidepressants: A meta-analysis. *Journal of General Internal Medicine, 15*(9), 659–666.

Ottani, A., Leone, S., Sandrini, M., et al. (2006). The analgesic activity of paracetamol is prevented by the blockade of cannabinoid CB1 receptors. *European Journal of Pharmacology, 531*, 280–281.

Oyler, J. M., Cone, E. J., Joseph, R. E., Jr., et al. (2000). Identification of hydrocodone in human urine following controlled codeine administration. *Journal of Analytical Toxicology, 24*, 530–535.

Passik, S. D., & Weinreb, H. I. (2000). Managing chronic nonmalignant pain: Overcoming obstacles to the use of opioids. *Advances in Therapy, 17*, 70–80.

Pesce, A., West, C., Rosenthal, M., et al. (2011). Illicit drug use in the pain patient population decreases with continued drug testing. *Pain Physician, 14*, 189–193.

Quigley, C. (2004). Opioid switching to improve pain relief and drug tolerability. *Cochrane Database Systemic Reviews, 3*, CD004847.

Rabbie, R., Derry, S., Moore, R. A., et al. (2010). Ibuprofen with or without an antiemetic for acute migraine headaches in adults. *Cochrane Database Systemic Reviews*, (10), CD008039.

Raffa, R. B., & Stone, D. J., Jr. (2008). Unexceptional seizure potential of tramadol or its enantiomers or metabolites in mice. *The Journal of Pharmacology and Experimental Therapeutics, 325*, 500–506.

Rahme, E., Pettitt, D., & LeLorier, J. (2002). Determinants and sequelae associated with utilization of acetaminophen versus traditional nonsteroidal anti-inflammatory drugs in an elderly population. *Arthritis and Rheumatism, 46*, 3046e54.

Ranoux, D., Attal, N., Morain, F., et al. (2008). Botulinum toxin type A induces direct analgesic effects in chronic neuropathic pain. *Annals of Neurology, 64*, 274–283.

Raskin, J., Smith, T. R., Wong, K., et al. (2006). Duloxetine versus routine care in the long-term management of diabetic peripheral neuropathic pain. *Journal of Palliative Medicine, 9*, 29–40.

Roelofs, P. D., Deyo, R. A., Koes, B. W., et al. (2008). Nonsteroidal anti-inflammatory drugs for low back pain: An updated Cochrane review. *Spine, 33*, 1766–1774.

Rowbotham, M. C., Twilling, L., Davies, P. S., et al. (2003). Oral opioid therapy for chronic peripheral and central neuropathic pain. *The New England Journal of Medicine, 348*, 1223–1232.

Russell, I. J., Kamin, M., Bennett, R. M., et al. (2000). Efficacy of tramadol in treatment of pain in fibromyalgia. *Journal of Clinical Rheumatology, 6*, 250–257.

Saarto, T., Wiffen, P. J. (2007). Antidepressants for neuropathic pain. *Cochrane Database Systemic Reviews, 17*(4), CD005454.

Sansone, R. A., & Sansone, L. A. (2009). Tramadol: Seizures, serotonin syndrome, and coadministered antidepressants. *Psychiatry (Edgmont), 6*, 17–21.

Simpson, D. M., Brown, S., Tobias, J., et al. (2008). Controlled trial of high-concentration capsaicin patch for treatment of painful HIV neuropathy. *Neurology, 70*, 2305–2313.

Simpson, D. M., Gazda, S., Brown, S., et al. (2010). Long-term safety of NGX-4010, a high-concentration capsaicin patch, in patients with peripheral neuropathic pain. *Journal of Pain and Symptom Management, 39*, 1053–1064.

Sindrup, S. H., Otto, M., Finnerup, N. B., et al. (2005). Antidepressants in the treatment of neuropathic pain. *Basic & Clinical Pharmacology & Toxicology, 96*, 399–409.

Skljarevski, V., Zhang, S., Desaiah, D., et al. (2010). Duloxetine versus placebo in patients with chronic low back pain: A 12-week, fixed-dose, randomized, double-blind trial. *The Journal of Pain, 11*, 1282–1290.

Smith, H. S. (2006). Goal-directed therapy agreements. *Journal of Cancer Pain & Symptom Palliation, 1*, 11–13.

Smith, H. S. (2007). Antidepressants: Classifications and implications for pain modulation. In Presented at the capital district pain research conference, Albany, NY.

Smith, H. S. (2008). Pre-opioid prescribing period. In H. S. Smith (Ed.), *Opioid therapy in the 21st century*. New York: Oxford University Press.

Smith, H. S. (2009). Potential analgesic mechanisms of acetaminophen. *Pain Physician, 12*, 269–280.

Stacey, B. R., Barett, J. A., Whalen, E., et al. (2008). Pregabalin for postherpetic neuralgia: Placebo controlled trial of fixed and flexible dosage regimens on allodynia and time to onset of pain relief. *The Journal of Pain, 9*, 1006–1017.

Temple, A. R., Lynch, J. M., Vena, J., et al. (2007). Aminotransferase activities in healthy subjects receiving three-day dosing of 4, 6, or 8 grams per day of acetaminophen. *Clinical Toxicology (Philadelphia), 45*, 36–44.

Tofferi, J. K., Jackson, J. L., & O'Malley, P. G. (2004). Treatment of fibromyalgia with cyclobenzaprine: A meta-analysis. *Arthritis and Rheumatism, 51*, 9–13.

Towheed, T. E. (2006). Pennsaid therapy for osteoarthritis of the knee: A systematic review and metaanalysis of randomized controlled trials. *The Journal of Rheumatology, 33*, 567–573.

Towheed, T. E., Maxwell, L., Judd, M. G., et al. (2006). Acetaminophen for osteoarthritis. *Cochrane Database Systemic Reviews,* (1), CD004257.

Tramer, M. R., Moore, R. A., Reynolds, D. J., et al. (2000). Quantitative estimation of rare adverse events which follow a biological progression: A new model applied to chronic NSAID use. *Pain, 85*, 169e82.

Vandevenne, M., Vandenbussche, H., & Verstraete, A. (2000). Detection time of drugs of abuse in urine. *Acta Clinica Belgica, 55*, 323–333.

Velly, A. M., Chen, H., Ferreira, J. R., & Friction, J. R. (2011). Temporomandibular disorders and fibromyalgia. In R. J. Moore (Ed.), *Handbook of pain and palliative care: Biobehavioral approaches for the life course*. New York: Springer.

Wade, W. E., & Spruill, W. J. (2009). Tapentadol hydrochloride: A centrally acting oral analgesic. *Clinical Therapeutics, 31*, 2804–2818.

Watkins, P. B., Kaplowitz, N., Slattery, J. T., et al. (2006). Aminotransferase elevations in healthy adults receiving 4 grams of acetaminophen daily: A randomized controlled trial. *Journal of American Medical Association, 296*, 87–93.

Webster, L. R., Malan, T. P., Tuchman, M. M., et al. (2010). A multicenter, randomized, double-blind, controlled dose finding study of NGX-4010, a high-concentration capsaicin patch, for the treatment of postherpetic neuralgia. *The Journal of Pain, 11*, 972–982.

Webster, L. R., & Webster, R. M. (2005). Predicting aberrant behaviors in opioid-treated patients: Preliminary validation of the Opioid Risk Tool. *Pain Medicine, 6*, 432–442.

Wiffen, P. J., McQuay, H. J., Edwards, J. E., et al. (2005). Gabapentin for acute and chronic pain. *Cochrane Database Systemic Reviews, 20*(3), CD005452.

World Health Organization. (2000). *Achieving balance in national opioids control policy: Guidelines for assessment.* Geneva: WHO.

Xiao, L., Mackey, S., Hui, H., et al. (2010). Subcutaneous injection of botulinum toxin a is beneficial in postherpetic neuralgia. *Pain Medicine, 11*, 1827–1833.

Zacny, J., Bigelow, G., Compton, P., et al. (2003). College on problems of drug dependence taskforce on prescription opioid non-medical use and abuse: Position statement. *Drug and Alcohol Dependence, 69*, 215–232.

Zhang, W., Doherty, M., Arden, N., et al. (2005). EULAR evidence based recommendations for the management of hip osteoarthritis: Report of a task force of the EULAR Standing Committee for International Clinical Studies Including Therapeutics (ESCISIT). *Annals of the Rheumatic Diseases, 64*, 669e81.

Zhang, W., Moskowitz, R. W., Nuki, G., et al. (2007). OARSI recommendations for the management of hip and knee osteoarthritis, Part I: Critical appraisal of existing treatment guidelines and systematic review of current research evidence. *Osteoarthritis and Cartilage, 15*, 981e1000.

Chapter 29
Chronic Pain and Opioids

Regina P. Szucs-Reed and Rollin M. Gallagher

Introduction

Chronic pain conditions are common and potentially disabling disorders, and it is estimated that between one-third and one-half of adults live with some form of daily or recurrent pain (Elliott et al. 1999). The *International Association for the Study of Pain* defines chronic pain as "pain that persists beyond normal tissue healing time, which is assumed to be three months" (Pain IAftSo 1986). Chronic pain conditions are rarely cured, and thus the focus becomes management in a chronic disease model. There are two main classifications of chronic pain: (1) nociceptive pain, which results from an injury or disease process that activates nociceptors (pain receptors) or (2) neuropathic pain, which results from injury to the central or peripheral nervous system. Pain has also traditionally been subdivided into pain associated with cancer or at the end of life and chronic non-cancer pain (CNCP), which is the focus of this chapter. The scope of CNCP is highlighted by the variety of conditions or syndromes associated with either nociceptive or neuropathic pain, including back pain, osteoarthritis, fibromyalgia, headache, and diabetic neuropathy. These disorders account for large costs to society. Low back pain, the most common of these conditions (Reid et al. 2002), alone has been estimated to account for $100 billion in health care expenditures in 2005 (Martin et al. 2008).

There is clearly a need for adequate treatment of the diverse and costly conditions associated with CNCP. Many of these treatments are covered in other chapters in this text. Opioid analgesics are widely accepted for the treatment of severe acute pain and chronic cancer-related pain, but until 1980, medical opinion held that opioids were not indicated for the treatment of CNCP (Jovey et al. 2003). Their use in CNCP remains more controversial than use in acute and cancer-related pain, but it has been acknowledged that opioid therapy may be a useful component of a treatment plan for CNCP (Jovey et al. 2003; Chou et al. 2009). However, opioid analgesics carry significant risks for adverse effects, including those that emerge with long-term therapy, as well as risks for abuse and dependence. The number of opioid prescriptions has increased dramatically over the past 20 years (Caudill-Slosberg et al. 2004; Olsen et al. 2006), a trend which has been accompanied by an increase in opioid misuse and mortality associated with opioid use (Office of Applied Studies SAaMHSA 2005). The risks and benefits of opioid therapy must be weighed for each patient, and there is

R.P. Szucs-Reed, MD, PhD (✉)
Penn Presbyterian Medical center, University of Pennsylvania, Philadelphia, PA, USA
e-mail: regina.szucs@uphs.upenn.edu

R.M. Gallagher, MD, MPH
Penn Pain Medicine Center, University of Pennsylvania, Philadelphia, PA, USA

R.J. Moore (ed.), *Handbook of Pain and Palliative Care: Biobehavioral Approaches for the Life Course*, 497
DOI 10.1007/978-1-4419-1651-8_29, © Springer Science+Business Media, LLC 2012

evidence that patients experience better outcomes if opioids are prescribed in a structured setting as part of a comprehensive treatment plan incorporating strategies to improve function and address psychosocial factors associated with CNCP (Nicholas et al. 2006; Wiedemer et al. 2007; Gallagher 2004).

History of Opioids

The analgesic properties of opioids have been known for millennia. The ancient Sumerians in Mesopotamia were among the first people to cultivate the poppy plant around 3,400 BC. They named it Hul Gil, or "the joy plant" (Booth 1986). It eventually spread to other civilizations in Europe and Asia and was used to treat pain and other ailments (Booth 1986; Askitopoulou et al. 2002; Dikotter et al. 2004). In 1680, Thomas Sydenham introduced laudanum, or the mixture of opium with sherry, which was used for pain relief (Meldrum 2003). In 1804, Friedrich Sertürner extracted morphine from crude opium (Schmitz 1985). Opium and alcohol-based compounds were unregulated and available over the counter during the nineteenth century (Meldrum 2003). In 1898, the Bayer company developed diacetylmorphine under the trade name Heroin as a cough remedy. By 1910, young Americans were crushing the pills into powder to achieve a euphoric effect. The spread of Heroin street use helped to generate support for the Harrison Narcotic Control Act, which passed in 1914 (Meldrum 2003). During most of the twentieth century, the U.S. medical profession widely believed that long-term use of opioids to treat CNCP was contraindicated due to the risk of addiction, increased disability, and lack of efficacy over time (Rosenblum et al. 2008). During the 1990s, the use of opioids for CNCP began to rise, and continues to increase (Rosenblum et al. 2008).

Pharmacology

Most of our knowledge about the use of opioids to treat pain has come from studies of patients with pain due to cancer; however, more recent studies suggest that the pharmacodynamic and pharmacokinetic properties of opioids derived from studies of cancer patients can be safely extended to those with CNCP (Inturrisi 2002) (see also Smith et al. 2011). Most of the available opioid analgesics act as agonists at one or more of three classical opioid receptor types (Guststein and Akil 2006): mu (μ), delta (δ) and kappa (κ). Three major classes of opioid peptides serve as the endogenous ligands for these receptors: endorphins (at μ receptos), enkephalins (at δ receptors) and dynorphin (at κ receptors). Stimulation of all three receptor types can contribute to analgesia (reviewed in Inturrisi 2002; Trescot et al. 2008). Different profiles of efficacy and adverse effects among the different opioid drugs may be related to differential affinity and intrinsic activity at the three main opioid receptors as well as non-opioid receptors. Pure μ opioid receptor agonists are generally the most effective analgesics. Most opioids are metabolized by glucuronidation or by the cytochrome P450 (CYP) system (Trescot et al. 2008), and thus, the metabolism of these compounds may be subject to individual variation. There is also evidence that a polymorphism in the μ-opioid receptor gene (OPRM1) encoding the μ opioid receptor may contribute to individual variation in opioid sensitivity, including opioid analgesia, tolerance, and dependence (Han et al. 2004). Indeed, individual variation in the response to different opioid analgesics has been reported, such that certain patients were able to achieve successful treatment with one opioid, but experienced intolerable side effects without sufficient analgesia with others (Galer et al. 1992).

Terminology

Some clinicians encounter confusion over the terminology of opioid analgesics. The term *opioid* is used to describe all compounds that bind to opioid receptors. The term *opiate* is more specific and refers only to those opioids that are alkaloids derived from the opium poppy (such as morphine and codeine). Thus, *opioids* include the *opiates* plus synthetic compounds (e.g., methadone and fentanyl) and semisynthetic compounds (e.g., heroin and oxycodone). The term *narcotic* is a legal rather than a clinical designation, and includes opioids and other drugs that are grouped with opioids by law enforcement.

Pharmacology of Commonly Prescribed Opioids

Morphine

Morphine is a full agonist at the μ opioid receptor. After oral administration, 40–50% of the administered dose reaches the central nervous system, within 30 min for the immediate-release preparation, and within 90 min for the delayed-release preparation (Stoelting 1991). The elimination half-life of morphine is 2–3.5 h, which is shorter than the duration of analgesia (for the immediate-release preparation). In addition to the immediate-release oral preparation, controlled-, extended-, and sustained-release preparations are available, which can be dosed between every 8 h and every 24 h. Morphine is metabolized to normorphine, and in small quantities it is also metabolized to hydromorphone. Hydromorphone is present in the urine of 66% of patients taking morphine, though this metabolite is usually observed at morphine doses higher than 100 mg daily (Wasan et al. 2006). These multiple metabolic pathways leading to various metabolites may confuse the interpretation of laboratory testing; thus, clinicians should be aware of the pathways of morphine metabolism.

Codeine

Codeine is an opioid analgesic with only weak affinity for the μ opioid receptor, and it is available either alone or in combination with non-opioid analgesics. Its elimination half-life is 2.5–3 h. Onset of analgesic action occurs within 30 min to 1 h following oral codeine, and its duration of action is 4–6 h. Codeine is a pro-drug; it is believed that its analgesic efficacy results from its metabolism to morphine. Thus, codeine may not be an effective analgesic in all populations due to heterogeneity in CYP enzymes leading to reduced conversion of codeine to morphine in some individuals.

Hydrocodone

Hydrocodone is the most commonly prescribed opioid. Like codeine, hydrocodone has weak affinity for the μ opioid receptor, and it is available either alone or in combination with non-opioid analgesics such as acetaminophen or ibuprofen. The half-life of hydrocodone is 2.5–4 h. Onset of action is between 10 and 20 min, and the duration of analgesic action is 6 h. It has also been proposed that hydrocodone is a pro-drug, as it is metabolized by CYP2D6 to hydromorphone, which has higher affinity for the μ opioid receptor.

Oxycodone

Oxycodone is active at multiple opioid receptors, including the κ receptor. It is available in both immediate-release and controlled-release preparations, and is also available at lower doses in combination with non-opioid analgesics. The OxyContin controlled-release preparation provides a biphasic absorption profile such that approximately 30–40% of the dose is released immediately, while a second component is released over approximately 12 h (Amabile and Bowman 2006). The elimination half-life of immediate-release oxycodone is 2–3 h, while for controlled-release preparations the half-life is approximately 5 h. The duration of analgesic action is 3–6 h for immediate-release preparations, and the duration of analgesia for controlled-release oxycodone is 8–12 h. Onset of action of immediate-release oxycodone is approximately 10–15 min.

Fentanyl

Fentanyl is a very potent and highly lipophilic opioid agonist. It undergoes extensive metabolism in the liver, and it is available in parenteral, transdermal, and transbuccal preparations. The most common preparation used in patients with CNCP is transdermal. Onset of action of the transdermal formulation occurs within 6–12 h after application, and its half-life is approximately 3–4 h (Trescot et al. 2008). For most patients, administration every 72 h controls pain, though some patients require dosing every 48 h. Transdermal fentanyl creates a subcutaneous reservoir; after discontinuation, approximately 17 h are required for a 50% reduction in fentanyl levels.

Methadone

Methadone is a synthetic μ opioid receptor agonist that is perhaps best known for its role in the treatment of opioid dependence. It is a racemic mixture of two enantiomers; the R enantiomer is a more potent μ opioid receptor agonist, while the S enantiomer acts as an N-methyl-D-aspartate (NMDA) receptor antagonist and inhibits the reuptake of serotonin and norepinephrine. The NMDA receptor antagonist properties of methadone make it potentially useful in the treatment of severe neuropathic pain, or in patients who do not respond to other opioids. It has also been suggested that NMDA receptor blockade may prevent opioid tolerance (Inturrisi 2002). Methadone has excellent, though highly variable oral bioavailability (ranging from 40 to 100%). It has a long half-life, which is also variable and generally estimated as ranging between 12 and 50 h, although its half-life has been reported to be as long as 120 h (Lynch 2005). However, the duration analgesic action of methadone is only 4–8 h (Inturrisi 2002). Cross-tolerance between methadone and morphine appears incomplete, such that patients receiving the highest doses of morphine are more sensitive to the effects of methadone, thus complicating the calculating of an equianalgesic dose when switching to methadone (Foley and Houde 1998). Methadone can induce the CYP3A4 enzyme for 5–7 days after initiation of therapy, which can lead to low initial blood levels, but unexpectedly high levels a week later if titration occurs rapidly. Thus, care must be taken in the titration of methadone and in patient education to prevent unintentional overdose. For example, evidence-based clinical guidelines from the Departments of Defense and Veterans Affairs health systems recommend waiting at least a week between dose increases when titrating methadone to effectiveness (The Management of Opioid Therapy for Chronic pain Working Group 2010).

Buprenorphine

Buprenorphine is approved for the treatment of opioid dependence, and it is probably best known in this capacity. However, there is also evidence that it can be effective in the treatment of pain (Rosenblum et al. 2008; Heit and Gourlay 2008; Vadivelu and Hines 2007). Buprenorphine is a unique drug in many ways. It is a semisynthetic opioid with partial agonist effects at the μ opioid receptor and antagonist effects at the κ opioid receptor. Due to the partial agonist properties of buprenorphine at the μ opioid receptor, it may block the effects of full μ opioid receptor agonists. It has low oral bioavailability due to extensive first-pass metabolism, but good absorption sublingually. Buprenorphine is primarily metabolized to inactive conjugated metabolites (Heit and Gourlay 2008). However, the metabolite norbuprenorphine is noted to have more potent respiratory depressive effects than the parent compound (Ohtani et al. 1995, 1997). Buprenorphine is available in the U.S. as a sublingual preparation with or without added naloxone; some other preparations have also recently been approved. The rationale behind the addition of naloxone is to prevent diversion in patients who attempt to crush and inject the drug. A transdermal formulation is available in Europe for the treatment of chronic pain (Griessinger et al. 2005), and has recently been approved for the same indication in the U.S. While buprenorphine is generally administered once daily when used to treat opioid dependence, it has been suggested that it may be necessary to administer sublingual buprenorphine 3 or 4 times daily if it is used off-label to treat pain (Heit and Gourlay 2008). The status of buprenorphine as a μ opioid receptor partial agonist may increase its safety profile, and makes it a potentially attractive medication to treat CNCP in patients with addictive disorders. Future studies would be beneficial in characterizing the optimal use of buprenorphine to treat CNCP.

Tramadol

Tramadol has modest affinity for the μ opioid receptor, and also acts as a serotonin and norepinephrine reuptake inhibitor. Like methadone, it is a racemic mixture of two enantiomers, which have differing profiles at μ opioid receptors and serotonin and norepinephrine transporters (Raffa et al. 1992). One of the metabolites of tramadol (M1) has been reported to have approximately 700-fold higher affinity for the μ opioid receptor than the parent compound, racemic tramadol (Gillen et al. 2000). A portion the analgesic action of tramadol appears result from stimulation of μ opioid receptors; however, the effects of tramadol are not completely reversed by naloxone (Grond and Sablotzki 2004). The antinociceptive properties of tramadol are thought to be multimodal (Grond and Sablotzki 2004), and thus tramadol has been classified as a non-traditional centrally acting analgesic. The half-life of tramadol is approximately 6–8 h. It is available in both immediate-release and extended-release formulations; immediate-release tramadol is usually administered every 4–6 h, while the extended-release preparation is usually administered daily. Toxic doses can cause CNS excitation and seizures; thus, unlike most opioid analgesics, maximum daily doses exist for tramadol. The daily dose should not exceed 400 mg for immediate-release tramadol, and should not exceed 300 mg for most extended-release preparations. Potentially important drug interactions with tramadol are discussed below in section "Adverse Effects and Drug Interactions Related to Specific Opioids." Tramadol is a non-scheduled drug federally, although some states have classified it as a schedule IV drug. Tramadol is generally reported to have lower abuse potential than more conventional opioid analgesics (Epstein et al. 2006), although its abuse liability is not zero (Epstein et al. 2006; Tjaderborn et al. 2009). Thus, tramadol may be a good choice for patients with a history of substance abuse; clinicians should continue to exercise caution when prescribing an agent with any degree of abuse liability to this patient population.

Imaging Studies

Neuroimaging studies have investigated the mechanisms of chronic pain and the actions of opioids. A detailed review of imaging studies related to pain is provided in Chap. 18 of this book; here we briefly review studies related to CNCP and the actions of opioids. Various CNCP conditions have been shown to produce alterations in brain structure and function. In one study, chronic back pain patients exhibited 5–11% less cortical gray matter volume than control subjects, a reduction equivalent to the gray matter volume lost in 10–20 years of normal aging (Apkarian et al. 2004). Another study showed decreased white matter integrity in patients with disabling chronic low back pain as compared with patients with non-disabling low back pain (Buckalew et al. 2010). Functional studies have highlighted the commonalities in brain regions implicated in chronic pain and emotions. For example, chronic osteoarthritic knee pain (as compared with experimental knee pain) was associated with increased activity in several brain regions that are implicated in emotional processing: the cingulate cortex, thalamus, and amygdala (Kulkarni et al. 2007). Another study showed that activation of the medial prefrontal cortex [including the rostral anterior cingulate cortex (ACC)] was strongly related to the intensity of chronic back pain (Baliki et al. 2006). Furthermore, in patients with fibromyalgia, the degree of depression was observed to be related to activation in the amygdala and anterior insula during experimental pain (Giesecke et al. 2005). It is intriguing that variation in the OPRM1 is associated with differential sensitivity to social rejection, which was accompanied by differential activation in two areas implicated in chronic pain: the dorsal ACC and anterior insula (Way et al. 2009), thus highlighting the relationships between pain, emotional processing, and the opioid system.

Most of our knowledge of the actions of opioids in the brain comes from studies of patients with opioid addiction. In these patients, opioids and visual stimuli related to opioids have been found to increase activation in parts of the brain reward circuitry, including the midbrain, anterior insula, and ACC (Sell et al. 1999). These increases in brain activation may relate to the abuse liability of opioid analgesics. In another study, opioid cue-induced increases in activation in the amygdala, hippocampus, and insula were acutely reduced by administration of the daily methadone dose in methadone-maintained patients (Langleben et al. 2008), suggesting that opioids can modulate brain activity in these regions. It is also interesting to note that the endogenous opioid system has been implicated in placebo analgesia (Lidstone and Stoessl 2007). Future studies are needed to directly investigate the effects of chronic opioid therapy on the brain in CNCP patients.

Benefits of Opioids in CNCP

As discussed above, the analgesic properties of opioids have long been known. Though the use of opioid analgesics has been better studied in the treatment of acute and cancer-related pain (Gordon et al. 2004; Trescot 2010), recent guidelines in the U.S. and Canada have recommended the use of opioids in the treatment of CNCP in certain cases (Jovey et al. 2003; Chou et al. 2009; The Management of Opioid Therapy for Chronic pain Working Group 2010). The negative impact of chronic pain on patients' lives, emerging evidence for long-term brain changes resulting from CNCP (Apkarian et al. 2004; Buckalew et al. 2010; Baliki et al. 2008; Tracey and Bushnell 2009), and the public health costs of pain argue for effective treatment of CNCP. The use of opioid analgesics in CNCP may be appropriate if the pain condition would not be treated more effectively with non-opioid therapy, or if there is no evidence for the availability of specific, curative interventions for the pain condition. Furthermore, as with all medications, a trial of opioid analgesics for CNCP should be undertaken only if the benefits of therapy are likely to outweigh the risks, and if there is no alternative therapy with a more favorable balance of benefits to harms.

Case series and randomized controlled trials have provided evidence that opioids can provide significant pain relief, improved function, and improved quality of life in CNCP (Jovey et al. 2003; Furlan et al. 2006; Kalso et al. 2004). Some of these studies differentiated more-or-less homogeneous groups such as neuropathic type (e.g., diabetic neuropathy), nociceptive type (e.g., osteoarthritis) or non-specific regional type (e.g., low back pain). One study reports that the number of patients needed to treat (NNT) to find one that responds to opioid therapy with at least a 50% reduction in pain was 2.7 (Raja et al. 2002), which is superior to the NNT reported for other analgesics (e.g., the NNT for tricyclic antidepressants was 4.0 (Raja et al. 2002), for capsaicin it was 5.3 (Sindrup and Jensen 1999), and for gabapentin it has been reported at either 3.2 (Rowbotham et al. 1998) or 5.0 (Rice and Maton 2001)). In a systematic review of randomized placebo-controlled trials of opioid therapy for CNCP, Kalso et al. (2004) report that the mean pain relief with opioid therapy was 30%. Another systematic review reports a similar average change from baseline in pain intensity of 27.8% (Bloodworth 2005). In a meta-analysis of randomized controlled trials of opioid therapy for CNCP, Furlan et al. (2006) report that opioids were superior to placebo in alleviating pain and improving functional outcomes. Furthermore, another structured review concluded that chronic opioid therapy can lead to significant functional improvement (Devulder et al. 2005). However, others did not observe improvement in various functional measures with opioid therapy (Caldwell et al. 2002; Gimbel et al. 2003; Moulin et al. 1996).

Others have reported lower levels of analgesia with opioid therapy for CNCP, which are similar to levels of pain relief obtained with non-opioid analgesics (pain relief of 8–12/100 units; Stein et al. 2010). Concerns have also been raised that the duration of most studies investigating opioid therapy for CNCP is not sufficient to properly evaluate long-term opioid therapy for these conditions (Furlan et al. 2006; Stein et al. 2010; Chapman et al. 2010). Thus, future studies evaluating the long-term effects of chronic opioid therapy would benefit clinical decision-making.

It is difficult to predict which individual patients will respond best to opioid therapy. Although it was previously believed that neuropathic pain does not respond to opioids (Arner and Meyerson 1988) recent studies indicate that both neuropathic and nociceptive pain conditions appear to respond to chronic opioid therapy (Furlan et al. 2006; Kalso et al. 2004). However, it has been suggested that neuropathic pain may require higher doses of opioids or the addition of adjuvant analgesics (Jovey et al. 2003). Randomized trials indicate that chronic opioid therapy may be more appropriate for patients with moderate or severe pain who have not responded to non-opioid therapies (Furlan et al. 2006; Kalso et al. 2004). The presence of poorly defined pain conditions, a probable somatoform disorder, or unresolved compensation or legal issues may predict poorer response to all therapies, including opioid analgesics (Pincus et al. 2002; Rohling et al. 1995). Perhaps the best-studied specific conditions associated with CNCP are osteoarthritis, back pain, and neuropathic pain (Caldwell et al. 1999; Dellemijn and Vanneste 1997; Jamison et al. 1998; Schnitzer et al. 2000; Watson et al. 2003), and it has been suggested that opioids may be preferentially effective for the treatment of pain associated with these conditions than other CNCP conditions (Stein et al. 2010). It is also possible that certain specific opioid analgesics may be more effective for some CNCP conditions than others. For example, tramadol reduced pain and improved functional outcomes in patients with fibromyalgia (Furlan et al. 2006; Russell et al. 2000). Future research may help clarify patient selection questions.

Risks of Opioids in CNCP

As is true for any medication, the use of opioid analgesics carries with it certain risks. For the purposes of this chapter, the term "adverse effect" refers to any unintended effect that can be associated with opioid analgesics. We describe adverse effects seen early in the course of opioid therapy (acute adverse effects) separately from those that either develop or become problematic during chronic opioid therapy. Common adverse effects that are encountered routinely in the course of opioid therapy are referred to as "common side effects." *Clinicians should note that the risks, including suicide, of untreated or poorly controlled pain are well-established and highly morbid. So that when making decisions about the use of opioids, some of the associational studies mentioned below often occur in patients with chronic pain or in patients with addiction disorders. Confounding is a common methodological problem in studies of causes of side effects and toxicity.*

Adverse Effects Seen Acutely

Common Side Effects

There are a number of side effects associated with opioid analgesics, many of which can develop early in the course of therapy. Indeed, tolerance may develop to some of the adverse effects that appear early in the course of therapy. Kalso et al. reported that 80% of patients receiving opioid therapy reported at least one side effect compared with 56% of those receiving placebo (Kalso et al. 2004). Common acute side effects of opioid analgesics include nausea and vomiting, sedation, dizziness, constipation, urinary retention, and pruritus. Of these, constipation, dry mouth sedation, and nausea may be the most frequent, followed by vomiting, dizziness, and pruritus (Kalso et al. 2004; Moore and McQuay 2005). Opioids cause constipation by decreasing peristalsis and intestinal secretions. Tolerance develops very slowly to the gastrointestinal effects of opioid analgesics, such that constipation usually persists throughout chronic treatment. Concurrent use of stool softeners and cathartics, as well as dietary modifications (e.g., addition of more fiber) can alleviate opioid-induced constipation. Opioid analgesics produce nausea and vomiting through actions at the medullary chemoreceptor trigger zone. For patients experiencing this adverse effect, antiemetics can be used in conjunction with opioids. Tolerance to the sedative effects of opioid analgesics usually develops within the first several days of treatment. If patients experience significant sedation, the opioid may be administered at a lower dose more frequently (Inturrisi 2002) to avoid large peaks in plasma concentration. Other CNS depressants including sedative-hypnotics (particularly benzodiazepines), which are frequently co-prescribed with opioids (Skurtveit et al. 2010) may potentiate the sedative and respiratory effects of opioids (Webster et al. 2008; Webster 2010), and should ideally be discontinued if possible. Opioids can cause bladder spasm and an increase in sphincter tone, leading to urinary retention, particularly in elderly patients. In some cases, catheterization may be required to alleviate urinary retention.

Respiratory Depression

The most serious potential adverse event associated with opioid therapy is respiratory depression. Opioid agonists act on brainstem respiratory centers to produce dose-dependent respiratory depression, and death due to overdose on an opioid agonist is almost always the result of respiratory depression (Inturrisi 2002). Tolerance to respiratory depression develops rapidly with chronic administration, allowing for relatively safe dose escalation over time. However, individuals with impaired respiratory function (e.g., COPD, asthma) are at greater risk of clinically significant respiratory depression even at usual doses of opioid analgesics, and thus caution should be exercised when prescribing opioids to these populations.

Adverse Effects and Drug Interactions Related to Specific Opioids

As fentanyl is usually administered as a transdermal patch in CNCP patients, there is a risk of local skin reactions. As stated above, CNS excitation and seizures can be seen with tramadol. In addition, because tramadol inhibits serotonin reuptake, it may induce serotonin syndrome, particularly in patients who are also taking other serotonergic medications such as SSRIs, SNRIs, or tricyclic anti-depressants. These potential interactions are of note because such medications are commonly used to treat neuropathic pain (e.g., TCAs and SNRIs) or to treat co-morbid depression which co-occurs frequently in patients with CNCP (Gallagher and Verma 1999; Mossey and Gallagher 2004). Methadone is associated with QTc prolongation (Chugh et al. 2008; Cruciani et al. 2005) and rarely with cardiac arrhythmias (particularly Torsades des Pointes; Krantz et al. 2002). It has been noted that the duration of analgesia from methadone is shorter than its effects on respiratory depression, which has been suggested to lead to potential intensification of respiratory depression risk (Beaver et al. 1967; Olsen et al. 1977). These risks of methadone may be greater in patients receiving higher doses. Epidemiologic studies have indicated a rise in methadone-related deaths in the United States (Gagajewski and Apple 2003; Maxwell et al. 2005; Piercefield et al. 2010), and it has been suggested that the risk of overdose toxicity may be greater for methadone than for other opioid analgesics (Twycross 1977). Thus, there is a need to titrate the methadone dose carefully, and monitor closely for adverse events.

Long-Term Consequences of Chronic Opioid Treatment

Opioid-Induced Hyperalgesia

It is well known that higher doses of opioids are required to produce the same analgesic effects when these medications are administered chronically. It could be assumed that these effects of opioids are solely the result of opioid tolerance. However, there is evidence suggesting that opioids can induce an increase in pain sensitivity through mechanisms distinct from tolerance. Animal data support the development of increased pain sensitivity with continuous opioid administration, including the compelling observation that thermal hyperalgesia and allodynia were observed even during active opioid infusion (Vanderah et al. 2000; Mao 2002). There is also evidence suggesting that similar opioid-induced hyperalgesia phenomena occur in humans (Chang et al. 2007; Fishbain et al. 2009), although these effects in humans are more controversial(Fishbain et al. 2009). For example, hyperalgesia upon cessation of chronic opioid administration has been considered a symptom of the opioid withdrawal syndrome (O'Brien 2006). A structured review by Fishbain and colleagues found that the best evidence to support the existence of opioid-induced hyperalgesia in humans comes from normal volunteers receiving opioid infusions; however, these authors also concluded that there was insufficient evidence to support or refute the existence of opioid-induced hyperalgesia in humans except in the case of normal volunteers (Fishbain et al. 2009). Nevertheless, some studies suggest opioid-induced hyperalgesia in clinical populations. For example, Guignard et al. reported increased opioid demand in patients who received intraoperative opioids as compared with matched patients. In this study, it was noted that the opioid-treated patients reported more pain than the matched controls (Guignard et al. 2000). In addition, sensitivity to experimental pain stimulation was found to be higher in former opioid addicts on methadone maintenance compared to matched former opioid addicts not receiving methadone maintenance (Compton et al. 2001). Perhaps more relevant for the management of CNCP patients, a small prospective study reported the development of opioid-induced hyperalgesia (as measured by the cold pressor test, but not the heat pain test) after 30 days of morphine therapy in six chronic back pain patients (Chu et al. 2006). The paucity of methodologically sound epidemiologic and clinical studies in well-defined clinical populations challenges pain medicine to establish a better understanding of the true prevalence of hyperalgesia and its phenomenology in specific patient populations. Until then its salience for opioid analgesia generally will remain speculative, and its clinical impact on the use of opioid analgesics for the treatment of persistent pain in any particular patient, will remain in domain of the clinical acumen of the individual physician.

Whereas tolerance is thought to result from a desensitization process, opioid-induced hyperalgesia is thought to be due to a sensitization process (Mao 2002), and both spinal and supraspinal systems have been proposed as neuroplastic sites of action (Bederson et al. 1990; Dogrul et al. 2005; Gardell et al. 2002; Kaplan and Fields 1991; King et al. 2005). It is thought that the glutamatergic system, and specifically the NMDA receptor system, is involved in the development of opioid-induced hyperalgesia (Laulin et al. 2002; Mao et al. 1994). Thus, it is possible that NMDA receptor blockade may prevent opioid-induced hyperalgesia (Celerier et al. 2000). It is interesting to note that the glutamate system is thought to be important in both opioid tolerance and opioid-induced hyperalgesia (Mao 2002). Various neuropeptides have also been implicated in the development of opioid-induced hyperalgesia. For example, there is evidence to support the involvement of spinal dynorphin in the expression of opioid-induced hyperalgesia (Vanderah et al. 2000; Gardell et al. 2002), and opioids have been shown to increase levels of the pro-nociceptive peptide CCK (Xie et al. 2005). Intriguingly, there is also evidence to suggest neuroimmune processes in the development of opioid-induced hyperalgesia (Leo et al. 2004; Watkins and Maier 2000).

Disentangling opioid tolerance, opioid-induced hyperalgesia, and disease progression can be challenging, as all of these phenomena would manifest as decreased opioid analgesic efficacy. The clinician must also consider opioid addiction and pseudoaddiction in patients who complain of diminished opioid efficacy or request higher opioid doses (discussed below in section "Addiction"). If there is no evidence to support disease progression, addiction, or pseudoaddiction, the clinical question becomes that of distinguishing between opioid tolerance and opioid-induced hyperalgesia. It has been suggested that the characteristics of opioid-induced hyperalgesia may be different from those of the underlying pain condition in that opioid-induced hyperalgesia is expected to be more diffuse, less defined in quality, and beyond the distribution of the pre-existing pain state (Mao 2002, 2006). Opioid tolerance would respond to dose escalation, whereas such an intervention may exacerbate opioid-induced hyperalgesia. In fact, dose reductions may improve pain sensitivity associated with opioid use. Rotation to a different opioid (discussed below in section "Opioid Rotation") may also be considered (Chang et al. 2007).

Effects of Opioids on Endocrine Systems

Opioids have been reported to affect multiple endocrine systems in both humans and animals, including LH/FSH and sex hormones, ACTH, growth hormone, prolactin, thyrotropin, arginine vasopressin, and oxytocin, and may also have effects related to obesity and diabetes. An exhaustive review of these endocrine effects is beyond the scope of this chapter; readers interested in the endocrine effects of opioids are referred to a recent review by Vuong et al. (2010). Here, we will highlight endocrine effects of particularly relevant clinical importance.

Effects of Opioids on Sex Steroids

A reduction in sex steroid hormone levels is perhaps the best known of the endocrine disturbances associated with chronic opioid use. These changes have been observed in both pre-clinical animal studies (Yilmaz et al. 1999) and human studies, and are thought to result from decreased LH levels (Vuong et al. 2010). In humans, studies have shown effects of opioids on sex steroids in both men and women. For example, in women, long-term intrathecal opioid administration led to a reduction in LH, FSH, estradiol, and progesterone levels in premenopausal women, which was in turn associated with amenorrhea or irregular menstruation (Abs et al. 2000). Similar results have also been demonstrated with oral and transdermal opioid administration (Daniell 2008).

The effects of opioids on sex hormones have been better studied in men, and indeed there is some evidence suggesting that these effects are more pronounced in men than in women (Fraser et al. 2009). Males with heroin dependence exhibit decreased testosterone levels compared to controls (Lafisca et al. 1985; Rasheed and Tareen 1995). Furthermore, male patients receiving opioid analgesics for CNCP showed dose-related reductions in total testosterone and free testosterone compared to controls (Daniell 2002). Male opioid-induced hypogonadism is associated with such side effects as delayed ejaculation, erectile dysfunction, and decreased libido (Daniell 2002; Paice et al. 1994). Hypogonadism in men can also lead to decreased bone mineral density, osteopenia, and osteoporosis (Fraser et al. 2009; Kinjo et al. 2005), and opioid administration has been reported to be associated with a 1.5- to 6-fold increase in osteoporotic fractures (Vestergaard et al. 2006). Opioid-induced male hypogonadism has also been reported to lead to increased depression (Daniell et al. 2006). These clinical effects of hypogonadism may be managed by a trial of reducing the opioid dose or even discontinuing opioid therapy, especially if analgesia is poor. In some cases, control of pain symptoms necessitates the use of opioids. Testosterone supplementation can be tried in these cases (Daniell et al. 2006), or patients may be switched to buprenorphine, which has been associated with higher testosterone levels and lower frequency of sexual dysfunction than methadone (Bliesener et al. 2005; Hallinan et al. 2008).

Effects of Opioids on Food Intake and Blood Glucose

Opioid analgesics may also affect food intake and blood sugar levels, though these effects are somewhat controversial. Some animal studies have found that direct administration of opioid peptides into the CNS increase food intake, while opioid antagonists decrease food intake (Baile et al. 1986; Levine et al. 1985), although other studies have reported that opioids cause decreased food intake (Vuong et al. 2010). Animal studies have also shown that opioid agonists induce hyperglycemia (Bailey and Flatt 1987; Sadava et al. 1997). In humans, opioids have also been associated with increased serum glucose and elevated risk for metabolic disorders (Karam et al. 2004). Opioids and opioid peptides have been hypothesized to act centrally through the sympathetic nervous system to induce hyperglycemia and impaired insulin secretion (Giugliano 1984). It is also interesting to note that the analgesic efficacy of opioids may be decreased in diabetic patients (Karci et al. 2004). Thus, more caution may be called for in prescribing opioids to diabetic patients with CNCP compared to non-diabetics. More research is needed to fully elucidate the relationship between diabetes and opioids.

Immunosuppression

Long-term use of opioid analgesics has been shown to interfere with immune function in both animals and humans (reviewed in Sacerdote 2006). There is evidence that opioids have inhibitory effects on both humoral and cellular immune responses (Vallejo et al. 2004), and morphine has been associated with increased morbidity and mortality related to experimentally induced infection in animals (Risdahl et al. 1998). Two mechanisms have been suggested to contribute to the immunosuppressive effects of opioids: (1) peripheral binding to μ opioid receptors on immune cells and (2) centrally mediated activation of the hypothalamic-pituitary-adrenal axis and sympathetic nervous system (Sacerdote 2006). Clinicians and patients should be aware of the potential immunomodulatory effects of opioids in making clinical decisions. There is some evidence suggesting that certain opioid analgesics (e.g., hydromorphone, oxycodone, and buprenorphine) produce less immunosuppression than others (Gomez-Flores and Weber 2000; Martucci et al. 2004; Sacerdote et al. 1997). Thus, these agents may be preferable for patients in whom immunosuppression is of particular concern (e.g., HIV and cancer patients).

Tolerance, Physical Dependence, and Addiction

Tolerance and Physical Dependence

Tolerance refers to a given dose of opioid producing a decreasing effect, or the requirement for larger doses of medication to maintain the same clinical effect. The neuroadaptations associated with tolerance act to maintain homeostasis by countering acute drug effects. The molecular mechanisms leading to the development of opioid tolerance are incompletely understood, but may involve reduced cell surface expression of opioid receptors, reduced capacity of opioid receptors to activate second messenger cascades, or increased activation of second messenger cascades that opioid agonists acutely suppress (Christie 2008; Koch and Hollt 2008). Some degree of tolerance can be expected among most patients receiving long-term opioid therapy (McQuay 1999), though the rate at which tolerance develops can vary greatly (Kanner and Foley 1981). Tolerant patients frequently complain of a decrease in the duration of effective analgesia, though sudden dramatic increases in opioid requirements may signal disease progression or development of a new problem rather than opioid tolerance. The rate of development of tolerance may be slowed by the use of combinations of opioids with non-opioids that enhance analgesia, as tolerance does not develop to the non-opioid component of the combination (Inturrisi 2002).

Physical dependence develops with long-term opioid use, and refers to the requirement to continue to take opioid analgesics to avoid physical withdrawal symptoms upon abrupt discontinuation or abrupt reduction in dose. The severity of withdrawal symptoms is proportional to the dose and duration of administration of the discontinued opioid, such that patients taking high doses of opioids for prolonged periods will exhibit more severe withdrawal symptoms. Common symptoms of opioid withdrawal include initial anxiety and irritability, salivation, lacrimation, rhinorrhea, diaphoresis, abdominal cramps, arthralgias and myalgias, vomiting and diarrhea (Jovey et al. 2003; O'Brien 2006). The time course of the withdrawal syndrome is related to the half-life of the opioid that has been chronically administered. For short half-life opioids such as morphine, abstinence symptoms will begin within 6–12 h and peak between 24 and 72 h of drug cessation. For longer half-life agents such as methadone, withdrawal symptoms may begin within 36 and 48 h and peak at approximately 5 days after drug cessation. Opioid withdrawal is very rarely life-threatening, though it is unpleasant for the patient. Thus, opioid doses should be tapered gradually if the need arises to discontinue therapy.

Addiction

In addition to their analgesic actions, opioids can also produce euphoric effects and stimulate reward centers in the brain (Kreek 2001), and thus, they carry abuse liability. One of the biggest concerns for physicians prescribing opioid analgesics is the risk of addiction associated with these medications. Addiction in the current psychiatric Diagnostic and Statistical Manual (DSM-IV) (American Psychiatric Association 1994) encompasses substance abuse and the more severe substance dependence. Criteria for these disorders are provided in Table 29.1. The upcoming DSM-5 proposes to rename both substance abuse and dependence under the same heading (Substance Use Disorder; criteria listed in Table 29.2; American Psychiatric Association 2011) which will have severity modifiers of moderate (two to three criteria met) and severe (four or more criteria met). Addiction specifically in the context of pain treatment with opioids has been defined as "a primary, chronic, neurobiological disease, with genetic, psychosocial, and environmental factors influencing its development and manifestations. It is characterized by behaviors that include one or more of the following: impaired control over drug use, compulsive use, continued use despite harm, and craving" (The American Academy of Pain Medicine tAPS and the American Society of Addiction Medicine 2001).

Table 29.1 Diagnostic and Statistical Manual (DSM-IV) criteria for substance abuse and substance dependence (American Psychiatric Association 1994)

Substance abuse: A maladaptive pattern of substance use leading to clinically significant impairment or distress, as manifested by *one (or more) of the following*, occurring within a 12-month period [*]
Recurrent substance use resulting in failure to fulfill major role obligations at work, school, or home (e.g., substance-related absences from school or work, neglect of children)
Recurrent substance use in situations in which it is physically hazardous (e.g., driving or operating machinery while impaired by substance use)
Recurrent substance-related legal problems (such as arrests for substance related disorderly conduct)
Continued substance use despite having persistent or recurrent social or interpersonal problems caused or exacerbated by the effects of the substance (e.g., arguments with spouse about the consequences of intoxication)
Substance dependence: A maladaptive pattern of substance use leading to clinically significant impairment or distress, as manifested by *three (or more) of the following*, occurring at any time in the same 12-month period
Tolerance, as defined by either of the following:
A need for markedly increased amount of the substance to achieve intoxication or desired effect or
Markedly diminished effect with continued use of the same amount of the substance
Withdrawal, as manifested by either of the following:
The characteristic withdrawal syndrome for the substance or
The same (or closely related) substance is taken to relieve or avoid withdrawal symptoms
The substance is often taken in larger amounts or over a longer period than intended
There is a persistent desire or unsuccessful efforts to cut down or control substance use
A great deal of time is spent in activities necessary to obtain the substance, use the substance or recover from its effects
Important social, occupational, or recreational activities are given up or reduced due to substance use
Substance use is continued despite knowledge of having a physical or psychological problem that is likely to have been caused or exacerbated by the substance (e.g., continued drinking despite recognition that ulcer that was made worse by alcohol consumption)

[*] Symptoms have never met criteria for substance dependence for this class of substance

Table 29.2 Proposed DSM-5 criteria for substance use disorder (American Psychiatric Association 2011)

Substance use disorder: A maladaptive pattern of substance use leading to clinically significant impairment or distress, as manifested by *two (or more) of the following*, occurring at any time in the same 12-month period
Recurrent substance use resulting in failure to fulfill major role obligations at work, school, or home (e.g., substance-related absences from school or work, neglect of children)
Recurrent substance use in situations in which it is physically hazardous (e.g., driving or operating machinery while impaired by substance use)
Continued substance use despite having persistent or recurrent social or interpersonal problems caused or exacerbated by the effects of the substance (e.g., arguments with spouse about the consequences of intoxication)
Tolerance, as defined by either of the following[a]:
A need for markedly increased amount of the substance to achieve intoxication or desired effect or
Markedly diminished effect with continued use of the same amount of the substance
Withdrawal, as manifested by either of the following[a]:
The characteristic withdrawal syndrome for the substance or
The same (or closely related) substance is taken to relieve or avoid withdrawal symptoms
The substance is often taken in larger amounts or over a longer period than intended
There is a persistent desire or unsuccessful efforts to cut down or control substance use
A great deal of time is spent in activities necessary to obtain the substance, use the substance or recover from its effects
Important social, occupational, or recreational activities are given up or reduced due to substance use
Continued substance use despite knowledge of having a physical or psychological problem that is likely to have been caused or exacerbated by the substance (e.g., continued drinking despite recognition that ulcer that was made worse by alcohol consumption)
Craving or a strong desire or urge to use a specific substance

[a] Tolerance and withdrawal are not counted for those taking medications under medical supervision
Severity specifiers:
Moderate: two to three criteria positive
Severe: four or more criteria positive

Table 29.3 Proposed criteria for problematic opioid Use (Chabal et al. 1997)

The patient displays an overwhelming focus on opioid issues that occupies a significant proportion of the pain clinic visit and impedes progress with other issues regarding the patient's pain. This behavior must persist beyond the third clinic treatment session
The patient has a pattern of early refills (three or more) or escalating drug use in the absence of an acute change in his or her medical condition
The patient generates multiple telephone calls or visits to the administrative office to request more opioids, early refills, or problems associated with the opioid prescription. A patient may qualify with fewer visits if he or she creates a disturbance with the office staff
There is a pattern of prescription problems for a variety of reasons that may include lost, spilled, or stolen medications
The patient has supplemental sources of opioids obtained from multiple providers, emergency rooms, or illegal sources

It should be emphasized that tolerance and the closely related phenomenon of physical dependence are distinct from addiction, which is characterized by a compulsive drive for drug use without regard to severe adverse consequences (Volkow and Li 2005). Most patients with opioid addiction will manifest some degree of tolerance and physical dependence, and it is certainly possible for a patient to be tolerant to and physically dependent on an opioid analgesic without being addicted. Thus, tolerance and physical dependence per se do not appear to be useful diagnostic criteria for prescription opioid addiction, as these phenomena cannot differentiate addiction from the normal consequences of treatment. In the proposed DSM-5 criteria, tolerance and withdrawal are excluded as criteria for a substance use disorder for medications taken under medical supervision, yet these aspects of prescribing opioids can still remain a source of confusion for physicians and patients alike. Due to some of these difficulties in applying current substance dependence criteria to CNCP patients, Chabal et al. (1997) proposed criteria specifically for opioid abuse in CNCP patients, which are listed in Table 29.3. These criteria notably include several aberrant drug-related behaviors (ADRB; discussed in more detail below), but do not include components relating to tolerance and withdrawal. Complicating the issue of diagnosing prescription opioid addiction in CNCP patients is the phenomenon of pseudoaddiction, in which patients with undertreated pain may appear to be drug-seeking or malingering (Elander et al. 2004; Gallagher and Rosenthal 2008; Lusher et al. 2006). Pseudoaddiction resolves once better pain control is achieved. It is important for clinicians to be aware of diagnostic pitfalls so that patients can be accurately diagnosed and managed appropriately.

Epidemiology of Prescription Opioid Addiction

Investigations of the epidemiology of prescription opioid addiction in CNCP have provided disparate estimates of the rates of this potential complication of chronic opioid therapy. A letter reporting addiction in only 4 hospitalized patients out of 11,882 treated with narcotics has been cited in support of low addiction rates in opioid-treated patients (Porter and Jick 1980). However, results observed in hospitalized patients may not generalize to an outpatient population; furthermore, this study documented opioid addiction only in patients with no prior addiction history, thereby potentially missing many addiction cases. An early study by Portenoy and Foley reported a 5% rate of addiction in CNCP patients (Portenoy and Foley 1986), while a prospective study of patients referred to an interventional pain clinic found the rate of opioid abuse to be 9% (Manchikanti et al. 2006). An early systematic review reported addiction rates of 3.2–18.9% in CNCP patients (Fishbain et al. 1992). A higher rate of opioid misuse (32%) was observed in a study of patients referred to a Veterans Administration (VA) primary pain clinic, with predictive factors being prior history of addiction or conviction on drug charges (Ives et al. 2006). Still higher levels of problematic opioid use among

CNCP patients were observed in two additional studies, which together reported rates of opioid misuse or dependence between 20 and 40% (Reid et al. 2002; Katz and Fanciullo 2002). The varied rates of opioid use disorders cited above likely reflect not only differences in study populations, but also differences in definitions of abuse, addiction and misuse, and in outcome measures used. Studies variously assessed opioid misuse, abuse, and dependence. The choice to measure different outcomes in these patient populations may in part reflect the difficulties and ambiguities in making opioid use diagnoses in CNCP patients. Clearly, there is a need for additional research to clarify the discrepancies in the epidemiology of opioid use disorders in CNCP patients.

Aberrant Drug-Related Behaviors

Clinicians have identified certain ADRB that are associated with opioid dependence (Fleming et al. 2008). Among these, it has been suggested that certain behaviors (forging prescriptions, stealing or borrowing drugs, frequently "losing" prescriptions, and resisting medication changes) are more predictive of opioid misuse than other behaviors (aggressive complaining about the need for more drugs, drug hoarding during periods of reduced symptoms, and unsanctioned dose escalations) as the latter may indicate poorly controlled pain (Portenoy 1996). There is some overlap between ADRB and DSM-IV criteria for opioid dependence (e.g., self-escalation in opioid dose may be analogous to more use than intended in DSM); however, not all patients with ADRB will meet criteria for DSM-IV opioid abuse or dependence. Thus, the presence of ADRB may alert clinicians to the presence of an opioid use disorder or may indicate *vulnerability* for developing an opioid use disorder.

Several scales and diagnostic tools have been developed to assess the presence of ADRB in patients receiving opioid analgesics. For example, the revised version of the Screener and Opioid Assessment for Patients with Pain (SOAPP-R) is a self-report questionnaire that includes questions about family and personal history of substance abuse problems, lost or stolen medications, legal problems, and medication craving (Butler et al. 2008). The same group developed another questionnaire, the Current Opioid Misuse Measure (COMM), which was designed to monitor the misuse of medication in patients who have been prescribed opioids for extended time periods (Butler et al. 2007). Another group developed a different questionnaire, the Opioid Risk Tool (ORT), which was developed to predict which patients will develop ADRB (Webster and Webster 2005). The ORT includes questions about family and personal history of substance abuse as well as questions about psychiatric diagnoses and history of sexual abuse. The Prescription Drug Use Questionnaire (PDUQ) is an interview screening tool created to stratify patients into three groups: those who are likely to be (1) non-addicted, (2) substance-abusing, and (3) substance-dependent (Compton et al. 1998). A limitation of the PDUQ is that it is designed to be used by a trained mental health professional, and thus may be difficult to incorporate into a primary care setting. Finally, the Diagnosis, Intractibility, Risk, and Efficacy (DIRE) Score is another clinician-scored tool that relies on chart review to assign scores based on diagnosis, engagement in treatment, history of psychiatric disorders and substance abuse, and functional status (Belgrade et al. 2006). The DIRE Score was developed with the aim of predicting compliance and efficacy with the ultimate goal of helping clinicians predict which patients would benefit most from opioid therapy.

Identifying Patients at Risk for Prescription Opioid Addiction

Efforts have been made to predict which CNCP patients are most at risk for prescription opioid addiction when prescribed opioid analgesics. Although these predictive factors are currently imperfect, certain risk factors for prescription opioid addiction have been identified. As might be expected, one of the most consistent predictors of prescription opioid misuse is a prior history of substance use disorders (Ives et al. 2006; Edlund et al. 2007; Turk et al. 2008). For example, a study conducted at a VA multidisciplinary opioid renewal clinic (ORC), a history of cocaine abuse was the most powerful predictor for failing the program, increasing the odds of program failure by approximately 5 times (odds ratio 4.97) (Meghani et al. 2009). In addition, tobacco smokers may be at greater risk for opioid misuse (Michna et al. 2004). A family history of substance abuse may also be predictive of opioid misuse (Schieffer et al. 2005). The clinical utility of self-reported history of substance use may be limited by patient reluctance to divulge these behaviors in themselves and in their significant others (Cook et al. 1995; Fishbain et al. 1999). Urine drug screens (UDS) can potentially address problems associated with relying on self-report, although they cannot provide diagnoses of substance abuse or dependence. A history of legal problems has also been observed to predict opioid misuse. For example, in one study a history of DUI or drug convictions were strong predictors of opioid misuse (Ives et al. 2006). Younger age may also predict greater risk for prescription opioid misuse (Turk et al. 2008).

The presence of ADRB can alert clinicians about the potential for opioid addiction. Fleming et al. (2008) showed that a significantly greater proportion of patients with four or more lifetime ADRBs (vs. those with one to three lifetime ADRBs) met DSM-IV criteria for opioid dependence. Even so, most patients who engage in ADRB do not appear to have opioid dependence, as this same study also reported that only 9.9% of patients with four or more lifetime ADRB met criteria for opioid dependence (Fleming et al. 2008). Furthermore, in a study of patients referred because of the presence of ADRB [performed at the PVAMC Opioid Renewal Clinic (ORC)], only 13% required referral for addiction treatment when provided a structured approach to opioid management that included opioid treatment agreements and UDSs (Wiedemer et al. 2007). It is possible that other patients with ADRB may have pseudoaddiction, or they engage in ADRB due to undertreatment of pain (Gallagher and Rosenthal 2008). It is also possible that certain ADRB are more predictive of substance use problems than others. For example, Fleming and colleagues propose that four specific behaviors appear useful as screening questions to predict patients at risk for a current substance use disorder based on the high proportion of positive responses in this group compared to low risk patients: (1) oversedated oneself, (2) felt intoxicated, (3) early refills, and (4) increased dose on own (Fleming et al. 2008). Another group reported that craving for an opioid medication predicted a higher incidence of physician-rated ADRB and more frequent positive UDS (Wasan et al. 2009).

Approach to Prescribing Opioid Analgesics for CNCP

As with all medications, clinicians must weigh the risks and benefits of opioid analgesic therapy for each individual patient. Balancing risks and benefits is particularly challenging in the case of opioid analgesics (Gallagher and Rosenthal 2008; Ballantyne 2007), as clinicians must not only consider benefits and traditional side effects/serious adverse events, but also the risk of addiction, which patients may not always recognize or divulge. These difficulties are compounded by lack of clarity in the terminology and diagnosis related to prescription opioid addiction, which results in a wide "gray area" between patients who clearly benefit from chronic opioid therapy vs. those who are clearly harmed.

Biopsychosocial Assessment of CNCP Patients

Any decision regarding the risks and benefits of chronic opioid therapy depends upon a proper assessment. In this regard, the use of biopsychosocial principles in the approach to the patient with CNCP has been advocated (Gallagher 2004). In this approach, clinicians asses not only the underlying physical condition associated with CNCP, but also any associated psychiatric conditions, stressors, and social factors that may exacerbate pain or contribute to poor function (Geisser et al. 2003). The level of suffering associated with CNCP and the outcome of treatment may be impacted by the patient's coping style (e.g., catastrophizing and external locus of control) or psychiatric comorbidities (Gallagher and Rosenthal 2008).

There is a complex relationship between pain and emotions, and a strong association between CNCP and both depressive and anxiety disorders has been described (Asmundson et al. 2002; Eisendrath 1995; Gallagher et al. 2000; McWilliams et al. 2008). Depression and anxiety disorders have been reported to be 2–3 times more prevalent among CNCP patients than in the general population, and for some disorders this ratio may be even higher (Asmundson and Katz 2009; Fishbain 1999). The causal relationships between CNCP and psychiatric comorbidities are under investigation. For example, seasonal co-variation between pain and depressed mood has been reported (Gallagher et al. 1995), and the stress of living with chronic pain increased the risk for depression even in persons without a personal or family history of depression (Dohrenwend et al. 1999), suggesting that at least in some cases the comorbidity between CNCP and depression may primarily result from stress of living with pain rather than familial risk. On the other hand, a shared pathogenesis between fibromyalgia and depression has been suggested, and it is possible that fibromyalgia is a depression spectrum disorder (Arnold et al. 2004; Raphael et al. 2004). Furthermore, exposure to the stress of a major life trauma (9/11 World Trade Center attack) did not increase rates of developing fibromyalgia, but was associated with increased pain in community subjects who had already been diagnosed with fibromyalgia (Raphael et al. 2002). These results highlight the complex relationships between CNCP and psychiatric comorbidities, and suggest that the causal relationships between pain and psychiatric disorders may be different among specific CNCP conditions. Regardless of causality, treating psychiatric comorbidities in CNCP patients may improve functioning and decrease reliance on opioid analgesics (Nickel et al. 2006). It is also possible that relief of pain with antidepressant treatment may lead to higher remission rates of depressive symptoms (Gallagher and Rosenthal 2008).

Principles of Prescribing Opioid Analgesics for CNCP

In general, opioids are not first line therapies for CNCP, and are only prescribed after trials of other agents have failed. It may be optimal to prescribe opioids in a multidisciplinary setting, which includes physical, vocational, or psychological components, and are provided by at least two healthcare professionals with different clinical backgrounds (Flor et al. 1992; Guzman et al. 2001). Because of the complexities of CNCP, opioids are often most effective when part of an individualized multiple component pain treatment plan. Some patients may benefit from cognitive-behavioral therapy (Chou et al. 2009; Hoffman et al. 2007; Morley et al. 1999; van Tulder et al. 2000) or other techniques such as progressive relaxation and biofeedback (van Tulder et al. 2000). In opioid-naïve patients, opioids should be started at a low dose and titrated slowly to minimize side effects. In patients with continuous pain, some authors recommend around-the-clock opioid dosing rather than an as-required (PRN) regimen (Jovey et al. 2003). The use of long-acting vs. short-acting opioids has also been advocated. It has been suggested that long-acting opioids may promote patients' focus on daily activities rather than on their pain, which may improve adherence and reduce pain-related anxieties (Jovey et al. 2003; Rauck 2009). However, long-term trials of these formulations are needed to draw firm conclusions regarding the relative risks and benefits of long-acting vs. short-acting opioids.

Certain standard practices regarding the prescribing of opioid analgesics to CNCP patients may help clinicians identify and respond to potential problems associated with these medications. The concept of "universal precautions," adopted from an infectious disease model, involves treating all patients as though they may be at risk for opioid addiction (Gourlay et al. 2005). This concept was developed in response to the difficulties in predicting which patients will demonstrate ADRB prior to beginning opioid therapy. Standardizing policies may prevent certain patients from feeling like they are being singled out. Adequate communication is key when prescribing opioids, so clinic policies should be clearly stated to help prevent any possible misunderstandings. The use of an opioid treatment agreement that is signed by the patient can be helpful in this regard. Additional measures to facilitate communication include telephone contacts and frequent visits (Wiedemer et al. 2007; Gallagher and Rosenthal 2008; Wasan et al. 2005). Monitoring is also an important aspect of opioid therapy. In addition to routinely monitoring treatment response and side effects, random UDS and pill counts have been advocated for patients receiving prescription opioids (Wiedemer et al. 2007; Gallagher and Rosenthal 2008). The utility of urine testing is enhanced by close attention to patients' behaviors; indeed, monitoring both UDS and behavior has been shown to identify more patients with ADRB than either strategy alone (Katz et al. 2003).

Some patients who are good candidates for a trial of opioid therapy may be reluctant to take opioid medications out of fear of side effects or addiction. If this occurs, clinicians can educate patients that tolerance develops to many of the side effects of opioids, and that effective treatments exist for those side effects that do not develop tolerance (e.g., fiber and stool softeners for constipation). Patients who are concerned about the risk of addiction may be educated that one of the most consistent predictors of prescription opioid addiction is personal history of substance use disorders. Thus, patients without a history of substance use disorders may be at relatively lower risk for the development of opioid misuse. Patients may also be confused about the difference between tolerance and addiction; therefore an explanation of these differences may be helpful, including an explanation that patients taking opioid analgesics are expected to develop some degree of tolerance to their medication, which is not the same as addiction. Finally, all patients should be reassured that they will be monitored carefully, and that treatment is available if they do develop opioid misuse or addiction.

Addressing Problems Associated with Chronic Opioid Therapy

Addiction

Many physicians have little training in addiction or dealing with difficult patient behavior (Wasan et al. 2005). A history of addiction or ADRB does not necessarily preclude the use of opioid analgesics, but it does indicate a need for practices that reduce risk in these patients (Wiedemer et al. 2007). Useful strategies to address ADRB and addiction problems in CNCP patients receiving opioids include increased structure and intensity of care, with increased frequency of visits, increased monitoring (e.g., UDS) and shorter-term opioid prescriptions (Gallagher and Rosenthal 2008). If a patient meets criteria for substance abuse or dependence (either for opioids or other drug classes), then referral to a clinician who specializes in the treatment of addictive disorders is also indicated. Some patients who are unable to be managed in a standard outpatient clinic may require treatment in a more supervised setting, such as a methadone program. Ultimately for some patients, it may be determined that the risks of opioid analgesics outweigh their benefits, and should thus be discontinued. Currently, there are no definitive guidelines regarding which specific behaviors warrant opioid taper (Chou et al. 2009); however, the seriousness of behavioral problems can suggest a course of action. If patients failed multiple attempts to treat opioid addiction, or if they engage in certain more serious ADRB (e.g., opioid diversion, forged prescriptions), then the use of chronic opioid therapy is generally not an appropriate treatment and in some guidelines, may be considered contraindicated (The Management of Opioid Therapy for Chronic pain Working Group 2010).

Opioid Rotation

Opioid rotation, or switching from one opioid to another is a potential strategy for patients who experience intolerable side effects or inadequate analgesia despite dose increases. The most frequent reason for opioid treatment failure is that a dose increase necessary for pain control is limited by intolerable side effects (Vissers et al. 2010). Some of the factors that may contribute to this phenomenon include pharmacological induction of opioid metabolism by other drugs (Trescot et al. 2008), opioid tolerance, and opioid-induced hyperalgesia (see above). The theory behind opioid rotation is thought to be based on incomplete cross-tolerance between different opioid analgesics (Chou et al. 2009; Vissers et al. 2010); individual differences in opioid responsiveness may also contribute to the success of opioid rotation (Smith 2008). A systematic review of opioid rotation in patients with cancer pain found that 50–70% of patients regained adequate pain control and/or experienced reduced side effects (McNicol et al. 2003). A study that included both patients with cancer pain and CNCP showed good pain control after opioid rotation preceded by a brief period of therapy with immediate-release morphine (Gatti et al. 2010). Studies performed in CNCP patients showed that opioid rotation from morphine to methadone or transdermal buprenorphine resulted in improved outcomes for a majority of patients (Fredheim et al. 2006a; Freye et al. 2007). Switching to methadone was also shown to result in a statistically significant (but not clinically significant) increase in QTc interval (Fredheim et al. 2006b).

Currently, there are no evidence-based guidelines for specific opioid choices with opioid rotation (Chou et al. 2009; Vissers et al. 2010). Dose conversion or equianalgesic tables are available (Vissers et al. 2010; Pereira et al. 2001); however, such conversion tables can only provide approximate guidelines for selecting appropriate doses due to individual differences in response and incomplete cross-tolerance (Galer et al. 1992; Vissers et al. 2010). It is generally recommended to start the new opioid at a dose lower than that theoretically calculated (e.g., 25–50%) from equianalgesic tables (Chou et al. 2009; Vissers et al. 2010). This general rule may need modification in the case of methadone due to its non-linear pharmacokinetics, large interindividual differences in drug clearance, and pharmacodynamic properties. The relative potency of methadone increases with increased morphine dose at the time of rotation (Gonzalez-Barboteo et al. 2008; Ripamonti et al. 1998). Methadone conversion ratios based on morphine dose equivalents have been recommended: 4:1 for a daily morphine equivalent of <90 mg, 5:1 for 90–400 mg morphine equivalent, and 10:1 for >400 mg daily morphine equivalent (Weschules and Bain 2008).

Discontinuation of Opioid Therapy

As mentioned above, the clinical decision may be made to discontinue opioid therapy if patients engage in repeated and serious ADRB. Opioids may also be discontinued if patients experience intolerable side effects or lack of progress toward therapeutic goals, and other measures such as opioid rotation or dose escalation have failed. There is insufficient evidence to guide specific discontinuation strategies; however, an opioid taper can usually be performed in an outpatient setting in patients without severe medical or psychiatric comorbidities (Chou et al. 2009). An inpatient setting may be necessary for patients who are unable to reduce their opioid use in a less structured setting. Few studies have examined the optimal rate of opioid taper; existing studies suggest that a slow taper (e.g., dose reduction of 10% per week) may reduce opioid withdrawal symptoms (Cowan et al. 2005; Ralphs et al. 1994; Tennant et al. 1983). Anecdotal evidence suggests that at higher opioid doses (e.g., over 200 mg/day of morphine equivalents) the initial taper can be more rapid, but when relatively low doses are reached (e.g., 60–80 mg/day of morphine equivalents), the rate of dose reduction may need to be slowed due to the occurrence of more withdrawal symptoms (Chou et al. 2009).

Summary

Opioid therapy can be a useful treatment strategy to improve pain symptoms and quality of life in some patients with CNCP. The risks and benefits of opioid therapy must be carefully weighed for each individual patient, and a trial of opioid analgesics begun in those patients for whom the likely benefits outweigh potential risks. This chapter presents the factors that clinicians must weigh in the decision to begin opioid therapy for CNCP conditions. In addition, we present some practical strategies for addressing problems that may arise in the course of opioid therapy. Though in some cases there is insufficient evidence for definitive guidance of clinical decisions, it is hoped that these questions will be addressed in future research.

Future Strategies

A number of issues show promise as potential areas of future research to improve the use of opioid analgesics to treat CNCP. For example, little is known about the effects of opioids on the brains of CNCP patients, or indeed about the long-term effects of opioids on the brain in general. Thus, more neuroimaging studies in these areas would be helpful. As mentioned above, there is substantial individual variability in response to opioids. In addition, there may be variability in response to opioids among different CNCP conditions. Predicting which patients are more likely to respond to opioid analgesics, and furthermore which patients will respond to specific opioids would help clinicians better guide treatment choices. Promising areas of future research also include the search for novel therapeutic compounds. For example, in 1995 a novel receptor with similarities to the known opioid receptors was identified (ORL-1, or "opioid-receptor-like 1" Chiou et al. 2007; Reinscheid et al. 1995; Meunier et al. 1995). Although there are no currently available medications that specifically target this receptor, it is possible that the ORL-1 receptor may become the target of novel analgesic medications.

References

Abs, R., Verhelst, J., Maeyaert, J., Van Buyten, J. P., Opsomer, F., et al. (2000). Endocrine consequences of long-term intrathecal administration of opioids. *The Journal of Clinical Endocrinology and Metabolism, 85*, 2215–2222.

Amabile, C. M., & Bowman, B. J. (2006). Overview of oral modified-release opioid products for the management of chronic pain. *The Annals of Pharmacotherapy, 40*, 1327–1335.

American Psychiatric Association. (1994). *Diagnostic and statistical manual of mental disorders*. Washington, DC: American Psychiatric Association.

American Psychiatric Association. (2011). *DSM-5 development proposed revisions: Substance-related disorders*. Washington, DC: American Psychiatric Association.

Apkarian, A. V., Sosa, Y., Sonty, S., Levy, R. M., Harden, R. N., et al. (2004). Chronic back pain is associated with decreased prefrontal and thalamic gray matter density. *The Journal of Neuroscience, 24*, 10410–10415.

Arner, S., & Meyerson, B. A. (1988). Lack of analgesic effect of opioids on neuropathic and idiopathic forms of pain. *Pain, 33*, 11–23.

Arnold, L. M., Hudson, J. I., Hess, E. V., Ware, A. E., Fritz, D. A., et al. (2004). Family study of fibromyalgia. *Arthritis and Rheumatism, 50*, 944–952.

Askitopoulou, H., Ramoutsaki, I. A., & Konsolaki, E. (2002). Archaeological evidence on the use of opium in the Minoan world. *International Congress Series, 1292*, 23–97.

Asmundson, G. J., Coons, M. J., Taylor, S., & Katz, J. (2002). PTSD and the experience of pain: Research and clinical implications of shared vulnerability and mutual maintenance models. *Canadian Journal of Psychiatry, 47*, 930–937.

Asmundson, G. J., & Katz, J. (2009). Understanding the co-occurrence of anxiety disorders and chronic pain: State-of-the-art. *Depression and Anxiety, 26*, 888–901.

Baile, C. A., McLaughlin, C. L., & Della-Fera, M. A. (1986). Role of cholecystokinin and opioid peptides in control of food intake. *Physiological Reviews, 66*, 172–234.

Bailey, C. J., & Flatt, P. R. (1987). Increased responsiveness to glucoregulatory effect of opiates in obese-diabetic ob/ob mice. *Diabetologia, 30*, 33–37.

Baliki, M. N., Chialvo, D. R., Geha, P. Y., Levy, R. M., Harden, R. N., et al. (2006). Chronic pain and the emotional brain: Specific brain activity associated with spontaneous fluctuations of intensity of chronic back pain. *The Journal of Neuroscience, 26*, 12165–12173.

Baliki, M. N., Geha, P. Y., Apkarian, A. V., & Chialvo, D. R. (2008). Beyond feeling: Chronic pain hurts the brain, disrupting the default-mode network dynamics. *The Journal of Neuroscience, 28*, 1398–1403.

Ballantyne, J. C. (2007). Opioid analgesia: Perspectives on right use and utility. *Pain Physician, 10*, 479–491.

Beaver, W. T., Wallenstein, S. L., Houde, R. W., & Rogers, A. (1967). A clinical comparison of the analgesic effects of methadone and morphine administered intramuscularly, and of orally and parenterally administered methadone. *Clinical Pharmacology and Therapeutics, 8*, 415–426.

Bederson, J. B., Fields, H. L., & Barbaro, N. M. (1990). Hyperalgesia during naloxone-precipitated withdrawal from morphine is associated with increased on-cell activity in the rostral ventromedial medulla. *Somatosensory and Motor Research, 7*, 185–203.

Belgrade, M. J., Schamber, C. D., & Lindgren, B. R. (2006). The DIRE score: Predicting outcomes of opioid prescribing for chronic pain. *The Journal of Pain, 7*, 671–681.

Bliesener, N., Albrecht, S., Schwager, A., Weckbecker, K., Lichtermann, D., et al. (2005). Plasma testosterone and sexual function in men receiving buprenorphine maintenance for opioid dependence. *The Journal of Clinical Endocrinology and Metabolism, 90*, 203–206.

Bloodworth, D. (2005). Issues in opioid management. *American Journal of Physical Medicine & Rehabilitation, 84*, S42–S55.

Booth, M. (1986). *Opium: A history*. New York, NY: St. Martin's Press.

Buckalew, N., Haut, M. W., Aizenstein, H., Morrow, L., Perera, S., et al. (2010). Differences in brain structure and function in older adults with self-reported disabling and nondisabling chronic low back pain. *Pain Medicine, 11*, 1183–1197.

Butler, S. F., Budman, S. H., Fernandez, K. C., Houle, B., Benoit, C., et al. (2007). Development and validation of the Current Opioid Misuse Measure. *Pain, 130*, 144–156.

Butler, S. F., Fernandez, K., Benoit, C., Budman, S. H., & Jamison, R. N. (2008). Validation of the revised Screener and Opioid Assessment for Patients with Pain (SOAPP-R). *The Journal of Pain, 9*, 360–372.

Caldwell, J. R., Hale, M. E., Boyd, R. E., Hague, J. M., Iwan, T., et al. (1999). Treatment of osteoarthritis pain with controlled release oxycodone or fixed combination oxycodone plus acetaminophen added to nonsteroidal antiinflammatory drugs: A double blind, randomized, multicenter, placebo controlled trial. *The Journal of Rheumatology, 26*, 862–869.

Caldwell, J. R., Rapoport, R. J., Davis, J. C., Offenberg, H. L., Marker, H. W., et al. (2002). Efficacy and safety of a once-daily morphine formulation in chronic, moderate-to-severe osteoarthritis pain: Results from a randomized, placebo-controlled, double-blind trial and an open-label extension trial. *Journal of Pain and Symptom Management, 23*, 278–291.

Caudill-Slosberg, M. A., Schwartz, L. M., & Woloshin, S. (2004). Office visits and analgesic prescriptions for musculoskeletal pain in US: 1980 vs. 2000. *Pain, 109*, 514–519.

Celerier, E., Rivat, C., Jun, Y., Laulin, J. P., Larcher, A., et al. (2000). Long-lasting hyperalgesia induced by fentanyl in rats: Preventive effect of ketamine. *Anesthesiology, 92*, 465–472.

Chabal, C., Erjavec, M. K., Jacobson, L., Mariano, A., & Chaney, E. (1997). Prescription opiate abuse in chronic pain patients: Clinical criteria, incidence, and predictors. *The Clinical Journal of Pain, 13*, 150–155.

Chang, G., Chen, L., & Mao, J. (2007). Opioid tolerance and hyperalgesia. *The Medical Clinics of North America, 91*, 199–211.

Chapman, C. R., Lipschitz, D. L., Angst, M. S., Chou, R., Denisco, R. C., et al. (2010). Opioid pharmacotherapy for chronic non-cancer pain in the United States: A research guideline for developing an evidence-base. *The Journal of Pain, 11*, 807–829.

Chiou, L. C., Liao, Y. Y., Fan, P. C., Kuo, P. H., Wang, C. H., et al. (2007). Nociceptin/orphanin FQ peptide receptors: Pharmacology and clinical implications. *Current Drug Targets, 8*, 117–135.

Chou, R., Fanciullo, G. J., Fine, P. G., Adler, J. A., Ballantyne, J. C., et al. (2009). Clinical guidelines for the use of chronic opioid therapy in chronic noncancer pain. *The Journal of Pain, 10*, 113–130.

Christie, M. J. (2008). Cellular neuroadaptations to chronic opioids: Tolerance, withdrawal and addiction. *British Journal of Pharmacology, 154*, 384–396.

Chu, L. F., Clark, D. J., & Angst, M. S. (2006). Opioid tolerance and hyperalgesia in chronic pain patients after one month of oral morphine therapy: A preliminary prospective study. *The Journal of Pain, 7*, 43–48.

Chugh, S. S., Socoteanu, C., Reinier, K., Waltz, J., Jui, J., et al. (2008). A community-based evaluation of sudden death associated with therapeutic levels of methadone. *The American Journal of Medicine, 121*, 66–71.

Compton, P., Charuvastra, V. C., & Ling, W. (2001). Pain intolerance in opioid-maintained former opiate addicts: Effect of long-acting maintenance agent. *Drug and Alcohol Dependence, 63*, 139–146.

Compton, P., Darakjian, J., & Miotto, K. (1998). Screening for addiction in patients with chronic pain and "problematic" substance use: Evaluation of a pilot assessment tool. *Journal of Pain and Symptom Management, 16*, 355–363.

Cook, R. F., Bernstein, A. D., Arrington, T. L., Andrews, C. M., & Marshall, G. A. (1995). Methods for assessing drug use prevalence in the workplace: A comparison of self-report, urinalysis, and hair analysis. *The International Journal of the Addictions, 30*, 403–426.

Cowan, D. T., Wilson-Barnett, J., Griffiths, P., Vaughan, D. J., Gondhia, A., et al. (2005). A randomized, double-blind, placebo-controlled, cross-over pilot study to assess the effects of long-term opioid drug consumption and subsequent abstinence in chronic noncancer pain patients receiving controlled-release morphine. *Pain Medicine, 6*, 113–121.

Cruciani, R. A., Sekine, R., Homel, P., Lussier, D., Yap, Y., et al. (2005). Measurement of QTc in patients receiving chronic methadone therapy. *Journal of Pain and Symptom Management, 29*, 385–391.

Daniell, H. W. (2002). Hypogonadism in men consuming sustained-action oral opioids. *The Journal of Pain, 3*, 377–384.

Daniell, H. W. (2008). Opioid endocrinopathy in women consuming prescribed sustained-action opioids for control of nonmalignant pain. *The Journal of Pain, 9*, 28–36.

Daniell, H. W., Lentz, R., & Mazer, N. A. (2006). Open-label pilot study of testosterone patch therapy in men with opioid-induced androgen deficiency. *The Journal of Pain, 7*, 200–210.

Dellemijn, P. L., & Vanneste, J. A. (1997). Randomised double-blind active-placebo-controlled crossover trial of intravenous fentanyl in neuropathic pain. *Lancet, 349*, 753–758.

Devulder, J., Richarz, U., & Nataraja, S. H. (2005). Impact of long-term use of opioids on quality of life in patients with chronic, non-malignant pain. *Current Medical Research and Opinion, 21*, 1555–1568.

Dikotter, F., Laaman, L., & Xun, Z. (2004). *Narcotic culture: A history of drugs in China*. Chicago, IL: University of Chicago Press.

Dogrul, A., Bilsky, E. J., Ossipov, M. H., Lai, J., & Porreca, F. (2005). Spinal L-type calcium channel blockade abolishes opioid-induced sensory hypersensitivity and antinociceptive tolerance. *Anesthesia and Analgesia, 101*, 1730–1735.

Dohrenwend, B. P., Raphael, K. G., Marbach, J. J., & Gallagher, R. M. (1999). Why is depression comorbid with chronic myofascial face pain? A family study test of alternative hypotheses. *Pain, 83*, 183–192.

Edlund, M. J., Steffick, D., Hudson, T., Harris, K. M., & Sullivan, M. (2007). Risk factors for clinically recognized opioid abuse and dependence among veterans using opioids for chronic non-cancer pain. *Pain, 129*, 355–362.

Eisendrath, S. J. (1995). Psychiatric aspects of chronic pain. *Neurology, 45*, S26–S34; discussion S35–S36.

Elander, J., Lusher, J., Bevan, D., Telfer, P., & Burton, B. (2004). Understanding the causes of problematic pain management in sickle cell disease: Evidence that pseudoaddiction plays a more important role than genuine analgesic dependence. *Journal of Pain and Symptom Management, 27*, 156–169.

Elliott, A. M., Smith, B. H., Penny, K. I., Smith, W. C., & Chambers, W. A. (1999). The epidemiology of chronic pain in the community. *Lancet, 354*, 1248–1252.

Epstein, D. H., Preston, K. L., & Jasinski, D. R. (2006). Abuse liability, behavioral pharmacology, and physical-dependence potential of opioids in humans and laboratory animals: Lessons from tramadol. *Biological Psychology, 73*, 90–99.

Fishbain, D. A. (1999). Approaches to treatment decisions for psychiatric comorbidity in the management of the chronic pain patient. *Medical Clinics of North America, 83*, 737–760, vii.

Fishbain, D. A., Cole, B., Lewis, J. E., Gao, J., & Rosomoff, R. S. (2009). Do opioids induce hyperalgesia in humans? An evidence-based structured review. *Pain Medicine, 10*, 829–839.

Fishbain, D. A., Cutler, R. B., Rosomoff, H. L., & Rosomoff, R. S. (1999). Validity of self-reported drug use in chronic pain patients. *The Clinical Journal of Pain, 15*, 184–191.

Fishbain, D. A., Rosomoff, H. L., & Rosomoff, R. S. (1992). Drug abuse, dependence, and addiction in chronic pain patients. *The Clinical Journal of Pain, 8*, 77–85.

Fleming, M. F., Davis, J., & Passik, S. D. (2008). Reported lifetime aberrant drug-taking behaviors are predictive of current substance use and mental health problems in primary care patients. *Pain Medicine, 9*, 1098–1106.

Flor, H., Fydrich, T., & Turk, D. C. (1992). Efficacy of multidisciplinary pain treatment centers: A meta-analytic review. *Pain, 49*, 221–230.

Foley, K. M., & Houde, R. W. (1998). Methadone in cancer pain management: Individualize dose and titrate to effect. *Journal of Clinical Oncology, 16*, 3213–3215.

Fraser, L. A., Morrison, D., Morley-Forster, P., Paul, T. L., Tokmakejian, S., et al. (2009). Oral opioids for chronic non-cancer pain: Higher prevalence of hypogonadism in men than in women. *Experimental and Clinical Endocrinology & Diabetes, 117*, 38–43.

Fredheim, O. M., Borchgrevink, P. C., Hegrenaes, L., Kaasa, S., Dale, O., et al. (2006a). Opioid switching from morphine to methadone causes a minor but not clinically significant increase in QTc time: A prospective 9-month follow-up study. *Journal of Pain and Symptom Management, 32*, 180–185.

Fredheim, O. M., Kaasa, S., Dale, O., Klepstad, P., Landro, N. I., et al. (2006b). Opioid switching from oral slow release morphine to oral methadone may improve pain control in chronic non-malignant pain: A nine-month follow-up study. *Palliative Medicine, 20*, 35–41.

Freye, E., Anderson-Hillemacher, A., Ritzdorf, I., & Levy, J. V. (2007). Opioid rotation from high-dose morphine to transdermal buprenorphine (Transtec) in chronic pain patients. *Pain Practice, 7*, 123–129.

Furlan, A. D., Sandoval, J. A., Mailis-Gagnon, A., & Tunks, E. (2006). Opioids for chronic noncancer pain: A meta-analysis of effectiveness and side effects. *The Canadian Medical Association Journal, 174*, 1589–1594.

Gagajewski, A., & Apple, F. S. (2003). Methadone-related deaths in Hennepin County, Minnesota: 1992–2002. *Journal of Forensic Sciences, 48*, 668–671.

Galer, B. S., Coyle, N., Pasternak, G. W., & Portenoy, R. K. (1992). Individual variability in the response to different opioids: Report of five cases. *Pain, 49*, 87–91.

Gallagher, R. M. (2004). Biopsychosocial pain medicine and mind-brain-body science. *Physical Medicine and Rehabilitation Clinics of North America, 15*, 855–882, vii.

Gallagher, R. M., Marbach, J. J., Raphael, K. G., Handte, J., & Dohrenwend, B. P. (1995). Myofascial face pain: Seasonal variability in pain intensity and demoralization. *Pain, 61*, 113–120.

Gallagher, R. M., & Rosenthal, L. J. (2008). Chronic pain and opiates: Balancing pain control and risks in long-term opioid treatment. *Archives of Physical Medicine and Rehabilitation, 89*, S77–S82.

Gallagher, R. M., & Verma, S. (1999). Managing pain and comorbid depression: A public health challenge. *Seminars in Clinical Neuropsychiatry, 4*, 203–220.

Gallagher, R. M., Verma, S., & Mossey, J. (2000). Chronic pain. Sources of late-life pain and risk factors for disability. *Geriatrics, 55*, 40–44, 47.

Gardell, L. R., Wang, R., Burgess, S. E., Ossipov, M. H., Vanderah, T. W., et al. (2002). Sustained morphine exposure induces a spinal dynorphin-dependent enhancement of excitatory transmitter release from primary afferent fibers. *The Journal of Neuroscience, 22*, 6747–6755.

Gatti, A., Reale, C., Luzi, M., Canneti, A., Mediati, R. D., et al. (2010). Effects of opioid rotation in chronic pain patients: ORTIBARN study. *Clinical Drug Investigation, 30*(Suppl 2), 39–47.

Geisser, M. E., Robinson, M. E., Miller, Q. L., & Bade, S. M. (2003). Psychosocial factors and functional capacity evaluation among persons with chronic pain. *Journal of Occupational Rehabilitation, 13*, 259–276.

Giesecke, T., Gracely, R. H., Williams, D. A., Geisser, M. E., Petzke, F. W., et al. (2005). The relationship between depression, clinical pain, and experimental pain in a chronic pain cohort. *Arthritis and Rheumatism, 52*, 1577–1584.

Gillen, C., Haurand, M., Kobelt, D. J., & Wnendt, S. (2000). Affinity, potency and efficacy of tramadol and its metabolites at the cloned human mu-opioid receptor. *Naunyn-Schmiedeberg's Archives of Pharmacology, 362*, 116–121.

Gimbel, J. S., Richards, P., & Portenoy, R. K. (2003). Controlled-release oxycodone for pain in diabetic neuropathy: A randomized controlled trial. *Neurology, 60*, 927–934.

Giugliano, D. (1984). Morphine, opioid peptides, and pancreatic islet function. *Diabetes Care, 7*, 92–98.

Gomez-Flores, R., & Weber, R. J. (2000). Differential effects of buprenorphine and morphine on immune and neuroendocrine functions following acute administration in the rat mesencephalon periaqueductal gray. *Immunopharmacology, 48*, 145–156.

Gonzalez-Barboteo, J., Porta-Sales, J., Sanchez, D., Tuca, A., & Gomez-Batiste, X. (2008). Conversion from parenteral to oral methadone. *Journal of Pain & Palliative Care Pharmacotherapy, 22*, 200–205.

Gordon, D. B., Dahl, J., Phillips, P., Frandsen, J., Cowley, C., et al. (2004). The use of "as-needed" range orders for opioid analgesics in the management of acute pain: A consensus statement of the American Society for Pain Management Nursing and the American Pain Society. *Pain Management Nursing, 5*, 53–58.

Gourlay, D. L., Heit, H. A., & Almahrezi, A. (2005). Universal precautions in pain medicine: A rational approach to the treatment of chronic pain. *Pain Medicine, 6*, 107–112.

Griessinger, N., Sittl, R., & Likar, R. (2005). Transdermal buprenorphine in clinical practice – A post-marketing surveillance study in 13,179 patients. *Current Medical Research and Opinion, 21*, 1147–1156.

Grond, S., & Sablotzki, A. (2004). Clinical pharmacology of tramadol. *Clinical Pharmacokinetics, 43*, 879–923.

Guignard, B., Bossard, A. E., Coste, C., Sessler, D. I., Lebrault, C., et al. (2000). Acute opioid tolerance: Intraoperative remifentanil increases postoperative pain and morphine requirement. *Anesthesiology, 93*, 409–417.

Guststein, H. B., & Akil, H. (2006). Opioid analgesics. In L. L. Brunton, J. S. Lazo, & K. L. Parker (Eds.), *Goodman and Gilman's the pharmacological basis of therapeutics* (11th ed., pp. 547–590). New York, NY: McGraw-Hill Medical.

Guzman, J., Esmail, R., Karjalainen, K., Malmivaara, A., Irvin, E., et al. (2001). Multidisciplinary rehabilitation for chronic low back pain: Systematic review. *British Medical Journal, 322*, 1511–1516.

Hallinan, R., Byrne, A., Agho, K., McMahon, C., Tynan, P., et al. (2008). Erectile dysfunction in men receiving methadone and buprenorphine maintenance treatment. *The Journal of Sexual Medicine, 5*, 684–692.

Han, W., Ide, S., Sora, I., Yamamoto, H., & Ikeda, K. (2004). A possible genetic mechanism underlying individual and interstrain differences in opioid actions: Focus on the mu opioid receptor gene. *Annals of the New York Academy of Sciences, 1025*, 370–375.

Heit, H. A., & Gourlay, D. L. (2008). Buprenorphine: New tricks with an old molecule for pain management. *The Clinical Journal of Pain, 24*, 93–97.

Hoffman, B. M., Papas, R. K., Chatkoff, D. K., & Kerns, R. D. (2007). Meta-analysis of psychological interventions for chronic low back pain. *Health Psychology, 26*, 1–9.

Inturrisi, C. E. (2002). Clinical pharmacology of opioids for pain. *The Clinical Journal of Pain, 18*, S3–S13.

Ives, T. J., Chelminski, P. R., Hammett-Stabler, C. A., Malone, R. M., Perhac, J. S., et al. (2006). Predictors of opioid misuse in patients with chronic pain: A prospective cohort study. *BMC Health Services Research, 6*, 46.

Jamison, R. N., Raymond, S. A., Slawsby, E. A., Nedeljkovic, S. S., & Katz, N. P. (1998). Opioid therapy for chronic noncancer back pain. A randomized prospective study. *Spine (Philadelphia, Pa 1976), 23*, 2591–2600.

Jovey, R. D., Ennis, J., Gardner-Nix, J., Goldman, B., Hays, H., et al. (2003). Use of opioid analgesics for the treatment of chronic noncancer pain – A consensus statement and guidelines from the Canadian Pain Society, 2002. *Pain Research & Management, 8*(Suppl A), 3A–28A.

Kalso, E., Edwards, J. E., Moore, R. A., & McQuay, H. J. (2004). Opioids in chronic non-cancer pain: Systematic review of efficacy and safety. *Pain, 112*, 372–380.

Kanner, R. M., & Foley, K. M. (1981). Patterns of narcotic drug use in a cancer pain clinic. *Annals of the New York Academy of Sciences, 362*, 161–172.

Kaplan, H., & Fields, H. L. (1991). Hyperalgesia during acute opioid abstinence: Evidence for a nociceptive facilitating function of the rostral ventromedial medulla. *The Journal of Neuroscience, 11*, 1433–1439.

Karam, G. A., Reisi, M., Kaseb, A. A., Khaksari, M., Mohammadi, A., et al. (2004). Effects of opium addiction on some serum factors in addicts with non-insulin-dependent diabetes mellitus. *Addiction Biology, 9*, 53–58.

Karci, A., Tasdogen, A., Erkin, Y., Aktas, G., & Elar, Z. (2004). The analgesic effect of morphine on postoperative pain in diabetic patients. *Acta Anaesthesiologica Scandinavica, 48*, 619–624.

Katz, N., & Fanciullo, G. J. (2002). Role of urine toxicology testing in the management of chronic opioid therapy. *The Clinical Journal of Pain, 18*, S76–S82.

Katz, N. P., Sherburne, S., Beach, M., Rose, R. J., Vielguth, J., et al. (2003). Behavioral monitoring and urine toxicology testing in patients receiving long-term opioid therapy. *Anesthesia and Analgesia, 97*, 1097–1102, table of contents.

King, T., Gardell, L. R., Wang, R., Vardanyan, A., Ossipov, M. H., et al. (2005). Role of NK-1 neurotransmission in opioid-induced hyperalgesia. *Pain, 116*, 276–288.

Kinjo, M., Setoguchi, S., Schneeweiss, S., & Solomon, D. H. (2005). Bone mineral density in subjects using central nervous system-active medications. *The American Journal of Medicine, 118*, 1414.

Koch, T., & Hollt, V. (2008). Role of receptor internalization in opioid tolerance and dependence. *Pharmacology and Therapeutics, 117*, 199–206.

Krantz, M. J., Lewkowiez, L., Hays, H., Woodroffe, M. A., Robertson, A. D., et al. (2002). Torsade de pointes associated with very-high-dose methadone. *Annals of Internal Medicine, 137*, 501–504.

Kreek, M. J. (2001). Drug addictions. Molecular and cellular endpoints. *Annals of the New York Academy of Sciences, 937*, 27–49.

Kulkarni, B., Bentley, D. E., Elliott, R., Julyan, P. J., Boger, E., et al. (2007). Arthritic pain is processed in brain areas concerned with emotions and fear. *Arthritis and Rheumatism, 56*, 1345–1354.

Lafisca, S., Bolelli, G., Franceschetti, F., Danieli, A., Tagliaro, F., et al. (1985). Free and bound testosterone in male heroin addicts. *Archives of Toxicology Supplement, 8*, 394–397.

Langleben, D. D., Ruparel, K., Elman, I., Busch-Winokur, S., Pratiwadi, R., et al. (2008). Acute effect of methadone maintenance dose on brain FMRI response to heroin-related cues. *The American Journal of Psychiatry, 165*, 390–394.

Laulin, J. P., Maurette, P., Corcuff, J. B., Rivat, C., Chauvin, M., et al. (2002). The role of ketamine in preventing fentanyl-induced hyperalgesia and subsequent acute morphine tolerance. *Anesthesia and Analgesia, 94*, 1263–1269, table of contents.

Leo, J. A., Tanga, F. Y., & Tawfik, V. L. (2004). Neuroimmune activation and neuroinflammation in chronic pain and opioid tolerance/hyperalgesia. *Neuroscentist, 10*, 40–52.

Levine, A. S., Morley, J. E., Gosnell, B. A., Billington, C. J., & Bartness, T. J. (1985). Opioids and consummatory behavior. *Brain Research Bulletin, 14*, 663–672.

Lidstone, S. C., & Stoessl, A. J. (2007). Understanding the placebo effect: Contributions from neuroimaging. *Molecular Imaging and Biology, 9*, 176–185.

Lusher, J., Elander, J., Bevan, D., Telfer, P., & Burton, B. (2006). Analgesic addiction and pseudoaddiction in painful chronic illness. *The Clinical Journal of Pain, 22*, 316–324.

Lynch, M. E. (2005). A review of the use of methadone for the treatment of chronic noncancer pain. *Pain Research & Management, 10*, 133–144.

Manchikanti, L., Cash, K. A., Damron, K. S., Manchukonda, R., Pampati, V., et al. (2006). Controlled substance abuse and illicit drug use in chronic pain patients: An evaluation of multiple variables. *Pain Physician, 9*, 215–225.

Mao, J. (2002). Opioid-induced abnormal pain sensitivity: Implications in clinical opioid therapy. *Pain, 100*, 213–217.

Mao, J. (2006). Opioid-induced abnormal pain sensitivity. *Current Pain and Headache Reports, 10*, 67–70.

Mao, J., Price, D. D., & Mayer, D. J. (1994). Thermal hyperalgesia in association with the development of morphine tolerance in rats: Roles of excitatory amino acid receptors and protein kinase C. *The Journal of Neuroscience, 14*, 2301–2312.

Martin, B. I., Deyo, R. A., Mirza, S. K., Turner, J. A., Comstock, B. A., et al. (2008). Expenditures and health status among adults with back and neck problems. *The Journal of American Medical Association, 299*, 656–664.

Martucci, C., Panerai, A. E., & Sacerdote, P. (2004). Chronic fentanyl or buprenorphine infusion in the mouse: Similar analgesic profile but different effects on immune responses. *Pain, 110*, 385–392.

Maxwell, J. C., Pullum, T. W., & Tannert, K. (2005). Deaths of clients in methadone treatment in Texas: 1994–2002. *Drug and Alcohol Dependence, 78*, 73–81.

McNicol, E., Horowicz-Mehler, N., Fisk, R. A., Bennett, K., Gialeli-Goudas, M., et al. (2003). Management of opioid side effects in cancer-related and chronic noncancer pain: A systematic review. *The Journal of Pain, 4*, 231–256.

McQuay, H. (1999). Opioids in pain management. *Lancet, 353*, 2229–2232.

McWilliams, L. A., Clara, I. P., Murphy, P. D., Cox, B. J., & Sareen, J. (2008). Associations between arthritis and a broad range of psychiatric disorders: Findings from a nationally representative sample. *The Journal of Pain, 9*, 37–44.

Meghani, S. H., Wiedemer, N. L., Becker, W. C., Gracely, E. J., & Gallagher, R. M. (2009). Predictors of resolution of aberrant drug behavior in chronic pain patients treated in a structured opioid risk management program. *Pain Medicine, 10*, 858–865.

Meldrum, M. L. (2003). A capsule history of pain management. *The Journal of American Medical Association, 290*, 2470–2475.

Meunier, J. C., Mollereau, C., Toll, L., Suaudeau, C., Moisand, C., et al. (1995). Isolation and structure of the endogenous agonist of opioid receptor-like ORL1 receptor. *Nature, 377*, 532–535.

Michna, E., Ross, E. L., Hynes, W. L., Nedeljkovic, S. S., Soumekh, S., et al. (2004). Predicting aberrant drug behavior in patients treated for chronic pain: Importance of abuse history. *Journal of Pain and Symptom Management, 28*, 250–258.

Moore, R. A., & McQuay, H. J. (2005). Prevalence of opioid adverse events in chronic non-malignant pain: Systematic review of randomised trials of oral opioids. *Arthritis Research & Therapy, 7*, R1046–R1051.

Morley, S., Eccleston, C., & Williams, A. (1999). Systematic review and meta-analysis of randomized controlled trials of cognitive behaviour therapy and behaviour therapy for chronic pain in adults, excluding headache. *Pain, 80*, 1–13.

Mossey, J. M., & Gallagher, R. M. (2004). The longitudinal occurrence and impact of comorbid chronic pain and chronic depression over two years in continuing care retirement community residents. *Pain Medicine, 5*, 335–348.

Moulin, D. E., Iezzi, A., Amireh, R., Sharpe, W. K., Boyd, D., et al. (1996). Randomised trial of oral morphine for chronic non-cancer pain. *Lancet, 347*, 143–147.

Nicholas, M. K., Molloy, A. R., & Brooker, C. (2006). Using opioids with persisting noncancer pain: A biopsychosocial perspective. *The Clinical Journal of Pain, 22*, 137–146.

Nickel, M. K., Lahmann, C., Muehlbacher, M., Nickel, C., Pedrosa Gil, F., et al. (2006). Change in instrumental activities of daily living disability in female senior patients with musculoskeletal pain: A prospective, randomized, controlled trial. *Archives of Gerontology and Geriatrics, 42*, 247–255.

O'Brien, C. P. (Ed.). (2006). *Drug addiction and drug abuse* (11th ed., pp. 607–625). New York, NY: McGraw-Hill.

Office of Applied Studies SAaMHSA. (2005). *Results from the 2004 national survey on drug use and health*. Rockville, MD: Department of Health and Human Services.

Ohtani, M., Kotaki, H., Nishitateno, K., Sawada, Y., & Iga, T. (1997). Kinetics of respiratory depression in rats induced by buprenorphine and its metabolite, norbuprenorphine. *The Journal of Pharmacology and Experimental Therapeutics, 281*, 428–433.

Ohtani, M., Kotaki, H., Sawada, Y., & Iga, T. (1995). Comparative analysis of buprenorphine- and norbuprenorphine-induced analgesic effects based on pharmacokinetic-pharmacodynamic modeling. *The Journal of Pharmacology and Experimental Therapeutics, 272*, 505–510.

Olsen, Y., Daumit, G. L., & Ford, D. E. (2006). Opioid prescriptions by U.S. primary care physicians from 1992 to 2001. *The Journal of Pain, 7*, 225–235.

Olsen, G. D., Wendel, H. A., Livermore, J. D., Leger, R. M., Lynn, R. K., et al. (1977). Clinical effects and pharmacokinetics of racemic methadone and its optical isomers. *Clinical Pharmacology and Therapeutics, 21*, 147–157.

Paice, J. A., Penn, R. D., & Ryan, W. G. (1994). Altered sexual function and decreased testosterone in patients receiving intraspinal opioids. *Journal of Pain and Symptom Management, 9*, 126–131.

Pain IAftSo. (1986). Classification of chronic pain: Descriptions of chronic pain syndromes and definitions of pain terms. International Association for the Study of Pain, Subcommittee on Taxonomy. *Pain. Supplement, 3*, S1–S226.

Pereira, J., Lawlor, P., Vigano, A., Dorgan, M., & Bruera, E. (2001). Equianalgesic dose ratios for opioids. A critical review and proposals for long-term dosing. *Journal of Pain and Symptom Management, 22*, 672–687.

Piercefield, E., Archer, P., Kemp, P., & Mallonee, S. (2010). Increase in unintentional medication overdose deaths: Oklahoma, 1994–2006. *American Journal of Preventive Medicine, 39*, 357–363.

Pincus, T., Burton, A. K., Vogel, S., & Field, A. P. (2002). A systematic review of psychological factors as predictors of chronicity/disability in prospective cohorts of low back pain. *Spine (Philadelphia, Pa 1976), 27*, E109–E120.

Portenoy, R. K. (1996). Opioid therapy for chronic nonmalignant pain: A review of the critical issues. *Journal of Pain and Symptom Management, 11*, 203–217.

Portenoy, R. K., & Foley, K. M. (1986). Chronic use of opioid analgesics in non-malignant pain: Report of 38 cases. *Pain, 25*, 171–186.

Porter, J., & Jick, H. (1980). Addiction rare in patients treated with narcotics. *The New England Journal of Medicine, 302*, 123.

Raffa, R. B., Friderichs, E., Reimann, W., Shank, R. P., Codd, E. E., et al. (1992). Opioid and nonopioid components independently contribute to the mechanism of action of tramadol, an 'atypical' opioid analgesic. *The Journal of Pharmacology and Experimental Therapeutics, 260*, 275–285.

Raja, S. N., Haythornthwaite, J. A., Pappagallo, M., Clark, M. R., Travison, T. G., et al. (2002). Opioids versus antidepressants in postherpetic neuralgia: A randomized, placebo-controlled trial. *Neurology, 59*, 1015–1021.

Ralphs, J. A., Williams, A. C., Richardson, P. H., Pither, C. E., & Nicholas, M. K. (1994). Opiate reduction in chronic pain patients: A comparison of patient-controlled reduction and staff controlled cocktail methods. *Pain, 56*, 279–288.

Raphael, K. G., Janal, M. N., Nayak, S., Schwartz, J. E., & Gallagher, R. M. (2004). Familial aggregation of depression in fibromyalgia: A community-based test of alternate hypotheses. *Pain, 110*, 449–460.

Raphael, K. G., Natelson, B. H., Janal, M. N., & Nayak, S. (2002). A community-based survey of fibromyalgia-like pain complaints following the World Trade Center terrorist attacks. *Pain, 100*, 131–139.

Rasheed, A., & Tareen, I. A. (1995). Effects of heroin on thyroid function, cortisol and testosterone level in addicts. *Polish Journal of Pharmacology, 47*, 441–444.

Rauck, R. L. (2009). What is the case for prescribing long-acting opioids over short-acting opioids for patients with chronic pain? A critical review. *Pain Practice, 9*, 468–479.

Reid, M. C., Engles-Horton, L. L., Weber, M. B., Kerns, R. D., Rogers, E. L., et al. (2002). Use of opioid medications for chronic noncancer pain syndromes in primary care. *Journal of General Internal Medicine, 17*, 173–179.

Reinscheid, R. K., Nothacker, H. P., Bourson, A., Ardati, A., Henningsen, R. A., et al. (1995). Orphanin FQ: A neuropeptide that activates an opioidlike G protein-coupled receptor. *Science, 270*, 792–794.

Rice, A. S., & Maton, S. (2001). Gabapentin in postherpetic neuralgia: A randomised, double blind, placebo controlled study. *Pain, 94*, 215–224.

Ripamonti, C., Groff, L., Brunelli, C., Polastri, D., Stavrakis, A., et al. (1998). Switching from morphine to oral methadone in treating cancer pain: What is the equianalgesic dose ratio? *Journal of Clinical Oncology, 16*, 3216–3221.

Risdahl, J. M., Khanna, K. V., Peterson, P. K., & Molitor, T. W. (1998). Opiates and infection. *Journal of Neuroimmunology, 83*, 4–18.

Rohling, M. L., Binder, L. M., & Langhinrichsen-Rohling, J. (1995). Money matters: A meta-analytic review of the association between financial compensation and the experience and treatment of chronic pain. *Health Psychology, 14*, 537–547.

Rosenblum, A., Marsch, L. A., Joseph, H., & Portenoy, R. K. (2008). Opioids and the treatment of chronic pain: Controversies, current status, and future directions. *Experimental and Clinical Psychopharmacology, 16*, 405–416.

Rowbotham, M., Harden, N., Stacey, B., Bernstein, P., & Magnus-Miller, L. (1998). Gabapentin for the treatment of postherpetic neuralgia: A randomized controlled trial. *The Journal of American Medical Association, 280*, 1837–1842.

Russell, I. J., Kamin, M., Bennett, R. M., Schnitzer, T. J., Green, J. A., et al. (2000). Efficacy of tramadol in treatment of pain in fibromyalgia. *Journal of Clinical Rheumatology, 6*, 250–257.

Sacerdote, P. (2006). Opioids and the immune system. *Palliative Medicine, 20*(Suppl 1), s9–s15.

Sacerdote, P., Manfredi, B., Mantegazza, P., & Panerai, A. E. (1997). Antinociceptive and immunosuppressive effects of opiate drugs: A structure-related activity study. *British Journal of Pharmacology, 121*, 834–840.

Sadava, D., Alonso, D., Hong, H., & Pettit-Barrett, D. P. (1997). Effect of methadone addiction on glucose metabolism in rats. *General Pharmacology, 28*, 27–29.

Schieffer, B. M., Pham, Q., Labus, J., Baria, A., Van Vort, W., et al. (2005). Pain medication beliefs and medication misuse in chronic pain. *The Journal of Pain, 6*, 620–629.

Schmitz, R. (1985). Friedrich Wilhelm Serturner and the discovery of morphine. *Pharmacy in History, 27*, 61–74.

Schnitzer, T. J., Gray, W. L., Paster, R. Z., & Kamin, M. (2000). Efficacy of tramadol in treatment of chronic low back pain. *The Journal of Rheumatology, 27*, 772–778.

Sell, L. A., Morris, J., Bearn, J., Frackowiak, R. S., Friston, K. J., et al. (1999). Activation of reward circuitry in human opiate addicts. *The European Journal of Neuroscience, 11*, 1042–1048.

Sindrup, S. H., & Jensen, T. S. (1999). Efficacy of pharmacological treatments of neuropathic pain: An update and effect related to mechanism of drug action. *Pain, 83*, 389–400.

Skurtveit, S., Furu, K., Bramness, J., Selmer, R., & Tverdal, A. (2010). Benzodiazepines predict use of opioids – A follow-up study of 17,074 men and women. *Pain Medicine, 11*, 805–814.

Smith, H. S. (2008). Variations in opioid responsiveness. *Pain Physician, 11*, 237–248.

Smith, H. S., Datta, S., & Manchikanti, L. (2011). Evidence-based pharmacotherapy of chronic pain. In R. J. Moore (Ed.), *Handbook of pain and palliative care*. New York, NY: Springer.

Stein, C., Reinecke, H., & Sorgatz, H. (2010). Opioid use in chronic noncancer pain: Guidelines revisited. *Current Opinion in Anaesthesiology, 23*, 598–601.

Stoelting, R. K. (1991). *Pharmacology, physiology, & anesthetic practice*. Baltimore, MD: Lippincott Williams & Wilkins.

Tennant, F. S., Jr., Rawson, R. A., Miranda, L., & Obert, J. (1983). Outpatient treatment of prescription opioid dependence: Comparison of two methods. *NIDA Research Monograph, 43*, 315–321.

The American Academy of Pain Medicine tAPS, American Pain Society, and the American Society of Addiction Medicine. (2001). *Definitions related to the use of opioids for the treatment of pain*.

The Management of Opioid Therapy for Chronic pain Working Group. (2010). *VA/DoD clinical practice guideline for management of opioid therapy for chronic pain*. Washington, DC: Department of Veteran Affairs.

Tjaderborn, M., Jonsson, A. K., Ahlner, J., & Hagg, S. (2009). Tramadol dependence: A survey of spontaneously reported cases in Sweden. *Pharmacoepidemiology and Drug Safety, 18*, 1192–1198.

Tracey, I., & Bushnell, M. C. (2009). How neuroimaging studies have challenged us to rethink: Is chronic pain a disease? *The Journal of Pain, 10*, 1113–1120.

Trescot, A. M. (2010). Review of the role of opioids in cancer pain. *Journal of the National Comprehensive Cancer Network, 8*, 1087–1094.

Trescot, A. M., Datta, S., Lee, M., & Hansen, H. (2008). Opioid pharmacology. *Pain Physician, 11*, S133–S153.

Turk, D. C., Swanson, K. S., & Gatchel, R. J. (2008). Predicting opioid misuse by chronic pain patients: A systematic review and literature synthesis. *The Clinical Journal of Pain, 24*, 497–508.

Twycross, R. G. (1977). A comparison of diamorphine with cocaine and methadone. *British Journal of Clinical Pharmacology, 4*, 691–693.

Vadivelu, N., & Hines, R. L. (2007). Buprenorphine: A unique opioid with broad clinical applications. *Journal of Opioid Management, 3*, 49–58.

Vallejo, R., de Leon-Casasola, O., & Benyamin, R. (2004). Opioid therapy and immunosuppression: A review. *American Journal of Therapy, 11*, 354–365.

van Tulder, M. W., Ostelo, R., Vlaeyen, J. W., Linton, S. J., Morley, S. J., et al. (2000). Behavioral treatment for chronic low back pain: A systematic review within the framework of the Cochrane Back Review Group. *Spine (Philadelphia, Pa 1976), 25*, 2688–2699.

Vanderah, T. W., Gardell, L. R., Burgess, S. E., Ibrahim, M., Dogrul, A., et al. (2000). Dynorphin promotes abnormal pain and spinal opioid antinociceptive tolerance. *The Journal of Neuroscience, 20*, 7074–7079.

Vestergaard, P., Rejnmark, L., & Mosekilde, L. (2006). Fracture risk associated with the use of morphine and opiates. *Journal of Internal Medicine, 260*, 76–87.

Vissers, K. C., Besse, K., Hans, G., Devulder, J., & Morlion, B. (2010). Opioid rotation in the management of chronic pain: Where is the evidence? *Pain Practice, 10*, 85–93.

Volkow, N., & Li, T. K. (2005). The neuroscience of addiction. *Nature Neuroscience, 8*, 1429–1430.

Vuong, C., Van Uum, S. H., O'Dell, L. E., Lutfy, K., & Friedman, T. C. (2010). The effects of opioids and opioid analogs on animal and human endocrine systems. *Endocrine Reviews, 31*, 98–132.

Wasan, A. D., Butler, S. F., Budman, S. H., Fernandez, K., Weiss, R. D., et al. (2009). Does report of craving opioid medication predict aberrant drug behavior among chronic pain patients? *The Clinical Journal of Pain, 25*, 193–198.

Wasan, A., Michna, E., Greenfield, S., & Jamison, R. (2006). Interpreting urine drug tests: Prevalence of morphine metabolites to hydromorphone in chronic pain patients treated with morphine. *Regional Anesthesia and Pain Medicine, 30*, A-7.

Wasan, A. D., Wootton, J., & Jamison, R. N. (2005). Dealing with difficult patients in your pain practice. *Regional Anesthesia and Pain Medicine, 30*, 184–192.

Watkins, L. R., & Maier, S. F. (2000). The pain of being sick: Implications of immune-to-brain communication for understanding pain. *Annual Review of Psychology, 51*, 29–57.

Watson, C. P., Moulin, D., Watt-Watson, J., Gordon, A., & Eisenhoffer, J. (2003). Controlled-release oxycodone relieves neuropathic pain: A randomized controlled trial in painful diabetic neuropathy. *Pain, 105*, 71–78.

Way, B. M., Taylor, S. E., & Eisenberger, N. I. (2009). Variation in the mu-opioid receptor gene (OPRM1) is associated with dispositional and neural sensitivity to social rejection. *Proceedings of the National Academy of Sciences of the United States of America, 106*, 15079–15084.

Webster, L. R. (2010). Considering the risks of benzodiazepines and opioids together. *Pain Medicine, 11*, 801–802.

Webster, L. R., Choi, Y., Desai, H., Webster, L., & Grant, B. J. (2008). Sleep-disordered breathing and chronic opioid therapy. *Pain Medicine, 9*, 425–432.

Webster, L. R., & Webster, R. M. (2005). Predicting aberrant behaviors in opioid-treated patients: Preliminary validation of the Opioid Risk Tool. *Pain Medicine, 6*, 432–442.

Weschules, D. J., & Bain, K. T. (2008). A systematic review of opioid conversion ratios used with methadone for the treatment of pain. *Pain Medicine, 9*, 595–612.

Wiedemer, N. L., Harden, P. S., Arndt, I. O., & Gallagher, R. M. (2007). The opioid renewal clinic: A primary care, managed approach to opioid therapy in chronic pain patients at risk for substance abuse. *Pain Medicine, 8*, 573–584.

Xie, J. Y., Herman, D. S., Stiller, C. O., Gardell, L. R., Ossipov, M. H., et al. (2005). Cholecystokinin in the rostral ventromedial medulla mediates opioid-induced hyperalgesia and antinociceptive tolerance. *The Journal of Neuroscience, 25*, 409–416.

Yilmaz, B., Konar, V., Kutlu, S., Sandal, S., Canpolat, S., et al. (1999). Influence of chronic morphine exposure on serum LH, FSH, testosterone levels, and body and testicular weights in the developing male rat. *Archives of Andrology, 43*, 189–196.

Chapter 30
Nerve Blocks, Trigger Points, and Intrathecal Therapy for Chronic Pain

Zirong Zhao and Doris K. Cope

Physiological Basis of Nerve Blocks, Trigger Points, and Intrathecal Therapy

Pain is an unpleasant sensory and emotional experience associated with actual or potential tissue damage, or described in terms of such damage (Siddall and Cousins 2009).

The techniques of nerve block, trigger point release and intrathecal therapy for chronic pain were introduced into the field of pain management based on the neurobiology of pain, pathophysiology of painful conditions and pain relief demonstrated by observational studies, case reports, and case series. The biological system that supports the process of transduction, transmission, and modulation of nociceptive signal or ectopic nerve impulse is quite complex (Siddall and Cousins 2009). It consists of primary afferent neuron in the dorsal root or trigeminal ganglion, second-order dorsal horn projection neurons, spinal local interneurons, ascending and descending tracts, neurons in the medulla, rostral pon, thalamus, and cortex. Nociceptors, $A\delta$-mechanothermal and C-polymodal, are nerve fibers of the primary afferent neuron that are capable of transducing mechanical, thermal, and chemical stimuli into nerve activities. This process can be enhanced by peripheral sensitization upon injury via "inflammatory mediators" such as hydrogen and potassium ions, prostaglandins, leucotrienes, nitric oxide, substance P, calcitonin-gene-related peptide (CGRP), bradykinin, histamine, 5-hydroxy tryptamine (5HT), and other cytokines and neuropeptides. The dorsal horn of the spinal cord is the center stage where complex interaction among primary afferent neurons, spinal interneurons, second-order projection neurons, and supraspinal neurons occur. Ion channels, neurotransmitters, neuromodulators, and receptors in the dorsal horn are players in this intricate and dynamic system. Nerve block, trigger point release, and intrathecal therapies target the various steps of the pain pathways. Our current understanding of the mechanisms of pain relieve from these treatment modalities are the following.

Z. Zhao, MD, PhD (✉)
Veterans Affairs Medical Center, Washington, DC, USA
e-mail: Zirong.zhao@va.gov

D.K. Cope, MD
Department of Anesthesiology, University of Pittsburgh Schools of Health Sciences, Pittsburgh, PA, USA

Interprofessional Program on Pain Research, Education and Health Care, University of Pittsburgh Schools of Health Sciences, Pittsburgh, PA, USA

R.J. Moore (ed.), *Handbook of Pain and Palliative Care: Biobehavioral Approaches for the Life Course*,
DOI 10.1007/978-1-4419-1651-8_30, © Springer Science+Business Media, LLC 2012

Trigger Point Release

Myofascial pain syndrome refers to one of the most common soft tissue regional pain disorders involving the muscle (Russell 2008). It is characterized by the identification of trigger points, "a hyperirritable spot in skeletal muscle that is associated with a hypersensitive palpable nodule in a taut band" (Simons and Simons 1999). Treatment is focused on trigger point release and needling therapy is one of the management options. According to Simons' integrated trigger point hypothesis, sustained contraction of muscle sarcomere results in increased local metabolic demand. Yet at the same time, the supply of oxygen and nutrients to this region is impaired because the muscular capillaries are closed from the compression of muscle contraction. Thus, there is a local energy crisis and consequently a group of substances are released from the cells. These substances are capable of sensitizing nociceptors in the region (Simons 1999). This hypothesis was supported by elegant in vivo microanalysis of biochemical melieu in the trigger points. Shah et al. (2005, 2008) demonstrated depressed pH and elevated levels of substance P, CGRP, bradykinin, tumor necrosis factor-α, interleukin-1β, interleukin-6, interleukin-8, serotonin, and norepinephrine in the micro environment of a trigger point. Moreover, after induction of a local twitch response, the levels of substance P and CGRP became lower than their baseline values and similar to that found in normal muscles. This observation correlated with clinical results of pain relief after inactivation of a trigger point.

Epidural Steroids

The application of epidural steroids to relieve pain associated with spinal nerve irritation from herniated discs or spinal stenosis has been a practice for over 50 years (Swerdlow and Sayle-Creer 1970). Although the precise mechanism by which epidural steroid reduces pain remains to be elucidated, it is widely accepted that the steroid anti-inflammatory property plays a key role. A histological study of spinal nerve roots taken during operation for sciatica reported instances of nerve fiber degeneration and mononuclear cell infiltration around the spinal ganglion cells (Lindahl and Rexed 1951). High levels of phospholipase A2 activity, prostaglandin E2, and cytokines were detected in human surgical lumbar disc samples (Saal et al. 1989; Takahashi et al. 1996; Kang et al. 1996; Olmarker and Larsson 1998). In a rat model of radiculopathy, phospholipase A2 activity was lower in the experimental group treated with epidural steroid than that in the controls (Lee et al. 1998). A lower amount of arachidonic acid is generated if phosphalipase A2 activity is low because arachidonic acid, the precursor of prostaglandins and leukotrienes, is freed from membrane phospholipid by the enzyme phosphalipase A2. This is consistent with the clinical outcome of less inflammation and less pain. Additionally, steroids also inhibit leukocytes adhesion to endothelium and blocks nociceptive C-fiber conduction (McLain et al. 2005).

Nerve Blocks

Pain relief from local anesthetics is the result of inhibition of generation and propagation of action potentials along a nerve fiber secondary to blockade of voltage-gated Na+ channels (Salinas et al. 2008). Aminoamide agents such as lidocaine, bupivacaine, and ropivacaine are the ones used commonly in pain management. Characteristically, lidocaine has rapid onset but short duration and poor sensorimotor differential block, whereas both bupivacaine and ropivacaine have longer duration and good separation of sensory and motor blockade. In comparison to bupivacaine, ropivacaine has an improved toxicity profile, particularly cardiac toxicity. Interruption of pain transmission for a longer time period can be achieved by destruction of nerve cells using alcohol, phenol, and glycerol (Molloy and Benzon 2008). Application of alcohol, 50–100%, to nerve cells, causes wallerian degeneration due to extraction of membrane lipid and precipitation of proteins. Phenol, 4–10%, causes segmental demyelination or wallerian degeneration from protein denaturation. Both alcohol and phenol can cause vascular injury.

Radiofrequency Treatments

An application of electric current at frequencies of 300–500 kHz, similar to that used in a radio transmitter, to nerve fibers or dorsal root ganglion has also been shown to produce durable pain relief (Zundert et al. 2008). The current is produced by a radiofrequency generator and oscillates in a closed circle consisting of the generator, lesion electrode, tissue, and a grounding pad. Currently there are two types of radiofrequency treatments based on the mode of delivery of the electric current, either continuous or pulsed. The mechanism(s) by which radiofrequency treatment reduces pain remains a subject of research and discussion. During radiofrequency treatment, there are two fields, namely electrical and magnetic, produced in the tissue around the tip of a lesion electrode (Cosman and Cosman 2005). The magnetic field is minute and insignificant, whereas the electrical field is the key to the biological effects of radiofrequency treatment. Heat is produced in the tissue around the lesion electrode as a result of friction generated during ion movement under the influence of the electrical field. Sustained temperatures that are equal or greater than 45–50°C for 20 s or more can cause cell damage, hence the term "lethal temperature." In routine clinical practice, temperatures are usually held at 80–85°C for 60–90 s during continuous radiofrequency treatment. Under this condition, ellipsoid tissue coagulation is noted around the lesion electrode with its long axis parallel to the length of the electrode (Govind and Bogduk 2010). The larger the diameter of a lesion electrode and the higher the temperature, the bigger the lesion size is. Thermal destruction of the nerve fibers and cells has been accepted as the mechanism of pain reduction by continuous radiofrequency treatment. However, when electrical current is applied in short bursts to nerve tissue as in pulsed radiofrequency treatment, there is still pain reduction despite no tissue coagulation that is observed. Therefore, other effects such as the disruption of neuronal membranes and function from an electrical field have been proposed to mediate pain reduction (Cosman and Cosman 2005).

Intrathecally Administered Drugs

The central nervous system is the primary target of intrathecally administered drugs. Opioid receptors are present in the peripheral tissues, spinal dorsal horn, midbrain periaqueductal gray, the nucleus raphe magnus, the rostral ventral medulla, thalamus, and cortex (Inturrisi and Lipman 2010). There are three types of opioid receptors, μ, κ, and δ, but analgesia from currently available agents is largely the result of drug interaction with the μ receptors (Carr and Cousins 2009). Opioid analgesia at the spinal dorsal horn is twofold. Presynaptically at the small C fiber terminal, opioids inhibit calcium channels which lead to decreased release of excitatory neurotransmitters (Carr and Cousins 2009; Yaksh 2008). Postsynaptically, opioids activate potassium channels which lead to membrane hyperpolarization and decreased excitation of the wide dynamic neurons. Additionally, opioid analgesia is mediated through ligand–receptor interaction at the supraspinal central nervous system, in particular at the midbrain periaqueductal gray, resulting in activation of the descending inhibitory pathway. Antinociception by clonidine is also achieved through receptor–ligand interaction at the pre- and post-synaptic sites between primary and secondary neurons as well as by the activation of descending inhibitory pathway. The effects of clonidine are mediated by α2 adrenergic receptors (Carr and Cousins 2009; Osenbach 2010; Warren and Liu 2008). Release of neurotransmitters from the presynaptic terminal is essential for the transmission of pain signals from primary to secondary neurons. This process is dependent on the influx of calcium through voltage-sensitive calcium channels and subject to blockade by agents such as zoconotide, a selective antagonist of N-type voltage-sensitive calcium channels (Seagrove and Dickenson 2009).

Common Peripheral Nerve, Neuraxial, and Sympathetic blocks, Trigger Point Injection, and Intrathecal Therapy for Chronic Pain

The Greater Occipital Nerve Block

Anatomy: Fibers of the dorsal rami of the second cervical nerve continue to form the greater occipital nerve (Brown 2006a; Ward 2003). It is deep to the cervical musculature while traveling upwards to the occipital area and becomes subcutaneous at the point that is just inferior to the superior nuchal line, about 2–3 cm lateral to the occipital protuberance and medial to the occipital artery. The greater occipital nerve innervates the medial portion of the posterior scalp (Candido and Batra 2008).

Indications: Occipital neuralgia, cervicogenic headache, migraine, and cluster headache (Tsui et al. 2009).

Block technique (Brown 2006a; Ward 2003; Candido and Batra 2008): The patient is placed in a sitting position with his/her head flexed forward and supported. The landmarks for this injection, the occipital protuberance, occipital artery, and superior nuchal line, are identified. The skin entry point, 2–3 cm lateral to the occipital protuberant, medial to the occipital artery and slightly inferior to the superior nuchal line, is cleaned and prepped in a sterile manner. A 25-G needle, either 3/8 or 1½ in., is used to penetrate the skin at a 90° toward the occiput until a bony endpoint is obtained. The needle is then withdrawn 1 mm and redirected upwards slightly. After negative aspiration for blood, 1–3 mL local anesthetic is injected. It is unclear if the addition of steroid to local anesthetic solution provides added benefit for pain reduction (Tobin and Flitman 2009).

Gasserian Ganglion and Trigeminal Nerve Block

Anatomy: The trigeminal (Gasserian or semilunar) ganglion is located in the Meckel's cave, a dural pouch that contains cerebral spinal fluid (CSF), in the middle cranial fossa (Surash and Jagannathan 2009). It is bounded medially by internal carotid artery and the cavenous sinus, superiorly by the temporal lobe, inferiorly by petrous bone and foramen lacerum, anterior by the three branches of the trigeminal nerve, and posterior by the pon (Candido and Batra 2008; Henderson 1965; Brown 2006b). Of the three divisions of the trigeminal nerve, the opthalmic and maxillary nerves are exclusively sensory, whereas the mandibular nerve is a mixed motor and sensory nerve. The opthalmic nerve enters the cranium through the superior orbital fissure and carries sensory information from the anterior scalp, forehead, eye brow, eye lid, cornea, conjuntiva, ciliary body, the iris, the lacrimal gland, and nasal mucosa (Surash and Jagannathan 2009). The maxillary nerve passes through the infraorbial foramen, pterygopalantine fossa and enters the cranium from the foramen rotundum. It receives sensory information from the upper lip, cheek, lower eyelid, area of the temple and zygomatic region, the side of the nose, upper jaw, teeth, gums, hard and soft palate, mucosa of the maxillary

Fig. 30.1 Gasserian ganglion block. Three-dimensional CT-view constructed after the needle (*yellow*) tip was advanced through the foramen ovale (Image reprinted with permission from Springer. The image was originally published in Koizuka et al. (2009), Figure 3)

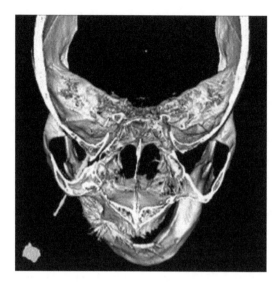

sinus, and dura matter of the middle cranial fossa (Erdine et al. 2008). The mandibular branch passes through foramen ovale and supplies the motor function of the muscles of mastication and relays sensory information from the chin, lower lip, lower jaw, and anterior two thirds of the tongue.

Indications: The gasserian ganglion is blocked for trigeminal neuralgia (Hickey et al. 2010) and tumor invasion of the gasserian ganglion, most commonly when neurosurgical management is not feasible (Candido and Batra 2008). The individual nerve branches are blocked for diagnosis of facial pain and surgical analgesia (Brown 2006c, d, e).

Block technique (Erdine et al. 2008): The block is performed with the patient in a supine position. Monitors of vital signs and cardiac rhythm are attached. Intravenous sedation with fentanyl and midazolam helps to reduce patient discomfort during the procedure. The procedure is performed under X-ray or CT fluoroscopy guidance. The landmark for needle entry for gasserian ganglion block is approximately 2–3 cm lateral to the corner of the mouth. The foramen ovale is noted by adjusting the fluoroscope to a lateral-caudal inclination. After preparation of a sterile field and anesthatizing the skin with 1% lidocaine, a 22-G 3.5-in. needle is directed towards the foramen ovale co-axial to the X-ray beam. Care must be taken so that the needle is not accidentally pushed into the oral cavity to reduce the complication of meningitis. Once the needle is in the foramen ovale, the fluroscope is turned laterally to guide the depth of needle placement. For a diagnostic block, local anesthetic up to 1 mL can be injected after negative aspiration for blood and CSF (Fig. 30.1). To obtain longer duration of pain relief, trigeminal rhizotomy can be completed by percutaneous approaches using radiofrequency, glycerol injection, or balloon compression (Assad and Eskandar 2010). Each of these techniques provides good initial pain relief but with a significant complication rate. For example, trigeminal motor dysfunction was noted in 24% of patients treated with percutaneous radiofrequency rhizotomy.

Sphenopalatine Ganglion Block

Anatomy: The sphenopalatine ganglion that is also known as the pterygopalatine ganglion resides in the pterygopalatine fossa, along with the maxillary artery and its branches (Erdine 2008; Moore et al. 2010). It is just behind the middle turbinate and below a depth of 1–1.5 mm mucosa/soft tissue

(Windsor and Jahnke 2004). It contains both sensory and autonomic neuronal components (Erdine 2008; Moore et al. 2010; Windsor and Jahnke 2004). The sensory nerves, that innervate the nasal membranes, the soft palate, and parts of the pharynx, pass through the ganglion and join the maxillary nerve just above the ganglion. Postganglionic sympathetic fibers pass through the ganglion and innervate the lacrimal gland and the nasal and palatine mucosa. Preganglionic parasympathtic fibers originate from the superior salivatory nucleus, travel with the facial nerve, the greater petrosal nerve and the vidian nerve, and synapse on their postganglionic cells in the ganglion. The postganglionic parasympathetic fibers innervate the nasal, paranasal sinus mucosa, and lacrimal gland.

Indications: Sphenopalatine neuralgia, trigeminal neuralgia, cluster headache, migraine, and atypical facial pain (Erdine 2008).

Block technique: There are three approaches namely transnasal, transoral, and lateral to block the sphenopalatine ganglion using local anesthetic (Tsui et al. 2009). Among these, the transnasal approach produces least patient discomfort. The patient is placed supine with monitors for vital signs and cardiac rhythm attached (Erdine 2008; Windsor and Jahnke 2004). To facilitate the insertion of a cotton-tip to the pterygopalatine fossa, the nasal mucosa is anesthetized with 2% viscous lidocaine. The cotton-tip that has been soaked with a local anesthetic, such as 4% lidocaine is slowly advanced to the posterior wall of the nasopharynx along the superior border of the middle turbinate. The cotton-tip is left in place for 20–45 min. An intravenous infusion tube can be slid over the cotton stick and attached to a syringe to allow for more precise instillation of local anesthetic (Windsor and Jahnke 2004). Pain reduction is short lived and periodic repetition of the procedure is common in order to maintain a sustained response (Erdine 2008). Longer pain relief for months to years has been reported after either pulsed radiofrequency or thermal radiofrequency treatment of the sphenopalatine ganglion.

Intercostal Nerve Block

Anatomy: There are 11 pairs of intercostal nerves derived from the anterior rami of thoracic spinal nerve T1–T11 (Gundamraj and Richeimer 2010). Each intercostal nerve has four branches, the white and gray sympathetic rami communicates, the lateral cutaneous branches and the anterior cutaneous branches (Brown 2006f). The lateral and anterior cutaneous branches along with posterior cutaneous branch from the posterior rami, collectively, provide innervation to the skin and muscles of the chest wall and abdomen. The intercostal nerves run inferior to the intercostal vein and artery as a neurovascular bundle. The common sites of needle entry for intercostal nerve block are the posterior angle of a rib and the posterior axillary line where the intercostal nerve is between the innermost intercostal muscle and internal intercostal muscle and in the intercostal groove (Brown 2006f; Nachi et al. 2008).

Indications: Relief of chest wall pain associated with surgery (i.e., thoracic and breast surgeries), tumor invasion, rib fracture, and postherpetic neuralgia (Gundamraj and Richeimer 2010; Nachi et al. 2008; Burton et al. 2009).

Block technique (Brown 2006f; Nachi et al. 2008; Waldman 2008): A patient is placed in a prone or seated or lateral position. Needle entry site is either the posterior angle of the rib or posterior or mid-axillary line at the level of the intercostal nerve corresponding to the location of the pain. The skin is prepared and draped according to usual sterile technique. Conscious sedation may be provided especially if blocks are placed in multiple intercostal levels. After infiltration of the skin and subcutaneous tissue with fast-acting local anesthetics such as lidocaine, a 22- or 25-gauge, 1½-in., short-beveled needle is inserted at the inferior edge of the rib until it reaches the bone. The needle is then walked off the rib into the intercostal grove. After negative aspiration for blood and air, 3–5 mL of local anesthetic is injected. The block can be performed under the guidance of fluoroscopy (Waldman 2008) or ultrasound (Harmon and Shorten 2009). To provide a longer duration of pain reduction, a neurolytic solution such as 10% phenol can be injected (Burton et al. 2009).

Lateral Femoral Cutaneous Nerve Block

Anatomy: The lateral femoral cutaneous nerve derives from the L2 and L3 spinal nerves (Enneking et al. 2009). It is a pure sensory nerve supplying the lateral aspect of the thigh from the ilioinguinal ligament to the knee. It emerges from the psoas muscle laterally, advancing between the iliac muscle and fascia, passing below the inguinal ligament and medial to the anterior superior iliac spine into the thigh. It is initially beneath the fascial lata, but pierces it about 7–9 cm from the anterior superior iliac spine and splits into anterior and posterior branches.

Indications: This block is a diagnostic tool for meralgia paresthetica and may also provide therapeutic value (Harney and Patijn 2007). It can also be used for analgesia during biopsy or skin graft harvesting (Enneking et al. 2009).

Block technique (Waldman 2008; Harney and Patijn 2007; Brown 2006g; Hadzic and Vloka 2004): To perform a lateral femoral cutaneous nerve block, one first identifies the anterior superior iliac spine. The needle entry point is approximately 2 cm medial to this landmark and just below the inguinal ligament. This block can be carried out using a 22–25-G 1½-in. needle. It is recommended using a needle with a short bevel to enhance the sensation of a "pop" when the needle passes through the fascia lata. Commonly injected anesthetics are 0.2–0.5% Ropivacaine or 0.25–0.5% bupivacaine or 1% lidocaine. The drug should be injected in a fanlike fashion as well above and below the fascia lata. If the procedure is carried out without a nerve stimulator or ultrasound guidance, an injection volume of around 10 mL is recommended due to the anatomical variation of the nerve as it emerges under the inguinal ligament.

Ilioinguinal/Iliohypogastrick Nerve Block

Anatomy: The iliohypogastric nerve derives from the T12 and L1 spinal nerves. It controls the motor function of the internal and external oblique muscles as well as the transverse abdominis at the anterior inferior abdominal wall (Enneking et al. 2009). It contains sensory innervation for the inferior abdominal wall and the upper lateral quadrant of buttock.

The ilioinguinal nerve derives from the L1 spinal nerve (Enneking et al. 2009). It controls the motor function of the internal oblique muscle and provides sensory innervation for inferior to medial aspect of the inguinal ligament. After leaving the lumbar plexus in the psoas muscle, the iliohypogasstric and ilioinguinal nerves extend laterally along the posterior lateral abdominal wall and in front of quadratus lumborum (Netter 1989). They then pierce the transverse abdominis, internal oblique and external oblique muscles while continuing to extend anteromedially in the anterior abdominal wall. At or near the anterior superior iliac spine, the iliohypogastric nerve lies between the internal and external oblique muscles, whereas the ilioinguinal nerve is between the transverse abdominis and internal oblique muscles. The ilioinguinal nerve pieces the internal oblique muscle at a more medial location in the anterior abdominal wall (Harmon and Shorten 2009).

Indications: Diagnosis and treatment of inguinal and suprapubic pain after inguinal hernia repair or lower abdominal surgery (Molloy and Benzon 2008).

Block technique (Waldman 2008; Harmon and Shorten 2009; Brown 2006h): To perform an ilioinguinal/iliohypogastric nerve block, one identifies the anterior superior iliac crest. According to different text books, the needle entry point is 1 cm (Harmon and Shorten 2009), or 3 cm (Brown 2006h), or 2 in. (Waldman 2008) medial and inferior to this landmark. Local anesthetic is then deposited between the internal oblique and external oblique muscles as well as between the transverse abdominis and internal oblique muscles. To improve block accuracy and success, the procedure can be carried out using ultrasonography that allows direct visualization of the fascia planes and nerves (Peng and Tumber 2008). Ultrasound guidance also helps to decrease complications such as puncturing the bowel.

Genitofemoral Nerve Block

Anatomy: The genitofemoral nerve derives from the L1 and L2 spinal nerves (Enneking et al. 2009). After it emerges from psoas major muscle, it descends behind the ureter and divides into a femoral branch and a genital branch just above the inguinal ligament (Waldman 2008). The femoral branch runs lateral to the external iliac artery in the femoral sheath and innervates the skin of the thigh just below the inguinal ligament. In the male, the genital branch runs inside the inguinal canal, exits the superficial inguinal ring, follows the spermatic cord, and innervates the cremaster muscle and skin of the scrotum. In the female, the genital branch runs with the round ligament and innervates the mons pubis and labia majora on the same side.

Indications: As a diagnostic tool for chronic inguinal pain, pain relief after the block supports a diagnosis of genitofemoral neuralgia (Nachi et al. 2008).

Block technique (Nachi et al. 2008): The landmarks for a genitofemoral nerve block include the pubic tubercle, inguinal ligament, inguinal crease, and femoral artery. To block the femoral branch, one inserts the needle lateral to the femoral artery at the inguinal crease and injects local anesthetic in a fanlike fashion into the subcutaneous tissue. The medication is injected laterally to the pubic tubercle below the inguinal ligament to block the genital branch.

Sacroiliac Joint Block

Anatomy: The sacroiliac joint is a large, synovial joint characterized by irregular contours of the sacrum and ileum that provide interlocking mechanisms (Cohen 2005). The joint has limited movement and its main function is stress-relieving (Bogduk 2005). The joint volume ranges from 0.8 to 2.5 mL with an average of 1.5 mL (Bogduk 2004f). The joint is stabilized by strong ligaments, including interosseous, posterior and anterior sacroiliac ligaments (Bogduk 2005). There have been variable descriptions of the spinal nerves that give rise to branches innervating this joint. The current thinking is that the posterior aspect of the joint is innervated by the lateral branches of the posterior rami of L4–S3 and the anterior aspect of the joint is innervated by nerves derived from the anterior rami of L2–S2. A recent study showed that local anesthetic blockade at L5 dorsal rami and S1–S3 lateral branches can render only insensitivity to painful stimulation applied to the interosseous and posterior sacroiliac ligament but not the sacroiliac joint (Dreyfuss et al. 2009).

Indications: Diagnosis of pain from sacroiliac joint (Bogduk 2004f).

Block technique (Bogduk 2004f): The patient is placed in a prone position and the skin overlying the target sacroiliac joint is prepared following the standard protocol for an aseptic procedure. Using a

Fig. 30.2 Sacroiliac joint injection. Anterior–posterior view of a fluoroscopic image shows the needle (*round shadow* with a *short black line* within) is directed to the joint

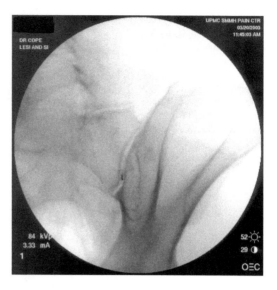

C-arm, a fluoroscopic view which displays the anterior and posterior margin of the joint is obtained. The goal is to obtain a maximally crisp medial cortical line of the posterior joint margin. A common needle entry point is where anterior and posterior joint margins overlap. A 22- to 25-G 3½-in. spinal needle is used most often to enter the joint (Fig. 30.2). Once the needle is inside the joint, 0.3–0.5 mL contrast medium can be injected to confirm placement. Local anesthetics are then injected. The total volume from contrast and local anesthetic should not exceed 2.5 mL maximally.

Medial Branch Nerve Block and Radiofrequency Treatment

Anatomy: Zygapophyseal or facet joints are synovial joints. Between the third cervical and first sacral level, they are formed by the inferior articular process of one vertebra and the superior articular process of the vertebra immediately below it (Cramer 2005; Boorstein and McGraw 2004). Each joint is innervated by two medial branch nerves, one that derives from the posterior ramus of the spinal nerve at the level of the joint and one from the level above.

In the lumbar region, the medial branches from the L1 to L4 dorsal rami run along the junction between the roots of subjacent transverse process and superior articular process, covered partially by the mamillo-accessory ligament (Fig. 30.3). Each medial branch nerve innervates two facet joints, the multifidus muscle, the interspinous muscle and ligaments (Bogduk 2005). The L5 dorsal ramus passes the groove where ala and superior articular process of the sacrum meet. It then gives rise to its medial branch nerve to innervate the L5–S1 facet joint and multifidus muscles.

In the cervical region, medial branches from the C4 to C7 dorsal rami run along the waist of its respective articular pillar (Bogduk 1982; Lord et al. 1995) (Fig. 30.4). Each medial branch gives rise rostral and caudal articular branches to innervate the facet joint above and below. For example, medial branch from the C5 dorsal ramus innervates C4–C5 and C5–C6 facet joints. This is different for the C3 dorsal ramus in that it gives rise to two medial branches. A larger one, the third occipital nerve, runs along the C2–C3 facet joint and gives rise to the articular branches to it. A deep one runs around the waist of C3 articular pillar just like the other cervical medial branch nerves below it and provides innervation to the C3–C4 facet joint.

Fig. 30.3 The lumbar medial branch nerves and targets (x) for anesthetic blocks of L4–L5 and L5–S1 zygapophysial joints. L2 the second lumbar vertebra, SAP superior articular process, SP spinous process, TP transverse process, L4–L5, L4–L5 zygapophysial joint, L5–S1, L5–S1 zygapophysial joint

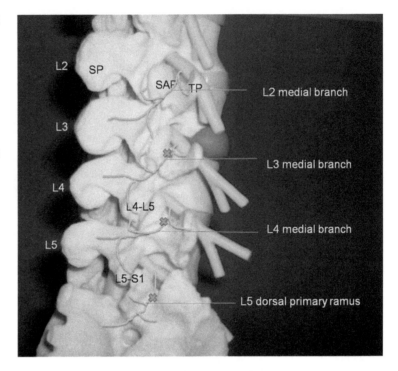

Fig. 30.4 The cervical medial branch nerves and third occipital nerve (TON). Targets (x, +) for anesthetic blocks. C2, the second cervical vertebra; SP, spinous process

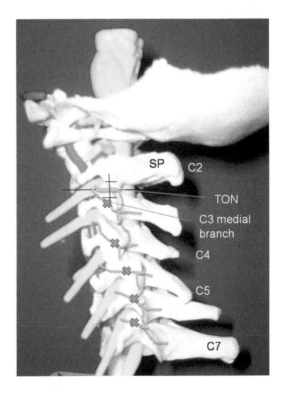

Fig. 30.5 A sketch of the medial branches of the thoracic dorsal rami viewed from behind. On the right side, the multifidus and lateral branches are not shown. *TP* transverse process; *MB* medial branch; *ZJ* zygapophysial joint; *SP* spinous process; *LB* lateral branch; *MF* multifidus; *ISL*, interspinous ligament; *C* cervical vertebra; *L* lumbar vertebra; *asterisk* atypical medial branch (Reprinted with permission from Springer-Verlag Wien. The image was originally published in Chua and Bogduk (1995))

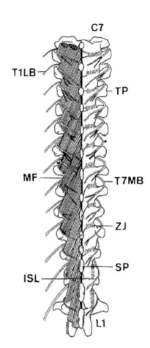

In the thoracic region, medial branches from the T1 to T4 and the T9 to T10 derive from the dorsal rami of their respective spinal nerves (Chua and Bogduk 1995) (Fig. 30.5). Each of them then runs posteriorly through the intertransverse space, reaches the superolateral corner of the respective transverse process, and continues caudally along the posterior surface of the tip of the transverse process. The medial branches of T5–T8 dorsal rami do not always come into contact with the transverse process. The medial branches of T11 and T12 dorsal rami runs within the junction of the superior articular process and the base of the transverse process, in a manner similar to that in the lumbar region.

Indications: Medial branch nerve blocks are used to determine if a facet joint is the pain generator and radiofrequency treatment of the medial branch nerves are used to treat facet joint pain (Bogduk 2004a, c).

Block technique: The skin over the injection site is prepared and draped according to the standard protocol for aseptic procedures.

To block lumbar medial branch nerves, the patient is placed in the prone position with a pillow under the abdomen to decrease lumbar lordosis (Bogduk 2004c). An oblique view of the ipsilateral lumbar spine is obtained using a C-arm fluoroscope (Fig. 30.6). The target point for the L1–L4 medial branch is the junction of the superior articular process and the transverse process (Fig. 30.7a–c). The target point for L5 dorsal ramus is the junction of the superior articular process of the sacrum and ala (Fig. 30.3).

To block cervical medial branch nerves, the patient is placed in either a prone or supine or lateral (affected site up) position. A true lateral view, the right and left articular pillars of cervical spine at the level to be blocked are superimposed, is obtained using a C-arm. To adequately block the third occipital nerve, it is recommended that local anesthetic be placed at three target points over the C2–C3 joint capsule. Precisely, one is to draw an imaginary vertical line bisecting the C2–C3 joint (Fig. 30.4). On this line, the highest target point is at the level of the tip of the C3 superior articular process, the middle line is at the level of the joint and the lowest point is at the level of the bottom of the C2–C3 intervertebral foramen. To block C3–C6 medial branch, the target point is at the middle

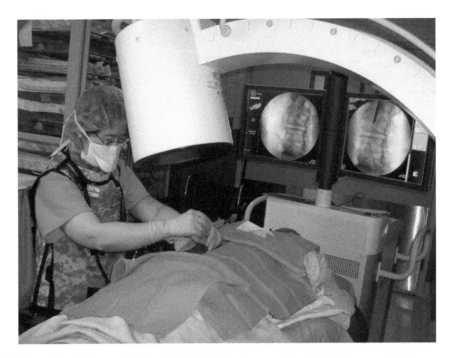

Fig. 30.6 The setting during a medial branch block. Needle placement is guided by fluoroscopic images

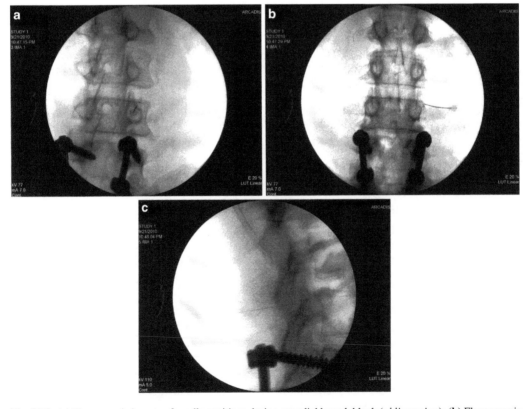

Fig. 30.7 (**a**) Fluoroscopic images of needle positions during a medial branch block (*oblique view*); (**b**) Fluoroscopic images of needle positions during a medial branch block (*anterior–posterior view*); (**c**) Fluoroscopic images of needle positions during a medial branch block, (*lateral view*)

Fig. 30.8 Fluoroscopic images of needle positions during cervical medial branch blocks (*oblique view*). The highest needle in this picture shows one of the positions for blocking TON. The next three needles are in positions to block C3, C4, and C5 medial branches

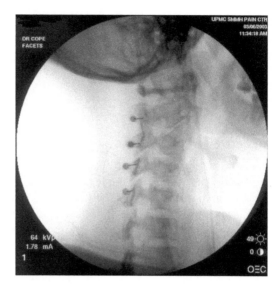

of the centroid of the articular pillar of the appropriate cervical vertebra (Fig. 30.8). To block the C7 medial branch nerve, the target point is at the apex of the C7 superior articular process.

To block the thoracic medial branch nerve, the patient is placed in a prone position. An oblique view of the ipsilateral thoracic spine is obtained using a C-arm. The target point for blocking a medial branch nerve derived from the T1 to T4 and T9 and T10 nerves is the superior lateral corner of the transverse process of the level to be blocked (Chua and Bogduk 1995; Nelson 2008). The target point for the T11 or 12 medial branch nerve is the junction of the superior articular process and transverse process. This is similar to that at the L1–L4 level. The target point for a medial branch block at the T5–T8 level is below the rib at the depth of the transverse process.

Local anesthetic is delivered to the target site using a 22- or 25-G spinal needle. In a retrospective evaluation of 500 consecutive patients with chronic neck, thoracic or low back pain, Manchukonda et al. (2007) reported that the false-positive rates after a single medial branch block at the cervical, thoracic, and lumbar spine were 45, 42, and 45% respectively. In order to reduce this false-positive response, comparative local anesthetic blocks have been advocated (Bogduk 2004a, c). This is accomplished by two injections separated by weeks. On one occasion the patient receives a local anesthetic such as lidocaine with a short duration of action. On another occasion, the patient receives a local anesthetic such as bupivacaine with a long duration of action. In general, a positive response constitutes 80% pain reduction with the ability to perform previously painful movements on both occasions (Manchukonda et al. 2007). Patients with positive responses can then be treated with radiofrequency therapy.

Continuous radiofrequency medial branch neurotomy (Bogduk 2004e): To perform a continuous radiofrequency medial branch neurotomy at either the cervical, thoracic, or lumbar spine, the patient is usually placed in a prone position. An appropriate size radiofrequency cannula depending on the anatomical characteristics (5–15 cm length, 18–22 G with a 5–10 mm active tip) is placed parallel to the target nerve under fluoroscopy guidance. The proximity of the electrode to the nerve can be estimated by sensory stimulation at 50 Hz and less than 0.5 V. Motor testing to ensure the electrode is placed sufficiently away from a motor nerve is conducted at 2 Hz and no less than three times the sensory threshold or 3 V (Rathmell 2006a). Once the position of the cannula is satisfactory, target site is anesthetized with local anesthetic and a thermal probe is placed into the cannula. Thermal lesioning is carried out at no less than 80°C and no more than 85°C for 60–90 s.

Pulsed radiofrequency of medial branch (Rathmell 2006a): To perform pulsed radiofrequency of medial branch at the various level of the spine, the radiofrequency cannula is placed perpendicular to the target nerve, in the same way as the needle placement for medial branch block. After sensory and motor testing, pulsed radiofrequency treatment is performed at 42°C with a voltage between 40 and 45 V for 120 s.

Stellate Ganglion Block

Anatomy: The stellate ganglion is the fusion of the inferior cervical ganglion and the first thoracic ganglion in most individuals (Erdine 2008). It is located at the vertebral level between C7 and T1. The surrounding structures include the longus colli muscle medially, scalene muscles laterally, subclavian and vertebral arteries anteriorly, transverse processes and prevertebral fascia posteriorly and posterior aspect of the pleura anterior and inferiorly. It is also near the phrenic nerve, recurrent laryngeal nerve, and brachial plexus (Molloy and Benzon 2008). As part of the sympathetic nervous system for the head and neck, all preganglionic fibers originate from the anterolateral horn of the first and second thoracic spinal cord segments (Erdine 2008). They either synapse or pass the inferior cervical ganglion. On the other hand, not all preganlionic fibers of the upper extremity sympathetic nerve system relay through the stellate ganglion. The upper extremity sympathetic preganglionic fibers originate from the T2 to T8 and sometimes the T9 anterolateral horn cells. These fibers synapse at the second thoracic ganglion, stellate ganglion, and sometimes the middle cervical ganglion. Postganglionic fibers from the stellate ganglion join gray rami communicates to enter C7, C8, and T1 spinal nerves to the upper extremity. Other postganglionic fibers from the stellate ganglion form a cardiac branch, ansa subclavius, and vertebral plexus (Darby 2005).

Indications: Relief sympathetically mediated pain in the upper extremities, head, and neck. The most common application is complex regional syndrome I and II of the upper extremity. Stellate ganglion block is also used to treat vascular insufficiency from occlusion and embolism, vasospasm, phantom limb pain, pain due to Paget disease, herpes zoster, postherpetic neuralgia, postradiation neuritis, intractable angina pectoris, frostbite, and hyperhidrosis (Erdine 2008; Rathmell 2006b; Breivik and Cousins 2009).

Block technique: Stellate ganglion block has been done for many years using anatomical landmarks without image guidance. The patient is placed in a supine position without a pillow and often with a towel roll under the shoulders to keep the neck in extension (Erdine 2008; Brown 2006i). The patient's head should be turned slightly to the contralateral site of the procedure. After skin preparation according to procedures for aseptic technique, the C6 vertebral tubercle (Chassaignac's), trachea and the carotid artery are identified. While keeping the carotid artery retracted laterally and the trachea medially, a 22- or 25-gauge needle is inserted through the skin until contacting the C6 transverse process. The needle is then pulled back 1–2 mm to have the needle tip outside of the longus coli muscle. After negative aspiration for blood and CSF, 0.5 mL of the anesthetic solution (such as 0.25% bupivacaine or 0.2% ropivacaine) is injected first. The patient should be told beforehand that he or she should avoid cough and speaking during the procedure. The patient is instructed to raise his/her thumb to request the procedure to be stopped. If no adverse reactions noted during the testing dose, additional anesthetics can be injected slowly in 3–4 mL interval. The total volume of anesthetic is usually 5–10 mL. Some use 1:200,000 epinephrine with local anesthetic as a test dose. Once the block is completed, the needle is removed, the patient should be observed for at least 30 min. To increase block accuracy and decrease complications, the use of fluoroscopic guidance (Abdi et al. 2004) or ultrasound guidance (Narouze et al. 2007; Gofeld et al. 2009) has been strongly advocated. When image guidance is available, the block can be done at the C7 level. This allows the needle to be placed at the location of the ganglion and decreases the volume of local anesthetic injection. However, this is associated with increased risk of pneumothorax and puncture of the vertebral artery (Erdine 2008; Abdi et al. 2004).

Celiac Plexus, Splanchnic Nerve Block, and Neurolysis

Anatomy: The celiac plexus is a network of nerve fibers and ganglia that are located anterior to the abdominal aorta and between the origin of the celiac and superior mesenteric arteries at the T12–L2 vertebral level (Darby 2005; Loukas et al. 2010). Sympathetic preganglionic fibers from the greater splanchnic nerves synapse on neurons in the celiac ganglia. The great splanchnic nerve derives from the T5 to T9 and sometimes the T10 thoracic sympathetic ganglia. The great splanchnic nerve descends obliquely along the lateral vertebral body and pieces the diaphragm to enter the abdominal cavity. Preganglionic sympathetic fibers in the lesser splanchnic nerve from the T9 and T10 or the T10 and T11 thoracic ganglia pierce the diaphragm with the greater splanchnic nerve and synapse at the aorticorenal ganglion, which is the lower, separate part of the celiac ganglia. The least splanchnic nerve that is present in 56% of cases derives from the T12 or the T11 and T12 thoracic ganglia. It synapses at the renal plexus after entering the abdomen. Postganglionic sympathetic fibers from the celiac plexus form downstream secondary plexuses near the target organs. These include hepatic, phrenic, gastric, splenic, testicular, ovarian, superior and inferior mesenteric, renal and abdominal aortic plexuses. Consequently, blockade of the celiac plexus can affect abdominal visceral pain.

Indications: Pain from abdominal viscera including pancreas, liver, gallbladder, omentum, mesentery and gastrointestinal tract from stomach to the transverse colon (Niv and Gofeld 2008; Rathmell 2006c).

Block technique: There are several approaches to perform a celiac plexus block. There are two large categories based on needle entry during the procedure, either posterior or anterior approaches. The classic description by Kappis employs a posterior approach which has been the basis for modern modifications in performing the block under fluoroscopy or CT guidance (Niv and Gofeld 2008; Rathmell 2006c). The patient is usually given intravenous conscious sedation with monitoring of cardiac rhythm, heart rate, blood pressure, and oxygen saturation. If using a fluoroscope to perform the procedure, the patient is placed prone on the procedure table. The scope is rotated to the ipsilateral site of needle entry until the tip of the transverse process of L1 overlies the anterolateral margin o f the L1 vertebral body. Frequently, the procedure is performed on the left side first. The skin and subcutaneous tissue that overlay the upper 1/3 of the lateral margin of the L1 vertebral body are anesthetized with 1% lidocaine, followed by insertion of a 22-gauge, 5–7-in. long spinal needle along the X-ray beam to contact the anterolateral margin of L1 vertebral body. The needle is then advanced 2–3 cm anterior to the anterior aspect of L1 vertebral body with the fluoroscope rotated to provide lateral views. Sometimes, the needle enters the aorta during the process. If this occurs, the needle should be advanced further until it completely penetrates through the aorta (this constitutes the transaortic approach). The needle position is verified on an AP view. One to two ml of radiographic contrast is injected after negative aspiration for blood, CSF, urine, and lymphatic fluid. The contrast may cover the left and right area anterior to the aorta. If this occurs, there is no need to perform a block on the right side. Otherwise, the procedure is repeated on the right side. For a celiac plexus block, 20–40 mL of local anesthetic, such as 0.25% bupivacaine or 0.2% ropivacaine is injected in increments of 5 mL with intermittent aspiration. If the procedure is repeated on the right side, 20–40 mL of local anesthetic is divided in half and distributed on each side. For neurolytic block, replace the local anesthetic with 50–100% alcohol or 6–10% phenol. A higher concentration of alcohol is often diluted with local anesthetics to a lower desired concentration. A higher concentration of phenol is often diluted with radiographic contrast. If a splanchnic nerve block or neurolysis is desired, the fluoroscope is tilted cephalocaudad to clear the 12th rib after lining up the tip of the L1 transverse process with the lateral margin of the L1 vertebra. The needle is then directed towards the anterolateral aspect of the T12 vertebra just below the 12th rib. This is also the end point for needle insertion during the retrocrural approach.

More recently, celiac plexus block/neurolysis has been completed by the guidance of endoscopic ultrasound (Wiersema and Wiersema 1996; Levy and Wiersema 2003). Although the celiac plexus cannot be visualized by ultrasound, its location in relation to celiac trunk is relatively stable. Vascular landmarks can be easily identified by color doppler. Using a transgastric anterior approach, access to the celiac plexus is much more direct than techniques guided by fluoroscopy or CT via either posterior or anterior approach. Because this approach avoids the retrocrural space, it may have lower risk of neurological and pulmonary complications (Levy and Wiersema 2003). The current, limited data suggest the efficacy of this approach is not inferior to other percutaneous methods (Chak 2009).

Lumbar Sympathetic Block

Anatomy: The lumbar sympathetic chain is part of the paravertebral sympathetic system that is situated at the anterolateral vertebral bodies bilaterally. It consists of ganglia, mostly four pairs at the level of the second to fourth lumbar vertebra, and connecting nerve fibers. The ganglia receive preganglionic fibers that originate from neurons in the lateral horn, intermediate nucleus, and paracentral nuclei of the thoracolumbar spinal cord via the white rami communicantes (Niv and Gofeld 2008). Postganglionic fibers join the lumbosacral plexus via the gray rami communicantes and the L1–L5 nerves.

Indications: Sympathetically mediated pain such as complex regional pain syndrome (CRPS) type I and type II, peripheral vascular insufficiency secondary to diffuse microvascular occlusion and other low extremity neuropathic pain may be reduced by this block (Rathmell 2006d).

Block technique (Niv and Gofeld 2008; Rathmell 2006d): Currently, a lumbar sympathetic block is carried out under fluoroscopic guidance. To perform the block, the patient is placed in a prone position. Lumbar vertebrae are identified under fluoroscopic image. The C-arm is oblique to the side to be blocked such that the lateral edge of the transverse process and lateral edge of the vertebral body are overlapped. This permits the needle entering the skin to reach the vertebra without bony structures in the way. For an anesthetic block, it is recommended to place the needle superior to the L3 transverse process in order to avoid the exiting spinal nerve root. Once the block needle touches the vertebra, the C-arm is rotated to a lateral view, the needle is then walked off laterally to reach the first 1/3 portion of the vertebra. The C-arm is then rotated to an anterior–posterior position. The block needle should be medial to the lateral margin of the vertebra. Nonionic contrast is injected to confirm needle position and rule out intravascular needle placement. Fifteen to twenty ml local anesthetic is injected, i.e., 0.25–0.5% bupivacaine. A minimal of 1–2°C rising in skin temperature of the lower extremity on the side of the block signifies a successful sympathetic block. Neurolysis with 10% phenol, or 50–100% ethyl alcohol or radiofrequency have been well described but is not done frequently in routine clinical practice due to post-sympathectomy pain.

Superior Hypogastric Plexus Block

Anatomy: The superior hypogastric plexus, an extension of the aortic plexus, is located anterior to the aorta and inferior to its bifurcation at the vertebra level of L5–S1 (Bosscher 2001). The lower two lumbar splanchnic nerves also send input to this plexus (Brown 2006j). The superior hypogastric plexus descends and divides along the internal iliac arteries to form the hypogastric nerve, which connects with inferior hypogastric plexus (Bosscher 2001). Most subsidiary plexuses to the pelvic organs originate from the inferior hypogastric plexus. Pelvic visceral pain afferent fibers, which have their cell bodies in the dorsal root ganglion, travel along the autonomic system. Therefore, blockade of the superior hypogastric plexus offers relief from pain originating from pelvic organs.

Indications: Pain from gynecological disorders, such as inflammatory pelvic disorders and adhesions, pelvic visceral pain due to nongynecological diseases, such as interstitial cystitis, irritable bowel syndrome and chronic pain after pelvic surgery, tumors of the pelvic organs. (Erdine and Ozyalcin 2008).

Block technique: The superior hypogastric block is performed with the aid of a fluoroscope. The patient is placed prone on the table. The skin overlaying the lumbosacral region is prepared and draped per routine for aseptic procedures (Stevens et al. 2000). After anesthetizing the skin and subcutaneous tissue, under fluoroscope guidance, a 7-in. 22-gauge spinal needle is inserted on one side of the L5 vertebra. The final tip position is just anterior to the L5 vertebra. Similar steps are then repeated on the other side. Radiographic contrast is injected after negative aspiration for blood to confirm the proper placement of the needle. This is followed by 6–8 mL of local anesthetic such as 0.25% bupivacaine or 0.2% ropivacaine on each site in the case of a diagnostic block. If longer-term relief is desired, neurolytic agents, 6–10% of phenol or 50% alcohol can be used instead (Erdine and Ozyalcin 2008).

Ganglion Impar Block

Anatomy: The ganglion impar, also known as the ganglion of Walther, is the union of the two sympathetic chains that located just anterior to the coccyx (Oh et al. 2004). Visceral afferents transmitting pain from the perineum, distal rectum, anus, distal urethra, vulva, and distal third of the vagina converge at this ganglion (de Médicis and de Leon-Casasola 2001).

Indications: Visceral or sympathetically mediated pain in the perineum, rectum, and genitalia (Erdine and Ozyalcin 2008).

Block technique: Several techniques have been described to block the ganglion impar under fluoroscopy guidance. These include the introduction of a bend needle through the anococcygeal ligament (Erdine and Ozyalcin 2008) or paracooccygeally (Foye and Patel 2009). Alternatively, a straight needle can be advanced through sacrococcygeal junction (Erdine and Ozyalcin 2008) or coccygeal joint (Hong and Jang 2006). Accurate needle placement is confirmed by radiographic contrast spreading along the anterior wall of sacrum and coccyx (Fig. 30.9). For diagnosis and temporary relief, 4–6 mL of local anesthetic such as 0.25% bupivacaine or 0.2% ropivacaine or 1% lidocaine can be injected. For longer-term relief, 4–6 mL of 6% phenol can be used (de Médicis and de Leon-Casasola 2001).

Epidural Steroid Injection

Anatomy: The epidural space is defined as the space outside the dura mater and within the bony spinal canal (Hogan 2009). The space starts superiorly from foramen magnum and ends inferiorly at sacral hiatus. The anterior boundary is the posterior longitudinal ligament, the vertebral body, and the intervertebral disc. Posteriorally, it is limited by the lamina, zygapophyseal joint, and ligament flavum. Laterally, the neural foramens allow the passage of nerves, vessels, and lymphatics, whereas pedicles protect the space. The epidural space is filled by areolar fat. It is largest in the mid-lumbar

Fig. 30.9 Ganglion impar
block. *Top image*, the
anterior–posterior view;
lower image, lateral view.
Contrast was spreading along
the anterior wall of sacrum
and coccyx

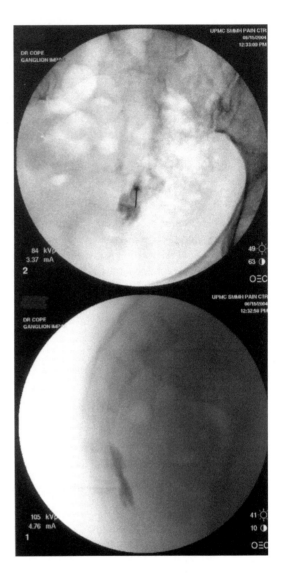

region and decreases progressively cephalad that it becomes a potential space above the C7 level.
The internal vertebral venus plexus, the spinal branches of the segmental arteries, lymphatics and
dura arachnoid projections that surround the spinal nerve are also found in the epidural space (Botwin
et al. 2004).

Indications: Radicular pain in cervical, thoracic, and lumbar regions due to disc pathology or spinal
stenosis (Bogduk 2010; Obray and Huntoon 2008).

Block technique: The epidural space can be accessed via the interlaminar, transforaminal, and caudal
route (Fig. 30.10). Although blind technique has been used for many years to place medication into
the epidural space via the interlaminar or caudal route, fluoroscopy guidance is highly recommended
because needle placements are not always in the epidural space even in experienced hands (Price
et al. 2000; Bartynski et al. 2005).

Interlaminar approach: The principles of interlaminar epidural steroid injection at the cervical, thoracic, and lumbar spine are the same. Technically, there are specifics for each level to accommodate

Fig. 30.10 Access the epidural space via the interlaminar or transforaminal route. *SAP* superior articular process; *SP* spinous process; *TP* transverse process

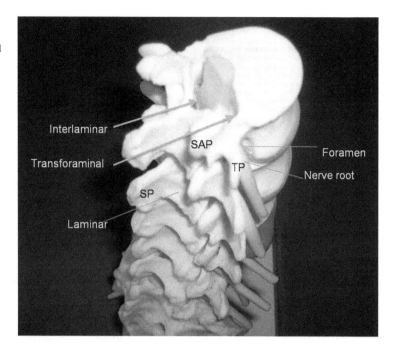

regional anatomy. In general, to perform an epidural steroid injection under fluoroscopic guidance in the cervical, thoracic, or lumbar spine, the patient is placed in a prone position. Skin overlaying the injection site is cleaned and draped according to standard practice for an aseptic procedure. An anterior–posterior fluoroscopic image is obtained and the C-arm is adjusted to maximize the target interlaminar space for needle access. Skin and subcutaneous tissue is anesthetized with 1% lidocaine. A 20-gauge 3½-in. or 18-gauge 5-in. Tuohy needle is inserted through the skin and gently pushed towards the epidural space with the guidance of intermittent anterior–posterior and lateral fluoroscopy. Loss of resistance to saline or air adds the identification of epidural space. The needle position is confirmed by 1–2 mL nonionic radiographic contrast medium (Fig. 30.11a, b). This also serves to rule out intrathecal or intravascular needle placement. Steroid diluted in preservative free saline is injected followed by removal of the needle and placement of a bandaid (Rathmell 2006e).

Transforaminal approach: The use of a fluoroscope is essential when this approach is utilized. In the lumbar region, the procedure is carried out with the patient in the prone position. After the skin is cleaned and draped according to protocol for aseptic procedure, an anterior–posterior fluoroscopic image is obtained. The C-arm is adjusted so that the anterior and posterior edges of the inferior vertebral end plate of the upper of the two vertebrae of the target segment are superimposed. The C-arm is then obliqued towards the site to be injected until the superior articular process of the lower vertebra is under the pedicle of the upper vertebra. There are two techniques, subpedicular and retroneural. In the subpedicular approach, the final position of the needle tip is above the nerve root and below the pedicle near the posterior vertebral surface (Fig. 30.12). In the retroneural technique, the needle entry point is slightly lateral to the tip of superior articular process of the lower vertebra. The final position of the needle tip is right behind the exiting nerve root (Fig. 30.12). Once the needle placement is in a satisfactory position as judged by fluoroscopy, a small amount of contrast is injected to ensure neither intrathecal nor intravascular injection occurs (Figs. 30.13). This is followed by the injection of a mixture of steroid and local anesthetic (Bogduk 2004d). To inject the S1 nerve root, the subpedicular technique is used.

Fig. 30.11 Interlaminar
epidural steroid injection.
Contrast pattern demonstrated
epidural spread

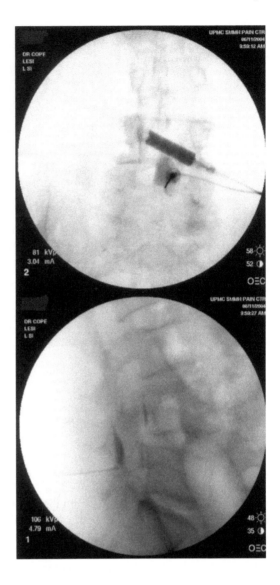

Cervical transforaminal epidural steroid injection is much more technically demanding. It is performed with the patient in supine, oblique, or lateral position (Bogduk 2004b; Rathmell 2006f). After preparation of the procedure field, the C-arm is obliqued towards the site to be treated, so that the intervertebral foramina are clearly visualized. The needle entry site is over the anterior half of the superior articular process that forms the posterior wall of the target intervertebral foramen. The needle is first placed on this bone and then readjusted to pass tangentialy into the intervertebral foramen by no more than 2–3 mm. Prior to injection of steroid and local anesthetic, the needle position is confirmed by fluoroscopy with contrast. Digital subtraction angiogram increased the sensitivity of detection of intravascular injection.

Thoracic transforaminal epidural steroid injection is also technically demanding and is performed much less frequently. Detailed descriptions can be found in the Practice Guidelines, Spinal Diagnostic and Treatment Procedures published by the International Spine Intervention Society (Bogduk 2004g).

Caudal approach: The patient is placed prone on the procedure table. After preparation of the procedure site, sacrum, sacral hiatus, and coccyx are examined from a lateral fluoroscopic view (Rathmell 2006e; Racz and Noe 2008). The skin entry site, subcutaneous tissue, and potential needle

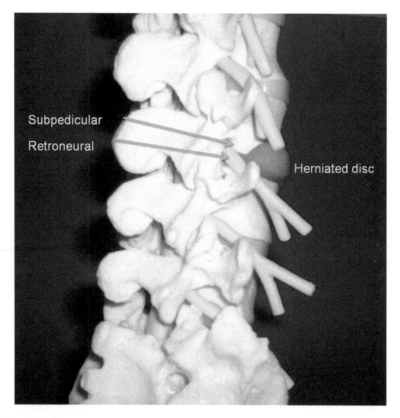

Fig. 30.12 Subpedicular or retroneural approach to perform transforaminal epidural steroid injections

path are infiltrated with local anesthetic. A 22-gauge, 3½-in. spinal needle is frequently used to access the epidural space. The needle is inserted at about 40° to the axial plane at the level of sacrococcygeal ligament. The needle is then lowered to lay closer to the plane of the sacrum. The needle is pushed 1–2 cm into the sacral spinal canal. Contrast is injected to confirm epidural needle placement and rule out intravascular or intrathecal injections (Fig. 30.14). A mixture of steroid and anesthetic is injected.

Trigger Point Injection

Anatomy: According to Travell and Simons, myofascial trigger point is "a cluster of electrically active loci each of which is associated with a contraction knot and a dysfunctional motor endplate in skeletal muscle" (Simons and Simons 1999). Clinically, a trigger point is a nodule in a taut muscle band that is tender when compressed. If the patient recognizes this pain as similar to his/her usual pain, the point is defined as an active trigger point (Simons 1999). Otherwise, it is a latent trigger point. Active trigger points occur frequently in postural muscles of the neck, upper trapezius, scalene, sternocleidomastoid, levator scapulae, quadratus lumborum, and the masticatory muscles. The development of trigger points is often the result of muscle overload from acute, sustained, and/or repetitive muscle use. Pain resulted from a myofascial trigger point is frequently reported as a poorly localized aching with referred pain pattern that is characteristic for an individual muscle. Pain and muscle dysfunction limit full stretch range of motion while reflex motor inhibition may cause weakness. The phenomena, spontaneous low-voltage motor endplate "noise" activity and high-voltage

Fig. 30.13 Fluoroscopic images of a transforaminal epidural steroid injection by retroneural approach. This is also termed selective nerve root block because the needle tip is outside the intervertebral foramen. *Top image*, anterior–posterior view; *lower image*, lateral view

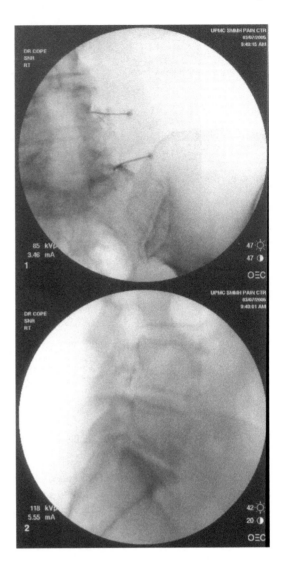

spike activity, in needle electromyography are considered characteristic of myofascial trigger points, but not pathognomonic. Local twitch response is a transient contraction of muscle fibers in the taut band, when a trigger point is stimulated by a penetrating needle or snapping palpation. It can be felt by palpation or seen as a twitch or dimpling of the skin near the terminal attachment of the fibers. This has also been observed on high-resolution ultrasound image.

Indication: Myofascial pain due to trigger points (Simons 1999).

Block technique: Trigger point injection is one of the methods that release a trigger point. It frequently provides immediate inactivation of trigger points. Injection with local anesthetic decreases post needling soreness in comparison to dry needling alone. Corticosteroid injection has been used to treat enthesopathy, but its use is not recommended for the inactivation of myofascial trigger points at the motor end-plate (Simons 1999). There is also no clear evidence to support the use of botulinum toxin A for trigger point injection (Ho and Tan 2007). To perform an injection, one gently rubs across the direction of the muscle fibers of a superficial muscle (Simons 1999). The taut muscle

Fig. 30.14 Caudal epidural steroid injection. *Top image*, lateral view; *lower image*, anterior–posterior view. Contrast shows epidural spread pattern

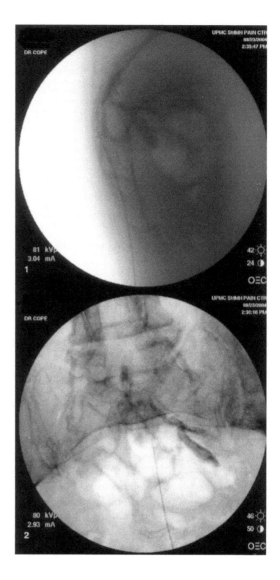

fibers are felt as a rope-like induration and the trigger point is a firm nodule in this taut band. The application of pressure to the nodule may elicit a pain sensation that the patient identifies as their familiar pain as well as a local twitch response may be elicited as confirmation. These points are marked and the skin is cleaned with povidone-iodine followed by alcohol. A trigger point is then positioned between one's index and middle fingers of the nondominant hand. While applying pressure using the index and middle finger, a needle is inserted quickly through the skin and into the trigger point, followed by injection of a small amount of local anesthetic (<1 mL at any one location). A 25-gauge, 1½-in. hypodermic needle is most commonly used. A longer needle may be necessary for deeper trigger points. A needle is never inserted all the way to the hub, as this is an area where needle breakage is most like to occur. A local twitch response and/or pain response that are familiar to the patient may be elicited. The needle is then pulled back but remains inside the skin. The needle is redirected to another trigger point. The needle is removed after all tender spots in that region are eliminated. To provide hemostasis, pressure is exerted by the fingers of the palpating hand over where the needle was and the track of needle when it is withdrawn.

Intrathecal Therapy

Anatomy: The intrathecal (subarachnoid) space is between the arachnoid and pia matter which ends at the lower border of the S2 vertebra in majority of individuals (Darby 2005). Naturally, arachnoid and dura matters are in close contact to each other and collectively form the dura (thecal) sac. Approximately 80–150 mL of CSF flows within the thecal sac. CSF is actively secreted by the choroid plexus within the brain ventricles at a rate of 0.3–0.4 mL/min (Ghafoor et al. 2007). This allows the total volume of CSF to be replaced 3–4 times a day. CSF is reabsorbed into the venous blood through arachnoid villi. Drugs in the intrathecal space can diffuse through pia matter with little resistance because pia matter is formed by one to two layers of cells joined by desmosones and gap junctions (Darby 2005). Intrathecal opioids must diffuse through pia matter and white matter to reach their final target location. White matter is composed of neuronal tracts with high content of lipids. Therefore, hydrophilic opioids, such as morphine has higher bioavailability in comparison to lipophilic molecules such as fentanyl (Ghafoor et al. 2007).

Indications: Chronic pain due to cancer or nonmalignant conditions in patients who have failed conservative therapies (either inadequate pain control or intolerable side effects) (Osenbach 2010).

Block technique (Osenbach 2010; Ghafoor et al. 2007; Staats 2008): Prior to permanent implantation of an intrathecal drug delivery system, a patient is evaluated by a multidisciplinary team. His/her history of pain, response to prior treatments, and psychological profile are thoroughly reviewed. A trial in which the medication is delivered by a single intrathecal injection or a temporary epidural or intrathecal catheter is conducted. Once a patient is determined to be appropriate for the therapy, an implantation is scheduled. Currently, the most common drug delivery device is a programmable infusion system with either 20 or 40 mL reservoir. The surgeon discusses the procedure with the patient and marks the location of the pump. Most frequently, the infusion pump is implanted in the lower abdomen subcutaneously. The procedure is done under general anesthesia or local anesthesia with monitoring. The patient is placed in the lateral decubitus position with the side of implantation up. Prophylactic antibiotics are given intravenously. The patient's back and abdomen are prepared and draped sterilely. The procedure is performed with fluoroscopic guidance. At the lumbar spine, an incision is made down to the dorso-lumbar fascia. The intrathecal space is accessed via a Tuohy needle, through which the intrathecal catheter is passed into the intrathecal space. The catheter is secured by anchors and sutured to the supraspinous ligament and dorsal lumbar fascia. This is followed by the creation of a subcutaneous pocket to accommodate the infusion pump and a subcutaneous tunnel to allow the passage of the catheter to the pump. The pump is programmed before it is connected to the catheter. Incisions are closed and infusion is started while the patient remains in the hospital for observation and drug titration.

Efficacy of Nerve Blocks, Trigger Points, and Intrathecal Therapy in Specific Diseases

The vast majority of procedures for the treatment of pain have sound physiological basis and are supported by case reports and case series, however, there is very limited randomized controlled studies to address the efficacy of them. Interventional pain procedures are analogous to surgeries in that their outcome is partially dependent on the experience and skill of the operator (Lenrow and Chou 2003). Just as in surgical treatment, blinding is frequently difficult to achieve. Additionally, pain is a presentation of diseases of heterogeneous etiology which may affect the response to a particular treatment and make conclusions on the efficacy of a specific pain procedure difficult.

Myofascial Pain Syndrome

Treatment for myofascial pain syndrome is focused on trigger point release and needling therapy is one of the management options. A recent systematic review by Scott et al. (2009) indicated that the efficacy of this treatment remains uncertain. It was not possible to synthesize the existing data due to heterogeneity among studies, small sample sizes, and incomplete reporting of study information. Consistently, it has observed that trigger point injection was safe if performed by appropriately trained providers. The therapy relieved pain regardless of injectant, however, injection using local anesthetic decreased pain associated with needling. The current evidence, as reviewed by various authors, does not support the use of botulinum toxin A for myofascial trigger point pain (Ho and Tan 2007; Scott et al. 2009; Kuan 2009).

Pain of Spinal Origin

Radicular Pain

Epidural steroid injection for lumbar sciatica was described in 1953 by Lievre via the sacral route (Swerdlow and Sayle-Creer 1970). This was followed by the publication of a case series of 113 patients with painful radiculopathy treated with procaine and hydrocortisone in 1961 by Goebert et al. (1961). Manchikanti et al. (2009) reported that 4,336 epidural procedures were performed per 100,000 Medicare beneficiaries in the fee-for-service program in 2006 according to analysis of the Centers for Medicare & Medicaid Services carrier claim records. Nevertheless, no long-term efficacy of epidural procedures for chronic spinal pain has been firmly established. Difficulties in drawing conclusions from the existing data lie in the heterogeneity of etiologies of spinal pain, techniques used to access the epidural space, medications injected, what and how the placebos were administered, post treatment time points when outcome data were collected, and parameters used to measure efficacy. The majority of the randomized controlled trials defined lumbar radicular pain from a herniated disc by clinical criteria, although more recent studies also provided magnetic resonance imaging (MRI) or computed tomography (CT) correlation. Data addressing the effects of epidural steroid injection on pain from spinal stenosis, low back pain without radicular pain and failed back surgery syndrome is sparse. When an interlaminar approach is used, nearly all studies access the lumbar epidural space using loss of resistance to saline or air technique without fluoroscopic guidance (Swerdlow and Sayle-Creer 1970; Dilke et al. 1973; Snoek et al. 1977; Klenerman et al. 1984; Cuckler et al. 1985; Carette et al. 1997; Valat et al. 2003; Arden et al. 2005). Similarly, older studies of caudal epidural steroid injections were done without radiological confirmation of the needle position (Bush and Hillier 1991). Transforaminal epidural steroid injections with fluoroscopic guidance are for precision needle placement (Karppinen et al. 2001; Ng et al. 2005; Ghahreman et al. 2010). In a prospective, randomized study examining the efficacy of transforaminal injection of steroid for lumbar radicular pain, Ghahreman et al. (2010) demonstrated a subgroup of patients responded with pain reduction more than 50% at 1 month after treatment. This subgroup constituted 54% of the patients in the transforaminal epidural steroid group. The percentage of patients who had similar pain reduction was much lower in the control groups which included transforaminal injection of local anesthetic (7% patients had pain reduction more than 50% at 1 month), transforaminal injection of saline (19%), intramusclular steroid injection (21%), and intramuscular saline injection (13%). The authors then analyzed the clinical and radiological features of these study participants. They found that the less compression of a nerve root, the more likely a patient will get pain relief from transforaminal injection of steriod Ghahreman and Bogduk (2011). The number of patients who maintained pain relief, however, diminished at 3, 6, and 12-month follow-up appointments. The question as to whether transforaminal epidural steroid injection is superior or equivalent to fluoroscopically guided interlaminar epidural steroid injection cannot be answered with certainty, in the absence of study results from prospective, controlled studies that compare the two approaches head-to-head. The consensus opinion reflected by guideline recommendations from the various medical societies including American Society of Anesthesiologists, American Pain Society, American Society of Interventional Pain Physicians, American Academy of Neurology, and American College of Occupational and Environmental Medicine is that epidural steroid injection with or without local anesthetics provide pain relief for a short period ranging from 2 weeks to 3 months in patients with radicular pain or radiculopathy (American Society of Anesthesiologists 2010; Chou et al. 2009; Manchikanti et al. 2009; Armon et al. 2007; American College of Occupational and Environmental Medicine 2007). The magnitude of pain reduction in lumbosacral radicular pain is modest and there is no consistent evidence that the treatment has impact on impairment of function, on need for surgery and on long-term pain relief beyond 3 months. Epidural steroid injection by transforaminal, interlaminar, or caudal route should be a part of a multimodal treatment regimen for the relief of chronic pain.

There are no randomized controlled trials to date that address the efficacy of interlaminar or transforaminal cervical epidural steroid injection. Some data suggesting cervical epidural steroid injections reduce radicular pain were taken from prospective, noncontrolled studies (Zundert et al. 2010).

A double blind sham-controlled randomized trial of pulsed radiofrequency treatment of cervical dorsal root ganglion for chronic cervical radicular pain was reported by Zundert et al. (2007). The study participants all had positive Spurling test on physical examination and a minimum of 50% pain reduction after diagnostic nerve block with local anesthetic. At 3 months after pulse radiofrequency treatment, 9 out of 11 patients (82%) reported a 50% or greater improvement as assessed by global perceived effect scale, whereas 4 out of 12 (33%) patients in the sham group reported the same. Additionally, 82% patients in the treatment group noted a 20-points or greater decrease in pain intensity measured by visual analog scale, whereas only 25% in the sham group achieved pain reduction to the same extent. There was no reduction in pain medication use, however. The sample size of this study was small, 11 patients in the treatment group and 12 patients in the sham group, despite screening 256 patients with cervicobrachialgia. There were 63 patients who did not give consent to participate in the study, which illustrated the difficult in recruiting patients for interventional pain trials.

Zygapophyseal Joint Pain

Pain originated from the zygapophyseal joint has been considered a source of chronic back pain including cervical, thoracic and lumbar regions (Manchikanti et al. 2004). The underlying pathologies are osteoarthrosis or chondromalacia facetae, and occult fractures (Schwarzer et al. 1994). In volunteers without low back pain, intra-articular or pericapsular injection of normal saline was capable of eliciting pain that was deep and away from the injection site (McCall et al. 1979). Pain from the L4/L5 facet joint is often referred to the buttocks and that from L1/L2 joint to the flank region. There is variation in the extent of individual referral pattern and referred pain overlapped at the posterior iliac crest and groin. Similarly, in the cervical spine, intra-articular injection of contrast dye produced pain in the neck, shoulder, and upper back in previously asymptomatic volunteers (Dwyer et al. 1988). There are no consistent clinical features that reliably diagnose facet joint pain (Schwarzer et al. 1994; Manchikanti et al. 2000). The diagnosis of a facet joint as the pain generator rests on anesthetizing the medial branch nerves innervating the joint by blocks. Utilizing comparative local anesthetic blocks, Manchikanti et al. (2004) reported the prevalence of facet joint pain in patients presented with cervical, thoracic, and lumbar spine pain in a non-university, private interventional pain clinic as 55, 42, and 31%, respectively. It is important to realize that among the 500 patients evaluated in this study, 140 had cervical facet joint pain, 30 had thoracic facet joint pain, and 124 had lumbar facet joint pain. Thoracic facet joint pain is much less common. Barnsley et al. (1995) reported that the prevalence of chronic cervical facet joint pain after whiplash was 54%. The prevalence of facet joint pain in the general population is unknown. The definitive treatment for facet joint pain is radiofrequency application to the medial branch nerve.

In the lumbar spine, randomized controlled trials yielded inconsistent results on pain reduction after radiofrequency treatment of the medial branch nerves (Van Kleef et al. 1999; Tekin et al. 2007; Nath et al. 2008; Leclaire et al. 2001; Van Wijk et al. 2005). Close examination of each studies reviewed that those studies that reported lack of efficacy had suboptimal placement of the radiofrequecy cannulae and patient selection was not based on outcome of comparative local anesthetic blocks (Leclaire et al. 2001; Van Wijk et al. 2005). To date, there is only one randomized controlled trial which selected patients based on an 80% pain reduction from comparative diagnostic blocks (Nath et al. 2008). This study had appropriate radiofrequency cannula placement and a patient population representative of everyday clinic practice. In this study, there was an average 2-point reduction in VAS in generalized pain and back pain, decrease in analgesic consumption, improved personal hygiene, better tolerance in sitting, standing, working, and improved subjective global assessment. However, the studies terminated at 6-month post treatment. Observational studies indicated that the effect of thermal radiofrequency persisted for 12 months and in a subset of patients continued to show improvement 24 months post treatment (Dreyfuss et al. 2000; Gofeld et al. 2007). Pulsed radiofrequecy of the lumbar medial branch did not yield as much pain reduction and the beneficial effected was lost at 6 months (Tekin et al. 2007). Radiofrequency neurotomy is not a curative procedure. After initial benefits dissipate, repeat treatments provide similar success rate and duration of pain reduction (Schofferman and Kine 2004). The American Society of Anesthesiologist Task Force on Chronic Pain Management and the American Society of Regional Anesthesia and Pain Medicine practice guideline recommends conventional (80°C) or thermal (67°C) medial branch radiofrequency ablation for facet joint mediated low back pain when there is good response to anesthetic medial branch nerve block (American Society of Anesthesiologists 2010).

In the cervical spine, there is only one randomized controlled trial completed to date to address the efficacy of thermal radiofrequency medial branch neurotomy in patients with whiplash-associated cervical facet joint pain (Lord et al. 1996). This meticulously conducted study demonstrated lasting, complete relief in a moderate percentage of patients identified by two comparative anesthetic block plus saline placebo block. Observational studies provided evidence for the effectiveness of this procedure in degenerative cervical facet joint pain with median duration of pain reduction lasting 31–36 weeks (McDonald et al. 1999; Barnsley 2005). A few patients had prolonged relief lasting for 2–3 years. Patient responses to subsequent treatments from recurrence of facet joint pain at the level were as good as the initial intervention (McDonald et al. 1999; Barnsley 2005; Husted et al. 2008).

Sacroiliac Joint Pain

Although there is no gold standard for the diagnosis of sacroiliac joint pain, it is accepted that low back pain could result from of pathological changes in the joint. The common etiologies include trauma, leg length discrepancy, spine pathology, pregnancy, inflammation from ankylosing spondylitis, metabolic dysfunction such as gout and pseudogout, osteoarthritis, infection, and tumor (Malik and Benzon 2008). Clinically, it appears that pain from the sacroiliac joint is predominantly located below the L5 spinous process and at the posterior superior iliac spine or within 2 cm of it (Cohen 2005; Murakami et al. 2008). The prevalence of sacroiliac joint pain in chronic low back pain population is estimated to be 15–25% (Cohen 2005). Although injection of the sacroiliac joint using steroid and local anesthetic is a frequently performed procedure in routine clinical practice, there is a lack of well-conducted studies to evaluate the effectiveness of this treatment (Rupert et al. 2009). Likewise, there is limited data for the evaluation of radiofrequency denervation for the treatment of sacroiliac joint pain (American Society of Anesthesiologists 2010; Rupert et al. 2009).

Complex Regional Pain Syndrome

CRPS is subdivided into type I (reflex sympathetic dystrophy) and type II (causalgia). There is an apparent nerve injury in causalgia. The diagnostic criteria for CRPS were established by The International Association for the Study of Pain in 1994 (Williams et al. 2008). The criteria have high sensitivity but low specificity. Therefore, it was modified in 2003 by a group of pain experts in a consensus meeting held in Budapest, Hungary. The "Budapest Criteria" are currently recommended for use in clinical practice and research according to its decision rules established for these two different settings (Harden et al. 2010). Historically, as early as in World War I, surgical sympathectomy was used to treat CRPS (Fechir et al. 2008). Studies in human and animals showed that there is an interaction between the sympathetic and sensory nervous system (Gibbs et al. 2008; De Mos et al. 2009). The active components of this interaction include inflammatory mediators, alpha-1 adrenergic receptors, and neuropeptides. Observational studies showed short-term pain reduction ranging from 1 to 4 weeks when lumbar sympathetic or stellate ganglion blocks were used to treat CRPS (American Society of Anesthesiologists 2010). No study addressed long-term efficacy of a series of lumbar sympathetic or stellate ganglion blocks in treating CRPS. So far, final results from only one published randomized controlled clinical trials addressed anesthetic sympathetic blockage on pain relief with comparison to normal saline. This trial has a small sample size (7 participants) and a short duration of study (7 days), but it confirmed what was noted in our daily practice that the effect of pain relief lasted longer than the expected duration of local anesthetics (Price et al. 1998). The expert opinion at this time is that lumbar sympathetic blocks or stellate ganglion blocks should be used as one of the treatment modalities in comprehensive, multidisciplinary approaches to the management of CRPS (American Society of Anesthesiologists 2010).

Intrathecal Therapy for Pain

Most intrathecal therapy pumps implanted in the United States are for the treatment of spine pain as a result of failed back surgery syndrome, compression fracture, spinal stenosis, radiculitis, spondylosis, and spondylolisthesis, with the most common diagnosis being post laminectomy pain (Deer 2008). In the context of cancer, cancer patients with pain refractory to medical management are often referred too late in their stages of diseases which render them poor candidates for this therapy. Morphine, zocinotide, and bacolfen are the only three agents that are approved by the Food and Drug Administration for use intrathecally, with the first two carrying the indication for pain management. Other drugs that are frequently used off-label include hydromorphone, fentanyl, sufentanil, bupivicaine, and clonidine. To help clinicians making decision on starting agent, dose titration, drug combination, spinal drug delivery experts have established an intrathecal drug treatment algorithm. Morphine intrathecal administration in humans was first reported in 1978 by Wang et al. (1979) who demonstrated a dramatic pain reduction without sedation, respiratory depression, and diminished neurological function in cancer patients after 0.5–1 mg single injection. Since then, morphine has been the cornerstone drug used in intrathecal drug infusion for pain. Hydromorphone is approximately 5–6 times more potent than morphine with lesser side effects (Osenbach 2010). There are less clinical data regarding the long-term use of fentanyl and sufentanil which are characteristically more lipophilic and potent (Osenbach 2010; Deer 2008). Among the local anesthetics, bupivacaine is the drug that is used most often and has strong clinical data support its safety and efficacy. When it is used in combination with other drugs intrathecally, bupivacaine improves pain control with less opioid dosage than that would be needed if opioid is used as a solo agent (Deer 2008). Its impact on neuropathic pain is greater than that on nociceptive pain (Osenbach 2010). Clonidine, an alpha-1 adrenergic agonist, relieves pain by postsynaptic activation of descending noradrenergic inhibitory system and therefore it works synergistically with opioids. Ziconotide, a N-type voltage-sensitive calcium channel antagonist, blocks neurotransmission at the primary nociceptive afferents. Two randomized, double-blind, placebo-controlled trials addressed the efficacy and safety of ziconotide when used as a solo intrathecal agent in chronic pain patients who are refractory to systemic or intrathecal opioid therapy. In ziconotide responders with pain secondary to cancer or AIDS, a pain reduction as expressed in percentage changes of mean visual analog scale of pain index was 51% in the treatment group and 18% in the placebo group at the end of 10-day study period (Staats et al. 2004). Rauck et al. (2006) examined patients mostly with nonmalignant pain (58% participants with failed back surgery syndrome) and extended the study period to 3 weeks. Their reported mean percentage change of visual analog scale of pain index was only 14.7% in the ziconotide-treated group and 7.2% in the placebo group. Both studies reported decreased opioid use in the treatment group. In a subsequent open-label study in patients with either malignant or nonmalignant pain, Webster et al. (2009) reported sustained pain reduction with relatively stable dosages in responders at 3 years after initiation of the treatment. The mean percentage change in visual analog scale of pain index from the beginning of the study was 22%.

Efficacy of intrathecal drug therapy in comparison to comprehensive medical management for refractory cancer pain was examined in a randomized clinical trial by Smith et al. (2002, 2005). All patients started with an opioid as the solo agent (94% morphine, 6% hydromorphone), but the investigators were allowed to modify the regimen to a combination of agents after the initial 4 weeks. The study showed better pain control in both the intrathecal drug therapy and comprehensive medical management groups at 4 and 12 weeks, however, the great advantage of intrathecal therapy over systemic medical therapy was significantly fewer drug side effects. Patient survival was also improved in the intrathecal group at the end of this 6-month trial.

There is no randomized control trial published to date that addresses the efficacy of intrathecal opioid therapy in nonmalignant pain patients. Observational studies consistently showed improved pain control, better overall patient satisfaction, and improved activity level (Patel et al. 2009; Thimineur et al. 2004; Deer et al. 2004; Roberts et al. 2001). These beneficial effects are sustained over several years. However, there is no change in return to work status. Although systemic use of opioid is reduced, the overall dose is not decreased when one considers the amount infused intrathecally. A range of 5–15 mg intrathecal morphine per day was reported by Roberts et al. (2001).

Abdominal Pain Associated with Pancreatic Cancer and Chronic Pancreatitis

Although celiac plexus block can be used to alleviate pain from pancreas, liver, gallbladder, omentum, mesentery, and gastrointestinal tract from stomach to the transverse colon, almost all studies on the efficacy of this procedure are conducted in patients with pain from pancreatic cancer or chronic pancreatitis (Bielefeldt and Gebhart 2008). Alcohol neurolytic blocks were performed in pancreatic cancer patients and the success of the block was irrespective of blocking techniques and means of needle guidance. (Ischia et al. 1992; Mercadante 1993; Kawamata et al. 1996; Polati et al. 1998; Wong et al. 2004; Lillemoe et al. 1993; Staats et al. 2001; Gunaratnam et al. 2001). In the posterior approach, a needle tip is placed in front of the aorta or retrocrural under fluoroscopy or CT guidance.

In the anterior approaches, a needle tip is always placed in front of the celiac plexus and is usually under endoscopic ultrasound guidance. After a neurolytic celiac plexus block, 70–90% of pancreatic cancer patients experienced pain relief as measured by visual analog scale (Ischia et al. 1992; Kaufman et al. 2010). Greater pain reduction was noted over the initial 4 weeks post block but it often lasted months until death (Ischia et al. 1992; Mercadante 1993; Kawamata et al. 1996; Gunaratnam et al. 2001). Two small studies, involving 20 and 24 patients, respectively, reported decreased opioid consumption in the neurolytic block group (Mercadante 1993; Polati et al. 1998). However, this was not confirmed in two larger studies, involving 66 and 101 patients (Wong et al. 2004; Gunaratnam et al. 2001). There is also no improvement in survival for patients treated with neurolytic celiac block except when the neurolysis was preformed intraoperatively (Wong et al. 2004; Lillemoe et al. 1993; Staats et al. 2001). At this time, neurolytic celiac plexus block is best used as an adjunctive analgesic modality in the overall pain management regimen of a patient whose pancreatic cancer is confined to the viscera.

Celiac plexus block with local anesthetic and steroid has been performed in patients with chronic pancreatitis. Limited data from prospective randomized studies showed that 50–60% of the patients reported temporary pain reduction (Kaufman et al. 2010). In the study by Gress et al. (2001), 55% patient reported less pain at 8 weeks post block, 26% at 16 weeks, and only 10% at 24 weeks. Additional studies are needed to determine the characteristics of patients who are likely to response to this treatment. At this time, celiac plexus block may be best used during an acute flare of chronic pancreatitis (Kaufman et al. 2010).

Complications Associated with Nerve Block, Trigger Point Injection, and Intrathecal Therapy

That which is necessary is never a risk (Brown 2007).

Like all interventions in medicine or surgery, there are benefits and risks associated with every procedure. Because there is not a system that mandates reporting of complications and the number of a specific procedure performed is unknown, the frequencies of various complications are estimated from case series. The probability of a complication occurring in a given patient is influenced by both patient and procedural factors. Examples of patient factors are age, medical co-morbidities, and individual anatomy. Certain procedures are riskier than others, for example, more serious complications have been reported from transforaminal epidural steroid injections than that from interlaminal epidural steroid injections. Complications are most often viewed from the aspect of vascular and neurological damages, infection, drug-related adverse effects, and procedural trauma.

The American Society of Anesthesiologists has a Closed Claim database (Fitzgibbon et al. 2004). During 1970–1999, there were 276 claims relating to interventional pain procedures according to professional liability companies that covered about 60% of the anesthesiologists in the United States. More than half of the complications occurred after discharge and the great majority of them were determined not preventable by better pre- or post-procedural care. Nerve injury, infection, and headache accounted for 64% of complications associated with epidural steroid injection. These included devastating paraplegia, quadriplegia, meningitis, epidural abscess, and osteomyelitis. Spinal cord infarction has been associated with the injection of particulate steroid into radicular arteries that feed into the anterior spinal arteries (Bogduk 2007). Postprocedural epidural hematoma, a neurosurgical emergency, is a rare but severe complication with an outcome ranging from complete recovery to permanent neurological deficit (Abbasi et al. 2007; Xu et al. 2009; Williams et al. 1990; Lee et al. 2007; Ghaly 2001). There is a higher occurrence in the cervical and thoracic spine. Antiplatelet therapy, multiple attempts of needle placement, and history of multiple cervical epidurals are risk factors.

However, there were instances in which antiplatelet agents or anticoagulation was held according to guidelines or there were no apparent risk factors (Abbasi et al. 2007; Xu et al. 2009; Ain and Vance 2005; Stoll and Sanchez 2002).

According to the ASA closed claim database, pneumothorax is the major complication associated with trigger point injections and nerve blocks in the lower neck and thorax (Fitzgibbon et al. 2004). Death or brain damage from cardiovascular and respiratory failure was associated with unintentional intrathecal injection of local anesthetic or epidural morphine administration and severe allergic reaction. Respiratory depression is delayed following epidural morphine injection. In patients with implanted pumps, death or brain damage occurred after opioid overdose due to pump programming error. A similar report by Coffey et al. (2009) showed that there is a higher mortality in intrathecal opioid-treated patients for chronic non-cancer pain as compared to those treated with spinal cord stimulation at 3, 30 days, and 1 year after implantation. When the cause of death was noted, almost half were due to confirmed or suspected drug overdose.

Other rare but severe vascular complications that have been reported include subdural hematoma (Reitman and Watters 2002), paratracheal hematoma with airway obstruction and death after a stellate block (Rauck and Rathmell 2007), and massive retroperioneal hematoma after lumbar sympathetic block while on anticoagulants (Maier et al. 2002).

The amount of local anesthetics injected during pain procedures are much less in comparison to regional anesthesia and toxicity is most commonly from direct intravascular injection. The incidence of intravascular injection during cervical transforaminal injections was 19.4% (Furman et al. 2003), whereas in the lumbar spine, similar incidence (19.9%) was only seen during S1 transforaminal injections (Sullivan et al. 2000). The incidence of intravascular uptake during L3, L4, and L5 transforaminal injections were 12.5, 9, and 6.9%, respectively. Seizures can occur immediately, if bupivacaine 2.5 mg (1 mL of the 0.25% solution) is injected into the vertebral or internal carotid artery (Rauck and Rathmell 2007).

Vasovagal reaction is a frequent but reversible cardiovascular complication with higher occurrence in procedures performed in the cervical spine (Trentman et al. 2009). In most cases, patients recover after conservative management such as cessation of the procedure, lying supine or in a trendelenburg position and administration of intravenous fluid and oxygen (Mahajan 2006).

Hypotension after sympathetic block is also common and expected. It was reported that 38% of cancer patients treated with neurolytic celiac plexus block were hypotensive post procedure in a meta-analysis (Wong 2007).

Glucoorticosteroids injected during pain procedures can cause hypercorticism and adrenal suppression and it may take 30 days for the system to return to normal (Abram 2007). In a diabetic patient, glucose level can be higher for 48 and 72 h post injection and require extra monitoring and treatment.

Postprocedure pain appears to be a significant side effect of cervical medial branch neurotomy with an observed frequency of 97% (Rathmell and Borgoy 2007). Cutaneous numbness and dysesthesia are also prevalent, especially after neurotomy of the third occipital nerve and C3 and C4 medial branches owing to the large sensory component in these nerves.

Summary

To date, good evidence support the efficacy of lumbar transforaminal epidural steroid for radicular pain from herniated disc, thermal radiofrequency neurotomy for zygapophyseal joint pain from arthropathy in the lumbar and cervical spine, intrathecal therapy for malignant pain and neurolytic celiac plexus block for abdominal pain secondary to pancreatic cancer. There is insufficient data to speak for the efficacy of many other commonly performed procedures, which is not to say that these procedures are not effective. To continue practicing them in this era of evidence-based medicine, it is our imminent task to prove or refute the utility of these procedures. Consistently, we observe a spectrum of response to an intervention even when patients are selected based on strict criteria during a clinical trial. Pain relief from interventional procedures is temporary ranging from days to years and beneficial effect can be prolonged by repeating procedures. Pain reduction does not necessarily translate into improved function and return to work. Pain procedures are quite safe considering the large numbers performed in everyday clinical practice, however, catastrophic events do occur. Therefore, it is imperative to balance the risk and benefit for each patient.

References

Abbasi, A., Malhotra, G., Malanga, G., Elovic, E. P., & Kahn, S. (2007). Complications of interlaminar cervical epidural steroid injections: A review of the literature. *Spine, 32*(19), 2144–2151.

Abdi, S., Zhou, Y., Patel, N., Saini, B., & Nelson, J. (2004). A new and easy technique to block the stellate ganglion. *Pain Physician, 7*, 327–331.

Abram, S. E. (2007). Complications associated with epidural, facet joint, and sacroiliac joint injections. In J. M. Neal & J. P. Rathmell (Eds.), *Complications in regional anesthesia and pain medicine*. Philadelphia: Saunders.

Ain, R., & Vance, M. (2005). Epidural hematoma after epidural steroid injection in a patient withholding enoxaparin per guidelines. *Anesthesiology, 102*(30), 701–703.

American College of Occupational and Environmental Medicine. (2007). Low back disorders. In *Occupational medicine practice guidelines: Evaluation and management of common health problems and functional recovery in workers*. www.guideline.gov June 5, 2010.

American Society of Anesthesiologists. (2010). Practice guidelines for chronic pain management. *Anesthesiology, 112*, 810–833.

Arden, N. K., Price, C., Reading, I., Stubbing, J., Hazelgrove, J., Dunne, C., et al. (2005). A multicentre randomized controlled trial of epidural corticosteroid injections for sciatica: The WEST study. *Rheumatology, 44*, 1399–1406.

Armon, C., Argoff, C. E., Samuels, J., & Backonja, M. M. (2007). Assessment: Use of epidural steroid injections to treat radicular lumbosacral pain: Report of the Therapeutics and Technology Assessment Subcommittee of the American Academy of Neurology. *Neurology, 68*(10), 723–729.

Assad, W. F., & Eskandar, E. N. (2010). The surgical management of trigeminal neuralgia. In S. M. Fishman, J. C. Ballantyne, & J. P. Rathmell (Eds.), *Bonica's management of pain* (4th ed.). Baltimore: Lippincott Williams & Wilkins.

Barnsley, L. (2005). Percutaneous radiofrequency neurotomy for chronic neck pain: Outcomes in a series of consecutive patients. *Pain Medicine, 6*(4), 282–286.

Barnsley, L., Lord, S. M., Wallis, B. J., & Bogduk, N. (1995). The prevalence of chronic cervical zygapophysical joint pain after whiplash. *Spine, 20*(1), 20–26.

Bartynski, W. S., Grahovac, S. Z., & Rothfus, W. E. (2005). Incorrect needle position during lumbar epidural steroid administration: Inaccuracy of loss of air pressure resistance and requirement of fluoroscopy and epidurography during needle insertion. *American Journal of Neuroradiology, 26*, 502–505.

Bielefeldt, K., & Gebhart, G. F. (2008). Visceral pain. In H. T. Benzon, J. P. Rathmell, C. L. Wu, D. C. Turk, & C. E. Argoff (Eds.), *Raj's practical management of pain* (4th ed.). Philadelphia: Mosby.

Bogduk, N. (1982). The clinical anatomy of the cervical dorsal rami. *Spine, 7*(4), 319–330.

Bogduk, N. (Ed.) (2004a). Cervical medial branch blocks. In *International spine intervention society practice guidelines for spinal diagnostic and treatment procedures* (1st ed.). San Francisco: International Spine Intervention Society.

Bogduk, N. (Ed.) (2004b). Cervical transforaminal injection of corticosteroids. In *International spine intervention society practice guidelines for spinal diagnostic and treatment procedures* (1st ed.). San Francisco: International Spine Intervention Society.

Bogduk, N. (Ed.) (2004c). Lumbar medial branch blocks. In *International spine intervention society practice guidelines for spinal diagnostic and treatment procedures* (1st ed.). San Francisco: International Spine Intervention Society.

Bogduk, N. (Ed.) (2004d). Lumbar transforaminal injection of corticosteroids. In *International spine intervention society practice guidelines for spinal diagnostic and treatment procedures* (1st ed.). San Francisco: International Spine Intervention Society.

Bogduk, N. (Ed.) (2004e). Percutaneous radiofrequency lumbar medial branch neurotomy. In *International spine intervention society practice guidelines for spinal diagnostic and treatment procedures* (1st ed.). San Francisco: International Spine Intervention Society.

Bogduk, N. (Ed.) (2004f). Sacroiliac joint blocks. In *International spine intervention society practice guidelines for spinal diagnostic and treatment procedures* (1st ed.). San Francisco: International Spine Intervention Society.

Bogduk, N. (Ed.) (2004g). Thoracic transforaminal injections. In *International spine intervention society practice guidelines for spinal diagnostic and treatment procedures* (1st ed.). San Francisco: International Spine Intervention Society.

Bogduk, N. (2005). The sacroiliac joint. In N. Bogduk (Ed.), *Clinical anatomy of the lumbar spine and sacrum* (4th ed.). Sydney: Elsevier.

Bogduk, N. (2007). Complications associated with transforaminal injections. In J. M. Neal & J. P. Rathmell (Eds.), *Complications in regional anesthesia and pain medicine*. Philadelphia: Saunders.

Bogduk, N. (2010). Epidural steroid injections. In S. M. Fishman, J. C. Ballantyne, & J. P. Rathmell (Eds.), *Bonica's management of pain* (4th ed.). Baltimore: Lippincott Williams & Wilkins.

Boorstein, J. M., & McGraw, J. K. (2004). Facet joint injections. In J. K. McGraw (Ed.), *Interventional radiology of the spine*. Totowa: Humana.

Bosscher, H. (2001). Blockade of the superior hypogastric plexus block for visceral pelvic pain. *Pain Practice, 1*(2), 162–170.

Botwin, K. P., Natalicchio, J., & Hanna, A. (2004). Fluoroscopic guided lumbar interlaminar epidural injections: A prospective evaluation of epidurography contrast patterns and anatomical review of the epidural space. *Pain Physician, 7*, 77–80.

Breivik, H., & Cousins, M. J. (2009). Sympathetic neural blockade of upper and lower extremity. In M. J. Cousins, D. B. Carr, T. T. Horlocker, & P. O. Bridenbaugh (Eds.), *Neural blockade in clinical anesthesia and pain medicine* (4th ed.). Philadelphia: Lippincott Williams & Wilkins.

Brown, D. L. (Ed.) (2006a). Occipital block. In *Atlas of regional anesthesia* (3rd ed.). Philadelphia: Saunders.

Brown, D. L. (Ed.) (2006b). Trigeminal block. In *Atlas of regional anesthesia* (3rd ed.). Philadelphia: Saunders.

Brown, D. L. (Ed.) (2006c). Maxillary block. In *Atlas of regional anesthesia* (3rd ed.). Philadelphia: Saunders.

Brown, D. L. (Ed.) (2006d). Mandibular block. In *Atlas of regional anesthesia* (3rd ed.). Philadelphia: Saunders.

Brown, D. L. (Ed.) (2006e). Distal trigeminal block. In *Atlas of regional anesthesia* (3rd ed.). Philadelphia: Saunders.

Brown, D. L. (Ed.) (2006f). Intercostal block. In *Atlas of regional anesthesia* (3rd ed.). Philadelphia: Saunders.

Brown, D. L. (Ed.) (2006g). Lateral femoral cutaneous block. In *Atlas of regional anesthesia* (3rd ed.). Philadelphia: Saunders.

Brown, D. L. (Ed.) (2006h). Inguinal block. In *Atlas of regional anesthesia* (3rd ed.). Philadelphia: Saunders.

Brown, D. L. (Ed.) (2006i). Stellate block. In *Atlas of regional anesthesia* (3rd ed.). Philadelphia: Saunders.

Brown, D. L. (Ed.) (2006j). Superior hypogastric plexus block. In *Atlas of regional anesthesia* (3rd ed.). Philadelphia: Saunders.

Brown, D. L. (2007). An overview of risk analysis. In J. M. Neal & J. P. Rathmell (Eds.), *Complications in regional anesthesia and pain medicine*. Philadelphia: Saunders.

Burton, A. W., Phan, P. C., & Cousins, M. J. (2009). Treatment of cancer pain: Role of neural blockade and neuromodulation. In M. J. Cousins, D. B. Carr, T. T. Horlocker, & P. O. Bridenbaugh (Eds.), *Neural blockade in clinical anesthesia and pain medicine* (4th ed.). Philadelphia: Lippincott Williams & Wilkins.

Bush, K., & Hillier, S. (1991). A controlled study of caudal epidural injections of triamcinolone plus procaine for the management of intractable sciatica. *Spine, 16*(5), 572–575.

Candido, K. D., & Batra, M. (2008). Nerve blocks of the head and neck. In H. T. Benzon, J. P. Rathmell, C. L. Wu, D. C. Turk, & C. E. Argoff (Eds.), *Raj's practical management of pain* (4th ed.). Philadelphia: Mosby.

Carette, S., Léclaire, R., Marcoux, S., Morin, F., Blaise, G. A., St. Pierre, A., et al. (1997). Epidural corticosteroid injections for sciatica due to herniated nucleus pulposus. *The New England Journal of Medicine, 336*(23), 1634–1640.

Carr, D. B., & Cousins, M. J. (2009). Spinal route of analgesia: Opioids and future options for spinal analgesic chemotherapy. In M. J. Cousins, D. B. Carr, T. T. Horlocker, & P. O. Bridenbaugh (Eds.), *Neural blockade in clinical anesthesia and pain medicine* (4th ed.). Philadelphia: Lippincott Williams & Wilkins.

Chak, A. (2009). What is the evidence for EUS-guided celiac plexus block/neurolysis? *Gastrointestinal Endoscopy, 69*(2 suppl), S172–S173. doi:10.1016/j.gie.2008.12.022.

Chou, R., Stlas, S. J., Stanos, S. P., & Rosenquist, R. W. (2009). Nonsurgical interventional therapies for low back pain: A review of the evidence for an American Pain Society Clinical Practice Guideline. *Spine, 34*(10), 1078–1093.

Chua, W. H., & Bogduk, N. (1995). The surgical anatomy of thoracic facet denervation. *Acta Neurochirurgica, 136*, 140–144.

Coffey, R. J., Owens, M. L., Broste, S. K., Dubois, M. Y., Ferrante, F. M., Schultz, D. M., et al. (2009). Mortality associated with implantation and management of intrathecal opioid drug infusion systems to treat noncancer pain. *Anesthesiology, 111*, 881–891.

Cohen, S. P. (2005). Sacroiliac joint pain: A comprehensive review of anatomy, diagnosis, and treatment. *Anesthesia and Analgesia, 101*, 1440–1453.

Cosman, E. R., Jr., & Cosman, E. R., Sr. (2005). Electric and thermal field effects in tissue around radiofrequency electrodes. *Pain Medicine, 6*(6), 405–424.

Cramer, G. D. (2005). General characteristics of the spine. In G. D. Cramer & S. A. Darby (Eds.), *Basic and clinical anatomy of the spine, spinal cord, and ANS* (2nd ed.). St. Louis: Mosby.

Cuckler, J. M., Bernini, P. A., Wiesel, S. W., Booth, R. E., Rothman, R. H., & Pickens, G. T. (1985). The use of epidural steroids in the treatment of lumbar radicular pain. A prospective, randomized, double-blind study. *The Journal of Bone Joint Surgery. American Volume, 67,* 63–66.

Darby, S. A. (2005). Neuroanatomy of the autonomic nervous system. In G. D. Cramer & S. A. Darby (Eds.), *Basic and clinical anatomy of the spine, spinal cord, and ANS* (2nd ed.). St. Louis: Mosby.

de Médicis, É., & de Leon-Casasola, O. A. (2001). Ganglion impair block: Critical evaluation. *Techniques in Regional Anesthesia and Pain Management, 5*(3), 120–122.

De Mos, M., Sturkenboom, M. C. J. M., & Huygen, F. J. P. M. (2009). Current understandings on complex regional pain syndrome. *Pain Practice, 9*(2), 86–99.

Deer, T. R. (2008). Intrathecal drug delivery: Overview of the proper use of infusion agents. In H. T. Benzon, J. P. Rathmell, C. L. Wu, D. C. Turk, & C. E. Argoff (Eds.), *Raj's practical management of pain* (4th ed.). Philadelphia: Mosby.

Deer, T., Chapple, I., Classen, A., Javery, K., Stoker, V., Tonder, L., et al. (2004). Intrathecal drug delivery for treatment of chronic low back pain: Report from the national outcomes registry for low back pain. *Pain Medicine, 5*(1), 6–13.

Dilke, T. F. W., Burry, H. C., & Grahame, R. (1973). Extradural corticosteroid injection in management of lumbar nerve root compression. *British Medical Journal, 2*(5867), 635–637.

Dreyfuss, P., Halbrook, B., Pauza, K., Joshi, A., McLarty, J., & Bogduk, N. (2000). Efficacy and validity of radiofrequency neurotomy for chronic lumbar zygapophysial joint pain. *Spine, 25*(10), 1270–1277.

Dreyfuss, P., Henning, T., Malladi, N., Goldstein, B., & Bogduk, N. (2009). The ability of multi-site, multi-depth sacral lateral branch blocks to anesthetize the sacroiliac joint complex. *Pain Medicine, 10*(4), 679–688.

Dwyer, A., Aprill, C., & Bogduk, N. (1988). Cervical zygapophyseal joint pain pattern I: A study in normal volunteers. *Spine, 15*(6), 453–457.

Enneking, F. K., Wedel, D. J., & Horlocker, T. T. (2009). The lower extremity: Somatic blockade. In M. J. Cousins, D. B. Carr, T. T. Horlocker, & P. O. Bridenbaugh (Eds.), *Neural blockade in clinical anesthesia and pain medicine* (4th ed.). Philadelphia: Lippincott Williams & Wilkins.

Erdine, S. (2008). Sympathetic blocks of the head and neck. In P. P. Raj, L. Lou, S. Erdine, P. S. Staats, S. D. Waldman, G. Racz, M. Hammer, D. Niv, R. Ruiz-Lopez, & J. E. Heavner (Eds.), *Interventional pain management: Image-guided procedures* (2nd ed.). Philadephia: Sauders.

Erdine, S., & Ozyalcin, S. (2008). Pelvic sympathetic blocks. In P. P. Raj, L. Lou, S. Erdine, P. S. Staats, S. D. Waldman, G. Racz, M. Hammer, D. Niv, R. Ruiz-Lopez, & J. E. Heavner (Eds.), *Interventional pain management: Image-guided procedures* (2nd ed.). Philadephia: Sauders.

Erdine, S., Racz, G. B., & Noe, C. E. (2008). Somatic blocks of the head and neck. In P. P. Raj, L. Lou, S. Erdine, P. S. Staats, S. D. Waldman, G. Racz, M. Hammer, D. Niv, R. Ruiz-Lopez, & J. E. Heavner (Eds.), *Interventional pain management: Image-guided procedures* (2nd ed.). Philadephia: Sauders.

Fechir, M., Geber, C., & Birklein, F. (2008). Evolving understanding about complex regional pain syndrome and its treatment. *Current Pain and Headache Reports, 12,* 186–191.

Fitzgibbon, D. R., Posner, K. L., Bomino, K. B., Caplan, R. A., Lee, L. A., & Cheney, F. W. (2004). Chronic pain management: American Society of Anesthesiologists Closed Claims Project. *Anesthesiology, 100,* 98–105.

Foye, P. M., & Patel, S. I. (2009). Paracoccygeal corkscrew approach to ganglion impar injections for tailbone pain. *Pain Practice, 9*(4), 317–321.

Furman, M. B., Giovanniello, M. T., & O'Brien, E. M. (2003). Incidence of intravascular penetration in transforaminal cervical epidural steroid injections. *Spine, 28*(1), 21–25.

Ghafoor, V. L., Epshteyn, M., Carlson, G. H., Terhaar, D. M., Charry, O., & Phelps, P. K. (2007). Intrathecal drug therapy for long-term pain management. *American Journal of Health-System Pharmacy, 64,* 2447–2461.

Ghahreman, A., Ferch, R., & Bogduk, N. (2010). The efficacy of transforaminal injection of steroids for the treatment of lumbar radicular pain. *Pain Medicine, 11,* 1149–1168.

Ghahreman, A. & Bogduk, N. (2011). Predictors of a favorable response to transforaminal injection of steroid in patients with lumbar radicular pain due to disc herniation. *Pain Medicine, 12*(6), 871–879.

Ghaly, R. F. (2001). Recovery after high-dose methylprednisolone and delayed evacuation: A case of spinal epidural hematoma. *Journal of Neurosurgery Anesthesiology, 13*(4), 323–328.

Gibbs, G. F., Drummond, P. D., Finch, P. M., & Phillips, J. K. (2008). Unravelling the pathophysiology of complex regional pain syndrome: Focus on sympathetically maintained pain. *Clinical and Experimental Pharmacology and Physiology, 35,* 717–724. doi:10.1111/j.1440-1681.2007.04862.x.

Goebert, H. W. Jr, Jallo, S. J., Gardner, W. J., & Wasmuth, C. E. (1961). Painful radiculopathy treated with epidural injection of procaine and hydrocortisone acetate: results in 113 patients. *Current Researches in Anesthesia and Analgesia, 40*(1), 130–134.

Gofeld, M., Bhatia, A., Abbas, S., Ganapathy, S., & Johnson, M. (2009). Development and validation of a new technique for ultrasound-guided stellate ganglion block. *Regional Anesthesia and Pain Medicine, 34*(5), 475–479.

Gofeld, M., Jitendra, J., & Faclier, G. (2007). Radiofrequency denervation of the lumbar zygapophysial joints: 10-year prospective clinical audit. *Pain Physician, 10*, 291–299.

Govind, J., & Bogduk, N. (2010). Neurolytic blockade for noncancer pain. In S. M. Fishman, J. C. Ballantyne, & J. P. Rathmell (Eds.), *Bonica's management of pain* (4th ed.). Baltimore: Lippincott Williams & Wilkins.

Gress, F., Schmitt, C., Sherman, S., Ciaccia, D., Ikenberry, S., & Lehman, G. (2001). Endoscopic ultrasound-guided celiac plexus block for managing abdominal pain associated with chronic pancreatitis: a prospective single center experience. *The American Journal of Gastroenterology, 96*(2), 409–416.

Gunaratnam, N. T., Sarma, A. V., Norton, I. D., & Wiersema, M. J. (2001). A prospective study of EUS-guided celiac plexus neurolysis for pancreatic cancer pain. *Gastrointestinal Endoscopy, 54*(3), 316–324.

Gundamraj, N. R., & Richeimer, S. (2010). Chest wall pain. In S. M. Fishman, J. C. Ballantyne, & J. P. Rathmell (Eds.), *Bonica's management of pain* (4th ed.). Baltimore: Lippincott Williams & Wilkins.

Hadzic, A., & Vloka, J. D. (Eds.) (2004). Cutaneous nerve blocks of the lower extremity. In *Peripheral nerve blocks: Principles and practice* (1st ed.). New York: McGraw-Hill.

Harden, R. N., Bruehl, S., Perez, R. S. G. M., Birklein, F., Marinus, J., Maihofner, C., et al. (2010). Validation of proposed diagnostic criteria (the "Budapest Criteria") for complex regional pain syndrome. *Pain, 150*(2), 268–274.

Harmon, D. C., & Shorten, G. D. (2009). Intercostal, intrapleural, and peripheral blockade of the thorax and abdomen. In M. J. Cousins, D. B. Carr, T. T. Horlocker, & P. O. Bridenbaugh (Eds.), *Neural blockade in clinical anesthesia and pain medicine* (4th ed.). Philadelphia: Lippincott Williams & Wilkins.

Harney, D., & Patijn, J. (2007). Meralgia paresthetica: Diagnosis and management strategies. *Pain Medicine, 8*(8), 669–677.

Henderson, W. R. (1965). The anatomy of the gasserian ganglion and the distribution of pain in relation to injections and operations for trigeminal neuralgia. *Annals of the Royal College of Surgeons of England, 37*(6), 346–373.

Hickey, A. H., Scrivani, S., & Bajwa, Z. (2010). Cranial neuralgias. In S. M. Fishman, J. C. Ballantyne, & J. P. Rathmell (Eds.), *Bonica's management of pain* (4th ed.). Baltimore: Lippincott Williams & Wilkins.

Ho, K., & Tan, K. (2007). Botulinum toxin A for myofascial trigger point injection: A qualitative systematic review. *European Journal of Pain, 11*, 519–527.

Hogan, Q. H. (2009). Anatomy of the neuraxis. In M. J. Cousins, D. B. Carr, T. T. Horlocker, & P. O. Bridenbaugh (Eds.), *Neural blockade in clinical anesthesia and pain medicine* (4th ed.). Philadelphia: Lippincott Williams & Wilkins.

Hong, J. H., & Jang, H. S. (2006). Block of the ganglion impar using a coccygeal joint approach. *Regional Anesthesia and Pain Medicine, 31*(6), 583–584. doi:10.1016/j.rapm.2006.08.009.

Husted, D. S., Orton, D., Schofferman, J., & Kine, G. (2008). Effectiveness of repeated radiofrequency neurotomy for cervical facet joint pain. *Journal of Spinal Disorders & Techniques, 21*(6), 406–408.

Inturrisi, C. E., & Lipman, A. G. (2010). Opioid analgesics. In S. M. Fishman, J. C. Ballantyne, & J. P. Rathmell (Eds.), *Bonica's management of pain* (4th ed.). Baltimore: Lippincott Williams & Wilkins.

Ischia, S., Ischia, A., Polati, E., & Finco, G. (1992). Three posterior percutaneous celiac plexus block techniques. *Anesthesiology, 76*, 534–540.

Kang, J. D., Georgescu, H. I., McIntyre-Larkin, L., Stefanovic-Racic, M., Donaldson, W. F., III, & Evans, C. H. (1996). Herniated lumbar intervertebral discs spontaneously produce matrix metalloproteinases, nitric oxide, interleukin-6 and prostaglandin E2. *Spine, 21*(3), 271–277.

Karppinen, J., Malmivaara, A., Kurunlahti, M., Kyllöen, E., Pienimäki, T., Nieminen, P., et al. (2001). Periradicular infiltration for sciatica: A randomized controlled trial. *Spine, 26*(9), 1059–1067.

Kaufman, M., Singh, G., Das, S., Concha-Parra, R., Erber, J., Micames, C., et al. (2010). Efficacy of endoscopic ultrasound-guided celiac plexus block and celiac plexus neurolysis for managing abdominal pain associated with chronic pancreatitis and pancreatic cancer. *Journal of Clinical Gastroenterology, 44*(2), 127–134.

Kawamata, M., Ishitani, K., Ishikawa, K., Sasaki, H., Ota, K., Omote, K., et al. (1996). Comparison between celiac plexus block and morphine treatment on quality of life in patients with pancreatic cancer pain. *Pain, 64*, 597–602.

Klenerman, L., Greenwood, R., Davenport, H. T., White, D. C., & Preskett, S. (1984). Lumbar epidural injections in the treatment of sciatica. *British Journal of Rheumatology, 23*, 35–38.

Koizuka, S., Saito, S., Sekimoto, K., Tobe, M., Obata, H., & Koyama, Y. (2009). Percutaneous radio-frequency thermocoagulation of the Gasserian ganglion guided by high-speed real-time CT fluoroscopy. *Neuroradiology, 51*, 565.

Kuan, T. (2009). Current studies on myofascial pain syndrome. *Current Pain Headache Reports, 13*, 365–369.

Leclaire, R., Fortin, L., Lambert, R., Bergeron, Y. M., & Rossignol, M. (2001). Radiofrequency facet joint denervation in the treatment of low back pain: A placebo-controlled clinical trial to assess efficacy. *Spine, 26*(13), 1411–1417.

Lee, J. Y., Nassr, A., & Ponnappan, R. K. (2007). Epidural hematoma causing paraplegia after a fluoroscopically guided cervical nerve-root injection. *The Journal of Bone Joint Surgery. American Volume, 89*, 2037–2039. doi:10.2106/JBJS.F.01332.

Lee, H., Weinstein, J. N., Meller, S. T., Hyashi, N., Spratt, K. F., & Gebhart, G. F. (1998). The role of steroids and their effects on phospholipase A₂: An animal model of radiculopathy. *Spine, 23*(11), 1191–1196.

Lenrow, D. A., & Chou, L. H. (2003). Randomized controlled trials in interventional spine: Perils and pitfalls. *Pain Physician, 6*, 83–87.

Levy, M. J., & Wiersema, M. J. (2003). EUS-guided celiac plexus neurolysis and celiac plexus block. *Gastrointestinal Endoscopy, 57*(7), 923–930.

Lillemoe, K. D., Carneron, J. L., Kaufman, H. S., Yeo, C. J., Pitt, H. A., & Sauter, P. K. (1993). Chemical splanchnicectomy in patients with unresectable pancreatic cancer. *Annals of Surgery, 217*(5), 447.

Lindahl, O., & Rexed, B. (1951). Histologic changes in spinal nerve roots of operated cases of sciatica. *Acta Orthopaedica Scandinavica, 20*, 215–225.

Lord, S. M., Barnsley, L., & Bogduk, N. (1995). Percutaneous radiofrequency neurotomy in the treatment of cervical zygapophysial joint pain: A caution. *Neurosurgery, 36*(4), 732–739.

Lord, S. M., Barnsley, L., Wallis, B. J., McDonald, G. J., & Bogduk, N. (1996). Percutaneous radio-frequency neurotomy for chronic cervical zygapophyseal-joint pain. *The New England Journal of Medicine, 335*(23), 1721–1726.

Loukas, M., Klaassen, Z., Merbs, W., tubs, R. S., Gielecki, J., & Zurada, A. (2010). A review of the thoracic splanchnic nerves and celiac ganglia. *Clinical Anatomy, 23*(5), 512–522.

Mahajan, G. (2006). Pain clinic emergencies. *Pain Medicine, 9*(S1), S113–S120.

Maier, C., Gleim, M., Weiss, T., Stachetzki, U., Nicolas, V., & Zenz, M. (2002). Severe bleeding following lumbar sympathetic blockade in two patients under medication with irreversible platelet aggregation inhibitors. *Anesthesiology, 97*(3), 740–743.

Malik, K., & Benzon, H. T. (2008). Low back pain. In H. T. Benzon, J. P. Rathmell, C. L. Wu, D. C. Turk, & C. E. Argoff (Eds.), *Raj's practical management of pain* (4th ed.). Philadelphia: Mosby.

Manchikanti, L., Boswell, M. V., Singh, V., Benyamin, R. M., Fellows, B., Abdi, S., et al. (2009). Comprehensive evidence-based guidelines for interventional techniques in the management of chronic spinal pain. *Pain Physician, 12*, 699–802.

Manchikanti, L., Boswell, M. V., Singh, V., Pampati, V., Damron, K. S., & Beyer, C. D. (2004). Prevalence of facet joint pain in chronic spinal pain of cervical, thoracic, and lumbar regions. *BMC Musculoskeletal Disorders, 5*, 15.

Manchikanti, L., Pampati, V., Fellows, B., & Baha, A. G. (2000). The inability of the clinical picture to characterize from facet joints. *Pain Physician, 3*(2), 158–166.

Manchikanti, L., Singh, V., Pampati, V., Smith, H., & Hirsch, J. (2009). Analysis of growth of interventional techniques in managing chronic pain in the medicare population: A 10-year evaluation from 1997–2006. *Pain Physician, 12*, 9–34.

Manchukonda, R., Manchikanti, K. N., Cash, K. A., Pampati, V., & Manchikanti, L. (2007). Facet joint pain in chronic spine pain: An evaluation of prevalence and false-positive rate of diagnostic blocks. *Journal of Spinal Disorders & Techniques, 20*(7), 539–545.

McCall, I. W., Park, W. M., & O'Brien, J. P. (1979). Induced pain referral from posterior lumbar elements in normal subjects. *Spine, 4*(5), 441–446.

McDonald, G. J., Lord, S. M., & Bogduk, N. (1999). Long-term follow-up of patients treated with cervical radiofrequency neurotomy for chronic neck pain. *Neurosurgery, 45*(1), 61–67.

McLain, R. F., Kapural, L., & Mekhail, N. A. (2005). Epidural steroid therapy for back and leg pain: Mechanisms of action and efficacy. *The Spine Journal, 5*, 191–201.

Mercadante, S. (1993). Celiac plexus block versus analgesics in pancreatic cancer pain. *Pain, 52*, 187–192.

Molloy, R. E., & Benzon, H. T. (2008). Neurolytic blocking agents: Uses and complications. In H. T. Benzon, J. P. Rathmell, C. L. Wu, D. C. Turk, & C. E. Argoff (Eds.), *Raj's practical management of pain* (4th ed.). Philadelphia: Mosby.

Moore, K. L., Dalley, A. F., Agur, & A. M. R. (Eds.) (2010) Pterygopalatine fossa. In *Clinically oriented anatomy* (6th ed.). Philadelphia: Lippincott Wiliams & Wilkins.

Murakami, E., Aizawa, T., Noguchi, K., Kanno, H., Okuno, H., & Uozumi, H. (2008). Diagram specific to sacroiliac joint pain site indicated by one-finger test. *Journal of Orthopaedic Science, 13*, 492–497.

Nachi, P., Singelyn, F., & Paqueron, X. (2008). Truncal blocks. In H. T. Benzon, J. P. Rathmell, C. L. Wu, D. C. Turk, & C. E. Argoff (Eds.), *Raj's practical management of pain* (4th ed.). Philadelphia: Mosby.

Narouze, S., Vydyanathan, A., & Patel, N. (2007). Ultrasound-guided stellate ganglion block successfully prevented esophageal puncture. *Pain Physician, 10*, 747–752.

Nath, S., Nath, C. A., & Pettersson, K. (2008). Percutaneous lumbar zygapophysial (facet) joint neurotomy using radiofrequency current, in the management of chronic low back pain: A randomized double-blind trial. *Spine, 33*(12), 1291–1297.

Nelson, J. W. (2008). Thoracic facet joint blocks and neurotomy. In P. P. Raj, L. Lou, S. Erdine, P. S. Staats, S. D. Waldman, G. Racz, M. Hammer, D. Niv, R. Ruiz-Lopez, & J. E. Heavner (Eds.), *Interventional pain management: Image-guided procedures* (2nd ed.). Philadephia: Sauders.

Netter, F. H. (1989). Psoas and iliacus muscles. In F. H. Netter (Ed.), *Atlas of human anatomy*. Summit, NJ: Ciba-Geigy.

Ng, L., Chaudhary, N., & Sell, P. (2005). The efficacy of corticosteroids in periradicular infiltration for chronic radicular pain. *Spine, 30*(8), 857–862.

Niv, D., & Gofeld, M. (2008). Lumbar sympathetic blocks. In P. P. Raj, L. Lou, S. Erdine, P. S. Staats, S. D. Waldman, G. Racz, M. Hammer, D. Niv, R. Ruiz-Lopez, & J. E. Heavner (Eds.), *Interventional pain management: Image-guided procedures* (2nd ed.). Philadephia: Sauders.

Obray, J. B., & Huntoon, M. A. (2008). Interlaminar and transforaminal epidural steroid injections. In H. T. Benzon, J. P. Rathmell, C. L. Wu, D. C. Turk, & C. E. Argoff (Eds.), *Raj's practical management of pain* (4th ed.). Philadelphia: Mosby.

Oh, C., Chung, H., Ji, H., & Yoon, D. (2004). Clinical implications of topographic anatomy on the ganglion impar. *Anesthesiology, 101*, 249–250.

Olmarker, K., & Larsson, K. (1998). Tumor necrosis factor [alpha] and nucleus-pulposus-induced nerve root injury. *Spine, 23*(23), 2538–2544.

Osenbach, R. K. (2010). Intrathecal drug delivery in the management of pain. In S. M. Fishman, J. C. Ballantyne, & J. P. Rathmell (Eds.), *Bonica's management of pain* (4th ed.). Baltimore: Lippincott Williams & Wilkins.

Patel, V. B., Manchikanti, L., Singh, V., Schultz, D. M., Hayek, S. M., & Smith, H. S. (2009). Systematic review of intrathecal infusion systems for long-term management of chronic non-cancer pain. *Pain Physician, 12*, 345–360.

Peng, P. W. H., & Tumber, P. S. (2008). Ultrasound-guided interventional procedures for patients with chronic pelvic pain – A description of techniques and review of literature. *Pain Physician, 11*, 215–224.

Polati, E., Finco, G., Gottin, L., Bassi, C., Pederzoli, P., & Ischia, S. (1998). Prospective randomized double-blind trial of neurolytic celiac plexus block in patients with pancreatic cancer. *British Journal of Surgery, 85*, 199–201.

Price, D., Long, S., Wilsey, B., & Rafii, A. (1998). Analysis of peak magnitude and duration of analgesia produced by local anesthetics injected into sympathetic ganglia of complex regional pain syndrome patients. *The Clinical Journal of Pain, 14*(3), 216–226.

Price, C. M., Rogers, P. D., Prosser, A. S. J., & Arden, N. K. (2000). Comparison of the caudal and lumbar approaches to the epidural space. *Annals of the Rheumatic Diseases, 59*, 879–882.

Racz, G. B., & Noe, C. E. (2008). Pelvic spinal neuroaxial procedures. In P. P. Raj, L. Lou, S. Erdine, P. S. Staats, S. D. Waldman, G. Racz, M. Hammer, D. Niv, R. Ruiz-Lopez, & J. E. Heavner (Eds.), *Interventional pain management: Image-guided procedures* (2nd ed.). Philadephia: Sauders.

Rathmell, J. P. (Ed.) (2006a). Facet injection: Intra-articular injection, medial branch block, and radiofrequency treatment. In *Atlas of image-guided intervention in regional anesthesia and pain medicine*. Philadelphia: Lippincott Wiliams & Wilkins.

Rathmell, J. P. (Ed.) (2006b). Stellate ganglion block. In *Atlas of image-guided intervention in regional anesthesia and pain medicine*. Philadelphia: Lippincott Wiliams & Wilkins.

Rathmell, J. P. (Ed.) (2006c). Celiac plexus block and neurolysis. In *Atlas of image-guided intervention in regional anesthesia and pain medicine*. Philadelphia: Lippincott Wiliams & Wilkins.

Rathmell, J. P. (Ed.) (2006d). Lumbar sympathetic block and neurolysis. In *Atlas of image-guided intervention in regional anesthesia and pain medicine*. Philadelphia: Lippincott Wiliams & Wilkins.

Rathmell, J. P. (Ed.) (2006e). Interlaminar epidural injection. In *Atlas of image-guided intervention in regional anesthesia and pain medicine*. Philadelphia: Lippincott Wiliams & Wilkins.

Rathmell, J. P. (Ed.) (2006f). Transforaminal and selective nerve root injection. In *Atlas of image-guided intervention in regional anesthesia and pain medicine*. Philadelphia: Lippincott Wiliams & Wilkins.

Rathmell, J. P., & Borgoy, J. (2007). Complications associated with radiofrequency treatment for chronic pain. In J. M. Neal & J. P. Rathmell (Eds.), *Complications in regional anesthesia and pain medicine*. Philadelphia: Saunders.

Rauck, R. L., & Rathmell, J. P. (2007). Complications associated with stellate ganglion and lumbar sympathetic blocks. In J. M. Neal & J. P. Rathmell (Eds.), *Complications in regional anesthesia and pain medicine*. Philadelphia: Saunders.

Rauk, R. L., Wallace, M. S., Leong, M. S., Mine-Hart, M., Webster, L. R., Charapata, S. G., et al. (2006). A randomized, double-blind, placebo-controlled study of intrathecal ziconotide in adults with severe chronic pain. *Journal of Pain and Symptom Management, 31*(5), 393–406.

Reitman, C. A., & Watters, W., III. (2002). Subdural hematoma after cervical epidural steroid injection. *Spine, 27*(6), E174–E176.

Roberts, L. J., Finch, P. M., Goucke, C. R., & Price, L. M. (2001). Outcome of intrathecal opioids in chronic non-cancer pain. *European Journal of Pain, 5*, 353–361. doi:10.1053/eujp. 2001.0255.

Rupert, M. P., Lee, M., Manchikanti, L., Datta, S., & Cohen, S. P. (2009). Evaluation of sacroiliac joint interventions: A systematic appraisal of the literature. *Pain Physician, 12*, 399–418.

Russell, I. J. (2008). Myofascial pain syndrome and fibromyalgia syndrome. In H. T. Benzon, J. P. Rathmell, C. L. Wu, D. C. Turk, & C. E. Argoff (Eds.), *Raj's practical management of pain* (4th ed.). Philadelphia: Mosby.

Saal, J. S., Franson, R. C., Dobrow, R., Saal, J. A., White, A. H., & Goldthwaite, N. (1989). High levels of inflammatory phospholipase A$_2$ activity in lumbar disc herniations. *Spine, 15*(7), 674–678.

Salinas, F. V., Malik, K., & Benzon, H. T. (2008). Local anesthetics for regional anesthesia and pain management. In H. T. Benzon, J. P. Rathmell, C. L. Wu, D. C. Turk, & C. E. Argoff (Eds.), *Raj's practical management of pain* (4th ed.). Philadelphia: Mosby.

Schofferman, J., & Kine, G. (2004). Effectiveness of repeated radiofrequency neurotomy for lumbar facet pain. *Spine, 29*(21), 2471–2473.

Schwarzer, A. C., April, C. N., Derby, R., Fortin, J., Kine, G., & Bogduk, N. (1994). Clinical features of patients with pain stemming from the lumbar zygapophysial joints: Is the lumbar facet syndrome a clinical entity? *Spine, 19*(10), 1132–1137.

Scott, N. A., Guo, B., Barton, P. M., & Gerwin, R. D. (2009). Trigger point injections for chronic non-malignant musculoskeletal pain: A systematic review. *Pain Medicine, 10*(1), 54–69.

Seagrove, L. C., & Dickenson, A. H. (2009). Pharmacologic substrates of pain: Peripheral voltage gated ion channels in pain. In M. J. Cousins, D. B. Carr, T. T. Horlocker, & P. O. Bridenbaugh (Eds.), *Neural blockade in clinical anesthesia and pain medicine* (4th ed.). Philadelphia: Lippincott Williams & Wilkins.

Shah, J. P., Danoff, J. V., Desai, M. J., Parikh, S., Nakamura, L. Y., Philips, T. M., et al. (2008). Biochemicals associated with pain and inflammation are elevated in sites near to the remote from active myofascial trigger points. *Archives of Physical Medicine and Rehabilitation, 89*, 16–23.

Shah, J. P., Phillips, T. M., Danoff, J. V., & Gerber, L. H. (2005). An in vivo microanalytical technique for measuring the local biochemical milieu of human skeletal muscle. *Journal of Applied Physiology, 99*, 1977–1984. doi:10.1152/japplphysiol.00419.2005.

Siddall, P. J., & Cousins, M. J. (2009). Introduction to pain mechanisms: Implications for neural blockade. In M. J. Cousins, D. B. Carr, T. T. Horlocker, & P. O. Bridenbaugh (Eds.), *Neural blockade in clinical anesthesia and pain medicine* (4th ed.). Philadelphia: Lippincott Williams & Wilkins.

Simons, D. G. (1999). General overview. In D. G. Simons, J. G. Travell, & L. S. Simons (Eds.), *Travell & Simons' myofascial pain and dysfundtion: The trigger point manual* (2nd ed.). Baltimore: Lippincott Williams & Wilkins.

Simons, D. G., & Simons, D. G. (1999). Glossary. In D. G. Simons, J. G. Travell, & L. S. Simons (Eds.), *Travell & Simons' myofascial pain and dysfundtion: The trigger point manual* (2nd ed.). Baltimore: Lippincott Williams & Wilkins.

Smith, T. J., Coyne, P. J., Staats, P. S., Deer, T., Stearns, L. J., Rauck, R. L., et al. (2005). An implantable drug delivery system (IDDS) for refractory cancer pain provides sustained pain control, less drug-related toxicity, and possibly better survival compared with comprehensive medical management (CMM). *Annals of Oncology, 16*, 825–833.

Smith, T. J., Staats, P. S., Deer, T., Stearns, L. J., Rauck, R. L., Boortz-Marx, R. L., et al. (2002). Randomized clinical trial of an implantable drug delivery system compared with comprehensive medical management for refractory cancer pain: Impact on pain, drug-related toxicity and survival. *Journal of Clinical Oncology, 20*(19), 4040–4049.

Snoek, W., Weber, H., & Jørgensen, B. (1977). Double blind evaluation of extradural methyl prednisolone for herniated lumbar discs. *Acta Orthopaedica Scandinavica, 48*, 635–641.

Staats, P. S. (2008). Intrathecal drug delivery systems. In P. P. Raj, L. Lou, S. Erdine, P. S. Staats, S. D. Waldman, G. Racz, M. Hammer, D. Niv, R. Ruiz-Lopez, & J. E. Heavner (Eds.), *Interventional pain management: Image-guided procedures* (2nd ed.). Philadephia: Sauders.

Staats, P. S., Hekmat, H., Sauter, P., & Lillemoe, K. (2001). The effects of alcohol celiac plexus block, pain, and mood on longevity in patients with unresectable pancreatic cancer: A double-blind, randomized, placebo-controlled study. *Pain Medicine, 2*(1), 28–34.

Staats, P. S., Yearwood, T., Charapata, S. G., Presley, R. W., Wallace, M. S., Byas-Smith, M., et al. (2004). Intrathecal ziconotide in the treatment of refractory pain in patients with cancer or AIDS: A randomized controlled trial. *JAMA: The Journal of American Medical Association, 291*(1), 63–70.

Stevens, D. S., Balatbat, G. R., & Lee, F. M. K. (2000). Coaxial imaging technique for superior hypogastric plexus block. *Regional Anesthesia and Pain Medicine, 25*(6), 643–647.

Stoll, A., & Sanchez, M. (2002). Epidural hematoma after epidural block: Implications for its use in pain management. *Surgical Neurology, 57*, 235–240.

Sullivan, W. J., Willick, S. E., Chira-Adisai, W., Zuhosky, J., Tyburski, M., Dreyfuss, P., et al. (2000). Incidence of intravascular uptake in lumbar spinal injection procedures. *Spine, 25*(4), 481–486.

Surash, S., & Jagannathan, N. (2009). Somatic blockade of the head and neck. In M. J. Cousins, D. B. Carr, T. T. Horlocker, & P. O. Bridenbaugh (Eds.), *Neural blockade in clinical anesthesia and pain medicine* (4th ed.). Philadelphia: Lippincott Williams & Wilkins.

Swerdlow, M., & Sayle-Creer, W. (1970). A study of extradural medication in the relief of the lumbosciatic syndrome. *Anesthesiology, 25*(3), 341–345.

Takahashi, H., Suguro, T., Okazima, Y., Motegi, M., Okada, Y., & Kakiuchi, T. (1996). Inflammatory cytokines in the herniated disc of the lumbar spine. *Spine, 21*(2), 218–224.

Tekin, I., Mirzai, H., Ok, G., Erbuyun, K., & Batansever, D. (2007). A comparison of conventional and pulsed radiofrequency denervation in the treatment of chronic facet joint pain. *The Clinical Journal of Pain, 23*(6), 524–529.

Thimineur, M. A., Kravitz, E., & Vodapally, M. S. (2004). Intrathecal opioid treatment for chronic non-malignant pain: A 3-year prospective study. *Pain, 109*, 242–249.

Tobin, J., & Flitman, S. (2009). Occipital nerve blocks: When and what to inject? *Headache, 49*, 1521–1533. doi:101 111/j.1526-4610.2009.01493.x.

Trentman, T. L., Rosenfeld, D. M., Seamans, D. P., Hentz, J. G., & Stanek, J. P. (2009). Vasovagal reactions and other complications of cervical vs. lumbar translaminar epidural steroid injections. *Pain Practice, 9*(1), 59–64.

Tsui, B. C. H., Dillane, D., & Finucane, B. T. (2009). Neural blockade for surgery to the head and neck. In M. J. Cousins, D. B. Carr, T. T. Horlocker, & P. O. Bridenbaugh (Eds.), *Neural blockade in clinical anesthesia and pain medicine* (4th ed.). Philadelphia: Lippincott Williams & Wilkins.

Valat, J., Giraudeau, B., & Rozenberg, S. (2003). Epidural corticosteroid injections for sciatica: A randomized, double blind, controlled clinical trial. *Annals of the Rheumatic Diseases, 62*, 639–643.

Van Kleef, M., Barendse, G. A. M., Kessels, A., Voets, H. M., Weber, W. E. J., & de Lange, S. (1999). Randomized trial of radiofrequency lumbar facet denervation for chronic low back pain. *Spine, 24*(18), 1937–1942.

Van Wijk, R. M. A. W., Geurts, J. W. M., Wynne, H. J., Hammink, E., Buskens, E., lousberg, R., et al. (2005). Radiofrequency denervation of lumbar facet joints in the treatment of chronic low back pain: A randomized, double-blind, sham lesion-controlled trial. *The Clinical Journal of Pain, 21*(4), 335–344.

Waldman, S. D. (2008). Somatic blocks of the thorax. In P. P. Raj, L. Lou, S. Erdine, P. S. Staats, S. D. Waldman, G. Racz, M. Hammer, D. Niv, R. Ruiz-Lopez, & J. E. Heavner (Eds.), *Interventional pain management: Image-guided procedures* (2nd ed.). Philadephia: Sauders.

Wang, J. K., Nauss, L. A., & Thomas, J. E. (1979). Pain relief by intrathecally applied morphine in man. *Anesthesiology, 50*(2), 149–151.

Ward, J. B. (2003). Greater occipital nerve block. *Seminars in Neurology, 23*(1), 59–61.

Warren, D. T., & Liu, S. S. (2008). Neuraxizl anesthesia. In H. T. Benzon, J. P. Rathmell, C. L. Wu, D. C. Turk, & C. E. Argoff (Eds.), *Raj's practical management of pain* (4th ed.). Philadelphia: Mosby.

Webster, L. R., Fisher, R., Charapata, S., & Wallace, M. S. (2009). Long-term intrathecal ziconotide for chronic pain: An open-label study. *Journal of Pain and Symptom Management, 37*(3), 363–372.

Wiersema, M. J., & Wiersema, L. M. (1996). Endosonography-guided celiac plexus neurolysis. *Gastrointestinal Endoscopy, 44*(6), 656–662.

Williams, K. A., Hurley, R. W., Lin, E. E., & Wu, C. L. (2008). Neuropathic pain syndromes. In H. T. Benzon, J. P. Rathmell, C. L. Wu, D. C. Turk, & C. E. Argoff (Eds.), *Raj's practical management of pain* (4th ed.). Philadelphia: Mosby.

Williams, K. N., Kackowski, A., & Evans, P. J. D. (1990). Epidural haematoma requiring surgical decompression following repeated cervical epidural steroid injections for chronic pain. *Pain, 42*, 197–199.

Windsor, R. E., & Jahnke, S. (2004). Sphenopalatine ganglion blockade: A review and proposed modification of the transnasal technique. *Pain Physician, 7*, 283–286.

Wong, G. Y. (2007). Complications associated with neurolytic celiac plexus block. In J. M. Neal & J. P. Rathmell (Eds.), *Complications in regional anesthesia and pain medicine*. Philadelphia: Saunders.

Wong, G. Y., Schroeder, D. R., Carns, P. E., Wilson, J. L., Martin, D. P., Kinney, M. O., et al. (2004). Effect of neurolytic celiac plexus block on pain relief, quality of life, and survival in patients with unresectable pancreatic cancer: A randomized controlled trial. *JAMA: The Journal of American Medical Association, 291*(9), 1092–1099.

Xu, R., Bydon, M., Gokaslan, Z. L., Wolinsky, J., Witham, T. F., & Bydon, A. (2009). Epidural steroid injection resulting in epidural hematoma in a patient despite strict adherence to anticoagulation guidelines. *Journal of Neurosurgery. Spine, 11*, 358–364.

Yaksh, T. L. (2008). A review of pain-processing pharmacology. In H. T. Benzon, J. P. Rathmell, C. L. Wu, D. C. Turk, & C. E. Argoff (Eds.), *Raj's practical management of pain* (4th ed.). Philadelphia: Mosby.

Zundert, J. V., Huntoon, M., Patijn, J., Lataster, A., Mekhail, N., & van Kleef, M. (2010). Cervical radicular pain. *Pain Practice, 10*(1), 1–17.

Zundert, J. V., Patijn, J., Kessels, A., Lamé, I., van Suijlekom, H., & van Kleef, M. (2007). Pulsed radiofrequency adjacent to the cervical dorsal root ganglion in chronic cervical radicular pain: A double blind sham controlled randomized clinical trial. *Pain, 127*, 173–182.

Zundert, J. V., Sluijter, M., & Van Keef, M. (2008). Thermal and pulsed radiofrequency. In P. P. Raj, L. Lou, S. Erdine, P. S. Staats, S. D. Waldman, G. Racz, M. Hammer, D. Niv, R. Ruiz-Lopez, & J. E. Heavner (Eds.), *Interventional pain management: Image-guided procedures* (2nd ed.). Philadephia: Sauders.

Chapter 31
Neurosurgical Interventions for the Control of Chronic Pain Conditions

Brittany L. Adler, Mark Yarchoan, and John R. Adler Jr.*

Introduction

There is a storied history of neurosurgical interventions developed to disrupt or alter pain signaling pathways. Despite this long history and demonstrated efficacy, the application of neurosurgical techniques for treating pain has declined, attributable in large part to advancements in the use of opiates and other systemic analgesics (Sundaresan and DiGiacinto 1987), (Sundaresan et al. 1989). In one study involving 1205 cancer patients, adequate pain relief was achieved in 98.7% (Hogan et al. 1991). Nevertheless, pain is often an undertreated condition and neurosurgical pain management remains relevant. In other studies involving cancer, 10–30% of patients fail to achieve adequate pain relief with pharmacotherapy alone or experienced undesirable side-effects (Hanks and Justins 1992; Smith et al. 2005). Meanwhile it has been reported that 25% of cancer patients die in pain (Stearns et al. 2005). While pharmacotherapy is the mainstay of pain control today, neurosurgical treatments should be considered whenever (1) pain control is considered to be inadequate by the patient and (2) further pharmacological pain relief cannot be achieved without incurring unacceptable side-effects. For some patients, a neurosurgical procedure may be the only effective method of achieving stable pain relief. The goal in such neurosurgical procedures should be to improve quality of life by relieving chronic pain and limiting the side-effects resulting from high-dose narcotics.

Neurosurgical pain interventions fall into three broad categories: destructive/ablative, neuropharmacological, and augmentative/neuromodulatory. The most commonly utilized procedures within these categories are reviewed.

Destructive/Ablative Surgeries for the Treatment of Pain

Cordotomy

The spinothalamic tract (anterolateral system) conducts ascending pain and temperature sensation. Fibers in this tract typically ascend ipsilaterally for one or more segments of the spinal cord before crossing in the anterior white commissure to ascend in the contralateral anterolateral quadrant.

---

*These authors contributed equally to this work

B.L. Adler, MD • M. Yarchoan, MD • J.R. Adler Jr., MD (✉)
Department of Neurosurgery Stanford University Medical Center, 300 Pasteur Drive, Stanford, CA 94305, USA
e-mail: jra@stanford.edu

R.J. Moore (ed.), *Handbook of Pain and Palliative Care: Biobehavioral Approaches for the Life Course*,
DOI 10.1007/978-1-4419-1651-8_31, © Springer Science+Business Media, LLC 2012

Fig. 31.1 Anatomic location
of cordotomy and other
destructive spinal cord
lesions for the treatment of
chronic pain. Figure by
Daniel Kramer, University of
Pennsylvania

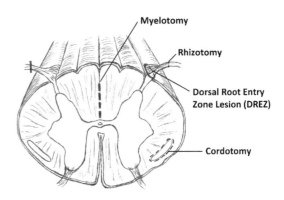

Cordotomy is a procedure in which the anterolateral quadrant of the spinal cord is lesioned, thereby blocking the spinothalamic tract and the transmission of pain (and temperature) sensation in a section of the body that is contralateral and inferior to the site of the lesion (Fig. 31.1).

Cordotomy was first devised by Spiller in 1905 when he studied a patient who had lost pain and temperature sensation in a section of his body secondary to a tuberculoma involving the anterolateral quadrant of the spinal cord. In 1912, Spiller convinced his colleague Martin to deliberately recreate this lesion to alleviate a patient's chronic leg pain, thereby performing the first cordotomy. Although initial results were disappointing, subsequent cordotomy attempts proved to be more successful. The modern technique is highly effective, and this procedure remains an important option for managing severe opiate-refractory cancer pain (Sundaresan et al. 1989).

Cordotomy may be considered for patients who have failed pharmacotherapy and have pain that is clearly transmitted by the spinothalamic tract. The best candidates for cordotomy include patients with intractable somatic pain below the C5 dermatome from unilateral cancer or compression of a nerve root or plexus, both of which can be effectively denervated by the procedure (Kanpolat 2004). Although bilateral cordotomy has been described for the treatment of visceral, bilateral, or midline pain, it is generally associated with a significantly higher rate of complications than unilateral cordotomy (Rosomoff 1969). Cordotomy is not effective in the treatment of deafferentation pain (Ischia et al. 1984).

Percutaneous cordotomy has largely replaced open cordotomy and carries significantly lower operative morbidity and mortality. The percutaneous method is minimally invasive, allows intraoperative feedback from the patient regarding pain relief, and is easily repeated if the desired result is not achieved after the first attempt. However, this method is limited to the cervical region; an open cordotomy must be performed if a lesion is needed elsewhere in the spinal cord (Jones et al. 2003).

The most common operative approach to the percutaneous cordotomy is a high cervical lateral approach through the C1–2 interspace. This technique was first described in detail by Rosomoff in 1965 and has not been modified substantially since this time (Rosomoff et al. 1965). With this technique, the patient lies in the supine position under regional or local anesthesia. The needle is introduced laterally using fluoroscopic guidance between C1 and C2 stopping at a point slightly anterior to the middle of the spinal canal. Intrathecal contrast material may be used at this time to accentuate the outline of the dentate ligament. An electrode is subsequently passed through the spinal needle and inserted into the spinothalamic tract, just anterior to the dentate ligament. The position of the electrode should be confirmed by passing a small current of approximately 50 Hz. If the placement is correct, the patient may report anesthesia on the contralateral side; incorrect placement may result in movement of the ipsilateral body, neck, or limbs. The electrode may be withdrawn after an appropriate lesion has been made and the patient reports adequate analgesia (Lipton 1968; Rosomoff et al. 1965; Foer 1971).

The historically reported effectiveness of cordotomy is in the range of 54–89% at the time of hospital discharge, and complete pain resolution has been reported in up to about half of all treated patients (Cetas et al. 2008; Sanders and Zuurmond 1995; Yegul and Erhan 2003). However, the success rate of cordotomy falls steadily over the course of months to years, and in time analgesia resulting from the procedure may be replaced with postcordotomy dysesthesias (Sanders and Zuurmond 1995). In one reported cohort, the initial cordotomy success rate of 84% fell to 43% in years 1–5, and 37% from years 5 to 10 (Bonica 1990). For this reason, use of cordotomy is typically reserved for terminally ill cancer patients with a life expectancy of less than 2 years (Jones et al. 2003).

The complication rate of cordotomy is related to the underlying pathology and both the size and location of the lesion that is produced. It is difficult to estimate the contemporary rate of complications resulting from cordotomy because most of the series reported in the literature date back more than two decades. In a single series of patients treated from 1977 to 1983, mortality rates of 6% were reported. The most frequently reported complications were Horner's syndrome (very commonly), ipsilateral leg weakness (69%), urinary retention rates requiring catheterization (20%), ipsilateral arm weakness (18%), and motor deficits (4%). In this same series, pinprick sensation deficits were also commonly observed, with almost half of patients reporting deficits in the upper quadrant and over a third of patients reporting pinprick sensation deficits in one-half of the body (Lahuerta et al. 1994).

New pain opposite to the original site of pain is another frequent complication of cordotomy. In a relatively recent study, 62% of patients who underwent a unilateral cordotomy reported new pain that mirrored the original site of pain, although such symptoms were often transient in nature, and in nearly all cases, the new pain was more moderate and easy to control than the original pain (Nagaro et al. 2001). Although the mechanism of postcordotomy mirror pain is unclear, it has been hypothesized that it might stem from lesioning inhibitory descending pain pathways or the unmasking of preoperative pain that was previously obscured by the more severe pain on the opposite side (Nagaro et al. 2001), (Sanders and Zuurmond 1995). Another risk of percutaneous cordotomy is pulmonary dysfunction, because of the close anatomical relationship of the reticulospinal tract carrying autonomic respiratory fibers to the lesion site. The unilateral loss of a reticulospinal tract is problematic, while a bilateral lesion of this tract may be fatal. For this reason cordotomy is generally contraindicated in patients with pulmonary dysfunction, a contralateral pulmonary lesion or hemi-diaphragm paralysis, or in patients with a partial oxygen concentration of less than 80% (Jones et al. 2003).

The safety and efficacy of percutaneous cordotomy may be significantly improved by the implementation of computed tomography (CT) guidance. The advent of CT-guided percutaneous cordotomy, first described by Kanpolat and colleagues in 1989, represents the first major advancement in the field of cordotomy in over 30 years. The reported success rates of CT-guided percutaneous cordotomy range from 89 to 97%, while the rate of complications is much lower than older series; an overall operative mortality rate of less than 1% is described (Yegul and Erhan 2003; Kanpolat et al. 1995). There are several advantages of CT guidance in percutaneous cordotomy that may improve outcomes. These include the possibility of measuring the spinal cord diameter at the lesion site, visualization of the electrode tip and its relation to the target, improved localization of the electrode within the spinothalamic tract, and the immediate identification of hematomas or other physical complications that can complicate cordotomy (Kanpolat et al. 1989).

While bilateral cordotomy is frequently avoided because of its much higher rate of complications, the inclusion of CT guidance during the procedure may significantly improve safety and efficacy. When performing bilateral cordotomies, it may be advisable to allow several days to pass before lesioning the opposite side of the spinothalamic tract. If 1 week is allowed to pass between the opposing first and second cordotomies, it has been shown with a relatively small sample that the success rate of the second procedure is similar to the first, with a similar overall rate of complications (Yegul and Erhan 2003). Thus CT guidance represents a major advancement in the field of cordotomy that may also allow bilateral cordotomy to be considered in more patients with bilateral or midline pain syndromes.

Myelotomy

Commissural myelotomy is an ablative neurosurgical procedure that blocks transmission of pain fibers crossing the midline from the dorsal horn to the contralateral spinothalamic pathway. The classical spinal commissural myelotomy is performed three spinal levels above the source of painful stimulus, reflecting the fact that pain fibers typically ascend two or more levels within the dorsal horn before crossing at the midline. The procedure was first proposed by Greenfield in 1926 as a means to address bilateral or midline pain without the morbidity and mortality of bilateral cordotomy. Armor reported on the first successful commissural myelotomy in 1927 and the general technique he proposed continues to be employed today (Gildenberg 2006) (Fig. 31.1).

In theory, sphincter disturbances and respiratory dysfunction are less likely to occur with myelotomy than with cordotomy. Given the attractiveness of a single procedure producing bilateral pain relief without high risk of damaging essential axonal tracts, one would expect the procedure to be of great interest to the neurosurgical community. However, in spite of its potential advantages, the procedure has never gained wide acceptance as compared to other ablative neurosurgical pain interventions. Commissural myelotomy was applied on a relatively wide scale in the 1940s and early 1950s by French and German neurosurgeons Wertheimer, Lecuire, Mansuy, and others. However, the procedure soon fell out of favor, and Wertheimer's group eventually abandoned the procedure in favor of unilateral or bilateral cordotomy (Papo and Luongo 1976). The procedure has endured periods of resurgence since this time, but only a few hundred myelotomies are reported in the literature.

A commissural myelotomy may be performed either percutaneously or open. The percutaneous method is less invasive but has only been described by a handful of surgeons. The more common open myelotomy technique is performed by means of a laminectomy. After making a midline incision in the dura, the midline septum of the dorsal spinal cord is exposed by laterally displacing, or where necessary, delicately dividing the network of overlying dorsal veins.

Success rates for commissural myelotomy of 60–70% have been reported, although the inclusion criteria, technique, and endpoints vary greatly among studies. Complications of commissural myelotomy include dysesthesias, bowel and bladder dysfunction, decreased proprioception, paralysis, and death. It is not uncommon for patients to report an "absent" sensation in their lower extremities that subsides within a few weeks of the operation (Sourek 1969; King 1977; Cook and Kawakami 1977). Pain may also recur with time; therefore, it may be advisable to select only patients with a relatively short life expectancy for this procedure. At the same time the open commissural myelotomy is a relatively invasive procedure requiring general anesthesia and, as such, may not be suitable for fragile patients in poor medical condition (Gybels and Sweet 1989).

The indications for high cervical myelotomy, performed at the C1-3 level, are more limited than for spinal commissurotomy. It has been suggested that high cervical myelotomy may be attempted to provide relief of shoulder, arm, and upper chest pain without the high rate of respiratory complications of high cervical cordotomy. Hitchcock showed in a series published in 1974 that such lesions may also relieve lower body pain. The finding that a focused central lesion could relieve upper and lower pain prompted the study of cervical lesions as an alternative to the longitudinal commissural procedures described above. However, the success rate of high cervical myelotomy reported in a small series by Papo was disappointing, as only three of ten patients had successful pain relief. Furthermore, pain returned to these patients within 4–6 weeks (Papo and Luongo 1976). Nonetheless, in cases where cordotomy is contraindicated because of respiratory impairment or a short life expectancy, a high cervical myelotomy may still be considered for patients with upper body bilateral or midline pain.

Since the advent of the classic commissural myelotomy, several modifications of this procedure have been developed. These modifications are intended to maintain similar visceral pain relief while potentially reducing the frequency of sensory perception disturbances. One such procedure, the limited midline myelotomy, was first described by Gildenberg and Hirshberg (Gildenberg and

Hirshberg 1984). With this procedure, a small laminectomy is performed at approximately the thoracolumbar junction. The vertical extent of the midline dissection within the adjacent dorsal spinal cord need only span 5–7 mm with a depth of 6 mm. The procedure provides remarkably widespread visceral pain relief, and the authors reported satisfactory results in ten of 14 patients treated. No reported sensory loss, weakness, or other complications were reported in this series. Gildenberg and Hirshberg proposed that the procedure interrupts a previously unrecognized ascending midline pain pathway (Gildenberg 2006; Gildenberg and Hirshberg 1984). Although this claim was met with controversy, subsequent postmortem specimens and animal experiments have since supported the existence of a long midline dorsal column pathway involved in the perception of pelvic visceral pain (Willis and Westlund 2001).

Building on the anatomical discovery of an ascending midline dorsal column visceral pain pathway, Nauta introduced the punctuate midline myelotomy, a minimally invasive procedure that specifically lesions this newly recognized pathway while sparing the crossing spinothalamic fibers. Nauta's punctuate midline myelotomy was produced with 5-mm deep puncture using a 16-gauge needle on either side of the median septum in the dorsal column of the spinal cord (T-8) in a patient with pelvic cancer pain (Nauta et al. 1997). Following Nauta's initial positive report, the procedure has been reproduced successfully in a dozen patients with a variety of sources of visceral pain (Nauta et al. 2000; Hwang et al. 2004). In each case the procedure provided immediate pain reduction without neurological side-effects. Because punctuate midline myelotomy deliberately spares crossing spinothalamic fibers, the success of this operation corroborates the existence of an ascending visceral nociceptive pathway in the midline of the dorsal column.

Dorsal Root Entry Zone Lesioning

Dorsal root entry zone (DREZ) lesioning is a neuroablative procedure of the posterolateral aspect of the spinal cord, including the medial portion of Lissauer's tract and the superficial five layers of Rexed's laminae, where sensory root fibers synapse with axons that join the spinothalamic tract (Nashold and Ostdahl 1979). The procedure has classically been used to treat deafferentation pain arising from a brachial plexus injury, a pain syndrome that may be poorly managed with other medical or surgical interventions (Nashold and Ostdahl 1980). DREZ-lesioning has also been used to treat other forms of chronic pain including spinal cord "end zone" pain, trigeminal neuralgia, phantom limb pain, and radiation plexopathy (Saris et al. 1985; Zeidman et al. 1993; Friedman et al. 1984) (Fig. 31.1).

The concept of DREZ-lesioning was first introduced by Sindou and colleagues in 1972. Sindou successfully used microsurgical incisions to lesion the dorsal root and a small portion of the lateral portion of the dorsal horn as a means to relieve pain in a patient suffering from a malignancy within the brachial plexus (Sindou 1972). In 1974, Nashold built on Sindou's experience and developed a wider and deeper lesion of the DREZ using radiofrequency thermocoagulation. Nashold greatly popularized the DREZ lesion and in time introduced the complete DREZ lesion as a means of controlling pain attributable to brachial plexus avulsion (Nashold and Ostdahl 1979). Nashold's procedure requires complete laminectomy extending three levels on either side of the affected spinal cord. After opening the midline dura, an electrode is inserted approximately 2 mm into the DREZ portion of the cord at a 25° angle to the vertical plane; multiple lesions are produced approximately 1–2 mm apart in the inferior–superior direction. Other successful modalities of lesioning the DREZ have been introduced including laser light (Levy et al. 1983) and ultrasound (Dreval 1993).

DREZ-lesioning provides long-term efficacy in the management of pain from brachial plexus avulsion. In one series of 55 patients who underwent treatment of a severe brachial plexus avulsion with Sindou's microsurgical DREZ technique, 95% reported excellent pain relief at discharge. At 3 months, 82% reported excellent or good pain relief, and at 29 months 66% of the patients not lost to follow-up had continued excellent or good pain relief, and 71% reported an improvement in activity level (Sindou et al. 2005). In a separate study, 77% of patients with brachial plexus avulsion treated by DREZ-lesioning had good or fair pain relief at 63 months (Thomas and Kitchen 1994). The success of DREZ-lesioning has been more varied when applied to other pain syndromes.

The introduction of the operating microscope and modern electrodes has greatly reduced complications of DREZ-lesioning. Nonetheless, neurological deficits remain a relatively common complication of the procedure, including ipsilateral lower-limb weakness, sensory changes, or both. These neurological deficits are typically mild and improve with time. Other reported complications include CSF leaks and transient loss of continence or bladder spasm (Thomas and Kitchen 1994), (Nashold and Ostdahl 1980).

Cingulotomy

The cingulate gyrus is a part of the limbic system and is involved in pain perception. The history of surgery in this brain region as a treatment for pain, i.e. cingulotomy, dates back to the mid-twentieth century discovery that prefrontal lobotomy often provides significant chronic pain relief (Foltz and White 1962). Although "lobotomy" lesions were relatively nonspecific and typically destroyed a large area of white matter tracts arising in the prefrontal cortex, the associated pain-reducing effects are now believed to stem from injury to the adjacent cingulate gyrus. Despite initial enthusiasm for prefrontal lobotomy as an innovative approach to managing severe pain, and even much more commonly treating disorders of the psyche, the lobotomy soon fell out of favor plagued by reports of devastating side-effects and changes in personality. After a period of dormancy, the field of psychosurgery was partially rejuvenated by the advent of stereotactic surgical method, which more accurately targets specific brain regions while simultaneously minimizes damage to adjacent structures (Brotis et al. 2009). Modern studies have clearly shown cingulotomy to be effective in the treatment of intractable pain when medical, surgical, and pharmacological interventions have failed (Wilkinson et al. 1999).

The cingulate gyrus is a paramedian cortical structure that is embedded deep within the interhemispheric fissure and wraps around the corpus collosum. A number of studies have implicated the cingulate gyrus in the perception of pain. Injection of lidocaine or morphine in the anterior cingulum of rats produces analgesia (Vaccarino and Melzack 1989), (LaGraize et al. 2006), and increased neuronal activity in areas of the cingulate gyrus of rabbits has been reported in response to noxious stimuli (Sikes and Vogt 1992). In particular, fibers of the cingulum bundle, which passes through the gyrus and connects the anterior and posterior cingulate cortex, appear to play a major role in pain perception (Vaccarino and Melzack 1989). Position emission tomography (PET) analysis of regional blood flow has confirmed these animal findings in humans. PET scans have identified the contralateral cingulate cortex as one of the centers in the brain that responds to a noxious, painful stimuli compared to a non-painful stimuli (Casey et al. 1994; Jones et al. 1991; Coghill et al. 1994).

Although it is clear that the cingulate cortex plays an important role in pain perception, its exact role remains poorly understood. The diffuse distribution of cortical and thalamic activation after a painful stimulus highlights the complex nature of pain and the difficulty in treating it (Coghill et al. 1994). The anterior cingulate cortex is highly interconnected with other limbic structures and cortical regions, which allows it to integrate affective, motor, and memory stimuli to modify the perception of a painful stimulus without actually changing the sensation itself. The region of the cingulate cortex responsible for this emotional component of pain has numerous connections with the amygdala, frontal cortex, and periaqueductal gray. Input from the hippocampus may allow the cingulate cortex to integrate nociceptive input with memory to evaluate the danger of a situation. The affective area of the anterior cingulate is implicated in conditioned emotional learning, vocalizations of emotion, motivation, and determining emotional relevance of stimuli. Another region of the cingulate cortex is the cognitive division, which is involved in information processing and determining appropriate motor responses to painful stimuli (Devinsky et al. 1995).

In 1962, Foltz and White reported the results from a study assessing the outcome of frontal cingulotomy in 16 patients with chronic, intractable pain. To test their hypothesis that chronic pain has a strong emotional component that is controlled by the cingulate, the authors chose a study population with intractable pain in whom emotional factors were thought to exacerbate their pain. The authors found that bilateral frontal cingulotomy in 12 of the 16 patients had a good or excellent outcome. Although the patients continued to sense pain, they did not react to the pain as strongly, saying that the pain "is not particularly bothersome" or "doesn't worry me anymore" (Foltz and White 1962). Hurt and Ballantine in 1974 found that 66–67% of a total of 68 patients with chronic pain experienced some degree of pain relief after stereotactic anterior cingulate lesions (Hurt and Ballantine 1974). In subsequent studies the percent of patients who experience pain relief after an anterior cingulotomy ranges from 45 to 67% (Faillace et al. 1971; Hurt and Ballantine 1974; Yen et al. 2005; Wilkinson et al. 1999; Wong et al. 1997). A recent report published in 1999 found that the majority of 18 patients who received a bilateral anterior cingulotomy for chronic noncancer pain experienced improvement in their pain, were no longer taking narcotics, noted improvements in their family life and social interactions, and thought that cingulotomy was beneficial (Wilkinson et al. 1999).

Hassenbusch was the first to propose using magnetic resonance-guided stereotaxis for cingulotomies. Prior to this, stereotactic localization had been achieved using air ventriculograms, which requires lumbar or cisternal puncture to inject filtered air into the ventricles and was associated with a higher risk of meningitis and hemorrhage. MRI-guided stereotaxis also has the benefit of not requiring general anesthesia, is more accurate because it images the cingulate gyrus directly, and is useful for postoperative follow-up of the lesion (Hassenbusch et al. 1990; Pillay and Hassenbusch 1992). Since the 1990s, MRI-guided stereotaxis is routinely used when performing cingulotomies (Brotis et al. 2009).

Despite recent improvements in technology that have made cingulotomies more accurate and less destructive, cingulotomy remains an invasive procedure that can have serious side-effects including seizures or lasting behavioral deficits. Neurocognitive function is generally preserved after cingulotomy, although some studies have reported deficits in focused and sustained attention (Yen et al. 2009; Cohen, Kaplan, Moser et al. 1999; Cohen, Kaplan, Zuffante et al. 1999), learning and organizing verbal material (Faillace et al. 1971), and self-initiated behaviour (Cohen, Kaplan, Zuffante et al. 1999). Another study reported altered emotional experiences of patients who underwent cingulotomy, especially in regards to emotional agitation and tension. Although family members often noted personality changes after the surgery and described the patients as being more "relaxed" (or even more apathetic in a few cases), the patients were not functionally crippled by these emotional changes. The patients felt less tension and anger, but did not report a significant reduction in self-perceived energy level (Cohen et al. 2001). Despite the severity of pre-existing pain and the subtle nature of possible changes, cingulotomy remains a controversial procedure; any risk of altering a patient's affect and personality appears to preclude widespread acceptance of this approach.

Hypophysectomy

Several methods of pituitary ablation, a procedure called hypophysectomy, have been described for the treatment of chronic pain. These include transcranial hypophysectomy and microsurgical hypophysectomy. The mechanisms underlying the analgesic effect of hypophysectomy are not completely understood. The pituitary gland secretes a number of essential endocrine hormones, but the analgesic effect does not appear to directly relate to the interruption of these hormones, leading some to postulate that a direct neuronal mechanism is involved. Another theory is that the analgesic effect of hypophysectomy is mediated by a change in hypothalamic-pituitary axis (HPA) peptides in the cerebrospinal fluid (Takeda et al. 1986).

Hypophysectomy has classically been used to relieve pain from severe and diffuse cancer such as seen with widely metastatic breast and prostate adenocarcinoma. Surgical and chemical hypophysectomy with injection of alcohol are fundamentally similar procedures that have been shown to produce comparable levels of pain relief (Ramirez and Levin 1984). Chemical hypophysectomy is carried out by introducing a needle through the nostril to puncture the sphenoid sinus. Once the sinus has been punctured and rinsed, a 19-gauge or 20-gauge needle is advanced using biplanar fluoroscopy guidance to the floor of the sella turcica. Once the needle is in place, 1–2 ml of absolute alcohol is slowly injected and the patient's pupillary reactions and body movements are closely monitored. Afterwards, the hole in the sella is sealed and the nasal cavity is packed (Ramirez and Levin 1984), (Lloyd et al. 1981).

Despite the unknown mechanism of action of hypophysectomy, it is highly effective, providing satisfactory or excellent relief of pain in 70–83% of patients with metastatic cancer (Ramirez and Levin 1984; Tindall et al. 1976; Lloyd et al. 1981). Interruption of normal pituitary function is a common complication of the procedure, resulting in the insufficiency of one or multiple pituitary hormones (Evans et al. 1982). In one published series, central diabetes insipidus occurred in 17% of patients, resulting from interruption of ADH secretion from the posterior pituitary gland. Prolonged visual disturbance was another frequent complication in this study (Lloyd et al. 1981).

Neuropharmacological

Intraspinal Pumps

Intraspinal analgesic pumps are the most commonly used alternative pain management approach in patients who cannot tolerate the side-effects or achieve adequate pain relief from systemic pharmacotherapy. The pumps deliver analgesics directly into the cerebrospinal fluid that engulfs the spinal cord. Because the drugs are delivered closer to their site of action in the dorsal horn, lower doses of analgesics can be administered as compared to systemic therapy, resulting in fewer systemic side-effects. Intraspinal pumps reduce the amount of systemic narcotic exposure by a factor of 30–300 depending on the route of spinal cord administration (Smith et al. 2005; Kim 2005). The device itself consists of a pump that stores the medication and can be refilled percutaneously, which is itself attached to an intraspinal catheter. Implantation of the pump is an invasive procedure that can cause serious side-effects and therefore is reserved for the minority of patients who do not achieve adequate pain control with traditional pharmacotherapy (Hogan et al. 1991).

Opiates can be delivered into either the intrathecal (subarachnoid) or epidural space to reach their site of action in the brain and the substantia gelatinosa of the spinal cord (Kedlaya et al. 2002). Both these methods of delivery can be equally effective. The advantage of intrathecal opioid delivery is that one-tenth the dose of analgesic is necessary to achieve the same degree of pain relief, which results in fewer systemic side-effects (Kim 2005). Epidural delivery is less potent but also causes less respiratory depression and somnolence. Intrathecal delivery is preferred for therapy longer than 3 months because of the association between long-term epidural drug delivery and catheter obstruction, fibrosis, and loss of analgesic efficacy (Aldrete 1995).

Physicians can choose the rate at which analgesics are delivered around the spinal cord. A fixed-rate pump delivers the medication at a constant rate, whereas a programmable pump delivers the medication at a rate pre-set by a computer program. In addition, patient-controlled analgesia systems allow the patient to deliver the bolus of drug based on their current state of pain (Rauck et al. 2003).

The physician's choice of drug delivery system should take into account the patient's predicted life-expectancy, cost-effectiveness, and the route of administration (whether epidural or intrathecal). Type 1 (percutaneous) catheters are designed for short-term use of less than 1 week, whereas Type 2 catheters are subcutaneous and are designed for outpatients. Type 3 catheters require a minor surgical procedure to implant the device and can be placed in the epidural or intrathecal space, while Type 4 catheters are totally implanted (Kim 2005). An external drug delivery system should be used if the patient has less than 3 months to live. Permanent implantation of the catheter under local anesthesia is preceded by a trial period with a temporary external pump (Kedlaya et al. 2002).

Morphine is the most commonly used analgesic in intraspinal pumps. Other opioids such as fentanyl, hydromorphine, sufentanil, methadone, and meperidine are also available if morphine fails or the patient does not tolerate morphine well. In addition, a number of conditions may respond poorly to morphine, in which case other nonopioid drugs such as local anesthetics may be substituted. If tolerance develops, another opioid can be used or the opioid can be used in combination with a co-analgesic, such as a local anesthetic (bupivicaine, tetracaine), calcium-channel blocker (ziconitide), alpha-2-agonist (clonidine), or gaba-B-agonist (baclofen) (Kim 2005).

Although intraspinal pumps are more targeted and therefore minimize systemic side-effects, many of the effects of morphine are mediated by the central nervous system and remain of primary concern. The patient must be monitored after initial implantation for signs of toxicity such as respiratory depression and hypotension. More common but less serious side-effects associated with morphine pump-use include nausea, vomiting, constipation, itching, edema, sexual dysfunction, and hyperalgesia (Ruan 2007). Prolonged use of an intraspinal pump is associated with complications such as pain on injection of the analgesic, hyperesthesia, infection, epidural abscess, and technical problems with the catheter and pump (Hogan et al. 1991). Catheter dislocation, obstruction, rupture, or disconnection occurred in 17 of 165 patients over the course of 3 years in one study by Koulousakis et al. (2007).

Despite the effectiveness in controlling chronic pain, the benefits of intraspinal drug delivery must be balanced with the side-effects from the drug and potential complications from the procedure itself. A randomized control trial involving 202 patients found that intraspinal pumps in combination with comprehensive pain management improved pain control compared to comprehensive pain management alone, and decreased the incidence of drug toxicities, fatigue, and depressed levels of consciousness. There was also a trend toward increased 6-month survival among patients receiving intraspinal drug delivery (Smith et al. 2002).

Augmentative/Neuromodulatory Surgeries for the Treatment of Pain

Spinal Cord Stimulation

Spinal cord stimulation (SCS) is an important technology for treating chronic, localized neuropathic pain. A device that contains a set of electrodes is implanted into the epidural space either percutaneously or by laminectomy, and delivers electrical impulses to a targeted area of the dorsal column of the spinal cord. A pulse generator implanted in the buttocks or abdomen generates the electrical current (Shealy, Mortimer et al. 1967; Shealy, Taslitz et al. 1967). This therapy is used to treat a wide variety of chronic pain conditions, including intractable low back pain, complex regional pain syndromes, phantom pain, diabetic neuropathy, and angina pectoris (North et al. 1993).

Little is known about the mechanism of action of SCS. The Gate Control Theory of pain, proposed in 1965 by Melzack and Wall, argues that excess stimulation of large afferent non-pain A-β fibers closes the "gate" in the dorsal horn of the spinal cord and therefore prevents the transmission of painful nociceptive signals in small afferent fibers (Krames 1999). Although this theory is commonly thought to be the primary mechanism of pain relief, it is an imperfect explanation because it fails to reconcile many clinical observations, such as why SCS is only effective in the treatment of chronic and not acute pain, or why activation of large afferent fibers can signal pain. Several other explanations have been proposed, and it is likely that multiple mechanisms interact in a complex and poorly understood way to result in pain relief (Oakley and Prager 2002). Other proposed theories that may explain the efficacy of SCS include inhibition of signal transmission in the spinothalamic tract, modulation of supraspinal neurons, inhibition of sympathetic efferent neurons, or the release of vasoactive substances such as vasoactive peptide and substance P (Krames 1999). In support of these other theories, patients often experience pain relief many hours after cessation of the stimulation, which suggests that long-lasting neural modulation occurs from SCS (Linderoth and Foreman 1999).

The sensation of pain is modified in many patients receiving SCS and is perceived as paresthesia, or a tingling sensation. The efficacy of SCS depends on the type of pain. SCS seems to specifically block continuous and induced pain such as tactile or thermal allodynia, but it has no effect on acute nociceptive pain (Meyerson and Linderoth 2000). While SCS is generally more effective at treating neuropathic pain than nociceptive pain, interestingly patients with peripheral vascular disease and angina pectoris also experience pain relief from SCS. Such benefits possibly stem from an inhibitory effect of SCS on the sympathetic nervous system, which in turn promotes vasodilation and reduces the noxious signals that underlie angina (Oakley and Prager 2002).

A large number of case and descriptive studies have been published that find SCS to be beneficial in relieving pain. In a study by North et al. 52% of the patients self-reported at least 50% pain relief from SCS, and 60% of the patients were satisfied enough with the treatment to be willing to repeat the implantation. However, not all patients benefit from SCS equally. In this same study, 22% of the patients did not experience at least 50% pain relief and 7% had no pain benefit at all (North et al. 1993).

The paucity of well-controlled studies evaluating SCS makes it difficult to arrive at any strong conclusions regarding its efficacy. To date there have been only a handful of randomized control trials. One well-designed study found that patients with Complex Regional Pain Syndrome that received SCS and physical therapy had a significant reduction in pain intensity and improved health-related quality of life at 6 and 12 months compared to those who only received physical therapy. However, there was no improvement in functional status after 6 months. Notably, only two-thirds of patients in this study who responded positively to a test stimulation went on to receive permanent implantations (Kemler et al. 2000). In a series of failed back syndrome patients, 15% of the patients who underwent SCS returned to work over the course of 5 years, compared to zero patients in the control group. This functional improvement was attributed to pain relief and reduction in drug usage. Moreover, patients in the SCS group reported a 27% improvement in quality of life over the 5 years of follow-up compared to only 12% in the control group (Kumar et al. 2002). Of note, SCS is rarely used in terminal cancer patients because of the high cost to the procedure and need for patient involvement in monitoring their pain. Nevertheless, SCS shows great promise in treating a variety of other chronic pain conditions.

Patients undergoing SCS are at risk for a number of complications, including infection, bleeding, pain in the region of the stimulator, spinal cord or nerve injury, equipment failure, and in some patients such symptoms can require stimulator removal. A metanalysis of 18 studies found an average complication rate of 34% from SCS (Turner et al. 2004). Because of the invasive nature of SCS, it should be reserved for patients who fail to respond to more conservative treatments. Although the complication rate will continue to drop as technology improves (Meyerson and Linderoth 2000), such a significant complication rate and the high price tag for both surgery and the implanted stimulator underscore the need for more long-term, randomized control trials to determine the true efficacy of SCS.

Despite its many limitations, the use of SCS in the clinic has increased significantly in the last decade as patient selection criteria and the technology of the device itself have improved

Fig. 31.2 A 3D schematic image demonstrating the basic location of a SCS generator with attached intraspinal electrodes. Figure courtesy of Medtronic, Inc

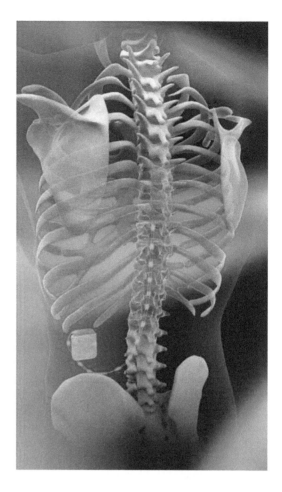

(North et al. 1993). Coinciding with these improvements, there has been a significant increase in the long-term efficacy of SCS from 40% in the 1970s and early 1980s to 70% today. Moreover, development of the temporary percutaneous electrode implantation has allowed patients to first try SCS for up to a few weeks to see if they respond (i.e.: have a greater than 50% improvement in pain) before a permanent device is implanted (Mailis-Gagnon et al. 2004). Even before better-designed and more definitive studies can determine the ultimate efficacy of SCS, the clinical use of this technology seems destined to increase, seemingly giving some chronic pain patients symptom relief and improving the quality of their lives (Figs. 31.2 and 31.3).

Deep Brain and Motor Cortex Stimulation

Deep brain stimulation (DBS) has been used for the relief of chronic pain symptoms for the past 50 years. The first reports that electrical stimulation can modulate pain sensation were in 1954 by Heath and Mickle and in 1956 by Pool et al. (Kumar et al. 1997). Since then, the indications for DBS have expanded to include a number of neurological and psychiatric conditions, including among others Parkinson's disease, Tourette's syndrome, obsessive-compulsive disease, and major depression. DBS can also benefit select patients with chronic pain that is refractory to more conservative treatments such as pharmacotherapy, physical therapy, psychiatric intervention, or even SCS (Kumar et al. 1997; Levy et al. 1987).

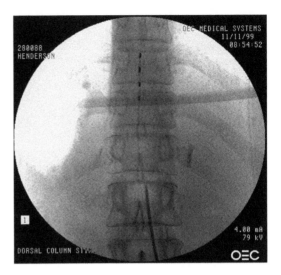

Fig. 31.3 An anterior–posterior x-ray of the spine depicting the position of SCS epidural electrodes within the spinal canal

DBS is a procedure that involves surgical implantation of electrodes that send impulses to targeted areas of the brain. The surgically implanted device includes a pulse-generator that is placed subcutaneously below the clavicle or in the chest or abdomen, which is capable of continuously delivering electrical impulses to precise regions of the brain. In general, neuropathic pain is best treated by thalamic stimulation, whereas nociceptive pain is treated by stimulation of the periaqueductal/periventricular gray matter (Awan et al. 2009). However, the majority of patients present with both nociceptive and neuropathic pain, and in these cases the surgeon attempts to stimulate both the thalamus and the periaqueducal/periventircular gray matter simultaneously (Levy et al. 1987).

During the implantation of the DBS brain electrode the patient is awake enough for the surgeon to assess the pain relieving benefits of stimulation. Equally important, the effect of stimulation on a variety of functions, including among others short-term memory, speech, swallowing, limb movement, and alertness (Hariz 2002) must be assessed. A few weeks after implantation surgery, the output from the device is carefully calibrated to optimize symptom relief and minimize side-effects. The non-ablative and reversible nature of DBS makes it an appealing treatment for many types of pain. Nevertheless, these same characteristics also represent inherent shortcomings of this approach.

Although the mechanism of action is uncertain, one study has shown that stimulation induces a reversible chemical blockade at the targeted area through the release of ATP and accumulation of adenosine, which binds to A1 receptors and suppresses excitatory transmission (Bekar et al. 2008). Meanwhile, in another study analgesia induced by stimulation of the midbrain central gray (Reynolds 1969) was shown to be reversed by nalaxone, suggesting that endogenous opioid transmission is involved in DBS (Akil et al. 1976). It is likely that a combination of mechanisms is responsible for the neuromodulation observed in DBS. Ultimately, four general theories have been proposed: (1) Depolarization blockade, which is the inhibition of activation of voltage-gated currents, (2) Synaptic inhibition of synapses connecting with neurons near the electrode, (3) synaptic depression from transmitter depletion, and (4) modulation of network activity (McIntyre et al. 2004).

Despite the surgical nature of DBS, it has a relatively low rate of peri-operative complications. Potential problems include paralysis, hematoma, and transient or permanent neurological deficits. However, hardware problems, electrode fracture, lead dislocation, and skin infection are not rare occurrences (Hariz 2002; Voges et al. 2006). The most common side-effects arise from chronic stimulation itself. Although most of these side-effects are reversible or adjustable, there have been reports of permanent damage, such as irreversible dementia in patients with impaired mental status who

Fig. 31.4 This AP x-ray of the head depicts the placement of bilateral DBS electrodes in a patient being treated for chronic pain

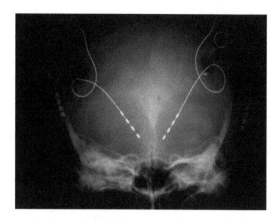

received substantia nigra stimulation. Meanwhile, side-effects from thalamic stimulation include decreased fine motor movement, parathesias, impaired proprioception, and dystonia (Hariz 2002).

Studies have shown variable effects of DBS on pain symptoms. However, most studies have found a 25–60% response rate among patients (Awan et al. 2009). Such variability stems largely from the wide variety of pain conditions treated by DBS and the variation in patient screening, selection criteria, and outcome measures. In a study by Levy et al., 141 patients with either nociceptive or neuropathic pain were assessed for self-reported pain relief after DBS. About 59% of the patients experienced initial pain relief that was significant enough to justify permanent implantation of the stimulator and in whom pain relief persisted up until the first post-operative visit after the surgery. Nevertheless, the percent of patients who still experienced pain relief after a mean follow-up period of 6.8 years dropped to 31%. Patients with peripheral neuropathies responded best to DBS with a long-term success rate of over 50%, while no patients with chronic pain from spinal cord injury responded to DBS (Levy et al. 1987). Similarly, Kumar et al. found a 62% response rate to DBS; patients with failed back syndrome, trigeminal neuropathy, and peripheral neuropathy had the highest response rates (Kumar et al. 1997).

Despite promising results in some DBS studies involving chronic pain patients, other trials have been disappointing, particularly two trials sponsored by Medtronic Inc. entitled Model 3380 and 3387. The 3387 trial was stopped early because of high patient drop-out and poor efficacy. Neither of these trials achieved their goal of pain relief in more than 50% of patients. The percent of patients achieving pain relief at 12 months was 46.1% in the Model 3380 and 16.2% in the Model 3387 study, whereas pain relief at 24 months fell to 17.8% in the Model 3380 and 13.5% in the Model 3387 study (Coffey 2001) (Fig. 31.4).

Motor cortex stimulation is an exciting but still investigational alternative to DBS. Tsubokawa first observed in 1991 that deafferentation of the spinothalamic tract in cats induced thalamic hyperactivity, and this burst hyperactivity was completely inhibited by stimulation of the motor cortex (Tsubokawa et al. 1991). Translating these findings into the clinic, Tsubokawa implanted electrodes to stimulate the motor cortex in a small cohort of patients with central pain from central nervous system lesions. About 67% of the patients in this cohort experienced effective pain relief at 1 year, 63% of whom reported complete pain relief (Tsubokawa et al. 1991). These pioneering trials paved the way for additional studies of motor cortex stimulation for treating a range of chronic pain indications. This procedure has been most extensively tested and validated for central and facial pain syndromes, conditions that respond poorly to pharmacotherapy or traditional stimulation techniques including DBS. Despite a strong selection bias towards using motor cortex stimulation in only those patients with the most refractory and debilitating pain conditions, published results to date have been particularly promising.

References

Akil, H., Mayer, D. J., & Liebeskind, J. C. (1976). Antagonism of stimulation-produced analgesia by naloxone, a narcotic antagonist. *Science, 191*(4230), 961–962.

Aldrete, J. A. (1995). Epidural fibrosis after permanent catheter insertion and infusion. *Journal of Pain and Symptom Management, 10*(8), 624–631.

Awan, N. R., Lozano, A., & Hamani, C. (2009). Deep brain stimulation: Current and future perspectives. *Neurosurgical Focus, 27*(1), E2.

Bekar, L., Libionka, W., Tian, G. F., Xu, Q., Torres, A., Wang, X., et al. (2008). Adenosine is crucial for deep brain stimulation-mediated attenuation of tremor. *Nature Medicine, 14*(1), 75–80.

Bonica, J. J. (1990). The management of pain. (2nd edn.). Philadelphia: Lea & Febiger. John J. Bonica with the collaboration of John D. Loeser, C. Richard Chapman, Wilbert E. Fordyce; illustrations by Majorie Domenowske.; 2v; Includes bibliographical references and index.

Brotis, A. G., Kapsalaki, E. Z., Paterakis, K., Smith, J. R., & Fountas, K. N. (2009). Historic evolution of open cingulectomy and stereotactic cingulotomy in the management of medically intractable psychiatric disorders, pain and drug addiction. *Stereotactic and Functional Neurosurgery, 87*(5), 271–291.

Casey, K. L., Minoshima, S., Berger, K. L., Koeppe, R. A., Morrow, T. J., & Frey, K. A. (1994). Positron emission tomographic analysis of cerebral structures activated specifically by repetitive noxious heat stimuli. *Journal of Neurophysiology, 71*(2), 802–807.

Cetas, J. S., Saedi, T., & Burchiel, K. J. (2008). Destructive procedures for the treatment of nonmalignant pain: A structured literature review. *Journal of Neurosurgery, 109*(3), 389–404.

Coffey, R. J. (2001). Deep brain stimulation for chronic pain: Results of two multicenter trials and a structured review. *Pain Medicine, 2*(3), 183–192.

Coghill, R. C., Talbot, J. D., Evans, A. C., Meyer, E., Gjedde, A., Bushnell, M. C., et al. (1994). Distributed processing of pain and vibration by the human brain. *Journal of Neuroscience, 14*(7), 4095–4108.

Cohen, R. A., Kaplan, R. F., Moser, D. J., Jenkins, M. A., & Wilkinson, H. (1999). Impairments of attention after cingulotomy. *Neurology, 53*(4), 819–824.

Cohen, R. A., Kaplan, R. F., Zuffante, P., Moser, D. J., Jenkins, M. A., Salloway, S., et al. (1999). Alteration of intention and self-initiated action associated with bilateral anterior cingulotomy. *Journal of Neuropsychiatry and Clinical Neurosciences, 11*(4), 444–453.

Cohen, R. A., Paul, R., Zawacki, T. M., Moser, D. J., Sweet, L., & Wilkinson, H. (2001). Emotional and personality changes following cingulotomy. *Emotion, 1*(1), 38–50.

Cook, A. W., & Kawakami, Y. (1977). Commissural myelotomy. *Journal of Neurosurgery, 47*(1), 1–6.

Devinsky, O., Morrell, M. J., & Vogt, B. A. (1995). Contributions of anterior cingulate cortex to behaviour. *Brain, 118*(Pt 1), 279–306.

Dreval, O. N. (1993). Ultrasonic DREZ-operations for treatment of pain due to brachial plexus avulsion. *Acta Neurochirurgica (Wien), 122*(1–2), 76–81.

Evans, P. J., Lloyd, J. W., Moore, R. A., & Smith, R. F. (1982). Pituitary function following hypophysectomy for pain relief. *British Journal of Anaesthesia, 54*(9), 921–925.

Faillace, L. A., Allen, R. P., McQueen, J. D., & Northrup, B. (1971). Cognitive deficits from bilateral cingulotomy for intractable pain in man. *Diseases of the Nervous System, 32*(3), 171–175.

Foer, W. H. (1971). Percutaneous cervical radiofrequency cordotomy: A modern method for relief of intractable pain. *Journal of the Medical Society of New Jersey, 68*(9), 737–741.

Foltz, E. L., & White, L. E., Jr. (1962). Pain "relief" by frontal cingulumotomy. *Journal of Neurosurgery, 19*, 89–100.

Friedman, A. H., Nashold, B. S., Jr., & Ovelmen-Levitt, J. (1984). Dorsal root entry zone lesions for the treatment of post-herpetic neuralgia. *Journal of Neurosurgery, 60*(6), 1258–1262.

Gildenberg, P. L. (2006). Evolution of spinal cord surgery for pain. *Clinical Neurosurgery, 53*, 11–17.

Gildenberg, P. L., & Hirshberg, R. M. (1984). Limited myelotomy for the treatment of intractable cancer pain. *Journal of Neurology, Neurosurgery, and Psychiatry, 47*(1), 94–96.

Gybels, J. M., & Sweet, W. H. (1989). Neurosurgical treatment of persistent pain. physiological and pathological mechanisms of human pain. *Pain and Headache, 11*, 1–402.

Hanks, G. W., & Justins, D. M. (1992). Cancer pain: Management. *Lancet, 339*(8800), 1031–1036.

Hariz, M. I. (2002). Complications of deep brain stimulation surgery. *Movement Disorders, 17*(Suppl 3), S162–S166.

Hassenbusch, S. J., Pillay, P. K., & Barnett, G. H. (1990). Radiofrequency cingulotomy for intractable cancer pain using stereotaxis guided by magnetic resonance imaging. *Neurosurgery, 27*(2), 220–223.

Hogan, Q., Haddox, J. D., Abram, S., Weissman, D., Taylor, M. L., & Janjan, N. (1991). Epidural opiates and local anesthetics for the management of cancer pain. *Pain, 46*(3), 271–279.

Hurt, R. W., & Ballantine, H. T., Jr. (1974). Stereotactic anterior cingulate lesions for persistent pain: A report on 68 cases. *Clinical Neurosurgery, 21*, 334–351.

Hwang, S. L., Lin, C. L., Lieu, A. S., Kuo, T. H., Yu, K. L., Ou-Yang, F., et al. (2004). Punctate midline myelotomy for intractable visceral pain caused by hepatobiliary or pancreatic cancer. *Journal of Pain and Symptom Management, 27*(1), 79–84.

Ischia, S., Luzzani, A., Ischia, A., Magon, F., & Toscano, D. (1984). Subarachnoid neurolytic block (L5-S1) and unilateral percutaneous cervical cordotomy in the treatment of pain secondary to pelvic malignant disease. *Pain, 20*(2), 139–149.

Jones, A. K., Brown, W. D., Friston, K. J., Qi, L. Y., & Frackowiak, R. S. (1991). Cortical and subcortical localization of response to pain in man using positron emission tomography. *Proceedings Biological Sciences, 244*(1309), 39–44.

Jones, B., Finlay, I., Ray, A., & Simpson, B. (2003). Is there still a role for open cordotomy in cancer pain management? *Journal of Pain and Symptom Management, 25*(2), 179–184.

Kanpolat, Y. (2004). The surgical treatment of chronic pain: Destructive therapies in the spinal cord. *Neurosurgery Clinics of North America, 15*(3), 307–317.

Kanpolat, Y., Caglar, S., Akyar, S., & Temiz, C. (1995). CT-guided pain procedures for intractable pain in malignancy. *Acta Neurochirurgica. Supplement (Wien), 64*, 88–91.

Kanpolat, Y., Deda, H., Akyar, S., & Bilgic, S. (1989). CT-guided percutaneous cordotomy. *Acta Neurochirurgica. Supplement (Wien), 46*, 67–68.

Kedlaya, D., Reynolds, L., & Waldman, S. (2002). Epidural and intrathecal analgesia for cancer pain. *Best Practice & Research. Clinical Anaesthesiology, 16*(4), 651–665.

Kemler, M. A., Barendse, G. A., van Kleef, M., de Vet, H. C., Rijks, C. P., Furnee, C. A., et al. (2000). Spinal cord stimulation in patients with chronic reflex sympathetic dystrophy. *The New England Journal of Medicine, 343*(9), 618–624.

Kim, P. S. (2005). Interventional cancer pain therapies. *Seminars in Oncology, 32*(2), 194–199.

King, R. B. (1977). Anterior commissurotomy for intractable pain. *Journal of Neurosurgery, 47*(1), 7–11.

Koulousakis, A., Kuchta, J., Bayarassou, A., & Sturm, V. (2007). Intrathecal opioids for intractable pain syndromes. *Acta Neurochirurgica. Supplement (Wein), 97*(Pt 1), 43–48.

Krames, E. (1999). Spinal cord stimulation: Indications, mechanism of action, and efficacy. *Current Review of Pain, 3*(6), 419–426.

Kumar, K., Malik, S., & Demeria, D. (2002). Treatment of chronic pain with spinal cord stimulation versus alternative therapies: Cost-effectiveness analysis. *Neurosurgery, 51*(1), 106,15. discussion 115–116.

Kumar, K., Toth, C., & Nath, R. K. (1997). Deep brain stimulation for intractable pain: A 15-year experience. *Neurosurgery, 40*(4), 736,46. discussion 746–747.

LaGraize, S. C., Borzan, J., Peng, Y. B., & Fuchs, P. N. (2006). Selective regulation of pain affect following activation of the opioid anterior cingulate cortex system. *Experimental Neurology, 197*(1), 22–30.

Lahuerta, J., Bowsher, D., Lipton, S., & Buxton, P. H. (1994). Percutaneous cervical cordotomy: A review of 181 operations on 146 patients with a study on the location of "pain fibers" in the C-2 spinal cord segment of 29 cases. *Journal of Neurosurgery, 80*(6), 975–985.

Levy, R. M., Lamb, S., & Adams, J. E. (1987). Treatment of chronic pain by deep brain stimulation: Long term follow-up and review of the literature. *Neurosurgery, 21*(6), 885–893.

Levy, W. J., Nutkiewicz, A., Ditmore, Q. M., & Watts, C. (1983). Laser-induced dorsal root entry zone lesions for pain control: Report of three cases. *Journal of Neurosurgery, 59*(5), 884–886.

Linderoth, B., & Foreman, R. (1999). Physiology of spinal cord stimulation: Review and update. *Neuromodulation: Technology at the Neural Interface, 2*(3), 150–164.

Lipton, S. (1968). Percutaneous electrical cordotomy in relief of intractable pain. *British Medical Journal, 2*(5599), 210–212.

Lloyd, J. W., Rawlinson, W. A., & Evans, P. J. (1981). Selective hypophysectomy for metastatic pain: A review of ethyl alcohol ablation of the anterior pituitary in a regional pain relief unit. *British Journal of Anaesthesia, 53*(11), 1129–1133.

Mailis-Gagnon, A., Furlan, A. D., Sandoval, J. A., & Taylor, R. (2004). Spinal cord stimulation for chronic pain. *Cochrane Database of Systematic Reviews, 3*, CD003783.

McIntyre, C. C., Savasta, M., Kerkerian-Le Goff, L., & Vitek, J. L. (2004). Uncovering the mechanism(s) of action of deep brain stimulation: Activation, inhibition, or both. *Clinical Neurophysiology, 115*(6), 1239–1248.

Meyerson, B. A., & Linderoth, B. (2000). Mechanisms of spinal cord stimulation in neuropathic pain. *Neurological Research, 22*(3), 285–292.

Nagaro, T., Adachi, N., Tabo, E., Kimura, S., Arai, T., & Dote, K. (2001). New pain following cordotomy: Clinical features, mechanisms, and clinical importance. *Journal of Neurosurgery, 95*(3), 425–431.

Nashold, B. S., Jr., & Ostdahl, R. H. (1979). Dorsal root entry zone lesions for pain relief. *Journal of Neurosurgery, 51*(1), 59–69.

Nashold, B. S., Jr., & Ostdahl, R. H. (1980). Pain relief after dorsal root entry zone lesions. *Acta Neurochirurgica Supplement (Wien), 30*, 383–389.

Nauta, H. J., Hewitt, E., Westlund, K. N., & Jr Willis, W. D. (1997). Surgical interruption of a midline dorsal column visceral pain pathway: Case report and review of the literature. *Journal of Neurosurgery, 86*(3), 538–542.

Nauta, H. J., Soukup, V. M., Fabian, R. H., Lin, J. T., Grady, J. J., Williams, C. G., et al. (2000). Punctate midline myelotomy for the relief of visceral cancer pain. *Journal of Neurosurgery, 92*(2 Suppl), 125–130.

North, R. B., Kidd, D. H., Zahurak, M., James, C. S., & Long, D. M. (1993). Spinal cord stimulation for chronic, intractable pain: Experience over two decades. *Neurosurgery, 32*(3), 384, 94. discussion 394–395.

Oakley, J. C., & Prager, J. P. (2002). Spinal cord stimulation: Mechanisms of action. *Spine (Phila Pa 1976), 27*(22), 2574–2583.

Papo, I., & Luongo, A. (1976). High cervical commissural myelotomy in the treatment of pain. *Journal of Neurology, Neurosurgery, and Psychiatry, 39*(7), 705–710.

Pillay, P. K., & Hassenbusch, S. J. (1992). Bilateral MRI-guided stereotactic cingulotomy for intractable pain. *Stereotactic and Functional Neurosurgery, 59*(1–4), 33–38.

Ramirez, L. F., & Levin, A. B. (1984). Pain relief after hypophysectomy. *Neurosurgery, 14*(4), 499–504.

Rauck, R. L., Cherry, D., Boyer, M. F., Kosek, P., Dunn, J., & Alo, K. (2003). Long-term intrathecal opioid therapy with a patient-activated, implanted delivery system for the treatment of refractory cancer pain. *The Journal of Pain, 4*(8), 441–447.

Reynolds, D. V. (1969). Surgery in the rat during electrical analgesia induced by focal brain stimulation. *Science, 164*(878), 444–445.

Rosomoff, H. L. (1969). Bilateral percutaneous cervical radiofrequency cordotomy. *Journal of Neurosurgery, 31*(1), 41–46.

Rosomoff, H. L., Brown, C. J., & Sheptak, P. (1965). Percutaneous radiofrequency cervical cordotomy: Technique. *Journal of Neurosurgery, 23*(6), 639–644.

Ruan, X. (2007). Drug-related side effects of long-term intrathecal morphine therapy. *Pain Physician, 10*(2), 357–366.

Sanders, M., & Zuurmond, W. (1995). Safety of unilateral and bilateral percutaneous cervical cordotomy in 80 terminally ill cancer patients. *Journal of Clinical Oncology, 13*(6), 1509–1512.

Saris, S. C., Iacono, R. P., & Nashold, B. S., Jr. (1985). Dorsal root entry zone lesions for post-amputation pain. *Journal of Neurosurgery, 62*(1), 72–76.

Shealy, C. N., Mortimer, J. T., & Reswick, J. B. (1967). Electrical inhibition of pain by stimulation of the dorsal columns: Preliminary clinical report. *Anesthesia and Analgesia, 46*(4), 489–491.

Shealy, C. N., Taslitz, N., Mortimer, J. T., & Becker, D. P. (1967). Electrical inhibition of pain: Experimental evaluation. *Anesthesia and Analgesia, 46*(3), 299–305.

Sikes, R. W., & Vogt, B. A. (1992). Nociceptive neurons in area 24 of rabbit cingulate cortex. *Journal of Neurophysiology, 68*(5), 1720–1732.

Sindou M. (1972). Etude de la jonction radiculo-médullaire postérieure: La radicellectomie postérieur sélective dans la chirurgie de la douleur. These Med., Lyon. 1–182.

Sindou, M. P., Blondet, E., Emery, E., & Mertens, P. (2005). Microsurgical lesioning in the dorsal root entry zone for pain due to brachial plexus avulsion: A prospective series of 55 patients. *Journal of Neurosurgery, 102*(6), 1018–1028.

Smith, T. J., Staats, P. S., Deer, T., Stearns, L. J., Rauck, R. L., Boortz-Marx, R. L., et al. (2002). Implantable drug delivery systems study group. Randomized clinical trial of an implantable drug delivery system compared with comprehensive medical management for refractory cancer pain: Impact on pain, drug-related toxicity, and survival. *Journal of Clinical Oncology, 20*(19), 4040–4049.

Smith, T. J., Swainey, C., & Coyne, P. J. (2005). Pain management, including intrathecal pumps. *Current Pain and Headache Reports, 9*(4), 243–248.

Sourek, K. (1969). Commissural myelotomy. *Journal of Neurosurgery, 31*(5), 524–527.

Stearns, L., Boortz-Marx, R., Du Pen, S., Friehs, G., Gordon, M., Halyard, M., et al. (2005). Intrathecal drug delivery for the management of cancer pain: A multidisciplinary consensus of best clinical practices. *Journal of Supportive Oncology, 3*(6), 399–408.

Sundaresan, N., & DiGiacinto, G. V. (1987). Antitumor and antinociceptive approaches to control cancer pain. *The Medical Clinics of North America, 71*(2), 329–348.

Sundaresan, N., DiGiacinto, G. V., & Hughes, J. E. (1989). Neurosurgery in the treatment of cancer pain. *Cancer, 63*(11 Suppl), 2365–2377.

Takeda, F., Uki, J., Fuse, Y., Kitani, Y., & Fujita, T. (1986). The pituitary as a target of antalgic treatment of chronic cancer pain: A possible mechanism of pain relief through pituitary neuroadenolysis. *Neurological Research, 8*(4), 194–200.

Thomas, D. G., & Kitchen, N. D. (1994). Long-term follow up of dorsal root entry zone lesions in brachial plexus avulsion. *Journal of Neurology, Neurosurgery, and Psychiatry, 57*(6), 737–738.

Tindall, G. T., Ambrose, S. S., Christy, J. H., & Patton, J. M. (1976). Hypophysectomy in the treatment of disseminated carcinoma of the breast and prostate gland. *Southern Medical Journal, 69*(5), 579–583.

Tsubokawa, T., Katayama, Y., Yamamoto, T., Hirayama, T., & Koyama, S. (1991a). Chronic motor cortex stimulation for the treatment of central pain. *Acta Neurochirurgica. Supplement (Wien), 52*, 137–139.

Tsubokawa, T., Katayama, Y., Yamamoto, T., Hirayama, T., & Koyama, S. (1991b). Treatment of thalamic pain by chronic motor cortex stimulation. *Pacing and Clinical Electrophysiology, 14*(1), 131–134.

Turner, J. A., Loeser, J. D., Deyo, R. A., & Sanders, S. B. (2004). Spinal cord stimulation for patients with failed back surgery syndrome or complex regional pain syndrome: A systematic review of effectiveness and complications. *Pain, 108*(1–2), 137–147.

Vaccarino, A. L., & Melzack, R. (1989). Analgesia produced by injection of lidocaine into the anterior cingulum bundle of the rat. *Pain, 39*(2), 213–219.

Voges, J., Waerzeggers, Y., Maarouf, M., Lehrke, R., Koulousakis, A., Lenartz, D., et al. (2006). Deep-brain stimulation: Long-term analysis of complications caused by hardware and surgery–experiences from a single centre. *Journal of Neurology, Neurosurgery, and Psychiatry, 77*(7), 868–872.

Wilkinson, H. A., Davidson, K. M., & Davidson, R. I. (1999). Bilateral anterior cingulotomy for chronic noncancer pain. *Neurosurgery, 45*(5), 1129, 34. discussion 1134–1136.

Willis, W. D., Jr., & Westlund, K. N. (2001). The role of the dorsal column pathway in visceral nociception. *Current Pain and Headache Reports, 5*(1), 20–26.

Wong, E. T., Gunes, S., Gaughan, E., Patt, R. B., Ginsberg, L. E., Hassenbusch, S. J., et al. (1997). Palliation of intractable cancer pain by MRI-guided cingulotomy. *The Clinical Journal of Pain, 13*(3), 260–263.

Yegul, I., & Erhan, E. (2003). Bilateral CT-guided percutaneous cordotomy for cancer pain relief. *Clinical Radiology, 58*(11), 886–889.

Yen, C. P., Kuan, C. Y., Sheehan, J., Kung, S. S., Wang, C. C., Liu, C. K., et al. (2009). Impact of bilateral anterior cingulotomy on neurocognitive function in patients with intractable pain. *Journal of Clinical Neuroscience, 16*(2), 214–219.

Yen, C. P., Kung, S. S., Su, Y. F., Lin, W. C., Howng, S. L., & Kwan, A. L. (2005). Stereotactic bilateral anterior cingulotomy for intractable pain. *Journal of Clinical Neuroscience, 12*(8), 886–890.

Zeidman, S. M., Rossitch, E. J., & Nashold, B. S., Jr. (1993). Dorsal root entry zone lesions in the treatment of pain related to radiation-induced brachial plexopathy. *Journal of Spinal Disorders, 6*(1), 44–47.

Chapter 32
Rehabilitation Treatments for Chronic Musculoskeletal Pain

Nalini Sehgal, Frank Falco, Akil Benjamin, Jimmy Henry, Youssef Josephson, and Laxmaiah Manchikanti

Introduction

The prevalence of chronic pain in the adult population ranges from 2 to 40%, with a median point prevalence of 15% (Manchikanti et al. 2009; Lihavainen et al. 2010). Amongst chronic pain the prevalence of chronic musculoskeletal pain is high, affecting one in four adults (Walsh et al. 2008). Musculoskeletal pain can arise from a variety of common conditions including osteoarthritis, rheumatoid arthritis, osteoporosis, surgery, low back pain, and bone fracture. It is estimated that among US adults, nearly 27 million have clinical osteoarthritis , 5.0 million have fibromyalgia, 4–10 million have carpal tunnel syndrome, 59 million have had low back pain in the past 3 months, and 30.1 million have had neck pain in the past 3 months (Lawrence et al. 2008). Chronic persistent low back and neck pain is seen in 25–60% of patients, 1-year or longer after the initial episode. A 1-year prevalence study of musculoskeletal pain in the Quebec working population found that for both men and women, back pain was the most frequent musculoskeletal symptom that had disturbed their activities during the past year (Leroux et al. 2005). Low back pain is the most prevalent of musculoskeletal conditions; it affects nearly everyone at some point in time and about 4–33% of the population at any given point (Woolf and Pfleger 2003).

Musculoskeletal conditions often manifest with the onset of pain and the resulting physical limitations and are the most common source of serious long-term pain and physical disability (Woolf and Pfleger 2003). Previous studies have demonstrated that highly repetitive work, heavy pushing or

N. Sehgal, MD (✉)
Department of Orthopedics and Rehabilitation, University of Wisconsin School of Medicine and Public Health, Madison, WI, USA
e-mail: sehgal@rehab.wisc.edu

F. Falco, MD
Temple University Medical School, Philadelphia, PA, USA

Temple University Hospital, Philadelphia, PA, USA

Mid Atlantic Spine and Pain Physicians, Newark, DE, USA

Mid Atlantic Spine and Pain Physicians, Elkton, MD, USA

A. Benjamin, DO • J. Henry, MD • Y. Josephson, DO
Temple University Hospital, Philadelphia, PA, USA

L. Manchikanti, MD
University of Louisville, Louisville, KY, USA

Pain Management Center of Paducah, Paducah, KY, USA

R.J. Moore (ed.), *Handbook of Pain and Palliative Care: Biobehavioral Approaches for the Life Course*, DOI 10.1007/978-1-4419-1651-8_32, © Springer Science+Business Media, LLC 2012

pulling, heavy lifting and prolonged standing, low job satisfaction, and high levels of fear avoidance predict musculoskeletal pain in working adults (Andersen et al. 2007). Factors that lead to worsening of activities of daily living (ADL's) in patients with osteoarthritis include increased pain, reduced range of motion (ROM), and decreased muscle strength at 1-year follow-up, higher morbidity count, and to a lesser extent poor cognitive functioning (Sharma et al. 2003; van Dijk et al. 2010). In decreasing order of importance the most significant predictors of disability in chronic low back pain (CLBP) patients are pain, psychological distress, fear avoidance beliefs, muscle activation levels, lumbar ROM, and gender (Mannion et al. 2001a, b). Musculoskeletal disorders are also associated with some of the poorest quality-of-life issues, particularly in terms of bodily pain and physical functioning, where quality of life is lower than that for gastrointestinal conditions, chronic respiratory diseases, and cardiovascular conditions (Reginster 2002).

Musculoskeletal conditions are a major burden on individuals, health systems, and social care systems, with indirect costs being predominant (Reginster 2002; Woolf and Pfleger 2003). The number of people in Western countries on long-term sick-leave and disability pension due to musculoskeletal complaints and psychological health problems is increasing (Mantyselka et al. 2002). American businesses face huge costs for work-related musculoskeletal pain, and according to a National Academy of Sciences study in 1999, the total cost is more than US dollar 1 trillion/year (USD). Important factors that independently predict work capacity in patients with musculoskeletal disorders include ability to undertake activities, quality of life, and fitness on exercise (Lydell et al. 2005). A large-scale population-based study investigated the association between self-reported physical exercise at baseline and the prevalence of chronic musculoskeletal complaints (CMSC) at follow-up. Individuals who exercised at baseline were less likely to report CMSC 11 years later (OR 0.91, 95% CI 0.85–0.97) than inactive persons. Among individuals who exercised more than 3 times/week, chronic widespread CMSC were 28% less common (OR 0.72, 95% CI 0.59–0.88) compared to inactive individuals (Holth et al. 2008).

Fear of movement or kinesiophobia is significantly associated with increased pain during activity, both general activity and exercise in chronic pain, and even in those with low psychological distress (Damsgard et al. 2010). Kinesiophobia must be taken into consideration when designing and performing rehabilitation programs for patients with musculoskeletal pain (Lundberg et al. 2006; Oyeflaten et al. 2008). Other factors that should be included during treatment planning are physical capacity, emotional distress, and coping skills of the individual with chronic pain. Factors that protect against a poor functional outcome include muscle strength, activity level measured by the amount of aerobic exercise per week, psychosocial factors, mental health, self-efficacy, and social support (Sharma et al. 2003). The identification of these factors provides possible targets for rehabilitative and self-management strategies to prevent disability. Rehabilitation treatments are an essential component of any well-designed pain treatment program and are believed to effectively target several of the factors that contribute to persistent pain, decreased function, and long-term disability. This chapter will briefly describe physical consequences of chronic pain on the individual as a whole and then discuss the role of rehabilitation therapies in chronic musculoskeletal pain.

Adverse Physical Consequences of Chronic Pain

Muscle Disuse and Deconditioning

Disuse is defined as decreased level of activity in physical life (Verbunt et al. 2010; Young 1946). Physical deconditioning implies cardiovascular and neuromuscular consequences of disuse (Young 1946). Bortz (1984) described the multidimensional effects of inactivity or disuse, which included: cardiovascular vulnerability, obesity, musculoskeletal fragility, depression, and premature aging

(Bortz 1984; Young 1946). Deconditioning is thought to be both a cause and consequence of chronic pain. In chronic painful states, muscle disuse is caused by avoidance of painful positions and/or depression (Young 1946; Vlaeyen and Crombez 1999; Vlaeyen and Linton 2000). For instance, avoidance of activity in the acute and subacute phases of back pain leads to muscle disuse and atrophy. Marked atrophy of lumbar multifidus and paraspinous muscles is not uncommon in patients with CLBP. A CT imaging study reported statistically significant atrophy of paraspinous muscles in the lower lumbar levels in backs of CLBP patients without history of surgery as compared to age matched controls (Danneels et al. 2000).

Bone Health

Patients with chronic pain often avoid weight bearing activities. Avoiding weight bearing activity has negative consequences on bone health and increases the likelihood of developing osteoporosis. Examination of active and sedentary populations at single points in time confirms a positive relationship between habitual activity and bone density (Whalen et al. 1988; Gaber et al. 2002). A prospective age matched study demonstrated that inactivity in CLBP patients predisposes them to develop osteopenia and osteoporosis (Gaber et al. 2002). This issue is especially important in women, who are at greater risk of osteoporosis. Prevention strategies for osteoporosis should encourage lifestyle modification and include measures to reduce falls risk and bone loss such as exercise, adequate dietary calcium and avoidance of smoking, and excessive alcohol consumption (McCloskey 2011). Exercise is important for the prevention of osteoporosis and the reduction of fracture risk because it improves muscle mass and strength, besides improving balance (Tolomio et al. 2010). Physical exercise is also known to strongly stimulate the endocrine system in both sexes, induce an increase in circulating androgens (Enea et al. 2011) and achieve optimal peak bone mass (Body et al. 2011). Observational studies have shown that a physically active lifestyle is associated with a 30–50% decrease in vertebral or hip fractures (Kemmler and Stengel 2011). While numerous studies have shown the beneficial effects of various types of exercise on bone mass, fracture data as an endpoint are scanty (Body et al. 2011).

Altered Biomechanics

Patients with chronic pain can also demonstrate fear of movement, termed as "kinesiophobia." They display several biomechanical abnormalities such as abnormal postures, aberrant muscle activation patterns, abnormally weak and tight muscles across joints, decreased muscle endurance and easy fatigability, joint stiffness, joint instability, and decreased ROM. Factors that alter ROM include muscle spasm, tendon contracture, capsular adhesions, and joint fluid (Hoffman 1997). Reduction in segmental stiffness, in conjunction with poor neuromuscular control, and reduction in muscle stiffness leads to clinical instability. Spinal instability resulting from osteoligamentous laxity, muscle dysfunction, or reduced neuromuscular control causes adaptive changes such as alteration in muscle recruitment patterns. These muscles become painful and show increased fatigability, as demonstrated on electromyography studies of erector spinae muscles in the thoracic and lumbar region in patients with CLBP (Sung et al. 2009). Increased activation of the abdominal muscles and altered synergist patterns has been demonstrated in CLBP patients and is hypothesized to represent a possible cause or consequence of continued dysfunction and chronic pain (Cholewicki and McGill 1996; Cholewicki et al. 1997; Silfies et al. 2005; Gardner-Morse and Stokes 1998). An association between muscle deconditioning and chronic spinal pain has been demonstrated in studies by Vlaeyen, and muscle deconditioning is considered to be a major predictor of failed treatments (Vlaeyen and

Crombez 1999; Vlaeyen and Linton 2000). A critical goal of any exercise program should be to restore normal joint mobility, improve flexibility and balance agonist and antagonist muscle activity across joints and thereby improve function.

Cardiovascular Fitness

Chronic pain patients have a lower level of aerobic fitness than healthy controls. Smeet observed a higher incidence of aerobic deconditioning in men compared to women with CLBP (Smeets et al. 2006). When compared with healthy individuals, patients with nonspecific CLBP demonstrate a reduced level of aerobic capacity and an increased body fat percentage (Hodselmans et al. 2010). Patients with chronic pain show increased muscle fatigability with "symptom limited effort" endpoints; an association is seen among the clinical endpoints and the VO_2 value achieved indicating aerobic deconditioning (Duque et al. 2009). Aerobic deconditioning is believed to be a consequence of low back pain (Mayer et al. 1987; Hultman et al. 1993; Zusman 1997). However recent studies, have found no association between pain intensity and aerobic fitness (Wittink et al. 2002). It is suggested that fear avoidance and overall disuse and lack of exercise may be the cause of aerobic deconditioning in CLBP.

Rehabilitation Treatments in Chronic Pain

Treatment principles that underlie rehabilitation-based approach to chronic pain include restoration of physical activity and function, reduction or elimination of factors that perpetuate chronic pain, and fostering a change towards active self management by the patient. General aims of rehabilitation treatments are to increase activity level, improve mobility, apply pain management techniques, improve coping, and return to productive life. The specific goals of the rehabilitation program include increasing the physical abilities (flexibility, strength, and endurance), educating on correct use of body mechanics and back protection techniques, decreasing analgesic use, decreasing dependency on the medical community, improving patients' own positive coping skills and levels of emotional control, increasing the patient's activity level at home and facilitating return to work, where indicated. A variety of physical modalities and therapeutic exercises are employed and combined with behavioral and psychological treatments and other treatments to meet these objectives within the setting of multidisciplinary or interdisciplinary pain programs. Several studies have discussed and evaluated value of these interventions in chronic musculoskeletal pain as discussed in this chapter. There is however a paucity of long-term evaluations on rehabilitation of musculoskeletal disorders.

Rehabilitation treatments are offered in a variety of clinical settings: multidisciplinary pain clinic, multidisciplinary pain center, pain clinic, and modality oriented clinic. Generally speaking, multidisciplinary treatment centers or clinics may or may not include a formal interdisciplinary collaboration model. Although often used interchangeably, they are fundamentally different concepts in nature. The term "multidisciplinary" refers to collaboration with members of different disciplines managed by a leader who directs a range of ancillary services. Team members assess and treat patients independently and then share information. In comparison, the term "interdisciplinary" refers to a deeper level of consensus-based collaboration where the entire process is orchestrated by the team, facilitated by regular face to face meetings, and primarily delivered within a single facility. The team is typically led by a physiatrist (physician trained in physical medicine and rehabilitation) or other pain specialist, and typically includes, a physical therapist, pain psychologist, and nurse educator. In selected cases, occupational therapist, vocational rehabilitation therapist, orthotist, social worker, and case manager join the team (Frymoyer 1988).

Rehabilitation Modalities

A wide range of physical modalities are employed by therapists in treating patients with both acute and chronic pain: thermal, electrotherapeutic, traction, orthoses (Table 32.1). Thermal modalities employ heat or cold energy to affect body part and may use hot or cold packs, water or paraffin baths, infrared bulbs, ultrasound or galvanic current. Depending on the modality used, the mode of energy transfer can be conduction (hot or cold pack), convection (water bath), radiation (infrared lamps), or conversion (ultrasound) of energy. Thermal modalities are commonly used to decrease pain, reduce edema and swelling, improve circulation, increase tissue flexibility, decrease soft tissue stiffness, and muscle spasms. These treatments however have limited application in chronic pain and are often used prior to therapeutic exercises, for example hot packs to facilitate stretching exercises or ROM exercises. Long-term use of thermal modalities should be discouraged because continued use confers no added benefit and may encourage continued dependence on passive therapies. Electro therapeutic modalities involve application of low intensity electrical stimulation to skin surface to stimulate nerve fibers and block transmission of nociceptive impulses, or stimulate muscle fibers to facilitate muscle contraction and strengthening. Traction is a method of mechanically distracting spinal segments in cervical and lumbar region to reduce pain and muscle spasm. Evidence demonstrating efficacy of these therapeutic modalities is sparse (Table 32.2) and hence their use should be limited to patients who have demonstrated evidence of ongoing clinical improvement and progress with rehabilitation treatment program. In some patients, splints, braces, rigid, or semi-rigid orthosis may be indicated to support a weak muscle or unstable joint, decrease pain, limit excessive motion or facilitate motion. Elastic or neoprene sleeves can be used to decrease edema and support affected limb.

Contrast Baths

Immersion in hot and cold water alternatively creates an alternating mechanical force. The procedure involves immersing the affected limb, 3–7 times, alternatively in a hot bath for 2–3 min followed by a cold bath with ice and water for 1–2 min. The methodology is not standardized and protocols may vary by temperature range, timing, and overall duration. Cold water temperatures can vary from 45 to 71.6°F and warm/hot water temperatures range from 80 to 113°F. Contrast baths are used to decrease edema, stiffness and pain in patients with rheumatoid arthritis, diabetes, foot or ankle injuries. Hand therapists may use contrast baths before and after surgery to reduce hand volume, alleviate pain, and decrease stiffness in affected limb. The benefit of contrast bath has been poorly substantiated and a systematic review failed to find evidence to support its use (Breger Stanton et al. 2009). A randomized controlled study demonstrated that contrast bath treatments, pre- and/or postoperatively, in Carpal Tunnel Syndrome patients had no significant effect on increase or decrease of hand volume (Janssen et al. 2009).

Heat Wraps

Heat wraps are disposable cloth like patches that heat up to 104°F within 30 min on exposure to air and last for at least 8 h. Continuous low level heat wrap therapy has been employed in treatment of acute low back pain alone or in combination with exercises in three large randomized control trials (Nadler et al. 2003a, b; Mayer et al. 2005). Heat wrap therapy resulted in greater pain relief, less muscle stiffness, increased flexibility and functional improvement with decreased disability in comparison with placebo, or control interventions. One study reported sustained positive effects of treatment 48 h later. No study has described utility of heat wraps in chronic pain. In patients with chronic pain, this modality may help manage an acute exacerbation of pain or pain flares.

Table 32.1 Rehabilitation modalities

Modality	Effects	Indications	Contraindications	Danger
Ultrasound	Thermal Increases local blood flow, and connective tissue extensibility Decreases pain	Muscle spasm Contusion	Acute phase of injury Pregnancy	Burns Avoid use over open epiphysis, broken skin, major nerves, fractures, cranium, eyes, or malignancy
	Decreases pain	Local inflammation: sprain, strains	DVT Acute infection Metal implants Pacemaker	
Transcutaneous electrical nerve stimulation (TENS)	Non thermal Micro-massage Decreases pain *High frequency*: pain relief is immediate and short term; muscle stimulation *Low frequency*: latent pain relief	Acute injuries Decrease pain and muscle spasm	Not directly over carotid sinus, pace maker	
Interferential stimulation	Pain relief Decrease edema Muscle stimulation	Acute soft tissue injury Swelling/edema Muscle spasm Deep pain (knee, ankle, shoulder)	Avoid direct use over carotid sinus, cardiac pacemaker, pregnancy, DVT, local infection, malignancy	Electrical burns
Cryotherapy	Decrease pain, swelling, edema, bleeding (vasoconstriction)	Muscle spasm, trigger point pain, acute swelling, injury, edema, inflammation	Cold hypersensitivity, Raynauds, disease, circulatory insufficiency, sensory deficits	Ice burns
Superficial heat	Pain relief Increase local blood flow	Pain Muscle spasm	Sensory deficits Circulatory d/o	Increased bleed and swelling if use in first 48 h after injury
Contrast baths	Pain relief Decrease swelling Decrease stiffness	Pain Edema	Sensory deficits Circulatory insufficiency Open skin lesions	

Table 32.2 Randomized clinical trials evaluating rehabilitation modalities

Diagnosis	Study (references)	Modality	Outcomes	Comments
Low back pain	RCT, single blind, N=60 (Schimmel et al. 2009)	Accu-SPINA traction device	Improved visual analog pain scale (VAS), SF-36 scores in active and sham groups; analgesic use decreased; no change in scores for kinesiophobia and coping	No additional benefit of adding axial, intermittent, mechanical traction
Shoulder pain	RCT, placebo control, N=221 (Ainsworth et al. 2007)	Ultrasound	There were no statistically significant differences at the 5% level between active and sham-treated groups	US was not superior to placebo in the short-term management of shoulder pain
Chronic shoulder pain (periarticular soft tissue disorders)	RCT, placebo control, N=40 (Kurtais Gursel et al. 2004)	Ultrasound	No significant differences between active and sham groups	No further benefit of true US as compared with sham US
Subacromial bursitis	RCT, double blind trial, N=20 (Downing and Weinstein 1986)	Ultrasound	No significant difference between the sham or true US groups	US is of little or no benefit when combined with ROM exercises and NSAIDs or ROM exercises
Osteoarthritis bilateral knee	RCT, single blind, N=100 women (Cetin et al. 2008)	Diathermy or TENS or ultrasound compared with exercise (control group)	Decrease in pain and disability in all groups except controls	Hot pack+TENS or short-wave diathermy before exercises reduced pain, improved exercise performance and function
Nonspecific neck pain	RCT multicenter, N=350 (Dziedzic et al. 2005)	Pulsed shortwave therapy	No statistically significant between groups differences	No additional benefits of adding pulsed shortwave or manual therapy to advice and exercise
Acute low back pain	RCT, multicenter, N=219 (Nadler et al. 2003a, b)	Heat wrap	Heat wrap group with greater pain relief, less muscle stiffness and disability, increase in flexibility	Continuous heat-wrap therapy is effective in acute, nonspecific LBP
Acute low back pain	RCT, N=100 (Mayer et al. 2005)	Heat wrap	Greater decrease in pain, disability, and improvement in function in heat+exercise group	Combined heat wrap therapy with directional preference-based exercise effective in acute low back pain
Acute low back pain	RCT, N=76 (Nadler et al. 2003a, b)	Heat wrap	Heat wrap decreased pain, stiffness, disability, and improved trunk flexibility for more than 48 h	Effective pain relief with heat-wrap therapy in acute low back pain
Acute traumatic pain	RCT, double blind, N=100 (Ordog 1987)	TENS	Significant pain relief differences between placebo and active TENS groups	TENS is effective acute traumatic pain

(continued)

Table 32.2 (continued)

Diagnosis	Study (references)	Modality	Outcomes	Comments
Postop pain after inguinal hernia repair	RCT double blind, placebo controlled, N=40 (DeSantana et al. 2008)	TENS	Compared to placebo significantly decreased pain in active TENS group and decreased analgesic requirements	TENS is beneficial for postoperative pain relief after inguinal herniorrhaphy
Postop pain after Laparoscopy for tubal ligation	RCT double blind, N=64 (Desantana et al. 2009)	TENS	Both high- and low-frequency TENS significantly decreased pain as compared with placebo TENS	TENS + standard analgesic treatment was effective in relief of postoperative pain after laparoscopy
Postop pain after C-section	RCT, single blind, N=18 (Smith et al. 1986)	TENS	TENS more effective in controlling cutaneous and movement-associated incisional pain	TENS decreases somatic pain from surgical incision but not deep visceral pain
Sickle cell pain crises	RCT, double blind, N=60 (Wang et al. 1988)	TENS	No difference in pain ratings or Analgesic use at 1 and 4 h from onset	Value of TENS not established
Chronic low back pain	RCT, double blind, N=120 (26 men, 94 women) (Zambito et al. 2006)	Interferential currents (IFT), horizontal therapy (HT)	Significantly improved pain and function at 2 weeks; pain and function continued to improve in IFT and HT groups ($p < 0.01$ vs. controls)	IFT and HT therapy provide significantly more relief of pain and disability in CLBP
Myofascial pain	RCT, single blind, N=10 (Kruger et al. 1998)	TENS	No relief	TENS did not decrease pain
Chronic pain	RCT: single blind, cross-over trial, N=180 (Koke et al. 2004)	TENS: compared three programs	No differences in pain indicating no superiority of one type of TENS	Not placebo controlled, no definite conclusions on effectiveness
Chronic pain	RCT, double blind, N=163 (Oosterhof et al. 2006)	TENS	No differences in pain intensity for patients treated with TENS or sham TENS	TENS not superior to sham treatments
Chronic low back pain	RCT, N=54 (Lehmann et al. 1986)	Electro-acupuncture or TENS	Less average pain in acupuncture group	Electro-acupuncture group had better outcome than TENS
Chronic low back pain	RCT, N=42 (Marchand et al. 1993)	TENS	TENS significantly more efficient in reducing pain intensity but not unpleasantness. Effect of TENS were additive on repetitive use	Significantly reduced pain at 1 week, but not at 3 and 6 months

Condition	Study	Intervention	Results	NMES/TENS treatment
Low back pain	measures comparison, N=24 (16 women and 8 men) (Moore and Shurman 1997)	stimulation (NMES)	tions in pain intensity. Combined treatment superior to placebo, and to both TENS and NMES	
	RCT, single blinded, sham-controlled cross-over study, N=60 (Ghoname et al. 1999a)	Percutaneous electrical nerve stimulation (PENS)	PENS is more effective in decreasing pain, analgesic use, improving physical activity, quality of sleep, well-being	PENS was more effective than TENS or exercise therapy in providing short-term pain relief and improved physical function in patients with long-term LBP
Chronic low back pain	Controlled trial, N=53 (Yokoyama et al. 2004)	PENS	PENS decreased pain, physical impairment and NSAIDs use. Effects were not sustained at 2-month follow-up	PENS is effective for CLBP; require continued treatments to sustain analgesia
Chronic low back pain	RCT, N=200 (65 years and over) (Weiner et al. 2008)	PENS	Significantly reduced pain, self-reported disability, improved gait velocity was sustained at 6 months	Control-PENS facilitated comparably reduced pain and improved function at 6 months as compared with PENS
Chronic low back pain	RCT, N=145 (Deyo et al. 1990)	TENS	At 1 month no clinically or statistically significant treatment effect	TENS is no more effective than placebo, and adds no apparent benefit to exercise alone
Sciatica due to lumbar disc herniation	Randomized, single blinded, cross-over study, N=64 (Ghoname et al. 1999b)	PENS or TENS	PENS (42%) and TENS (23%) were more effective than sham (8%) treatments in decreasing VAS pain scores	PENS was better than TENS in providing short-term pain relief and improved function
Postamputation limb pain	RCT, N=51 (Finsenet al. 1988)	Active low-frequency TENS	Fewer surgeries and more rapid healing in active TENS group	
Spinal cord injury neuropathic pain	Non RCT, N=24 (Norrbrink 2009)	HF (80 Hz) or LF (burst of 2 Hz) TENS	No differences between the two modes of stimulation	TENS may be considered as a complementary treatment in patients with SCI and neuropathic pain
Chronic low-back pain in multiple sclerosis	RCPT, N=90 with probable or definite MS (Warke et al. 2006)	TENS: low-frequency or high-frequency or placebo	No significant differences in both active treatment groups	No statistically significant effects
Vestibulodynia	RCT, N=40 (Murina et al. 2008)	TENS	VAS and SF-MPQ improved in the active TENS group	Effective and safe short-term (3 months) treatment effect
Patellofemoral pain	RCT, N=20 (Eng and Pierrynowski 1993)	Soft foot orthotics	Significantly decreased pain in treatment group	Soft foot orthotics is an effective in treatment of patellofemoral pain syndrome

Ultrasound

Ultrasound (US) is a commonly used modality in the treatment of soft tissue injury and musculoskeletal pain. Therapeutic ultrasound involves application of high frequency acoustic energy to produce thermal and mechanical effects in tissues. Phonophoresis is use of ultrasound energy in combination with an analgesic or anti-inflammatory medication. As yet the clinical effects of this method of treatment are uncertain. The value of ultrasound in chronic pain has also been questioned. A randomized control study of 221 patients with shoulder pain demonstrated that ultrasound was not superior to placebo in short-term management of shoulder pain (Ainsworth et al. 2007). Two other randomized control studies on patients with periarticular soft tissue disorder and subacromial bursitis found no significant differences between sham and true ultrasound groups for improvements in pain, ROM, and function (Downing and Weinstein 1986; Kurtais Gursel et al. 2004).

Electrotherapeutic Modalities

A large number of electrotherapeutic modalities are available for treating pain. Their use varies widely and is based on clinical experience or anecdotal evidence rather than actual scientific evidence. Some of the modalities have an important role to play in treating pain, but should not be used in isolation. These modalities are combined with other therapies to improve outcomes. For example, application of hot packs combined with short wave diathermy, or transcutaneous electrical nerve stimulation (TENS) prior to isokinetic exercises has been shown to augment exercise performance, reduce pain and improve function in patients with osteoarthritis of the knee joints (Cetin et al. 2008).

- *Shortwave diathermy and microwave*: Diathermy and microwave devices use high frequency electromagnetic waves to create heat in superficial muscles. Pulsed short wave diathermy is used in sports injuries, when intermittent short duration pulses are delivered and produce a relatively short duration thermal effect. In nonspecific neck disorders, addition of pulsed short wave or manual therapy to education and exercise does not provide any additional benefits (Dziedzic et al. 2005).
- *Transcutaneous electrical nerve stimulation (TENS)*: TENS involves applying a direct current across the skin to cause electrical stimulation. High frequency current (conventional TENS) stimulates large afferent nerve fibers and provides rapid pain relief but has a short duration. It is perceived as comfortable pins and needles sensation with no motor response. Low frequency TENS (acupuncture like) stimulates larger motor fibers, eliciting a motor response. Pain relief is longer and thought to be mediated by beta-endorphins. It is used to stimulate trigger points or acupuncture points. A randomized cross-over study reported no difference in outcomes with high frequency low intensity TENS, high frequency high intensity TENS, and control TENS (Koke et al. 2004). The utility of TENS in controlling acute and chronic pain has been investigated in several randomized controlled studies. TENS has been shown to relieve acute traumatic pain (Ordog 1987), and postoperative pain (Smith et al. 1986; DeSantana et al. 2008, 2009) especially cutaneous and movement associated incision pain. It is not as effective in controlling deep visceral pain (due to uterine contractions; gas pains associated with decreased peristalsis) (Smith et al. 1986). TENS decreases pain intensity (sensory discriminative component of pain) without decreasing pain unpleasantness (motivational-affective component of pain) (Marchand et al. 1993). In the treatment of chronic pain, the results are not consistent, some trials have demonstrated TENS to be superior to control or placebo treatments (Marchand et al. 1993; Moore and Shurman 1997), while other studies have questioned utility of TENS and demonstrated it to be no more effective than treatment with placebo (Deyo et al. 1990; Kruger et al. 1998; Oosterhof et al. 2006). In one study, only patients satisfied with treatment, noticed gradual decrease in pain intensity with

repeated application; both groups i.e., conventional TENS and sham TENS, reported pain relief equally, suggesting patient satisfaction was an important factor (Oosterhof et al. 2006). The role of TENS in patients with postamputation and phantom limb pain (Finsen et al. 1988), spinal cord injury pain (Norrbrink 2009), pain in multiple sclerosis (Warke et al. 2006), vestibulodynia (Murina et al. 2008), chronic pelvic pain and prostatitis (Sikiru et al. 2008), and sickle cell pain crises (Wang et al. 1988) has not been established . A comparison study of TENS and electroacupuncture showed that average pain relief is better with electroacupuncture than low intensity TENS (Lehmann et al. 1986).

- *Interferential stimulation*: This is a form of TENS in which two alternating medium frequency currents are simultaneously applied to the skin. Interferential therapy stimulates muscle in a manner similar to normal voluntary muscle contraction, its effect on pain is similar to conventional TENS, and effects on circulation vary depending on frequency used. Vasodilatation occurs at 90–100 Hz , while at a frequency of 0–10 Hz muscle stimulation occurs to assist removal of fluid in venous and lymph channels. Interferential currents (IFT) and horizontal therapy (HT) significantly improved pain and function in 120 subjects with CLBP when compared with sham treatments in a randomized double blind study (Zambito et al. 2006).
- *Percutaneous electrical nerve stimulation (PENS)*: Placebo controlled studies have compared PENS to TENS in patients with low back pain, with or without sciatica, and reported overall treatment outcomes to be superior with PENS in controlling pain and improving function; Weiner et al. however reported that pain reduction and improved function at 6 months was comparable in group treated with PENS and control-PENS (Ghoname et al. 1999a, b; Yokoyama et al. 2004; Weiner et al. 2008).

Traction

Traction is used in treatment of spinal pain. It involves intermittent or sustained pressure in a direction to distract vertebral bodies, or facet joints, widen (open) intervertebral foramen, and stretch spinal muscles. Traction may be manual or delivered by a traction apparatus, either with weights or an electric machine. In patients with neck pain, addition of mechanical cervical traction to a multimodal treatment program of manual therapy and exercise did not yield any significant additional benefit with respect to improvements in pain, function, or disability in cervical radiculopathy patients (Young et al. 2009). A randomized single blind study in low back pain patients compared lumbar traction to sham traction and found that low back pain scores, Oswestry disability scores, and SF-36 scores improved significantly in both groups at 14 weeks follow-up. The addition of intermittent mechanical lumbar traction (Accu-SPINA) to a standard graded activity program was of no added benefit (Schimmel et al. 2009).

Bracing

Bracing with splints or orthotics is used to support or reorient moving body parts (joints, tendons), control or guide direction of movement, align a body part into more stable or less painful position, limit or stop excessive motion, and facilitate or correct motion. Semi-rigid cervical collars have been shown to decrease acute neck pain. In a randomized controlled study of 205 patients with acute cervical radiculopathy of <1 month duration, semi-hard cervical collar and rest significantly decreased pain and improved neck disability index; pain relief was comparable to that obtained by physical therapy and home exercises (Kuijper et al. 2009). In another study, significantly greater pain relief was reported by patients with patellofemoral syndrome and excessive forefoot varus or calcaneovalgus deformity, when a soft foot orthotics was added to the exercise program (Eng and Pierrynowski 1993).

Rehabilitation Exercises

Physicians who prescribe exercise therapy must understand the basics of exercise physiology and training principles and recognize that treatment must be tailored to the disease and its stage, the baseline fitness level of the patient, and the goals of the program mutually established with the patient (Kujala 2004, 2006). As a therapeutic modality, exercise has a primary goal of improving functioning of targeted tissues, that is, tissue length, tissue resilience, muscle strength, and endurance. From a cognitive standpoint, successful completion of exercise in the presence of chronic pain lessens patients' fears and concerns, improves self-efficacy and confidence for performing daily activities, thereby decreasing disability. At the cornerstone of any rehabilitation exercise regime is the requirement that function be quantified so that progress towards this goal can be measured. For instance, in the case of chronic back pain baseline measurements of trunk and lower extremity flexibility, trunk strength, lifting capacity and cardiovascular endurance should be recorded at onset of treatment. Quantification initially serves to identify baseline impairments and guide clinicians in the selection of an appropriate level of exercise. Provided that there are no contraindications to aggressive exercise, patients are assigned to an exercise level based on measured impairments. During the initial therapy evaluation, instructions are provided regarding a home stretching program specific for measured impairments in flexibility. Stretching at the physiological limits of flexibility is performed at least twice per day. Following assessment of strength, treatment goals are established according to a patient's age, gender, and ideal body weight (IBW). Patients are carefully instructed on the correct set-up and use of all exercise equipment. The next 1–2 weeks is dedicated towards acquiring proper exercise technique and diminishing fear of physical exertion. The second phase of treatment generally lasts between 2 and 4 weeks, during which rapid progression towards treatment goals is expected. Patients generally meet with their therapist 2–3 times/week with sessions lasting between 1 and 2.5 h. Patients who are highly motivated and experienced with exercise require only one weekly therapy session and exercise independently several more times per week. Exercise sessions involve supervised stretching, aerobic conditioning, general strengthening, specific back strengthening, and lifting. Repeat quantification is performed every 2 weeks to monitor progress, provide feedback, and document treatment outcomes. Patients are encouraged to achieve their pre-established goals by increasing their repetitions and/or weights with each session. Exercise must provide sufficient physiologic overload to produce improvements in physical abilities. In the presence of chronic pain, this intensity of exercise will often stimulate abnormally sensitive nociceptors associated with the chronic pain symptoms and exacerbate pain complaints. These exacerbations are usually tolerable, brief and do not represent tissue damage. As training progresses, tissue function improves and the sensitivity of abnormal nociceptors tends to decrease.

Data from prospective and retrospective studies utilizing aggressive exercise as treatment for patients with CLBP reveal that within a period of 6–8 weeks, it is possible to improve trunk flexibility by 20%, trunk strength and lifting capacities by 50%, and endurance by 20–60%. Pain-related disability as determined by the Oswestry scale reduced by 50%, on average, and pain severity by 30% in one study (Cohen and Rainville 2002). Exercise is important for the prevention of osteoporosis and the reduction of fracture risk because it improves muscle mass and strength, besides improving balance. One study evaluated the effect of a specific exercise program on bone mass and quality and physical function capacity in postmenopausal women with low bone mineral density and found that the group that took part in an 11-month exercise program, consisting of a multicomponent (strength, aerobic capacity, balance, joint mobility) dual-modality (on ground and in the water; alternating group and home-based exercise periods) exercise regimen showed significantly improved femoral neck *T*-score as compared to the control group that did not exercise. After the training program osteosonography showed no differences in exercise group and significantly decreased all bone quality parameters in control group (Tolomio et al. 2010).

Flexibility Exercises

Adequate soft tissue extensibility is essential for pain free movements. Inflammation, swelling, pain, muscle spasm and stiffness inhibit normal muscle function, decrease musculotendinous flexibility, increase joint pressure, and decrease the ability to move the joint. A decrease in joint ROM adversely affects the health of articular cartilage. Prolonged immobilization due to pain also leads to adaptive tightening of joint capsule and pericapsular tissues (ligament, muscles, and tendons). Kinesiophobia, exhibited by chronic pain patients, compounds this problem, culminating in stiffness, contractures, altered biomechanics, and more pain. Improving soft tissue flexibility and thereby function becomes a major treatment goal. Maximizing flexibility or ROM of joints and soft tissues must be instituted as early as possible. Both joint and surrounding soft tissues are gradually mobilized and stretched after surgery or trauma. Joint mobilization regains joint ROM and stretching exercises regain flexibility of musculotendinous unit.

Joint ROM can be improved by various techniques: continuous passive motion (CPM), passive mobilization, active exercises, active assisted exercises, and passive exercises. CPM is usually instituted after surgery or in postinjury stage to reduce joint stiffness. ROM should always be pain free and increased progressively. Passive mobilization is employed when active movement cannot be performed due to pain or when active movements are insufficient to fully mobilize the joint. Mobilization should be gentle in early stages, and can be vigorous in later stages. Active ROM exercises are commenced as soon as possible, within limits of pain, and with goal of increasing ROM progressively without increasing pain. During active assisted exercises, the joint is actively moved through the available ROM with assistance from opposite limb or with the help of a therapist or a pulley system. Passive ROM exercises are indicated, when active exercises are too painful or when end range is restricted. The joint is moved through available ROM with assistance of gravity and using other limb or an outside force.

Loss of musculotendinous flexibility is associated with specific injuries. For instance, Achilles tendinitis is associated with tight soleus muscle; in patellofemoral syndrome, vastus lateralis, iliotibial band and tensor fascia lata muscles lose flexibility; patellar tendinitis is associated with tight quadriceps muscle and hamstring injuries are common in the presence of psoas muscle inflexibility. Stretching of musculotendinous unit increases muscle flexibility, causes muscles to relax, decreases muscle pain, improves circulation, and prevents formation of adhesions. There is lengthening of muscle tendon unit, which then decreases spinal reflex excitability, reducing passive tension, and increasing joint ROM (Guissard and Duchateau 2006). Three different methods of stretching are described: static, ballistic, and proprioceptive neuromuscular facilitation (PNF). Static stretching applies slow controlled tension on the muscle unit that is held for several seconds. Ballistic stretching uses the momentum of repetitive bouncing movements to elicit a rapid stretch, but may put the patient at risk for injury during the early rehabilitative phase and therefore not recommended in early stages. PNF techniques cause reciprocal inhibition of stretched muscles. Active contraction followed by passive stretch results in inhibition of the stretch reflex and facilitates incremental increases in ROM. A 4–8 week program of PNF in patients with CLBP, produces significant gains in dynamic trunk muscle endurance, lumbar flexibility, and functional performance (Kofotolis and Kellis 2006). The inclusion of a shortening contraction of the opposing muscle in order to place the target muscle on stretch, followed by a static contraction of the target muscle, achieves the greatest increase in joint ROM (Sharman et al. 2006). Which stretching technique is superior? A randomized controlled study of 132 subjects with bilateral knee osteoarthritis compared the effects of different stretching techniques on the outcomes of isokinetic muscle strengthening exercises and demonstrated that although stretching therapy increase the effectiveness of isokinetic exercise in terms of functional improvement in patients with knee osteoarthritis, PNF techniques are more effective than static stretching (Weng et al. 2009).

Stretching is more effective if (a) preceded by warm ups (jogging, cycling, swimming) or topical heat, these activities increase tissue temperatures and facilitate stretching; (b) performed in correct position for the particular muscle; (c) stretches are slow and sustained for minimum 15 s; (d) patient is able to feel the stretch in appropriate area (Oakley et al. 2005); (e) antigravity reflexes are eliminated to relax the muscle e.g., lumbar stretch in sitting or lying down position are pain free. Routine flexibility exercises should be performed in a controlled, deliberate manner in order to minimize injury and maximize results. In a study of healthy volunteers, two 30-s bouts of constant-torque passive stretching caused a significant decrease in musculotendinous stiffness of the plantar flexor muscles and remained depressed following the third and fourth stretches, but did not decrease any further (Ryan et al. 2009). Stretching daily for 1 min over a period of 3 weeks can increase tolerance to the discomfort associated with stretch in patients with chronic musculoskeletal pain (Law et al. 2009). Intermittent stretching (i.e., 2 or 3 days/week) is sufficient to maintain ROM gains acquired from a prior static stretching program (Rancour et al. 2009). Stretching is based on overload principle i.e., it is a function of intensity, duration, frequency, and type of stretch. There is a risk of overstretching and subsequent injury, depending on the intensity, duration, velocity, and number of movements in a given period. Stretching is contraindicated in individuals with hypermobility syndromes or in the presence of instability.

Muscle Conditioning Exercises

There are four components of muscle conditioning: (1) muscle strength; (2) muscle power; (3) muscle endurance; and (4) motor reeducation. Each of these components is necessary for ADL's and essential to protect the body and preventing injury. These components are adversely affected by injury, pain and disuse and therefore need to be assessed and rehabilitated accordingly.

Strength training: Muscle strength is the ability of muscle to exert force. Increases in muscle strength and muscle hypertrophy are stimulated by conditioning. An initial improvement in strength in response to exercise is related to neuromuscular facilitation, and strength gains occur before hypertrophy. Three main types of exercises are used in muscle conditioning: isometric, isotonic, and isokinetic (Table 32.3). Isometric exercises are instituted after injury or surgery. A typical protocol consists of isometric contractions held for 5–6 s with a rest of 10–20 s, and performed frequently during the day, in sets of 10–20 repetitions. Isometric exercises should be carried out at varying angles, because strength gain is fairly specific to angle of exercise. Patients progress from submaximal to maximal isometric exercises slowly within limitations of pain. Once multiple isometrics are tolerated at multiple joint angles the patient is advanced to dynamic exercises. Training in dynamic exercise begins with concentric exercises and progresses to eccentric exercises (EE). EE should commence at very low levels and gradually progress to higher intensity and volume. If used inappropriately they can result in delayed onset muscle soreness and cause muscle damage. EE have proved successful in the management of chronic tendinopathy, particularly of the Achilles and patellar tendons, where they have been shown to be effective in controlled trials. However, numerous questions regarding EE remain. The standard protocols are time-consuming and require very motivated patients. EE are effective in some tendinopathies but not others. Furthermore, the location of the lesion can have a profound effect on efficacy; for example, standard EE in insertional lesions of the Achilles are ineffective (Rees et al. 2009). Standardized eccentric loading training combined with repetitive low-energy shock-wave treatment (SWT) in patients suffering from chronic midportion Achilles tendinopathy showed that at 4-month follow-up, eccentric loading alone was less effective when compared with a combination of eccentric loading and repetitive low-energy SWT (Rompe et al. 2009). Isokinetic exercises have substantially superior measurability and reliability, but require sophisticated and expensive training equipment and therefore cannot be performed at home. It is ultimately desirable to develop exercise programs that can be continued by the patient outside the

Table 32.3 Muscle conditioning exercises

Type of exercise	Definition	Indication	Benefits
Isometric	Static exercise; muscle contracts without moving the joint on which the muscle acts	After injury or joint surgery Inflammatory joint d/o Muscle is too weak for ROM exercise	Prevent muscle atrophy Decrease swelling by pumping action of muscle
Isotonic	Muscle contracts against a constant resistance or weight and moves the joint through its ROM Two types: a. Concentric: shortening muscle contraction results in decrease in muscle length from approximation of its origin and insertion; individual muscle fibers shorten b. Eccentric: lengthening muscle contraction, origin and insertion separate and individual muscle fiber lengthens	High resistance and low repetition exercises increase muscle fiber size and density; best in later stages of rehabilitation Eccentric exercises indicated in management of tendinopathy and preventing recurrence of musculotendinous injuries	Eccentric exercises produce greater intramuscular force per unit motor unit
Isokinetic	Muscle contracts at fixed speed and variable resistance, that accommodates to individual throughout the ROM	Specialized equipment such as Kin Com or Cybex Used primarily to assess progress of rehabilitation, determine muscle weakness or imbalance Exercises are not functional and therefore not of much use in chronic pain setting	Superior measurability and reliability

clinical setting. In addition to specific resistance training all round physical exercise must be included in the treatment protocol. A single blind randomized controlled study measured effects of specific neck/shoulder resistance training, all-round physical exercise, and a reference intervention on musculoskeletal pain symptoms in 549 office workers. Both specific resistance training and all-round physical exercise for office workers caused better effects than a reference intervention in relieving musculoskeletal pain symptoms in exposed regions of the upper body (Andersen et al. 2010).

Power training: Power is the muscle's rate of doing work and is equivalent to explosive strength. When deficits of muscle power occur as a result of injury, especially in athletes, power training is emphasized in later stages of rehabilitation in the form of fast speed isotonic or isokinetic exercises, increased speed of functional exercises and plyometrics. These exercises must be specific to a given sport activity or job activity.

Endurance training: Muscle endurance is the muscle's ability to sustain contraction or perform repeated contractions. Endurance training is pivotal in counteracting the deconditioning associated with chronic pain. Chronic pain patients demonstrate easy fatigability and the maximal voluntary contraction and endurance time during submaximal contractions is reduced in musculoskeletal pain (Graven-Nielsen and Arendt-Nielsen 2008). As activity is encouraged and activity tolerance improves, oftentimes pain decreases. Endurance conditioning should be included in conjunction with strengthening program. Endurance exercises are low load, high repetition exercises that stress the aerobic pathways, improve the oxidative enzyme capacity of slow twitch muscle fibers and increase the density of mitochondria in the muscle fibers. The amount of resistance is gradually increased to allow for cellular adaptation to occur and to facilitate strength gains. Exercises that increase endurance include riding a stationary bike, swimming, specific low load, high repetition isotonic or isokinetic exercise or circuit training. The muscular endurance response to training occurs only in specific muscles used in the exercise, and there is no cross-over effect. Exercise intensity should be determined by the fitness level and functional ability of the patient. High intensity exercise can be continued for only short durations, whereas low intensity exercise can be sustained for relatively longer periods of time. A shortened rest interval between exercises improves endurance and aerobic capacity. An exercise program should progress gradually from a strictly low intensity regimen to incorporating more challenging high intensity exercise, as endurance allows, in order to avoid overuse injury.

Motor re-education: Fatigue and failure of specific muscle groups also contribute to musculoskeletal pain. In patients with chronic pain, dynamic exercises reveal muscular dyssynergy and incoordination, which are maladaptive responses to pain. A typical maladaptive response is characterized by inhibition of agonist muscles and increase in activity of antagonist muscles acting on a joint, which in turn reduces joint force and velocity (Lund et al. 1991). For example, in chronic shoulder impingement, the scapular stabilizers are weak and the timing and order of muscle recruitment is altered and unsynchronized. The scapula protracts and elevates excessively, reducing the leverage of the long muscles attached to the scapula, decreasing the size of the sub-acromial space and further increasing impingement of the rotator cuff tendons. Similarly, patients with nonspecific low back pain demonstrate differences in trunk muscle activation timing as compared to asymptomatic controls during a self-initiated postural challenge. There is significantly delayed trunk muscle onset latency, shorter bursts, and co-contraction durations suggesting that these patients may be inefficient in regulating trunk posture during voluntary extremity movements or have developed a compensatory control pattern to avoid pain (Mehta et al. 2010). Evidence of atrophy of deep trunk muscles in the form of decreased muscle fiber diameter and increased intramuscular fat is seen on MRI images of lumbar spine in patients with CLBP. Motor reeducation and motor control exercise is designed to improve motor function, coordination, and movement of specific muscle groups, which may potentially aid in recovery and prevention of injury. Motor control exercise, alone or as a supplement to another therapy, is superior to minimal intervention or manual therapy in reducing pain and disability (Macedo et al. 2009). It confers benefit when added to other therapies for pain at all time points and for disability at long-term follow-up. For example, combining neuromuscular electrical stimulation and voluntary muscular contractions is more effective than either therapy alone in inducing corrective muscular adaptations during recovery, improving the performance of complex dynamic movements, and accelerating recovery of muscle contractility during rehabilitation (Paillard 2008). Some studies have also shown that motor control exercise is not more effective than manual therapy or other forms of exercise (Macedo et al. 2009). In patients with CLBP, motor reeducation retrains the paraspinous muscles to regain the optimal control and coordination of the spine. Compared to placebo or general exercise, motor control exercise produces short-term improvements in patient's global impression of recovery and activity for people with CLBP (Ferreira et al. 2007; Costa et al. 2009).

Proprioceptive Training

Proprioception or position sense provides valuable information on the body's coordinates in space. Afferent input is conducted from several structures acting in concert, including muscles, joint capsules, ligaments, and skin. Inability to obtain or perceive this information may predispose one to undue injury, either directly through inadvertent joint destruction or indirectly through increased risk of falls. Chronic musculoskeletal pain and a decline in proprioception are associated with an increased occurrence of falls in the elderly, especially if multiple painful sites are identified (Leveille et al. 2009). In patients with stroke, poststroke shoulder pain is related to altered proprioception and kinematics in the affected limb, and the risk of shoulder pain is increased if there is preexisting dysfunction as demonstrated by examining the unaffected limb (Niessen et al. 2009). Decreased joint proprioception also contributes to the progressive joint deterioration observed in patients with osteoarthritis, rheumatoid arthritis, and Charcot's disease (Hoffman 1997). However proprioceptive dysfunction may not necessarily correlate with the presence of radiographic osteoarthritis (Felson et al. 2009).

Measures of postural sway, passive joint position sense testing, or active joint repositioning following passive displacement may provide some objective evidence of proprioceptive functioning (Hoffman 1997). Early and comprehensive proprioceptive training improves proprioception and reduces rate of recurrence of injuries. Proprioceptive exercises act to restore kinesthetic awareness, not stressful to healing tissues and enhance general coordination as well as facilitate effectiveness of strength and endurance exercises. Simple proprioceptive exercises such as on one leg stands are introduced and more complex tasks added as simple tasks are mastered. Later on dynamic training using uni- or multi-directional tilt boards, wobble boards, or balance trainers is introduced to improve proprioceptive feedback. In a clinical trial of patients with osteoarthritis, proprioceptive training was found to be as effective as strength training in improving knee pain scores following an 8 week rehabilitation program (Shakoor et al. 2008; Lin et al. 2009).

Functional Exercises

Once a reasonable level of strength, power, endurance, flexibility, and proprioception has been achieved, functional exercises are gradually introduced. While traditional strength training will improve isolated weaknesses, the addition of functional exercises will aid to address functional weaknesses that may not be readily apparent. Functional training programs should be tailored to the specific functional needs of the patient, and based on the occupational requirements and ADL's. These activities prepare to cope with the demands of the job. Functional exercises simultaneously employ multiple muscles and joints to improve muscular endurance, overall strength, coordination, balance, posture, and agility. They require neural communication between muscles and promote coordinated use of multiple-joint movements (Hoffman 1997). These exercises dynamically integrate several basic functional movement patterns such as squatting, lunging, bending, lifting, pushing, pulling, and twisting in order to train muscle groups together rather than in isolation. There is emphasis on replication of movements associated with practical daily activities which cannot be achieved with a standard exercise machine. Movements are incorporated in combination with cables, dumbbells, medicine balls, and physioballs in a functional and integrative way that is especially challenging to the core musculature of the patient. In addition to the increased efficiency of simultaneously activating multiple muscle groups, functional exercises are easily transferable from the outpatient to the home setting.

Cardiovascular Fitness Exercises

A normal physiologic response to exercise is increased heart rate, initially due to decreased parasympathetic activity followed by an increase in sympathetic tone, which also augments cardiac contractility and redistributes circulation to metabolically active tissues. An increase in preload translates to increased stroke volume. Combined with the aforementioned increase in heart rate, cardiac output rises significantly with maximal output. It is therefore essential that, the exercise prescription is tailored to the functional level of the patient, especially those with concomitant cardiovascular disease. Usually, it is advisable to obtain baseline measurements of cardiovascular fitness in the at-risk patient. Aerobic capacity, expressed as milliliters of oxygen per kilogram of body weight per minute (mL O_2/kg/min) or as metabolic equivalents (METs; 1 MET 3.5 mL O_2/kg/min) is best assessed by VO_{2max} (Franklin 2009). VO_{2max} is defined as the product of maximal cardiac output and maximal arteriovenous oxygen difference. A submaximal step test is used to measure the VO_2 using a portable breath by breath metabolic system and a telemetric heart rate monitor. VO_{2max} can be estimated by : (1) a direct measurement of VO_2, (2) estimation by heart rate, and (3) a step test method using predetermined charts (Uth et al. 2004; Balderrama et al. 2010). VO_{2max} can be used to monitor changes in endurance and cardiovascular fitness (Hoffman 1997). The intensity, duration, and frequency of exercise should progress in a gradual stepwise fashion. The recommended exercise intensity range is 55–90% of maximal heart rate, depending on fitness level (Hoffman 1996, 1997). Beginners may train as little as 3 times a week for 20 min and see results, whereas the more advanced may train up to 5 times a week and for significantly longer duration. Care must be taken not to ramp activity too quickly as this may precipitate noncompliance or injury. Ideally, cardiovascular fitness should be combined with strength and endurance training to achieve optimal results, namely functional recovery and pain relief.

Correcting Abnormal Biomechanics

An understanding of the kinetic chain helps the clinician to interpret the patient's deficits and to develop a treatment regimen. The kinetic chain concept is based on the fundamental premise that for functional movement in space, each link of the body must move in a coordinated manner. The sequence of the links and the inter-relationship of muscle activation and of translation of forces within the body are referred to as the kinetic chain (Kibler 1990; Kibler et al. 1992, 2006). Each link of this system creates force and energy that are ultimately transferred from the proximal core stabilizing link to the distal peripheral link. When one link is weak or injured, other links compensate. Distal links typically compensate for proximal links, and the added stress and loads result in further injury. For instance, if a patient has weak hip abductors, the knee often has to absorb more of the forces during gait. If the patient also has a tendency to over pronate (flat-foot position), then the forces in the knee are increased. Malalignment of the foot may lead to changes at the knee such as excessive patellofemoral joint pressures and abnormal patellar tracking. Patellar tracking is described as dynamic movement of the kneecap, with its insertion to the tibia and muscle attachment to the quadriceps during extension and flexion of the knee. Hence, proper rehabilitation of patellofemoral joint pain will need to address factors along the kinetic chain that is, proximal to the knee (strengthening of the quadriceps, gluteus muscle groups, and hip external rotators) and distally (correcting pronation at the foot).

In the area of spine rehabilitation, it is understood that spinal function is directly related to spinal structure, as has been proven for the cervical and lumbar spinal regions. With mal-alignment in neutral posture, static and especially dynamic function from this mal-alignment dictates altered stress/strain relationships of associated spinal structures, including the bones, intervertebral discs, facet joints, musculotendinous tissues, ligamentous tissues, and neural elements. Postural alterations are known to be associated with problems in specific joints such as the hip and the knee, and to problems with specific spinal regions such as the flat-back syndrome and cervical kyphosis. A typical kinetic chain biomechanical evaluation looks at leg lengths, pelvic alignment, hip and knee ROM and stability, ankle ROM and stability as well as how the body moves while walking and running. When abnormal motions are noted specific recommendations can be made to correct the abnormal biomechanics. Assessment is also made of the musculature of the body because biomechanical abnormalities often produce muscular imbalances and significant improvements in biomechanics can be made from strengthening and or stretching certain muscle groups.

Work Hardening

Work hardening programs aim to improve the work status for workers on sick-leave. According to the Department of Labor and Industries, work hardening is defined as an interdisciplinary, individualized, job specific program of activity with the goal of return to work (see also http://www.lni.wa.gov/ClaimsIns/Files/ReturnToWork/WhStds). Work hardening provides a transition between acute care and successful return to work and is designed to improve the biomechanical, neuromuscular, cardiovascular, and psychosocial functioning of the worker. Programs are also designed to treat the entire spectrum of disability preventing a return to work. This contrasts with traditional rehabilitation programs, which focus on anatomic impairment. Functional capacity evaluations of strength, endurance, coordination, pace, and safety are included. The program should incorporate a customized obstacle course that includes lifting, carrying, twisting, crawling, bending, stooping, and other movements peculiar to a job. Normal performance levels are established by the therapist. The patient is observed and timed moving through the course, and deviations from the norm are quantified so that they can be identified. Work hardening programs use real or simulated work tasks and progressively graded conditioning exercises that are based on the individual's measured tolerances. Because the program is goal oriented and job specific, the program must be intensive, operating 5 days/week for 4–8 h daily. Work hardening is costly, with programs costing between $5,000 and $15,000, per patient and is more appropriate when physical deconditioning and behavioral changes are preventing job return. This is typically about 4 months after an injury. When a patient is referred, the diagnosis must be firmly established and no further treatment, such as surgical procedure, is anticipated. The programs usually last about 3 weeks. About 10–15% of participants dropout due to lack of motivation. Encouragement and support from the referring physician and the insurance company are important. Specific goals should be set, and progress measured objectively. The physician and clinical team must clearly convey and patient must clearly understand that this is the most appropriate treatment and possibly the last chance for a return to gainful employment (Mooney and Hughson 1992).

The effectiveness of work conditioning programs in reducing sick-leave when compared to usual care or other exercises in workers with back pain still remains uncertain. A Cochrane Review of 23 randomized control trials compared effectiveness of physical conditioning programs in reducing time lost from work for 3,676 workers with back pain. Physical conditioning programs were compared to usual care in 14 studies. In workers with acute back pain, there was no effect on sickness absence; results were conflicting in subacute back pain, but a subgroup analysis showed a positive effect of interventions with workplace involvement. In workers with chronic back pain, pooled results of five studies showed a small effect on sickness absence at long-term follow-up (SMD: −0.18 (95% CI: −0.37 to 0.00). Six studies compared physical conditioning programs to other exercise therapy in workers with chronic back pain and reported conflicting results. The addition of cognitive behavioral therapy to physical conditioning programs was not more effective than the physical conditioning alone. A better understanding of the mechanism behind physical conditioning programs and return-to-work is required to develop more effective interventions (Schaafsma et al. 2010).

Functional Restoration Programs

Functional restoration programs (FRP) have been developed to promote the socio-professional reintegration of patients with significant work absenteeism. One study determined the long-term effectiveness of FRP in a group of 105 chronic low-back pain patients with over 1 month of work absenteeism. Fifty-five percent of the patients returned to work after mean follow-up time of 3.5 years, compared with 9% of the patients at work at baseline. Quality of life, functional disability, psychological factors, and fear and avoidance beliefs were all significantly improved. Three predictive factors were found: younger age at the onset of low-back pain, practice of sports, and shorter duration of sick-leave at baseline. FRP show positive results in terms of return to work for CLBP patients with prolonged work absenteeism (Mayer et al. 1987, 1994; Gatchel and Mayer 2008; Poulain et al. 2010).

Exercise Programs for Chronic Low Back Pain

McKenzie Method: The McKenzie method for CLBP has two components: an initial assessment of lumbar movements followed by an intervention based on the results of the assessment. The objective of assessment is to identify a direction of movement that centralizes pain. The term "centralization" refers to a pattern of pain response whereby a single direction of repeated movements or sustained postures produces sequential and lasting abolition of all distal referred symptoms and subsequent abolition of any remaining spinal pain. The assessment may uncover a "directional preference," which refers to a particular direction of lumbosacral movement or sustained posture that cause symptoms to centralize, decrease, or even abolish while the individual's limited range of spinal movement simultaneously returns to normal. The overall objective of the McKenzie method is patient self-management that includes three important phases: (1) demonstrating and educating patients about the beneficial effects of positions and end-range movements on their symptoms, and the aggravating effects of the opposite movements and postures; (2) educating patients in how to maintain the reduction and abolition of their symptoms; and (3) educating patients in how to restore full function to the lumbar spine without symptom recurrence (May and Donelson 2008).There is limited evidence for the use of McKenzie method in CLBP (Machado et al. 2006). However one study did conclude that McKenzie treatment and strengthening training were equally effective in the treatment of patients with CLBP at the 14-month follow-up (Petersen et al. 2007).

Core Stabilization: The core is the center of the functional kinetic chain, and seen as a muscular corset that works as a unit to stabilize the body, in particular the spine, both with and without limb movement. Kibler et al. stressed the importance of the core in providing local strength and balance, in decreasing back injury and in maximizing force control (Kibler et al. 2006). The core of the body includes both passive and active structures: the passive structures are the osseoligamentous components of the thoracolumbar spine and pelvis and the active structures are the muscles of the trunk. If any of the active or passive components are impaired in function, instability of the spine may occur. It has been shown that the musculature is most important in maintaining spinal stability under various conditions. In addition, to muscle strength, muscular endurance and, in particular, sensory-motor control is important in providing sufficient core stability (Anderson and Behm 2005). One of the greatest challenges in training the core is the integration of specific training regimens into functional activities. Isolation of specific muscles or joints should be avoided in core stabilization exercises and the emphasis should be on the training of muscle activation sequences in functional positions and motions. In this way, normal biomechanical motions are restored through normal physiological activations. The eventual goal is to make the required muscle recruitment automatic and to achieve an adequate coordination of activation of the segments that are part of the kinetic chain (Kibler et al. 2006). Core Stability training occurs in four phases – (1) alignment, (2) lower quarter dynamic stability, (3) upper core dynamic stability, (4) posterior core stability-trunk extensors. Exercises that target agonist–antagonist muscle coactivation are ideal for injury prevention and rehabilitation. These exercises promote the kinesthetic awareness necessary to maintain a safe "neutral" spine. Stabilization exercises can be progressed from a beginner level to more advanced levels. The most accepted program includes components from the Saal and Saal seminal dynamic lumbar stabilization efficacy study (Saal 1990, 1992). Dynamic muscular stabilization techniques as well as conventional treatments are more effective in males than females with LBP (Kumar et al. 2010). A favorable long-term outcome at 1-year follow-up was observed after functional multidisciplinary rehabilitation in a randomized controlled trial with 1-year follow-up on patients with CLBP randomized to an exercise program or routine follow-up (Henchoz et al. 2010). A very popular mode of training in recent years has been the use of instability devices and exercises to train the core musculature. Instability training is viewed by many as the most effective way to train the core; however, evidence suggests instability training can increase core muscle activation, but it may not be the best choice in all situations (Behm et al. 2010). More research is needed to establish the effectiveness of instability training in preventing injury, enhancing sport performance, or for use in various clinical situations outside of rehabilitation for low back pain (Fowles 2010).

Hydrotherapy

Several properties of water make hydrotherapy an attractive treatment modality: (1) immersion in water exerts an upward force on the body (buoyancy), which decreases ground reaction forces by half, and reduces stress on painful joints; (2) hydrostatic pressure of water exerts an external compressive force and aids with resolution of edema in injured body part; (3) improved circulation and oxygen delivery increases tissue perfusion and healing; (4) immersion to chest level increases endurance, cardiac output, and cardiovascular conditioning; (5) viscosity of water (internal friction) provides resistance to motion, and allows for gentle resistance to exercise that is self-mediated and can be tailored to the fitness level of the patient (Becker 2009). Hydrotherapy is commonly employed in rehabilitation of rheumatologic disorders. The degenerative cascade of inflammation in osteoarthritis and inflammatory arthropathy leads to decreased strength, joint mobility, and functional capacity. Aquatic physical therapy significantly reduces pain and improves physical function, strength and quality of life in patients with symptomatic osteoarthritis of hip and knee (Hinman et al. 2007) and is shown to be superior to land based exercises (Silva et al. 2008). Patients are transitioned later to a surface program, once they are able to handle gravitational loads and are prepared to progress towards functional goals. In a meta-analysis of 19 randomized controlled trials in adults with neurological or musculoskeletal disease, aquatic exercise achieved comparable pain-relieving effects to land-based exercise, while attaining only a modest post-treatment effect in relieving pain compared with no treatment (Hall et al. 2008). A systematic review of controlled trials revealed that therapeutic aquatic exercise is potentially beneficial in CLBP and pregnancy-related low back pain, however, they are no better than other interventions. Evidence synthesis is limited due to the low methodological quality of available studies; high-quality trials are needed to substantiate the use of therapeutic aquatic exercise in a clinical setting (Waller et al. 2009). A structured therapeutic exercise program in an aquatic environment also improves aerobic and functional capacity (Bunning and Materson 1991; Hampson et al. 1993). There is evidence that aquatic exercises and deep water running improve physical function, body pain, and general health perception in patients with fibromyalgia; however, few of these gains are maintained on follow up at 3–6 months (Tomas-Carus et al. 2007; Assis et al. 2006; Gusi et al. 2006). Hydrotherapy is proven to be at least as beneficial as land-based programs and should be strongly considered, especially in the chronic pain patient unable to tolerate land-based activity. However, the effectiveness of hydrotherapy in curing disease or improving health remains unclear (Kamioka et al. 2010).

Cost-Effectiveness of Rehabilitation Treatments

Exercise interventions are cost-effective in musculoskeletal disorders (54% cases), cardiac disorders (60% cases), and in patients with rheumatic diseases (75% cases). The evidence is most convincing for rehabilitation of cardiac and back pain patients (Roine et al. 2009). There is however no consensus on what is an optimum exercise regimen. Both manual therapy and exercises are associated with significant improvement but exercise therapy is reported to be 40% more cost effective than individual manual therapy (Lewis et al. 2005). A randomized controlled trial compared physician consultation alone with combined manipulation, stabilization exercises, and physician consultation in CLBP patients and found that physician consultation alone is more cost-effective for both health care use and work absenteeism, and led to equal improvement in disability and health-related quality of life. Patients in combined treatment group reported a slightly more significant reduction in visual analog pain scale (VAS) ($p = 0.01$, analysis of variance) but clearly higher patient satisfaction ($p = 0.001$, Pearson chi2) at 2 years. Incremental analysis showed that the cost of a one-point change in VAS was \$512 for the combined group (Niemisto et al. 2005). Cost effectiveness studies have also indicated that multidisciplinary rehabilitation is relatively costly and unless it achieves return to work in people in the working-age group, or averts the need for residential care in frail older people, it is not likely to be cost effective (Cameron 2004). A study from Sweden estimated the net economic gain of an 8-week multidisciplinary rehabilitation for patients with persistent pain by comparing reduction in production losses due to sick-leave with the actual cost of the program. The estimated benefit of the program was €3,799–€7,515 per treated patient and year, and the total cost of the program was €5,406 per patient. Based on these figures the total cost of the program, including costs for patients remaining on sick-leave, had been recovered when the successfully rehabilitated patients had worked for 9–17 months. Any additional work after that yielded net economic benefits (Norrefalk et al. 2008). A light multidisciplinary treatment model was found to be a cost-effective treatment for men with CLBP. Productivity gains from light multidisciplinary treatment vs. "treatment as usual" in male patients with low back pain during the first 2 years were estimated to accumulate to U.S. \$852.000 (Skouen et al. 2002). In the case of women working in blue-collar or service/care occupations and suffering from back/neck pain, a full-time behavioral medicine program is a cost-effective method for improving health and increasing return to work (Jensen et al. 2005). A rehabilitation program consisting of physiotherapy + cognitive behavioral therapy reduced sick-leave by about two-thirds of a working year compared to "treatment-as-usual" control group and had a substantial impact on costs for production losses (Jensen et al. 2005). Taylor et al. showed that rehabilitation program had a significant impact in getting compensation claimants back to work. At a median of 5 months vocational success was achieved in 75%, and of those in work, 48% went back to the same job, 7% went back to the same job but with a different employer and 15% went to a different job that used the same skills. Only a minority required substantive retraining and early intervention was associated with a better outcome (Taylor et al. 2001). There is evidence that patient education with exercise is effective in osteoarthritis and CLBP, including occupational low back pain. Exercise, supported by advice and education should therefore be at the core of self-management strategies for CLBP and osteoarthritis (Niemisto et al. 2005; May 2010). Sjostrom et al. reported that multidisciplinary rehabilitation consisting of physical activity, relaxation, education and individual guidance decreased full-time sick-leave by 37% ($p < 0.0001$) in women, and by 25% ($p < 0.05$) in men with neck and back pain. At 2 years follow-up majority of the participants were still physically active, their QOL was increased, and most participants had returned to work (Sjostrom et al. 2008). There was no improvement reported in the group with more severe pain and greater physical disability at end of 2 year (Sjostrom et al. 2009).

Conclusions

The primary goal of rehabilitation-based treatments for chronic musculoskeletal pain is to maximize and maintain physical activity and function and reduce pain intensity and pain perception by employing therapeutic exercises as one component of a multimodal treatment program. Rehabilitation treatments in combination with behavioral interventions seek to reduce analgesic use, decrease need for invasive procedures and surgeries, discourage maladaptive pain behaviors, and dependence on passive modalities. Patient education is an essential element of rehabilitation treatments and patients learn to actively self-manage pain. The ultimate objective of treatment is to return the patient to previous levels of activity at home, in the workplace and in leisure pursuits and to obtain resolution and/or closure of contentious work related or litigation aspects of the pain condition. Outcome studies that demonstrate rehabilitation treatments actually achieve these objectives are lacking. Most studies have shown that exercise decreases pain and improves activity in the short-term. However, there are no high-quality long-term studies and no study has investigated if rehabilitation treatments actually reduce analgesic consumption, or decrease need for invasive pain procedures or surgical procedures. Large-scale, longitudinal studies are needed to determine long-term efficacy of rehabilitation treatments and to compare outcomes with other treatments.

In the future, research may show whether muscle conditioning exercises and core stabilization exercises prevent or reverse atrophy of deep trunk muscles, increase muscle fiber diameter and/or decrease intramuscular fat seen on MRI images of lumbar spine in patients with CLBP. Gender studies may disclose why dynamic muscular stabilization techniques as well as conventional treatments are more effective in males than females with LBP and possibly guide development of an optimal exercise program for women. A better understanding of the mechanism behind physical conditioning programs and return-to-work is also required to develop more effective interventions for long-term effectiveness of FRPs. More research is needed to establish the effectiveness of instability training in preventing injury, enhancing performance, or for use in various clinical situations outside of rehabilitation for low back pain (Fowles 2010). High-quality trials are needed to substantiate the use of therapeutic aquatic exercise in a clinical setting (Waller et al. 2009). There is evidence that patient education and advice combined with exercise is effective in management of osteoarthritis and CLBP, however it is not known if the same is true for other pain disorders, for instance in patients with whiplash injures and chronic neck pain.

Rehabilitation treatments for chronic pain are practiced in many different models ranging from biomedical to bio-psychosocial assessment and treatments. The traditional biomedical model is criticized for placing too much focus on the identification and treatment of a specific anatomic pain generator and failing to address/or account for the psychosocial aspects of the chronic pain paradigm. Proponents of the bio-psychosocial model believe that a functional cognitive behaviorally mediated therapeutic approach is necessary to maximize outcomes, help foster patient optimism, decrease fear of reinjury and maximize patient compliance. No study has conclusively demonstrated superiority of one approach over the other and there is no evidence that the two approaches are mutually exclusive and cannot be applied in the same patient. The premise of multimodal pain treatment is that there is no single stand-alone treatment that can adequately control pain and normalize function and activity in patients with persistent pain. Optimal pain management mandates a multimodality treatment approach that combines analgesic pharmacotherapy with rehabilitation and behavioral approaches, and judicious application of interventional pain procedures and surgical treatments in an appropriate clinical situation to improve outcomes. An individualized rehabilitation program must be developed based on the specific pain condition, the baseline fitness level of the patient, and the goals of the program mutually established with the patient. Exercise must provide sufficient physiologic overload to produce improvements in physical abilities. Treatment outcomes, must be quantified, so that they are amenable to analysis using statistical databases. By tracking treatment outcomes, information can be derived to modify treatment regimens, with the goal of improving patient care

References

Ainsworth, R., Dziedzic, K., et al. (2007). A prospective double blind placebo-controlled randomized trial of ultrasound in the physiotherapy treatment of shoulder pain. *Rheumatology (Oxford, England), 46*(5), 815–820.

Andersen, L. L., Christensen, K. B., et al. (2010). Effect of physical exercise interventions on musculoskeletal pain in all body regions among office workers: A one-year randomized controlled trial. *Manual Therapy, 15*(1), 100–104.

Andersen, J. H., Haahr, J. P., et al. (2007). Risk factors for more severe regional musculoskeletal symptoms: A two-year prospective study of a general working population. *Arthritis and Rheumatism, 56*(4), 1355–1364.

Anderson, K., & Behm, D. G. (2005). The impact of instability resistance training on balance and stability. *Sports Medicine, 35*(1), 43–53.

Assis, M. R., Silva, L. E., et al. (2006). A randomized controlled trial of deep water running: Clinical effectiveness of aquatic exercise to treat fibromyalgia. *Arthritis and Rheumatism, 55*(1), 57–65.

Balderrama, C., Ibarra, G., et al. (2010). Evaluation of three methodologies to estimate the VO2max in people of different ages. *Applied Ergonomics, 42*(1), 162–168.

Becker, B. E. (2009). Aquatic therapy: Scientific foundations and clinical rehabilitation applications. *PM&R: The Journal of Injury, Function, and Rehabilitation, 1*(9), 859–872.

Behm, D. G., Drinkwater, E. J., et al. (2010). The use of instability to train the core musculature. *Applied Physiology, Nutrition, and Metabolism, 35*(1), 91–108.

Body, J. J., Bergmann, P., et al. (2011). Non-pharmacological management of osteoporosis: A consensus of the Belgian Bone Club. *Osteoporosis International, 22*(11):2769–2788.

Bortz, W. M., II. (1984). The disuse syndrome. *The Western Journal of Medicine, 141*(5), 691–694.

Breger Stanton, D. E., Lazaro, R., et al. (2009). A systematic review of the effectiveness of contrast baths. *Journal of Hand Therapy, 22*(1), 57–69; quiz 70.

Bunning, R. D., & Materson, R. S. (1991). A rational program of exercise for patients with osteoarthritis. *Seminars in Arthritis and Rheumatism, 21*(3 Suppl 2), 33–43.

Cameron, I. D. (2004). How to manage musculoskeletal conditions: When is 'rehabilitation' appropriate? *Best Practice & Research. Clinical Rheumatology, 18*(4), 573–586.

Cetin, N., Aytar, A., et al. (2008). Comparing hot pack, short-wave diathermy, ultrasound, and TENS on isokinetic strength, pain, and functional status of women with osteoarthritic knees: A single-blind, randomized, controlled trial. *American Journal of Physical Medicine & Rehabilitation, 87*(6), 443–451.

Cholewicki, J., & McGill, S. M. (1996). Mechanical stability of the in vivo lumbar spine: Implications for injury and chronic low back pain. *Clinical Biomechanics (Bristol, Avon), 11*(1), 1–15.

Cholewicki, J., Panjabi, M. M., et al. (1997). Stabilizing function of trunk flexor-extensor muscles around a neutral spine posture. *Spine (Philadelphia, Pa 1976), 22*(19), 2207–2212.

Cohen, I., & Rainville, J. (2002). Aggressive exercise as treatment for chronic low back pain. *Sports Medicine, 32*(1), 75–82.

Costa, L. O., Maher, C. G., et al. (2009). Motor control exercise for chronic low back pain: A randomized placebo-controlled trial. *Physical Therapy, 89*(12), 1275–1286.

Damsgard, E., Thrane, G., et al. (2010). Activity-related pain in patients with chronic musculoskeletal disorders. *Disability and Rehabilitation, 32*(17), 1428–1437.

Danneels, L. A., Vanderstraeten, G. G., et al. (2000). CT imaging of trunk muscles in chronic low back pain patients and healthy control subjects. *European Spine Journal, 9*(4), 266–272.

DeSantana, J. M., Santana-Filho, V. J., et al. (2008). Hypoalgesic effect of the transcutaneous electrical nerve stimulation following inguinal herniorrhaphy: A randomized, controlled trial. *The Journal of Pain, 9*(7), 623–629.

Desantana, J. M., Sluka, K. A., et al. (2009). High and low frequency TENS reduce postoperative pain intensity after laparoscopic tubal ligation: A randomized controlled trial. *The Clinical Journal of Pain, 25*(1), 12–19.

Deyo, R. A., Walsh, N. E., et al. (1990). A controlled trial of transcutaneous electrical nerve stimulation (TENS) and exercise for chronic low back pain. *The New England Journal of Medicine, 322*(23), 1627–1634.

Downing, D. S., & Weinstein, A. (1986). Ultrasound therapy of subacromial bursitis. A double blind trial. *Physical Therapy, 66*(2), 194–199.

Duque, I. L., Parra, J. H., et al. (2009). Aerobic fitness and limiting factors of maximal performance in chronic low back pain patients. *Journal of Back and Musculoskeletal Rehabilitation, 22*(2), 113–119.

Dziedzic, K., Hill, J., et al. (2005). Effectiveness of manual therapy or pulsed shortwave diathermy in addition to advice and exercise for neck disorders: A pragmatic randomized controlled trial in physical therapy clinics. *Arthritis and Rheumatism, 53*(2), 214–222.

Enea, C., Boisseau, N., et al. (2011). Circulating androgens in women: Exercise-induced changes. *Sports Medicine, 41*(1), 1–15.

Eng, J. J., & Pierrynowski, M. R. (1993). Evaluation of soft foot orthotics in the treatment of patellofemoral pain syndrome. *Physical Therapy, 73*(2), 62–68; discussion 68–70.

Felson, D. T., Gross, K. D., et al. (2009). The effects of impaired joint position sense on the development and progression of pain and structural damage in knee osteoarthritis. *Arthritis and Rheumatism, 61*(8), 1070–1076.

Ferreira, M. L., Ferreira, P. H., et al. (2007). Comparison of general exercise, motor control exercise and spinal manipulative therapy for chronic low back pain: A randomized trial. *Pain, 131*(1–2), 31–37.

Finsen, V., Persen, L., et al. (1988). Transcutaneous electrical nerve stimulation after major amputation. *The Journal of Bone and Joint Surgery (British Volume), 70*(1), 109–112.

Fowles, J. R. (2010). What I always wanted to know about instability training. *Applied Physiology, Nutrition, and Metabolism, 35*(1), 89–90.

Franklin, B. A. (2009). Exercise capacity: A crystal ball in forecasting future health outcomes? *The Physician and Sportsmedicine, 37*(4), 154–156.

Frymoyer, J. W. (1988). Back pain and sciatica. *The New England Journal of Medicine, 318*(5), 291–300.

Gaber, T. A., McGlashan, K. A., et al. (2002). Bone density in chronic low back pain: A pilot study. *Clinical Rehabilitation, 16*(8), 867–870.

Gardner-Morse, M. G. & Stokes, I. A. (1998). *The effects of abdominal muscle coactivation on lumbar spine stability.* Spine (Phila Pa 1976), 23(1): p. 86–91; discussion 91–92.

Gatchel, R. J., & Mayer, T. G. (2008). Evidence-informed management of chronic low back pain with functional restoration. *The Spine Journal, 8*(1), 65–69.

Ghoname, E. A., Craig, W. F., et al. (1999a). Percutaneous electrical nerve stimulation for low back pain: A randomized crossover study. *Journal of American Medical Association, 281*(9), 818–823.

Ghoname, E. A., White, P. F., et al. (1999b). Percutaneous electrical nerve stimulation: An alternative to TENS in the management of sciatica. *Pain, 83*(2), 193–199.

Graven-Nielsen, T., & Arendt-Nielsen, L. (2008). Impact of clinical and experimental pain on muscle strength and activity. *Current Rheumatology Reports, 10*(6), 475–481.

Guissard, N., & Duchateau, J. (2006). Neural aspects of muscle stretching. *Exercise and Sport Sciences Reviews, 34*(4), 154–158.

Gusi, N., Tomas-Carus, P., et al. (2006). Exercise in waist-high warm water decreases pain and improves health-related quality of life and strength in the lower extremities in women with fibromyalgia. *Arthritis and Rheumatism, 55*(1), 66–73.

Hall, J., Swinkels, A., et al. (2008). Does aquatic exercise relieve pain in adults with neurologic or musculoskeletal disease? A systematic review and meta-analysis of randomized controlled trials. *Archives of Physical Medicine and Rehabilitation, 89*(5), 873–883.

Hampson, S. E., Glasgow, R. E., et al. (1993). Self-management of osteoarthritis. *Arthritis Care and Research, 6*(1), 17–22.

Henchoz, Y., de Goumoens, P., et al. (2010). Role of physical exercise in low back pain rehabilitation: A randomized controlled trial of a three-month exercise program in patients who have completed multidisciplinary rehabilitation. *Spine (Philadelphia, Pa 1976), 35*(12), 1192–1199.

Hinman, R. S., Heywood, S. E., et al. (2007). Aquatic physical therapy for hip and knee osteoarthritis: Results of a single-blind randomized controlled trial. *Physical Therapy, 87*(1), 32–43.

Hodselmans, A. P., Dijkstra, P. U., et al. (2010). Nonspecific chronic low back pain patients are deconditioned and have an increased body fat percentage. *International Journal of Rehabilitation Research, 33*(3), 268–270.

Hoffman, M. D. (1996). Name of the game: A healthy lifestyle. *Wisconsin Medical Journal, 95*(6), 331.

Hoffman, M. D. (1997). Principles of musculoskeletal sports injury rehabilitation. *Wisconsin Medical Journal, 96*(12), 38–48.

Holth, H. S., Werpen, H. K., et al. (2008). Physical inactivity is associated with chronic musculoskeletal complaints 11 years later: Results from the Nord-Trondelag Health Study. *BMC Musculoskeletal Disorders, 9*, 159.

Hultman, G., Nordin, M., et al. (1993). Body composition, endurance, strength, cross-sectional area, and density of MM erector spinae in men with and without low back pain. *Journal of Spinal Disorders, 6*(2), 114–123.

Janssen, R. G., Schwartz, D. A., et al. (2009). A randomized controlled study of contrast baths on patients with carpal tunnel syndrome. *Journal of Hand Therapy, 22*(3), 200–207; quiz 208.

Jensen, I. B., Bergstrom, G., et al. (2005). A 3-year follow-up of a multidisciplinary rehabilitation programme for back and neck pain. *Pain, 115*(3), 273–283.

Kamioka, H., Tsutani, K., et al. (2010). Effectiveness of aquatic exercise and balneotherapy: A summary of systematic reviews based on randomized controlled trials of water immersion therapies. *Journal of Epidemiology, 20*(1), 2–12.

Kemmler, W., & Stengel, S. (2011). Exercise and osteoporosis-related fractures: Perspectives and recommendations of the sports and exercise scientist. *The Physician and Sportsmedicine, 39*(1), 142–157.

Kibler, W. B. (1990). Clinical aspects of muscle injury. *Medicine and Science in Sports and Exercise, 22*(4), 450–452.

Kibler, W. B., Chandler, T. J., et al. (1992). Principles of rehabilitation after chronic tendon injuries. *Clinics in Sports Medicine, 11*(3), 661–671.

Kibler, W. B., Press, J., et al. (2006). The role of core stability in athletic function. *Sports Medicine, 36*(3), 189–198.

Kofotolis, N., & Kellis, E. (2006). Effects of two 4-week proprioceptive neuromuscular facilitation programs on muscle endurance, flexibility, and functional performance in women with chronic low back pain. *Physical Therapy, 86*(7), 1001–1012.

Koke, A. J., Schouten, J. S., et al. (2004). Pain reducing effect of three types of transcutaneous electrical nerve stimulation in patients with chronic pain: A randomized crossover trial. *Pain, 108*(1–2), 36–42.

Kruger, L. R., van der Linden, W. J., et al. (1998). Transcutaneous electrical nerve stimulation in the treatment of myofascial pain dysfunction. *South African Journal of Surgery, 36*(1), 35–38.

Kuijper, B., Tans, J. T., et al. (2009). Cervical collar or physiotherapy versus wait and see policy for recent onset cervical radiculopathy: Randomised trial. *British Medical Journal, 339*, b3883.

Kujala, U. M. (2004). Evidence for exercise therapy in the treatment of chronic disease based on at least three randomized controlled trials – Summary of published systematic reviews. *Scandinavian Journal of Medicine & Science in Sports, 14*(6), 339–345.

Kujala, U. M. (2006). Benefits of exercise therapy for chronic diseases. *British Journal of Sports Medicine, 40*(1), 3–4.

Kumar, S., Sharma, V. P., et al. (2010). Comparative efficacy of two multimodal treatments on male and female subgroups with low back pain (part II). *Journal of Back and Musculoskeletal Rehabilitation, 23*(1), 1–9.

Kurtais Gursel, Y., Ulus, Y., et al. (2004). Adding ultrasound in the management of soft tissue disorders of the shoulder: A randomized placebo-controlled trial. *Physical Therapy, 84*(4), 336–343.

Law, R. Y., Harvey, L. A., et al. (2009). Stretch exercises increase tolerance to stretch in patients with chronic musculoskeletal pain: A randomized controlled trial. *Physical Therapy, 89*(10), 1016–1026.

Lawrence, R. C., Felson, D. T., et al. (2008). Estimates of the prevalence of arthritis and other rheumatic conditions in the United States. Part II. *Arthritis and Rheumatism, 58*(1), 26–35.

Lehmann, T. R., Russell, D. W., et al. (1986). Efficacy of electroacupuncture and TENS in the rehabilitation of chronic low back pain patients. *Pain, 26*(3), 277–290.

Leroux, I., Dionne, C. E., et al. (2005). Prevalence of musculoskeletal pain and associated factors in the Quebec working population. *International Archives of Occupational and Environmental Health, 78*(5), 379–386.

Leveille, S. G., Jones, R. N., et al. (2009). Chronic musculoskeletal pain and the occurrence of falls in an older population. *Journal of American Medical Association, 302*(20), 2214–2221.

Lewis, J. S., Hewitt, J. S., et al. (2005). A randomized clinical trial comparing two physiotherapy interventions for chronic low back pain. *Spine (Philadelphia, Pa 1976), 30*(7), 711–721.

Lihavainen, K., Sipila, S., et al. (2010). Contribution of musculoskeletal pain to postural balance in community-dwelling people aged 75 years and older. *The Journals of Gerontology. Series A, Biological Sciences and Medical Sciences, 65*(9), 990–996.

Lin, D. H., Lin, C. H., et al. (2009). Efficacy of 2 non-weight-bearing interventions, proprioception training versus strength training, for patients with knee osteoarthritis: A randomized clinical trial. *The Journal of Orthopaedic and Sports Physical Therapy, 39*(6), 450–457.

Lund, J. P., Donga, R., et al. (1991). The pain-adaptation model: A discussion of the relationship between chronic musculoskeletal pain and motor activity. *Canadian Journal of Physiology and Pharmacology, 69*(5), 683–694.

Lundberg, M., Larsson, M., et al. (2006). Kinesiophobia among patients with musculoskeletal pain in primary healthcare. *Journal of Rehabilitation Medicine, 38*(1), 37–43.

Lydell, M., Baigi, A., et al. (2005). Predictive factors for work capacity in patients with musculoskeletal disorders. *Journal of Rehabilitation Medicine, 37*(5), 281–285.

Macedo, L. G., Maher, C. G., et al. (2009). Motor control exercise for persistent, nonspecific low back pain: A systematic review. *Physical Therapy, 89*(1), 9–25.

Machado, L. A., de Souza, M. S., et al. (2006). The McKenzie method for low back pain: A systematic review of the literature with a meta-analysis approach. *Spine (Philadelphia, Pa 1976), 31*(9), E254–E262.

Manchikanti, L., Singh, V., et al. (2009). Comprehensive review of epidemiology, scope, and impact of spinal pain. *Pain Physician, 12*(4), E35–E70.

Mannion, A. F., Junge, A., et al. (2001a). Active therapy for chronic low back pain: Part 3. Factors influencing self-rated disability and its change following therapy. *Spine (Philadelphia, Pa 1976), 26*(8), 920–929.

Mannion, A. F., Muntener, M., et al. (2001b). Comparison of three active therapies for chronic low back pain: Results of a randomized clinical trial with one-year follow-up. *Rheumatology (Oxford, England), 40*(7), 772–778.

Mantyselka, P. T., Kumpusalo, E. A., et al. (2002). Direct and indirect costs of managing patients with musculoskeletal pain-challenge for health care. *European Journal of Pain, 6*(2), 141–148.

Marchand, S., Charest, J., et al. (1993). Is TENS purely a placebo effect? A controlled study on chronic low back pain. *Pain, 54*(1), 99–106.

May, S. (2010). Self-management of chronic low back pain and osteoarthritis. *Nature Reviews. Rheumatology, 6*(4), 199–209.

May, S., & Donelson, R. (2008). Evidence-informed management of chronic low back pain with the McKenzie method. *The Spine Journal, 8*(1), 134–141.

Mayer, T. G., Gatchel, R. J., et al. (1987). A prospective two-year study of functional restoration in industrial low back injury. An objective assessment procedure. *Journal of American Medical Association, 258*(13), 1763–1767.

Mayer, J. M., Ralph, L., et al. (2005). Treating acute low back pain with continuous low-level heat wrap therapy and/or exercise: A randomized controlled trial. *The Spine Journal, 5*(4), 395–403.

Mayer, T., Tabor, J., et al. (1994). Physical progress and residual impairment quantification after functional restoration. Part I: Lumbar mobility. *Spine (Philadelphia, Pa 1976), 19*(4), 389–394.

McCloskey, E. (2011). Preventing osteoporotic fractures in older people. *Practitioner, 255*(1736), 19–22, 12–13.

Mehta, R., Cannella, M., et al. (2010). Altered trunk motor planning in patients with nonspecific low back pain. *Journal of Motor Behavior, 42*(2), 135–144.

Mooney, V., & Hughson, W. G. (1992). Resurgence of work-hardening programs. *The Western Journal of Medicine, 156*(4), 410.

Moore, S. R., & Shurman, J. (1997). Combined neuromuscular electrical stimulation and transcutaneous electrical nerve stimulation for treatment of chronic back pain: A double-blind, repeated measures comparison. *Archives of Physical Medicine and Rehabilitation, 78*(1), 55–60.

Murina, F., Bianco, V., et al. (2008). Transcutaneous electrical nerve stimulation to treat vestibulodynia: A randomised controlled trial. *British Journal of Obstetrics and Gynaecology, 115*(9), 1165–1170.

Nadler, S. F., Steiner, D. J., et al. (2003a). Continuous low-level heatwrap therapy for treating acute nonspecific low back pain. *Archives of Physical Medicine and Rehabilitation, 84*(3), 329–334.

Nadler, S. F., Steiner, D. J., et al. (2003b). Overnight use of continuous low-level heatwrap therapy for relief of low back pain. *Archives of Physical Medicine and Rehabilitation, 84*(3), 335–342.

Niemisto, L., Rissanen, P., et al. (2005). Cost-effectiveness of combined manipulation, stabilizing exercises, and physician consultation compared to physician consultation alone for chronic low back pain: A prospective randomized trial with 2-year follow-up. *Spine (Philadelphia, Pa 1976), 30*(10), 1109–1115.

Niessen, M. H., Veeger, D. H., et al. (2009). Relationship among shoulder proprioception, kinematics, and pain after stroke. *Archives of Physical Medicine and Rehabilitation, 90*(9), 1557–1564.

Norrbrink, C. (2009). Transcutaneous electrical nerve stimulation for treatment of spinal cord injury neuropathic pain. *Journal of Rehabilitation Research and Development, 46*(1), 85–93.

Norrefalk, J. R., Ekholm, K., et al. (2008). Evaluation of a multiprofessional rehabilitation programme for persistent musculoskeletal-related pain: Economic benefits of return to work. *Journal of Rehabilitation Medicine, 40*(1), 15–22.

Oakley, P. A., Harrison, D. D., et al. (2005). Evidence-based protocol for structural rehabilitation of the spine and posture: Review of clinical biomechanics of posture (CBP) publications. *Journal of the Canadian Chiropractic Association, 49*(4), 270–296.

Oosterhof, J., De Boo, T. M., et al. (2006). Outcome of transcutaneous electrical nerve stimulation in chronic pain: Short-term results of a double-blind, randomised, placebo-controlled trial. *The Journal of Headache and Pain, 7*(4), 196–205.

Ordog, G. J. (1987). Transcutaneous electrical nerve stimulation versus oral analgesic: A randomized double-blind controlled study in acute traumatic pain. *The American Journal of Emergency Medicine, 5*(1), 6–10.

Oyeflaten, I., Hysing, M., et al. (2008). Prognostic factors associated with return to work following multidisciplinary vocational rehabilitation. *Journal of Rehabilitation Medicine, 40*(7), 548–554.

Paillard, T. (2008). Combined application of neuromuscular electrical stimulation and voluntary muscular contractions. *Sports Medicine, 38*(2), 161–177.

Petersen, T., Larsen, K., et al. (2007). One-year follow-up comparison of the effectiveness of McKenzie treatment and strengthening training for patients with chronic low back pain: Outcome and prognostic factors. *Spine (Philadelphia, Pa 1976), 32*(26), 2948–2956.

Poulain, C., Kerneis, S., et al. (2010). Long-term return to work after a functional restoration program for chronic low-back pain patients: A prospective study. *European Spine Journal, 19*(7), 1153–1161.

Rancour, J., Holmes, C. F., et al. (2009). The effects of intermittent stretching following a 4-week static stretching protocol: A randomized trial. *Journal of Strength and Conditioning Research, 23*(8), 2217–2222.

Rees, J. D., Wolman, R. L., et al. (2009). Eccentric exercises; why do they work, what are the problems and how can we improve them? *British Journal of Sports Medicine, 43*(4), 242–246.

Reginster, J. Y. (2002). The prevalence and burden of arthritis. *Rheumatology (Oxford, England), 41*(Supp 1), 3–6.

Roine, E., Roine, R. P., et al. (2009). Cost-effectiveness of interventions based on physical exercise in the treatment of various diseases: A systematic literature review. *International Journal of Technology Assessment in Health Care, 25*(4), 427–454.

Rompe, J. D., Furia, J., et al. (2009). Eccentric loading versus eccentric loading plus shock-wave treatment for mid-portion achilles tendinopathy: A randomized controlled trial. *The American Journal of Sports Medicine, 37*(3), 463–470.

Ryan, E. D., Herda, T. J., et al. (2009). Determining the minimum number of passive stretches necessary to alter musculotendinous stiffness. *Journal of Sports Sciences, 27*(9), 957–961.

Saal, J. A. (1990). Dynamic muscular stabilization in the nonoperative treatment of lumbar pain syndromes. *Orthopaedic Review, 19*(8), 691–700.

Saal, J. A. (1992). The new back school prescription: Stabilization training. Part II. *Occupational Medicine, 7*(1), 33–42.

Schaafsma, F., Schonstein, E., et al. (2010). Physical conditioning programs for improving work outcomes in workers with back pain. *The Cochrane Database of Systematic Reviews, (1)*, CD001822.

Schimmel, J. J., de Kleuver, M., et al. (2009). No effect of traction in patients with low back pain: A single centre, single blind, randomized controlled trial of Intervertebral Differential Dynamics Therapy. *European Spine Journal, 18*(12), 1843–1850.

Shakoor, N., Furmanov, S., et al. (2008). Pain and its relationship with muscle strength and proprioception in knee OA: Results of an 8-week home exercise pilot study. *Journal of Musculoskeletal & Neuronal Interactions, 8*(1), 35–42.

Sharma, L., Cahue, S., et al. (2003). Physical functioning over three years in knee osteoarthritis: Role of psychosocial, local mechanical, and neuromuscular factors. *Arthritis and Rheumatism, 48*(12), 3359–3370.

Sharman, M. J., Cresswell, A. G., et al. (2006). Proprioceptive neuromuscular facilitation stretching: Mechanisms and clinical implications. *Sports Medicine, 36*(11), 929–939.

Sikiru, L., Shmaila, H., et al. (2008). Transcutaneous electrical nerve stimulation (TENS) in the symptomatic management of chronic prostatitis/chronic pelvic pain syndrome: A placebo-control randomized trial. *International Brazilian Journal of Urology, 34*(6), 708–713; discussion 714.

Silfies, S. P., Squillante, D., et al. (2005). Trunk muscle recruitment patterns in specific chronic low back pain populations. *Clinical Biomechanics (Bristol, Avon), 20*(5), 465–473.

Silva, L. E., Valim, V., et al. (2008). Hydrotherapy versus conventional land-based exercise for the management of patients with osteoarthritis of the knee: A randomized clinical trial. *Physical Therapy, 88*(1), 12–21.

Sjostrom, R., Alricsson, M., et al. (2008). Back to work–evaluation of a multidisciplinary rehabilitation programme with emphasis on musculoskeletal disorders. A two-year follow-up. *Disability and Rehabilitation, 30*(9), 649–655.

Sjostrom, R., Alricsson, M., et al. (2009). Back to work – A two-year outcome of a multidisciplinary rehabilitation programme focused on physical function and pain. *Disability and Rehabilitation, 31*(3), 237–242.

Skouen, J. S., Grasdal, A. L., et al. (2002). Relative cost-effectiveness of extensive and light multidisciplinary treatment programs versus treatment as usual for patients with chronic low back pain on long-term sick leave: Randomized controlled study. *Spine (Philadelphia, Pa 1976), 27*(9), 901–909; discussion 909–910.

Smeets, R. J., Wittink, H., et al. (2006). Do patients with chronic low back pain have a lower level of aerobic fitness than healthy controls?: Are pain, disability, fear of injury, working status, or level of leisure time activity associated with the difference in aerobic fitness level? *Spine (Philadelphia, Pa 1976), 31*(1), 90–97; discussion 98.

Smith, C. M., Guralnick, M. S., et al. (1986). The effects of transcutaneous electrical nerve stimulation on post-cesarean pain. *Pain, 27*(2), 181–193.

Sung, P. S., Lammers, A. R., et al. (2009). Different parts of erector spinae muscle fatigability in subjects with and without low back pain. *The Spine Journal, 9*(2), 115–120.

Taylor, W., Simpson, R., et al. (2001). Rehabilitation that works – Vocational outcomes following rehabilitation for occupational musculoskeletal pain. *The New Zealand Medical Journal, 114*(1130), 185–187.

Tolomio, S., Ermolao, A., et al. (2010). The effect of a multicomponent dual-modality exercise program targeting osteoporosis on bone health status and physical function capacity of postmenopausal women. *Journal of Women & Aging, 22*(4), 241–254.

Tomas-Carus, P., Hakkinen, A., et al. (2007). Aquatic training and detraining on fitness and quality of life in fibromyalgia. *Medicine and Science in Sports and Exercise, 39*(7), 1044–1050.

Uth, N., Sorensen, H., et al. (2004). Estimation of VO2max from the ratio between HRmax and HRrest – The Heart Rate Ratio Method. *European Journal of Applied Physiology, 91*(1), 111–115.

van Dijk, G. M., Veenhof, C., et al. (2010). Prognosis of limitations in activities in osteoarthritis of the hip or knee: A 3-year cohort study. *Archives of Physical Medicine and Rehabilitation, 91*(1), 58–66.

Verbunt, J. A., Smeets, R. J., et al. (2010). Cause or effect? Deconditioning and chronic low back pain. *Pain, 149*(3), 428–430.

Vlaeyen, J. W., & Crombez, G. (1999). Fear of movement/(re)injury, avoidance and pain disability in chronic low back pain patients. *Manual Therapy, 4*(4), 187–195.

Vlaeyen, J. W., & Linton, S. J. (2000). Fear-avoidance and its consequences in chronic musculoskeletal pain: A state of the art. *Pain, 85*(3), 317–332.

Waller, B., Lambeck, J., et al. (2009). Therapeutic aquatic exercise in the treatment of low back pain: A systematic review. *Clinical Rehabilitation, 23*(1), 3–14.

Walsh, N. E., Brooks, P., et al. (2008). Standards of care for acute and chronic musculoskeletal pain: The Bone and Joint Decade (2000-2010). *Archives of Physical Medicine and Rehabilitation, 89*(9), 1830–1845.

Wang, W. C., George, S. L., et al. (1988). Transcutaneous electrical nerve stimulation treatment of sickle cell pain crises. *Acta Haematologica, 80*(2), 99–102.

Warke, K., Al-Smadi, J., et al. (2006). Efficacy of transcutaneous electrical nerve stimulation (TENS) for chronic low-back pain in a multiple sclerosis population: A randomized, placebo-controlled clinical trial. *The Clinical Journal of Pain, 22*(9), 812–819.

Weiner, D. K., Perera, S., et al. (2008). Efficacy of percutaneous electrical nerve stimulation and therapeutic exercise for older adults with chronic low back pain: A randomized controlled trial. *Pain, 140*(2), 344–357.

Weng, M. C., Lee, C. L., et al. (2009). Effects of different stretching techniques on the outcomes of isokinetic exercise in patients with knee osteoarthritis. *The Kaohsiung Journal of Medical Sciences, 25*(6), 306–315.

Whalen, R. T., Carter, D. R., et al. (1988). Influence of physical activity on the regulation of bone density. *Journal of Biomechanics, 21*(10), 825–837.

Wittink, H., Michel, T. H., et al. (2002). The association of pain with aerobic fitness in patients with chronic low back pain. *Archives of Physical Medicine and Rehabilitation, 83*(10), 1467–1471.

Woolf, A. D., & Pfleger, B. (2003). Burden of major musculoskeletal conditions. *Bulletin of the World Health Organization, 81*(9), 646–656.

Work Hardening Program Standards. United States Department of Labor and Industries. *Work Hardening Program Standards* Retrieved from http://www.lni.wa.gov/ClaimsIns/Files/ReturnToWork/WhStds.pdf.

Yokoyama, M., Sun, X., et al. (2004). Comparison of percutaneous electrical nerve stimulation with transcutaneous electrical nerve stimulation for long-term pain relief in patients with chronic low back pain. *Anesthesia & Analgesia, 98*(6), 1552–1556; table of contents.

Young, J. Z. (1946). Effects of use and disuse on nerve and muscle. *The Lancet, 2*, 109–113.

Young, I. A., Michener, L. A., et al. (2009). Manual therapy, exercise, and traction for patients with cervical radiculopathy: A randomized clinical trial. *Physical Therapy, 89*(7), 632–642.

Zambito, A., Bianchini, D., et al. (2006). Interferential and horizontal therapies in chronic low back pain: A randomized, double blind, clinical study. *Clinical and Experimental Rheumatology, 24*(5), 534–539.

Zusman, M. (1997). Instigators of activity intolerance. *Manual Therapy, 2*(2), 75–86.

Part VI
Psychosocial, Complementary and Alternative (CAM) and Spiritual Approaches for the Control of Symptoms

Chapter 33
Pain, Depression, and Anxiety in Cancer

Kristine A. Donovan, Lora M.A. Thompson, and Paul B. Jacobsen

Pain in Cancer Patients

Pain is one of the most common and distressing symptoms experienced by cancer patients. Cancer pain has been shown to have adverse effects on quality of life in all domains, including physical, psychological, social, and spiritual well-being (Padilla et al. 1990). Cancer pain can interfere significantly with daily life while psychological factors, including depression, anxiety, and the meaning attributed to the pain can intensify the experience of pain (Breitbart et al. 2010) (see also Ransom et al. 2011).

Etiology of Pain

Cancer pain is typically divided into three major categories based on etiology (McGuire 2004). The first category is pain caused by direct tumor involvement. Examples of this include pain resulting from nerve or plexus compression or infiltration of the tumor into pain-sensitive structures such as bone or soft tissue (Foley 1996). The second category is pain caused by diagnostic or therapeutic procedures. Examples of this include pain resulting from fine needle aspiration and pain after thoracotomy. The third category is pain caused by side effects or toxicities of cancer treatment. Examples of this include chemotherapy-related pain such as peripheral neuropathy and radiation fibrosis of the lumbosacral plexus (Foley 1996). Pain may wax and wane over the course of the cancer trajectory, and patients commonly have more than one type of pain at the same time (Caraceni and Weinstein 2001; McGuire 2004).

K.A. Donovan, PhD, MBA (✉) • L.M.A. Thompson, PhD
Moffitt Cancer Center and Research Institute, Department of Health Outcomes and Behavior,
Tampa, FL, USA

Moffitt Cancer Center and Research Institute, Psychosocial and Palliative Care Department,
Tampa, FL, USA
e-mail: Kristine.donovan@moffitt.org

P.B. Jacobsen, PhD
Moffitt Cancer Center and Research Institute, Department of Health Outcomes and Behavior,
Tampa, FL, USA

Department of Psychology, University of South Florida, Tampa, FL, USA

R.J. Moore (ed.), *Handbook of Pain and Palliative Care: Biobehavioral Approaches for the Life Course*,
DOI 10.1007/978-1-4419-1651-8_33, © Springer Science+Business Media, LLC 2012

Prevalence of Pain

Published prevalence rates of pain in cancer patients vary widely; according to previous reviews, between 14 and 100% of cancer patients report pain at some time during the cancer trajectory (McGuire 2004). Among patients with advanced cancer the overall prevalence of pain ranges from 62 to 86% (Teunissen et al. 2007b; van den Beuken-van Everdingen et al. 2007). The wide variability in prevalence rates is attributable to a number of factors including differences across studies in the demographic, disease, and treatment characteristics of the samples studied, study design and methodology, and the methods used to assess pain. A recent systematic review by van den Beuken-van Everdingen et al. (2007) of studies published between 1966 and 2005 identified 160 studies reporting on the prevalence of cancer pain in an adult cancer population. The demographic and clinical characteristics of the patients included in these studies varied widely. Pain prevalence was documented via study reports of pain prevalence and pain severity. The recall periods also varied widely and included, for example, pain at the time of assessment and pain in the past week, month, or year. The instrumentation used to assess pain was diverse; pain was assessed using visual analog scales, numerical ratings scales, verbal ratings scales, and "yes/no." Fifty-two of the studies met quality criteria for inclusion and provided data sufficient for meta-analyses. Pooled prevalence rates for pain, yes or no, were calculated for four patient groups. In those studies that included only patients after curative treatment, the pooled prevalence rate was 33%. In studies among patients in active cancer treatment, the pooled prevalence rate was 59%. In those studies that included only patients with advanced, metastatic, or terminal disease, the pooled prevalence rate was 64%. Finally, in studies that included patients at all disease stages, the pooled prevalence rate was 53%. With respect to pain severity, more than one-third of patients with pain rated their pain as moderate to severe; approximately 45% of patients with advanced cancer reported moderate to severe pain. This is generally consistent with a recent study by Wilson et al. (2009) that found approximately 34% of cancer patients receiving palliative care near the end of life reported moderate to extreme pain. Generally, these findings indicate that the prevalence of pain is high in cancer patients at all disease stages and that pain remains a significant problem for patients who are receiving palliative care at the end of life.

Depression in Cancer Patients

Etiology of Depression

Depression in the general population is often associated with significant disability, impairments in quality of life, and increased health care utilization (Rodin et al. 2007). In some adults with cancer, symptoms of depression may predate the diagnosis of cancer. In others, depressive symptoms may occur as a psychological response to a serious, potentially life-threatening diagnosis and the experience of unpleasant symptoms, including pain. Cancer patients commonly experience concerns about diminished quality of life, disruption of life plans and role responsibilities, and cancer recurrence or disease progression. Such concerns have the potential to produce in patients a wide range of emotional reactions, including depression. High rates of depression associated with some cancers suggest that depression may be caused by changes induced by the tumor in the neuroendocrine system. Depression has been shown to be associated with pancreatic cancer before diagnosis (Krouse 2010). Depression is also more common in pancreatic cancer than in other gastrointestinal cancers (Holland et al. 1986; Joffe et al. 1986). It is worth noting, however, that pain with pancreatic cancer is common and so may be a causative factor in the development of depression (Shakin and Holland 1988). Potential biological mechanisms by which pancreatic cancer may result in depressive symptoms include the theory that pancreatic tumors secrete serotonin in sufficient quantities to deplete central nervous system stores of serotonin, thereby resulting in depression (Brown and Parakevas 1982). Another theory is that pancreatic tumor cells secrete antibodies that either block central nervous system receptors for serotonin or reduce the synaptic availability of serotonin (Jacobsson 1971). Certain cancer treatments also may result in depression via biological mechanisms. The administration of exogenous cytokines, including interferon-alpha, has been found to produce a "sickness syndrome," with many symptoms, including anhedonia, fatigue, insomnia, and psychomotor retardation, that overlap with depression (Capuron et al. 2002, 2000; Raison and Miller 2003). Studies suggest that 30–45% of patients will develop symptoms consistent with major depressive disorder during treatment with interferon-alpha (Musselman et al. 2001). Other anti-cancer drugs, such as corticosteroids and tamoxifen, have also been associated with depression (Miller and Massie 2010).

Assessment of Depression

Depression in cancer patients has been assessed using a single symptom approach, a multi-symptom approach, and a clinical syndrome approach (Hotopf et al. 2002; Jacobsen et al. 2006b). The single symptom approach refers to assessment methods that generally focus on measuring depressed mood as a continuous variable (e.g., visual analog scales assessing severity of depressed mood) or as a categorical variable (e.g., clinical interview questions assessing the presence or absence of depressed mood). The advantages of the single symptom approach are its brevity and the absence of item content (e.g., low energy or loss of appetite) that might reflect disease symptoms or treatment side effects rather than the presence of adverse emotional states. The disadvantages include the potential for single-item measures to yield unreliable findings, the limited information they yield about depression, and the challenge of identifying clinically significant problems based solely on information about mood. Nevertheless, the single symptom approach may be an effective means of screening for depression. In a study of patients receiving palliative care for advanced terminal cancer, Chochinov et al. (1997) used a single-item screening measure "are you depressed?" and correctly identified the eventual diagnostic outcome of every patient.

The multi-symptom approach refers to assessment methods that focus on measuring constellations of depressive symptoms. This typically involves the use of self-report scales, such as the Center for Epidemiologic Studies Depression Scale (CES-D) (Radloff 1977) and the Depression Subscale of the Hospital Anxiety and Depression Scale (HADS-D) (Zigmond and Snaith 1983). The advantages of this approach include the established psychometric properties of these measures and the ability to compare scores across a variety of medical and nonmedical populations. Disadvantages include the presence on some measures of item content that might reflect disease symptoms or treatment side effects rather than the presence of adverse emotional states. Other measures have little or no item content which overlaps with disease symptoms or treatment side effects but, as a consequence, do not include somatic symptoms generally considered to be key features of depression. Another disadvantage of many of these measures is the lack of well-validated cut-off scores for identifying clinically significant depression in cancer patients.

The clinical syndrome approach refers to assessment methods used to detect the presence of a mood disorder (e.g., major depressive disorder). This approach typically involves the application of criteria identified in the fourth edition of the American Psychiatric Association's Diagnostic and Statistical Manual of Mental Disorders (DSM-IV) (American Psychiatric Association 1994). In research studies, the application of these criteria is typically conducted using interview schedules, such as the Structured Clinical Interview for DSM Disorders (SCID) (First et al. 1996). The advantage of this approach is its utility in identifying the presence of clinically significant depression. Disadvantages include the presence of criteria (e.g., fatigue) that might reflect disease symptoms or treatment side effects, rather than the presence of emotional difficulties, and the relatively high threshold that presence of a mood disorder poses for identifying individuals who may be experiencing emotional difficulties.

Prevalence of Depression

Prevalence rates for depression in cancer patients vary widely. A recent review reports that between 10 and 25% of adult cancer patients are affected by depression (Pirl 2004). Another review reports prevalence rates for depression ranging from 0 and 58% (Massie 2004). In a recent study of cancer patients receiving palliative care, 21% met diagnostic criteria for a depressive disorder, and the most frequent individual diagnosis was major depressive disorder (Wilson et al. 2007). The variability in prevalence rates is due, in part, to differences in patient factors, such as age, gender, ethnicity, disease severity, heterogeneity in cancer types, treatments received, and time since diagnosis. Higher rates of depression are seen in younger patients (Fallowfield et al. 2001), patients with decreased performance status (Bukberg et al. 1984; Chen et al. 2000; Wilson et al. 2007), certain tumor sites (Carlson et al. 2004), and particular treatment modalities (e.g., interferon, corticosteroids) (Miller and Massie 2010). Greater disease burden, including pain, has also been associated with the occurrence of depressive symptoms (Chen et al. 2000; Harter et al. 2001; Wilson et al. 2007). Finally, patients with more advanced disease have demonstrated higher rates of depression (Hotopf et al. 2002). Evidence for gender differences in prevalence of depression is seemingly inconclusive; published reviews have highlighted both differences and no differences in depression between men and women (Massie 2004). Relatively few studies have examined prevalence rates in ethnic or racial minority samples although results suggest that these groups may have higher rates of depression (Agarwal et al. 2010; Middlecamp Kodl et al. 2006; Nelson et al. 2010). Variability in prevalence rates is also attributable to different criteria used to conceptualize depression and the manner in which prevalence is estimated. In general, higher rates of depression are reported in studies using less stringent assessment methods of criteria; that is the use of cut-off scores on continuous measures of depressive symptomatology as opposed to diagnostic clinical interviews (Pirl 2004).

Relationship of Depression and Pain in Cancer Patients

Psychiatric disorders, including depression, are more common in cancer patients with pain. In the Psychosocial Oncology Group study on the prevalence of psychiatric disorders in cancer patients, 39% of patients with a psychiatric diagnosis reported significant pain compared with 19% of patients who did not have a psychiatric disorder (Derogatis et al. 1983). Fifteen percent of patients with pain had major depression (Derogatis et al. 1983). Consistent with this, Chen et al. (2000) found that prevalence rates of depression based on responses to the HADS were higher in patients with pain than in patients without pain. Other researchers (Ciaramella and Poli 2001) found similar results using the Structured Clinical Interview for DSM-III-R, Endicott Criteria (which substitutes psychological symptoms for somatic symptoms), and the Hamilton Depression Rating Scale. Independent of assessment approach, patients who were depressed had more metastasis and pain than nondepressed patients.

Certainly, pain and depression may occur independently in patients with cancer (Valentine 2003). Cleeland (1984) found that among cancer patients with moderate to severe pain, there were no differences between depressed and nondepressed patients in pain intensity and function status. However, depressed patients did report more interference with mood and activity than nondepressed patients. The relatively high comorbidity of depression in chronic pain patients is suggestive, however, and exceedingly, researchers have attempted to clarify the relationship between pain, pain characteristics and depression in the general population and in cancer and other medical illnesses. In general, evidence that depression causes pain is lacking (Wurzman et al. 2008). However, researchers (Spiegel and Bloom 1983) have demonstrated that psychological factors, including depressed mood, are factors that contribute to the variance in pain experienced by cancer patients. That is, depression may increase the intensity of pain, a suggestion that has empirical support in the literature (Ciaramella and Poli 2001; Cleeland 1984; Lin et al. 2003; Zimmerman et al. 1996).

The more compelling evidence suggests that pain is more likely to cause depression. Spiegel et al. (1994) found that the rate of depressive disorders was higher in a group with more severe pain than in a group with less severe pain but that the more severe pain group had a lower rate of history of depression. Spiegel et al. (1994) concluded that pain plays a causal role in depression. Similarly, Ciaramella and Poli (2001) found a higher rate of depression in patients with pain than in patients without pain but increased intensity of pain in patients who were depressed compared to nondepressed patients. The depressed patients did not have higher lifetime rates of depression, and the authors argued that depression follows pain.

Laird et al. (2009) identified 14 studies that met criteria for inclusion in a systematic review of the evidence available to support a causal relationship between cancer pain and depression. None of the studies that met criteria for inclusion were longitudinal studies, however. Twelve studies were cross-sectional studies, and two were cohort studies. Thus, causality could not be determined. Instead, Laird et al. (2009) focused on the interdependent nature of the association between pain and depression as well as the relationships between pain characteristics and depression. Laird et al. (2009) identified four studies examining the combined prevalence of depression and pain. Among cancer patients with pain, the mean prevalence rate of depression was 36.5% and ranged from 22 to 49%. Interestingly, across studies, depression was less prevalent when multi-symptom assessment tools were used and more prevalent when the SCID was used. A statistically significant association between pain and depression was demonstrated in 9 of 14 studies. Laird et al. (2009) concluded that, although it was not feasible to establish the interdependence of pain and depression, the evidence that the two are closely linked is compelling.

Studies included in the review by Laird et al. (2009) also evidenced relationships between specific pain characteristics and depression. In general, greater pain severity and intensity has been shown to be significantly associated with worse depression (Ciaramella and Poli 2001; Kelsen et al. 1995; Sist et al. 1998; Wilson et al. 2009). Patients who are depressed tend to report a higher intensity of pain than patients who are not depressed (Sist et al. 1998). In a study of cancer patients receiving palliative care, Wilson et al. (2009) found that patients with moderate to extreme pain were approximately twice as likely to meet DSM-IV criteria for major depression. Overall, the rates of any diagnosed depressive disorder were approximately two times those in the high pain group compared to the low pain group (Wilson et al. 2009). Similarly, the longer the duration of pain, the higher the risk of depression (Glover et al. 1995; Kelsen et al. 1995). Researchers have also found that pain perception differs between depressed and nondepressed patients. For example, in a study of metastatic breast cancer patients, Spiegel and Bloom (1983) found that women with metastatic breast cancer who were depressed and believed their pain was indicative of disease progression reported more intense pain. Mood disturbance and belief about the meaning of pain were stronger predictors of pain level than number or site of metastases.

In summary, there is good evidence for a relationship between cancer pain and depression. Although one may not cause the other, it is reasonable to suggest that one may exacerbate the other. Similarly, it may be that palliation of each may make management of the other more effective (Valentine 2003). Nevertheless, it does not necessarily follow that successful pain management is always associated with a reduction in depressive symptoms or, similarly, that depression treatment will result in a reduction in pain. It is certainly the case though that each symptom warrants treatment and supportive care.

Management of Depression in Cancer Patients

Clinical Practice Guidelines for Management of Depression in Cancer Patients

Clinical practice guidelines for the psychosocial care of cancer patients have been proposed by several organizations in recent years (Turner et al. 2005). In 2004, the National Institute for Clinical Excellence in the United Kingdom published guidelines on psychosocial aspects of cancer care entitled *Improving Supportive and Palliative Care for Adults with Cancer* (National Institute for Clinical Excellence 2004). The publication's focus is on models of service delivery, and the manual includes recommendations, policy statements, and economic evaluation, supported by reviews of the available scientific literature. Topic areas covered include psychological support services, general and specialist palliative care services, and complementary therapy services. Specific clinical interventions (e.g., for pain control or management of depression) are not recommended; rather the manual defines service models likely to ensure that cancer patients receive the care necessary to help them cope with cancer and its treatment, from diagnosis to survivorship and palliative care. The chapter on psychological support services, for example, outlines a four-level model of professional psychological assessment and intervention encompassing the range and diversity of skills and expertise reflected in different professional disciplines and the variety of psychological and psychiatric interventions available to manage different emotional states, including depression.

The National Breast Cancer Centre (NBCC) and the National Cancer Control Initiative in Australia published the first edition of *Clinical Practice Guidelines for the Psychosocial Care of Adults with Cancer* in 2003 (National Breast Cancer Centre and National Cancer Control Initiative 2003). The guidelines are presented as a series of recommendations with supporting evidence and detailed references. The recommendations are based predominantly on higher level evidence from meta-analyses and randomized controlled trials (RCTs). The recommendations for management of depression in cancer patients include antidepressant medication, the provision of education and information, cognitive-behavioral therapy (CBT), supportive therapy, and psychoeducation.

In the United States, the National Comprehensive Cancer Network (NCCN) publishes and updates annually the NCCN *Clinical Practice Guidelines in Oncology: Distress Management* (National Comprehensive Cancer Network 2010). The guidelines provide recommendations for evaluation and treatment of emotional distress as well as follow-up care organized as clinical pathways. These recommendations are based on lower-level evidence, such as clinical experience and uniform consensus among members of an expert panel. Recommendations for the management of symptoms of depression appear primarily in the sections of the guidelines devoted to mood disorder. For patients with a mood disorder, the initial recommendation is for evaluation, diagnostic studies, and modification of factors, such as pain, fatigue, or medications, that may be contributing to mood disorder symptoms. Thus, the presence of uncontrolled or poorly managed pain should be addressed before or concurrently with treatment for depression. Based on the results of the psychological or psychiatric evaluation, recommendations for the management of depression include antidepressant medication and psychotherapy.

Pharmacologic Approaches

Antidepressants

Antidepressants are routinely recommended to treat depression in cancer patients. Trials of antidepressants in cancer patients in which the medications were dosed adequately and administered for sufficient duration have generally demonstrated benefit (Carr et al. 2002; Patrick et al. 2004). The selection of a specific antidepressant is guided by the patients' presenting symptoms, the side effect profile of the antidepressant, the patient's clinical status, and potential drug interactions (Schwartz et al. 2002; Valentine 2003). No antidepressant or class of antidepressants has been shown to have greater efficacy in the management of depression in cancer patients (Valentine 2003). Several antidepressants have a specific analgesic activity and so are also recommended for the management of pain (Breitbart et al. 2010; Green et al. 2010); the effect on pain is independent of the effect on mood, the onset of the analgesic effect is generally faster than in depression, and the analgesic effect occurs at lower doses (Berney et al. 2000). In palliative care, the main pain management indication for antidepressants is neuropathic pain (Berney et al. 2000; Valentine 2003).

Tricyclic antidepressants (TCAs) are reportedly the most well studied antidepressant class in terms of pain control and, in cancer, are used most often in combination with opioids. The main side effects of TCAs are related to their anticholinergic and antihistamine properties and include sedation, dry mouth, constipation, urinary retention, orthostatic hypotension, cognitive impairment or acute confusional states (Berney et al. 2000; Valentine 2003). These effects may be exacerbated in the elderly and in patients who have advanced disease or are being managed with opioids and other drugs (see also Szucs-Reed and Gallagher 2011; Smith et al. 2011). TCAs are thought to be particularly helpful in patients with combinations of symptoms, such as pain, depression, insomnia, and agitation (Berney et al. 2000).

Selective serotonin reuptake inhibitors (SSRIs) and serotonin norepinephrine reuptake inhibitors (SNRIs) are typically first-line antidepressants. Their more favorable side effect profiles make them generally well tolerated by patients, and evidence suggests they are equally efficacious in improving depressive symptoms (Miller and Massie 2010). Side effects include gastrointestinal disturbances, nausea, anxiety or agitation, insomnia, headaches, weight changes, sedation and sexual dysfunction. Although there are relatively few RCTs of antidepressants in cancer patients (Braun and Pirl 2010; Miller and Massie 2010), SSRIs appear to have been evaluated more extensively than other classes of antidepressants (Carr et al. 2002; Rodin et al. 2007; Williams and Dale 2006). In general, results suggest that SSRIs are effective for depression. Relative to SSRIs, newer and atypical antidepressants, including SNRIs (e.g., venlafaxine), noradrenergic and specific serotoninergic antidepressants (e.g., mirtazapine), and norepinephrine/dopamine reuptake inhibitors (e.g., bupropion) are prescribed less frequently than the SSRIs. There is less information available about their use in cancer patients with depression. Most of the studies in cancer have reportedly focused on the use of venlafaxine for hot flashes and neuropathic pain and duloxetine, TCAs and mirtazapine for pain (Braun and Pirl 2010; Valentine 2003).

Psychostimulants

Psychostimulants have energizing effects, may stimulate appetite, and improve concentration and so are considered to be useful in the management of depression in cancer patients (Braun and Pirl 2010; Orr and Taylor 2007). The rapid onset of antidepressant action of these medications make them particularly useful for the depressed patient in the period before an antidepressant takes full clinical effect or in terminally ill cancer patients with a short life expectancy (Berney et al. 2000; Braun and Pirl 2010). In cancer patients with pain, psychostimulants can reduce opioid-induced sedation and may provide some analgesic effect (Bruera et al. 1992; Bruera and Neumann 1998). Studies of the effects of psychostimulants in cancer patients have also demonstrated improvements in symptoms, such as anorexia, fatigue, concentration, and sedation, as well as pain (Orr and Taylor 2007). Side effects include agitation, anxiety, and insomnia. Although scientific evidence from RCTs of psychostimulants are lacking, in general, nonrandomized studies suggest these medications are effective as antidepressants, particularly in patients in palliative care.

A review of recent systematic reviews (Carr et al. 2002; Rodin et al. 2007; Williams and Dale 2006) suggests that there have been relatively few RCTs of pharmacologic interventions for depression in cancer patients and virtually no such trials for depression in cancer patients with pain. To date, trials have evaluated different classes of medications including antidepressants, psychostimulants, anxiolytics, and corticosteroids for depression. In general, the results support the use of pharmacotherapy, especially antidepressants for depression in cancer patients; hence the recommended use of these agents in the various clinical practice guidelines currently available for the psychosocial support of cancer patients.

Although there are seemingly no RCTs of pharmacologic interventions for depression in cancer patients with pain, it seems reasonable to suggest that pain and depression may each serve as an obstacle to the effective management of the other. Similarly, the successful treatment of pain or depression will likely serve to make the treatment of the other more effective (Valentine 2003). Certainly, both pain and depression must be adequately managed to reduce suffering and improve quality of life in cancer patients. To this end, researchers used a collaborative care model in the Indiana Cancer Pain and Depression (INCPAD) trial to identify and treat cancer patients with depression, pain, or both (Kroenke et al. 2009, 2010). The intervention consisted of centralized telephone-based care management by a nurse trained in assessing symptom response and medication adherence, providing pain and depression-specific education, and making adjustments to treatment consistent with evidence-based treatment guidelines working in collaboration with the treating oncology practitioner and a consulting psychiatrist with pain management expertise. Scheduled telephone contacts by the nurse care manager took place at baseline, and 1, 4, and 12 weeks later and when automated monitoring indicated inadequate symptom improvement, nonadherence to medication, adverse effects, suicidal ideation, or patient request. Automated symptom monitoring took place at routine intervals throughout the 12 months of the trial. Medication management was informed by previous randomized trials and published clinical practice guidelines in cancer and pain.

The efficacy of the telecare management intervention was evaluated against a usual care condition using a randomized controlled design. Patients were eligible if they screened positive for depression that was at least moderately severe, screened positive for pain that was cancer-related, persistent despite a trial of at least one analgesic, and at least moderately severe, or screened positive for both depression and pain. Study findings showed that pain-specific outcomes were significantly improved in the intervention group relative to the usual care group at all times points over the 12 months of the trial. This was also the case for depression-specific outcomes as well; significantly fewer patients in the intervention group had major depressive disorder at the 3- and 12-month assessments.

This study provides strong evidence that a collaborative care model that includes telephone-based centralized symptom management can effectively treat depression and pain in cancer patients. Further, the results support pain and depression symptom management based on regular symptom monitoring combined with treatments according to evidence-based treatment guidelines.

Psychosocial Approaches

In general, recent systematic reviews and meta-analyses (Barsevick et al. 2002; Bottomley 1998; Devine and Westlake 1995; Leubbert et al. 2001; Lovejoy and Matteis 1997; Newell et al. 2002; Osborn et al. 2006; Rodin et al. 2007; Sellick and Crooks 1999; Sheard and Maguire 1999; Uitterhoeve et al. 2004; Williams and Dale 2006) provide broad support for psychosocial interventions for reducing depressive symptoms in cancer patients. Although fewer randomized controlled intervention trials have involved cancer patients with clinically diagnosed depression, the limited evidence suggests that psychosocial interventions may be effective in treating diagnosed depression. Across reviews, these conclusions must be interpreted with caution, however. Differences in the scope of the reviews, the methods used to summarize findings across identified studies and the rationale upon which recommendations are based limit any conclusions that can be made from existing reviews. Systematic reviews and meta-analyses (Akechi et al. 2008; Uitterhoeve et al. 2004), focused exclusively on cancer patients with advanced or terminal disease broadly support the effectiveness of psychosocial interventions for improving depressive symptoms. In their review of interventions for depression in patients with incurable cancer, Akechi et al. (2008) identified ten RCTs that met inclusion criteria for review. The interventions evaluated in the studies varied widely and included supportive therapy, specific behavioral therapies, problem-solving therapy, and CBT. Only six of the studies provided data required for meta-analyses. Based on these six studies, the authors observed a significant effect for psychosocial interventions. They noted, however, that none of the six studies included patients with clinically diagnosed depression. Thus, they concluded that psychosocial interventions were useful in treating depressive states in advanced cancer patients and that such interventions should be combined with routine patient care of patients with advanced cancer. However, there was little evidence to support their use in treating clinically diagnosed depression in advanced cancer patients.

Psychosocial approaches for the treatment of depression in cancer patients involve a wide variety of interventions including psychoeducation, supportive therapy, and CBT. Cognitive-behavioral interventions are typically considered any approaches based on the assumption that thoughts, feelings, and behaviors can be identified, monitored, and altered and that this will effect change in a clinical outcome. These interventions are usually brief, goal-oriented, and designed to teach specific coping skills. Cognitive-behavioral interventions are widely recommended for treatment of depression in cancer patients, and there is evidence for their effectiveness (Lovejoy and Matteis 1997; Osborn et al. 2006). For example, Edelman et al. (1999) evaluated a manualized group CBT program in a RCT with patients with metastatic breast cancer. The intervention consisted of 8 weekly sessions of group CBT. Each session focused on instruction and practice related to cognitive skills (e.g., how to identify and challenge maladaptive thoughts and beliefs) and behavioral skills (e.g., meditation), and homework was assigned between sessions. A part of each session was also devoted to a particular theme (e.g., managing depression, interpersonal relationships). Post-treatment, patients who participated in the intervention showed significant improvements in depression relative to those in the usual care condition. There was no difference between the groups at the 3- and 6-month follow-ups, however. As one possible explanation for the lack of sustained benefit, the researchers suggested that advanced cancer patients may need more individualized therapy, rather than group therapy. They also suggested that CBT might have limited efficacy in patients with advanced disease and that more supportive therapy focusing on the individual patient's emotional needs might produce better or more sustained benefits.

To this end, Savard et al. (2006) evaluated the efficacy of cognitive therapy, a type of CBT, in reducing depression in patients with metastatic cancer. Beck's cognitive therapy (Beck et al. 1979) for depression in the general population was adapted to meet the needs of women with metastatic breast cancer. The ultimate goal of the therapy was to foster an optimistic but realistic attitude toward the patients' situation, as opposed to a negative (e.g., only thinking about death) or overly positive (e.g., hoping for a cure) attitude. Therapy sessions focused on participants' maintaining an appropriate level of daily pleasant and energizing activities and modifying dysfunctional or irrational thoughts about cancer and other situations in their life.

The efficacy of the intervention was evaluated in a RCT. The individually administered intervention consisted of 8 weekly sessions followed by three booster sessions every 3 weeks. Patients with metastatic breast cancer who met criteria for clinically significant depressive symptoms were randomized to the cognitive therapy intervention or a wait-list control condition. Findings indicated that patients who received the cognitive therapy intervention demonstrated significant reductions in depressive symptoms from pre- to post-treatment. This effect was sustained at follow-up 3 and 6 months after the intervention. The researchers suggested that the longer-term beneficial effect of the intervention was attributable to the individual therapy sessions which facilitated tailoring of the intervention to the patient's needs. As noted previously, relatively few RCTs have been conducted with patients who have clinically significant depressive symptoms; thus, the study by Savard et al. (2006) is noteworthy not only for administering an intervention individualized to the patient's needs but also for testing its efficacy in patients with pre-existing clinically significant depression.

Supportive therapies have also been widely used to treat depressive symptoms in cancer patients and have also demonstrated beneficial effects (Devine and Westlake 1995). In the context of cancer, supportive interventions are designed to provide patients the opportunity to express feelings and concerns about their cancer and the effect that the cancer has had on their lives in a supportive environment. For example, Goodwin et al. (2001) evaluated the benefit of supportive-expressive psychotherapy in patients with metastatic cancer. The therapy was intended to foster support and to encourage the expression of feelings and thoughts about cancer and its effect on the physical, emotional, social, and spiritual lives. Participants were encouraged to interact with each other and to support each other outside of the sessions. The effectiveness of the intervention was evaluated in a RCT. The therapy was administered in a group format and consisted of weekly sessions for at least 1 year. Patients with metastatic breast cancer were randomized to the supportive expressive therapy or usual care. Patients with untreated major depression were not eligible to participate. Patient-reported outcomes were assessed prior to therapy and at 4, 8, and 12 months after the therapy commenced. These follow-up scores were averaged, and baseline scores were subtracted from these averages. Results indicated that patients who participated in the intervention demonstrated a greater improvement in psychological symptoms, including depressive symptoms, than patients in the usual care condition. Patients who were initially more depressed benefited from the intervention; patients who were less depressed did not. Patients in the intervention condition also reported less pain. Although baseline pain scores were reportedly low, patients in the intervention condition reported less worsening of pain over the course of the study. Patients in the intervention condition reportedly benefited only if their baseline pain scores were high. Although described as a supportive intervention, each group session in this intervention ended with a self-hypnosis and relaxation exercise. The researchers speculated that the beneficial effect of the intervention on patients' experience of pain might be attributable to the exercise, one that is commonly employed in cognitive-behavioral interventions for pain and depression. These findings support the growing awareness that cancer patients experience clusters of symptoms rather than symptoms in isolation (Miaskowski et al. 2004) and that effective interventions will treat symptom clusters (Williams 2007).

Systematic reviews and meta-analyses (Allard et al. 2001; Devine 2003) of psychosocial interventions for relieving cancer pain generally support their effectiveness. Although limited, there is evidence for the use of cognitive-behavioral strategies, psychoeducational interventions, and supportive therapies for pain in cancer. Studies evaluating psychosocial interventions in cancer patients with pain and depression as primary outcomes are not readily available in the existing literature. It is not uncommon for studies evaluating pain management interventions also to assess the effects of the intervention on depression as a secondary outcome, however. For example, Yates et al. (2004) examined the effects of a nurse-administered psychoeducational intervention for improving cancer pain management in patients with breast, colorectal, lung, or head and neck cancer. The aim of the intervention was to improve patients' knowledge and attitudes regarding pain management, increase patients' ability to communicate with health care providers about pain management, and decrease patients' reluctance to take analgesia via education, instruction and training in problem solving. The intervention was administered using an individual format in two sessions 1 week apart. Participants were randomized to the intervention condition or to an educational intervention about cancer that was equivalent in time to the intervention. One week post-intervention, participants in the intervention reported a greater increase in self-reported pain knowledge, perceived control over pain, and number of pain treatments recommended by health care professionals relative to participants in the control condition. Gains in certain pain management-related factors were sustained 2 months postintervention. There were no differences between the intervention and control conditions on depression, a secondary outcome. Similarly, a RCT of a brief cognitive-behavioral intervention for pain control in metastatic breast cancer patients who were experiencing pain demonstrated the effectiveness of the intervention in ability to decrease pain; there was no effect on depressed mood.

Findings from RCTs of psychosocial interventions for either pain or depression highlight several important points: (1) pain and depression are both complex and multidimensional in nature with numerous potential etiologies; (2) optimal treatments for one do not necessarily result in successful management of the other; (3) there are a variety of treatment options available to treat pain and depression and a combination of treatments may be necessary for effective management; and (4) treatment effectiveness may depend, at least in part, on tailoring the interventions to individual needs to provide support and enhance coping.

Anxiety in Cancer Patients

Etiology of Anxiety

Anxiety is a predictable response to the diagnosis of cancer, as it represents a threat to social roles, interpersonal relationships, future health, and life plans. However, symptoms that cause significant distress and interfere with functioning may suggest the presence of an anxiety disorder. For some people, a cancer diagnosis may reawaken or exacerbate symptoms of a pre-existing anxiety disorder. An example is the patient with a history of panic disorder who begins to have panic attacks during confining procedures, such as MRIs or radiation therapy. For others, anxiety symptoms are a psychological reaction to cancer and its treatment and may vary depending on disease or treatment status. Anxiety is typically higher during the evaluation and diagnosis of cancer (Fallowfield et al. 1994), prior to surgery (Tjemsland et al. 1998), and during chemotherapy or radiotherapy treatment (Miller and Massie 2006; Stark and House 2000). Increased anxiety is also associated with more advanced disease (Miovic and Block 2007; Roth and Massie 2007; Stark and House 2000). Completion of treatment may lead to increased anxiety as patients may feel more vulnerable due to less frequent monitoring and contact with the treatment team. Anxiety may be caused or exacerbated by medications used to treat cancer, such as corticosteroids, which may be provided to reduce nausea and vomiting during chemotherapy. High doses or rapid tapering of this medication is likely responsible for the development of anxiety symptoms. Medications, such as psychostimulants used to treat fatigue, depressed mood and other symptoms, can cause irritability, restlessness and tremulousness (Miller and Massie 2006). Other cancer or treatment-related conditions that are associated with increased anxiety include pain and endocrine and metabolic changes, such as hypoglycemia and hypoxia (Miller and Massie 2006; Roy-Byrne et al. 2008). Among terminally ill patients, anxiety may also be a symptom of depression or delirium (Roth and Massie 2007).

Assessment of Anxiety

Anxiety in people with cancer has also been assessed using various approaches focusing on a single symptom, multiple symptoms, and the presence of a clinical syndrome (Jacobsen et al. 2006b). The single symptom approach generally focuses on measuring anxious mood as a continuous variable (e.g., visual analog scales assessing severity of anxious mood) or as a categorical variable (clinical interview questions assessing presence/absence of anxious mood). As with depression, there are advantages and disadvantages to this approach. Single-item measures, while focused and brief, provide limited information and may yield unreliable findings. In a study of hospitalized palliative care cancer patients, asking the question, "Are you anxious," had a positive predictive value of 46%, indicating inadequate ability of this item to screen out those who were not distressed (Teunissen et al. 2007a). The multi-symptom assessment approach to anxiety focuses on measuring constellations of anxious symptoms, including for example, shakiness, numbness or tingling, nervousness, and fear. Self-report scales representative of this approach are the State-Trait Anxiety Inventory (STAI) (Spielberger 1983), the Anxiety Subscale of the HADS-A (Zigmond and Snaith 1983), and the Beck Anxiety Inventory (BAI) (Beck and Steer 1990). Perhaps, the greatest advantage of this approach over other methods of assessing anxiety is the well established psychometric properties of these commonly used measures. The greatest disadvantages are perhaps the lack of well-validated cut-off scores for identifying clinically significant anxiety and the inability of these measures to adequately distinguish among the various types of anxiety disorders (e.g., generalized anxiety disorder vs. specific phobia). Finally, the clinical syndrome approach to assessing anxiety, like that for assessing depression, typically involves applying the criteria set forth in the DSM-IV and the use of interview schedules, such as the Clinician-Administered PTSD Scale (CAPS) (Blake et al. 1990) or the Acute Stress Disorder Interview (ASDI) (Bryant et al. 1998). The advantages and disadvantages of this approach for assessing anxiety mirror those for assessing depression using this approach. The clinical syndrome approach enables one to more accurately gauge the presence of clinically significant anxiety and to distinguish among types of anxiety disorders. However, it includes criteria (e.g. heart palpitations) that might reflect disease symptoms or treatment-related side effects rather than emotional difficulties. Further, the threshold for presence of an anxiety disorder based on diagnostic criteria is relatively high. A cancer patient who does not meet criteria for an anxiety disorder may nevertheless be experiencing emotional difficulties worthy of clinical attention.

Prevalence of Anxiety

Between 19 and 44% of cancer patients report significant anxiety symptoms (Brintzenhofe-Szoc et al. 2009; Dahl et al. 2005; Stark and House 2000), while prevalence rates for diagnosable anxiety disorders range from 10 to 30% (Roy-Byrne et al. 2008). Rates of diagnosable anxiety disorders in advanced cancer patients range from a low of 6% to a high of 35% (Miovic and Block 2007; Spencer et al. 2010). The comorbidity of depression and anxiety may be a complicating factor when examining rates of anxiety. However, studies have shown that at least one-third of individuals with anxiety do not report depressive symptoms (Brintzenhofe-Szoc et al. 2009; Stark et al. 2002), suggesting that anxiety can be a distinct emotional problem experienced by cancer patients. Variation in prevalence rates of symptoms as well as diagnosable anxiety disorders across studies may be attributed to differences in the clinical characteristics of the samples, including cancer site and stage, treatment type, and time since diagnosis (Harter et al. 2001; Roy-Byrne et al. 2008). Difference in the methodologies used to assess anxiety and to estimate prevalence (Harter et al. 2001; Roy-Byrne et al. 2008) are also a contributing factor. Two studies, which have estimated prevalence based on cut-off scores on a continuous multi-symptom measure of anxiety, have reported rates of 19% (Dahl et al. 2005) and 48% (Stark et al. 2002). Prevalence rates varied by disorder in studies assessing cancer patients using a standardized clinical interview based on DSM-IV or International Classification of Disorders, 10th Revision (ICD-10) criteria (Harter et al. 2001; Spencer et al. 2010; Stark et al. 2002). Specific phobia was the most prevalent disorder (12–14%) while rates of other anxiety disorders were below 10%. Although most studies of prevalence have been cross-sectional, findings from a prospective study by Kangas et al. (2005) are generally consistent with cross-sectional prevalence studies. As few studies have assessed anxiety based on diagnostic criteria, it is difficult to draw more definitive conclusions from the existing research in cancer.

Relationship of Anxiety and Pain in Cancer Patients

The relationship between psychological distress and pain has been well established in the literature, with earlier studies finding a positive relationship between pain and anxiety in cancer outpatients (Glover et al. 1995), cancer inpatients (Strang and Qvarner 1990), and terminally ill cancer patients (Kane et al. 1985). Studies have also found similar results for patients with specific disease sites, including breast cancer (Vahdaninia et al. 2010) and pancreatic cancer (Kelsen et al. 1995). In a mixed sample of outpatients with a prevalence rate of anxiety of 11.8% based on responses to the HADS, patients with pain had a higher prevalence of anxiety than those without pain (Chen et al. 2000). Wilson et al. (2009) examined the prevalence of anxiety disorders among cancer patients receiving palliative care. Data were collected as part of the Canadian National Palliative Care Survey. Based on responses to the Structured Interview of Symptoms and Concerns and selected items from the Primary Care Evaluation of Mental Disorders, significantly more patients with moderate to severe pain met criteria for an anxiety disorder as compared to patients with no pain or mild pain (24 vs. 8.7% respectively).

Several studies using the multi-symptom approach to assess anxiety have shown low to modest but significant correlations between pain intensity and anxiety (Glover et al. 1995; Lin et al. 2003; Zimmerman et al. 1996). However, inconsistent results emerged when cancer patients with pain were compared to those without pain in these studies. While Glover et al. (1995) reported a significant difference in anxiety between pain patients and pain-free patients, both Zimmerman et al. (1996) and Lin et al. (2003) found no difference between pain and pain-free groups on the level of anxiety. When the clinical syndrome approach was utilized to assess anxiety in one study by Stark et al. (2002), there was no significant difference in the level of pain between cancer outpatients who met ICD-10 criteria for an anxiety disorder and those who did not have an anxiety disorder. Possible reasons for these inconsistent results could be different measures used to assess anxiety as well as differences in sample characteristics.

One possibility to consider is that anxiety and cancer pain may occur independently. Chen et al. (2000) compared hospitalized cancer patients with pain to those without pain. Initial analyses indicated a significant relationship between pain intensity and anxiety symptoms and greater anxiety in patients with pain compared to patients without pain. However, when Karnofsky functional status and treatment effect (i.e., whether patients perceived improvement due to treatment) were controlled in the regression analyses, pain status no longer predicted anxiety. Similar results were found by Lin et al. (2003) which demonstrated that pain did not predict anxiety after controlling for gender, presence of metastatic disease, and inpatient vs. outpatient recruitment site. Thus, demographic and clinical characteristics may explain some of the variability in the relationship between pain and anxiety.

It may be that the higher anxiety observed in cancer pain patients is related to cognitive factors rather than pain intensity. Cancer patients with increased anxiety have reported more interference with enjoyment of life (Zimmerman et al. 1996), with relations with other people (Mystakidou et al. 2006), and with overall daily activities (Lin et al. 2003). Greater anxiety symptoms have also been reported by cancer pain patients who perceived their pain to be a sign of disease progression compared to cancer pain patients who did not have this fear (Ahles et al. 2003). Consistent with this finding, pain patients with cancer reported more anxiety and fear of pain than pain patients who did not have cancer (Turk et al. 1998). Catastrophizing is a cognitive coping strategy that has often been linked to increased pain in cancer patients (Jacobsen and Butler 1996). Studies have also shown that cancer patients with greater anxiety are also more likely to engage in catastrophizing about pain (Bishop and Warr 2003; Fischer et al. 2010; Prasertsri et al. 2011). Taken together, these results suggest that cognitive factors may play a role in influencing anxiety in cancer patients with pain.

Management of Anxiety in Cancer Patients

Clinical Practice Guidelines for Management of Anxiety in Cancer Patients

Published clinical practice guidelines for the psychosocial care of cancer patients are available and include recommendations for the pharmacological and psychological management of anxiety (Turner et al. 2005). Organizations, such as the National Institute for Clinical Excellence in the United Kingdom (National Institute for Clinical Excellence 2004) and the National Cancer Control Initiative (NCCI)/NBCC in Australia (National Breast Cancer Centre and National Cancer Control Initiative 2003), have published guidelines that summarize recommendations for supportive and palliative cancer care based on reviews of the research literature and consumer input. As noted previously, in the United States, The NCCN publishes the *NCCN Clinical Practice Guidelines in Oncology: Distress Management* (National Comprehensive Cancer Network 2010), which includes a clinical pathway for referring anxious patients for assessment by a mental health provider. The pathway directs the provider to select the appropriate treatment option depending on the severity of anxiety. Individuals with lower levels of anxiety may be adequately treated with social work or chaplaincy interventions. For mild adjustment disorders, psychological therapy only is the first-line treatment, while moderate to severe adjustment disorders are initially treated with a combination of medication and counseling. Psychological therapy with or without medication is recommended for those with anxiety disorders after contributing factors, such as pain, have been addressed. Follow-up and reevaluation is recommended to insure that treatment is adjusted for patients who experience worsening symptoms or no response to initial treatment. Although these guidelines were created based on the agreement of experts with psycho-oncology experience rather than high-level evidence, such as RCTs, they are a useful tool for healthcare professionals working with cancer patients (Jacobsen et al. 2006a; Turner et al. 2005), including those working with patients with advanced disease and pain.

Pharmacologic Approaches

Much of the evidence for the use of specific medications is based on studies of anxiety disorders in noncancer populations, which have found that antidepressant medications are indicated for the treatment of panic disorder (Mitte 2005; van Balkom et al. 1997), generalized anxiety disorder (Rickels et al. 2000, 2003), and post-traumatic stress disorder (Stein et al. 2006). Although not given as a treatment for anxiety, antidepressants have been prescribed to cancer patients and were found to be well-tolerated (Holland et al. 1998). The SSRIs and SNRIs are favored over older antidepressants because they lead to fewer side effects than the other classes of antidepressants (Bakker et al. 2002). However, they should still be prescribed with caution in the cancer setting due to potential drug–drug interactions (Braun and Pirl 2010). In addition, patients taking SSRIs may experience short-term side effects, such as sleep difficulty, dizziness, or jitteriness when first starting an SSRI, which could be misinterpreted as symptoms of anxiety (Ravindran and Stein 2010). Although these side effects are likely to remit with continued use, they may have an impact on patients' willingness to continue taking the medication until the desired reduction in anxiety is achieved. Some antidepressants, such as the SNRI duloxetine, have analgesic effects and may be appropriate for use with patients requiring treatment for both anxiety and neuropathic pain (Roth and Massie 2007).

Another frequently used type of medication to treat anxiety is the benzodiazepines, such as lorazepam or alprazolam (Ravindran and Stein 2010). There are several advantages to using this class of medications with cancer patients. These medications have a rapid onset and can provide more immediate relief of anxiety symptoms than antidepressant medications (Braun and Pirl 2010). Other advantages include the varied forms of administration (Levin and Alici 2010) and its potential usefulness as an adjunct treatment for chemotherapy-related nausea and vomiting (Feyer and Jordan 2011) and dyspnea (Simon et al. 2010). Benzodiazepines are not recommended for cancer patients with impaired hepatic function, and they may increase the risk of falls or delirium in elderly cancer patients due to oversedation (Levin and Alici 2010). Tolerance and dependence may develop with long-term use of benzodiazepines, and therefore, buspirone, a nonbenzodiazepine anxiolytic, may be a better choice when treating anxiety in a patient with a history of substance abuse (Levin and Alici 2010). Despite the common use of benzodiazepines, a Cochrane review (Jackson and Lipman 2004) concluded that there is not enough evidence to support their use in palliative care settings. Further, nonpharmacological alternatives to the use of benzodiazepines exist, which can offer patients relief without bothersome side effects. In a RCT of alprazolam and relaxation training, cancer patients randomized to either group demonstrated significant reductions in anxiety symptoms after 10 days of treatment (Holland et al. 1991).

There are a number of alternatives, which can be considered when other symptoms are present in addition to anxiety. For example, mirtazapine may be prescribed for the cancer patient with anxiety who is also experiencing insomnia and anorexia (Roth and Massie 2007). Antipsychotics, such as haloperidol, may be prescribed to treat anxiety in cancer patients with delirium or risk of mental status changes (Mazzocato et al. 2000). Anticonvulsants may be effective for cancer patients with neuropathic pain in addition to anxiety, but evidence for their use is limited (Buclin et al. 2001).

In summary, there are several factors to consider when selecting medication, including compromised hepatic, renal, or pulmonary function, potential for abuse, side effect profile, and drug–drug interactions (Braun and Pirl 2010; Levin and Alici 2010) (see also Ransom et al. 2011; Smith et al. 2011). For terminally ill patients, the selection of a medication may depend on how long the individual has to live (Roth and Massie 2007). Although there are a few medications that are indicated for both anxiety and pain, providers may follow the same prescribing guidelines used for treating anxiety in anxious cancer patients without pain after careful consideration of the risks and benefits of pharmacotherapy.

Psychosocial Approaches

Evidence to support the use of psychological approaches to treat anxiety in cancer patients is based on several meta-analyses (Devine and Westlake 1995; Leubbert et al. 2001; Osborn et al. 2006; Sheard and Maguire 1999). Although significant, the degree of the effects found in these meta-analyses ranged in size from small ($d=0.36$) to large ($g=1.99$). The wide range of effect sizes reported may be due to differences in study inclusion criteria, as some examined studies of a specific intervention type (Leubbert et al. 2001; Osborn et al. 2006), while others examined a variety of intervention types including CBT and psychoeducation (Sheard and Maguire 1999) or relaxation therapy and psychoeducation (Devine and Westlake 1995). Included studies also varied by quality (RCT vs. pre–post design) and quantity, with one meta-analysis conducted on only four studies (Osborn et al. 2006). In a more critical review, which excluded methodologically poor studies, Newell et al. (2002) concluded that the existing evidence is insufficient to make a judgment about intervention effectiveness. A systematic review of only studies of advanced cancer patients similarly concluded that too few good quality RCTs targeting anxiety have been conducted among palliative care populations (Uitterhoeve et al. 2004). Despite these limitations, several intervention types have been recommended to treat anxiety in cancer patients, including CBT and psychoeducation (Jacobsen and Jim 2008).

Cognitive-behavioral interventions targeting distress in general have led to reductions in anxiety symptoms in cancer patients with a life expectancy greater than 1 year (Greer et al. 1992). Moorey et al. (2009) found similar positive results for CBT delivered in a palliative care setting. Hospice nurse specialists providing home care to cancer patients were randomly selected to undergo CBT training or no training. CBT trained nurses learned how to use skills, such as problem solving and thought reframing, to address hopelessness, worry, sleep difficulty and other typical problems. They received weekly supervision for over 1 year before subject recruitment began. Patients who were enrolled in the study had to be experiencing distress, defined as a score above 8 on the HADS anxiety or depression subscales. There was a significant group by time interaction effect, such that patients ($N=24$) receiving care from CBT trained nurses reported significantly less anxiety by the 16-week follow-up than patients ($N=22$) who received care from nurses without CBT training. Further, there was a significant difference in the number of anxiety cases at 16 weeks, with 19% of CBT care patients meeting HADS case criteria compared to 56% of the standard care patients. However, the researchers suggest caution in interpreting these results as their study had a number of limitations, including a recruitment rate of less than 10%, an attrition rate of over 50%, randomization by treatment provider rather than at the patient level, and no standardization of the CBT techniques delivered to patients (Moorey et al. 2009).

Several studies have examined cognitive-behavioral interventions designed to target anxiety as a primary outcome. Relaxation techniques, such as progressive muscle relaxation or guided imagery, have often been the main component of these interventions, and there is evidence to support the efficacy of these techniques in reducing anxiety (Cheung et al. 2003; Leon-Pizarro et al. 2007; Redd et al. 2001). However, some studies have developed interventions, which consist of relaxation techniques in combination with other cognitive techniques. One example is a study by Antoni et al. (2006), which was designed to test the effects of an intervention on cancer-specific anxiety and general anxiety. Nonmetastatic breast cancer patients undergoing treatment were randomized to participate in a group CBT intervention or psychoeducation. The intervention participants met for 10 weekly 2 h groups to learn relaxation techniques, cognitive restructuring, and coping skills. Women in the control group participated in a 5–6 h psychoeducation program, which consisted of information about the techniques taught in the group intervention. Participants completed the Impact of Event Scale (Horowitz et al. 1979) prior to group assignment and at 3 and 6 months after completion of the intervention. The intervention group had a more significant decline in intrusive thoughts about cancer than the control group. It should be noted that patients with a history of psychiatric treatment for a serious disorder, including panic attacks, were excluded from participation. Thus, it is not known whether this intervention would be effective for patients with diagnosed anxiety disorders.

A more recent RCT by DuHamel et al. (2010) also examined anxiety as a primary outcome. Hematopoietic stem-cell transplant survivors who were experiencing symptoms of PTSD were randomized to participate in a ten-session telephone intervention or no treatment control condition. The intervention consisted of PTSD and CBT education, skills training (e.g., relaxation, communication), guided exposure, and cognitive modification. Patients were ineligible to participate if they had current psychosis, suicidal ideation, or substance dependence but previous history of an anxiety disorder was not one of the exclusion criteria. To be eligible, patients had to be experiencing clinical or sub-clinical symptoms of PTSD based on PTSD Checklist – Civilian Version (PCL-C) scores or some PTSD symptoms in combination with two or more scores exceeding the clinical cutoff on measures of general distress. The Clinician Administered PTSD Scale for DSM-IV (CAPS) and the PCL-C were administered at four intervals. Intervention participants reported less intrusive thoughts and less avoidance at all follow ups, and they were less likely to have a PTSD diagnosis at the 12-month follow-up than control participants. Prevalence rates of the disorder were not reported. Anxiety has also been examined in studies of cognitive-behavioral interventions for pain in metastatic breast cancer patients (Arathuzik 1994) and in cancer patients with mixed diagnoses (Dalton et al. 2004), but these studies did not demonstrate any effect on anxiety in these samples.

Psychoeducation is another psychological approach that has demonstrated positive results in reducing anxiety in newly diagnosed patients (McQuellon et al. 1998; Orringer et al. 2005) and patients who have completed or are undergoing treatment (Jacobs et al. 1983). Katz and colleagues pilot tested a psychoeducational booklet plus support with 19 patients scheduled to undergo potentially disfiguring surgery for oral cancer. The booklet contained general information about oral cancer and the effects of surgery as well as information about coping with anxiety and depression. A significant reduction in anxiety was reported by those who were randomized to the intervention as compared to standard care, but this was only true for 1 out of 2 measures of anxiety. In a study of advanced cancer patients with pain conducted by Lovell et al. (2010), participants were randomized to receive standard care or 1 of 3 interventions delivered in a booklet and/or video format. The content of the materials focused on pain management, which included a description of emotional responses to pain. The presence of anxiety was not one of the eligibility criteria, but 32% of participants were reporting baseline HADS scores in the clinically significant range. Although the decrease in pain scores was significantly greater in the participants who received the combined booklet and video intervention compared to the standard care participants, there was no significant difference in anxiety between groups from baseline to follow-up. These results suggest information about pain management is not sufficient to address anxiety in this population.

Complementary therapies, such as massage, yoga, or meditation, are increasingly being used as adjuncts to standard care for treating symptoms experienced by cancer patients (Cassileth et al. 2007) (see also Kutner and Smith 2011). Although the quality of previous research on complementary therapies has been questionable, more recent research is of higher quality. In a within-subjects study, cancer patients in a palliative care center who were referred for massage were asked to complete before and after measures of anxiety. The primary reasons for referral were anxiety (59%) and pain (32%). Anxiety significantly decreased after massage. RCTs have also demonstrated that anxiety is reduced in early breast cancer patients who practiced yoga during cancer treatment (Rao et al. 2009) and in patients with advanced cancer who received partner delivered foot reflexology (stimulation of specific areas of the foot) (Stephenson et al. 2007). The addition of mindfulness meditation to cognitive therapy, for example, resulted in a reduction in anxiety in a mixed group of cancer patients participating in weekly group sessions (Foley et al. 2010).

In summary, there is evidence to support the use of cognitive-behavioral or psychoeducational interventions to reduce anxiety in cancer patients. Many of these studies have targeted anxiety as a secondary outcome and have not made the presence of a diagnosed anxiety disorder part of the eligibility criteria. There is less evidence to support the use of these interventions to reduce anxiety in cancer patients with advanced disease or those with pain. Emerging evidence suggests that complementary therapies may also have some usefulness in reducing anxiety symptoms. Additional well-designed studies are needed before any firm conclusions can be drawn.

Conclusions and Future Directions

Pain is highly prevalent among cancer patients and remains a significant problem for many patients receiving palliative care (see also Ransom et al. 2011). Pain is associated with higher rates of depression and anxiety in cancer patients at all points along the cancer trajectory; research suggests that among patients with advanced disease and patients receiving palliative care, patients with pain are more likely to have clinically significant depression and anxiety. Whether there is a causal relationship between pain and depression and anxiety remains to be determined. Much of the evidence for the relationship stems from cross-sectional studies; future research should include prospective studies that enable the examination of temporal associations between pain, depression and anxiety. There is limited evidence suggesting that effectively managing pain will result in a reduction in symptoms of depression and anxiety. A number of pharmacologic and psychosocial interventions are available to treat depression and anxiety in cancer patients, and several of these have been shown to be useful in the management of pain in cancer patients. RCTs of these interventions for the treatment of depression and anxiety in cancer patients with pain and in palliative care patients are lacking. More research is needed to evaluate the efficacy of these interventions in these patients. To date, relatively few studies have included racially and ethnically diverse samples of cancer patients with pain. Thus, future research should examine depression and anxiety in racial or ethnic minority cancer populations with pain and in palliative care to more accurately assess and meet the needs of these groups (Green 2011, This Volume). Compassionate and comprehensive care of the cancer patient with pain requires that depression and anxiety be recognized, assessed, and treated.

References

Agarwal, M., Hamilton, J. B., Moore, C. E., & Crandell, J. L. (2010). Predictors of depression among older African American cancer patients. *Cancer Nursing, 33*, 156–163.

Ahles, T. A., Saykin, A. J., Noll, W. W., Furstenberg, C. T., Guerin, S., Cole, B., & Mott, L. A. (2003). The relationship of APOE genotype to neuropsychological performance in long-term cancer survivors treated with standard dose chemotherapy. *Psycho-Oncology, 12*, 612–619.

Akechi, T., Okuyama, T., Onishi, J., Morita, T., & Furukawa, T. A. (2008). Psychotherapy for depression among incurable cancer patients. *Cochrane Database Systemic Reviews, 2*, CD005537.

Allard, P., Maunsell, E., Labbe, J., & Dorval, M. (2001). Educational interventions to improve cancer pain control: A systematic review. *Journal of Palliative Medicine, 4*, 191–203.

American Psychiatric Association. (1994). *Diagnostic and statistical manual of mental disorders*. Washington: American Psychiatric Association.

Antoni, M. H., Wimberly, S. R., Lechner, S. C., Kazi, A., Sifre, T., Urcuyo, K. R., Phillips, K., Smith, R. G., Petronis, V. M., Guellati, S., Wells, K. A., Blomberg, B., & Carver, C. S. (2006). Reduction of cancer-specific thought intrusions and anxiety symptoms with a stress management intervention among women undergoing treatment for breast cancer. *The American Journal of Psychiatry, 163*, 1791–1797.

Arathuzik, D. (1994). Effects of cognitive-behavioral strategies on pain in cancer patients. *Cancer Nursing, 17*, 207–214.

Bakker, A., van Balkom, A. J., & Spinhoven, P. (2002). SSRIs vs. TCAs in the treatment of panic disorder: A meta-analysis. *Acta Psychiatrica Scandinavica, 106*, 163–167.

Barsevick, A. M., Sweeney, C., Haney, E., & Chung, E. (2002). A systematic qualitative analysis of psychoeducational interventions for depression in patients with cancer. *Oncology Nursing Forum, 29*, 73–84. quiz 77–85.

Beck, A. T., Rush, A. J., Shaw, B. F., & Emery, G. (1979). *Cognitive therapy of depression*. New York: Guilford Press.

Beck, A. T., & Steer, R. A. (1990). *Manual for the Beck Anxiety Inventory*. San Antonio: Psychological Corporation.

Berney, A., Stiefel, F., Mazzocato, C., & Buclin, T. (2000). Psychopharmacology in supportive care of cancer: A review for the clinician. III. Antidepressants. *Supportive Care in Cancer, 8*, 278–286.

Bishop, S. R., & Warr, D. (2003). Coping, catastrophizing and chronic pain in breast cancer. *Journal of Behavioral Medicine, 26*, 265–281.

Blake, D. D., Weathers, F., Nagi, L. M., Kaloupek, D. G., Klauminzer, G., Charney, D. S., & Keane, T. M. (1990). A clinician's rating scale for assessing current and lifetime PTSD: The CAPS 1. *Behavior Therapist, 13*, 187–188.

Bottomley, A. (1998). Depression in cancer patients: A literature review. *European Journal of Cancer Care, 7*, 181–191.

Braun, I. M., & Pirl, W. F. (2010). Psychotropic medications in cancer care. In J. C. Holland, W. S. Breitbart, P. B. Jacobsen, M. S. Lederberg, M. J. Loscalzo, & R. McCorkle (Eds.), *Psycho-oncology* (pp. 378–385). New York: Oxford University Press.

Breitbart, W. S., Park, J., & Katz, A. M. (2010). Pain. In J. C. Holland, W. S. Breitbart, P. B. Jacobsen, M. S. Lederberg, M. J. Loscalzo, & R. McCorkle (Eds.), *Psycho-oncology* (pp. 215–228). New York: Oxford University Press.

Brintzenhofe-Szoc, K. M., Levin, T. T., Li, Y., Kissane, D. W., & Zabora, J. R. (2009). Mixed anxiety/depression symptoms in a large cancer cohort: Prevalence by cancer type. *Psychosomatics, 50*, 383–391.

Brown, J. H., & Parakevas, F. (1982). Cancer and depression: Cancer presenting with depressive illness: An autoimmune disease? *The British Journal of Psychiatry, 141*, 227–232.

Bruera, E., Miller, M. J., Macmillan, K., & Kuehn, N. (1992). Neuropsychological effects of methylphenidate in patients receiving a continuous infusion of narcotics for cancer pain. *Pain, 48*, 163–166.

Bruera, E., & Neumann, C. M. (1998). The uses of psychotropics in symptom management in advanced cancer. *Psycho-Oncology, 7*, 346–358.

Bryant, R. A., Harvey, A. G., Dang, S. T., & Sackville, T. (1998). Assessing acute stress disorder: Psychometric properties of a structured clinical interview. *Psychological Assessment, 10*, 215–220.

Buclin, T., Mazzocato, C., Berney, A., & Stiefel, F. (2001). Psychopharmacology in supportive care of cancer: A review for the clinician. IV. Other psychotropic agents. *Supportive Care in Cancer, 9*, 213–222.

Bukberg, J., Penman, D., & Holland, J. C. (1984). Depression in hospitalized cancer patients. *Psychosomatic Medicine, 46*, 199–212.

Capuron, L., Gumnick, J. F., Musselman, D. L., Lawson, D. H., Reemsnyder, A., Nemeroff, C. B., & Miller, A. H. (2002). Neurobehavioral effects of interferon-alpha in cancer patients: Phenomenology and paroxetine responsiveness of symptom dimensions. *Neuropsychopharmacology, 26*, 643–652.

Capuron, L., Ravaud, A., & Dantzer, R. (2000). Early depressive symptoms in cancer patients receiving interleukin 2 and/or interferon alfa-2b therapy. *Journal of Clinical Oncology, 18*, 2143–2151.

Caraceni, A., & Weinstein, S. M. (2001). Classification of cancer pain syndromes. *Oncology (Williston Park), 15*, 1627–1640. 1642; discussion 1623–1642, 1627–1646.

Carlson, L. E., Angen, M., Cullum, J., Goodey, E., Koopmans, J., Lamont, L., MacRae, J. H., Martin, M., Pelletier, G., Robinson, J., Simpson, J. S., Speca, M., Tillotson, L., & Bultz, B. D. (2004). High levels of untreated distress and fatigue in cancer patients. *British Journal of Cancer, 90*, 2297–2304.

Carr, D., Goudas, L., Lawrence, D., Pirl, W., Lau, J., DeVine, D., et al. (2002). Management of cancer symptoms: Pain, depression, and fatigue. Evidence report/technology assessment No. 61. (Prepared by the New England Medical center evidence-based practice center under contract No. 290-97-0019). AHRQ publication no. 02-E032. Rockville, MD: Agency for Health care research and quality. July 2002.

Cassileth, B. R., Deng, G. E., Gomez, J. E., Johnstone, P. A., Kumar, N., & Vickers, A. J. (2007). Complementary therapies and integrative oncology in lung cancer: ACCP evidence-based clinical practice guidelines (2nd edition). *Chest, 132*, 340S–354S.

Chen, M.-L., Chang, H.-K., & Yeh, C.-H. (2000). Anxiety and depression in Taiwanese cancer patients with and without pain. *Journal of Advanced Nursing, 32*, 944–951.

Cheung, Y. L., Molassiotis, A., & Chang, A. M. (2003). The effect of progressive muscle relaxation training on anxiety and quality of life after stoma surgery in colorectal cancer patients. *Psycho-Oncology, 12*, 254–266.

Chochinov, H. M., Wilson, K. G., Enns, M., & Lander, S. (1997). "Are you depressed?" screening for depression in the terminally ill. *The American Journal of Psychiatry, 154*, 674–676.

Ciaramella, A., & Poli, P. (2001). Assessment of depression among cancer patients: The role of pain, cancer type and treatment. *Psycho-Oncology, 10*, 156–165.

Cleeland, C. S. (1984). The impact of pain on the patient with cancer. *Cancer, 54*, 2635–2641.

Dahl, A. A., Haaland, C. F., Mykletun, A., Bremnes, R., Dahl, O., Klepp, O., Wist, E., & Fossa, S. D. (2005). Study of anxiety disorder and depression in long-term survivors of testicular cancer. *Journal of Clinical Oncology, 23*, 2389–2395.

Dalton, J. A., Keefe, F. J., Carlson, J., & Youngblood, R. (2004). Tailoring cognitive-behavioral treatment for cancer pain. *Pain Management Nursing, 5*, 3–18.

Derogatis, L. R., Morrow, G. R., Fetting, J., Penman, D., Piasetsky, S., Schmale, A. M., Henrichs, M., & Carnicke, C. L., Jr. (1983). The prevalence of psychiatric disorders among cancer patients. *Journal of American Medical Association, 249*, 751–757.

Devine, E. C. (2003). Meta-analysis of the effect of psychoeducational interventions on pain in adults with cancer. *Oncology Nursing Forum, 30*, 75–89.

Devine, E. C., & Westlake, S. K. (1995). The effects of psychoeducational care provided to adults with cancer: Meta-analysis of 116 studies. *Oncology Nursing Forum, 22*, 1369–1381.

DuHamel, K. N., Mosher, C. E., Winkel, G., Labay, L. E., Rini, C., Meschian, Y. M., et al. (2010). Randomized clinical trial of telephone-administered cognitive-behavioral therapy to reduce post-traumatic stress disorder and distress symptoms after hematopoietic stem-cell transplantation. *Journal of Clinical Oncology, 28*, 3754–3761.

Edelman, S., Bell, D. R., & Kidman, A. D. (1999). A group cognitive behaviour therapy programme with metastatic breast cancer patients. *Psycho-Oncology, 8*, 295–305.

Fallowfield, L., Ratcliffe, D., Jenkins, V., & Saul, J. (2001). Psychiatric morbidity and its recognition by doctors in patients with cancer. *British Journal of Cancer, 84*, 1011–1015.

Fallowfield, L. J., Hall, A., Maguire, P., Baum, M., & A'Hern, R. P. (1994). Psychological effects of being offered choice of surgery for breast cancer. *British Medical Journal, 309*, 448.

Feyer, P., & Jordan, K. (2011). Update and new trends in antiemetic therapy: The continuing need for novel therapies. *Annals of Oncology, 22*(1), 30–38.

First, M. B., Gibbons, M., & Spitzer, R. L. (1996). *Users guide for the structured clinical interview for DSM-IV axis I disorders: Research version*. New York: Biometrics Research.

Fischer, D. J., Villines, D., Kim, Y. O., Epstein, J. B., & Wilkie, D. J. (2010). Anxiety, depression, and pain: Differences by primary cancer. *Supportive Care in Cancer, 18*, 801–810.

Foley, E., Bailie, A., Huxter, M., Price, M., & Sinclair, E. (2010). Mindfulness-based cognitive therapy for individuals whose lives have been affected by cancer: A randomized controlled trial. *Journal of Consulting and Clinical Psychology, 78*, 72–79.

Foley, K. M. (1996). Pain syndromes in patients with cancer. In R. K. Portenoy & R. M. Kanner (Eds.), *Pain management: Theory and practice* (pp. 191–216). Philadelphia: F. A. Davis Company.

Glover, J., Dibble, S. L., Dodd, M. J., & Miaskowski, C. (1995). Mood states of oncology outpatients: Does pain make a difference? *Journal of Pain and Symptom Management, 10*, 120–128.

Goodwin, P. J., Leszcz, M., Ennis, M., Koopmans, J., Vincent, L., Guther, H., Drysdale, E., Hundleby, M., Chochinov, H. M., Navarro, M., Speca, M., & Hunter, J. (2001). The effect of group psychosocial support on survival in metastatic breast cancer. *The New England Journal of Medicine, 345*, 1719–1726.

Green, E., Zwaal, C., Beals, C., Fitzgerald, B., Harle, I., Jones, J., Tsui, J., Volpe, J., Yoshimoto, D., & Wiernikowski, J. (2010). Cancer-related pain management: A report of evidence-based recommendations to guide practice. *The Clinical Journal of Pain, 26*, 449–462.

Greer, S., Moorey, S., Baruch, J. D., Watson, M., Robertson, B. M., Mason, A., Rowden, L., Law, M. G., & Bliss, J. M. (1992). Adjuvant psychological therapy for patients with cancer: A prospective randomised trial. *British Medical Journal, 304*, 675–680.

Harter, M., Reuter, K., Aschenbrenner, A., Schretzmann, B., Marschner, N., Hasenburg, A., & Weis, J. (2001). Psychiatric disorders and associated factors in cancer: Results of an interview study with patients in inpatient, rehabilitation and outpatient treatment. *European Journal of Cancer, 37*, 1385–1393.

Holland, J. D., Korzun, A. H., Tross, S., Silberfarb, P., Perry, M., Comis, R., & Oster, M. (1986). Comparative psychological disturbance in patients with pancreatic and gastric cancer. *The American Journal of Psychiatry, 143*, 982–986.

Holland, J. C., Morrow, G. R., Schmale, A., Derogatis, L., Stefanek, M., Berenson, S., Carpenter, P. J., Breitbart, W., & Feldstein, M. (1991). A randomized clinical trial of alprazolam versus progressive muscle relaxation in cancer patients with anxiety and depressive symptoms. *Journal of Clinical Oncology, 9*, 1004–1011.

Holland, J. C., Romano, S. J., Heiligenstein, J. H., Tepner, R. G., & Wilson, M. G. (1998). A controlled trial of fluoxetine and desipramine in depressed women with advanced cancer. *Psycho-Oncology, 7*, 291–300.

Horowitz, M., Wilner, N., & Alvarez, W. (1979). Impact of Event Scale: A measure of subjective stress. *Psychosomatic Medicine, 41*, 209–218.

Hotopf, M., Chidgey, J., Addington-Hall, J., & Ly, K. L. (2002). Depression in advanced disease: A systematic review Part 1. Prevalence and case finding. *Palliative Medicine, 16*, 81–97.

Jackson, K. C., Lipman, A. G. (2004). Drug therapy for delirium in terminally ill patients. *Cochrane Database Systemic Reviews, 2*, CD004770.

Jacobs, C., Ross, R. D., Walker, I. M., & Stockdale, F. E. (1983). Behavior of cancer patients: A randomized study of the effects of education and peer support groups. *American Journal of Clinical Oncology, 6*, 347–353.

Jacobsen, P., Donovan, K., Scwaine, Z., & Watson, I. (2006a). *Management of anxiety and depression: Toward an evidence-based approach*. New York: Springer.

Jacobsen, P. B., & Butler, R. W. (1996). Relation of cognitive coping and catastrophizing to acute pain and analgesic use following breast cancer surgery. *Journal of Behavioral Medicine, 19*, 17–29.

Jacobsen, P. B., Donovan, K. A., Swaine, Z. N., & Watson, I. S. (2006b). Management of anxiety and depression in adult cancer patients: Toward an evidence-based approach. In A. E. Change, P. A. Ganz, D. F. Hayes, et al. (Eds.), *Oncology: An evidence-based approach* (pp. 1552–1579). New York: Springer.

Jacobsen, P. B., & Jim, H. S. (2008). Psychosocial interventions for anxiety and depression in adult cancer patients: Achievements and challenges. *CA: A Cancer Journal for Clinicians, 58*, 214–230.

Jacobsson, L. O. (1971). Initial mental disorders in carcinoma of pancreas and stomach. *Acta Psychiatrica Scandinavica, 220*, 120–127.

Joffe, R., Rubinow, D., Demicoff, K., Maher, M., & Sindelar, W. F. (1986). Depression and carcinoma of the pancreas. *General Hospital Psychiatry, 8*, 241–245.

Kane, R. L., Berstein, L., Wales, J., & Rothenberg, R. (1985). Hospice effectiveness in controlling pain. *Journal of American Medical Association, 253*, 2683–2686.

Kangas, M., Henry, J., & Bryant, R. (2005). The course of psychological disorder in the 1st year after cancer diagnosis. *Journal of Consulting and Clinical Psychology, 73*, 763–768.

Kelsen, D. P., Portenoy, R. K., Thaler, H. T., Niedzwiecki, D., Passik, S. D., Tao, Y., Banks, W., Brennan, M. F., & Foley, K. M. (1995). Pain and depression in patients with newly diagnosed pancreas cancer. *Journal of Clinical Oncology, 13*, 748–755.

Kroenke, K., Theobald, D., Norton, K., Sanders, R., Schlundt, S., McCalley, S., Harvey, P., Iseminger, K., Morrison, G., Carpenter, J. S., Stubbs, D., Jacks, R., Carney-Doebbeling, C., Wu, J., & Tu, W. (2009). The Indiana Cancer Pain and Depression (INCPAD) trial: Design of a telecare management intervention for cancer-related symptoms and baseline characteristics of study participants. *General Hospital Psychiatry, 31*, 240–253.

Kroenke, K., Theobald, D., Wu, J., Norton, K., Morrison, G., Carpenter, J., & Tu, W. (2010). Effect of telecare management on pain and depression in patients with cancer: A randomized trial. *Journal of American Medical Association, 304*, 163–171.

Krouse, R. S. (2010). Gastrointestinal cancer. In J. C. Holland, W. S. Breitbart, P. B. Jacobsen, M. S. Ledoux, M. J. Loscalzo, & R. McCorkle (Eds.), *Psycho-oncology*. New York: Oxford University Press.

Kutner, J. S., & Smith, M. C. (2011). CAM in chronic pain and palliative care. In R. J. Moore (Ed.), *Handbook of pain and palliative care: Biobehavioral approaches for the life course*. New York: Springer.

Laird, B. J., Boyd, A. C., Colvin, L. A., & Fallon, M. T. (2009). Are cancer pain and depression interdependent? a systematic review. *Psycho-Oncology, 18*, 459–464.

Leon-Pizarro, C., Gich, I., Barthe, E., Rovirosa, A., Farrus, B., Casas, F., Verger, E., Biete, A., Craven-Bartle, J., Sierra, J., & Arcusa, A. (2007). A randomized trial of the effect of training in relaxation and guided imagery techniques in improving psychological and quality-of-life indices for gynecologic and breast brachytherapy patients. *Psycho-Oncology, 16*, 971–979.

Leubbert, K., Dahme, B., & Hasenbring, M. (2001). The effectiveness of relaxation training in reducing treatment-related symptoms and improving emotional adjustment in acute non-surgical cancer treatment: A meta-analytical review. *Psycho-Oncology, 10*, 490–502.

Levin, T. T., & Alici, Y. (2010). Anxiety disorders. In J. C. Holland, W. S. Breitbart, P. B. Jacobsen, M. S. Ledoux, M. J. Loscalzo, & R. McCorkle (Eds.), *Psycho-oncology* (pp. 324–331). New York: Oxford University Press.

Lin, C. C., Lai, Y. L., & Ward, S. E. (2003). Effect of cancer pain on performance status, mood states, and level of hope among Taiwanese cancer patients. *Journal of Pain and Symptom Management, 25*, 29–37.

Lovejoy, N. C., & Matteis, M. (1997). Cognitive-behavioral interventions to manage depression in patients with cancer: Research and theoretical initiatives. *Cancer Nursing, 20*, 155–167.

Lovell, M. R., Forder, P. M., Stockler, M. R., Butow, P., Briganti, E. M., Chye, R., Goldstein, D., & Boyle, F. M. (2010). A randomized controlled trial of a standardized educational intervention for patients with cancer pain. *Journal of Pain and Symptom Management, 40*, 49–59.

Massie, M. J. (2004). Prevalence of depression in patients with cancer. *Journal of the National Cancer Institute. Monographs, 32*, 57–71.

Mazzocato, C., Stiefel, F., Buclin, T., & Berney, A. (2000). Psychopharmacology in supportive care of cancer: A review for the clinician: II. Neuroleptics. *Supportive Care in Cancer, 8*, 89–97.

McGuire, D. B. (2004). Occurrence of cancer pain. *Journal of the National Cancer Institute Monographs, 32*, 51–56.

McQuellon, R. P., Wells, M., Hoffman, S., Craven, B., Russell, G., Cruz, J., Hurt, G., DeChatelet, P., Andrykowski, M. A., & Savage, P. (1998). Reducing distress in cancer patients with an orientation program. *Psycho-Oncology, 7*, 207–217.

Miaskowski, C., Dodd, M., & Lee, K. (2004). Symptom clusters: The new frontier in symptom management research. *Journal of the National Cancer Institute Monographs, 32*, 17–21.

Middlecamp Kodl, M., Lee, J. W., Matthews, A. K., Cummings, S. A., & Olopade, O. I. (2006). Correlates of depressive symptoms among women seeking genetic counseling and risk assessment at a high-risk cancer clinic. *Journal of Genetic Counseling, 15*, 267–276.

Miller, K., & Massie, M. J. (2006). Depression and anxiety. *Cancer Journal, 12*, 388–397.

Miller, K., & Massie, M. J. (2010). Depressive disorders. In J. C. Holland (Ed.), *Psycho-oncology* (pp. 311–318). New York: Oxford University Press.

Miovic, M., & Block, S. (2007). Psychiatric disorders in advanced cancer. *Cancer, 110*, 1665–1676.

Mitte, K. (2005). A meta-analysis of the efficacy of psycho- and pharmacotherapy in panic disorder with and without agoraphobia. *Journal of Affective Disorders, 88*, 27–45.

Moorey, S., Cort, E., Kapari, M., Monroe, B., Hansford, P., Mannix, K., Henderson, M., Fisher, L., & Hotopf, M. (2009). A cluster randomized controlled trial of cognitive behaviour therapy for common mental disorders in patients with advanced cancer. *Psychological Medicine, 39*, 713–723.

Musselman, D. L., Lawson, D. H., Gumnick, J. F., Manatunga, A. K., Penna, S., Goodkin, R. S., Greiner, K., Nemeroff, C. B., & Miller, A. H. (2001). Paroxetine for the prevention of depression induced by high-dose interferon alfa. *The New England Journal of Medicine, 344*, 961–966.

Mystakidou, K., Tsilika, E., Parpa, E., Katsouda, E., Galanos, A., & Vlahos, L. (2006). Psychological distress of patients with advanced cancer: Influence and contribution of pain severity and pain interference. *Cancer Nursing, 29*, 400–405.

National Breast Cancer Centre and National Cancer Control Initiative. (2003). *Clinical practice guidelines for the psychosocial care of adults with cancer*. Camperdown, Australia: National Breast Cancer Centre.

National Comprehensive Cancer Network. (2010). *NCCN clinical practice guidelines in oncology: Distress management Version 1.2011*. Washington: National Comprehensive Cancer Network.

National Institute for Clinical Excellence. (2004). *Improving supportive and palliative care for adults with cancer. The manual*. London: National Institute for Clinical Excellence.

Nelson, C. J., Balk, E. M., & Roth, A. J. (2010). Distress, anxiety, depression, and emotional well-being in African-American men with prostate cancer. *Psycho-Oncology, 19*, 1052–1060.

Newell, S. A., Sanson-Fisher, R. W., & Savolainen, N. J. (2002). Systematic review of psychological therapies for cancer patients: Overview and recommendations for future research. *Journal of the National Cancer Institute, 94*, 558–584.

Orr, K., & Taylor, D. (2007). Psychostimulants in the treatment of depression: A review of the evidence. *CNS Drugs, 21*, 239–257.

Orringer, J. S., Fendrick, A. M., Trask, P. C., Bichakjian, C. K., Schwartz, J. L., Wang, T. S., Karimipour, D. J., & Johnson, T. M. (2005). The effects of a professionally produced videotape on education and anxiety/distress levels for patients with newly diagnosed melanoma: A randomized, prospective clinical trial. *Journal of the American Academy of Dermatology, 53*, 224–229.

Osborn, R. L., Demoncada, A. C., & Feuerstein, M. (2006). Psychosocial interventions for depression, anxiety, and quality of life in cancer survivors: Meta-analyses. *International Journal of Psychiatry in Medicine, 36*, 13–34.

Padilla, G. V., Ferrell, B., Grant, M. M., & Rhiner, M. (1990). Defining the content domain of quality of life for cancer patients with pain. *Cancer Nursing, 13*, 108–115.

Patrick, D. L., Ferketich, S. L., Frame, P. S., Harris, J. J., Hendricks, C. B., Levin, B., Link, M. P., Lustig, C., McLaughlin, J., Reid, L. D., Turrisi, A. T., III, Unutzer, J., & Vernon, S. W. (2004). National institutes of health state-of-the-science conference Statement: symptom management in cancer: Pain, depression, and fatigue, July 15–17. *Journal of the National Cancer Institute Monographs, 2002*, 9–16.

Pirl, W. F. (2004). Evidence report on the occurrence, assessment, and treatment of depression in cancer patients. *Journal of the National Cancer Institute Monographs, 32*, 32–39.

Prasertsri, N., Holden, J., Keefe, F. J., & Wilkie, D. J. (2011). Repressive coping style: Relationships with depression, pain, and pain coping strategies in lung cancer out patients. *Lung Cancer, 71*(2), 235–240.

Radloff, L. S. (1977). The CES-D Scale: A self-report depression scale for research in the general population. *Applied Psychological Measurement, 1*, 385–401.

Raison, C. L., & Miller, A. H. (2003). Depression in cancer: New developments regarding diagnosis and treatment. *Biological Psychiatry, 54*, 283–294.

Ransom, S., Pearman, T. P., Philip, E., & Anwar, D. (2011). Adult cancer-related pain. In R. J. Moore (Ed.), *Handbook of pain and palliative care: Biobehavioral approaches for the life course*. New York: Springer.

Rao, M. R., Raghuram, N., Nagendra, H. R., Gopinath, K. S., Srinath, B. S., Diwakar, R. B., Patil, S., Bilimagga, S. R., Rao, N., & Varambally, S. (2009). Anxiolytic effects of a yoga program in early breast cancer patients undergoing conventional treatment: A randomized controlled trial. *Complementary Therapies in Medicine, 17*, 1–8.

Ravindran, L. N., & Stein, M. B. (2010). The pharmacologic treatment of anxiety disorders: A review of progress. *The Journal of Clinical Psychiatry, 71*, 839–854.

Redd, W. H., Montgomery, G. H., & DuHamel, K. N. (2001). Behavioral intervention for cancer treatment side effects. *Journal of the National Cancer Institute, 93*, 810–823.

Rickels, K., Pollack, M. H., Sheehan, D. V., & Haskins, J. T. (2000). Efficacy of extended-release venlafaxine in non-depressed outpatients with generalized anxiety disorder. *The American Journal of Psychiatry, 157*, 968–974.

Rickels, K., Zaninelli, R., McCafferty, J., Bellew, K., Iyengar, M., & Sheehan, D. (2003). Paroxetine treatment of generalized anxiety disorder: A double-blind, placebo-controlled study. *The American Journal of Psychiatry, 160*, 749–756.

Rodin, G., Lloyd, N., Katz, M., Green, E., Mackay, J. A., & Wong, R. K. (2007). The treatment of depression in cancer patients: A systematic review. *Supportive Care in Cancer, 15*, 123–136.

Roth, A. J., & Massie, M. J. (2007). Anxiety and its management in advanced cancer. *Current Opinion in Supportive and Palliative Care, 1*, 50–56.

Roy-Byrne, P. P., Davidson, K. W., Kessler, R. C., Asmundson, G. J., Goodwin, R. D., Kubzansky, L., Lydiard, R. B., Massie, M. J., Katon, W., Laden, S. K., & Stein, M. B. (2008). Anxiety disorders and comorbid medical illness. *General Hospital Psychiatry, 30*, 208–225.

Savard, J., Simard, S., Giguere, I., Ivers, H., Morin, C. M., Maunsell, E., Gagnon, P., Robert, J., & Marceau, D. (2006). Randomized clinical trial on cognitive therapy for depression in women with metastatic breast cancer: Psychological and immunological effects. *Palliative & Supportive Care, 4*, 219–237.

Schwartz, L., Lander, M., & Chochinov, H. M. (2002). Current management of depression in cancer patients. *Oncology (Williston Park), 16*, 1102–1110. discussion 1110, 1105–1114.

Sellick, S. M., & Crooks, D. L. (1999). Depression and cancer: An appraisal of the literature for prevalence, detection, and practice guideline development for psychological interventions. *Psycho-Oncology, 8*, 215–333.

Shakin, E. J., & Holland, J. (1988). Depression and pancreatic cancer. *Journal of Pain and Symptom Management, 3*, 194–198.

Sheard, T., & Maguire, P. (1999). The effect of psychological interventions on anxiety and depression in cancer patients: Results of two meta-analyses. *British Journal of Cancer, 80*, 1770–1780.

Simon, S. T., Higginson, I. J., Booth, S., Harding, R., Bausewein, C. (2010). Benzodiazepines for the relief of breathlessness in advanced malignant and non-malignant diseases in adults. *Cochrane Database Systemic Reviews, 1*, CD007354.

Sist, T. C., Florio, G. A., Miner, M. F., Lema, M. J., & Zevon, M. A. (1998). The relationship between depression and pain language in cancer and chronic non-cancer pain patients. *Journal of Pain and Symptom Management, 15*, 350–358.

Smith, H. S., Datta, S., & Manchikanti, L. (2011). Evidence-based pharmacotherapy of chronic pain. In R. J. Moore (Ed.), *Handbook of pain and palliative care: Biobehavioral approaches for the life course*. New York: Springer.

Spencer, R., Nilsson, M., Wright, A., Pirl, W., & Prigerson, H. (2010). Anxiety disorders in advanced cancer patients: Correlates and predictors of end-of-life outcomes. *Cancer, 116*, 1810–1819.

Spiegel, D., & Bloom, J. R. (1983). Group therapy and hypnosis reduce metastatic breast carcinoma pain. *Psychosomatic Medicine, 45*, 333–339.

Spiegel, D., Sands, S., & Koopman, C. (1994). Pain and depression in patients with cancer. *Cancer, 74*, 2570–2578.

Spielberger, C. D. (1983). *Manual for the State-Trait Anxiety Inventory*. Palo Alto: Consulting Psychologists Press.

Stark, D., Kiely, M., Smith, A., Velikova, G., House, A., & Selby, P. (2002). Anxiety disorders in cancer patients: Their nature, associations, and relation to quality of life. *Journal of Clinical Oncology, 20*, 3137–3148.

Stark, D. P. H., & House, A. (2000). Anxiety in cancer patients. *British Journal of Cancer, 83*, 1261–1267.

Stein, D. J., Zungu-Dirwayi, N., van der Linden, G. J. H., Seedat, S. (2006). Pharmacotherapy for post traumatic stress disorder (PTSD). Cochrane database of systematic reviews 2006, Issue 1. Art No. CD002795. DOI: 10.1002/14651858.

Stephenson, N. L., Swanson, M., Dalton, J., Keefe, F. J., & Engelke, M. (2007). Partner-delivered reflexology: Effects on cancer pain and anxiety. *Oncology Nursing Forum, 34*, 127–132.

Strang, P., & Qvarner, H. (1990). Cancer-related pain and its influence on quality of life. *Anticancer Research, 10*, 109–112.

Szucs-Reed, R. P., & Gallagher, R. M. (2011). Chronic pain and opioids. In R. J. Moore (Ed.), *Handbook of pain and palliative care: Biobehavioral approaches for the life course*. New York: Springer.

Teunissen, S. C., de Graeff, A., Voest, E. E., & de Haes, J. C. (2007a). Are anxiety and depressed mood related to physical symptom burden? A study in hospitalized advanced cancer patients. *Palliative Medicine, 21*, 341–346.

Teunissen, S. C. C. M., Wesker, W., Kruitwagen, C., de Haes, H. C. J. M., Voest, E. E., & de Graeff, A. (2007b). Symptom prevalence in patients with incurable cancer: A systematic review. *Journal of Pain and Symptom Management, 34*, 94–104.

Tjemsland, L., Soreide, J. A., & Malt, U. F. (1998). Posttraumatic stress symptoms in operable breast cancer III: Status one year after surgery. *Breast Cancer Research and Treatment, 47*, 141–151.

Turk, D. C., Sist, T. C., Okifuji, A., Miner, M. F., Florio, G., Harrison, P., Massey, J., Lema, M. L., & Zevon, M. A. (1998). Adaptation to metastatic cancer pain, regional/local cancer pain and non-cancer pain: Role of psychological and behavioral factors. *Pain, 74*, 247–256.

Turner, J., Zapart, S., Pedersen, K., Rankin, N., Luxford, K., & Fletcher, J. (2005). Clinical practice guidelines for the psychosocial care of adults with cancer. *Psycho-Oncology, 14*, 159–173.

Uitterhoeve, R. J., Vernooy, M., Litjens, M., Potting, K., Bensing, J., De Mulder, P., & van Achterberg, T. (2004). Psychosocial interventions for patients with advanced cancer – A systematic review of the literature. *British Journal of Cancer, 91*, 1050–1062.

Vahdaninia, M., Omidvari, S., & Montazeri, A. (2010). What do predict anxiety and depression in breast cancer patients? A follow-up study. *Social Psychiatry and Psychiatric Epidemiology, 45*, 355–361.

Valentine, A. D. (2003). Cancer pain and depression: Management of the dual-diagnosed patient. *Current Pain and Headache Reports, 7*, 262–269.

van Balkom, A. J., Bakker, A., Spinhoven, P., Blaauw, B. M., Smeenk, S., & Ruesink, B. (1997). A meta-analysis of the treatment of panic disorder with or without agoraphobia: A comparison of psychopharmacological, cognitive-behavioral, and combination treatments. *The Journal of Nervous and Mental Disease, 185*, 510–516.

van den Beuken-van Everdingen, M. H., de Rijke, J. M., Kessels, A. G., Schouten, H. C., van Kleef, M., & Patijn, J. (2007). Prevalence of pain in patients with cancer: A systematic review of the past 40 years. *Annals of Oncology, 18*, 1437–1449.

Williams, L. A. (2007). Clinical management of symptom clusters. *Seminars in Oncology Nursing, 23*, 113–120.

Williams, S., & Dale, J. (2006). The effectiveness of treatment for depression/depressive symptoms in adults with cancer: A systematic review. *British Journal of Cancer, 94*, 372–390.

Wilson, K. G., Chochinov, H. M., Allard, P., Chary, S., Gagnon, P. R., Macmillan, K., De Luca, M., O'Shea, F., Kuhl, D., & Fainsinger, R. L. (2009). Prevalence and correlates of pain in the Canadian National Palliative Care Survey. *Pain Research & Management, 14*, 365–370.

Wilson, K. G., Chochinov, H. M., Skirko, M. G., Allard, P., Chary, S., Gagnon, P. R., Macmillan, K., De Luca, M., O'Shea, F., Kuhl, D., Fainsinger, R. L., & Clinch, J. J. (2007). Depression and anxiety disorders in palliative cancer care. *Journal of Pain and Symptom Management, 33*, 118–129.

Wurzman, R., Jonas, W., & Giordano, J. (2008). Chronic pain and depression: A spectrum disorder? *The Pain Practitioner, 18*(2), 48–54.

Yates, P., Edwards, H., Nash, R., Aranda, S., Purdie, D., Najman, J., Skerman, H., & Walsh, A. (2004). A randomized controlled trial of a nurse-administered educational intervention for improving cancer pain management in ambulatory settings. *Patient Education and Counseling, 53*, 227–237.

Zigmond, A. S., & Snaith, R. P. (1983). The hospital anxiety and depression scale. *Acta Psychiatrica Scandinavica, 67*, 361–370.

Zimmerman, L., Story, K. T., Gaston-Johansson, F., & Rowles, J. R. (1996). Psychological variables and cancer pain. *Cancer Nursing, 19*, 44–53.

Chapter 34
Support Groups for Chronic Pain

Penney Cowan

Why Peer Lead Groups Are Needed

Imagine if your life were stopped short by an injury or illness that prevented you from doing your daily routine. Living with any chronic disease or illness can be difficult at best. The inability to maintain a normal lifestyle prevents the normal daily interactions that fill the days with meaningful activities. When one loses their ability to function, they lose all hope that there is anything beyond the day-to-day suffering. Their entire being becomes lost in the veil of pain that seems to fall over even the smallest hopes and abilities. They lose their identity. While there are many things that might help, knowing that you are not alone is critical. Being able to identify with someone else is comforting and the most important components of a peer lead group. The aim of this chapter is to help you understand the value of peer groups, how to establish a group including such things as governance, funding, publicizing the groups, meeting formats, and maintaining a group.

The Problem of Pain

The annual total of both direct and indirect costs for chronic pain are estimated to be as high as $294.5 billion per year (National Academies of Sciences and Institute of Medicine 2001), with back pain alone estimated to cost in excess of $100 billion per year (Katz 2006) (see also May 2011).

While the enormity and the cost of chronic pain of these numbers may be surprising, to people who must live with pain the numbers validate that they are not alone and the problem of pain. What the numbers do not provide, however, are the human costs of pain (see also Palermo 2011). A person with pain finds that every plan they make is controlled by the fear of not knowing; not knowing how they will feel, the intensity of their pain, how well they will sleep and if they will have the energy to follow through with their plans. Fear of the pain controls the person and it is vital that the fear is addressed (see also Donovan et al. 2011; Palermo 2011). There is no one better to understand these fears than another person with pain.

Many of us define ourselves by what we can accomplish in a day. As our ability to function decreases, so does our self-esteem. There is a point in the long difficult road from a functional person to a dependent patient that any hope for a better tomorrow disappears. In some ways, we believe that we have failed; failed to benefit from all that our health care providers have done for us. Many lose

P. Cowan (✉)
American Chronic Pain Association, Rocklin, CA, USA

R.J. Moore (ed.), *Handbook of Pain and Palliative Care: Biobehavioral Approaches for the Life Course,*   639
DOI 10.1007/978-1-4419-1651-8_34, © Springer Science+Business Media, LLC 2012

all hope that life will improve so they seek out a way to relieve their pain. They are willing to do almost anything if someone promises a cure or relief.

More than anything, a person with pain needs validation; to have his or her health care provider believe their level of pain, their desire for relief and hope for tomorrow (see also Palermo 2011, This Volume). One experiences many feelings when pain invades our life. Pain is invisible and it is not always at the same level of intensity. Having good days intermingled with more difficult days where abilities are greatly reduced creates a sense of self-doubt and fear. It is these feelings of self-doubt and fear that needs to be addressed if any type of improvement is possible.

Window of Hope

As pain consumes our very being, hope can die (see also, Coulehan 2011; Penson et al. 2011). While we try to make others understand the impact the pain has on our very being – both body and mind – no one can really understand. That is unless they also are living a life filled with pain. There is a connection that happens when there is a common denominator that brings them together, even if it is chronic pain. Suddenly there is no need to explain. No need to explain why you can function 1 day and then are unable to do anything for the next 3 days. When you are in a group of your peers – people with pain – you are immediately validated no matter what you may be able to do at any given moment. You realize, perhaps for the first time in a very long time that you are not the only one who is trying to live with persistent pain. There is a real sense of relief to know that there is another person who you can talk with that will understand how some of the most remedial task can turn into overwhelming obstacles. There is a real sense of hope in listening to other in the group talk about how far they have come that provides a sense of hope that perhaps tomorrow could be better.

Value of Peer Support Groups

Being part of peer lead support group means that you no longer have to defend your pain, how you look, or your fluctuation in your ability to function. Defenses that have become a part of you are no longer necessary. Everyone in the group understands the confusion of long-term pain. They are accepting of you no matter what your ability. It is the validation that they provide that, for many, allows them to take their first steps on their journey from patient to person.

When pain becomes the unwelcomed guest in your life it can eat away at your ability to function. With each activity that you erase from your life, a small part of who you thought were also disappears. At some point, you find that you define yourself by your disabilities rather than your abilities. However, when you become part of a peer group of others who understand what it is like to live with pain, you feel a sense of belonging. In watching other members focus on their abilities rather than talking about their disabilities, one can find encouragement to at least try moving forward one step at a time.

The simple act of being in a group provides a sense of community and belonging that was lost long ago. You are now part of a community of like-minded people who are willing to work within your limits to ensure that you are included in activities. Being part of a group of friends is something that the pain took away a long time ago. There is no need to justify any of your actions, they understand. The isolation that your pain created fades as you become a more active part of a group of your peers. This may being you one step closer on as you travel on your journey from patient to person.

Peers understand the challenges the simplest of tasks can become. They can share their real life knowledge and experience of how to accomplish the task, even if it takes longer. It is the change in how one begins to approach life. Instead of focusing on all the disabilities the pain has created, with the help of peers who understand the challenges of living with pain can help others look at their abilities. A positive attitude can be one of the most important outcomes in being involved with a peer support group.

Types of Groups

There are a number of different types of groups that are available today. Each one has its own advantages and some disadvantages.

- *Peer lead groups* provide a level playing field. What that means is that each person who is a part of the group shares the same concerns as all the other members. These groups can focus on the issues that brought them together and exploring way they can begin to manage all the obstacles created because of the pain. There tends to be less focus on specific pain problems and more focus on managing the pain. There is usually no cost to attend these groups.
- *Pain specific groups* are designed to bring people together that all have the same condition. This means that everyone in the group may all have fibromyalgia. While it provides the validation and support a person needs, it can also provide specific information about the condition. Group members can share resources they have found to better understand the current research and treatments offered. The one drawback to this kind of group is that because they all share the same condition they often compare their progress, medication and treatment with each other. It is important to make sure that each person in the group understands that they are all individuals and what works for one may not work for the other. There is usually no cost to attend these groups.
- *Therapy groups* are usually facilitated by a health care professional. While they bring together groups of people who share a common bond, the tone of the group is often very different from a peer lead groups. People who attend therapy groups usually have different expectations. They attend these groups as part of their treatment plan. While they are in a group of their peers it is a completely different atmosphere. In peer lead groups there should be no medical advice or treatments offered. Therapy groups are just that, therapy be it to change behaviors or attitudes. There may be a cost for attending this type of group.
- *Educational groups* that meet for a set number of weeks are typically part of a pain management program that are taught by hospital or clinical staff. They have a set curriculum and once the sessions are over, there is rarely any other support group available to them. These groups are useful as first steps in the journey from patient to person, but too often only scratch the surface of what is really needed for a person to better manage their pain. There is usually a cost for this.
- *Aftercare groups* can be an important part of one's ability to maintain all that they learned and the progress they made during educational groups. They are usually open-ended and are available to anyone who has completed a pain program for as long as they feel they need it. There is often a cost to attend these groups, but they may be available without any charges.
- *Groups based on demographics* are not as common as the other types of groups, however they do provide a unique connection for its members. These types of groups focus on a specific health problem that is shared but is also limited by a specific demographic such as age, vocation or gender. However, when it comes to living with pain there is such a strong identification with each other that age, gender or any other issues never really prevents the group from moving forward.

Governance of Group

Having a strong foundation for any group is important to its ongoing success. Before any decisions are made, it needs to be determined how you want to structure the group. If the idea is to establish a community-based group that will meet to discuss, share and encourage each other through difficult times, then governance is not so important. However, if you want to formalize the group and grow into a recognized organization that can develop as the need arises, then it is important to begin to build a foundation. One way to build this foundation is to develop a board of directors. Establishing a board of directors for a group designed to help people with pain can be problematic. People who are already struggling with managing their pain have limited energy so the best rule of thumb is to keep the board as simple as possible.

A board of 3 of 4 people would be significant to begin. The people establishing the group will be the ones to determine what they want to see over time with the group as it grows. It is helpful to have people with a variety of skills that will support the needs of the group. Some of the skills to consider are people who are good with finances, writing letters, knowing who and how to reach the other community and perhaps a health care provider that would be available to provide support to the board members.

Funding

Funding the group will again depend on what the needs of the group are. The need for funds will also be a determining factor in the governance of the group. If you only want to have a free will offering to cover incidental costs, then the offering would support the effort. However, if funds are needed for rental fees on a meeting room, supplies, postage and copying, then funding the group becomes more difficult. This group may have to look to the community for support through donations and small fundraising activities. It is only when you have large expenses that one would think about obtaining a formal tax-exempt status. With that comes a great deal of responsibility and might be more than the members are willing to do. Affiliating with another established organization might be the best alternative.

How to Form a Peer Lead Support Group

The first step in forming a peer lead support group is to define a mission. State clearly and simply what it is you want to accomplish. Keep it short and to the point so that it will be clear to anyone that reads it exactly what your mission is. For the remainder of this chapter we will discuss the steps for establishing and maintaining a peer lead support group.

You need to establish guidelines for the group to ensure that the meeting will run smoothly and there will be no questions about what is acceptable behavior and what is not acceptable in group meetings. Trusting each member of the group is vital for its survival. Keep in mind that most people with pain have been through a great deal and are not only hurting physically but quite often are emotionally drained. For this reason each person in the group should hold what it shared in group in the strictest confidence at all times. Understanding that what is said in group will remain in group will help members to openly share issues they have been struggling with. It is very beneficial to have a place that a person can go to talk freely and openly about what they are feeling and the impact the pain has on his or her life is priceless.

At the initial meeting it is important to explain that the group does not provide any type of medical advice or treatment. The group is designed to provide an atmosphere of understanding and a means to gain support from their peers. Each person who attends the group will get as much out of the group as he or she invests. While there is a designated facilitator of the group, each member of the group should share in the responsibility to ensure that it holds to its mission. And because there are no health care providers involved in the meetings, be very clear that there will be no therapy of any kind provided during the meetings or among members outside of meetings.

Peer lead groups should realize that their most valuable resource is the group members. Placing the needs of those attending meetings should always remain the number one priority. As members begin to share problems they are having it is easy to want to provide advice on what they should do. The problem with giving advice is that essentially you will be taking responsibility for others' actions. It is always advised to ask them what they think they should do. The group can openly discuss possible opinions to provide some alterative solutions, but in the end it is the individuals' decision to determine what will be best for him or her.

Identify the Goals of the Group

It is important to learn coping skills so that members may begin to regain some control over their lives. While it is important to focus on the needs of individuals attending the group, having materials to help them address the many obstacles that pain presents can help the group stay on track. The American Chronic Pain Association has a workbook, *From Patient to Person: First Steps* which provides a number of learned skills to help each member as they move forward in their journey form patient to person. It is critical that it is clearly understood that the goal of the group is to help individuals improve the quality of his or her life, increase their level of functioning and reduce their sense of suffering. The goal of the group is not to eliminate their pain, however they may find as they apply some of the coping skills to their daily life their pain levels are reduced.

Establishing the Logistics

Three questions you need to answer: where, when, and how often. A group designed for people with pain has special needs. One of the factors that must be taken into account is where to hold the meetings. Is the location centrally located and easy to get to from various parts of the community?

Of course finding a meeting space that is provided free of charge is the ideal solution. But there are other factors that must be considered. Where to meet given the needs of members must take into consideration if the location is handicap accessible. Are their stairs that will prevent some from getting to the meeting room? Is there plenty of space for parking that is free of charge? Keep in mind that people with pain often have limited resources and parking fees may determine whether or not they will be able to attend meetings.

Another consideration when thinking about starting a group is what time of the day the meeting will be held? If there are a number of members who are older adults they may not want to drive at night. For those who are still able to work, it might be better to have an evening meeting. And for some it really won't matter. It is important to understand the best time of day to meet. Also what day would work best? Weekdays usually are the preference, but there are groups that prefer to meet on weekends when family can watch small children, be free to drive the person with pain to group, or perhaps simply because that may be the only time the facility has free meeting space. Then you have to consider how many times during a month does the group want to meet. The usual choice is twice a month, but for some it is better to meet every week. The members seem to need the support and count on the group to help them through the week. Other groups may meet only once a month. Again it depends on the members but it may also be controlled by the availability of the meeting room.

Who should attend the group meetings? As stated earlier people with pain share a common bond that breaks down many barriers such as age, socioeconomic considerations, and gender. The group should be open to anyone who has pain and is willing to take an active role in regaining some control of his or her life. Age is rarely a factor. The only factor that the majority of the group has is if the person lives with chronic pain. Health care providers should not be part of the ongoing meetings out of concern that the groups will become therapy groups where members are looking to the health care provider for individual health questions. It is also important to not have family members or significant others attend the meetings with the person with pain. Usually there are many issues that would not be addressed with a family members present. The groups need to provide a risk-free place to speak openly and free without fear of repercussions from families. If there are several family members who feel they need support, it helps to establish a separate meeting space and time for them. Families and significant others experience many if not all of the same things as a person with pain. The only difference is they do not feel the pain, but their lives are very much controlled by their loved one's pain.

Publicizing Group Meetings

How to reach prospective members can be difficult but it is important to the establishment and growth of the group. There are several ways to create awareness in the community.

- Public service announcements (PSA) are brief messages placed in community papers and radio stations that provide information about when, where and who to contact about the meetings. With the extensive use of the Internet today it is better to place a PSA on-line rather than in newspapers.
- Building relationships with health care professionals within the community is another good way to make the service of a support group known. These are the folks that have daily encounters with people with pain who not only need peer support but also can identify those who are interested and have a desire to take an active role in the recovery process. Contacting local hospitals, rehabilitation clinics and other health care facilities and talking with the social service department is the best place to start. Always have a brief one page overview of objectives and goals for the group when meeting with any health care professional.
- Outreach to other community groups is another way to let the community know about the group and services it offers. There are usually local clubs like the Lions Club, Rotary and civic organizations that are always looking for speakers.

Having Meaningful Meetings

Anyone who attends a support group designed to meet the needs of people with pain already knows what it is like to live with pain. Spending a large portion of the meeting time allowing each member to talk about their physical symptoms only focuses on pain reinforcing the negatives leaving little time for problem solving. To avoid this trap, it is important to keep in mind the mission statement. Why is this group meeting? Staying true to the mission will not only keep the group focused, but maintain the integrity of the organization.

It is also important to have a meeting format and stick to it so that the majority of time is constructive. It is important for each new person to tell their story, but it should be very limited with the understanding that as they get more involved in the meetings their story will become more evident. Members need to know that each meeting they attend will provide them with an important take-away message that will help them better manage their pain. For that reason it is important to have a plan in place from the beginning. An open format that touches on many of the coping skills, if only briefly, will provide the positive reinforcement that members need to maintain their wellness.

It is always nice to be able to have as many people as possible access the services you provide. However, it is not always possible to have large numbers respond to your efforts. What is important is to have a solid core group of 2 or 3 people. For the facilitator, starting out small allows them to "grow" into the role of facilitating the group and having the ability to grow with the group in understanding and knowledge about the group process and the subject matter. The core group will be the foundation of the group moving forward. As new members attend the meeting it will be the core members who can help by working with them individually to answer questions and provide background information that the group has already reviewed. The core members will be able to share the responsibility of welcoming new members into the group at any time.

Establishing ground rules at the beginning of the group experience is necessary to inform members of what is appropriate and what is not. Providing a list of written do's and don'ts will help reinforce the rules. When it comes to groups for people with pain one issue that always comes up is medication. Each person will respond differently to medications and may have an other health care issues. It is best to always encourage members to discuss any questions or issues that they might have with their health care provider or pharmacist. They are the only ones who really know your medical history and can advice you on any medications. Other rules like not talking about physical symptoms, not giving advice, being respectful of other's point of view are but a few. Work with members to determine what rules they might like to see put into place for the group.

No one said that living with pain is easy. Going to a support group for people with pain can be downright impossible. There is something about asking for help when life is out of control and the body hurts so much it can hurt to breath. Ones sense of hope vanished long ago. So, the act of going to a group takes a huge amount of courage. Acknowledging their courage while making a new member comfortable is paramount to whether or not they will return. There is a fine balance between making them feel welcome and providing them with a sense that they are not alone. The group can simply accomplish this by providing validation that their pain is real and there is no longer a need to be defensive. The first group session will set the frame of mind for the future sessions. Having a welcoming kit that includes the mission statement, an overview of what the group has to offer, and what is expected from the new member is very beneficial. Paring the new member with an established member to contact in-between meetings will help "fill in the gaps" that may happen at group. Any group that meets for a long period of time will have covered topics that new members are not aware of. It would be counterproductive to review the basics over and over so for a new member to have someone to help them understand is critical.

One concern that people with pain have is how comfortable the chairs will be no matter where they go. Like many other areas of living with pain, the questions of comfort and access are critical to their decision to attend. No matter where the meeting is, comfort has to be considered. Anyone who might be considering attending the meeting needs to know that the room can accommodate their special needs. While no one expects lush sofa and chairs, they do need sturdy chairs that support the back. It is also important to let prospective members know that they can bring pillows if they need them for added comfort and that sitting on the floor or standing during the meeting is not a problem. Don't forget to let them know that dress is casual and comfort is the first priority.

Traps

Establishing and maintaining a peer lead support group is one of the most rewarding experiences a person can have. It can, however, be very frustrating for a variety of traps that can occur. When thinking about forming a peer lead group many people believe that they need help, however, it is important that they don't give away the control of the group to a member. Keep in mind that staying true to the mission is critical to long-term success of the group. Maintaining control of the group is important while still sharing some of the responsibility. Defining the areas where help is needed and asking members to help will allow control to remain with the facilitator.

When a group of people come together because their lives are controlled by pain it can be difficult to stay on topic. From time to time the conversation may get off of the topic and a member will redirect the discussion. The key is to recognize that the conversation has strayed off topic and knowing how to direct it back. It is helpful to have a few statements to help accomplish this. One way is to acknowledge that the conversation is important and the group understands how important to share but we need to get back to the topic for today. It is important to let the member know that if necessary they can stay after group and continue to conversation.

Subgroups are another trap that groups can fall into. From time to time members will pair off in smaller groups that share common interest. The problem is when these smaller groups become established within a group. It can make other members feel like outsiders, misfits, or resentful. They may feel as if the group creates more stress and pain than they are getting out of it and simply stop attending the meetings. To avoid this it is important to keep the conversation open to all members. If a member is not taking part in the discussion, make a point of drawing them into the conversation by asking their opinion in the form of a question related to the topic.

Funding the group should not be a main topic of discussion. Always asking members for financial support can misdirect the focus of the group. People with pain already struggle with their personal finances, they don't need to cope with it at every meeting or they will stop attending. Some donations may be necessary from time to time, but be careful not to make it the main topic of the group. If a person ask if there is a cost to attending the group, it is important to let them know that the most costly part of the group is the investment of their time to help him or herself.

Maintaining the Group Long Term

Communications with members between meetings is important. Calling members who didn't make it to a meeting to ask if they are okay can make a difference in their attitude toward the group. It lets them know that they were missed and they are important enough for someone to take the time to call and make sure they are alright.

Sharing responsibility of the group will prevent burnout of the facilitator and allow the members feel as if they are giving back. Initially, the person who established the group will be baring the bulk of the responsibility for the group. Once a few people attend on a regular basis, it is important to ask them to help with the group. Overall there is not a lot to do to maintain a peer lead support group, but if one person bears the burden for the entire group, they may become burned out over time. Knowing that they can look to the members to help is important to the longevity of the group.

Introduce new materials whenever possible in group. Part of keeping a group together is to keep it fresh. People are attending the meeting for peer support but they also are looking for a means to manage their pain. Each person learns in different ways so having the ability to provide new information in a variety of formats will help members better understand their role. In addition, the field of pain management has many resources available that can easily be accessed and introduced to the group.

Welcoming new members can be difficult. Those attending the meeting for the first time have not had the benefit of learning with the rest of the group. They feel as if they came in the middle of the "story." It is important that new members are provided with the basics of pain management but it is unfair to members who have been attending for some time. A sponsor program can provide a support system for anyone who is involved in the group. It will benefit both the new member as well as established members. For the first time the new member will have someone to talk with who understands what it is like to live with pain. Having one person to work with, learn from and most importantly trust will help new members. Instead of constantly reviewing materials with the entire group, the sponsor can work one-to-one with a new member to provide information already discussed in meetings. The sponsor program also helps the established member by reinforcing what they have already covered. Learning to live with pain is an on-going process and the basics are important to keep fresh.

Types of Meetings

There are a number of ways that you can keep the group fresh and offer new materials and information. The most important component of the group is to allow members time to talk about issues they are struggling with and discuss coping skills that will help them address these problems. However, there is also a need to provide a variety of information, resources and social activities.

A peer lead group should never offer any type of medical advice, however, members need to have information so that they can make informed decisions. To help members learn more about all aspects of pain management you can invite a guest speaker. It is important to make sure that the members are interested in the topic and are comfortable having the speaker attend their meeting. Depending on the speaker and the topic it may also be possible to open the meeting up to the public. The speakers can range from physicians, physical therapists and pharmacists to cooking demonstrations and craft lessons. Not all meetings need to be focused on pain. Keep in mind that a key component for managing pain is redirecting your thoughts off the pain and onto things that you may have more control over.

Keeping with the theme of focusing on things other than pain recreational meetings can be a wonderful way to help members experience how to redirect their focus from their pain. They can be as simple as going to a movie as a group to having members make collages using magazines to reflect their personalities and interests. Ask members if they have any special talents they would be willing to share with the group or teach them a skill. Even a meeting where members meet for lunch or dinner can be very helpful. The act of being involved in the everyday occurrences that most people take for granted can be a major hurtle for a person with pain. Doing simple things as a group helps members to see that they still have the ability to enjoy life and take part in normal activities.

Another way to introduce new materials into the group and at the same time share responsibility for the meeting with the members is a book study group. There are numerous books available that would be appropriate for a peer group. In each meeting, a member would lead a discussion of one of the chapters in the book. The topics could range from nutrition and diet to self-awareness and sleep hygiene. There is no limit to the types of books that the group could select.

It is never wise to have family members attend group meetings. It makes it difficult for member to be open and honest about their feelings, especially when they may be having trouble with a family member. If there is an interest from family members to have access to others who live with a person with pain, they can start a group that will meet their needs. The American Chronic Pain Association has a manual especially designed for those living with a person with pain. While they do not experience the physical pain, they must deal with many of the same feelings and often need peers to talk with.

Resources for Starting and Maintain a Support Group

Developing a peer lead support group is one thing, but getting the word out so that people are aware of its existence is another matter. It can take time and effort to establish a group in the community. Identifying the media outlets in the local area and sending regular meeting announcements about the meeting can help reach people. Remember, simply having an announcement in a local paper one time does not mean everyone will see it. It takes repeated announcements in local papers and other media outlets to ensure that the information about the group reaches the people intended. Posters placed in pharmacies, churches, community centers, and health club is another way to get the word out about group meetings.

In addition to raising awareness about the group, there will be as many issues that people with pain deal with as there are people. For some, pain is not the main problem. It is important to develop a list of resources on a variety of organizations and agencies within the community. People with pain often need help in the following areas:

- Health insurance
- Access to health care provider
- Physiological help
- Financial assistance
- Transportation assistance
- Home care
- Crisis intervention

Establishing the group means that those in need will look to the group and the resources that are available to provide support, direction and information. It is important to ensure that you have access to community resources. One place that can provide a variety of information about community agencies is the local United Way. They work with other organizations keeping up-to-date records of services provided. Local hospitals also can be helpful in directing group members to services that can help them address their individual problems. Usually the Social Service Department is the starting place in accessing information about available resources. Some community churches and houses of worship can also offer help for a variety of problems listed above. If you do not know the answer to questions or concerns, don't be afraid to admit that you don't know but let them know that you will make every effort to find out and get back to them.

As we move forward with both our understanding for managing chronic pain and knowledge of how to reduce suffering while improving quality of life, there will always be a place for peer support. The most effective approach would be for the health care community and people with pain to work together to bridge the gap in understanding and acceptance of the needs of both sides. Teamwork is the key to a positive future in the field of pain management. No one can do it alone, it takes all involved to become active participants. For many there may always be some level of pain, but that does not mean that they have to relinquish their life to the pain. There is hope and life after pain.

References

Coulehan, J. (2011). Suffering, hope, and healing. In R. J. Moore (Ed.), *Handbook of pain and palliative care: Biobehavioral approaches for the life course*. New York: Springer.

Donovan, K. A., Thompson, L. M. A., & Jacobsen, P. B. (2011). Pain, depression and anxiety in cancer. In R. J. Moore (Ed.), *Handbook of pain and palliative care: Biobehavioral approaches for the life course*. New York: Springer.

Katz, J. N. (2006). Lumbar disc disorders and low-back pain: socioeconomic factors and consequences. *Journal of Bone and Joint Surgery, 88*(Suppl 2), 21–24.

May, S. (2011). Chronic low back pain. In R. J. Moore (Ed.), *Handbook of pain and palliative care: Biobehavioral approaches for the life course*. New York: Springer.

National Academies of Sciences and Institute of Medicine. (2001). *Musculoskeletal disorders and the workplace: Low back pain and upper extremities*. Washington: National Academies Press.

Ngo Su-Mien, L., Geet Yi, G. L., & Penson, R. T. (2011). Hope in the context of pain and palliative care. In R. J. Moore (Ed.), *Handbook of pain and palliative care: Biobehavioral approaches for the life course*. New York: Springer.

Palermo, Y. (2011). The art of pain: The patient's perspective of chronic pain. In R. J. Moore (Ed.), *Handbook of pain and palliative care: Biobehavioral approaches for the life course*. New York: Springer.

Chapter 35
CAM in Chronic Pain and Palliative Care

Jean S. Kutner and Marlaine C. Smith

Complementary and Alternative Medicine (CAM)

What Is Complementary and Alternative Medicine (CAM)?

Complementary and alternative medicine (CAM) encompasses diverse medical and health care systems, practices, and products that are not generally considered part of conventional medicine. Conventional medicine (also called Western or allopathic medicine) is medicine as practiced by holders of M.D. (medical doctor) and D.O. (doctor of osteopathy) degrees and by allied health professionals, such as physical therapists, psychologists, and registered nurses. The boundaries between CAM and conventional medicine are not absolute, and specific CAM practices may, over time, become widely accepted. "Complementary medicine" refers to use of CAM together with conventional medicine, such as using acupuncture in addition to usual care to help lessen pain. "Alternative medicine" refers to use of CAM instead of conventional medicine. The characterization of specific health systems, practices, and products as within the purview of CAM changes continually as new CAMs are introduced and therapies with scientifically demonstrated safety and efficacy are integrated into conventional medical care (http://nccam.nih.gov/health/whatiscam/).

The National Center for Complementary and Alternative Medicine (NCCAM) groups CAM into *three primary categories*: (1) natural products, which includes use of a variety of herbal medicines (also known as botanicals), vitamins, minerals, and other "natural products" as well as probiotics; (2) *mind–body practices,* which focus on the interactions among the brain, mind, body, and behavior, with the intent to use the mind to affect physical functioning and promote health. Many CAM practices embody this concept, including meditation, yoga, acupuncture, deep-breathing exercises, guided imagery, qi gong, and tai chi. Of note, while acupuncture is considered to be a part of mind–body medicine, it is also a component of energy medicine, manipulative and body-based practices, and traditional Chinese medicine; and (3) manipulative and body-based practices, which include spinal manipulation (chiropractic) and massage therapy (MT). *Other CAM practices* include: (1) manipulation of energy fields to influence health (e.g., healing touch, Reiki, therapeutic touch (TT), magnet therapy); (2) movement therapy (e.g., pilates); (3) traditional healers (e.g., Native American

J.S. Kutner, MD, MSPH
Division of General Internal Medicine, Department of Medicine, University of Colorado
School of Medicine, Aurora, CO, USA

M.C. Smith, RN, PhD, AHN-BC, FAAN
Christine E. Lynn College of Nursing, Florida Atlantic University, Boca Raton, FL, USA

R.J. Moore (ed.), *Handbook of Pain and Palliative Care: Biobehavioral Approaches for the Life Course*,
DOI 10.1007/978-1-4419-1651-8_35, © Springer Science+Business Media, LLC 2012

healers); and (4) whole medical systems, which are complete systems of theory and practice that have evolved over time in different cultures and apart from conventional medicine (e.g., traditional Chinese medicine, Ayurvedic medicine) (http://nccam.nih.gov/health/whatiscam/).

How Prevalent Is Use of CAM?

Despite the fact that rigorous, well-designed clinical trials for many CAM therapies are often lacking and, therefore, the safety and effectiveness of many CAM therapies are uncertain, CAM use is common, particularly among individuals with chronic pain and advanced illness. Use of CAM therapies is gaining acceptance in mainstream venues. In 2002, the White House Commission on Complementary and Alternative Medicine recommended integration of CAM therapies that are considered safe and effective into health care throughout the nation (White House Commission on Complementary and Alternative Medicine 2010).

The 2007 National Health Interview Survey (NHIS) found that CAM use is prevalent and increasing. Thirty-eight percent of U.S. adults and 12% of children reported CAM use in 2007, up from 36% of adults surveyed in the 2002 NHIS (Barnes et al. 2007). In 1996, there were an estimated 630 million visits to CAM providers, exceeding the number of visits to primary care physicians (Eisenberg 2005). A survey of patients hospitalized on surgical services in Adelaide, South Australia revealed that 90% acknowledged using some CAM modality, with the most commonly used modalities being biologically based therapies, including herbal and nonherbal preparations (69%) and mind–body interventions (65%), followed by manipulative and body-based methods (63%) (Shoroni and Abron 2010).

Use of CAM is more prevalent among those with advanced or chronic illnesses than is seen in the general public. One review found that CAM use in cancer patients has been reported to be between 7 and 64% with an average of 31% (Eliott et al. 2008). Sixty-nine percent of oncology patients at one cancer center reported having used CAM (excluding use of spiritual practices and psychotherapy) in a study published in 2000 (Richardson et al. 2000). The most commonly used CAM modalities among cancer patients are massage, nutrition, aromatherapy, relaxation, and reflexology (Lewith et al. 2002). In a study of patients undergoing radiation therapy for various cancers at rural cancer centers in Minnesota, CAM use was reported by 95% of respondents when including prayer and exercise and 92% when these modalities were excluded. The five most commonly used CAM approaches were spiritual healing/prayer (62%), exercise (20%), music (18%), chiropractics (16%), and meditation (13%) (Rausch et al. 2011). Similar prevalence of CAM use has been found in other studies (Lim et al. 2010; Ndao-Brumblay and Green 2010). Patients with cancer report using CAM for boosting the immune system, relieving pain, and controlling side effects related to the cancer itself or its treatment (Mansky & Wallerstedt 2006).

Despite evidence of common use of CAM by cancer patients, oncologists refer patients for CAM therapy less often than physicians from other specialties and patients report that they do not disclose use of CAM to their health care providers (Rausch et al. 2011; Lee et al. 2008). This disconnect raises the concern that the use of CAM therapies by patients with cancer is likely occurring outside the setting of oncology care centers and without the knowledge of or approval by oncologists. There are multiple barriers to integrating CAM with conventional medical care (Ben-Arye et al. 2008). Patients themselves may hinder this integration, feeling that CAM "efficacy intrinsically requires faith, that CAM is solely for cure, that it is for specific types of people, or that it implies a lack of faith in the medical profession" (Eliott et al. 2008).

Health care providers' attitudes may impede integration of CAM into conventional medical care. Fadlon et al. found physicians had respect for what CAM could provide but were often concerned about hazards of CAM as well as ulterior motives of CAM practitioners (Fadlon et al. 2008).

Indeed, some CAM therapies may interact with other more conventional therapies. For example, St John's wort, Ginkgo biloba, and ginseng have been shown to have potentially adverse interactions with chemotherapeutic agents as well as other pharmaceuticals commonly used for patients with cancer, such as warfarin, cyclosporin, and anxiolytics (Lee et al. 2008). Health care providers also report concern about potential liability they may face as a consequence of providing or referring CAM therapies for patients (Hirschkorn & Bourgeault 2008). Evidence-based guidelines recommend that patients be asked about use of CAM and that evidence-based advice be given about the advantages and disadvantages of CAM therapies (Cassileth et al. 2007). Proposed recommendations for effectively discussing CAM with patients include ten steps: (1) understand, (2) respect, (3) ask, (4) explore, (5) respond, (6) discuss, (7) advise, (8) summarize, (9) document, and (10) monitor. A critical feature of this recommended strategy is that the health care provider does not have to be an expert in CAM in order to have an effective discussion about CAM with patients (Schofield et al. 2010).

Insurance coverage may influence whether or not patients pursue CAM therapies. The NHIS 2007 survey found that for adults younger than age 65 years, those with private health insurance were more likely than those with public health insurance or those without health insurance to use biologically based, body-based, and mind–body therapies (Barnes et al. 2007). In addition, organizational factors, such as lack of space or resources, as well as organizational policies which preclude incorporation of CAM practices have been cited as barriers to integration of CAM into hospice (Hirschkorn & Bourgeault 2008).

Despite these barriers, Lewis et al. found that a wide variety of CAM therapies can be successfully integrated into hospice settings, with preliminary data suggesting positive outcomes for patients and family members (Lewis et al. 2003). More than 80% of respondents to a national survey of hospices reported that they would support integration of CAM into their organization if not already present (Corbin).

Evidence for Use of CAM in Chronic Pain and Palliative Care

This section presents evidence regarding selected CAM modalities in the settings of chronic pain and palliative care. The modalities discussed were selected so as to not substantially overlap with other chapters in this edited volume. The presentation of the evidence is organized according to the following NCCAM-specified categories: (1) mind–body practices, (2) manipulative and body-based practices, (3) manipulation of energy fields, and (4) biologically based therapies. Where sufficient data are available, the evidence is presented in table format. For some modalities, little evidence is available. For these modalities, the existing evidence is described in the text only.

Despite many years of CAM practice and common usage, rigorous scientific research on CAM therapies has occurred only relatively recently. CAM research is also limited by methodologic and ethical issues. Gaps in research are thus the norm and the current evidence base is insufficient.

Mind–Body Practices

A number of practices may be considered under the umbrella of "mind–body" practice, including biofeedback, progressive muscle relaxation, meditation, guided imagery, and hypnosis, as well as yoga and acupuncture. A structured review of mind–body interventions for older adults with chronic nonmalignant pain found that there were few randomized clinical trials with small numbers of participants. This review notes that while these interventions are feasible in this population and likely safe, with modifications tailored for older adults, there is not yet sufficient evidence to conclude that such interventions reduce chronic nonmalignant pain in older adults (Morone & Greco 2007). A summary of 28 systematic reviews found strong evidence for the use of mind–body therapies as adjunctive therapy for cancer patients given demonstrated efficacy in improving mood, quality of life, and coping with both the disease and treatment-related side effects. The same summary found strong evidence for use of mind–body therapies as adjunctive or stand-alone therapies for recurrent migraine and tension headaches and as adjunctive therapies in medical management of chronic low back pain (Astin et al. 2003).

Meditation

Meditation entails a systematic mental focus on particular aspects of inner or outer experience. Meditation encompasses practices to increase mental awareness and clarity of mind (concentrative meditation), quiet the ordinary stream of internal mental dialogue (transcendental meditation), or focus attention on the flow of sensations experienced from moment to moment (mindfulness meditation) (Cassileth et al. 2007; Astin et al. 2003). The most commonly studied meditation practice appears to be the Mindfulness-Based Stress Reduction (MBSR) program developed by Jon Kabat-Zinn, usually operationalized as 8–10 weeks of weekly 2½h sessions. A review of experimental and nonexperimental studies of meditation, such as mindfulness meditation and transcendental meditation for chronic pain, concluded that the limited available data seems to indicate that meditation programs may ease the burden of chronic pain with both short- and long-term effects (Teixeira 2008).

Given limitations of existing data (few randomized clinical trials with small sample sizes and variable control groups), it appears that meditation is a safe, well-accepted intervention for chronic pain and in the palliative care setting, and may have benefits on pain intensity, functional status, quality of life, function, sleep quality, well-being, and mood (anxiety and depression) (Table 35.1). Pending additional research evidence, meditation is likely a viable option for patients with chronic pain or palliative care needs. The American College of Chest Physicians (ACCP) recommends mind–body modalities as part of a multidisciplinary approach to reduce anxiety, mood disturbance, or chronic pain among patients with lung cancer (Cassileth et al. 2007).

Yoga

Yoga combines physical movement, breath control, and meditation with the goal of uniting the mind, body, and spirit for health and self-awareness. Studies of yoga for chronic low back pain and knee osteoarthritis suggest that it may be effective for decreasing pain and fatigue and improving function (Table 35.2). A clinical practice guideline on the diagnosis and treatment of low back pain issued by the American College of Physicians (ACP) and the American Pain society weakly recommends, based on moderate-quality evidence, yoga for patients with chronic or subacute low back pain (Chou et al. 2007). A systematic review of literature examining the impact of yoga on psychological adjustment of cancer patients identified ten studies, six of which were RCTs. Overall study quality was high; limiting factors included lack of long-term data and small sample size. Studies demonstrated improvements in sleep, stress levels, and mood. While a number of positive results were found, the authors concluded that the variability across studies and methodologic drawbacks limit the extent to which yoga can be considered effective for managing psychological symptoms associated with cancer (Smith & Pukall 2009). Yoga thus appears to be a promising intervention for improving psychological symptoms among cancer patients and for improving function among persons with chronic pain.

Table 35.1 Meditation evidence

References	Measurement	Participants population & N	Design and control group for RCTs	Findings/notes
Ando et al. (2009)	HADS FACIT-Sp (sense of meaning) Measured pre-/post-intervention	N = 28 outpatients receiving anticancer chemotherapy, radiation, or medication at a general hospital in Western Japan, age > 20 years. Excluded if experiencing severe pain or other symptoms (>8 on 0–10 numeric rating scale)	Intervention: Mindfulness-Based Stress Reduction (MBSR) – two sessions	HADS: Anxiety and Depression and total scores significantly decreased FACIT-Sp scores increased
Bruce & Davies (2005)	Qualitative interviews	Hospice in which Western palliative care and Zen Buddhist philosophy are integrated Nine participants (four volunteer caregivers, three staff caregivers, two community members living with HIV/AIDS) who had regular meditation practice × >6 months	Narrative inquiry – in-depth unstructured conversations exploring participants' experiences of mindfulness awareness and its impact on providing hospice care	Four themes Hospice care as meditation in action: considered caregiving as a significant aspect of their meditation practice Abiding in liminal spaces Seeing differently Resting with groundlessness Argue that mindfulness meditation helps caregivers create a better environment for hospice care
Carson et al. (2005)	Chronic low back pain (present for at least 6 months) McGill Pain Questionnaire Brief Pain Inventory State-Trait Anger Expression Inventory-II (STAXI-II) Brief Symptom Inventory Daily treatment diary – pain, anger, and tension Measured pre/post and 3 months later	N = 43 patients with chronic low back pain	Randomized to intervention or standard care Intervention: Loving-Kindness Meditation Program – 8 weekly 90-min group sessions that aim to facilitate a positive affective shift	Greater improvements in pain and psychological adjustment in intervention group Dose–response relationship: those who practiced longer with loving-kindness meditation more likely to experience lower pain and less anger

(continued)

Table 35.1 (continued)

References	Measurement	Participants population & N	Design and control group for RCT's	Findings/notes
Morone et al. (2008a)	Chronic low back pain Measures at baseline, postintervention, and 3-months Pain intensity: McGill Pain Questionnaire Short Form (MPQ-SF) Pain acceptance: Chronic Pain Acceptance Questionnaire (CPAQ) Quality of life (QOL): SF-36 Health Status Inventory Physical function: Roland and Morris Questionnaire; Short Physical Performance Battery; SF-36 Physical Function scale	Community-dwelling English-speaking older adults (age ≥65 years) with chronic moderate low back pain occurring daily or almost every day for at least the past 3 months	Randomized wait-list controlled trial of mindfulness meditation modeled on work of Jon Kabat-Zinn and the Mindfulness-Based Stress Reduction Program (MBSR) Intervention: (n=19) 8 weekly 90-min mindfulness meditation sessions and meditation homework assignments Controls: (n=18) no intervention initially – crossed over after 8 weeks	Chronic Pain Acceptance Questionnaire total score significantly improved for meditation group while control group worsened. Activities Engagement subscale of the CPAQ also significantly improved Mean pain scores changed in the expected direction for meditation group for the McGill Pain Questionnaire and the SF-36 Pain Scale, although not significantly Significant improvement in Physical Function Scale of SF-36 Roland Disability Questionnaire changed in expected direction, although not significantly No significant change on Short Physical Performance Battery QOL (summary scores and SF-36) in expected direction, but not significant Majority continued to meditate at 3 month follow-up
Morone et al. (2008b)	Chronic low back pain	N=27 adults ≥ age 65 years with chronic low back pain of at least moderate intensity × at least 3 months	Grounded theory to analyze diary entries of participants in an RCT who recorded information about their experiences with mindfulness meditation modeled on work of Jon Kabat-Zinn and the Mindfulness-Based Stress Reduction Program (MBSR)	Findings Pain reduction Improved attention skills Improved sleep resulting from meditation Achieved well-being

| Rosenzweig et al. (2010) | Chronic pain patients SF-36 (HRQoL) Symptom Checklist-90-Revised (SCL-90-R) Administered pre- and post 8-week MBSR intervention | $N = 133$ patients with chronic pain (6 months or longer): chronic neck/back pain, chronic headaches/migraines, arthritis, fibromyalgia, other. 111 were women | Prospective cohort design Intervention: 8-week MBSR program modeled after Kabat-Zinn | HRQoL outcomes differed substantially across chronic pain conditions – arthritis showed greatest improvements; migraine/headache patients showed least improvement SCL-90-R: chronic pain subgroups experienced medium to large magnitude reductions in psychological distress (except fibromyalgia group which had small to medium reductions) Better adherence to formal home meditation practice associated with reduced overall psychological distress and somatic symptoms, and improvement in self-rated health Chronic back/neck pain and those with two or more comorbid pain conditions experienced largest average improvement in pain severity and functional limitations due to pain |

(continued)

Table 35.1 (continued)

References	Measurement	Participants population & N	Design and control group for RCTs	Findings/notes
Schechter et al. (2007)	Functional back pain Pain intensity (VAS) QOL (RAND SF-12) Medication usage Activity level Follow up at least 3–12 months after treatment	$N=51$ patients with "functional" back pain	Case series in single physician's office Program of office visits, written educational materials, structured workbook and educational audio CDs, individual psychotherapy (some cases)	Mean VAS scores for average pain and worst pain and least pain decreased SF-12 Physical health scores increased Medication usage decreased Activity levels increased Participants aged >47 years and in pain for >3 years benefited most
Zautra et al. (2010)	Thermal pain threshold assessment Visual analogue pain scale (0–10) Positive and negative affect (PANAS)	$N=25$ age-matched healthy women $N=27$ women with physician-confirmed fibromyalgia	2×2 repeated measures nested design Breathe at normal rate or ½ normal rate during four blocks of four trials	Overall reduction in pain intensity among healthy controls when paced to breathe slowly Greatest effects on ratings of pain stimuli of moderate in comparison to mild intensity Fibromyalgia participants benefited less – ratings of pain intensity unaffected by slow breathing

Table 35.2 Yoga evidence

References	Measurement	Participants population & N	Design and control group for RCTs	Findings/notes
Galantino et al. (2004)	Chronic low back pain Oswestry Disability Index (ODI) at 6 weeks	N=22 adults with chronic low back pain	Randomized controlled trial Intervention: 1 h of immediate Iyengar yoga-based intervention twice weekly for 6 weeks Control: usual activities during observation period; delayed yoga training	Improved balance and flexibility and decreased disability and depression in yoga group Study not powered to reach statistical significance
Groessl et al. (2008)	Chronic back pain Outcomes measured at baseline and 10 weeks Pain: single visual numeric scale (0–10) and 5-question severity scale modified from Medical Outcomes Study pain severity scale Energy/fatigue using modified items from Medical Outcomes Study Depression: Center for Epidemiologic Studies Short Depression Scale (CESD-10) Health-Related Quality of Life (HRQOL) – Short-From 12 version 2 (SF12v2)	N=33 Veterans Administration (VA) patients with chronic back pain	Single group pre–post design Intervention: Weekly yoga sessions×8 weeks	Significant improvements in pain, depression, energy/fatigue, and SF-12
Sapir et al. (2009)	Chronic low back pain Outcome data collected at 6, 12, and 26 weeks Feasibility outcomes Two primary efficacy outcomes at 12 weeks Average pain level for the previous week using 11-point numerical rating scale Back-related function using modified Roland–Morris Disability Questionnaire Secondary outcomes Use of pain medication during the preceding week Global improvement Health-related quality of life (SF-36)	N=30 adults with chronic low back pain recruited from two community health centers	Pilot randomized controlled trial 12-week protocol of weekly 75-min hatha yoga classes + home practice 30 min daily vs. usual care waitlist control group	Intervention group attended a median of 8 classes; 13 practiced at least once at home One reported increase in back pain with yoga Yoga participants had statistically significant greater reduction in pain intensity and pain medication use at 12 weeks compared to control group Longer term retention and adherence poor

(continued)

Table 35.2 (continued)

References	Measurement	Participants population & N	Design and control group for RCTs	Findings/notes
Sherman et al. (2005)	Chronic low back pain Outcomes measured at 12 and 26 weeks Roland–Morris Disability Questionnaire (RDQ) Symptom bothersomeness score Medication use Back pain-related health care provider visits	$N = 101$ adults with chronic low back pain	Three-arm randomized controlled trial comparing 6 weeks of Viniyoga, conventional exercise, and a self-care book	RDQ: Viniyoga slightly superior to conventional exercise and moderately superior to a self-care education book at 12 weeks, but only superior to the self-care book at 26 weeks Symptom bothersomeness: Effects similar at 12 weeks for all three interventions; yoga substantially superior to self-care book at 26 weeks Medication use: Yoga associated with decreased use at week 26 No difference in back pain-associated health care provider visits
Tekur et al. (2008)	Chronic low back pain Outcomes measured within 7 days of intervention Spinal mobility Functional Disability Index (Oswestry low-back pain Disability Index (ODI)	$N = 80$ women with chronic low back pain	Wait-list randomized controlled trial Intervention: ($n = 40$) 1-week intensive residential yoga program composed of asanas (physical postures), pranayamas (breathing practices), meditation and didactic and interactive sessions on philosophical concepts of yoga Control: ($n = 40$) physical exercises under trained physiatrist + didactic and interactive sessions on lifestyle change	Significant reduction (49%) in disability (ODI) in yoga group Spinal flexion improved in both groups – higher effect sizes in yoga group
Williams et al. (2005a)	Chronic low back pain Outcomes measured baseline, posttreatment, and at 3 months Present Pain Index Pain Disability Index Pain on visual analogue scale	$N = 60$ adults with chronic low back pain	Randomized controlled trial Intervention: 1½h Iyengar yoga class weekly × 16 weeks Control: exercise education × 16 weeks	Significant reductions in pain intensity, functional disability, and pain medication usage in the yoga group posttreatment and at 16 months

Acupuncture

Acupuncture, a CAM modality that originated from traditional Chinese medicine, is based on the theory that one can regulate the flow of "Qi" (vital energy) by stimulation of certain points on the body with needles, heat, or pressure. Stimulation of specific points along the 12 primary and 8 secondary meridians is believed to restore the proper flow of Qi. It appears that the effects of acupuncture are mediated by the nervous system. Evidence includes observations that administration of local anesthesia at acupuncture needle insertion sites completely blocks the immediate analgesic effects of acupuncture and documented neurotransmitter release and changes in brain functional MRI signals during acupuncture (Han 2003; Wu et al. 1999; Berman et al. 2010).

Systematic reviews of the use of acupuncture for chronic low back pain have concluded that while real acupuncture was no more effective than sham acupuncture, both real and sham acupuncture were more effective than no treatment and that acupuncture can be a useful supplement to other forms of conventional treatment for low back pain (Yuan et al. 2008; Rubinstein et al. 2010; Chou & Huffman 2007). A clinical practice guideline on the diagnosis and treatment of low back pain issued by the ACP and the American Pain Society weakly recommends, based on moderate-quality evidence, acupuncture for patients with chronic or subacute low back pain (Chou et al. 2007). The North American Spine Society concluded that acupuncture provides better short-term pain relief and functional improvement than no treatment and that the addition of acupuncture to other treatments provides a greater benefit than other treatments alone (Ammendolia et al. 2008). The U.K. National Institute for Health and Clinical Excellence has recommended acupuncture as a treatment option for patients with low back pain (Royal College of General Practitioners 2009).

A systematic review of seven systematic reviews of acupuncture as a treatment for cancer palliation and supportive care found that acupuncture as a treatment of chemotherapy-induced nausea and vomiting is backed by good evidence. Evidence is lacking as to whether acupuncture is superior to other interventions available for treatment of chemotherapy-induced nausea and vomiting (Ernst & Lee 2010). The ACCP recommends acupuncture as a complementary therapy for patients with lung cancer when pain is poorly controlled or when side effects such as neuropathy or xerostomia from other modalities are clinically significant as well as for poorly controlled nausea and vomiting associated with chemotherapy. A trial of acupuncture is recommended by the ACCP for patients with lung cancer who have symptoms such as fatigue, dyspnea, chemotherapy-induced neuropathy, or postthoracotomy pain. The ACCP notes that acupuncture should be performed by qualified practitioners and used cautiously in patients with bleeding tendencies (Cassileth et al. 2007). A Cochrane Review concluded that there is insufficient evidence to recommend the routine use of acupuncture/acupressure for relief of dyspnea in advanced stages of malignant and nonmalignant diseases, recommending further study before they are routinely used in clinical practice (Bausewein et al. 2008). A systematic review of acupressure for symptom management in end-stage renal disease (ESRD) found few well-designed trials. The authors conclude that the small number and suboptimal methodological quality of available studies preclude determination of the therapeutic effects of acupressure for ESRD patients (Kim et al. 2010). Table 35.3 details relevant available evidence.

Manipulative and Body-Based Practices

Manipulative and body-based practices focus on moving the bones, joints, and soft tissues of the body and, in doing so, affect the circulatory, lymphatic, neuroendocrine, and musculoskeletal systems. Manipulative/body-based practices are relatively familiar to and commonly accessed by the American public. In the National Health Interview Survey (2007), 8.6% of adults and 2.8% of children indicated that they used some form of osteopathic manipulation or chiropractic care, while

Table 35.3 Acupuncture evidence

References	Measurement	Participants population & N	Design and control group for RCTs	Findings/notes
Brinkhaus et al. (2006)	Chronic low back pain Outcomes measured at baseline, 8, 26, and 52 weeks Pain intensity Back function Pain Disability Index Emotional aspects of pain Depression scale SF-36	$N = 301$ adults with chronic low back pain >6 months, average pain intensity ≥ 40 on a 100-mm visual analogue scale in past 7 days	Multicenter, randomized controlled trial Intervention ($n = 147$): 12 sessions of 30 min duration, each administered over 8 weeks Controls: (1) ($N = 75$) Sham acupuncture (minimal acupuncture) of same number, frequency, and duration as real acupuncture: and (2) ($N = 79$) no acupuncture waiting list	Acupuncture more effective in improving pain than no acupuncture No significant differences between acupuncture and sham (minimal) acupuncture
Jobst et al. (1986)	Modified Borg Scale Oxygen Cost Diagram Shortness of Breath Score 6-min walk mean Measured at baseline and after 3 weeks.	$N = 24$ adults with chronic obstructive pulmonary disease (COPD) and disabling breathlessness for at least 5 years severely limiting exercise tolerance and compromising performance of activities of daily living	Randomized controlled trial Intervention ($n = 12$): acupuncture (according to traditional Chinese principles), over 3 weeks, on 13 occasions Control ($n = 12$): same number of treatments as intervention, needles inserted into nonacupuncture "dead" points	Intervention group demonstrated significantly greater benefit in all subjective scores and in distance walked at 6 min
Lewith et al. (2004)	Daily breathlessness visual analogue scale at baseline, during first treatment, at washout, and during second treatment St. George's Respiratory Questionnaire (SGRQ) at baseline and at end of each of the two 3-week treatment periods	$N = 36$ adults with chronic lung disease ($n = 33$ with COPD, one with pulmonary fibrosis, two with cystic fibrosis), receiving home care and baseline breathlessness > 60 mm on visual analogue scale	Single-blind, placebo-controlled randomized study with cross-over design. Six treatments over 3 weeks with a 2-week washout period prior to second treatment phase Intervention ($n = 16$): acupuncture × 20 min plus stud insertion Control ($n = 16$): Mock TENS at same points for same duration as real acupuncture	Worse breathlessness improved significantly during the study; no significant differences between acupuncture and control
Maa et al. (1997)	Visual analogue scale breathlessness Borg Scale Bronchitis Emphysema Checklist (BESC) Dyspnea Scale Measured at weeks 1, 6, and 12	$N = 31$ adults with COPD beginning a 12-week pulmonary rehabilitation program	Randomized, single-blind pretest-posttest cross-over design Intervention ($n = 19$): acupressure for 6 weeks, then sham acupressure for 6 weeks Control ($n = 12$): sham acupressure for 6 weeks, then acupressure for 6 weeks	Real acupressure more effective than sham acupressure for reducing dyspnea

Study	Outcome measures	Sample	Design/Intervention	Results
Vickers et al. (2005)	Numeric Rating Scale every 15 min for 75 min immediately before and 1 h after acupuncture	N=47 adults with lung or breast cancer and subjective complaint of shortness of breath and ATS Breathlessness Scale >2	Randomized controlled trial. Intervention (n=25): true acupuncture (single treatment × 15 min) followed by true acupressure 1 h after removal of needles. Control (n=20): placebo acupuncture (single treatment × 15 min using placebo needles) and placebo acupressure	Improvement in NRS in both groups; no differences between the groups
Witt et al. (2006)	Chronic low back pain. Outcomes measured at baseline, 3 and 6 months. Back Function (Hannover Function Ability Questionnaire – HFAQ). Low Back Pain Rating Scale. Medical Outcomes Study 36-Item Short Form (SF-36). Adjunctive use of analgesics. Costs	N=3,093 adults with chronic low back pain >6 months	Multicenter, randomized controlled trial with a nonrandomized cohort. Intervention (n=1,549): immediate acupuncture; maximum of 15 sessions. Control (n=1,544) delayed acupuncture 3 months later	Acupuncture group demonstrated significant improvements in symptoms and quality of life compared to those who received routine care alone. Acupuncture associated with higher costs but considered cost effective
Wu et al. (2004) Wu et al. (2007)	Visual Analogue Scale. Pulmonary Function Status and Dyspnea Questionnaire (PFDQ-M). Geriatric Depression Scale	N=44 adults with COPD	Randomized clinical trial. Intervention (n=22): 20 a 16-min acupressure sessions, 5 times per week for 4 weeks. Control (n=22): sham acupressure with same duration and frequency as intervention	Dyspnea and depression scores of true acupressure group improved significantly compared to the control group

8.3% of adults and 1% of children used some form of MT for health or healing (National Health Interview Survey 2010). Massage is defined as "pressing, rubbing and moving muscles and other soft tissues of the body, primarily by using the hands and finge" (http://nccam.nih.gov/health/whatiscam/). In this section, manipulation and massage will be discussed separately, including the proposed mechanisms of action, summary of evidence, and recommendations for use for management of chronic pain and other symptoms in chronic, life-limiting illnesses. NCCAM defines spinal manipulation as "the application of controlled force to a joint, moving it beyond the normal range of motion in an effort to aid in restoring health. Manipulation may be performed as a part of other therapies or whole medical systems, including chiropractic medicine, massage and naturopathy" (http://nccam.nih.gov/health/whatiscam/). Practitioners such as chiropractors, osteopathic physicians, and physical therapists perform manipulative procedures on the body. Insufficient data regarding craniosacral therapies were identified to warrant a separate discussion.

Massage and Lymphatic Drainage

Massage therapy (MT) is one of the oldest of the identified complementary-alternative therapies with references to its use appearing in Chinese texts at least 4,000 years ago. There are more than 80 different methods classified as massage including Swedish, sports, deep tissue, neuromuscular, trigger point, shiatsu, and manual lymph drainage. Massage can be full body or provided locally to specific areas of the body including the neck, shoulders, hands, and feet. In the mid-1800s, Swedish massage was imported to the USA, named as such by two physicians who learned the techniques in Sweden. This common form of massage includes smooth, gliding strokes over the body (effleurage), firm kneading of soft tissues (petrissage), and tapping or vibrating areas of the body (tapotement).

There are multiple hypotheses related to the mechanisms of action of MT for relief of chronic pain and other symptoms. The palliative effects of massage are proposed to be related to: an increase in blood flow and lymph drainage reducing the accumulation of metabolites in the tissues; muscle relaxation through the manual release of muscle tension; the generalized relaxation response; release of increased serotonin that decreases noxious pain impulses to the brain; increased release of somatostatin promoting restorative sleep and decreased release of substance P secreted in deep sleep deprivation (Field 1998); endorphin release from the pleasant sensation of touch; overriding pain signals (gate control theory); and energy transfer and energy field repatterning. However, the actual mechanisms of action have not been established.

Massage with common maneuvers such as effleurage and petrissage and delivered by trained professionals is a safe therapy. There are a few reports of adverse reactions to MT; however, for the most part these are related to more exotic types of manual therapies delivered by the lay public (Ernst 2003a; Grant 2003). Massage is contraindicated in persons with clotting disorders, taking anticoagulant medications, with potential or known thrombus, and at risk for fracture and over any lesions.

Research on the effects of massage related to pain and palliative care has proliferated over the past 25 years. (Field 1998; Ernst 1999, 2002, 2003a, 2004, 2009a; Cherkin et al. 2003; Fellowes et al. 2004; Furlan et al. 2002, 2008, 2009; Hughes et al. 2008; Jane et al. 2008; Lafferty et al. 2006; National Guidelines Clearinghouse 2010; Natural Standard 2010a; Pan et al. 2000; Russell et al. 2008; Tan et al. 2007; Wilkinson et al. 2008a). Two meta-analyses of massage research have been published (Fellowes et al. 2004; Moyer et al. 2004). Fellowes et al. reported on eight RCTs of MT in patients with cancer published before 2002. A 19–32% reduction in anxiety was reported in four studies. Pain was an outcome in three studies and a decrease in pain occurred in one. Two studies showed a reduction in nausea and another revealed an effect on sleep (Fellowes et al. 2004). Moyer et al. (2004) included 37 trials with statistically significant overall effect sizes in categories of state anxiety, immediate assessment of pain, and delayed assessment of pain among others; the findings support the conclusion that MT is effective.

A number of reviews have found that massage has demonstrated benefits for improving symptoms and functions those for those with subacute and chronic nonspecific low back pain (Cherkin et al. 2003; Ernst 1999, 2004; Furlan et al. 2002, 2008, 2009). For those with chronic low back pain the effects were long lasting (at least a year after the end of sessions). The greatest benefit seemed to come from massage delivered by professional massage therapists with many years of experience and when massage was combined with stretching exercises and education. These reviews conclude that massage is effective for persistent low back pain and has the potential to reduce costs of care after an initial course of therapy but more and stronger investigations are needed (Cherkin et al. 2003; Ernst 2009a).

There appears to be consistent common findings across MT studies, including decreases in anxiety, depression, and stress hormones and an increase in parasympathetic activity (Field 1998). Since pain is exacerbated by stress and tension, this is an important consideration. MT has been found to be "useful for pain relief in numerous chronic pain conditions" (Tan et al. 2007). There is less support for its efficacy for neck pain and fibromyalgia.

Several reviews focus specifically on massage for cancer, cancer pain and palliative care at end of life. These reviews conclude that there is support for the use of massage for relief from cancer pain in those at end of life (Lafferty et al. 2006; Pan et al. 2000). The Natural Standard Database rated the evidence that massage improved quality of life at a "B" or good rating; all other outcomes including for pain and anxiety were rated "C" or inconclusive (Natural Standard 2010a). In his review of 14 trials of massage for cancer palliation and supportive care, Ernst (2009a) reported "encouraging evidence." He stated that the effect sizes for massage were small to moderate, but added that these effects can be beneficial for this population. Finally, he noted the methodological flaws and pitfalls of the studies and pointed to the Kutner et al. (2008) study as a model for future research. While it is difficult to compare across studies because of variation related to type of massage, dosage, control conditions, and outcomes, there is a trend that massage has more positive effects than controls for decreasing pain intensity, nausea, fatigue, distressing symptoms, anxiety, and enhancing relaxation. The most inconsistent outcomes are related to sleep, analgesic consumption, quality of life, and depression/mood disturbance (Jane et al. 2008; Wilkinson et al. 2008a). It appears that MT has an immediate or short-term (5–20 min) effect on symptoms, but there is no evidence that these effects are sustained over hours or days even with multiple treatments (Russell et al. 2008). MT can be safely integrated into the care of children with cancer, and that it can be beneficial for managing side effects and the emotional turbulence of the experience (Hughes et al. 2008).

Table 35.4 summarizes the research in MT for chronic pain and palliative care. The table includes randomized controlled trials (RCTs) and some quasi-experimental designs without controls or randomization. Only studies of chronic pain, those conditions that are persistent, recurring, and not self-limiting were included. For this reason, studies of episodic pain syndromes such as acute back pain, postoperative pain, and tension headaches were not included.

Many of the studies listed have methodological weaknesses, and a quality analysis was not conducted for this review. For example, small sample sizes are the norm, possibly because a considerable portion of the studies listed were unfunded or underfunded. Research related to MT can be expensive because of the cost of administering massage. These small sample sizes compromise the ability to detect actual differences that may exist. The intensity and duration of the intervention varies widely, so it is challenging to compare results. Some studies examine the effects of a few treatments while others use ten or more treatments over weeks or months. Many studies have no follow up. The control conditions vary from usual care, exercise, relaxation, or other therapies. Many reports lack adequate descriptions of outcome variables. All this compromises the ability to draw evidentiary conclusions.

Types and dosages of the MT varied across the studies. Pain was most frequently measured using a visual analogue or numeric rating scale, with immediate and follow-up measures variably present. Based on these data, MT provides some degree of efficacy, if only short term, for a variety of chronic pain syndromes. This conclusion is consistent with other reviews of MT for back pain.

Table 35.4 Massage evidence table

References	Measurement	Participants population & N	Design and control group	Findings/notes
Ahles et al. (1999)	HR, RR, BP, pain, anxiety, emotional distress, nausea, fatigue	Bone marrow transplant patients during 3-week hospital stay, N=33	RCT comparing MT (upper body; 20 min; nine sessions) to quiet time control	Immediate effects for BP, anxiety, emotional distress nausea, HR, RR, pain, and fatigue. Longer term effects for anxiety, depression, mood disturbance
Billhult et al. (2007)	VAS for anxiety and nausea; Hospital Anxiety and Depression Scale	Women with breast cancer, N=39	RCT comparing MT (20 min; five sessions) to 20 attention control (visits)	Significantly greater decrease in nausea for MT compared to control. No differences in anxiety and depression
Brattberg (1999)	VAS and use of analgesics measured during treatment and at 6 month follow-up	Adults with fibromyalgia, N-48	RCT comparing massage (connective tissue massage, 15 treatments for 10 weeks) to routine care	Reported a reduction in pain, depression, and use of analgesics, and improved quality of life. Incomplete statistical analysis
Campeau et al. (2007)	Anxiety VAS (immediate effects) and STAI (intermediate effects)	Adult cancer patients undergoing radiation therapy, N=100	RCT comparing MT (ten sessions) to usual care control	Significant decrease on immediate anxiety scores by 45%; no significant decrease on intermediate anxiety
Cassileth & Vickers (2004)	Symptom rating scales 0–10 for pain, fatigue, stress/anxiety, nausea, depression, and "other"	Adult patients with cancer in treatment at a Cancer Center, N=1290	Pre–post intervention measurement of symptoms; no control group	Symptom scores reduced by 50% even for patients reporting high baseline scores
Cherkin et al. (2001)	NRS 0–10 for pain and other symptoms and 0–23 rating scale for dysfunction. Follow up at 4, 10, and 52 weeks. Interviewers blinded to treatment group. Follow up at 4, 10, and 52 weeks	Adults with persistent low back pain, N=262 (acupuncture N=94; MT N=78; self-care N=90)	RCT comparing massage; <10 treatments of unspecified length over 10 weeks to acupuncture and self-care	MT significantly superior to self-care at 10 weeks for pain and disability. MT superior to acupuncture on disability scale. After 1 year MT was not better than self-care but better than acupuncture for pain and dysfunction. MT group used least medications and had lowest medical costs
Corner et al. (1995)	Anxiety, depression, quality of life symptom distress assessed twice weekly, before massage and 24 h later	Adults with cancer, N=52	RCT comparing MT with essential oils to massage with carrier oil (eight massages)	Immediate effects included decreased anxiety for MT with essential oils as compared to without essential oils. Significant improvements in pain, mobility, fatigue, and function from first to last assessment for those receiving aromatherapy massage. No significant difference between groups

Author	Population	Measures	Design	Results
Ferrell-Torry & Glick (1993)	Adult veterans, N=9 with solid tumor or hematologic cancer with moderate pain or generalized discomfort	VAS for pain intensity, STAI for anxiety, VAS for relaxation. Measurements immediately after treatment	Massage consisted of 30 min of effleurage and petrissage to feet, back, neck, and shoulders using warm cocoa butter. Myofacial trigger point stimulation of 6 TP in upper, middle, and lower trapezius muscle region. Concluded with 3 min light effleurage and cupping over sacral area. Pre–post intervention measurement of pain, HR, RR BP, and MAP. 7/9 had two trials on consecutive evenings	Significant decreases immediately after MT for pain intensity and anxiety. Significant increase in relaxation immediately after massage. Inconsistent findings with physiological measures
Field et al. (1997)	Children with rheumatoid arthritis	Pain reported by children, parents, and physicians	Quasi-experimental design comparing massage to progressive muscle relaxation	Those in MT group had decreased anxiety and cortisol after first and last sessions and decreased pain and pain limitations on activities over 1 month
Field (2002)	Adults with fibromyalgia, N=24	Physician reports of pain and number of tender points	RCT comparing MT to guided relaxation therapy	Physician's ratings of pain, disease, and number of tender points decreased significantly in MT group
Godfrey et al. (1984)	Adults with low back pain, N=81	Pain VAS, mobility, functional ability	RCT comparing MT (light effleurage for 10 min, five treatments in 2 weeks) to chiropractic and electrostimulation	No significant differences between groups; improvements noted in all
Grealish et al. (2000)	Hospitalized cancer patients, N=87	VAS for pain, nausea, and relaxation	Foot massage, 5 min/foot Pre–post single group design	Significant immediate effect on pain, nausea, and relaxation post foot massage
Hasson et al. (2004)	Adults with chronic musculoskeletal pain, N=129	Muscle pain rated before, during, and after treatment	RCT comparing MT to mental relaxation group	Significant improvement in pain during treatment; this was not sustained at the 3 month follow-up
Hernandez-Reif et al. (2001)	Adults with chronic low back pain, N=24	Self-reports of pain, anxiety, and range of motion measurement	Quasi-experiment comparing MT (30 min, 2 times/week for 5 weeks) to progressive muscle relaxation	MT group had significant improvement in range of motion and reported less pain and anxiety; MT group had lower depression and higher serotonin and dopamine levels

(continued)

Table 35.4 (continued)

References	Measurement	Participants population & N	Design and control group	Findings/notes
Hoehler et al. (1981)	VAS, follow up after 3 weeks	Adults with acute or chronic low back pain, N=95	RCT comparing MT (soft tissue massage of the lumbosacral area, about 4 treatments in 20 days) to rotational manipulation (5 treatments in 30 days)	No significant differences between groups at the end of the treatment period; improvements noted in both groups
Hsieh et al. (1992)	VAS for pain; measures of confidence, strength, range of motion; follow up after 4 weeks	Chronic low back pain, N=63	RCT comparing MT (gentle stroking back massage 3 times/week for 3 weeks) to chiropractic, corset, and TC muscle stimulation	Significantly greater improvement in chiropractic group as compared to MT
Irnich et al. (2001)	Pain related to motion. Measured immediately after 1st and last treatments and 3 weeks after 1st and last treatments	Adults with chronic neck pain, N=177	RCT comparing massage (5 treatments of 30 min each over 3 weeks; conventional Western massage including effleurage, petrissage, friction, tapotement, and vibration) to acupuncture and sham laser	Reduction in pain significantly greater in the acupuncture group as compared with the massage group but not compared with the sham laser. Pain improved by greater than 50% compared with baseline in 57% of patients who received acupuncture compared to 32% who received sham laser and 25% who received massage
Konrad et al. (1992)	VAS, analgesic use, mobility, and functional ability	Adults with subacute or chronic low back pain, N=158	RCT comparing MT (underwater massage; 3 for 15 min for 4 weeks) with balneotherapy, traction and no-treatment control	No significant differences between treatment group; MT was significantly superior to no treatment at end of treatment period
Kutner et al. (2008)	Brief pain inventory, Memorial Symptom Distress Scale, McGill Quality of Life Questionnaire, use of pain medications; pain and mood measured before and after massage with Memorial Symptom Assessment Card	Adults with advanced cancer and moderate pain enrolled in hospice or palliative care, N=380	Multisite RCT comparing MT (massage, 30 min, 3 massages/week for 2 weeks; effleurage, petrissage, and myofascial trigger point therapy provided by massage therapist) to simple touch	Significantly greater decrease in pain and increase in mood for MT group immediately after treatment compared to simple touch. No significantly greater decrease in pain, symptom distress, or mood for MT vs. simple touch. Improvements noted over time in pain and symptom distress for both groups. No increase in parenteral morphine equivalent use over time

Study	Measures	Population	Intervention	Results
Meek Spring (1993)	Measures of relaxation: HR, BP, skin temp. immediately and 5 min after MT. Repeated 24 h later	Persons with terminal illness enrolled in hospice, N = 30	Slow stroke back massage; 60 strokes/min with Biotone massage oil on 2-in.-wide areas on both sides of spinous processes from crown of head to sacral area for 3 min; Pre–post intervention measures on two consecutive days of treatment	Significant changes in HR, BP, and skin temperature on both days with increased relaxation indicators on the second day
Myers et al. (1999)	VAS; McGill Pain Questionnaire before and after session	Adults with sickle cell pain, N = 16	RCT comparing MT (six sessions) to relaxation training	No significant differences between groups. Both groups showed decrease in pain dimensions
Perlman et al. (2006)	VAS and Western Ontario and McMaster Universities Osteoarthritis Index	Adults with osteoarthritis of the knee	RCT comparing MT (1 h full body Swedish, twice/week for 4 weeks and once/week for 4 weeks) to usual care delayed intervention control	MT group had significant improvements in WOMAC scores and in VAS of pain
Phipps et al. (2005)	VAS for distress and mood	Children undergoing bone marrow transplant, N = 50	RCT comparing parent massage (parent-provided massage and control-provided massage, three massage sessions for 4 weeks) and standard care	No significant differences for distress and mood between groups
Plews-Ogan et al. (2005)	Numeric Rating Scale (0–10); pain unpleasantness and pain sensation	Adults with chronic musculoskeletal pain, N = 30	RCT comparing massage (1 h sessions, once a week for 8 weeks. Techniques used at discretion of therapist included Swedish, deep-tissue, neuromuscular, and pressure point) and mindfulness-based stress reduction to standard care	At week 8 MT group had mean change score in pain unpleasantness of 2.9 compared to standard care group mean change score of 0.13. These were not statistically significant

(continued)

Table 35.4 (continued)

References	Measurement	Participants population & N	Design and control group	Findings/notes
Post-White et al. (2003)	Pain index, analgesic usage, mood and fatigue	Adults with cancer, N=164 (N=77 HT or MT; N=75 control); 33.6% drop out	Randomized two period cross-over comparing massage Rx and HT to no-treatment control; self-control (attention control – sitting). HT; four sessions of control and four sessions of massage Rx; 45 min/session	No differences in pain reduction between MT and control group. Mean difference: 0.0. Pain reduction, fatigue reduction, and improved mood for both HT and MT groups
Puustjarvi et al. (1990)	VAS and incidence of pain over 2-week period; range of motion, ENMG; Beck Depression Index	Adult females with chronic tension headaches	Single group pre–post design Upper body MT with deep tissue techniques. Trigger point therapy	Range of motion increased after MT, VAS, and days with neck pain decreased significantly. Significant change in ENMG and depression improved
Sims (1986)	Symptom distress assessed four times (before and after MT and rest periods)	Adults with breast cancer, N=6	Randomized crossover massage (gentle, 3 consecutive days) and rest period	Control group showed no differences after crossover. MT group showed improvement then significant increase in symptom distress after crossover
Smith et al. (2002a)	VAS for pain, VSH for sleep, STAI for anxiety and McCorkle & Young's Symptom Distress Scale measured at baseline and after 1 week	Adults with cancer hospitalized for chemotherapy or radiation therapy, N=41 (20 MT, 21 control)	Quasi-experimental design; pretest–posttest control group design without random assignment comparing MT (using Swedish techniques delivered by nurse massage therapist, 30 min, three massages over 1 week period) to therapeutic nurse presence group	Statistically significant interactions were found for pain, symptom distress, and sleep. Sleep improved slightly for those in the MT group and deteriorated significantly for those in the control group. There were statistically significant differences in improved pain and symptom distress for those in the MT group
Soden et al. (2004)	Pain and anxiety measured by VAS of pain intensity, Verran and Snyder-Halpern sleep scale and Hospital Anxiety and Depression scale, and Rotterdam Symptom Checklist	Cancer patients, N=42	RCT comparing weekly massage with aromatherapy, massage without aromatherapy, and no-treatment control	No significant long-term benefits of aromatherapy massage or massage in improving pain control, anxiety, or quality of life

Study	Measure	Population	Design	Results
Sunshine et al. (1996)	Dolimeter and self-reports of pain and symptoms	Adults with fibromyalgia syndrome	Quasi-experiment comparing MT (30 min treatment, two times/week for 5 weeks) to TENS and sham TENS	MT group reported lower anxiety and depression and lower immediate cortisol levels. MT had greater improvement on dolimeter and reported less pain, stiffness, fatigue, and fewer nights of difficult sleeping
van den Dolder & Roberts (2003)	SF McGill Pain Questionnaire and Patient Specific Functional Disability Measure	Adults with chronic shoulder pain, N=29 (N=15 MT; N=14 control)	RCT comparing MT (soft tissue massage around the shoulder, six treatments for 2 weeks) to waitlist control	Significant improvements in range of motion, pain, and functional ability for MT group
Walach et al. (2003)	Pain rating using a 9-point Likert-type scale. Measures posttreatment and 3 month follow up	Adults with chronic pain conditions of back, shoulders, head and limbs, N=29 (N=19 in MT and N=10 in SMC)	RCT of MT vs. standard medical care	Pain improved significantly in both groups, but only MT group sustained improvement at 3 months
Weinrich & Weinrich (1990)	VAS immediately after MT	Adults receiving radiation, chemotherapy, or both, N=28	Swedish massage, 10 min given by seven senior nursing students. Slow, continuous strokes with lotion RCT with verbal visit control group	Results varied for males and females. No analysis of significant differences between groups. Males showed decrease after massage
Wilcock et al. (2004)	Mood, quality of life, symptom intensity, symptom bother	Adults with cancer in palliative day care, N=29	RCT comparing MT (aromatherapy massage; 30 min/weekly for 4 weeks) with standard care control	No significant differences between MT and control groups
Wilkie et al. (2000)	Pain intensity, prescribed IM morphine equivalent doses, hospital admissions, and quality of life. Measures before first and after fourth massage	Adults with cancer pain, N=29 (MT N=14 and control N=15)	RCT comparing massage (four sessions (2 per week for 2 weeks) administered by licensed therapists) to usual hospice care	Pain intensity, pulse rate, and respiratory rate decreased significantly immediately after massages. Mixed results related to pain medication use
Wilkinson (1995)	Physical symptoms, quality of life	Adults with cancer, N=51 (N=26 AM; N=25 control)	Randomized case series comparing aromatherapy massage with massage without essential oils	Significant decrease in physical symptoms and fewer and less severe symptoms; significant increase in quality of life after aromatherapy massage; significant decrease in physical symptoms for aromatherapy massage compared to massage

(continued)

Table 35.4 (continued)

References	Measurement	Participants population & N	Design and control group	Findings/notes
Wilkinson et al. (2007)	Anxiety, depression measured at 6 and 10 weeks	Adults with cancer, $N=144$	RCT comparing aromatherapy massage with usual care control	Significant decrease in anxiety and depression at 6 weeks; no significant decrease in anxiety and depression at 10 weeks; significant decrease in self-reported anxiety at 6 and 10 weeks
Williams et al. (2005b)	Missoula-Vitas Quality of Life Index measured at baseline and 8 weeks	Adults with late stage AIDS	RCT comparing MT (30 min/day/5 days/week for 1 month), Metta meditation, both MT and meditation and routine care	Combined group demonstrated improvement in QOL from baseline to 8 weeks

Twenty-one studies of MT for palliative care are given in Table 35.4. A variety of outcomes were measured including pain; distress from symptoms such as nausea, fatigue, and dyspnea; quality of life; anxiety; mood; sleep; and physiological measures of arousal. The most consistent improvement was in anxiety or enhanced indicators of relaxation. Immediate effects were more frequent than any sustained effects. Based on these data, MT can provide comfort and relief for those experiencing pain and distress related to symptoms from cancer and side effects related to treatment. The effects of massage may be temporary; however, even this temporary relief is significant. The consistency of the findings supports the use of MT for palliative and end-of-life care.

A clinical practice guideline on the diagnosis and treatment of low back pain issued by the ACP and the American Pain society weakly recommends, based on moderate-quality evidence, massage for patients with chronic or subacute low back pain (Chou et al. 2007). The ACCP recommends MT delivered by a massage therapist trained in oncology as part of a multimodality treatment approach for lung cancer patients experiencing anxiety or pain. The ACCP cautions that the application of deep or intense pressure is not recommended near cancer lesions or anatomic distortions and in patients with bleeding tendencies (Cassileth et al. 2007).

In summary, there has been profound increase in research related to outcomes of MT for chronic pain and palliative care over the past 25 years. While the methodological quality of the studies is variable, with small sample sizes and inadequate control groups, the overall consistency of effects is compelling. There is sufficient evidence to support the use of MT for chronic low back pain and there is potential for its use for other chronic pain syndromes. In addition, there is evidence to support the use of massage for supportive, palliative care for those with cancer. Reviews have supported the efficacy of MT for chronic low back pain especially when combined with stretching and education and when provided by experienced therapists, and it may be cost effective. Future RCTs should follow the CONSORT guidelines for reporting. A focus on the theoretical foundations to determine mechanisms of action should be a focus of future studies. The question of the length of time that effects deserves attention in future studies.

Chiropractic

Chiropractic practice is based on creating optimum structure for the support of the nervous system. D. D. Palmer originated the practice in Davenport, Iowa in 1895. The most common use of chiropractic treatment is for back and neck pain; however, many chiropractors extol the virtues of the practice for maintaining a healthy nervous system and healing other organs. The foundation of chiropractic care is spinal manipulation; however, many practitioners add other forms of physical therapy/massage such as application of heat and ultrasound as well as counseling regarding nutrition, exercise, and lifestyle change.

While spinal manipulation is used safely by osteopathic physicians and chiropractors for the treatment of low back pain, there are questions about the safety of cervical adjustments, and spinal manipulation is not safe for persons with metastatic cancer to the spine or osteoporosis of the spine. In addition, chiropractic should be used cautiously for people with arthritis or osteoporosis, migraines, blood clotting disorders or with those on anticoagulant therapy, vertebrobasilar vascular insufficiency, or arteritis (Natural Standard 2010b).

The theory underpinning chiropractic care is that vertebral subluxation (misalignment) interrupts the flow of impulses (Palmer called it "innate intelligence") through the nervous system. These blockages create disturbances that result in disease. Another theory is that spinal adjustments break down adhesions that develop in the hypomobile or fixed Z joints, and the adjustments create space and promote physiological range of motion.

A considerable amount of research on chiropractic has been conducted for tension and migraine headaches, low back pain, carpal tunnel syndrome, dysmenorrhea, fibromyalgia, hip pain, infantile colic, temporomandibular joint disorder, neck pain, pelvic pain, and shoulder pain. The quality of studies varies; methodological problems include the lack of an appropriate control group, lack of blinding, small sample sizes, and variable dosages and types of manipulation, making comparisons across trials difficult.

Systematic reviews have been completed for chiropractic treatment for headache pain, low back pain, neck pain, dysmenorrhea, and infantile colic (Bronfort 1999). For this chapter, only the evidence related to chronic pain syndromes for headache, low back pain, and neck pain will be addressed because these are the three areas for which there is credible and consistent evidence of efficacy. There have been no studies focusing on spinal manipulation or chiropractic treatment for palliative care, that is, symptoms produced by life-limiting illnesses. Moreover, given the volume of clinical trials and the number of systematic reviews, only a selected number of relevant RCTs for the chronic pain syndromes are included in Table 35.5.

Two reviews specifically addressed chronic headache pain (Bronfort et al. 2004, 2001a). In the first Cochrane Review, 22 studies were analyzed. The authors concluded that spinal manipulation was an effective prophylactic treatment for chronic migraine headaches, but the effect was not long lasting and was similar to the preferred pharmacotherapy for migraines. In the second review of nine RCTs, the authors reported that spinal manipulation was better than massage for chronic cervical headache.

Four RCTs of chiropractic spinal manipulation for chronic headache pain are summarized in Table 35.5 (Boline et al. 1995; Haas et al. 2010; Nelson et al. 1998; Nilsson et al. 1997). These were selected for their quality; all four examined chiropractic spinal manipulation for the treatment of chronic headache pain (migraine, cervicogenic and chronic tension type). SMT was compared to amitriptyline, the medication of choice for headache pain, light massage, deep friction massage with laser, and a combination of amitriptyline and SMT. Across these four studies there was a small effect in favor of chiropractic spinal manipulation. There was not a significant clinical effect when compared to medication. Based on these reviews, there is evidence that chiropractic spinal manipulation has some benefit for a variety of chronic headache syndromes. The benefit may not be dramatic, is similar to medication, and may not be as cost effective or convenient as amitriptyline. Even so, SMT can be a choice for those suffering from chronic headaches.

Four meta-analyses and 12 reviews were published for chiropractic treatment of low back pain. Some reviews did not specify the focus on acute, subacute, or chronic low back pain, although the differences in outcomes by type were reported in some (Bronfort et al. 1996; Shekelle et al. 1992). One meta-analysis based on 23 RCTs of variable quality concluded that spinal manipulation therapy (SMT) was better than the comparison treatments for low back pain based on calculated effect sizes (Anderson et al. 1992). Bronfort et al.'s (2004) systematic review concluded that there is moderate evidence that SMT provides a similar effect to NSAIDS and is better than physical therapy and exercises. In a review of nine trials on chronic low back pain, van Tulder concluded that there was strong evidence in favor of SMT over placebo, and moderate evidence that SMT was better than usual care, bed rest, analgesics, and massage (van Tulder et al. 2003). Walker et al. (2010) conducted a review of 12 studies of combined chiropractic interventions (other than spinal manipulation) on pain, disability, back-related function, overall improvement, and patient satisfaction in adults with low back pain, finding that there was no difference between chiropractic and the comparison group treatments, and there was no difference for combined chiropractic treatments for chronic low back pain. In a review of 64 RCTs, 12 guidelines, 13 systematic reviews/meta-analyses, and 11 cohort studies, Lawrence et al. (2008) concluded that the evidence for the use of spinal manipulation is as strong for chronic low back pain as it is for acute and subacute LBP. These researchers state that exercise with manipulation may improve outcomes and minimize recurrence. There was less evidence for LBP with leg pain and sciatica. Based on these reviews, there is good evidence for the use of chiropractic spinal manipulation for the treatment of chronic low back pain.

Table 35.5 Manipulation/chiropractic evidence

References	Measurement	Participants population & N	Design and control group	Findings/notes
Boline et al. (1995)	VAS for pain intensity, h/day with headache and use of pain medications measured at 4 and 6 weeks posttreatment	Adults with chronic and episodic tension type headache, N=150	RCT comparing chiropractic SMT with amitriptyline	Medication group had greater pain reduction after 6 weeks of treatment; SMT group had greater decrease in pain intensity, hours with headache, and pain medications used after 4 weeks of treatment
Bronfort et al. (1996)	Pain VAS and analgesic use in past week Measured at 3, 5, and 11 weeks	Adults with chronic LBP, N=174	RCT comparing SMT and strengthening (20 supervised sessions, ten sessions of 10–15 min duration and ten sessions 1 h for 6 weeks) to NSAIDS and strengthening exercises (20 sessions) and SMT and stretching exercises	No differences in pain between the groups
Bronfort et al. (2001b)	VAS for neck pain measured at 3, 6, and 12 months	Adults with chronic mechanical neck pain, N=191	RCT comparing SMT to SMT with rehabilitative neck exercise to rehabilitative neck exercise for 11 weeks (20 sessions)	Other than for patient satisfaction in which the SMT + exercise was superior, there were no significant differences between groups
Cambron et al. (2006)	Pain VAS; followed for 1 year	Adults with chronic low back pain, N=235	RCT comparing chiropractic care using flexion/distraction to an exercise control	Both groups had a decrease in pain following the interventions; those who received chiropractic care had significantly lower pain than those who had the physical therapy exercise program
Evans et al. (2002)	VAS for pain	Adults with chronic neck pain, N=191	RCT comparing SMT with exercise, SMT alone, to rehabilitation exercise	Significant differences among the groups in patient rated pain; those in the groups with exercise had significantly less pain
Giles et al. (2003)	VAS of pain intensity administered at 2, 5, and 9 weeks after treatment	Adults with chronic low back pain, N=115	RCT comparing spinal manipulation to medication and acupuncture	Manipulation achieved the best results with 50% improvement on the VAS for back pain. Acupuncture showed a better result on the VAS for neck pain
Gudavalli et al. (2006)	Pain VAS measured after 4 weeks and 1 year follow up	Adults with chronic LBP, N=235	RCT comparing flexion-distraction, ultrasound, cold with exercise, ultrasound and cold; 2–4 times/week for 4 weeks	No significant differences between the groups

(continued)

Table 35.5 (continued)

References	Measurement	Participants population & N	Design and control group	Findings/notes
Haas et al. (2010)	Von Korff pain and disability scales, no headaches in past 4 weeks, medication use. Data collected every 4 weeks for 24 weeks	Adults with chronic cervicogenic headache, N=80	RCT comparing spinal manipulation (8 or 16 sessions; treated once or twice/week for 8 weeks) to a light massage control	Small dose effects for both 8 and 16 sessions and an advantage for spinal manipulation over the control group. The advantage increased with dose. Those with SMT were more likely to have 50% reduction in pain at 12 and 24 weeks
Hurwitz et al. (2002)	VAS	Adults with chronic neck pain, N=336	RCT comparing SMT with and without heat and electrical muscle stimulation and mobilization with and without heat and electrical muscle stimulation	No significant differences between the groups
Murphy et al. (2010)	VAS; Neck Disability Index (NDI) measured at week 4 and 12	Adults with chronic nonspecific neck pain, N=40	RCT comparing chiropractic care (4 weeks) with exercise to exercise alone; 8 weeks of exercise	Significant decreases in the NDI and VAS in both groups but no between group differences
Nelson et al. (1998)	Headache pain index	Adults with chronic migraine headaches, N=218	RCT comparing chiropractic SMT with chiropractic SMT with amitriptyline and amitriptyline alone	Small group differences in pain index after 2 months of treatment; SMT group had greater pain reduction but difference was not significant
Nilsson et al. (1997)	Headache pain index	Adults with chronic cervicogenic headache, N=53	RCT comparing chiropractic SMT with deep friction massage/placebo laser	Significant reduction in headache pain intensity and frequency with group receiving chiropractic SMT after 3 weeks of treatment
Palmieri & Smoyak (2002)	Numeric Pain Scale after procedure and 4 weeks later	Adults with chronic low back pain	RCT comparing chiropractic manipulation under anesthesia to traditional chiropractic treatment	The MUA group reported greater pain relief than the control
Savolainen et al. (2004)	VAS	Adults with chronic neck pain, N=75	RCT comparing thoracic manipulation with physiotherapeutic exercises	Manipulation more effective than the exercise program
Wilkey et al. (2008)	Pain NRS (current pain and average pain over past 2, 3, 6, and 8 weeks)	Adults with chronic LBP, N=48	RCT comparing the chiropractic treatments (at the discretion of practitioner (SMT), flexion, distraction drop technique, dry needling, exercise) to pain clinic treatment at discretion of consultant	No significant differences between the groups

Six RCTs of chiropractic therapy for low back pain are included in Table 35.5 (Bronfort et al. 1996; Cambron et al. 2006; Giles et al. 2003; Gudavalli et al. 2006; Palmieri & Smoyak 2002; Wilkey et al. 2008). The chiropractic therapies tested in these studies were either SMT, flexion-distraction, or manipulation under anesthesia. The results were mixed. In three of the six studies, there were no significant differences in pain between the treatment and control groups. In one study manipulation under anesthesia was superior to routine chiropractic care, and in the other two there were significant benefits to chiropractic care when compared to physical therapy exercise and acupuncture and medication. The results of these selected studies are overshadowed by the strength of the reviews; there is good evidence to support the use of chiropractic care for the treatment of chronic low back pain.

One meta-analysis and six reviews were conducted on chiropractic treatment for neck pain. The meta-analysis (Aker et al.) of nine studies showed some small effect (Aker et al. 1996). Vernon et al. (2007) reviewed 19 clinical trials and reported that there is "moderate to high quality evidence" that those with chronic neck pain that is not from whiplash benefit from a course of spinal manipulation or mobilization at 6, 12, and up to 201 weeks after treatment. Bronfort et al. (2004) concluded that for chronic neck pain there is moderate evidence that spinal manipulation and mobilization were more effective than general practitioner management, but that the effect was short term and no better than rehabilitative approaches. Other reviewers drew similar conclusions that spinal manipulation and mobilization when combined with exercise were beneficial, but without exercise were not (Gross et al. 2004). Other reviewers reported that there was no evidence that spinal manipulation was effective for the relief of chronic neck pain (Ernst 2003b; Hurwitz et al. 1996; Shekelle & Coulter 1997).

Five RCTs testing the effects of chiropractic spinal manipulation and/or mobilization on chronic neck pain are included in Table 35.5. The frequency and duration of treatments varied. The evidence from the aforementioned reviews and these selected RCTs are inconclusive for the use of chiropractic treatment for chronic neck pain.

One Cochrane Review of three studies on manipulation for dysmenorrhea was published (Proctor et al. 2006). Spinal manipulation was no more effective than the sham; it was more effective than no treatment at all. A review of chiropractic manipulation in the treatment of colic in infants revealed no benefit over placebo to support its use (Hughes & Bolton 2002). There is no evidence to support the use of chiropractic treatment for these or any other chronic pain syndromes.

Based on this analysis chiropractic care can be beneficial for the treatment of chronic headache pain (tension-type, migraine, or cervicogenic) and for chronic low back pain. The evidence is contradictory and inconclusive for the use of chiropractic treatment for chronic neck pain. There is no evidence to support the use of chiropractic spinal manipulation for any other chronic pain syndromes. Even for headache and low back pain the effects may be small and comparable to medication. Cost effectiveness of chiropractic care for headache and low back pain is important to consider given the small differences in clinical significance.

Reflexology

Reflexology is defined by the Reflexology Association of America as "the systematic, manual stimulation of the reflex maps located on the feet, hands and outer ears that resembles a shape of the human body" (http://www.reflexology-usa.org/articles/definitions_of_reflexology.html). Few studies of the efficacy or effectiveness of reflexology for chronic pain or palliative care have been published (Table 35.6). Those that have been published tend to be small and demonstrate mixed results. Methodological quality of these studies is often poor; and most high quality trials did not generate positive findings. Further complicating interpretation of the evidence is that published studies used different intensity and duration of treatment. The studies that did find positive effects demonstrated beneficial effects on pain and on mood (primarily anxiety) immediately following the reflexology session. Longer term effects are less certain. Patients seem to demonstrate satisfaction with reflexology

Table 35.6 Reflexology evidence

References	Measurement	Participants population & N	Design and control group for RCTs	Findings/notes
Gambles et al. (2002)	Qualitative care patients undergoing course of reflexology treatments	Thirty-four hospice patients	Questionnaire distributed within 1 week of completion of course of reflexology: at least four sessions and up to six sessions	All patients satisfied or very satisfied with treatment *Emotional benefits* Relaxation (91%): relief from tension and anxiety Soothing and calming Perceived reductions in anxiety and tension Help with "coming to terms" Lifting the emotional burden "Time out" Relaxation *Physical benefits* Improved sleep Improved appetite Help with treatment side effects
Gunnarsdottir & Peden-McAlpine (2010)	Changes in pain or other symptoms Data collected with observation, interviews, and symptom diary for 13 weeks; analyzed within cases and across cases Diary: quality of sleep, medication intake and any sensations of pain or any other symptoms/benefits. If pain experienced, marked sites of pain on a body diagram of a body and evaluated pain intensity at each site using a 0–10 Numerical Rating Scale (NRS)	Six women with fibromyalgia	Multiple case study 10 weekly sessions: 45 min of reflexology and 10–15 min of relaxation	Pain started to isolate and decrease as intervention progressed in four of six cases In those who showed decreased pain, pain increased after first session; decreased substantially after six or seven sessions Patterns of sleep did not change. Five did not feel as fatigued Migraine headaches, edema, and fecal elimination problems were better. Some pain in certain areas was not affected

Hodgson & Andersen (2008)	Primary: reduction of physiologic distress as measured by salivary-amylase Secondary observed pain Data collected: (1) saliva samples from which salivary-amylase (sAA) was measured; (2) 5-min observations of affect (e.g., anger, depression, anxiety) using the Apparent Affect Rating Scale (AARS); (3) pain using the checklist of nonverbal pain indicators (CNPI); (4) other demographic and physiologic measures (e.g., blood pressure, pulse, mental status)	Twenty-one nursing home residents over age of 75 with mild to moderate dementia	Experimental, repeated-measures, crossover design study Randomly assigned to two groups: (1) 4 weeks of weekly 30-min reflexology and 4 weeks of friendly visits; (2) 4 weeks of friendly visits and 4 weeks of weekly 30-min reflexology Data collected at four timepoints: (1) early morning: 7 AM–7:30 AM, (2) midmorning: 11 AM–11:30 AM, (3) early afternoon: 1 PM–1:30 PM, and (4) late afternoon: 3:30 PM–4 PM	Significant reduction in observed pain and salivary-amylase when receiving the reflexology treatment condition as compared to the control condition Statistically significant decline in pain (F 5.45, p 0.031), and sAA (F 4.37, p 0.049), with borderline improvements in sadness (F 4.06, p 0.069)
Kohara et al. (2004)	Fatigue: Cancer Fatigue Scale (CFS) just before, 1 and 4 h after treatment	Twenty terminally ill cancer patients	Pre–post design Aromatherapy with footsoak in warm water containing lavender essential oil for 3 min, followed by reflexology treatment with jojoba oil containing lavender for 10 min	Total CFS scores improved significantly from 25.6 ± 11.0 to 18.1 ± 10.0, $p < 0.001$ Among three CFS subscales, physical and cognitive subscale scores were reduced significantly (11.3 ± 6.1 to 6.7 ± 6.1, $p < 0.001$; 4.5 ± 3.2 to 2.4 ± 2.4, $p < 0.001$) No adverse effects
Ross et al. (2002)	Quality of life, well-being, cancer symptoms Hospital Anxiety and Depression Scale (HADS) Symptom Distress: 10-point rating scale of the severity of ten common symptoms Each scale was completed prior to the first treatment and repeated within 24 h of each session Short semistructured interview	Seventeen individuals with advanced cancer	Randomized controlled design One session weekly for 6 weeks (reflexology vs. foot massage)	Neither treatment had a significant effect on mood or common symptoms

(continued)

Table 35.6 (continued)

References	Measurement	Participants population & N	Design and control group for RCTs	Findings/notes
Stephenson et al. (2007)	Pain and anxiety Brief Pain Inventory (BPI) (short form) Short-Form McGill Pain Questionnaire (SF-MPQ) Visual Analog Scale for Anxiety	Forty-two experimental and 44 control subjects Patients with metastatic cancer and their partners	Experimental pretest/posttest design included patient-partner dyads randomly assigned to an experimental or control group Intervention: 15- to 30-min teaching session on foot reflexology to the partner by a certified reflexologist, an optional 15- to 30-min foot reflexology session for the partner, and a 30-min, partner-delivered foot reflexology intervention for the patient. Relaxing techniques for 10 min at the beginning five 5 min at end of the session Control: 30-min reading session from their partners	Following initial partner-delivered foot reflexology, patients experienced a significant decrease in pain intensity and anxiety After adjusting for preintervention pain, significant differences in postintervention pain between the intervention and control groups. Moderate effect in the subgroups with moderate to severe preintervention pain Experimental group experienced 62% decrease in anxiety from baseline to postintervention, Control: 23% After adjusting for preintervention anxiety, significant differences in postintervention anxiety between intervention and control groups
Stephenson et al. (2003)	Duration of effect of reflexology Yes/no response to the statement: "I believe that foot reflexology will help relieve my pain related to cancer"	Thirt-six oncology inpatients with metastasis with pain ≥ 2 on a 0–10 self-report pain scale Nineteen treatment Seventeen control	Experimental repeated-measures design Stratified random sample; selected from a predetermined random schedule of control or experimental subjects Stratified by scores of low pain (2–4) or high pain (5 and above) Foot reflexology delivered two times, 24 h apart	Pain scores lower by 2.4 points in the treatment group than in the control group immediately after intervention Adjusting for baseline pain levels, no statistically significant effect at 3 h after intervention nor significant effect at 24 h after intervention Prior beliefs in reflexology/immediate effects: no significant difference
Tsay et al. (2008)	Pain and anxiety postoperatively Short-form McGill Pain Questionnaire, visual analog scale for pain, summary of pain medications consumed, and the Hospital Anxiety and Depression Scale (HADS)	Sixty-one Postoperative patients with gastric cancer and hepatocellular cancer	Double-blind, randomized, controlled trial (intervention $n=30$, control $n=31$) Stratified block randomization procedure, with stratification for diagnosis of gastric or liver cancer Intervention group: usual pain management plus 10 min of foot reflexotherapy on each foot for a total of 20 min once/day for 3 consecutive days Control group: usual pain management	Using generalized estimation equations and controlling for confounding variables, less pain and anxiety reported by the intervention group compared with the control group Patients in the intervention group also received significantly less opioid analgesics than the control group

treatments. While reflexology would appear to have minimal risks, in one study patients described the reflexology treatment as painful, at least initially. Three systematic reviews of reflexology concluded that the evidence to date does not demonstrate convincingly that reflexology is an effective treatment (Ernst 2009b; Wang et al. 2008; Wilkinson et al. 2008b).

Manipulation of Energy Fields

Perhaps the most controversial category of therapies is energy medicine or biofield therapies. These therapies continue to be used by health care professionals and the public for the alleviation of chronic pain and for palliation of symptoms related to chronic illnesses, and they deserve attention. Energy medicine was one of NCCAM's five categories, but recently, with a new classification system, "biofield therapies" replaced "energy medicine," has been located within the category of "Other CAM Practices." NCCAM describes "biofield therapies" as "manipulation of various energy fields to affect health," and these energy fields are characterized as veritable (measurable) or putative (yet to be measured). Those therapies involving electromagnetic fields such as magnet and light therapies are considered veritable. Practices based on putative energy fields include qi gong, Reiki, TT, and healing touch (http://nccam.nih.gov/health/whatiscam/). In this section each of the relevant therapies in this category will be described, along with the purported mechanism of action, the synthesis of evidence, and recommendations for use for chronic pain and palliative care.

Table 35.7 summarizes research in biofield therapies for chronic pain and palliative care. The table includes randomized controlled trials (RCTs) and some trials without randomization. Only studies of chronic pain, those conditions that are persistent, recurring, and not self-limiting were included. For this reason, studies of episodic pain syndromes such as migraines and tension headaches were not included. Thirty-five studies of TT, magnets, healing touch, Reiki, Qigong, and spiritual healing are included. The decision was made to exclude studies related to pulsed electromagnetic fields (PEMF), cranial electrotherapy stimulation (CES), and transcutaneous electrical nerve stimulation (TENS) in this review because they are less consistent with the definition of biofield therapies, and may be classified as conventional therapies using electrical stimulation. Spiritual healing was included because the mechanism of action is consistent with the definition of biofield therapies.

In 2008, a systematic review of touch therapy studies for pain relief was conducted by The Cochrane Collaboration. Twenty-four studies with 1,153 participants were included in this review. Of these studies, 5 focused on healing touch, 16 on TT, and 3 on Reiki. On average, participants experiencing the touch therapies had a 0.83 unit (on a 0–10 point scale) lower pain intensity than those not exposed to these therapies (95% confidence interval: −1.16 to −0.50) (So et al. 2008). The ACCP does not recommend therapies based on manipulation of energy fields for patients with lung cancer (Cassileth et al. 2007).

Magnetic Therapy

Magnets have been marketed and used by the public for the relief of chronic pain. They have been applied as insoles to relieve foot pain, attached to localized areas like lower back and joints, worn as wrist bracelets, or used in mattress pads for more generalized pain. The purported mechanism of action is that the magnetic field increases blood flow to the area/s causing pain, thereby enhancing the body's ability to heal. Others suggest that the magnetic field increases the release of endorphins, altering pain perception and tolerance. Another hypothesis is that the electromagnetic field of the magnet may change the biofield in some way that promotes healing.

Table 35.7 Manipulation of energy fields evidence

References	CAM modality	Measurement	Participants POPULATION & N	Design and control group for RCTs	Findings/notes
Abbot et al. (2001)		Primary Total Pain Rating (PRIT) Index of McGill Pain Questionnaire; VAS	Adults with chronic pain, N=120 (N=25 SH, N=25 NLSH, N=27 sham SH, N=28 control)	RCT comparing local and nonlocal spiritual healing to sham spiritual healing and control (30 min/session; 8 weeks, 1×/week for local and sham groups)	All four arms showed decrease in PRIT over 8 weeks. No differences in VAS
Alfano et al. (2001)		Fibromyalgia Impact Questionnaire	Adults with fibromyalgia, N=119	RCT comparing magnetic mattress pad with weak magnetic mattress pad used for sleeping for 6 months	Significant difference in pain reduction between magnetic mattress pad group and placebo
Assefi et al. (2008)		VAS	Adults with fibromyalgia N=100 (four groups: direct Reiki N=23, distant Reiki N=24, direct sham N=23, distant sham N=23)	RCT comparing Reiki (both direct touch and distant); twice weekly Rx; for 8 weeks) to sham control	No differences in pain within or between groups
Brown et al. (2002)		McGill Pain Inventory	Adults with chronic pelvic pain, N=32 (N=32 for 2 weeks, N=19 for 4 weeks)	RCT comparing magnets (bipolar permanent magnets; either 2 or 4 weeks of Rx to abdominal trigger points 24 h/day) to placebo	No significant differences in pain
Castronova & Oleson (1991)		VAS	Adults with back pain, N=24 (N=12 TT and N=12 NT control)	RCT comparing TT (eight sessions; 50 min/session, weekly interval) to no treatment	Significantly greater pain reduction between TT and control group. Mean difference: −2.13
Colbert et al. (1999)		VAS, Body pain	Adults with fibromyalgia, N=30	RCT comparing magnetic therapy with placebo magnetic mattress pad used for 16 weeks at night	Significant difference in pain reduction between magnetic therapy group and placebo
Collacott et al. (2000)		McGill Pain Inventory	Adults back pain, N=20	RCT with crossover comparing magnet (applied to back for 6 h/day for 3 days) with placebo	No significant difference in pain reduction between magnet and placebo
Denison (2004)		Fibromyalgia Health Assessment Questionnaire	Adults with fibromyalgia, N=15 (N=10 TT and N=5 control) 6.67% drop out rate	RCT comparing TT (six sessions; 11–14 min/session; weekly intervals) to no-treatment control	Significantly greater pain reduction between TT and control group. Mean difference: 0.12
Dressen & Singg (1998)		McGill Pain Questionnaire	Adults with pain for >1 year, n=120 (n=30 Reiki, n=30 PMR, n=30 NT, n=30 sham)	RCT comparing Reiki (ten sessions; 30 min/session; twice/week interval; Reiki master treated) to sham, PMR, and no treatment	Significantly greater pain reduction between Reiki and control. Mean difference: −1.94

Study	Rating tool	Sample	Design	Results
Gehlart et al. (2000)	Rating tool	Older adults in long-term care setting, $n=23$ ($n=19$ HT, $n=4$ control)	RCT comparing HT (20–30 min; weekly interval to no-treatment control	Significant differences between HT and control. Only percent differences reported
Giasson & Bouchard (1998)	Well-being Scale	Terminally ill patients with cancer in palliative care, $N=20$ ($N=10$ TT, $N=10$ control)	Quasi-experiment (control/no randomization) comparing TT (three sessions, 15–20 min/ session; consecutive days) to a rest period control	Well-being increased significantly and was higher than control
Gillespie et al. (2007)	McGill Pain Questionnaire	Type II diabetics with neuropathic pain, $N=207$ ($N=93$ Reiki, $N=88$ sham, $N=26$ no treatment) Stopped randomizing to control due to dropout rate	RCT comparing Reiki (25 min/session; 12 weeks with two sessions week 1, and one session weeks 2–12) to sham and control	Significant within-group pain reduction for Reiki and sham Reiki, but no between-group differences for Reiki vs. sham Reiki
Gordon et al. (1998)	VAS and West Haven-Yale Multidimensional Pain Inventory	Adults with osteoarthritis of the knee, $N=27$ ($N=8$ TT, $N=11$ placebo, $N=8$ no treatment)	RCT comparing TT (six sessions; weekly intervals) to no-treatment control and sham placebo	Significantly greater pain reduction in TT group as compared to control Mean difference: -0.92
Harlow et al. (2004)	VAS and WOMAC	Adults with hip or knee pain, $N=193$	RCT comparing magnetic wrist bracelet with placebo (weak magnet) for 12 weeks	Significant difference in pain reduction between magnet and placebo group
Lee et al. (2001)	VAS	Elders with chronic pain, $N=40$ ($N=20$ qigong, $N=20$ no-treatment control)	RCT comparing qi therapy to no-treatment control	Significantly greater pain reduction between qi therapy and no-treatment control
Lee et al. (2003)	VAS	Elders with chronic pain, $N=84$	RCT comparing qi therapy (one session for 10 min) to sham qi therapy control	Significantly greater pain reduction between qi therapy and sham control
Lin & Taylor (1998)	Numerical Rating Scale	Elders with chronic musculoskeletal pain, $N=95$ ($N=33$ TT, $N=30$ placebo, $N=32$ no treatment)	RCT comparing TT (three sessions, 20 min/ session, daily) to sham and no-treatment control	Significantly greater pain reduction with TT as compared to control Mean difference: -0.98
Olson et al. (2003)	VAS, analgesic usage, vital signs	Adults with advanced cancer, $N=24$ ($N=13$ Reiki, $N=11$ control)	RCT comparing Reiki (90 min/session, two sessions with Rx on first and fourth day; Reiki Masters treated) to no treatment	Significantly greater pain reduction between Reiki and control. Mean difference: -0.69

(continued)

Table 35.7 (continued)

References	CAM modality	Measurement	Participants POPULATION & N	Design and control group for RCTs	Findings/notes
Peck (1997)		VAS	Elders with degenerative arthritis, $N=82$ ($N=45$ TT, $N=37$ PMR)	RCT comparing TT (six sessions) to progressive relaxation	Significant pain reduction with TT and PMR. PMR produced greater pain reduction than TT
Philcox et al. (2002)		VAS, vital signs	Adult amputees with phantom limb pain or stump pain/9 (3 TT, 3 control, 3 sham)	RCT comparing TT (12 sessions; 20 min/session, 3 times/week interval) to no treatment and sham control; participants blinded	None reported
Post-White et al. (2003)		Pain index, analgesic usage, mood and fatigue	Adults with cancer, $N=164$ ($N=77$ HT or MT, $N=75$ control); 33.6% drop out	Randomized two period cross-over comparing massage Rx and HT (four sessions of control and four sessions of Rx; 45 min/session) to no-treatment control; self-control (attention control – sitting)	No differences in pain reduction between HT and control group. Mean difference: 0.0. Pain reduction, fatigue reduction, and improved mood for both HT and MT groups
Redner et al. (1991)		McGill Pain Questionnaire	Adults with arthritis, headache, or low back pain, $N=47$ ($N=23$ TT, $N=24$ placebo); 4.26% drop out	RCT comparing TT (35-min session; at least level 2 practitioner) to sham control; treating practitioner served as the sham practitioner by stopping energy flow	Significantly greater pain reduction between TT and control. Mean difference: –0.58
Segal et al. (2001)		VAS	Adults with rheumatoid arthritis	RCT comparing magnetic therapy ((Magno Bloc device) wearing continuously for 1 week) with placebo (weak magnet)	No significant differences in pain reduction between magnetic Rx group and control
Slater (1996)		McGill Pain Questionnaire	Adults with chronic postsurgery pain	Quasi-experiment (control/no randomization) comparing HT by experienced practitioner to HT by someone without training	Significant decrease in pain for both the treatment and control groups. Relief lasted longer for those in group with experienced HT practitioner
Smith et al. (2002b)		VAS	Adults with pain >4 months, $N=12$ ($N=$TT and $N=5$ control)	RCT comparing TT to no-treatment control	Significantly greater pain reduction between TT and control. Mean difference: –1.20

Author (year)	Measure	Sample	Design	Results
Sundblom et al. (1994)	Hopkins Symptom Checklist	Adults with idiopathic chronic pain, N=24 (N=12 spiritual healing, N=12 no-treatment control)	RCT comparing spiritual healing from a prominent healer; 3–8 sessions within 2 weeks, 40 min/session to no-treatment control	No differences noted
Tsang et al. (2007)	Subscale of Functional Assessment of Cancer Therapy	Adults with stage I–IV cancer recently completing chemotherapy, N=32 (N=16 Reiki, N=16 control)	Randomized cross-over comparing Reiki (seven sessions; 45 min/session, treatments on first and fifth day; after washout two sessions; Reiki Master treated) to no treatment	Mean difference: −0.79
Vallbona et al. (1997)	McGill Pain Questionnaire	Adults with postpolio syndrome, N=50	RCT comparing magnetic therapy at pain site with placebo	Significant difference in pain reduction between magnet Rx and placebo group
Weintraub et al. (2003)	VAS	Adults with diabetic peripheral neuropathy foot pain, N=259	RCT comparing magnetic insoles 4 months of continuous use to placebo insoles	No significant difference in pain reduction between groups
Weymouth & Sandberg-Lewis (2000)	VAS	Adults with chronic low back pain, N=20s	Quasi-experiment (control/no randomization) comparing HT to chiropractic	Significant pain reduction in both groups; no differences between groups for pain
Winemiller et al. (2005)	VAS	Adults with foot pain, N=83	RCT comparing magnetic insoles with placebo insoles worn 4–8 weeks	No significant difference in pain reduction for magnet group
Wolsko et al. (2004)	VAS, WOMAC	Adults with osteoarthritis of the knee, N=26	RCT comparing magnetic knee sleeve to weak magnetic knee sleeve worn for 6 weeks	No significant differences in pain reduction
Yang et al. (2005)	VAS	Elders with chronic pain, N=40	RCT comparing qigong (20 min/session; Twice/week for 4 weeks) with no-treatment control	Significant reduction in pain for qi therapy compared to control
Ziembroski et al. (2003)	Quality of life; Missoula VITAS	Terminally ill persons enrolled in hospice, N=55 (N=29 HT, N=26 control)	RCT comparing HT to no-treatment control	No significant differences between the two groups

Ten studies listed in Table 35.7 focus on the use of magnets for chronic back pain, pelvic pain, hip, knee, or joint pain from osteoarthritis or rheumatoid arthritis, foot pain from diabetic neuropathy, and pain from postpolio syndrome. All those included in this review were double-blind RCTs with a placebo magnet used as the control. There is doubt about the ability of participants to remain blinded since it would be easy to test whether the device used had magnetic properties. The magnets were used for several days up to 6 months. In 4 of the 10 studies, there were significant differences in pain reduction between those in the magnet therapy group and those in the placebo group; in the other six there were not. Therefore, there is insufficient evidence to support the use of magnets for relief of chronic pain, especially insoles for foot pain or localized magnets to relieve back or joint pain (Pittler et al. 2007). In two studies persons with fibromyalgia had significantly greater pain reduction after sleeping on a magnetic mattress pad for 4 and 6 months, respectively (Colbert et al. 1999; Harlow et al. 2004). Since there are no adverse effects associated with the use of magnets, this particular use is promising. There is beginning evidence to support the prolonged use of a magnetic mattress pad to relieve pain for persons with fibromyalgia. More research is needed; studies with larger sample sizes and prolonged magnet use are desirable to continue the research in targeted, areas with potential.

Therapeutic Touch

Therapeutic touch (TT) is a biofield therapy that has been used since the early 1970s by nurses and other health professionals to promote generalized health and healing. The therapy was developed by a healer named Dora Kunz, and investigated and explicated by Dolores Krieger, RN, PhD, a professor at New York University. Because of this, the particular practice is often referred to as the Kunz–Krieger method to differentiate it from similar touch therapies. Because of its roots in a university, there have been more studies of TT than others testing putative biofield interactions. TT is defined as an intentionally directed process during which the practitioner uses hands to facilitate the healing process (Krieger 1975a; b). The practice was associated with Ayurvedic cultural beliefs about healing, but was formally linked to the tenets of Rogers' (1970) Science of Unitary Human Beings, a nursing conceptual model. The conceptual system purports that both giver and receiver of TT are energy fields that are integral with each other and the environment; that patterns of imbalance in the field can lead to symptoms and disease; that this imbalance can be sensed in part with the hands; and that the field can be balanced through intention and modulation of this energy leading to objective and subjective changes.

The practice involves five steps: centering (calming, focusing, and setting an intention to help or heal); assessing the field (using the hands to sense any disturbances in the recipient's energy field by scanning the body with the hands about 4 in. above the skin); unruffling the field (moving stagnant energy by sweeping the hands over the recipient's body), repatterning the field (using the hands, usually 4 in. away from the skin, to balance the recipient's energy field through channeling energy to areas of imbalance); and recognizing completion (ending the process when balance is sensed). An average treatment is 20–30 min.

TT is an innate human potential; the process can be learned through a training workshop (http://www.therapeutic-touch.org/newsarticle.php?newsID=1). There are TT practitioners throughout the world; many are health professionals who integrate TT as part of their practice in acute, long term, or community-based settings.

The practice of TT became controversial after a research study conducted by a 14 year old for her science project was published in JAMA (Rosa et al. 1998), and was widely publicized by the media as scientific refutation of TT. Several credible critiques (Achterberg 1998a, b; Leskowitz 1998; Smith 1998; Cox 2003) have challenged the results of this study by pointing out fatal conceptual and methodological flaws.

Approximately 100 studies of TT have been published using a variety of designs and methods, with diverse populations and investigating a range of outcomes from anxiety, pain, depression, and general well-being to hemoglobin, wound healing, immunological markers, stress hormones, and engraftment following bone marrow transplant. While methodological quality varies, strength in design and methods has been encouraged by published Standards for Conducting Clinical Biofield Energy Healing Research (Warber et al. 2003). An analysis of a sample of 47 of the studies revealed that researchers reported changes in at least one of the outcome variables in 35 of the studies; some research focused on several outcomes with mixed results (Smith 2005).

Nine of the studies in Table 35.7 focus on TT for chronic pain or palliative care. Populations include those with fibromyalgia, back pain, chronic musculoskeletal pain, amputees with limb/stump pain, or cancer pain. All but the one related to palliative care are RCTs. Control conditions are either a sham TT treatment (a treatment that appears authentic to the recipient) or standard care except for one study that used a comparison group of progressive muscle relaxation. Sample sizes are generally small.

In seven studies there was a significantly greater reduction in pain in the TT group as compared to the control. In the palliative care study there was a greater increase in well-being in the group receiving TT as compared to the control. The only study without significant results was the phantom limb pain study in which the sample size was too small for any meaningful conclusions to be drawn. The number of sessions and the length of each session varied, but for the most part, there were multiple sessions over a period of weeks with each session lasting about 20 min.

There are no adverse effects of TT reported in the literature, and there is good evidence for the use of TT as a complementary therapy for management of chronic pain. The reviewers for the National Standard database (2010) (www.naturalstandard.com) concluded that the use of TT for pain has "good scientific evidence. Studies suggest that TT may reduce pain…in patients with osteoarthritis…and may improve chronic muscle and joint pain in elderly patients. Preliminary research reports that those treated with TT need less pain medication following surgery. The early research is suggestive." There is limited evidence for its use in other forms of symptom management in palliative care, although there is evidence that TT increases relaxation and decreases anxiety in other populations. Research related to the most efficacious dosage for relief of various chronic pain syndromes and relief of other symptoms associated with palliative care must continue. Studies with larger sample sizes, using sham controls and following the standards for biofield research are important for the future. This means that funding of TT studies by NIH will continue to be essential.

Healing Touch

Healing touch (HT) has similarities to TT, but specific techniques vary. The premise for healing touch is that the "body is a complex energy system that can be affected by another to promote well-being" (Wardell & Weymouth 2004). Healing touch was originated in the 1980s by a nurse, Janet Mentgen. She formalized education and practice in the modality, and in 2004 there were over 75,000 healing touch practitioners who had taken at least the first level training. It is likely that this number has at least doubled today. Practitioners are trained formally in a certificate program offered through Healing Touch International, Inc. www.healingtouchinternational.org and offer healing touch in a variety of settings such as pain clinics, hospices, private practices, and nursing homes.

Five studies in Table 35.7 focus on healing touch. Chronic pain reduction was the focus of four of the studies. Two studies were RCTs comparing HT to a no-treatment control, and two were quasi-experimental designs comparing HT to chiropractic, or HT provided by an experienced vs. a novice practitioner. One RCT revealed no differences in cancer pain in terminally ill adults, and the other reported significant differences in chronic pain in nursing home residents who received HT compared to the controls; however, only percent changes were reported. In the two quasi-experimental studies, there were no differences in pain reduction between the treatment and control groups. In the two studies focused on palliative care, HT was not significantly better than the controls. In one study HT was compared to MT, and the findings revealed decreased pain and fatigue and improved mood for both groups. In the other study, there were no differences in quality of life between those receiving HT and a no-treatment control. Based on these results, there is no evidence that HT is an efficacious treatment for chronic pain or palliative care. Strong research designs with randomization, sham controls, and sample sizes to produce adequate statistical power need to be employed in future research studies.

Reiki

Reiki is a biofield therapy that balances life force energy through aligning it with universal energy. In this way, Reiki is considered to be a spiritual practice. In a Reiki treatment, there is a purported transfer of energy between the practitioner and the recipient through laying on of hands. A particular series of hand placements are taught as the therapist channels Reiki energy to the recipient through direct touch or with the hand/s above the skin. An assessment energy using the hands is conducted prior to the treatment to identify areas on which the practitioner focuses treatment. Reiki can be directed to persons, animals, or things at a distance as well.

The practice of Reiki was developed in 1922 by a Japanese Buddhist monk, Mikao Usui, from ancient Tibetan Buddhist healing practices (Koopsen & Young 2009). Reiki principles and practices vary depending on the lineage of the teacher. The practice is passed down from master to disciples who receive attunements for channeling Reiki energy. There are three levels of training, with Reiki Master as the highest level. Practitioners place their hands on the recipient on specific body parts in a specific sequence. There are no known adverse reactions to any of the biofield therapies. Reiki is used for self-care, health promotion, and healing.

Five studies in Table 35.7 focus on Reiki for chronic pain; there were no studies related to palliative care, although two studies (Olson et al. 2003; Tsang et al. 2007) enrolled persons with advanced cancer. The populations of the other three studies were adults with fibromyalgia, chronic pain for more than a year, and diabetics with neuropathic pain. RCTs and a randomized cross-over were designs used. The number of sessions varied from 2 to 24 over several days to 12 weeks. Sham controls were used in three studies. There was a significantly greater pain reduction in Reiki treatment groups in three studies. In two of those the difference was between the Reiki group and a no-treatment control group. In one study there were no within or between group differences in chronic pain for adults with fibromyalgia. In another study, there were significant within-group differences in neuropathic pain over a 12-week period, but no differences between the Reiki and sham control.

There are no known adverse effects of Reiki. While there have been only a few studies, several studies produced promising results, and the study of Reiki for chronic pain and palliative care deserves continued attention. Evidence that Reiki is an effective therapy for chronic pain is inconclusive. Future research should focus on the minimum efficacious dose for pain relief (number of treatments, length of treatments, and spacing of treatments), and should incorporate sham control groups and sufficient sample sizes.

Qi Therapy

Qigong is a component of Traditional Chinese Medicine (TCM). The movements associated with Qigong are practiced by many to strengthen internal Qi, the dynamic life force and to create balance within the life force. Medical Qigong has internal and external components. Internal Qi is developed by Qigong; when practitioners develop their internal Qi through this process they are able to share it with others, externally, in the healing process (Lee et al. 2001). The practice of internal Qi therapy or Qigong involves a series of prescribed movements. Qi therapy using external Qi is shared through a transfer of life force energy.

According to TCM, disease and symptoms such as pain are manifestations of disturbances in the flow and balance of Qi. Qi therapy (both internal and external) can restore the flow of Qi and enhance balance and harmony, thus relieving the symptoms associated with these disturbances (Lee et al. 2001).

Three studies in Table 35.7 are RCTs of Qi therapy for chronic pain in elders. One study employed a sham control while the other two used a no-treatment control. Samples range from 40 to 84 and the therapy ranged from one to eight sessions. In all three studies, those in the treatment group had a significantly greater reduction in pain as measured by a Visual Analogue Scale than the control group.

With only three small studies it is not possible to draw conclusions. However, Qi therapy is safe and may be comforting and meaningful to those who ascribe to the cultural beliefs about health and illness that are part of TCM.

The use of the therapy can be supported in this context. There is some evidence to support its use for chronic pain; however, with three studies the evidence is tentative. There needs to be additional well-designed studies to further explore Qi therapy for chronic pain and palliative care in more diverse populations.

Spiritual Healing

Spiritual healing has been included in this category of biofield therapies because it involves treating locally or at a distance through prayer or intentions. There can be multiple forms of spiritual healing and competing hypotheses related to the mechanism of action from divine intervention to the creation of changes in the biofield through the intentionality of consciousness.

In Table 35.7, there are two studies of spiritual healing for chronic pain. Abbott et al. (2001) examined both local and nonlocal forms of spiritual healing with adults with chronic pain. Both local and nonlocal sham treatments were used as controls. There was a decrease in pain in all study arms with no differences between the treatment and control groups. The second study of a prominent spiritual healer using chronic pain showed no differences in pain between the treatment and control groups Sundblom et al. 1994). Based on these two studies, there is no evidence to support the use of spiritual healing for chronic pain. Additional research must be conducted before any definitive conclusions can be drawn.

In summary, there has been significant research on the efficacy of biofield therapies for chronic pain and very little research that has specifically focused on palliative care. There is good evidence that TT is an effective treatment for chronic pain. Results of research in the other biofield therapies are less conclusive although there are some promising results for Reiki and Qi therapy for treatment of chronic pain. There is no evidence that the biofield therapies of magnetic therapy, healing touch, or spiritual healing are effective except for possible use of magnetic mattress pads for pain associated with fibromyalgia. Future research should focus on well-designed RCTs that might use multiple outcome variables from biomarkers of inflammation or stress to qualitative descriptions of pain and comfort. New measures that are sensitive to energy such as nitric oxide might be considered as an outcome. Additional studies that examine the mechanism of action and dosage of biofield therapies are needed.

Biologically Based Therapies

Biologically based therapies include a variety of herbal medicines, or "botanicals," vitamins, minerals, and other "natural products." Such products are popular but can be problematic. The ACCP recommends that dietary supplements, in particular herbal products, be evaluated for side effects and potential interactions with other drugs. In addition, the ACCP recommends that, for lung cancer patients who either do not respond to or decline antitumor therapies, use of botanical agents occur only in the context of clinical trials (Cassileth et al. 2007). Given lack of evidence and potential to interact with prescription medications, botanicals should be used with caution, if at all, and only under the guidance of a health care provider knowledgeable in their use (Mansky & Wallerstedt 2006; Deng et al. 2004).

Summary

CAM therapies are used by a significant and growing number of people seeking relief from chronic pain and other symptoms of life-limiting illnesses and have the potential to decrease suffering and maximize quality of life for these individuals. Some of these therapies have promising and even compelling results supporting their efficacy, and health care providers should refer their patients to these therapies if they are acceptable, accessible, and affordable. Health care providers should encourage open communication with their patients regarding CAM use, both to facilitate referrals where appropriate and to protect patients from ineffective, or even potentially harmful, therapies. Patients who request advice about the use of CAM therapies should receive accurate, evidence-based information about their efficacy, utilizing reliable information such as that provided by NCCAM or databases such as Natural Standard (www.naturalstandard.com). Rigorous clinical trials are needed to determine the efficacy of many CAM therapies, particularly in the setting of life-limiting illness.

References

Abbot, N. C., Harkness, E. F., Stevinson, C., Marshall, F. P., Conn, D. A., & Ernst, E. (2001). Spiritual healing as a therapy for chronic pain: A randomized, clinical trial. *Pain, 91*(1–2), 79–89.

Achterberg, J. (1998a). Between lightning and thunder: The pause before the shifting paradigm. *Alternative Therapies in Health and Medicine, 4*(3), 62–66.

Achterberg, J. (1998b). Clearing the air in the therapeutic touch controversy. *Alternative Therapies, 4*(4), 100–101.

Ahles, T. A., Tope, D. M., Pinkson, B., et al. (1999). Massage therapy for patients undergoing autologous bone marrow transplantation. *Journal of Pain and Symptom Management, 18*(3), 157–163.

Aker, P. D., Gross, A. R., Goldsmith, C. H., & Peloso, P. (1996). Conservative management of mechanical neck pain: Systematic overview and meta-analysis. *British Medical Journal, 313*(7068), 1291–1296.

Alfano, A. P., Taylor, A. G., Foresman, P. A., et al. (2001). Static magnetic fields for treatment of fibromyalgia: A randomized controlled trial. *Journal of Alternative and Complementary Medicine, 7*(1), 53–64.

Ammendolia, C., Furlan, A. D., Imamura, M., Irvin, E., & Van Tulder, M. (2008). Evidence-informed management of chronic low back pain with needle acupuncture. *The Spine Journal, 8*(1), 160–172.

Anderson, R., Meeker, W. C., Wirick, B. E., Mootz, R. D., Kirk, D. H., & Adams, A. (1992). A meta-analysis of clinical trials of spinal manipulation. *Journal of Manipulative and Physiological Therapeutics, 15*(3), 181–194.

Ando, M., Morita, T., Akechi, T., et al. (2009). The efficacy of mindfulness-based meditation therapy on anxiety, depression, and spirituality in Japanese patients with cancer. *Journal of Palliative Medicine, 12*(12), 1091–1094.

Assefi, N., Bogart, A., Goldberg, J., & Buchwald, D. (2008). Reiki for the treatment of fibromyalgia: A randomized controlled trial. *Journal of Alternative and Complementary Medicine, 14*(9), 1115–1122.

Astin, J. A., Shapiro, S. L., Eisenberg, D. M., & Forys, K. L. (2003). Mind-body medicine: State of the science, implications for practice. *The Journal of the American Board of Family Practice, 16*(2), 131–147.

Barnes, P., Bloom, B., & Nahin, R. (2007). Complementary and alternative medicine use among adults and children: United States. National Center for Health Station and National Center for Complementary and Alternative Medicine, National Institute of Health (reprint).

Bausewein, C., Booth, S., Gysels, M., & Higginson, I. (2008). Non-pharmacological interventions for breathlessness in advanced stages of malignant and non-malignant diseases. *Cochrane Database of Systemic Reviews.* (2), CD005623.

Ben-Arye, E., Frenkel, M., Klein, A., & Scharf, M. (2008). Attitudes toward integration of complementary and alternative medicine in primary care: Perspectives of patients, physicians and complementary practitioners. *Patient Education and Counseling, 70*(3), 395–402.

Berman, B. M., Langevin, H. M., Witt, C. M., & Dubner, R. (2010). Acupuncture for chronic low back pain. *New England Journal of Medicine, 363*(5), 454–461.

Billhult, A., Bergbom, I., & Stener-Victorin, E. (2007). Massage relieves nausea in women with breast cancer who are undergoing chemotherapy. *Journal of Alternative and Complementary Medicine, 13*(1), 53–57.

Boline, P. D., Kassak, K., Bronfort, G., Nelson, C., & Anderson, A. V. (1995). Spinal manipulation vs. amitriptyline for the treatment of chronic tension-type headaches: A randomized clinical trial. *Journal of Manipulative and Physiological Therapeutics, 18*(3), 148–154.

Brattberg, G. (1999). Connective tissue massage in the treatment of fibromyalgia. *European Journal of Pain, 3*(3), 235–244.

Brinkhaus, B., Witt, C. M., Jena, S., et al. (2006). Acupuncture in patients with chronic low back pain: A randomized controlled trial. *Archives of Internal Medicine, 166*(4), 450–457.

Bronfort, G. (1999). Spinal manipulation: Current state of research and its indications. *Neurologic Clinics, 17*(1), 91–111.

Bronfort, G., Assendelft, W. J., Evans, R., Haas, M., & Bouter, L. (2001a). Efficacy of spinal manipulation for chronic headache: A systematic review. *Journal of Manipulative and Physiological Therapeutics, 24*(7), 457–466.

Bronfort, G., Evans, R., Nelson, B., Aker, P. D., Goldsmith, C. H., & Vernon, H. (2001b). A randomized clinical trial of exercise and spinal manipulation for patients with chronic neck pain. *Spine (Phila Pa 1976), 26*(7), 788–797. discussion 798–789.

Bronfort, G., Goldsmith, C. H., Nelson, C. F., Boline, P. D., & Anderson, A. V. (1996). Trunk exercise combined with spinal manipulative or NSAID therapy for chronic low back pain: A randomized, observer-blinded clinical trial. *Journal of Manipulative and Physiological Therapeutics, 19*(9), 570–582.

Bronfort, G., Haas, M., Evans, R. L., & Bouter, L. M. (2004). Efficacy of spinal manipulation and mobilization for low back pain and neck pain: A systematic review and best evidence synthesis. *The Spine Journal, 4*(3), 335–356.

Brown, C. S., Ling, F. W., Wan, J. Y., & Pilla, A. A. (2002). Efficacy of static magnetic field therapy in chronic pelvic pain: A double-blind pilot study. *American Journal of Obstetrics and Gynecology, 187*(6), 1581–1587.

Bruce, A., & Davies, B. (2005). Mindfulness in hospice care: Practicing meditation-in-action. *Qualitative Health Research, 15*(10), 1329–1344.

Cambron, J. A., Gudavalli, M. R., Hedeker, D., et al. (2006). One-year follow-up of a randomized clinical trial comparing flexion distraction with an exercise program for chronic low-back pain. *Journal of Alternative and Complementary Medicine, 12*(7), 659–668.

Campeau, M. P., Gaboriault, R., Drapeau, M., et al. (Fall 2007). Impact of massage therapy on anxiety levels in patients undergoing radiation therapy: Randomized controlled trial. *Journal of the Society for Integrative Oncology, 5*(4), 133–138.

Carson, J. W., Keefe, F. J., Lynch, T. R., et al. (2005). Loving-kindness meditation for chronic low back pain: Results from a pilot trial. *Journal of Holistic Nursing, 23*(3), 287–304.

Cassileth, B. R., Deng, G. E., Gomez, J. E., Johnstone, P. A., Kumar, N., & Vickers, A. J. (2007). Complementary therapies and integrative oncology in lung cancer: ACCP evidence-based clinical practice guidelines (2nd edition). *Chest, 132*(3 Suppl), 340S–354S.

Cassileth, B. R., & Vickers, A. J. (2004). Massage therapy for symptom control: Outcome study at a major cancer center. *Journal of Pain and Symptom Management, 28*(3), 244–249.

Castronova, J., & Oleson, T. (1991). A comparison of supportive psychotherapy and laying-on of hands healing for chronic back pain patients. *Alternative Medicine, 3*(4), 217–226.

Cherkin, D. C., Eisenberg, D., Sherman, K. J., et al. (2001). Randomized trial comparing traditional Chinese medical acupuncture, therapeutic massage, and self-care education for chronic low back pain. *Archives of Internal Medicine, 161*(8), 1081–1088.

Cherkin, D. C., Sherman, K. J., Deyo, R. A., & Shekelle, P. G. (2003). A review of the evidence for the effectiveness, safety, and cost of acupuncture, massage therapy, and spinal manipulation for back pain. *Annals of Internal Medicine, 138*(11), 898–906.

Chou, R., & Huffman, L. H. (2007). Nonpharmacologic therapies for acute and chronic low back pain: A review of the evidence for an American Pain Society/American College of Physicians clinical practice guideline. *Annals of Internal Medicine, 147*(7), 492–504.

Chou, R., Qaseem, A., Snow, V., et al. (2007). Diagnosis and treatment of low back pain: A joint clinical practice guideline from the American College of Physicians and the American Pain Society. *Annals of Internal Medicine, 147*(7), 478–491.

Colbert, A. P., Banerji, M., & Pilla, A. A. (1999). Magnetic matress pad use in patients with fibromyalgia: A randomised double-blind pilot study. *Journal of Back and Musculoskeletal Rehabilitation, 13*, 19–31.

Collacott, E. A., Zimmerman, J. T., White, D. W., & Rindone, J. P. (2000). Bipolar permanent magnets for the treatment of chronic low back pain: A pilot study. *Journal of American Medical Association, 283*(10), 1322–1325.

Corbin, L. W., Mellis, K. B., Beaty, B .L., & Kutner, J. S. (2010). The use of complementary and Alternative Medicine Theraphies by Patients with Advanced Cancer in a hospice setting: A Multicentered Description Study. *I Palliative Medicine, 12*(1), 7–8.

Corner, J., Cawley, N., & Hildebrand, S. (1995). An evaluation of the use of massage and essential oils on the wellbeing of cancer patients. *International Journal of Palliative Nursing, 1*(2), 67–73.

Cox, T. (2003). A nurse-statistician reanalyzes data from the Rosa therapeutic touch study. *Alternative Therapies in Health and Medicine, 9*(1), 58–64.

Deng, G., Cassileth, B. R., & Yeung, K. S. (2004). Complementary therapies for cancer-related symptoms. *Journal of Supportive Oncology, 2*(5), 419–426. discussion 427–419.

Denison, B. (2004). Touch the pain away: New research on therapeutic touch and persons with fibromyalgia syndrome. *Holistic Nursing Practice, 18*(3), 142–151.

Dressen, L. J., & Singg, S. (1998). Effects of Reiki on pain and selected affective and personality variables of chronically ill patients. *Subtle Energies & Energy Medicine, 9*(1), 51–82.

Eisenberg, D. M. (2005). The Institute of Medicine report on complementary and alternative medicine in the United States–personal reflections on its content and implications. *Alternative Therapies in Health and Medicine, 11*(3), 10–15.

Eliott, J. A., Kealey, C. P., & Olver, I. N. (2008). (Using) complementary and alternative medicine: The perceptions of palliative patients with cancer. *Journal of Palliative Medicine, 11*(1), 58–67.

Ernst, E. (1999). Massage therapy for low back pain: A systematic review. *Journal of Pain and Symptom Management, 17*(1), 65–69.

Ernst, E. (2002). Complementary and alternative medicine for pain management in rheumatic disease. *Current Opinion in Rheumatology, 14*(1), 58–62.

Ernst, E. (2003a). The safety of massage therapy. *Rheumatology, 49*(9), 1101–1106.

Ernst, E. (2003b). Chiropractic manipulation for non-spinal pain–A systematic review. *New Zealand Medical Journal, 116*(1179), U539.

Ernst, E. (2004). Manual therapies for pain control: Chiropractic and massage. *The Clinical Journal of Pain, 20*(1), 8–12.

Ernst, E. (2009a). Massage therapy for cancer palliation and supportive care: A systematic review of randomised clinical trials. *Supportive Care in Cancer, 17*(4), 333–337.

Ernst, E. (2009b). Is reflexology an effective intervention? A systematic review of randomised controlled trials. *The Medical Journal of Australia, 191*(5), 263–266.

Ernst, E., & Lee, M. S. (2010). Acupuncture for palliative and supportive cancer care: A systematic review of systematic reviews. *Journal of Pain and Symptom Management., 40*(1), e3–e5.

Evans, R., Bronfort, G., Nelson, B., & Goldsmith, C. H. (2002). Two-year follow-up of a randomized clinical trial of spinal manipulation and two types of exercise for patients with chronic neck pain. *Spine (Phila Pa 1976), 27*(21), 2383–2389.

Fadlon, J., Granek-Catarivas, M., Roziner, I., & Weingarten, M. A. (2008). Familiarity breeds discontent: Senior hospital doctors' attitudes towards complementary/alternative medicine. *Complementary Therapies in Medicine, 16*(4), 212–219.

Fellowes, D., Barnes, K., & Wilkinson, S. (2004). Aromatherapy and massage for symptom relief in patients with cancer. *Cochrane Database of Systemic Reviews.* (2), CD002287.

Ferrell-Torry, A. T., & Glick, O. J. (1993). The use of therapeutic massage as a nursing intervention to modify anxiety and the perception of cancer pain. *Cancer Nursing, 16*(2), 93–101.

Field, T. M. (1998). Massage therapy effects. *American Psychology, 53*(12), 1270–1281.

Field, T. M. (2002). Massage therapy better than relaxation therapy for fibromyalgia. *Journal of Clinical Rheumatology, 8*(2), 72–76.

Field, T. M., Hernandez-Reif, M., & Seligman, S. (1997). Juvenile rheumatoid arthritis: Benefits from massage therapy. *Journal of Pediatric Psychology, 22*(5), 607–617.

Furlan, A. D., Brosseau, L., Imamura, M., & Irvin, E. (2002). Massage for low-back pain: A systematic review within the framework of the Cochrane Collaboration Back Review Group. *Spine (Phila Pa 1976)., 27*(17), 1896–1910.

Furlan, A. D., Imamura, M., Dryden, T., & Irvin, E. (2008). Massage for low-back pain. *Cochrane Database of Systemic Reviews.* (4), CD001929.

Furlan, A. D., Imamura, M., Dryden, T., & Irvin, E. (2009). Massage for low back pain: An updated systematic review within the framework of the Cochrane Back Review Group. *Spine (Phila Pa 1976)., 34*(16), 1669–1684.

Galantino, M. L., Bzdewka, T. M., Eissler-Russo, J. L., et al. (2004). The impact of modified Hatha yoga on chronic low back pain: A pilot study. *Alternative Therapies in Health and Medicine, 10*(2), 56–59.

Gambles, M., Crooke, M., & Wilkinson, S. (2002). Evaluation of a hospice based reflexology service: A qualitative audit of patient perceptions. *European Journal of Oncology Nursing, 6*(1), 37–44.

Gehlart, C., Forbes, M. A., & Schmid, M. M. (2000). The effect of healing touch on pain and mood in institutionalized elders. *Healing Touch Newsletter, 10*(3), 8.

Giasson, M., & Bouchard, L. (1998). Effect of therapeutic touch on the well-being of persons with terminal cancer. *Journal of Holistic Nursing, 16*(3), 383–398.

Giles, L. G., Muller, R., Giles, L. G., & Muller, R. (2003). Chronic spinal pain: A randomized clinical trial comparing medication, acupuncture, and spinal manipulation. *Spine (Phila Pa 1976)., 28*(14), 1490–1502. discussion 1502–1493.

Gillespie, E. A., Gillespie, B. W., & Stevens, M. J. (2007). Painful diabetic neuropathy: Impact of an alternative approach. *Diabetes Care, 30*(4), 999–1001.

Godfrey, C. M., Morgan, P. P., & Schatzker, J. (1984). A randomized trial of manipulation for low-back pain in a medical setting. *Spine (Phila Pa 1976), 9*(3), 301–304.

Gordon, A., Merenstein, J. H., D'Amico, F., & Hudgens, D. (1998). The effects of therapeutic touch on patients with osteoarthritis of the knee. *Journal of Family Practice, 47*(4), 271–277.

Grant, K. E. (2003). Massage safety: Injuries reported in Medline relating to the practice of therapeutic massage: 1965–2003. *Journal of Bodywork and Movement Therapy, 7*(4), 207–212.

Grealish, L., Lomasney, A., & Whiteman, B. (2000). Foot massage. A nursing intervention to modify the distressing symptoms of pain and nausea in patients hospitalized with cancer. *Cancer Nursing, 23*(3), 237–243.

Groessl, E. J., Weingart, K. R., Aschbacher, K., Pada, L., & Baxi, S. (2008). Yoga for veterans with chronic low-back pain. *Journal of Alternative and Complementary Medicine, 14*(9), 1123–1129.

Gross, A. R., Hoving, J. L., Haines, T. A., et al. (2004). A Cochrane review of manipulation and mobilization for mechanical neck disorders. *Spine (Phila Pa 1976), 29*(14), 1541–1548.

Gudavalli, M. R., Cambron, J. A., McGregor, M., et al. (2006). A randomized clinical trial and subgroup analysis to compare flexion-distraction with active exercise for chronic low back pain. *European Spine Journal, 15*(7), 1070–1082.

Gunnarsdottir, T. J., & Peden-McAlpine, C. (2010). Effects of reflexology on fibromyalgia symptoms: A multiple case study. *Complementary Therapies in Clinical Practice, 16*(3), 167–172.

Haas, M., Spegman, A., Peterson, D., Aickin, M., & Vavrek, D. (2010). Dose response and efficacy of spinal manipulation for chronic cervicogenic headache: A pilot randomized controlled trial. *Spine Journal., 10*(2), 117–128.

Han, J. S. (2003). Acupuncture: Neuropeptide release produced by electrical stimulation of different frequencies. *Trends in Neurosciences, 26*(1), 17–22.

Harlow, T., Greaves, C., White, A., Brown, L., Hart, A., & Ernst, E. (2004). Randomised controlled trial of magnetic bracelets for relieving pain in osteoarthritis of the hip and knee. *British Medical Journal, 329*(7480), 1450–1454.

Hasson, D., Arnetz, B., Jelveus, L., & Edelstam, B. (2004). A randomized clinical trial of the treatment effects of massage compared to relaxation tape recordings on diffuse long-term pain. *Psychotherapy and Psychosomatics, 73*(1), 17–24.

Hernandez-Reif, M., Field, T., Krasnegor, J., & Theakston, H. (2001). Lower back pain is reduced and range of motion increased after massage therapy. *International Journal of Neuroscience, 106*(3–4), 131–145.

Hirschkorn, K. A., & Bourgeault, I. L. (2008). Structural constraints and opportunities for CAM use and referral by physicians, nurses, and midwives. *Health (London, England), 12*(2), 193–213.

Hodgson, N. A., & Andersen, S. (2008). The clinical efficacy of reflexology in nursing home residents with dementia. *Journal of Alternative and Complementary Medicine, 14*(3), 269–275.

Hoehler, F. K., Tobis, J. S., & Buerger, A. A. (1981). Spinal manipulation for low back pain. *JAMA, 245*(18), 1835–1838.

Hsieh, C. Y., Phillips, R. B., Adams, A. H., & Pope, M. H. (1992). Functional outcomes of low back pain: Comparison of four treatment groups in a randomized controlled trial. *Journal of Manipulative and Physiological Therapeutics, 15*(1), 4–9.

Hughes, S., & Bolton, J. (2002). Is chiropractic an effective treatment in infantile colic? *Archives of Disease in Childhood, 86*(5), 382–384.

Hughes, D., Ladas, E., Rooney, D., & Kelly, K. (2008). Massage therapy as a supportive care intervention for children with cancer. *Oncology Nursing Forum, 35*(3), 431–442.

Hurwitz, E. L., Aker, P. D., Adams, A. H., Meeker, W. C., & Shekelle, P. G. (1996). Manipulation and mobilization of the cervical spine. A systematic review of the literature. *Spine (Phila Pa 1976), 21*(15), 1746–1759. discussion 1759–1760.

Hurwitz, E. L., Morgenstern, H., Harber, P., Kominski, G. F., Yu, F., & Adams, A. H. (2002). A randomized trial of chiropractic manipulation and mobilization for patients with neck pain: Clinical outcomes from the UCLA neck-pain study. *American Journal of Public Health, 92*(10), 1634–1641.

Irnich, D., Behrens, N., Molzen, H., et al. (2001). Randomised trial of acupuncture compared with conventional massage and "sham" laser acupuncture for treatment of chronic neck pain. *British Medical Journal, 322*(7302), 1574–1578.

Jane, S. W., Wilkie, D. J., Gallucci, B. B., & Beaton, R. D. (2008). Systematic review of massage intervention for adult patients with cancer: A methodological perspective. *Cancer Nursing, 31*(6), E24–E35.

Jobst, K., Chen, J. H., McPherson, K., et al. (1986). Controlled trial of acupuncture for disabling breathlessness. *Lancet, 2*(8521–8522), 1416–1419.

Kim, K. H., Lee, M. S., Kang, K. W., & Choi, S. M. (2010). Role of acupressure in symptom management in patients with end-stage renal disease: A systematic review. *Journal of Palliative Medicine, 13*(7), 885–892.

Kohara, H., Miyauchi, T., Suehiro, Y., Ueoka, H., Takeyama, H., & Morita, T. (2004). Combined modality treatment of aromatherapy, footsoak, and reflexology relieves fatigue in patients with cancer. *Journal of Palliative Medicine, 7*(6), 791–796.

Konrad, K., Tatrai, T., Hunka, A., Vereckei, E., & Korondi, I. (1992). Controlled trial of balneotherapy in treatment of low back pain. *Annals of the Rheumatic Diseases, 51*(6), 820–822.

Koopsen, C., & Young, C. (2009). *Integrative health: A holistic approach for health professionals*. Boston: Jones & Bartlett.

Krieger, D. (1975a). Therapeutic touch: The imprimatur of nursing. *The American Journal of Nursing, 75*(5), 784–787.

Krieger, D. (1975b). Therapeutic touch; an ancient, but unorthodox nursing intervention. *The Journal of the New York State Nurses' Association, 6*(2), 6–10.

Kutner, J. S., Smith, M. C., Corbin, L., et al. (2008). Massage therapy versus simple touch to improve pain and mood in patients with advanced cancer: A randomized trial. *Annals of Internal Medicine, 149*(6), 369–379.

Lafferty, W. E., Downey, L., McCarty, R. L., Standish, L. J., & Patrick, D. L. (2006). Evaluating CAM treatment at the end of life: A review of clinical trials for massage and meditation. *Complementary Therapies in Medicine, 14*(2), 100–112.

Lawrence, D. J., Meeker, W., Branson, R., et al. (2008). Chiropractic management of low back pain and low back-related leg complaints: A literature synthesis. *Journal of Manipulative and Physiological Therapeutics, 31*(9), 659–674.

Lee, R. T., Hlubocky, F. J., Hu, J. J., Stafford, R. S., & Daugherty, C. K. (2008). An international pilot study of oncology physicians' opinions and practices on complementary and alternative medicine (CAM). *Integrative Cancer Therapies, 7*(2), 70–75.

Lee, M. S., Jang, J. W., Jang, H. S., & Moon, S. R. (2003). Effects of Qi-therapy on blood pressure, pain and psychological symptoms in the elderly: A randomized controlled pilot trial. *Complementary Therapies in Medicine, 11*(3), 159–164.

Lee, M. S., Yang, K. H., Huh, H. J., et al. (2001). Qi therapy as an intervention to reduce chronic pain and to enhance mood in elderly subjects: A pilot study. *The American Journal of Chinese Medicine, 29*(2), 237–245.

Leskowitz, E. (1998). Un-debunking therapeutic touch. *Alternative Therapies, 4*(4), 101–102.

Lewis, C. R., de Vedia, A., Reuer, B., Schwan, R., & Tourin, C. (2003). Integrating complementary and alternative medicine (CAM) into standard hospice and palliative care. *The American Journal of Hospice & Palliative Care, 20*(3), 221–228.

Lewith, G. T., Broomfield, J., & Prescott, P. (2002). Complementary cancer care in Southampton: A survey of staff and patients. *Complementary Therapies in Medicine, 10*(2), 100–106.

Lewith, G. T., Prescott, P., & Davis, C. L. (2004). Can a standardized acupuncture technique palliate disabling breathlessness: A single-blind, placebo-controlled crossover study. *Chest, 125*(5), 1783–1790.

Lim, C. M., Ng, A., & Loh, K. S. (2010). Use of complementary and alternative medicine in head and neck cancer patients. *Journal of Laryngology & Otology, 124*(5), 529–532.

Lin, Y.-S., & Taylor, A. G. (1998). Effects of therapeutic touch in reducing pain and anxiety in an elderly population. *Integrative Medicine, 1*(4), 155–162.

Maa, S. H., Gauthier, D., & Turner, M. (1997). Acupressure as an adjunct to a pulmonary rehabilitation program. *Journal of Cardiopulmonary Rehabilitation, 17*(4), 268–276.

Mansky, P. J., & Wallerstedt, D. B. (2006). Complementary medicine in palliative care and cancer symptom management. *Cancer Journal, 12*(5), 425–431.

Meek, S. S. (Spring 1993). Effects of slow stroke back massage on relaxation in hospice clients. *Image: Journal of Nursing Scholarship, 25*(1), 17–21.

Morone, N. E., & Greco, C. M. (2007). Mind-body interventions for chronic pain in older adults: A structured review. *Pain Medicine, 8*(4), 359–375.

Morone, N. E., Greco, C. M., & Weiner, D. K. (2008a). Mindfulness meditation for the treatment of chronic low back pain in older adults: A randomized controlled pilot study. *Pain, 134*(3), 310–319.

Morone, N. E., Lynch, C. S., Greco, C. M., Tindle, H. A., & Weiner, D. K. (2008b). "I felt like a new person." the effects of mindfulness meditation on older adults with chronic pain: Qualitative narrative analysis of diary entries. *The Journal of Pain, 9*(9), 841–848.

Moyer, C. A., Rounds, J., & Hannum, J. W. (2004). A meta-analysis of massage therapy research. *Psychological Bulletin, 130*(1), 3–18.

Murphy, B., Taylor, H. H., & Marshall, P. (2010). The effect of spinal manipulation on the efficacy of a rehabilitation protocol for patients with chronic neck pain: A pilot study. *Journal of Manipulative and Physiological Therapeutics, 33*(3), 168–177.

Myers, C. D., Robinson, M. E., Guthrie, T. H., et al. (1999). Adjunctive approaches for sickle cell chronic pain. *Alternaticw Health Practioners, 5*(3), 203–212.

National Guidelines Clearinghouse. (2010). *Chronic pain.* Retrieved 7 October, 2010, from www.guidelines.gov/popups/printview.aspx?id=14284.

National Health Interview Survey. Retrieved 2010, from http://www.cdc.gov/nchs/nhis.htm.

Natural Standard. (2010). *Monograph on massage therapy.* Reteieved 8 January, 2010, from www.naturalstandard.com.

Natural Standard. (2010). *Chiropractic.* Retrieved 2010, from www.naturalstandard.com.

Ndao-Brumblay, S. K., & Green, C. R. (2010). Predictors of complementary and alternative medicine use in chronic pain patients. *Pain Medicine, 11*(1), 16–24.

Nelson, C. F., Bronfort, G., Evans, R., Boline, P., Goldsmith, C., & Anderson, A. V. (1998). The efficacy of spinal manipulation, amitriptyline and the combination of both therapies for the prophylaxis of migraine headache. *Journal of Manipulative and Physiological Therapeutics, 21*(8), 511–519.

Nilsson, N., Christensen, H. W., & Hartvigsen, J. (1997). The effect of spinal manipulation in the treatment of cervicogenic headache. *Journal of Manipulative and Physiological Therapeutics, 20*(5), 326–330.

Olson, K., Hanson, J., & Michaud, M. (2003). A phase II trial of Reiki for the management of pain in advanced cancer patients. *Journal of Pain and Symptom Management, 26*(5), 990–997.

Palmieri, N. F., & Smoyak, S. (2002). Chronic low back pain: A study of the effects of manipulation under anesthesia. *Journal of Manipulative and Physiological Therapeutics, 25*(8), E8–E17.

Pan, C. X., Morrison, R. S., Ness, J., Fugh-Berman, A., & Leipzig, R. M. (2000). Complementary and alternative medicine in the management of pain, dyspnea, and nausea and vomiting near the end of life. A systematic review. *Journal of Pain and Symptom Management, 20*(5), 374–387.

Peck, S. D. E. (1997). The effectiveness of therapeutic touch for decreasing pain in elders with degenerative arthritis. *Journal of Holistic Nursing, 15*(2), 176–198.

Perlman, A. I., Sabina, A., Williams, A. L., Njike, V. Y., & Katz, D. L. (2006). Massage therapy for osteoarthritis of the knee: A randomized controlled trial. *Archives of Internal Medicine, 166*(22), 2533–2538.

Philcox, P., Rawlins, L., & Rodgers, L. (2002). Therapeutic touch and its effects on phantom limb and stump pain. *Journal of the Australian Rehabilitation Nursing Association, 5*(1), 17–21.

Phipps, S., Dunavant, M., Gray, E., et al. (2005). Massage therapy in children hematopoietic stem cell transplant: Results of a pilot trial. *Journal of Cancer Integrated Medicine, 3*(2), 62–70.

Pittler, M. H., Brown, E. M., & Ernst, E. (2007). Static magnets for reducing pain: Systematic review and meta-analysis of randomized trials. *Canadian Medical Association Journal, 177*(7), 736–742.

Plews-Ogan, M., Owens, J. E., Goodman, M., Wolfe, P., & Schorling, J. (2005). A pilot study evaluating mindfulness-based stress reduction and massage for the management of chronic pain. *Journal of General Internal Medicine, 20*(12), 1136–1138.

Post-White, J., Kinney, M. E., Savik, K., Gau, J. B., Wilcox, C., & Lerner, I. (2003). Therapeutic massage and healing touch improve symptoms in cancer. *Integrative Cancer Therapies, 2*(4), 332–344.

Proctor, M. L., Hing, W., Johnson, T. C., & Murphy, P. A. (2006). Spinal manipulation for primary and secondary dysmenorrhoea. *Cochrane Database of Systemic Reviews.* (3), CD002119.

Puustjarvi, K., Airaksinen, O., & Pontinen, P. J. (1990). The effects of massage in patients with chronic tension headache. *Acupuncture & Electro-Therapeutics Research, 15*(2), 159–162.

Rausch, S. M., Winegardner, F., Kruk, K. M., et al. (2011) Complementary and alternative medicine: Use and disclosure in radiation oncology community practice. *Support Care Cancer, 19*(4), 521–529.

Redner, R., Briner, B., & Snellman, L. (1991). Effects of bioenergy healing technique on chronic pain. *Subtle Energies, 2*(3), 43–68.

Retrieved 10 October, 2010, from http://www.reflexology-usa.org/articles/definitions_of_reflexology.html.

Retrieved October 3, 2010, from http://nccam.nih.gov/health/whatiscam/.

Richardson, M. A., Sanders, T., Palmer, J. L., Greisinger, A., & Singletary, S. E. (2000). Complementary/alternative medicine use in a comprehensive cancer center and the implications for oncology. *Journal of Clinical Oncology, 18*(13), 2505–2514.

Rosa, L., Rosa, E., Sarner, L., & Barrett, S. (1998). A close look at therapeutic touch. *Journal of American Medical Association, 279*(13), 1005–1010.

Rosenzweig, S., Greeson, J. M., Reibel, D. K., Green, J. S., Jasser, S. A., & Beasley, D. (2010). Mindfulness-based stress reduction for chronic pain conditions: Variation in treatment outcomes and role of home meditation practice. *Journal of Psychosomatic Research., 68*(1), 29–36.

Ross, C. S., Hamilton, J., Macrae, G., Docherty, C., Gould, A., & Cornbleet, M. A. (2002). A pilot study to evaluate the effect of reflexology on mood and symptom rating of advanced cancer patients. *Palliative Medicine, 16*(6), 544–545.

Royal College of General Practitioners. (2009). *Low back pain; early management of persistent non-specific low back pain. Clinical guideline no. 88.* London: Royal College of General Practitioners.

Rubinstein, S. M., van Middelkoop, M., Kuijpers, T., et al. (2010). A systematic review on the effectiveness of complementary and alternative medicine for chronic non-specific low-back pain. *European Spine Journal, 19*(8), 1213–1228.

Russell, N. C., Sumler, S. S., Beinhorn, C. M., & Frenkel, M. A. (2008). Role of massage therapy in cancer care. *Journal of Alternative and Complementary Medicine, 14*(2), 209–214.

Sapir, R. B., Sherman, K. J., Cullum-Dugan, D., Davis, R. B., Phillips, R. S., & Culpepper, L. (2009). Yoga for chronic low back pain in a predominantly minority population: A pilot randomized controlled trial. *Alternative Therapies in Health and Medicine, 15*(6), 18–27.

Savolainen, A., Ahlberg, J., Nummila, H., & Nissinen, M. (2004). Active or passive treatment for neck-shoulder pain in occupational health care? A randomized controlled trial. *Occupational Medicine, 54*(6), 422–424.

Schechter, D., Smith, A. P., Beck, J., Roach, J., Karim, R., & Azen, S. (2007). Outcomes of a mind-body treatment program for chronic back pain with no distinct structural pathology–a case series of patients diagnosed and treated as tension myositis syndrome. *Alternative Therapies in Health and Medicine, 13*(5), 26–35.

Schofield, P., Diggens, J., Charleson, C., Marigliani, R., & Jefford, M. (2010). Effectively discussing complementary and alternative medicine in a conventional oncology setting: Communication recommendations for clinicians. *Patient Education & Counselling, 79*(2), 143–151.

Segal, N. A., Toda, Y., Huston, J., et al. (2001). Two configurations of static magnetic fields for treating rheumatoid arthritis of the knee: A double-blind clinical trial. *Archives of Physical Medicine and Rehabilitation, 82*(10), 1453–1460.

Shekelle, P. G., Adams, A. H., Chassin, M. R., Hurwitz, E. L., & Brook, R. H. (1992). Spinal manipulation for low-back pain. *Annals of Internal Medicine, 117*(7), 590–598.

Shekelle, P. G., & Coulter, I. (1997). Cervical spine manipulation: Summary report of a systematic review of the literature and a multidisciplinary expert panel. *Journal of Spinal Disorders, 10*(3), 223–228.

Sherman, K. J., Cherkin, D. C., Erro, J., Miglioretti, D. L., & Deyo, R. A. (2005). Comparing yoga, exercise, and a self-care book for chronic low back pain: A randomized, controlled trial. *Annals of Internal Medicine, 143*(12), 849–856.

Shoroni, S., & Abron, P. (2010). Complementary and alternative medicine (CAM) among hospitalised patients: An Australian study. *Complementary Therapies in Clinical Practice, 16*, 86–91.

Sims, S. (1986). Slow stroke back massage for cancer patients. *Nursing Times, 82*(47), 47–50.

Slater, V. (1996). *Safety, elements and effects of healing touch on chronic non-malignant abdominal pain.* Knoxville: University of Tennessee.

Smith, M. C. (1998). Researching integrative therapies. *Journal of Emergency Nursing, 24*, 609–613.

Smith, M. C. (2005). Complementary-alternative therapies: From pseudo to serious science. *Communicating Nursing Research, 38*, 23–38.

Smith, D. W., Arnstein, P., Rosa, K. C., & Wells-Federman, C. (2002a). Effects of integrating therapeutic touch into a cognitive behavioral pain treatment program. Report of a pilot clinical trial. *Journal of Holistic Nursing, 20*(4), 367–387.

Smith, M. C., Kemp, J., Hemphill, L., & Vojir, C. P. (2002b). Outcomes of therapeutic massage for hospitalized cancer patients. *Journal of Nursing Scholarship, 34*(3), 257–262.

Smith, K. B., & Pukall, C. F. (2009). An evidence-based review of yoga as a complementary intervention for patients with cancer. *Psycho-Oncology, 18*(5), 465–475.

So, P. S., Jiang, Y., & Qin, Y. (2008). Touch therapies for pain relief in adults. *Cochrane Database of Systemic Reviews.* (4), CD006535.

Soden, K., Vincent, K., Craske, S., Lucas, C., & Ashley, S. (2004). A randomized controlled trial of aromatherapy massage in a hospice setting. *Palliative Medicine, 18*(2), 87–92.

Stephenson, N., Dalton, J. A., & Carlson, J. (2003). The effect of foot reflexology on pain in patients with metastatic cancer. *Applied Nursing Research, 16*(4), 284–286.

Stephenson, N. L., Swanson, M., Dalton, J., Keefe, F. J., & Engelke, M. (2007). Partner-delivered reflexology: Effects on cancer pain and anxiety. *Oncology Nursing Forum, 34*(1), 127–132.

Sundblom, D. M., Haikonen, S., Niemi-Pynttari, J., & Tigerstedt, I. (1994). Effect of spiritual healing on chronic idiopathic pain: A medical and psychological study. *The Clinical Journal of Pain, 10*(4), 296–302.

Sunshine, W., Field, T. M., Quintino, O., et al. (1996). Fibromyalgia benefits from massage therapy and transcutaneous electrical stimulation. *Journal of Clinical Rheumatology, 2*(1), 18–22.

Tan, G., Craine, M. H., Bair, M. J., et al. (2007). Efficacy of selected complementary and alternative medicine interventions for chronic pain. *Journal of Rehabilitation Research and Development, 44*(2), 195–222.

Teixeira, M. E. (2008). Meditation as an intervention for chronic pain: An integrative review. *Holistic Nursing Practice, 22*(4), 225–234.

Tekur, P., Singphow, C., Nagendra, H. R., & Raghuram, N. (2008). Effect of short-term intensive yoga program on pain, functional disability and spinal flexibility in chronic low back pain: A randomized control study. *Journal of Alternative and Complementary Medicine, 14*(6), 637–644.

Tsang, K. L., Carlson, L. E., & Olson, K. (2007). Pilot crossover trial of Reiki versus rest for treating cancer-related fatigue. *Integrative Cancer Therapies, 6*(1), 25–35.

Tsay, S. L., Chen, H. L., Chen, S. C., Lin, H. R., & Lin, K. C. (2008). Effects of reflexotherapy on acute postoperative pain and anxiety among patients with digestive cancer. *Cancer Nursing, 31*(2), 109–115.

Vallbona, C., Hazlewood, C. F., & Jurida, G. (1997). Response of pain to static magnetic fields in postpolio patients: A double-blind pilot study. *Archives of Physical Medicine and Rehabilitation, 78*(11), 1200–1203.

van den Dolder, P. A., & Roberts, D. L. (2003). A trial into the effectiveness of soft tissue massage in the treatment of shoulder pain. *The Australian Journal of Physiotherapy, 49*(3), 183–188.

van Tulder, M., Furlan, A., Bombardier, C., & Bouter, L. (2003). Updated method guidelines for systematic reviews in the cochrane collaboration back review group. *Spine (Phila Pa 1976), 28*(12), 1290–1299.

Vernon, H., Humphreys, K., & Hagino, C. (2007). Chronic mechanical neck pain in adults treated by manual therapy: A systematic review of change scores in randomized clinical trials. *Journal of Manipulative and Physiological Therapeutics, 30*(3), 215–227.

Vickers, A. J., Feinstein, M. B., Deng, G. E., & Cassileth, B. R. (2005). Acupuncture for dyspnea in advanced cancer: A randomized, placebo-controlled pilot trial [ISRCTN89462491]. *BMC Palliative Care, 4*, 5.

Walach, H., Guthlin, C., & Konig, M. (2003). Efficacy of massage therapy in chronic pain: A pragmatic randomized trial. *Journal of Alternative and Complementary Medicine, 9*(6), 837–846.

Walker, B. F., French, S. D., Grant, W., & Green, S. (2010). Combined chiropractic interventions for low-back pain. *Cochrane Database of Systemic Reviews*. (4), CD005427.

Wang, M. Y., Tsai, P. S., Lee, P. H., Chang, W. Y., & Yang, C. M. (2008). The efficacy of reflexology: Systematic review. *Journal of Advanced Nursing, 62*(5), 512–520.

Warber, S. L., Gordon, A., Gillespie, B. W., Olson, M., & Assefi, N. (2003). Standards for conducting clinical biofield energy healing research. *Alternative Therapies in Health and Medicine, 9*(3 Suppl), A54–A64.

Wardell, D. W., & Weymouth, K. F. (2004). Review of studies of healing touch. *Journal of Nursing Scholarship, 36*(2), 147–154.

Weinrich, S. P., & Weinrich, M. C. (1990). The effect of massage on pain in cancer patients. *Applied Nursing Research, 3*(4), 140–145.

Weintraub, M. I., Wolfe, G. I., Barohn, R. A., et al. (2003). Static magnetic field therapy for symptomatic diabetic neuropathy: A randomized, double-blind, placebo-controlled trial. *Archives of Physical Medicine and Rehabilitation, 84*(5), 736–746.

Weymouth, K., & Sandberg-Lewis, S. (2000). Comparing the efficacy of healing touch and chiropractic adjustment in treating chronic low back pain: A pilot study. *Healing Touch Newsletter, 00*(3), 7–8.

White House Commission on Complementary and Alternative Medicine. (2010). Retrieved 2010, from http://www.whccamp.hhs.gov.

Wilcock, A., Manderson, C., Weller, R., et al. (2004). Does aromatherapy massage benefit patients with cancer attending a specialist palliative care day centre? *Palliative Medicine, 18*(4), 287–290.

Wilkey, A., Gregory, M., Byfield, D., & McCarthy, P. W. (2008). A comparison between chiropractic management and pain clinic management for chronic low-back pain in a national health service outpatient clinic. *Journal of Alternative and Complementary Medicine, 14*(5), 465–473.

Wilkie, D. J., Kampbell, J., Cutshall, S., et al. (2000). Effects of massage on pain intensity, analgesics and quality of life in patients with cancer pain: A pilot study of a randomized clinical trial conducted within hospice care delivery. *The Hospice Journal, 15*(3), 31–53.

Wilkinson, S. (1995). Aromatherapy and massage in palliative care. *International Journal of Palliative Nursing, 1*(1), 21–30.

Wilkinson, S., Barnes, K., & Storey, L. (2008a). Massage for symptom relief in patients with cancer: Systematic review. *Journal of Advanced Nursing, 63*(5), 430–439.

Wilkinson, S., Lockhart, K., Gambles, M., Storey, L., Wilkinson, S., Lockhart, K., Gambles, M., & Storey, L. (2008b). Reflexology for symptom relief in patients with cancer. *Cancer Nursing, 31*(5), 354–360. quiz 361–352.

Wilkinson, S. M., Love, S. B., Westcombe, A. M., et al. (2007). Effectiveness of aromatherapy massage in the management of anxiety and depression in patients with cancer: A multicenter randomized controlled trial. *Journal of Clinical Oncology, 25*(5), 532–539.

Williams, K. A., Petronis, J., Smith, D., et al. (2005a). Effect of Iyengar yoga therapy for chronic low back pain. *Pain, 115*(1–2), 107–117.

Williams, A. L., Selwyn, P. A., Liberti, L., et al. (2005b). A randomized controlled trial of meditation and massage effects on quality of life in people with late-stage disease: A pilot study. *Journal of Palliative Medicine, 8*(5), 939–952.

Winemiller, M. H., Billow, R. G., Laskowski, E. R., & Harmsen, W. S. (2005). Effect of magnetic vs sham-magnetic insoles on nonspecific foot pain in the workplace: A randomized, double-blind, placebo-controlled trial. *Mayo Clinic Proceedings, 80*(9), 1138–1145.

Witt, C. M., Jena, S., Selim, D., et al. (2006). Pragmatic randomized trial evaluating the clinical and economic effectiveness of acupuncture for chronic low back pain. *American Journal of Epidemiology, 164*(5), 487–496.

Wolsko, P. M., Eisenberg, D. M., Simon, L. S., et al. (2004). Double-blind placebo-controlled trial of static magnets for the treatment of osteoarthritis of the knee: Results of a pilot study. *Alternative Therapies in Health and Medicine, 10*(2), 36–43.

Wu, M. T., Hsieh, J. C., Xiong, J., et al. (1999). Central nervous pathway for acupuncture stimulation: Localization of processing with functional MR imaging of the brain–preliminary experience. *Radiology, 212*(1), 133–141.

Wu, H. S., Lin, L. C., Wu, S. C., & Lin, J. G. (2007). The psychologic consequences of chronic dyspnea in chronic pulmonary obstruction disease: The effects of acupressure on depression. *Journal of Alternative and Complementary Medicine, 13*(2), 253–261.

Wu, H. S., Wu, S. C., Lin, J. G., & Lin, L. C. (2004). Effectiveness of acupressure in improving dyspnoea in chronic obstructive pulmonary disease. *Journal of Advanced Nursing, 45*(3), 252–259.

Yang, K. H., Kim, Y. H., & Lee, M. S. (2005). Efficacy of Qi-therapy (external Qigong) for elderly people with chronic pain. *International Journal of Neuroscience, 115*(7), 949–963.

Yuan, J., Purepong, N., Kerr, D. P., Park, J., Bradbury, I., & McDonough, S. (2008). Effectiveness of acupuncture for low back pain: A systematic review. *Spine, 33*(23), E887–E900.

Zautra, A. J., Fasman, R., Davis, M. C., & Craig, A. D. (2010). The effects of slow breathing on affective responses to pain stimuli: An experimental study. *Pain, 149*(1), 12–18.

Ziembroski, J., Gilbert, N., Bossarte, R., & Guldberg, G. (2003). Healing touch and hospice care: Examining outcomes at the end of life. *Alternative & Complementary Therapies, 9*(3), 146–151.

Chapter 36
Spiritual Dimensions of Pain and Suffering

Amy Wachholtz and Suzana Makowski

Spiritual Dimensions of Pain and Suffering

Pain is a multi-dimensional, complex experience. It is a struggle to adequately identify and meet the needs of patients experiencing pain in a bio-psycho-social–spiritual context. In this chapter we explore the relationship between the spiritual dimensions of suffering and the experience of physical pain. By intertwining research with clinical case studies, the chapter reviews definitions, the relationship between spiritual anguish and physical pain, and finally interdisciplinary approaches to alleviating suffering.

Multiple Dimensions of Pain

The Concept of Total Pain

Dame Cicely Saunders, a physician, nurse and social worker, and founder of the modern hospice movement, coined the term "total pain," describing this phenomenon as early as 1964, after years of researching the experience of pain among her patients at St. Christopher's Hospice. In her early years, she focused on assessing and treating cancer pain pharmacologically, demonstrating that pain can be controlled with routine, rather than "prn" (as needed), medications of appropriate strength. Narratives of patients' pain reports upon admission to St. Christopher's hospice revealed qualities of the pain experience that existed beyond the physiologic clinical descriptors of intensity, location, nociceptive, or neuropathic. She discovered that pain is not merely an experience of the body but is often influenced by spiritual and psychosocial factors. In 1959, she began to write about the indivisibility of physical and mental pain, on how analgesics alone could not always alleviate pain. She coined the term *total pain* "which was presented as a complex of physical, emotional, social, and spiritual elements. The whole experience for a patient includes anxiety, depression, and fear; concerns for the family who will become bereaved; and often a need to find some meaning or purpose in the situation, some deeper reality in which to trust" (Clark 1999; Saunders 1996).

A. Wachholtz, PhD, MDIV (✉) • S. Makowski, MD, MMM, FACP
Dept of Psychiatry, University of Massachusetts Medical School, UMass Memorial Medical Center,
55 Lake Ave North, Worcester, MA 01545, USA
e-mail: amy.wachholtz@umassmemorial.org

R.J. Moore (ed.), *Handbook of Pain and Palliative Care: Biobehavioral Approaches for the Life Course*,
DOI 10.1007/978-1-4419-1651-8_36, © Springer Science+Business Media, LLC 2012

One of the most commonly quoted Saunders' excerpts describes a patient's answer to the question about her pain:

> "Well doctor, the pain began in my back, but now it seems that all of me is wrong." She gave a description of various symptoms and ills and then went on to say, "My husband and son were marvelous but they were at work and they would have had to stay off and lose their money. I could have cried for the pills and injections although I knew I shouldn't. Everything seemed to be against me and nobody seemed to understand." And then she paused before she said, "But it's so wonderful to begin to feel safe again." Without any further questioning she had talked of her mental as well as physical distress, of her social problems and of her spiritual need for security. (Saunders 1996, p. viii)

Saunders' work demonstrated, for the first time, the utility of appropriate use of opioids, their limitations, and the potential role of eliciting patient narratives as a means to alleviate "total pain." (Clark 1999)

Case Study 1: Ritual and Prayer

Rose is a lively Italian-American woman, raised a strict Catholic, who – whenever she feels well enough – wears bright red lip-stick and carefully places blush on her cheeks whenever she expects visitors. She was admitted to an inpatient hospice for pain related to metastatic breast cancer. Her pain is principally in her low back, at the site of some bony-metastases, with nociceptive quality that did not radiate. The intensity is difficult to assess at the onset, since some days she seems to be relatively pain free and required virtually no breakthrough morphine, while other days she is in severe pain despite escalating doses. During an inter-disciplinary team meeting, we discussed this pattern of pain intensity. It was the Chaplain who noted that the days she receives communion from her parish Priest she is pain free. Each day after that, no matter the dose of morphine, her pain intensity score increases by 1 point; so if she does not receive communion for a week, her pain is 7/10.

1. As communion was more effective than morphine in controlling pain for this patient, what are the ethics in reducing the opioid analgesic but increasing visits by the patient's priest?
2. Can/should physicians "prescribe" communion in this scenario?
3. What role should chaplains and outside spiritual providers play on a hospice team?
4. How might this patient's spiritual needs have been identified earlier?

Hierarchy of Needs Applied to Palliative Care

In order to meet Saunders' challenge to assess pain with "the same analysis and consideration as an illness itself," (Clark 1999, p 733) many interdisciplinary palliative care teams adapted the "hierarchy of human needs" originally conceptualized by Abraham H. Maslow, an American Psychologist, the founder of Humanist Psychology. Just as Saunders' patient so succinctly described her needs for security, physical, social, and spiritual comfort, Maslow outlined a process toward self-actualization that acknowledges the requirements that each one of these dimensions of humanity to be met. Maslow's model, as you shall see, creates a structure whereby the interdisciplinary team can organize the multi-model assessment of each patient's "total pain" experience. Unlike other models such as the Kubler-Ross Stages of Grief, the steps of the Maslow model must be achieved sequentially. In other words, someone cannot reach the next level without fully achieving all of the levels below. However, people can move backward. Significant stressors, such as severe pain, may make a person move backward to be more focused on the basic need of pain relief than self-actualization.

Fig. 36.1 Maslow's heirarchy
of needs

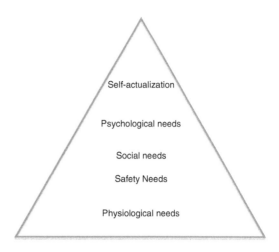

The most basic of needs according to Maslow's model are considered to be physiologic: eating, sleeping, breathing, and excreting. Physical comfort, or the absence of pain (and other symptoms), could be added to this list of basic needs. Yet, as patients approach the end of life, certain needs are threatened. Pain aside, constipation, urinary retention, breathlessness, etc., are all common symptoms. Patients often complain about sleeping too much or too little. Whether due to underlying nausea, intra-abdominal process, or perhaps terminal (or cancer-induced) anorexia, patients also tend to eat less as they approach the end of life (Plonk and Arnold 2005). Alleviating reversible symptoms, in Maslow's model, is critical to allowing patients to address higher levels of need and experiencing a decent quality of life. In the interdisciplinary palliative care model, physicians, nurses, and other members of the multidisciplinary team oversee the care of patients to assure physical comfort (physical symptom relief).

Safety, including physical, practical, and financial security, is the next motivator in human behavior, according to Maslow. Palliative care teams often turn to social workers as the experts who address this realm of patient need. In their discussion about how to apply Maslow's hierarchy of needs to hospice and palliative care, Zalenski and Raspa also noted that fear of abandonment also fits into this stage of motivation. For example, patients who have long been cared for by a particular physician or nurse may choose more aggressive care out of motivation toward non-abandonment and safety over other important end-of-life needs (Parks and Winter 2009; Winter et al. 2007). Patients who lack access to safe housing, food, or medical care often experience increased levels of pain either due to the added stress of the uncertainty, or more commonly through a lack of access to adequate health care (Fig. 36.1).

Love and connection is the next motivator in Maslow's model. While being loved interacts with the sense of safety, the act of loving, of caring for others, also feeds the drive toward the "expansive self" or being part of something larger than oneself, including belonging to a marriage, school, team, country, or religion. Relationships are crucial to human well-being at all the stages of life, and the threat to these connections can impair not only psychological health but also physical (Cacioppo et al. 2009; Christakis and Allison 2006). This domain is usually overseen by experienced social workers or psychologists on the palliative or hospice interdisciplinary teams.

Once a person has their basic physical, safety, and relationship needs met, Maslow postulates that needs defined by esteem and self-respect emerge. Self-esteem, according to this model, arises from firmly based achievement and respect earned from others. It is influenced by how others treat and interact with the person. Max Harvey Chochinov explores this level in depth in his studies of dignity at the end of life (Chochinov et al. 2008). Negative emotions, such as shame and guilt, may come into play during this life transition. Exploring this domain of Maslow's hierarchy could also shed some light on "situational pain," when patients' pain intensity seems to escalate in the presence of a parent or spouse. Social workers, psychologists, bereavement counselors, and chaplains all play an important role to alleviate suffering due to loss of self-esteem in the contexts of chronic pain, suffering and at the end of life by facilitating the patient's life-review, facilitating the potential for reconciliation, or the development of an "ethical will." An ethical will originated as Jewish tradition of *Zevaoth*, and more recently has been adapted the general public as a means to document ethical values or family and cultural history from one generation to the next.

Once these four levels have been achieved, a person seeks to become self-actualized. Maslow describes this process as the way humans discover and engage their full potential. Essentially, self-actualization is the merging of sense of purpose and recognized capacity with the realization of that one has potential (Maslow 1954). The loss of one's sense of meaning or the loss of ability to fulfill that sense of purpose, as seen in the context of chronic pain and illness, can lead to significant distress. Meaning and purpose have become recognized as aspects of a person's spiritual domain and thus is an important domain that can best be addressed by chaplains and psychologists. Laurel Herbst, a hematology–oncology and palliative medicine physician, notes that demands for chaplaincy support increased dramatically with the simple shift of inquiry from "do you want a chaplain?" to "one of our team members can help you explore your questions of meaning and value" (Herbst (2006)).

The benefits of this model have been outlined in case reports that show how the identification of suffering in this manner can effectively help, not only patients and significant others but also engage different members of an interdisciplinary team in addressing different faces of a patient's experience of "total pain" (Clark 1999).

Case Study 2: Truncated Life

Jose is a 37-year-old immigrant from Central America admitted to hospital once again for recurrent severe abdominal pain in the context of locally recurrent gastric cancer, status post-resection. He is found to have a malignant bowel obstruction and peritoneal carcinomatosis. Despite aggressive medical and surgical interventions for pain and symptom control, he remains in significant distress. After conversations about worsening prognosis, he asks whether we can help bring his family in from Central America to see him once again before he dies.

He and his wife moved to the USA 6 years prior to admission to hospital with the dream of working hard, earning a green card and bringing his mother and four children to the United States. He has not seen his mother or children since he left his home country, and he told us that his youngest is now 12 years old, and his oldest daughter is 22 and soon to marry. Further discussion reveals a deep faith linked to an evangelical church. On occasion parishioners from his church visit and hold prayer ceremonies at his bedside, praying that he will rediscover the depth of his faith he once had in order to enable healing.

1. What is the likely impact of a truncated life on this patient's pain?
2. How do you help family members understand the difference between healing and curing?
3. What plan would you adopt to help Jose begin the process of finding meaning despite the loss of his dreams?

Pain, Personhood, and Suffering

Eric Cassell's work further delved into this concept, recognizing suffering as anything that threatens the integrity of the person, in all or any its manifestations – body, mind, relationship, and existential

(Cassell 1991). In his landmark NEJM 1982 article, he explores the different dimensions of suffering and challenges the clinician to lend strength and tend to the suffering of the patient – by first acknowledging that suffering is a phenomena not solely defined as physical pain and not occurring due to infractions of a linear or progressive fashion (Cassel 1982). Cassell challenged clinicians to recognize the complexity of the personal and human experience of suffering, as one that involves both the physical experience of pain, as well as any form of severe distress that threatens the integrity of the person in their physical, spiritual, relational, cultural, political, behavioral, historical, transpersonal, and transcendent selves that suffer. While we all face challenges to our personhood on an almost daily basis without experiencing persistent suffering, we mitigate the experience of suffering by adapting or by rebuilding our sense of self. When, however, the threat to self is large enough, as is the case of unremitting chronic pain and illness, when suffering is intense, Cassel states that recovery requires help from others, finding meaning in the suffering, and ultimately, transcending. This transcendence is a deeply spiritual experience that may, or may not, include formal religion (Cassel 1982). He thus reminds clinicians to assess not only the physical aspects of pain, but to assess and make appropriate referrals for the treatment of the multiple dimensions of suffering, or "total pain."

Meaning and Suffering

Overcoming suffering through finding meaning and transcendence in the experience was perhaps most thoroughly explored by Viktor Frankl, a physician, Holocaust, survivor and founder of the field of Existential Psychology. In his treatise, *Man's Search for Meaning*, Frankl outlined three primary types of suffering, physical (pain, somatic diseases), psychological (emotional hardship, psychological disorders), and spiritual (lack of a meaningful life, moral dilemmas). During his imprisonment in Auschwitz, Frankl observed that prisoners who found a reason to live and those who died with lack of meaning proved the truth of Nietzche's statement: "if we possess the *why* of life then we can put up with almost any *how*" (Nietzsche and Hollingdale 1968, p. 74). From this, Frankl developed the psychotherapeutic approach known as logotherapy, from the Greek word *logos*, which means study, word, spirit, God, or meaning. Like Saunders, Frankl was also concerned about the prevailing reductionist biomedical model of medicine that tended to value only the physiologic processes of human experience. He saw the need to humanize both medicine and psychology through the recognition of a balance between the biopsychosocial including the physical, mental, emotional, and spiritual dimensions of humankind. This perspective was solidified in Auschwitz where he saw prisoners' physiology weaken to the point of death when the spirit or person lost their sense of purpose. In amazement, he also noted the ability of those who held on to their search for meaning also maintained their physical and psychological resilience (Frankl 2006).

Meaning can be found, according to Frankl, through experienced values (what we receive from the world, i.e. love), creative values (what we contribute to the world), or attitudinal values (which may be obtained through unavoidable suffering). He quoted one boy prisoner of Auschwitz, Yehudi Bacon, who said, "suffering can have a meaning if it changes you for the better" (Frankl 2006, p. 67). These three values, however, which Frankl postulates are but initial steps toward transcendence or supra-meaning, which relies on something greater than our selves. "In spite of all the enforced physical and mental primitiveness of the life in a concentration camp, it was possible for spiritual life to deepen. [...] They were able to retreat from their terrible surroundings to a life of inner riches and spiritual freedom" (Frankl 2006, p. 34).

Max Harvey Chochinov, a contemporary palliative psychiatrist, recently confirmed these observations in numerous studies, including one where he evaluated 253 patients receiving palliative care with the 25-item, self-report Patient Dignity Inventory (PDI) to assess the spiritual "landscape of distress in the terminally ill." He noted an inverse correlation between "sense of meaning" and "intensity of distress" (Chochinov et al. 2009). Chochinov has continued to incorporate this concept of assessing suffering and resilience to distress through an assessment of the "whole person," rather than the purely physical point of view more commonly found in traditional biomedical practice. The presence of hope (see also Coulehan, This volume) and a sense of meaning both consistently correlate with measurable improvements in the sense of well-being among patients facing the end of life and associated lack of hope and purpose, with distress (Thompson and Chochinov 2010).

Thus, per both Frankl and Chochinov's work, logotherapy, or exploring a patient's sense of meaning, is not postulated to directly affect pain pathways. Instead, that sense of meaning and the exploration of meaning seem to help patients with life-limiting illness cope with and to some degree, transcend pain and suffering. In these studies, the primary tool for understanding issues of pain was through patients' stories and narrative (see also Morris, This Volume). Hospice and palliative care teams can also apply a modified model of Maslow's Hierarchy of Needs to the interdisciplinary meeting to help delineate roles each team-member might play in the alleviation of pain and suffering.

The Bio-Psycho-Social–Spiritual Model of Pain

Dr. George Engel first described the bio-psycho-social model of disease in the 1970s (Engel 1977). This model quickly became the standard model through which many mental health clinicians came to view disease, illness, and treatment (Schwartz 1982), although the process of adoption was somewhat slower by the biomedical field (Engel 1989; Engel 1992). This model recognizes that the individual self is multi-faceted and it describes a framework for understanding how the biological, psychological, and social factors of an individual's life affect the experience and meaning of medical illness and pain. In addition, this model also recognizes that bidirectional pathways exist between the three domains (biological, psychological, social), and each domain can positively or negatively impact other domains. Disease/illness conceptualizations that incorporate the bio-psycho-social model can also explain how individuals may experience pain without a specific etiology, or how individuals may experience varying levels of pain within the context of a recognized disease or injury process. As the bio-psycho-social model seeks to understand the interaction between an individual's medical status, mental health status (including cognitive appraisals of his/her medical status), and sociological factors all interact to impact a patient's overall well-being.

The Gate Control/Neuromatrix theory of pain (Melzack 1999; Melzack and Wall 1965) builds upon the biopsychosocial model with a direct application to the pain experience. It describes the relationship between the biological, psychological, and social aspects of the individual pain experience and how each domain may influence an increase or decrease in the pain experience for the individual via descending pathways from the brain (Eippert et al. 2009). This model also continues to inform multi-factorial and multidisciplinary pain management and treatment.

Over time the empirical research evidence has supported the Bio-Psycho-Social and Gate/ Neuromatrix models' thesis that psychological states impact the level of pain experienced by the individual (Middleton and Pollard 2005). Some of those psychological factors mediating the pain experience that have been identified by the research include negative mood, anxiety, social support, sense of self-efficacy and control, and adaptive coping strategies (Covic et al. 2003; French et al. 2000; Keefe et al. 1997; Lefebvre et al. 1999). However, these factors still fail to completely explain the observed variability across individuals' experiences with pain.

In an attempt to create a more comprehensive model, researchers have also begun to incorporate spirituality into the biopsychosocial model (McKee and Chappel 1992; Sulmasy 2002; Wachholtz et al.

2007). The resulting biopsychosocial–spiritual model acknowledges the potential impact of spiritual and religious variables in mediating the biological and psychological experience of pain and illness (Wachholtz and Keefe 2006). The addition of spiritual coping mechanisms is still congruent with the Gate/Neuromatrix model since spirituality also affects the individual's experience of pain and his/her social, psychological, and physical environment.

Culture and religion-specific factors may also play a role in patient's experience and interpretation of chronic pain and suffering. The clinician, therefore, must also consider the patient's cultural and religious beliefs about death and dying when evaluating factors influencing the experience of pain, identifying treatment needs, and developing appropriate interventions. This is a topic that will be more extensively addressed in other chapters of this series (See also Hallenbeck, This Volume; Coulehan, This Volume). Because it is so important to identify the potential interplay between pain, suffering, and spirituality, we have included a brief table (Table 36.1), to address the role of suffering, images, and potential cultural symbols of suffering in each of the five major world religions.

Case Study 3: Opioids and Clarity of Mind

Mr. Tsong is a 79-year-old Buddhist grandfather with end-stage metastatic prostate cancer, and is cared for by his family at home, with the support of hospice. The patient has been agitated, crying out in pain, and unable to sleep due to the severity of his pain. The family meeting is held with the hospice team: physician, nurse, and chaplain are present.

Everybody present (patient, family, and hospice team) agrees that the patient is suffering from severe pain in his shoulder, spine, and left hip, due to the painful bony metastases. He is taking dexamethasone, ibuprofen and acetaminophen, but these medications are not alleviating his pain, described as an intensity of 9/10. He has thus far refused to try morphine because while he acknowledges that he is nearing his death, his family wants to avoid opioids in order to allow him to have a clear mind and thought at the time of his death.

Consider the following approaches to this challenge.

(a) "We will support your decision to avoid opioids, including morphine, and provide you with more chaplaincy support to engage meditation and ritual to help you confront your suffering and pain."

(b) "We understand your fear of morphine, but would you consider the following: Would you consider trying a small dose of morphine that could help you have clearer mind once your pain is better controlled and you have been able to have more restful sleep? We will use the lowest dose possible to avoid confusion."

What roles each of the following members of an interdisciplinary team might help this family and patient?

(a) Physician
(b) Nurse
(c) Pharmacist
(d) Chaplain
(e) Pain Psychologist
(f) Social worker

Table 36.1 Images and symbols related to religious dimensions of suffering

	Origin/Sacred text/ Exemplar of suffering	Core principles	Potential issues at end of life	Fear of Afterlife
Western origin	Judaism	Monotheistic Torah	There is one God who is transcendent and omnipresent;	The belief in the sanctity of life may lead to continue aggressive care.	Due to intense debate among Rabbinical scholars, fear of the afterlife generally revolved around its uncertainty.
		Job	Hebrews are God's chosen people; Failure to obey God is a sin; Life is sacred.	The belief in the sanctity of the body, especially at death, may lead to avoidance of interventions (i.e. surgery, intubation, feeding tubes).	
	Christianity	Bible Jesus	Humans are sinful Jesus Christ is the Savior, who died on the cross and was resurrected. Salvation is obtained through either faith or good deeds	The belief in the possibility of a miracle to save lives sometimes leads to decisions to prolong aggressive medical interventions.	Guilt and unresolved sin and issues of forgiveness and absolution can effect how the soul experiences the afterlife
	Islam	Monotheistic Koran	Islam means submission (to the will of God) There is one God, Allah, the creator of all. Mohammed is his prophet. *Five pillars of Islam:* 1. Shahad – Confession of faith 2. Salat – Prayer toward Mecca 3. Zakat – Almsgiving 4. Sawm – Fasting during the month of Ramadan 5. Haji – Pilgrimage to Mecca	Sanctity of life is paramount and its importance overrides obligations to the Five Pillars of Islam.	After death, humans rest in the grave until the Day of Judgment, when Allah determines who will go to Paradise or Hell.
		Job			

Eastern origin	Hinduism	Polytheistic Vedas Yogis	Five basic principles: 1. Samsara – All beings are reincarnated until they reach nirvana 2. Karma – deeds of prior lives affect future lives 3. Dukkha – Suffering infuses reincarnated lives 4. Moksha – Enlightenment (spiritual knowledge) is the only means to become free from suffering.	Some patients may fear anything that may cloud judgment at the end of life, as they are supposed to focus on sacred things at the moment of death in order to ensure rebirth to a higher form of being. Disease states such as delirium or medications such as opioids or benzodiazepines may be of concern to patient/family.	Rebirth to a lower order being due to bad karma or clouded state of mind at time of death.
	Buddhism	Nontheistic Boddhisattva	Ultimate goal is to obtain enlightenment, to end suffering, and end the cycle of reincarnation. Four noble truths of Buddhism: 1. Life means suffering 2. The origin of suffering is attachment 3. The cessation of suffering is attainable through nirodha (disengagement) 4. The path to cessation of suffering is by the "Middle Road" between self-indulgence and asceticism, the Eightfold Path.	Patients may fear lack of clarity of mind during the dying process, as the soul may get lost in transition to the next life. Concerns may arise around opioids, benzodiazepines, and in disease states such as delirium and dementia.	Fear of the soul getting lost in transition from this life to the next, especially if the mind is unclear. Buddhists believe that souls temporarily reside in one of six realms until their rebirth: heaven, human life, Asura (demi-god), animal life, hungry ghost, hell, etc.

Stages of Grief

Dr. Elizabeth Kubler-Ross is probably the most well-known and most cited figure in palliative care medicine. Through her qualitative research using interviews with terminally ill patients, she identified the now-classic five stages of grief: (1) denial and isolation, (2) anger, (3) bargaining, (4) depression, and (5) acceptance (Kubler-Ross 2009; Kübler-Ross 1997). These stages are not a one-way track. Individuals may move forward, backward, or skip stages altogether as they process their upcoming loss of life. The majority of the research supporting Kubler-Ross' stages of grief has used qualitative methods (Kubler-Ross 2009). The limited quantitative research in this area also supports this model (Maciejewski et al. 2007). In a study of 270 oncology patients treated for mental health via a psychiatry consultation liaison team, individuals who were at the "acceptance" stage had fewer mental health disorders, better compliance with treatment, and more coping resources compared with individuals at the anger/aggression stage (Grube 2006). While we can identify what is healthy coping in relation to stages of grief, to the best of our knowledge, there is no empirical research on how progression through the stages of grief affects the patient's experience of pain. We suspect there are probably changes that occur in the perception of pain, after adjusting for disease progression, when patients are in the different stages (e.g. higher in the anger stage; lower in the acceptance stage). However, despite the frequency that the Stages of Grief Model is used as a basis for psychotherapy treatment plans for palliative care patients, and our suspicions that these stages are related to pain, to the best of our knowledge, no empirical data exists to support this finding. Additional qualitative and quantitative research needs to be done in this field to estimate timelines for the stages, differentiate between normal and abnormal grieving processes, identify key information that would allow physicians to make more timely referrals to a mental health specialist, and assess the appropriateness of this model across different cultures and generations.

Case Study 4: Ritual at the End of Life

Meira is a 72-year-old woman with severe congestive heart failure. Despite the significant limitations placed on her life by this disease, she still attends her local Hindu temple as often as possible or worships at her home shrine. On her "good days" she will ask her nursing assistant to push her wheelchair through the park. She has signed a DNR/DNI, but does not have a medical bracelet. As her CNA left her at the edge of the park and went to get the car, Meira collapsed in her wheelchair. A bystander called 911 and she was transported to a local ER. The ER team intubated her. As Meira's breathing was severely impaired, it was unlikely she would survive the night without the intubation. When the family arrived with the DNR/DNI, they asked that she be extubated and no further heroic measures be performed. The family also asked that they be able to prepare her for death, by placing ritual objects in her line of vision and be allowed to chant at her bedside so that she is thinking holy thoughts at the time of her death.

1. How would you respond to the patient's family?
2. What barriers might prevent a family to engage in end-of-life rituals with their loved one?
3. How would you react if you were asked to participate in the chanting ritual with the family?
4. What if you were asked to chant as a form of apology to the patient as a member of the medical team that (albeit unknowingly) did not abide by the patient's wishes and prolonged her life?

Adaptive and Maladaptive Religious–Spiritual Coping

Although spirituality and religion are powerful forces, their observable effect is not always advantageous. While the popular media has primarily focused on the beneficial effects of religion and spirituality on health, it is also important to understand that there can be both positive and negative effects. It is the valence of the spiritual practice that strongly influences the outcome on health and pain. Positive (adaptive) spiritual practices have been shown to reduce the experience of pain. The positive influence on descending/central modulating pain pathways may include reducing stress, pain distraction, higher power support, and providing a supportive social environment. On a biobehavioral neuroscientific level, there is evidence that serotonin receptor densities are correlated with spiritual proclivities which suggests that spiritual practices may actually influence serotonin pathways that regulate mood and pain (Borg et al. 2003). Contrary to positive spiritual practices, negative (or maladaptive) spiritual practices can increase pain sensitivity (Rippentrop et al. 2005). For example negative spiritually related thoughts (e.g. "God is punishing me") can increase pain sensitivity and heighten the pain experience (Rippentrop et al. 2005). In the past, spiritual activity was viewed as a passive coping resource and equivalent to "hoping" (Covic et al. 2003). Yet ongoing research has shown that spirituality is actually an active resource that can be a tool to help or hinder the healing process, through multiple pathways including spiritual meaning making, spiritual growth, religious reappraisal, and spiritual support (see Wachholtz et al. 2007 for more details on the complex spiritual pathways that link to pain). Given the obvious impact that religion and spirituality can have on the pain experience and the viable neurological, psychological, and spiritual pathways support this effect on the pain experience, it is critical that we understand how our patients' spirituality may influence their bio-psycho-social–spiritual health, particularly in the context of chronic pain at the end of life.

While spiritual coping cannot simply be reduced to a variety of biological, psychological, and social factors (Pargament 2002), spiritual coping can cause positive changes in a constellation of other factors that have been shown to enhance pain tolerance. One of the critical areas of psycho-social pain management is the concept of self-efficacy and control over the pain (Ai et al. 2005; French et al. 2000; Keefe et al. 1997; Lefebvre et al. 1999). When individuals have some level of control over the pain, they are better able to engage in activities of daily living (ADL), participate in social activities, and enjoy the small pleasures of life.

Three forms of religious coping related to locus-of-control have been identified (Pargament et al. 1988). The first form of religious coping is "Deferred" coping in which the patient defers all aspects of his/her health care to their higher power (e.g. "I'm leaving it in God's hands"). The second form is "Collaborative" where the patients share responsibility for their health with their higher power (e.g. "God and I will get through this together. God will watch over me and it's my responsibility to go to my doctor's appointments/check blood sugars/get annual mammograms"). The third type is "Self-Directed" in which the patient does not rely on a higher power at all (e.g. "I'm on my own to make sure I stay healthy"). A fourth form of coping was more recently identified by Phillips and colleagues (Phillips et al. 2004). The fourth type is "Abandoned" in which the person must take care of their own health because their higher power has abandoned them (e.g. "God won't help me because I'm a bad person so I have to deal with it on my own"). Of these four coping styles involving locus of control, generally the Collaborative form of coping is associated with better mental and physical health outcomes (Hathaway and Pargament 1990, 1992; McIntosh and Spilka 1990; Pargament et al. 1988). Although the Self-directed coping has been shown to have mixed results, those who feel abandoned by their higher power often have strong negative outcomes (Phillips et al. 2004). Deferred coping has generally been associated with more negative outcomes; although in situations where there is more limited control, such as in palliative care, deferred coping appears to be related to decreased agitation and increased peace (Bickel et al. 1998; Pargament 2001; Pargament et al. 2005).

Case Study 5: Shame/Guilt vs. Forgiveness/Absolution

Shirley is a 44-year-old married African American woman with AIDS, who has a strong Christian spiritual background but has not attended church since she was diagnosed with HIV. Shirley contracted HIV when she had an extra-marital affair. Her husband forgave her, and the couple reconciled. Shirley, however, continues to have overwhelming feelings of guilt. Due to this guilt she ignored the symptoms of HIV and significantly delayed treatment once diagnosed. She was recently transferred to palliative care in a hospice facility. Her husband is emotionally devastated, but he is supportive and visits her every evening. She experiences significant neuropathic pain around the time of her husband's visits. Changes in timing and dosages of medications have not alleviated the pain.

1. What factors may be impacting the patient's mental and physical health?
2. Identify the differences between pain and suffering in this scenario.
3. Given the patient's spiritual background, what steps might you take to reduce the patient's pain and suffering?

Pain severity vs. Pain Tolerance

Religion and spirituality do not generally make the pain "disappear." The research suggests that religious and spiritual practices have a greater influence on pain tolerance than on pain sensitivity (Keefe et al. 1997; Wachholtz and Pargament 2005; Wachholtz and Pearce 2009). In other words, while the patients may not say that their pain level is reduced, they may require less pain medication because they have developed a greater tolerance for that level of pain. Positive spiritual practices have also been shown to increase tolerance in both chronic pain (Keefe et al. 1997; Wachholtz and Pargament 2008) and in acute pain situations (Wachholtz and Pargament 2005).

Clinical Assessment of Spirituality and Pain

Spiritual Well-Being Assessment Tools

Although a number of spiritual assessment tools exist for use in a clinical setting, few have been empirically validated. In the context of a spiritual assessment, the physician is not expected to be a spiritual director or a psychologist; rather they are responsible for assessing these needs and consulting with the appropriate professionals to ensure that the patients receive the treatment they need. Although the physicians should not be expected to meet the spiritual needs of the patients, they can facilitate access to the treatment or services that the patients require just as they would make referrals to psychologists, physical therapists, dieticians, or other treatment providers.

Qualitative Spiritual Assessments

HOPE. The HOPE survey uses an acronym which serves as a reminder to providers on how to walk a patient through the four-step spiritual assessment interview (Anandarajah and Hight 2001). Conceptually, the HOPE is similar to the FICA (below). That said, the language of the HOPE is more comfortable to use in a patient setting for some clinicians because it does not assume a faith or spiritual belief system. Other clinicians disagree and while they feel these questions are considered valuable to ask, the entry point for the measure is not explicitly spiritual and therefore is less of a spiritual assessment and more of a strengths assessment. The HOPE is a structured format for taking a spiritual history, therefore there are no explicit validation studies for this measure and limited empirically validated recommendations based on the results of this interview assessment (Anandarajah and Hight 2001).

In the HOPE spiritual assessment H stands for sources of *H*ope. This may include asking questions about where the patient finds hope, strength, comfort, peace, or feelings of connectedness. This helps the provider identify the patient's basic spiritual resources without the assumption of a theistic faith. The second letter of the acronym "O" stands for *O*rganized religion. This topic is concerned with religious and spiritual social support and includes questions such "Do you belong to an organized religious group?" and "How active are you in that group?" The third letter, "P," stands for *P*ersonal spirituality and practices and includes any private spiritual activities. This may include questions about use of prayer, music, meditation, etc. The provider may also wish to ask if the patients have specific spiritual/religious practices related to their health issues such as faith healing or acupuncture. In addition, this question may also include use of herbal supplements that religious groups may include as part of a healing ritual. The final letter "E" discusses the *E*ffects on medical and end-of-life issues. In this section the provider can focus the discussion back onto clinical management of the medical issues and identify how a patient's medical care may be affected by his/her spiritual or religious beliefs. This format allows the provider to ask information about the patients' religious and spiritual beliefs while simultaneously gathering critical information about how the patients would like to integrate this information into their care.

FICA. The FICA (Puchalski 2001) spiritual assessment uses an acronym to help the provider recall each of the four steps of this assessment. F stands for *F*aith/beliefs and encourages the provider to use an unstructured statement to assess the patient's current faith system (e.g. "Tell me something about your faith or beliefs"). I stands for *I*mportance/*I*nfluence and asks if the patients' belief systems have any impact on their lives (e.g. "How does this influence your health and well-being?"). The C stands for *C*ommunity and asks about religiously based social support versus only engaging in individual spiritual practice (e.g. "Are you part of a supportive community?"). The final letter A reminds the practitioner to explore *A*pplication of this information and how the patients use their spiritual beliefs in their healthcare (e.g. "How would you like me to address these issues in your health care?"). This four-step assessment provides for an open evaluation while also providing the health care provider with an exit point if the patient does not appear interested in discussing his/her religion/spirituality. This formal framework for spiritual history taking was recently empirically validated as correlating strongly with quantitative assessments of spiritual quality of life in palliative care patients (Borneman et al. 2010).

OASIS. The OASIS project is a 7-step assessment of patient spirituality that has been taught to oncologists and evaluated for the ease of use among the physicians as well as the patient's response to the inquiry (Kristeller et al. 2005). It is one of the very few qualitative spiritual assessments empirically validated in *both* physicians and patients. It was specifically validated on oncologists and oncology patients. Due to space constraints we cannot fully describe the seven steps and conversational algorithm. This assessment is described in greater detail in the work of Kristeller et al. (2005). Briefly, the seven-step spiritual assessment includes (1) Neutral inquiry, (2) Inquire further based on patient's initial response, (3) Continue to explore, (4) Inquire about meaning and sources of peace, (5) Inquire about spiritual resources (including spiritual social support), (6) Offer referral assistance to help access spiritual resources, (7) Bring inquiry to a close. This format allows physicians to gain a further understanding of the patients' religious and spiritual coping mechanisms, and provide a way to end the conversation in a timely manner (Kristeller et al. 2005). A significant strength of the measure is that immediately following the assessment and at a series of follow-ups, patients never expressed a negative response to the assessment, even if they did not endorse any spiritual/religious beliefs. And, although physicians were not initially comfortable with the interview procedures, they also came to recognize that their patients had positive responses to the assessment. As a consequence, many endorsed the continued use of this assessment.

Case Study 6: Religious vs. Medical Mandates

Hakim is a 52-year-old man of Middle Eastern descent who closely follows Islamic tradition. As he was driving home from work one evening he was in a serious automobile accident. He was rushed to surgery and appeared that he would make a full recovery. When he awoke after surgery, he was informed about his multiple injuries, and spoke with a dietician about his critical nutrition requirements during recovery from surgery. The patient was receptive to the recommendations, but stated he could not consume any food or receive total parenteral (IV) nutrition (i.e. TPN) nutrition during the day as it was currently Ramadan.

1. How would you react to this situation?
2. What resources might you use to help a patient who felt conflicted between their medical requirements and their religious beliefs?
3. Are there any tenants of Islam that might reduce this patient's feeling of conflict?

Quantitative Spiritual Assessments and Pain

In addition to qualitative assessment tools, it should be noted that a number of quantitative tools may also be useful to assess patient coping in a clinical setting. Some of the most empirically validated and widely used tools include (1) Religious/spiritual coping long form (RCOPE); (2) Religious/spiritual coping short form (Brief RCOPE); and (3) Functional Assessment of Chronic Illness Therapy - Spiritual Well- Being (FACIT-SP).

The *RCOPE* was designed by Pargament and colleagues (Pargament et al. 2000) and identified the 3 (and later 4) methods of religious/spiritual coping that was described earlier in this chapter. This is a 100+ question survey; it is somewhat time consuming for patients, but it can provide important information on spiritual coping methods.

The *Brief RCOPE* was also developed by Pargament and colleagues (Pargament et al. 1998). This shorter (14 item) version of the RCOPE will not provide as much detail but will indicate whether a patient is using positive or negative spiritual/religious coping techniques and will help the provider to determine if a chaplaincy or mental health referral is needed.

The *FACIT-SP* (Peterman et al. 2002) is a 12-item survey that has both long and short versions that can be used to assess a patient's spiritual well-being specifically in relationship to his/her illness and quality of life. The FACIT-SP has been validated in cross-cultural populations (Ando et al. 2009).

Another quantitative tool that can be used in patients' nearing the end of life is the Patient Dignity Inventory (PDI), a brief but comprehensive assessment of psychosocial, spiritual, and existential sources of distress that could be addressed in the clinical setting (Chochinov et al. 2008). The PDI is a 25-item measure to assess dignity-related distress associated with five primary areas: Symptom distress, Existential distress, Dependency, Peace of mind, and Social support. While this survey is relatively new and not widely used yet, it does have excellent internal consistency (Chronbach's $\alpha = 0.93$) and reliability (test-retest $r = 0.85$). The individual subscales have been validated with other known measures within their respective fields (Chochinov et al. 2008).

While this is far from a complete list, it does provide a brief understanding of which tools are available to identify how pain may be related to spiritual distress and where interdisciplinary interventions may be necessary for patients with chronic pain and in palliative care populations. Qualitative assessments have less empirically validated research connecting spirituality to the pain experience. Research based on the first three quantitative surveys (RCOPE, Brief RCOPE, FACIT) also indicates a strong connection between spiritual coping and the patients' pain experience (Bush et al. 1999; Wachholtz et al. 2007). Additional evidence using the PDI shows that dignity and pain are closely correlated when age is not a factor (Chochinov et al. 2008). That said, additional research using both qualitative and quantitative methods is required to better understand the association between spirituality, dignity, and pain.

Summary and Conclusion

Pain is a complex and multidimensional experience that encompasses biological, psychological, social, and spiritual factors (Wachholtz et al. 2007). Traditional biomedicine is historically focused on the biological aspects of pain management at the expense of the psychosocial or spiritual aspects of the experience (Engel 1992). As a consequence, there has been a tendency to under-assess and under-treat other areas that also contribute to the experience of pain and related suffering. By improving awareness on how to identify the multiple potential sources of pain in our patients, we then have the new opportunity to potentially alleviate some of that pain and related suffering. This includes the 3-As to treating multidimensional pain: Awareness, Assessment, and Alleviation. By integrating the resources of a multi-dimensional treatment team into palliative care practice, we will be able to provide a higher level of service to our patients and improve pain management at the end of life.

As palliative care experts of all disciplines gain increased recognition and presence in hospitals and healthcare settings, early spiritual assessment and care will become more common in the care of patients with pain, suffering, or facing end of life. With increasing focus on spirituality in the management of pain and suffering, more evidence will certainly emerge through both qualitative and quantitative research exploring the impact of early assessment and intervention, identifying best practices for intervention (including timing, type, and discipline of provider), understanding the roles that different disciplines play in addressing and alleviating spiritual sources of suffering, Of course the challenge to improve the empirically validated care of our patients, especially in the realm of spirituality, is the access to funding for research and personnel. As a result, research exploring the impact of spiritual interventions linking cost-effectiveness, quality of life outcomes, and hospital or insurer quality metrics will likely play a key role in defining the direction of this field.

While acknowledging the critical importance of future research, we must also recognize the limitations of current methodology that cannot adequately quantify the boundlessness of the soul. For the reasons we have outlined throughout this chapter, we need to broaden the challenge against the rigid Cartesian dualism approach to the management of pain and suffering that has ruled healthcare for so long and instead begin to reintegrate science with the esthetic, the spiritual, and the philosophical aspects of humanity.

References

Ai, A. L., Peterson, C., Rodgers, W., & Tice, T. N. (2005). Effects of faith and secular factors on locus of control in middle-aged and older cardiac patients. *Aging and Mental Health, 9*(5), 470–481.

Anandarajah, G., & Hight, E. (2001). Spirituality and medical practice: Using the HOPE questions as a practical tool for spiritual assessment. *American Family Physician, 62*(1), 81–89.

Ando, M., Morita, T., Ahn, S., Marquez-Wong, F., & Ide, S. (2009). International comparison study on the primary concerns of terminally ill cancer patients in short-term life review interviews among Japanese, Koreans, and Americans. *Palliatiative and Supportive Care, 7*(3), 349–355.

Bickel, C., Ciarrocchi, J., Sheers, N., Estadt, B., Powell, D., & Pargament, K. (1998). Perceived stress, religious coping styles, and depressive affect. *Journal of Psychology and Christianity, 17*(1), 33–42.

Borg, J., Andree, B., Soderstrom, H., & Farde, L. (2003). The serotonin system and spiritual experiences. *American Journal of Psychiatry, 160*(11), 1965–1969.

Borneman, T., Ferrell, B., & Puchalski, C. M. (2010). Evaluation of the FICA tool for spiritual assessment. *Journal of Pain and Symptom Management, 40*(2), 163–173. doi:10.1016/j.jpainsymman.2009.12.019.

Bush, E., Rye, M., Brant, C., Emery, E., Pargament, K., & Riessinger, C. (1999). Religious coping with chronic pain. *Applied Psychophysiology and Biofeedback, 24*(4), 249–260.

Cacioppo, J. T., Fowler, J. H., & Christakis, N. A. (2009). Alone in the crowd: The structure and spread of loneliness in a large social network. *Journal of Personality and Social Psychology, 97*(6), 977–991.

Cassel, E. J. (1982). The nature of suffering and the goals of medicine. *The New England Journal of Medicine, 306*(11), 639–645.

Cassell, E. J. (1991). Recognizing suffering. *The Hastings Center Report, 21*(3), 24–31.

Chochinov, H. M., Hassard, T., McClement, S., Hack, T., Kristjanson, L. J., Harlos, M., et al. (2008). The patient dignity inventory: A novel way of measuring dignity-related distress in palliative care. *Journal of Pain and Symptom Management, 36*(6), 559–571. http://www.virtualhospice.ca/Assets/the%20patient%20dignity%20inventory_20090427102735.pdf.

Chochinov, H. M., Hassard, T., McClement, S., Hack, T., Kristjanson, L. J., Harlos, M., et al. (2009). The landscape of distress in the terminally ill. *Journal of Pain and Symptom Management, 38*(5), 641–649.

Christakis, N. A., & Allison, P. D. (2006). Mortality after the hospitalization of a spouse. *The New England Journal of Medicine, 354*(7), 719–730.

Clark, D. (1999). 'Total pain,' disciplinary power and the body in the work of Cicely Saunders, 1958–1967. *Social Science and Medicine, 49*(6), 727–736.

Covic, T., Adamson, B., Spencer, D., & Howe, G. (2003). A biopsychosocial model of pain and depression in rheumatoid arthritis: A 12-month longitudinal study. *Rheumatology, 42*(11), 1287–1294.

Eippert, F., Finsterbusch, J., Bingel, U., & Buchel, C. (2009). Direct evidence for spinal cord involvement in placebo analgesia. *Science, 326*, 404.

Engel, G. L. (1977). The need for a new medical model: A challenge for biomedicine. *Science, 196*, 129–136.

Engel, G. L. (1989). The need for a new medical model: A challenge for biomedicine. *Journal of Interprofessional Care, 4*(1), 37–53.

Engel, G. L. (1992). How much longer must medicine's science be bound by a seventeenth century world view? *Psychotherapy and Psychosomatics, 57*, 3–16.

Frankl, V. E. (2006). *Man's search for meaning*. Boston: Beacon.

French, D., Holroyd, K., Pinell, C., Malinoski, P., Odonnell, F., & Hill, K. (2000). Perceived self-efficacy and headache-related disability. *Headache: The Journal of Head and Face Pain, 40*(8), 647–656.

Grube, M. (2006). Compliance and coping potential of cancer patients treated in liaison-consultation psychiatry. *International Journal of Psychiatry in Medicine, 36*(2), 211–229.

Hathaway, W. L., & Pargament, K. I. (1990). Intrinsic religiousness, religious coping, and psychosocial competence: A covariance structure analysis. *Journal for the Scientific Study of Religion, 29*, 423–441.

Hathaway, W., & Pargament, K. (1992). The religious dimensions of coping: Implications for prevention and promotion. In K.I. Pargment, K.I. Maton, & R.E. Hess (Eds.), *Religion and prevention in mental health: Research, vision, and action*, (pp. 129–154). New York: Haworth Press.

Herbst, L. (2006). Applying the concepts from Maslow in a large U.S. hospice program. *Journal of Palliative Medicine, 9*(5), 1049–1052.

Keefe, F. J., Lefebvre, J. C., Maixner, W., Salley, A. N., Jr., & Caldwell, D. S. (1997). Self-efficacy for arthritis pain: Relationship to perception of thermal laboratory pain stimuli. *Arthritis Care and Research, 10*(3), 177–184.

Kristeller, J. L., Rhodes, M., Cripe, L. D., & Sheets, V. (2005). Oncologist assisted spiritual intervention study (OASIS): Patient acceptability & initial evidence of effects. *International Journal of Psychiatry in Medicine, 35*(4), 329–347.

Kubler-Ross, E. (2009). *On death and dying: 40th anniversary edition*. Abingdon: Routledge.

Kübler-Ross, E. (1997). *On death and dying*. Nebraska: Scribner.

Lefebvre, J. C., Keefe, F. J., Affleck, G., Raezer, L. B., Starr, K., Caldwell, D. S., et al. (1999). The relationship of arthritis self-efficacy to daily pain, daily mood, and daily pain coping in rheumatoid arthritis patients. *Pain, 80*(1–2), 425–435. 10.1016/S0304-3959(98)00242-5.

Maciejewski, P., Zhang, B., Block, S., & Prigerson, H. (2007). An empirical examination of the stage theory of grief. *Journal of the American Medical Association, 297*(7), 716.

Maslow, A. (1954). *Motivation and personality*. New York: Harper.

McIntosh, D. N., & Spilka, B. (1990). Religion and physical health: The role of personal faith and control. In M. L. Lynn & D. O. Moberg (Eds.), *Research in the social scientific study of religion* (Vol. 2, pp. 167–194). Greenwich: JAI.

McKee, D., & Chappel, J. (1992). Spirituality and medical practice. *Journal of Family Practice, 35*(2), 201.

Melzack, R. (1999). From the gate to the neuromatrix. *Pain, 6*(S1), S121–S126.

Melzack, R., & Wall, P. D. (1965). Pain mechanisms: a new theory. *Science, 150*(3699), 971–979.

Middleton, P., & Pollard, H. (2005). Are chronic low back pain outcomes improved with co-management of concurrent depression? *Chiropractic and Osteopathy, 13*(1), 8.

Nietzsche, F. W., & Hollingdale, R. J. (1968). *Twilight of the idols and penguin: The anti-christ.* Harmondsworth: Penguin Classics.

Pargament, K. (2001). *The psychology of religion and coping: Theory, research, practice.* New York: Guilford.

Pargament, K. I. (2002). Is religion nothing but ...? explaining religion versus explaining religion away. *Psychological Inquiry, 13*(3), 239–244.

Pargament, K. I., Ano, G., & Wachholtz, A. B. (2005). Religion and Coping. In R. Paloutzian & C. Park (Eds.), *The Handbook of the Psychology of Religion.* New York: Guilford.

Pargament, K. I., Kennell, J., Hathaway, W., Grevengoed, N., Newman, J., & Jones, W. (1988). Religion and the problem solving process: Three styles of coping. *Journal for the Scientific Study of Religion, 27,* 90–104.

Pargament, K. I., Koenig, H. G., & Perez, L. M. (2000). The many methods of religious coping: Development and initial validation of the RCOPE. *Journal of Clinical Psychology, 56*(4), 519–543.

Pargament, K., Smith, B., Koenig, H., & Perez, L. (1998). Patterns of positive and negative religious coping with major life stressors. *Journal for the Scientific Study of Religion, 37*(4), 710–724.

Parks, S. M., & Winter, L. (2009). End of life decision-making for cancer patients. *Primary Care, 36*(4), 811–823. table of contents.

Peterman, A., Fitchett, G., Brady, M., Hernandez, L., & Cella, D. (2002). Measuring spiritual well-being in people with cancer: The functional assessment of chronic illness therapy-spiritual well-being scale (FACIT-Sp). *Annals of Behavioral Medicine, 24*(1), 49–58.

Phillips, R. E., Pargament, K. I., Lynn, Q. K., & Crossley, C. D. (2004). Self-directing religious coping: A deistic god, abandoning god, or no god at all? *Journal for the Scientific Study of Religion, 43*(3), 409–418.

Plonk, W. M., Jr., & Arnold, R. M. (2005). Terminal care: The last weeks of life. *Journal of Palliative Medicine, 8*(5), 1042–1054.

Puchalski, C. (2001). Spirituality and health: The art of compassionate medicine. *Hospital Physician, 37*(3), 30–36.

Rippentrop, E., Altmaier, E. M., Chen, J. J., Found, E. M., & Keffala, V. J. (2005). The relationship between religion/spirituality and physical health, mental health, and pain in a chronic pain population. *Pain, 116*(3), 311–321.

Saunders, C. (1964). Care of patients suffering from terminal illness at St. Joseph's Hospice. *Nursing Mirror,* vii–x.

Saunders, C. (1996). A personal therapeutic journey. *British Medical Journal, 313*(7072), 1599–1601.

Schwartz, G. (1982). Testing the biopsychosocial model: The ultimate challenge facing behavioral medicine? *Journal of Consulting and Clinical Psychology, 50*(6), 1040–1053.

Sulmasy, D. P. (2002). A biopsychosocial-spiritual model for the care of patients at the end of life. *Gerontologist, 42*(90003), 24–33.

Thompson, G. N., & Chochinov, H. M. (2010). Reducing the potential for suffering in older adults with advanced cancer. *Palliative and Supportive Care, 8*(1), 83–93.

Wachholtz, A. B., & Keefe, F. J. (2006). What physicians need to know about spirituality and chronic pain. *Southern Medical Journal, 99*(10).

Wachholtz, A., & Pargament, K. (2005). Is spirituality a critical ingredient of meditation? comparing the effects of spiritual meditation, secular meditation, and relaxation on spiritual, psychological, cardiac, and pain outcomes. *Journal of Behavioral Medicine, 28*(4), 369–384.

Wachholtz, A., & Pargament, K. (2008). Migraines and meditation: Does spirituality matter? *Journal of Behavioral Medicine, 31*(4), 351–366.

Wachholtz, A., & Pearce, M. (2009). Does spirituality as a coping mechanism help or hinder coping with chronic pain? *Current Pain and Headache Reports, 13*(2), 127–132.

Wachholtz, A. B., Pearce, M. J., & Koenig, H. G. (2007). Exploring the relationship between spirituality, coping, and pain. *Journal of Behavioral Medicine, 30*(4), 311–318.

Winter, L., Parker, B., & Schneider, M. (2007). Imagining the alternatives to life prolonging treatments: Elders' beliefs about the dying experience. *Death Studies, 31*(7), 619–631.

Part VII
Perspectives on Pain from the Humanities and Social Sciences

Chapter 37
Suffering, Hope, and Healing

Jack Coulehan

What Is Suffering?

The words "pain" and "suffering" are so often used together in clinical practice they sometimes seem to merge into a single concept, with clinicians simply referring to "pain-and-suffering." Writing in the early 1980s, Eric Cassell bemoaned the fact that the medical literature contained very few studies that specifically addressed suffering, although there were hundreds of reports that focused on all aspects of physical pain (Cassell 1982). Since then, the study of human suffering has advanced considerably, in large part due to the development of palliative medicine as a clinical specialty. Nonetheless, controversy about the primacy of pain and other physical and emotional symptoms as the causes of suffering in illness remains. Some observers argue that such symptoms are the central feature of suffering, even though emotional and cultural factors also play a role (Wall 1999). Most, however, focus their attention on existential factors not directly dependent on the experience of physical pain (Kellehear 2009).

Suffering represents a dimension of personal distress that goes far beyond physical, or even emotional, pain. There is no consensus on a single, precise, and comprehensive definition of human suffering (Wilkinson 2005). However, virtually all definitions focus on one or more of a cluster of related characteristics. According to Eric Cassell, suffering occurs when illness or other circumstances threaten a person's intactness (Cassell 2004). He defines the concept as "a specific state of severe distress induced by the loss of integrity, intactness, cohesiveness, or wholeness of the person, or by a threat that the person believes will result in the dissolution of his or her integrity" (Cassell 1995). An Irish palliative care physician, substitutes the term "soul pain" for suffering and defines it as "the experience of an individual who has become disconnected and alienated from the deepest and most fundamental aspects of him or herself." The psychotherapist Viktor Frankl identifies suffering with perceived loss of meaning in one's life (Frankl 2006). Arthur Frank views suffering as a person's experiential response to the loss of his or her sense of being "myself," which leads the person to mourn for their previous identity (Frank 2001). In an editorial entitled "Suffering and healing – our core business," George concludes that suffering results from an attack on "integrity of, or sense of, self, dissociation or otherness, a loss of dignity – the draining of events upon one's sense of worth or value" (George 2009).

J. Coulehan, MD, MPH (✉)
Center for Medical Humanities, Compassionate Care, and Bioethics, Stony Brook University, Stony Brook, NY 11794-8335, USA
e-mail: jcoul44567@aol.com

R.J. Moore (ed.), *Handbook of Pain and Palliative Care: Biobehavioral Approaches for the Life Course*, 717
DOI 10.1007/978-1-4419-1651-8_37, © Springer Science+Business Media, LLC 2012

Thus, the core concept of suffering involves dissolution, alienation, loss of personal identity, and/or a sense of meaninglessness. The onset of severe symptoms triggers suffering when a person interprets these symptoms as threats to his or her selfhood: What is happening to me? Will my future be cut short? Can anything be done? This existential crisis may occur even when the illness is not life-threatening (e.g., unexplained and uncontrolled migraine headaches) or, if threatening can be treated successfully (e.g., pneumonia or early-stage cancer). In these cases, much of the suffering resolves when the patient realizes that the condition can be cured or at least integrated into the patient's self-identified life narrative.

Such a resolution cannot occur when the illness is progressive or terminal. Thus, in palliative medicine, clinicians distinguish between the physical pain and other symptoms of seriously ill and dying patients, and their existential suffering. The former obviously contribute to, and interact with, the latter. In most cases severe symptoms can be substantially relieved by medical treatment, and this, in turn, may well reduce suffering; e.g., symptom-free patients are better able to address their suffering by generating hopefulness and participating in meaningful relationships. Cicely Saunders coined the term "total pain," equivalent to *pain plus suffering*, to indicate the comprehensive distress or suffering of dying patients (Saunders 1984). Even with complete symptomatic relief, however, patients still experience the suffering component of total pain.

Phenomenology of Suffering

We can learn much about the phenomenology of suffering from the accounts of writers who carefully observed and described their own experiences. For example, the late nineteenth century French novelist and playwright Alphonse Daudet wrote a series of notes documenting his suffering from tabes dorsalis, a form of tertiary syphilis (Daudet 2002). Here are three examples of Daudet's reflections:

> Very strange, the fear that pain inspires these days – or rather, this pain of mine. It's bearable, and yet I cannot bear it. It's sheer dread: and my resort to anesthetics is like a cry for help, the squeal of a woman before danger actually strikes (p. 9).

> Pain in the country: a veil over the horizon. Those roads, with their pretty little bends – all they provoke in me now is the desire to flee. To run away, to escape my sickness (p. 45).

> I've passed the stage where illness brings any advantage, or helps you understand things; also the stage where it sours your life, puts a harshness in your voice, makes every cogwheel shriek. Now there's only a hard, stagnant, painful torpor, and an indifference to everything. Nada! Nada! (p. 65).

These excerpts reflect three responses to suffering that in Daudet's case occurred sequentially: the cry for help, the desire to flee, and, finally, the development of indifference and immobilization.

Anna Akhmatova, a great twentieth century Russian poet, spent most of her life victimized by official Soviet disapproval. Her husband was executed, her son imprisoned, and for decades Akhmatova endured a marginal hand-to-mouth existence, her poetry suppressed by the government. After her son was arrested in 1938, Akhmatova, along with hundreds of other women, waited in line every week for 17 months at the prison gates, hoping to obtain some news about her son's fate. She later wrote a long poem entitled "Requiem," as an expression of her suffering during that period (Akhmatova 2004):

> Today there's so much I must do:
> Must smash my memories to bits,
> Must turn my heart to stone all through,
> And must relearn how one must live (p. 137).

> Admit it—fighting back's absurd,
> My own will just a hollow joke,
> I hear my broken babbling words
> As if some other person spoke (p. 140).

Do what you please, take any shape that comes to mind,
Burst on me like a shell of poison gas,
Or creep up like a mugger, club me from behind,
Or let the fog of typhus do the task (p. 139).

These excerpts evoke three stages of suffering somewhat different from Daudet's. The first communicates a recognition that action is preferable to passivity. In this case, the action is not a cry for help, perhaps because such an outburst would have been useless in Soviet Russia. Instead, Akhmatova commits herself to life changes – smashing memories, turning her heart, relearning how to live. In the next excerpt, she gives up. The poem turns passive and cynical. In the final stage, Akhmatova appears to welcome annihilation. Her numbness mutates into a strong, yet still confrontational, desire for nothingness.

Poet and novelist D.H. Lawrence provides a third example. As he was dying of tuberculosis in late 1929 and 1930, he wrote and rewrote "The Ship of Death," a poem that serves as a form of *ars moriendi*, a testament to his suffering and preparation for dying. One of Lawrence's central metaphors imagines the dying person as an unwilling voyager who sets out to search for an unknown and inexplicable shore:

Now launch the small ship, now as the body dies
and life departs, launch out, the fragile soul
in the fragile ship of courage, the ark of faith… (Lawrence 1947, p. 149).

However, Lawrence's persona evokes the possibility of redemption from suffering by making appropriate preparations for the voyage and maintaining one's integrity in the face of the "dark flight down oblivion":

O build your ship of death, your little ark
and furnish it with food, with little cakes, and wine
for the dark flight down oblivion (p. 139).

with its store of food and little cooking pans
and change of clothes,
upon the flood's black waste,
upon the waters of the end
upon the sea of death, where still we sail
darkly, for we cannot steer, and have no port (p. 149)

According to Lawrence's *ars moriendi*, the suffering of dissolution and incipient oblivion can be alleviated by personal agency. By building a "ship of death" and stocking it with provisions we impose order on the experience and make it comprehensible.

The examples quoted suggest that sustained suffering may have two quite different outcomes. The sufferer either ends up in a "hard, stagnant painful torpor" with "my own will just a hollow joke," or he or she transforms himself or herself into a "fragile ship of courage, the ark of faith." Reich (1989) identifies three stages in the arc of suffering. These are not quantitative stages (i.e., each progressively worse), but rather temporal changes that occur as a person successfully confronts and overcomes suffering. According to Reich, when an individual experiences catastrophic illness or loss, he or she initially responds with silence, shock, and immobilization. The sufferer is struck dumb, unable to make informed decisions because loss overwhelms agency. Autonomy diminishes. Imagination implodes. Reich identifies this as *mute suffering*, or speechlessness in the face of catastrophe. Persons who never move beyond this state remain locked in a "hard, stagnant painful torpor."

In the stage of *expressive suffering*, the sufferer seeks to understand the experience by finding a language in which to express it. Daudet accomplishes this in journal entries, while Akhmatova and Lawrence employ a structured literary approach. The literary control achieved in their poetry parallels an internal process of finding a voice to articulate and, thus, gain influence over, their suffering. This suggests a more universal process, documented in these cases by artistic creation, but available to all sufferers through reflection and self-expression. For example, a patient with cancer may learn to express his or her deepest fears and sense of loss to family members, or to a chaplain or health professional, in a manner that encourages conversation. The expressive sufferer "speaks" in his or her own style, using personal resources and coping skills. In fact, expressive suffering always requires the participation of others, if only as listeners (Reich, pp. 86–91).

Akhmatova speaks directly to her suffering, "Do what you please, take any shape that comes to mind." She announces this sentiment defiantly, the words of a tough woman who has survived decades of persecution. Daudet, on the other hand, describes his reaction to syphilitic pain with a finely wrought image: "the squeal of a woman before danger actually strikes." He distances himself from the crisis by implying that his cries are premature, even though his pain is severe. In another part of "The Ship of Death," Lawrence elsewhere a rotting fruit metaphor that acknowledges that he has dropped off the tree of life; his soul has fallen to the ground and begun to rot.

Reich calls his third and final stage *a new identity in suffering*. Here, the sufferer discovers a new self, or a new understanding of self. The old self may well have been beaten up beyond recognition, but in some important sense a resurrected self, or character, has emerged. The new self may manifest itself in outward activities, as, for example, Lawrence's admonition to stock the ship of death "with food, with little cakes and wine," but such pragmatic behaviors reflect a deeper personal transition (Reich 1989, pp. 86–91). In the next section, I discuss hope – specifically, deep hope – as the process by which one can forge a new identity in suffering.

In summary, existential suffering occurs when a person is threatened by, or experiences, the loss of identity, dignity, and/or life meaning. The initial response to this calamity is shock and silence (mute suffering), followed by attempts to understand and articulate the experience (expressive suffering). Such self-expression can itself be therapeutic, but the circumstances associated with severe illness often make reflection and conversation difficult (e.g., pain, isolation, anxiety, depression, low energy level, social, or cultural barriers). However, even in the face of incurable illness, amelioration of suffering is possible.

Suffering and Dignity

For many, an important component of suffering near the end of life is the perception that physical and mental deterioration result in the loss of dignity. They believe that the process of terminal illness is undignified in at least two ways. First, the suffering person may appear weak, vulnerable, even repulsive, to others. Dementia, delirium, incontinence, odors, enfeeblement: all of these seem inconsistent with human dignity. Second, progressive illness threatens, and often obliterates, autonomy, or self-determination. In our secular society, many consider moral agency (autonomy) to be the *sine qua non* of human dignity. Thus, diminished autonomy is equivalent to loss of dignity. Those who argue for the legalization of medically assisted death (physician-assisted suicide and euthanasia) argue that they are supporting "death with dignity." *This phrase implies that lack of choice over when and how your death will occur* (i.e. *the* "right to die") *means loss of dignity.*

The dignity-as-choice proposition discounts the relational and social dimensions of personhood. A dignified death in most cultures throughout most of human history was and is predicated on relationships between the individual and others. Dying must be viewed as both a personal challenge and a social role; in fact, these are two faces of the same process. For example, in traditional Chinese culture the dying patient suppresses self-efficacy in favor of family efficacy. She abdicates responsibility for decision making, while representative family members take charge of her final drama (Galanti 1997). It is considered rude and undignified even to mention death in the presence of the dying person, although the patient herself is well aware of the cultural liturgy in which she is playing a role. On the contrary, in American culture we focus the responsibility on the dying person himself or herself, insisting on his or her choosing among the options for treatment, although we often mask the meaninglessness of the options we offer (Holstein 1997). A more robust concept of human dignity would place self-determination into a dynamic relationship with other important social values, as many religious and existential writers do in their reflections on dignity (Mendiola 1996).

Chochinov et al. (2002a) conducted a cross-sectional study of perceived dignity in 213 palliative care patients, all of whom had cancer and were expected to die within 6 months. The great majority of these patients indicated that they maintained a strong sense of personal dignity, with only 16 (7.5%) reporting that they experience "fractured" dignity. The authors concluded, "The finding suggests that a person's sense of dignity is a particularly resilient construct and, in most instances, able to withstand the various physiological and psychological challenges that face patients who are terminally ill" (Chochinov et al. 2002a, p. 2028). Interestingly, "fractured" dignity was associated with hospitalization, but not with acuity of illness or proximity of death. These investigators have subsequently developed an empirical model for dignity at the end of life and devised a program of "dignity-conserving therapy" for palliative care patients (Chochinov et al. 2002b, 2005; Chochinov 2007). It is important not to generalize from the relative lack of dignity-loss in these studies because all patients were enrolled in palliative care settings, while only a small minority of Americans receives palliative care in the final months of their lives. They are much more likely to be subjected to fragmented and invasive care that may, in fact, contribute to the loss of dignity that many fear.

It appears that the excess suffering caused by loss of dignity at the end of life may be less common than those who fear it perceive to be the case. In most cases dignity seems to be resilient and able to reframe itself in a broader, more relational, context when faced with the "indignities" of terminal illness. In particular, the phrase "death with dignity" should not be trivialized as a euphemism for physician-assisted death.

Hope: An Antidote for Suffering

Medical Beliefs About Hope

As Claudio observes in *Measure for Measure*, "The miserable have no other medicine, but only hope" (Shakespeare 1952, p. 1116). Like Claudio, doctors have long looked upon hope as a universal balm. Thus, physicians have generally considered it their duty to assure that patients remained hopeful, even in the face of incurable disease or fatal injury (Groopman 2004). Promoting hopefulness usually involved manipulating the truth, or telling outright lies, about the patient's condition. This practice was grounded in two assumptions. First, the empirical assumption that knowledge of a terminal condition would destroy the patient's hope, and, second, the moral assumption that promotion of patient welfare trumps respect for patient self-determination (autonomy) in medical practice.

They argued that candor with terminally ill patients was usually unethical because "the most disastrous results may follow a tactless warning" (Hertzler 1940, p. 98). Physicians frequently shared anecdotes about patients who became hopeless, depressed, and suicidal upon learning their prognoses.

This attitude toward truthfulness has changed radically during the last 4 or 5 decades. In 1961, 90% of surveyed oncologists reported that they did not disclose cancer diagnoses to their patients (Oken 1961), but less than 2 decades later, 97% of physicians believed it was preferable to disclose a diagnosis of cancer (Novack et al. 1979). There are many reasons for this reversal of belief, some of them external to medicine, such as changes in social mores and patient expectations (Kodish and Post 1995). We now know that most people do, in fact, want to know the extent and prognosis of their disease. Moreover, experience in palliative medicine teaches us that it is often quite possible – even natural – for patients to remain deeply hopeful, even in the full awareness of impending death.

The development of palliative medicine as a medical specialty and the growth of hospice and palliative care services have led to a more scientific and humane approach to the suffering of terminal illness (Cherny 2004). Palliative care clinicians have reframed the traditional medical approach to hope in light of two important realizations. First, the goals of therapeutic hope need not involve disease remission or cure, or even prolongation of life, but rather they may include smaller, more focused objectives, such as resolution of family conflict or a picnic with friends at a cherished place. Thomas Warr writes, "As active treatment fails, hope can take on another form. Hope is that the remaining days of life will be happy ones that tasks at the end of life can be addressed, relationships mended and finalized, and every moment treasured" (Warr 1999). In other words, hope for a cure may transmute into hope for more realistic objectives. As one approaches death, hope endures, but with new aspirations. The physician's role in this process is "setting goals to maintain hope" (Von Roenn and von Gunten 2003).

In their article entitled, "Hope for the best, and prepare for the worst," Beck et al. (2003) provide us with a useful way of analyzing this situation. They argue that terminally ill patients often exist in a state of "middle knowledge," in which they alternate between planning for continued life and preparing for death (Weisman 1972, McCormick and Conley 1995). The dynamic between these poles allows physicians to encourage the dual agendas of hoping for the best (gently supporting a milieu of hopefulness) and, at the same time, doing the work of preparation (providing information, addressing fears, encouraging relationships). In this framework the patient does, in fact, prepare for death, while also maintaining hope.

The second realization of palliative care clinicians is that hope is much more resilient than physicians once thought. Hope can bounce back in the face of bad news and disappointment, even repeated disappointment. In fact, there appears to be a form of hope that underlies "hoping for" specific goals and that persists even after seemingly attainable objectives (e.g., a granddaughter's graduation, the enjoyment of a hamburger, a pain-free day) become unlikely. Many commentators have identified this phenomenon and suggested various names for it. I will discuss this form of "hoping against hope" it in the next section, but first must differentiate it from what physicians commonly refer to as *false hope*.

False Hope

Palliative care physicians speak of false hope or the "dark side of hope" in cases where a patient's treatment goals are unrealistic and his or her embrace of those goals leads to additional suffering to himself or herself and his or her family. For example, a patient with terminal pancreatic cancer might choose to undergo repeated courses of aggressive chemotherapy that cause him or her violent side effects, rather than choosing a palliative regimen that could minimize symptoms and maximize quality of life. Moreover, this patient's seemingly hopeful choices might put his or her family under severe psychological and financial stress. Although real hope is therapeutic, physicians argue, false hope is damaging (Snyder et al. 2002). But what, precisely, is the distinction?

In some cases the distinction might turn on the characteristics of the physician–patient–family relationship than on the extravagance of the hope. Is the patient interesting and pleasant, or demanding and manipulative? Is the family supportive or disruptive? Are clinical interactions fraught with tension or confrontation? Helwick quotes with approval one clinician's description of a terminal leukemia patient's "endless hope": "He had a tremendous amount of optimism… and he inspired the oncology team" (Helwick 2010). In this case the physician saw himself as an advocate for the patient, a character in his story, and affirmed his endless hope. However, when a patient is less inspiring and more disruptive, or causes pain in those around him, endless hope may morph into false hope. In other cases false hope might actually be generated by the physician, the result of miscalculation, over-optimistic promises, and manipulation of information about the prognosis or treatment. In other words, physicians may be responsible for false hope by acting under the guise of "therapeutic privilege" (Pellegrino and Thomasma 1996).

Perhaps the best conceptual way of approaching false hope is via Beck, Quill, and Arnold's framework of "hoping for the best, preparing for the worst" (Beck et al. 2003). In this context, the hope part of the equation need not be scaled down or realistic. Why not hope for a miracle cure? Why not have endless hope? The impression of "falseness" arises only when the patient's hope is unassociated with the mind-set of, and activities involved in, preparing for the worst.

Deep Hope: The Song Without Words

Dickinson (1960), a poet whose life was chock full of frustrated goals, wrote several poems about hope. This one is perhaps the most well-known:

"Hope" is the thing with feathers—
That perches in the soul—
And sings the tune without the words—
And never stops—at all—

And sweetest—in the Gale—is heard—
And sore must be the storm—
That could abash the little Bird
That kept so many warm—

I've heard it in the chilliest land—
And on the strangest sea—
Yet, never in Extremity,
it asked a crumb—of Me (p. 116).

Dickinson's observations that hope has "kept so many warm" and is "sweetest" during the worst of times coincide with traditional medical beliefs. She also highlights hope's endurance: a bird that "perches in the soul" and continues singing, despite the storms and extremities of life. Hope never asks for payment in return for its faithful service. However, the bird metaphor suggests another insight about hope: its sweet song is wordless, a melody without lyrics. What can this mean? Is the Amherst poet implying that the cognitive content of hope (i.e. the object hoped for) is not essential? Indeed, she seems to suggest a natural outpouring of song (hopefulness) that underlies whatever words we may attach to it. In a letter to his friend Joseph Goodman, Samuel Clemens offered a different image from nature to capture the ubiquity and naturalness of hope: "God save us," he wrote, "… from a hope-tree that has lost its faculty for putting out blossoms" (Ober 2003).

The existentialist philosopher Gabriel Marcel distinguished between two different forms of hope as expressed in the statements, "I hope…" and "I hope that…" (Marcel 1960). The latter corresponds to the usual understanding of hope as having a specific goal, whether superficial ("I hope that it doesn't rain tomorrow") or profound ("I hope that the bone marrow transplant will cure my leukemia"). However, the former statement "I hope…" is "a more general cosmic conviction affirming human life or being in general. This is the hope about the meaningfulness and purpose of human existence" (Pellegrino and Thomasma 1996, p. 57).

Pellegrino and Thomasma use the term *transcendental hope* for Marcel's second, deeper form of hope and they relate it closely to religious, specifically Christian, belief (Pellegrino and Thomasma 1996, p. 64). However, it is unnecessary to postulate transcendence or religious dogma to maintain a conviction that one's life has meaning and purpose, even in the face of imminent dissolution. Viktor Frankl provides an example of an immanent, psychological formulation. In *Man's Search for Meaning*, he directly confronts the problem of suffering. We experience suffering when illness or catastrophe threatens our integrity. We encounter our own vulnerability to destruction, the negation of everything that is meaningful to us. Yet, suffering also provides us with a profound opportunity to *discover meaning* in our lives. For Frankl, Thomasma and Pellegrino's *transcendent hope* might be recast as *having-agency-to-discover-meaning*.

The clinical literature includes a number of attempts to capture the distinction between hoping-for a specific outcome and a deeper, more existential form of hope. Like Frankl, Miller characterized the deepest level of hope as the experience of finding meaning in loss or suffering (Miller 1985). DuFault and Martoocchio (1985) contrasted *particularized hope*, which is related to specific desired objectives, to *generalized hope*, which is the "intangible inner experience of hope." In a longitudinal study of 30 dying patients, Herth (1990) defined deep hope as an "inner power directed toward enrichment of being." In a study of 11 palliative care patients in Sweden, Benzein et al. (2001) described their reports of experiencing tension between the two states of "hoping for something" and "living in hope." All these dichotomies appear to express the same notion: the existence of a level of hopefulness that underlies and sustains hoping-for-a-specific-future-goal. I call this *deep hope*.

Between Clinician and Patient

Physicians and other clinicians who treat seriously ill patients aim to relieve suffering by curative or remissive measures, i.e., directed toward curing or diminishing the disease process; and palliative measures, i.e., directed toward relieving symptoms and enhancing quality of life. Yet suffering may, and often does, elude these medically oriented approaches because they fail to address the existential core of suffering. Deep hope serves to ameliorate suffering, but clinicians may not understand how to facilitate their patients' hope, or enhance their patients' dignity, or even encourage them to express their suffering, beyond giving appropriate disease-specific diagnosis and treatment.

Several investigators have examined personal and clinical correlates of deep hope. Herth (1990), who, as noted earlier, defined deep hope as an "inner power directed toward enrichment of being," studied palliative care patients and identified seven "hope fostering" characteristics: interpersonal connectedness, attainable goals, spiritual base, personal attributes, lightheartedness, uplifting memories, and affirmation of worth. As the patients moved closer to dying, several of these dropped out, but interpersonal connectedness, spiritual base, and attainable aims remained significant. Herth also noted three "hope-hindering" characteristics: uncontrollable pain, abandonment–isolation, and devaluation of personhood.

In a later study of 32 oncology patients, Post-White et al. (1996) identified similar clusters of hope-enhancing and hope-hindering features. Among hope-enhancing strategies, they listed finding meaning, affirming relationships, and "living in the present." Benzein and Savemen (1998) discovered that patient hope was positively correlated with good nurse–patient relationships. Herth (1993) also studied geriatric persons living in institutions and in community settings. She found several hope-enhancing features were similar to those in her earlier investigation (interpersonal connectedness, spiritual base, lightheartedness, uplifting memories, and attainable goals), but, aside from uncontrolled pain, hope-hindering factors were different: hopelessness in others, depleted energy, and impaired cognition (Herth and Cutcliffe 2002).

These studies are, of course, only suggestive, and the noted correlations do not necessarily imply causal relationships. However, it is interesting that a large number of the identified factors can be influenced, either positively or negatively, by physicians and other healthcare professionals. Obviously, medical treatment can control pain. The clinician–patient relationship can help prevent abandonment and isolation, affirm worth, ensure respect for the suffering person, foster connectedness, suggest attainable goals, and, where appropriate, facilitate lightheartedness. This cluster of factors intimates that clinicians can relieve suffering by fostering deep hope.

To achieve this goal it is necessary: (a) to avoid the trap of detached concern, (b) to develop and practice the skills of clinical empathy, (c) to understand the power of compassion, and (d) to develop the bond of compassionate solidarity.

Detached Concern

Contemporary medical beliefs throw up a roadblock when it comes to understanding and treating suffering. Medical educators typically recommend emotional detachment or *detached concern* as the clinician's proper stance toward suffering patients. In the last 50 years, detached concern has evolved from a simple descriptive term used by medical sociologists recording their observations of medical students (Lief and Fox 1963; Becker et al. 1961) to a prescriptive or normative concept that identifies the *proper* attitude of doctors toward their patients. As part of this process, educators linked detached concern with William Osler's famous medical virtue, *aequanimitas*. In his essay of that name, Osler (2001) warned medical students that "a calm equanimity is the desirable attitude" and encouraged them to develop "such a judicious measure of obtuseness as will enable you to meet the exigencies of practice with firmness and courage." Late twentieth century medical education co-opted these sentiments and identified them with detached concern.

Educators give two reasons for the belief that professionalism demands substantial emotional and psychological distance between physician and patient. First, detachment protects the physician from being overwhelmed and paralyzed by pain and suffering. Second, detachment protects the patient. Medical decisions ought to be objective, uninfluenced by feelings and biases. Blumgart, for example, wrote that detachment is necessary to prevent "loss of objectivity and perspective" (Blumgart 1964). Thus, an emotional connection with the patient may bias clinical judgment and compromise patient care.

Such beliefs both reflect and support today's prevalent model of disease and medical intervention, in which disease can, in principle, be completely understood in anatomical, physiological, biochemical, or even molecular terms. The suffering that results from disease or trauma is considered an epiphenomenon, expected to resolve when the condition is cured, alleviated, or controlled. This version of the biomedical framework limits the scope of medical concern to aspects of suffering considered "fixable" (Gunderman 2002). It also implies that the catastrophic effect of illness on conceptions of personhood and self-worth is somehow mistaken or illegitimate; if an existential crisis occurs, it is not a problem to be addressed by medicine. As theologian Stanley Hauerwas writes, "The ideology… institutionalized in modern medicine requires that we interpret all illness as pointless" (1990, p. 69).

So much for the detachment part of detached concern. The "concern" component is intended to express the residual commitment that physicians should have to their patients, given their professional detachment. Concern is a weaker and more ambiguous word than "care" or "compassion." In other contexts the statement, "I am concerned about you" is open to both positive (looking out for his or her welfare) or negative (questioning his or her behavior) interpretations. In either case the phrase is cautious and less open-ended than the alternate sentiment, "I care for you," which seemingly violates the professional requirement for detachment. Detached concern opens medicine to Cynthia Ozick's indictment in "Metaphor and Memory"; physicians cultivate detachment from their patients because they are afraid of finding themselves "too frail … to enter into psychological twinship with the even frailer souls of the sick" (Ozick 1989).

Surprisingly, despite their profession's orthodox model of detached concern, physicians almost universally agree that *relationships* are significant in medical practice. Most physicians also assert that they practice the "art of medicine," which is far more than the sum of medicine's biological sciences. This "art," they contend, includes, among other components, compassion, responsiveness, clinical judgment, advocacy, rapport, and bedside manner. In other words, the majority of physicians seem simultaneously to hold (and compartmentalize) two conflicting beliefs: doctors should be detached and doctors should be connected.

Clinical Empathy

Empathy is a hard nut to crack because it challenges the conventional medical opinion that thinking is thinking, and feeling is feeling, and never the twain shall meet. *Clinical empathy is the ability to understand the patient's situation, perspective, and feelings, and to communicate that understanding to the patient.*

This definition has three important implications. First, empathy has a cognitive focus. The clinician enters into the perspective and experience of the other individual by means of verbal and nonverbal cues, but does not in the process lose her own perspective. Hojat emphasizes this cognitive aspect in his *Empathy in Patient Care*, a comprehensive survey of clinical empathy, including its history, development, scope, methodologies, and results of empirical studies (Hojat 2009; Hojat et al. 2002). Second, empathy also has an affective or emotional focus. To "know" emotions we have to feel them. Jodi Halpern uses the term *resonance emotions* to describe these feelings generated in the clinician as she practices empathy (Halpern 1992, 2007). She writes, "The special professional skill of clinical empathy is distinguished by the use of this subjective, experiential input for specific, cognitive aims. Empathy has as its goal imagining how it feels to be in another person's situation" (Halpern 2003). Psychiatrist Robert Coles uses the term *moral imagination* to designate this capacity for empathic understanding (Coles 1989).

Finally, the definition requires that clinical empathy has an action component. The practitioner communicates understanding by checking-back with the patient, using, for example, statements like "let me see if I have this right" or "I want to be sure I understand what you mean" (Coulehan et al. 2001). Thus, clinical empathy is a positive feedback loop in which the physician titrates his or her understanding by checking back with the patient in an iterative process. This gives the patient opportunities to correct or modulate the physician's formulation. At the same time it expresses the physician's desire to listen deeply, thereby reinforcing a bond or connection between clinician and patient (Coulehan and Block 2006).

In Howard Spiro's essay "What is empathy and can it be taught?," he answers the second question with a qualified yes, noting that "a better question might be, 'Can we recover the empathy we once had?'" (Spiro 1992). Arguing that the process of medical education tends to diminish our openness to others' feelings and experience, Spiro believes that enhancing clinical empathy is more of a restoration project, rather than a pedagogical one. Perhaps he overstates the case, but it is clear that medical education tends to narrowly focus students' attention on patients-as-objects, thus down-regulating their receptors for experiencing patients-as-subjects. In particular, concepts such as detachment and detached concern create barriers to the development of clinical empathy.

From Empathy to Compassion

The words "patient," "patience," and "compassion" derive from the Latin stem *pass-*, "to suffer." Patience refers to the calm endurance of inconvenience, pain, or suffering. A patient is a person who endures suffering. Compassion means to suffer with. To claim that compassion is a medical virtue is to assert that doctors ought to *suffer with* their patients. This is a far cry from detached concern.

Compassion is impossible without empathy, because only through empathic understanding can we recognize other persons as subjects like ourselves. Experiencing another person's suffering by means of empathy, resonance emotions, and the moral imagination creates an experiential bond quite different from the attitude of pity, which carries the connotation of separateness and condescension. Pity is often associated with detached concern; after all, who would not be moved to pity by the unfortunate cases physicians encounter? In fact, the word "unfortunate" is often used in medicine as a code word to indicate patients who are deserving of pity, as in the following: "This unfortunate 47-year-old man with anaplastic adenocarcinoma of unknown origin…" Or, "This unfortunate 16-year-old girl with Down syndrome and acute leukemia…." In such cases, the speaker indicates to his or her colleagues that it is appropriate for them to look with pity upon the patient.

Warren Reich defines compassion as "the virtue by which we have a sympathetic consciousness of sharing the distress or suffering of another person and on that basis are inclined to offer assistance in alleviating and/or living through that suffering" (Reich 1989, p. 85). Leonard Blum offers a second, synergistic definition: compassion is "a complex emotional attitude toward another, characteristically involving imaginative dwelling on the condition of the other person, an active regard for his or her good, a view of him or her as a fellow human being, and emotional responses of a certain degree of intensity" (Blum 1980, p. 509). It is clear from these definitions that compassion involves (a) a sympathetic awareness of the others' distress, (b) a sense of sharing that distress in some manner; and (c) an inclination to offer assistance. Writing specifically about medicine, Sulmasy contends that a compassionate physician addresses his or her patient's suffering at three levels: (a) the objective level, by recognizing suffering, (b) the subjective level, by internally responding to the suffering, and (c) the operative level, by performing concrete healing actions (Sulmasy 1997, p. 103).

Sulmasy's objective level may at first suggest the same concept of objectivity so highly valued in detached concern. However, in the case of compassion, the observing instrument (i.e. the physician) is sensitive to a wider spectrum of data. By practicing clinical empathy, he or she identifies the character and magnitude of suffering, in addition to symptoms and signs of disease processes. Self-awareness is a prerequisite for Sulmasy's subjective or internal response to suffering. Many commentators stress the need for physicians to better understand their own beliefs, feelings, attitudes, and response patterns (Kearney et al. 2009; Meier et al. 2001; Novack et al. 1997; Coulehan and Williams 2003; Frankel et al. 2003). Today's narrative medicine movement responds to this need by teaching self-awareness, clinical empathy, and reflective practice (Charon 2001a, b, 2004; DasGupta and Charon 2004; Morris 2001; Bolton 1999; Coulehan 2005). Students enhance their repertoire of life experience through narratives of illness and patient care, and enhance their professional identities by reflecting upon, and writing about, their clinical experiences (Coulehan and Clary 2005; DasGupta and Charon 2004). Sulmasy's third level of compassionate response, concrete healing acts, takes place in the context of compassionate solidarity with the patient.

Compassionate Solidarity

The objective and subjective components of compassion find their fulfillment in action directed toward alleviating suffering. This action, of course, includes efforts to cure the disease and suppress the symptoms. However, the creation of an empathic connection is in itself a healing action. Being present to, listening, affirming, and witnessing are actions that help relieve the patient's suffering by demonstrating respect and facilitating deep hope (Coulehan 2011). I call this type of therapeutic relationship *compassionate solidarity*. Unlike detached concern, its focus is on the patient as a person, rather than on the disease.

In his *Autobiography* (1951, p. 356), the American physician–poet William Carlos Williams wrote that he often began his evening office hours feeling totally exhausted, but as soon as he began seeing his patients, "I lost myself in the very properties of their minds: for the moment at least I actually became them, whoever they should be, so that when I detached myself from them… it was as though I were awakening from a sleep." Williams (1951) describes a state of immersion in which the "I" perspective remains intact (e.g., "in a flash the details of the case would begin to formulate themselves into a recognizable outline"), but stays in the background. He is entirely present to the situation, thus bridging the gap between subject and object. Nouwen et al. (1982) capture this sense of immersion in their statement, "Compassion requires us to be weak with the weak, vulnerable with the vulnerable, and powerless with the powerless. Compassion means full immersion in the condition of being human."

Summary and Conclusion

Suffering is the experience of distress or disharmony caused by the loss, or threatened loss, of what we most cherish. Suffering involves dissolution, alienation, loss of personal identity, and/or a sense of meaninglessness. It results from the stripping away of beliefs and symbols by which we construct a meaningful narrative of human life in general and our own lives in particular. Suffering is often compounded by a sense of threatened or lost dignity.

Hopelessness is an extreme manifestation of suffering. However, hope is a natural human resource that can palliate and contribute to healing. Hope is also more flexible and resilient that physicians, who traditionally withheld or manipulated the truth about dire prognoses, believed it to be. Maintaining hope, especially deep hope, is an antidote to suffering.

The vocation of physicians and other health professionals is, insofar as possible, to relieve suffering caused by illness, trauma, and bodily degeneration. However, since suffering is an existential state that may not parallel physical or emotional states, health professionals cannot rely solely on knowledge and skills that address physiological dysfunction to be effective at relieving suffering. Rather, clinicians must learn to engage the patient at an existential level and to engender hope.

For several decades detached concern has been the standard approach to patients taught by medical educators. This term was initially employed by sociologists to characterize students' and physicians' observed detachment and their inclination to treat patients as objects, rather than as subjects of experience. Later, medical educators adopted detached concern as a normative relationship, because they believed it promoted objectivity and protected the physician's emotional resources, while acknowledging medicine's beneficent motivation (concern). However, in reality, contemporary medical education and practice favor a process of progressive detachment from patients that devalues subjectivity, emotion, solidarity, and relationship as irrelevant and harmful. Such an ideal – fortunately not achieved by most clinicians – almost ensures that practitioners lose the ability to fully appreciate and respond to human suffering, or to facilitate hope. The term *compassionate solidarity* summarizes an alternate model of the physician–patient relationship. Compassionate solidarity begins with empathic listening and responding, which facilitate objective assessment of the others' subjective state; requires the physician to develop reflectivity and self-understanding; and is in itself a healing, hope-promoting act.

References

Akhmatova, A. (2004). *The word that causes death's defeat. Poems of memory (N. K. Anderson, Trans.).* New Haven: Yale University Press.

Beck, A. L., Arnold, R. M., & Quill, T. E. (2003). Hope for the best, and prepare for the worst. *Annals of Internal Medicine, 138*(3), 439–443.

Becker, H. S., Geer, B., Hughes, E., & Strauss, A. (1961). *Boys in White: Student culture in medical school.* Chicago: University of Chicago Press.

Bennett, M. J. (2001). *The empathic healer: An endangered species?* New York: Academic.

Benzein, E., Norberg, A., & Saveman, B. (2001). The meaning of the lived experience of hope in patients with cancer in palliative home care. *Palliative Medicine, 15*, 117–126.

Benzein, E., Saveman, B. (1998). "http://search.ebscohost.com.ezproxy.hsclib.sunysb.edu/login.aspx?direct=true& AuthType=ip,url,cookie,uid&an=1998019982&db=rzh&scope=site&site=ehost" \t "_blank" Nurses' perception of hope in patients with cancer: a palliative care perspective. *Cancer Nursing, 21*, 10–16.

Blum, L. C. (1980). In A. O. Rorty (Ed.), *Explaining emotions*. Berkeley: University of California Press, pp. 507–517.

Blumgart, H. L. (1964). Caring for the patient. *The New England Journal of Medicine, 270*, 449–456.

Bolton, G. (1999). Stories at work: Reflective writing for practitioners. *The Lancet, 354*, 243–245.

Cassell, E. J. (1982). The nature of suffering and the goals of medicine. *The New England Journal of Medicine, 306*(11), 639–645.

Cassell, E. J. (1995). Pain and suffering. In W. T. Reich (Ed.), *Encyclopedia of bioethics* (2nd ed., pp. 1897–1904). New York: Simon & Schuster.

Cassell, E. J. (2004). *The nature of suffering and the goals of medicine*. New York: Oxford University Press.

Charon, R. (2001a). Narrative medicine. A model for empathy, reflection, profession, and trust. *Journal of American Medical Association, 286*, 1897–1902.

Charon, R. (2001b). Narrative medicine: Form, function, and ethics. *Annals of Internal Medicine, 134*, 83–87.

Charon, R. (2004). Narrative and medicine. *The New England Journal of Medicine, 350*(9), 862–864.

Cherny, N. I. (2004). The challenge of palliative medicine: The problem of suffering. In D. Doyle, G. Hanks, N. Cherny, & K. Calman (Eds.), *Oxford textbook of palliative medicine* (pp. 7–14). Oxford: Oxford University Press.

Chochinov, H. M. (2007). Dignity and the essence of medicine: The A, B, C, and D of dignity conserving care. *British Medical Journal, 335*, 184–187.

Chochinov, H. M., Hack, T., Hassard, T., Kristjanson, L. J., McClement, S., & Harlos, M. (2002a). Dignity in the terminally ill: A cross-sectional, cohort study. *The Lancet, 360*, 2026–2030.

Chochinov, H. M., Hack, T., Hassard, T., Kristjanson, L. J., McClement, S., & Harlos, M. (2005). Dignity therapy: A novel psychotherapeutic intervention for patients near the end-of-life. *Journal of Clinical Oncology, 23*, 5520–5524.

Chochinov, H. M., Hack, T., McClement, S., Kristjanson, L. J., & Harlos, M. (2002b). Dignity in the terminally ill: A developing empirical model. *Social Science & Medicine, 54*, 433–443.

Coles, R. (1989). *The call of stories: Teaching and the moral imagination* (p. 179). Boston: Houghton Mifflin.

Coulehan, J. (2005). Today's professionalism: Engaging the mind, but not the heart. *Academic Medicine, 80*, 892–898.

Coulehan, J. (2011). On hope in palliative medicine. In J. Malpais & N. Lickiss (Eds.), *Perspectives on suffering*. New York: Springer.

Coulehan, J., & Block, M. R. (2006). *The medical interview: Mastering skills for clinical practice* (5th ed., pp. 29–44). Philadelphia: F.A. Davis Company.

Coulehan, J., & Clary, P. (2005). Healing the healer: Poetry in palliative care. *Journal of Palliative Care, 8*(2), 382–389.

Coulehan, J., Platt, F. W., Frankl, R., Salazar, W., Lown, B., & Fox, L. (2001). Let me see if I have this right: Words that build empathy. *Annals of Internal Medicine, 135*, 221–227.

Coulehan, J., & Williams, P. C. (2003). Conflicting professional values in medical education. *Cambridge Quarterly of Healthcare Ethics, 12*, 7–20.

DasGupta, S., & Charon, R. (2004). Personal illness narratives: Using reflective writing to teach empathy. *Academic Medicine, 79*(4), 351–356.

Daudet A. (2002). *In the land of pain*. J. Barnes (Ed.), New York: Alfred A. Knopf.

Dickinson E. (1960). *The complete poems of Emily Dickinson*. T. H. Johnson (Ed.), Boston: Little, Brown and Company, New York, p. 116.

DuFault, K., & Martoocchio, B. (1985). Hope: Its spheres and dimensions. *Nursing Clinics of North America, 20*, 379–391.

Farber, N. J., Novack, D. H., & O'Brien, M. K. (1997). Love, boundaries, and the patient physician relationship. *Archives of Internal Medicine, 157*, 2291–2294.

Frank, A. (2001). Can we research suffering? *Qualitative Health Research, 11*, 353–362.

Frankel, R. M., Quill, T. E., & McDaniel, S. H. (Eds.). (2003). *The biopsychosocial approach: Past, present, future*. Rochester: University of Rochester Press.

Frankl, V. (2006). *Man's search for meaning*. Boston: Beacon.

Galanti, G. A. (1997). *Caring for patients from different cultures. Case Studies from American Hospitals*. Philadelphia: University of Pennsylvania Press.

George, R. (2009). Suffering and healing – Our core business. *Palliative Medicine, 23*, 385–387.

Groopman, J. (2004). *The anatomy of hope. How people prevail in the face of illness*. New York: Random House.

Gunderman, R. B. (2002). Is suffering the enemy? *The Hastings Center Report, 32*(2), 40–44.

Halpern, J. (1992). Empathy: Using resonance emotions in the service of curiosity. In H. Spiro et al. (Eds.), *Empathy and the practice of medicine* (pp. 160–173). New Haven: Yale University Press.

Halpern, J. (2003). What is clinical empathy? *Journal of General Internal Medicine, 18*, 670–674.

Halpern, J. (2007). Empathy and patient-physician conflicts. *Journal of General Internal Medicine, 22*, 696–700.

Hauerwas, S. (1990). *God, medicine, and suffering* (p. 69). Grand Rapids: William B. Eerdmans.

Helwick, C. (2010). Fostering hope in hopeless situations. *MD Consult News, 24*, 2010.

Herth, K. (1990). Fostering hope in terminally ill people. *Journal of Advanced Nursing, 15*, 1250–1259.

Herth, K. (1993). Hope in older adults in community and institutional settings. *Issues in Mental Health Nursing, 14*, 139–156.

Herth, K. A., & Cutcliffe, J. R. (2002). The concept of hope in nursing 3: Hope and palliative care nursing. *British Journal of Nursing, 11*, 977–983.

Hertzler, A. E. (1940). *The horse and buggy doctor* (p. 322). Garden City: Blue Ribbon Books.

Hojat, M. (2009). *Empathy in patient care* (pp. 10–15). Springer: New York.

Hojat, M., Gonnella, J. S., Nasca, T. J., Mangione, S., Vergare, M., & Magee, M. (2002). Physician empathy: Definition, components, measurement, and relationship to gender and specialty. *The American Journal of Psychiatry, 159*, 1563–1569.

Holstein, M. (1997). Reflections on death and dying. *Academic Medicine, 72*, 848–855.

Kearney, M. (2000). *A place of healing: Working with suffering in living and dying.* Oxford: Oxford University Press.

Kearney, M. K., Weininger, R. B., Vachon, M. L. S., Harrison, R. I., & Mount, B. M. (2009). Self-care of physicians caring for patients at the end of life. "Being connected… A key to my survival". *Journal of American Medical Association, 301*, 1155–1164.

Kellehear, A. (2009). On dying and human suffering. *Palliative Medicine, 23*, 388–397.

Kodish, E., & Post, S. G. (1995). Oncology and hope. *Journal of Clinical Oncology, 13*(7), 1817–1822.

Lawrence, D. H. (1947). *Selected poems. Introduction by Kenneth Rexroth* (pp. 138–140). New York: New Directions.

Lief, H. I., & Fox, R. (1963). Training for "detached concern" in medical students. In H. I. Lief & N. R. Lief (Eds.), *The psychological basis for medical practice.* New York: Harper & Row.

Marcel, G. (1960). *Fresh hope in the world.* London: Longmans.

McCormick, T. R., & Conley, B. J. (1995). Patient perspectives on dying and on the care of dying patients. *The Western Journal of Medicine, 163*, 236–243.

Meier, D. E., Back, A. L., & Morrison, R. S. (2001). The inner life of physicians and care of the seriously ill. *Journal of American Medical Association, 286*, 3007–3014.

Mendiola, M. M. (1996). Overworked, but uncritically tested: Human dignity and the aid-in-dying debate. In E. E. Shelp (Ed.), *Secular bioethics in theological perspective* (pp. 129–143). New York: Kluwer Academic Publishers.

Miller, J. (1985). Hope. *American Journal of Nursing, 85*, 23–25.

Morris, D. B. (2001). Narrative, ethics, and thinking with stories. *Narrative, 9*, 55–77.

Nouwen, H. J. M., McNeill, D. P., & Morrison, D. A. (1982). *Compassion.* New York: Image Books.

Novack, D. H., Plumer, R., Smith, R. L., et al. (1979). Changes in physician attitudes toward telling the cancer patient. *Journal of American Medical Association, 241*, 897–900.

Novack, D. H., Suchman, A. L., Clark, W., Epstein, R. M., Najberg, E., & Kaplan, M. D. (1997). Calibrating the physician. Personal awareness and effective patient care. *Journal of American Medical Association, 278*, 502–509.

Ober, K. P. (2003). *Mark twain and medicine "Any mummery will cure".* Columbia: University of Missouri Press.

Oken, D. (1961). What to tell cancer patients: A study of medical attitudes. *Journal of American Medical Association, 175*, 1120–1128.

Osler, W. (2001). Aequanimitas. In S. Hinohara & H. Niki (Eds.), *Osler's "a way of life" & other addresses with commentary & annotations* (pp. 21–29). Durham: Duke University Press.

Ozick, C. (1989). Metaphor and memory. *Metaphor and memory: Essays.* New York: Knopf, pp. 265–283.

Pellegrino, E. D., & Thomasma, D. C. (1996). *The Christian virtues in medical practice.* Washington: Georgetown University Press.

Post-White, J., Ceronsky, C., & Kreitzer, M. (1996). Hope, spirituality, sense of coherence, and quality of life in patients with cancer. *Oncology Nursing Forum, 23*, 1571–1579.

Reich, W. T. (1989). Speaking of suffering. A moral account of compassion. *Soundings, 72*(1), 83–108.

Saunders, C. (1984). The philosophy of terminal care. In C. Saunders (Ed.), *The management of terminal malignant disease.* London: Edward Arnold.

Shakespeare, W. (1952). *Measure for measure act III, scene 1. The complete works* (p. 1116). New York: Harcourt Brace.

Snyder, C. R., Rand, K. L., King, E. A., Feldman, D. B., & Woodward, J. T. (2002). "False" hope. *Journal of Clinical Psychology, 58*, 1003–1022.

Spiro, H. (1992). What is empathy and can it be taught? In H. Spiro et al. (Eds.), *Empathy and the practice of medicine.* New Haven: Yale University Press.

Sulmasy, D. P. (1997). *The healer's calling. Spirituality for physicians and other health care professionals*. New York: Paulist Press.

Von Roenn, J. H., & von Gunten, C. F. (2003). Setting goals to maintain hope. *Journal of Clinical Oncology, 21*(3), 570–574.

Wall, P. (1999). *Pain: The science of suffering*. London: Weidenfield and Nicholson.

Warr, T. (1999). The physician's role in maintaining hope and spirituality. *Bioethics Forum, 15*(1), 31–37.

Weisman, A. (1972). *On Dying and Denying: A Psychiatric Study of Terminality*. New York, Behavioral Publications.

Wilkinson, I. (2005). *Suffering: A sociological introduction*. Cambridge: Polity Press.

Williams, W. C. (1951). *The autobiography of William Carlos Williams* (p. 356). New York: New Directions.

Chapter 38
Narrative and Pain: Towards an Integrative Model

David B. Morris

The brain is the organ responsible for all pain.

John D. Loeser (1991)

Introduction: Narrative and Cognition

The medical interest in narrative coincides with new attention to the narrative quality of human cognition. Human neurobiology, according to this line of inquiry, equips us with an inherently "narrative brain" (Newman 2005). An emerging scholarly consensus finds narrative indispensable to mind or consciousness (Bruner 1990; Turner 1996; Michael and Sengers 2003; Fireman et al. 2003; Gottschall and Wilson 2005). More precisely, narrative proves indispensable to mind or consciousness as they are dominated by the language-rich left hemisphere of the human brain. Brain neuroanatomist Jill Bolte Taylor, after suffering a massive left-hemispheric stroke, discovered during her 8-year recovery that the "most prominent" functions of her left hemisphere included "its ability to weave stories" (Taylor 2006). She fondly refers to her left brain as "my storyteller." Stories kept pouring forth without her intent. Taylor was not telling stories: rather, storytelling is what human brains, left to their own biological and cultural devices, just *do*.

The neurobiology of narrative remains imperfectly understood, as do the complex relationships among narrative, health, and illness. Certain stories—erotic or comic tales—implicitly affirm the interrelations between minds and bodies, as evidenced in the effect of laughter on vascular and respiratory systems or in the biology of sexual arousal. "Narrative therapy" holds a respected place among recent innovations in clinical psychology, Family dynamics, and community work (White and Epson 1990; White 2007; Madigan 2010). Mind/body medicine, however, rarely focuses on narrative, and pain medicine--with a few exceptions (Carretal 2005)--mostly ignores it in favor of a scientific knowledge of neurons, neurotransmitters, opiates, and analgesics. It is still unclear what exactly narrative has to do with pain. This chapter, in posing neglected questions about the intersection of pain and narrative, explores not only how narrative influences pain but also how narrative, in its largest medical application, might provide an analogy for the invention of a new and integrative model of pain.

A new integrative model of pain will have to encompass a role for narrative, and narrative offers a useful analogy (no more, no less) for thinking about a new integrative model of pain. Narrative

D.B. Morris (✉)
University Professor University of Virginia

R.J. Moore (ed.), *Handbook of Pain and Palliative Care: Biobehavioral Approaches for the Life Course*, DOI 10.1007/978-1-4419-1651-8_38, © Springer Science+Business Media, LLC 2012

thus holds at least indirect relevance to the professional thinking that relies on mental maps and models. The key point: narrative is not trouble free, and therefore an integrative model of pain that accounts for narrative cannot be trouble free. Pain and narrative are both irreducible to certainties. Quantitative analysis alone cannot master the open-ended matrix of variables at stake in pain (Carr 2005). In fact, core uncertainties make fully objective knowledge of pain a pipedream. Uncertainty is constitutive of pain—especially chronic pain—much as it is a constitutive principle in quantum mechanics. (Simply put, if you measure the position of an electron, you cannot know its velocity; if you measure velocity, you cannot know position: uncertainty is built in.) A new integrative model is valuable not because it is trouble free but because it seeks to account for the uncertainties intrinsic to pain as the experience of a brain-based, culturally inflected, and narrative-driven human consciousness.

What Is Narrative?

Narrative, while open to endless complications in the hands of skilled narratologists (Hyvärinen 2006; Herman 2007), lends itself to a straightforward definition useful in medical settings. Philosopher and novelist Richard Kearney (2002) reminds us of its basic communicative function when he defines narrative—from the Latin *narro* = to tell—as "someone telling something to someone about something...." Kearney's approach is significant for defining narrative through its function, and his functional definition helps move the discussion of narrative beyond a narrow concern with fiction. "Tellings" occur in nonfiction and in everyday lifes as well as in stories, and (in preference to the more restricted concept "story") *narrative* extends to various communicative forms and practices from dialogue to description. Narrative thus makes immediate contact with pragmatic everyday activities clearly relevant to medicine in which, despite charts and tests and a preference for evidence-based data, someone is forever just telling something to someone about something.

A definition of narrative restricted to its communicative function nonetheless fails to encompass its widest social and personal significance. Narrative matters finally because people do not just tell stories. We *live* stories (Eakin 1999; Holstein and Gubrium 2000). Physician and therapist Rachel Remen makes the strongest case when she writes, "Everybody is a story" (1996). The deceptively simple statement merits a second look: it does not say that everbody *has* a story but that everybody *is* a story. Storytelling, as Remen describes it, is not only something we do. Stories are not only something we possess, like a credit history. In Remen's account, the performative activity of storytelling *constitutes* the self. We are stories, stories are us. Narrative, in this sense, can offer clinical insights especially relevant to the lives of chronic pain patients, who regularly adopt a strategy of silence to conceal their day-to-day condition even from close friends and family members. Even the absence of story—beyond any difficulties in communication—may in fact prove an important clinical observation that exposes the erosion selfhood so common and perilous among people in pain.

Narrative, to summarize, is increasingly regarded as a basic human cognitive activity. Its biology, involving networks concerned with language, memory, time, and causation, among others, is centered in the left hemisphere, and its communicative function holds implicit, if unacknowledged, relevance to standard medical practices from patient histories to interviews and "clinical tales" (Sacks 1985). Modern medicine, despite its close association with scientific and technological change, has always been a cryptonarrative enterprise in which stories contributed implicitly to the structure of medical knowledge (Hunter 1991). The recent narrative turn, by contrast, brings an explicit focus to medical communication and to the uses of narrative in diagnosis, treatment, and beyond (Green halgh and Hurwitz 1998). Its serious challenge to traditional medical education and practice is well represented by the Program in Narrative Medicine, founded in 2000 by Rita Charon at the Columbia University College of Physicians and Surgeons.

What Is Narrative Medicine?

Narrative medicine, as Rita Charon describes it in her ground-breaking JAMA article (2001), is medicine practiced with "narrative competence." Narrative competence, as Charon defines it in a strategic move, complements (rather than disrupts or calls into question) standard Western biomedical procedures. It is an add-on, reformist rather than revolutionary, improving what already exists. This strategy serves a useful purpose in recommending narrative within the pages of a medical journal dedicated to scientific studies and to evidence-based claims. Charon's argument challenges standard biomedical thinking, however, in its departure from the usual patronizing medical-humanist claims that reading so-called great literature somehow (in ways unspecified) produces better doctors. Narrative, as she recommends it, offers medicine a fresh vision.

The importance of narrative for understanding medical issues is a persistent, if minor, theme in recent scholarship (Kleinman 1988; Mattingly and Garro 2000; DasGupta and Hurst 2007; Diedrich 2007). Doubtless it is more accurate to refer to narrative "medicines," Plural indiegnous and ongoing as well as postindustrial and newfangled (Morris 2008). Charon's crucial innovation, however, is to identify "narrative competence" as a specific medical skill. Moreover, she bases the argument for narrative medicine on two fundamental principles: epistemological and educational.

The epistemological foundation of narrative medicine identifies narrative as a form of knowledge. Knowledge is the key term. That is, narrative can no longer be erroneously identified with fiction alone. Charon's account defines narrative competence as a specific means of knowing, and it defines narrative knowing as a distinctive kind of knowledge. The emphasis on knowledge effectively disarms long-standing dismissals that impugn narrative as inherently resistant to scientific analysis. Instead, narrative competence and narrative knowledge assume a complementary position alongside the traditional data-driven, high-tech, medical knowledge that Charon calls "logicoscientific." This new epistemic status for narrative as a form of knowledge that *complements* logoscientific knowledge, however, accomplishes only the conceptual reform. Its implementation in reforming the practice of doctors requires significant changes in medical education.

Narrative competence requires, Charon argues, that doctors and health professionals learn the specific skills and ways of thinking necessary to access narrative knowledge. It is the job of medical education to teach such skills in narrative competence. The specific skills—not relevant to describe in this chapter—all of course support the implicit argument that narrative is worth attending to. But is it?

Almost all pain patients have personal stories to tell about their pain. Cultural stories also abound. For example, many patients openly believe the discredited story that pain holds a one-to-one relationship with tissue damage. They may also be unaware of the economic narratives at play, including possibly harmful links between pain in the workplace and disability payments (Mendelson 1992; Fordyce 1995). If narrative knowledge is to be as valid by its own standards as logicoscientific knowledge, gaining new skills is indispensable. In particular, medical practitioners must learn to deal with the two most significant sources of predictable uncertainties basic to every narrative encounter and basic to every valid claim of narrative knowledge: interactivity and intersubjectivity.

Predictable Uncertainties: Interactive and Intersubjective

Certainty in medical matters comforts patients as much as it reassures doctors, but second options and false positives indicate how often in practice medicine must deal with real-world uncertainties. *Complication* is already a familiar medical term, referring to extrinsic morbid processes or events that arise during the course of a disease or its treatment: in short, to predictable uncertainties. Pain is a magnet for complications and uncertainties. Appropriately, in *Complications*: *A Surgeon's Notes on an Imperfect Science*, Atul Gawande (2002) devotes an entire chapter to pain. It is thus not a fatal objection to observe that narrative (like pain, disease, and medical treatment) requires professional vigilance to monitor uncertainties that are built into the structure that makes its knowledge possible.

One main source of predictable uncertainties in narrative (which makes it such an irritant within logicoscientific or strongly science-based disciplines) is a human interactive structure. Unlike a moon rock or an inflamed tendon, narrative requires at least two human parties who interact. This interactive structure—requiring teller plus receiver (or an implied receiver)—proves at least as important as whatever is said. When someone tells something to someone, the narrative content (the "something") varies with tellers or tales, but the interactive structure remains constant. Any account of narrative content is flawed, then, if it ignores the interactive process between teller and receiver that ultimately produces the content. Narrative theorists in recognizing the importance of receivers invented a new subdiscipline known as "reader-response" criticism (Tompkins 1980), and renewed attention to the act of reading typifies late twentieth-century literary analysis from various schools of thought (Iser 1978; Jauss 1982; Miller 1998). While narrative content varies, then, from Greek myths to medical case histories, the stable narrative structure of teller-plus-receiver makes storytelling always (as Kearney puts it) a "quintessentially communicative act."

Communicative action adds predictable uncertainties to narrative, since communicative acts (unlike physical actions such as a bike ride) cannot be performed alone. Narrative, as Kearney insists, is "intrinsically interactive"—and for Rita Charon the pluralized two-person interactive process means that narrative knowledge cannot be reduced to objective data. "Narrative considerations," she writes, emphasizing a social, multivariant, interactive process, "probe the intersubjective domains of human knowledge and activity, that is to say, those aspects of life that are enacted in the relation between two persons." *Persons* here is a structural term indicating not two actual humans but rather the dual narrative positions of *teller* and of *receiver*. Uncertainties multiply with multiple actual receivers, as any group watching a film (and disagreeing about it) attests.

Predictable uncertainties implicit in its interactive structure mean that narrative resembles a verb as much as a noun, like the tango. It takes two to story. The intersubjectivity of narrative knowledge can introduce significant complications in medical settings, but it is important to distinguish intersubjectivity from the scarecrow *subjectivity*. Intersubjective knowledge differs fundamentally from subjective knowledge because it escapes from solipsism: individual claims enter a social realm where they are tested and contested alongside other evidence, as in a courtroom. Medicine, in its reliance on more than objective data, is learning to deal with inescapable forms of intersubjective knowledge, as when doctors need translators to communicate with nonnative-speaking patients. The predictable uncertainties that arise (is a family member translating correctly? does depression carry the same values or meanings in Asian and in Anglo cultures?) make uncertainties about meaning impossible to foreclose. Medicine regularly deals with the unforecloseable idiosyncrasies of organic life, however, as when doctors encounter a woman with two wombs (Bates 2009), and the narrative uncertainties predictable in an intersubjective and interactive communicative process assume, by comparison, a modest place amid the unruly scene of human illness.

The uncertainties native to narrative, as well as to pain, cannot be safely ignored. A patient's illness narrative simply cannot be extracted quickly, cleanly, completely, like an impacted wisdom tooth, as if the receiver now possessed an objective fact. Narrative just does not work that way. Its inherent intersubjective and interactive structure means that narrative is irreducible to an objective stable content: a story told today may change tomorrow, or a nurse may learn significant details withheld from the doctor. In addition, narratives are never mere containers for meanings. Words and images may carry an emotional charge far in excess of their social meanings. Emotions, like a personal subtext or supplement, may prove far more important and inexplicable than thoughts, just as certain myths invite centuries of reinterpretation by receivers from renaissance neoplatonists to contemporary Jungians and poststructuralists.

Narrative texts, then, always include predictably unstable elements—emotional nuance, words, metaphors, symbols, sounds, or sheer mumbo-jumbo—that open up meaning to a conflict of interpretations. The importance of linguistic texture and its uncertainties applies even to the verbal codes that narrative analysts assign to themes and content. Agreement about such codes already requires an intersubjective and interactive process among researchers, open to the human variables of institutional power, personal schedules, and funding guidelines. Such processes open narrative to uncertainties, but they do not disable understanding. In fact, language, despite its inherent slipperiness, is a rich field of clinical observations, as when a chronic pain patient describes her experience in a punitive religious vocabulary (Morris 2009). Inescapable uncertainties in interpretation are testable by—however radical it sounds—asking the patient (Cassel 1982). The exchange will fail to produce certainty, but it does create an intersubjective knowledge, and it may well advance treatment.

Pain and Narrative: Predictable Uncertainties

Pain specialists, in particular, might benefit from an attention to narrative and to its implicit uncertainties, for several reasons. First, narrative, like pain, always comes with filaments attaching it to the social world. Moreover, patients may conceal or remain unaware of filaments they find shameful or distressing, such as chaotic families or spouse abuse. Social differences of age or race or gender can also inflect narrative toward silence or oblique disclosure. Individual narratives too often reproduce patterns circulating within a culture. Patients may unknowingly produce personal narratives that, without conscious intent, replicate patterns from an episode on Oprah or from an article in *People* magazine. The point is not to debunk patient accounts as unreliable but to stress that narrative interactions—even and especially in pain medicine—always reflect, if indirectly, specific sociocultural circumstances (Morris 2010b).

Second, narrative uncertainties mirror and help explicate the predictable uncertainties implicit in pain. Is reflex sympathetic dystrophy a meaningful diagnosis, or is it destined to occupy the limbo of exploded diseases like the nineteenth-century pain syndrome "railway spine?" A professional task force asserts that pain is "always unpleasant and therefore also an emotional experience" (Merskey and Bogduk 1994). How far do nebulous or compounded emotional states—grief, guilt, loneliness—alter or interpenetrate pain? Meanings also possess the capacity to slide away from clear and distinct ideas. In an assisted care facility, an elderly arthritis-ridden patient with a touch of dementia keeps repeating that she wants to go home. Her family brings her home for Thanksgiving. She walks inside, looks around, and says, "I want to go home." Content analysis alone will not dissolve the uncertainties, cognitive and emotional. No authority can say exactly what this mini-narrative means. Pain specialists face such problems daily in understanding not only people with special difficulties in communication (such as the elderly, children, Alzheimer's patients, and nonnative speakers) but also people whose pain entails difficult personal or social circumstances (such as torture victims, HIV/AIDS patients, incest survivors, and the poor).

Everyone (it seems) has a story to tell about pain. The stories, however, usually do not treat pain as an object of description—in the manner of the famous McGill Pain Questionnaire (1971), which regards pain as a noun-like state knowable (or at least trackable) through its location on a grid of adjectival descriptors. In narrative contexts, by contrast, pain emerges mainly as a verbal, lived experience situated within a complex social world with filaments that reach beyond job, family, and substance abuse. Further, such narratives may infiltrate and modify the very pain they describe, much as a victim-narrative or disability-narrative can modify pain by enlisting it within a specific social practice or individual form of life. Pain is among the more elusive human experiences and changes not only over a day or year but also within particular social situations (worse at a lecture, say, better at a concert). Pain specialists are de facto clinicians and scientists of the uncertain.

Narrative competence is a skill useful especially for its power to articulate and to anticipate relevant uncertainties predictable in the experience of pain.

Narrative in Pain Medicine: What Good Is It?

Narrative competence is not yet a skill required for pain specialists, but narrative already holds a firm, if often unappreciated, presence within pain medicine. Interviews, for example, are a standard source for data in the recent medical literature on pain, especially semistructured, unstructured, and open-ended interviews. Researchers often study such interview data through qualitative "narrative analysis." The recent medical literature on pain contains specific studies of patients' stories (Werner et al. 2004; Winslow et al. 2005; Råheim and Håland 2006; Corbett et al. 2007; McGowan et al. 2007; Morone et al. 2008; Steihaug and Malterud 2008). There is even one study of physicians' stories (Vegni et al. 2005). These published studies do not reflect the largely undocumented use of oral patient narratives within support groups at pain management programs. Narrative thus already makes a solid if somewhat secretive contribution to pain medicine, both in research and in treatment.

The relatively low profile of narrative within pain medicine, despite increasing numbers of studies that employ it, suggests the need to address openly a basic pragmatic question. What, in particular, can narrative *do* for pain medicine? Bluntly, what *good* is it? What, specifically, is it good *for*? Rita Charon has discussed possible contributions of narrative in pain medicine (2005). Here, as a supplement, it seems worthwhile to examine the value of narrative to pain medicine in five specific areas: communication, diagnosis, treatment, ethics, and education. A brief survey of each area can suggest how and where narrative performs specific, valuable work.

Communication

Communication in medicine is a perennial problem, much discussed, but pain medicine faces problems in communication that are distinctive if not unique. Clinical medicine depends on a gaze that penetrates into the body and effectively engineers out narrative (Foucault 1973). A formerly narrative, dialogical encounter between physician and patient (beginning with the open-ended invitation *what is the matter?*) shrinks into a closed-off query that can be answered with one finger (*where does it hurt?*). Attention to the interactive and intersubjective structure of narrative, then, offers to help pain specialists develop the communication skills crucial for dealing with patients for whom lesions and organic signs often correlate poorly (or not at all) with their lived experience. Narrative competence can uncover data otherwise inaccessible in standard interview questions whose results are interpreted regularly by erroneous assumptions about patient subjectivity and medical objectivity.

Narrative competence enriches clinical data in pain medicine, then, by opening up the field of discourse, but it does more. It directs attention. While listening to patients is a skill regularly lamented as missing or badly flawed, effective listening requires more than good will: it requires skills in identifying specific types of recurrent narratives. Sociologist Arthur Frank (1995) shows how individual patient narratives tend to fall into general types, such as chaos narratives (about lives falling apart) or restitution narratives (about unexpected gains that accompany illness and its losses). The medical literature already identifies some specific types of pain narratives, such as women's pain narratives (McGowan et al. 2007), survivor pain narratives (Markovic et al. 2008), and stigma narratives of pain (Holloway et al. 2007; Goldberg 2010). The narrative payoff for pain medicine lies not only in a general improvement of listening skills but also in the competence to know what, specifically, to listen *for*.

Narrative inescapably raises questions about point of view (McKee 1997), and narrative competence holds proven value in addressing difficult questions that can be answered only from the patient's point of view. What, for example, do victims of domestic violence want physicians to understand? Narrative has proved the right tool for addressing this question (Nicolaidis 2002). Narrative holds similar value for pain specialists not only in situations, such as sexual abuse, where secrecy or shame impedes communication but also where the patient alone knows the facts. Or in working with children, whose point of view does not necessarily coincide with adult vision (Carter 2004; Meldrum et al. 2009). Narrative has a proven track record too as a resource for understanding and for addressing the needs of patients in palliative care—where pain control is a primary objective and where the patient's speech and point of view may be irretrievably compromised (Barnard et al. 2000). Narrative skills cannot offer access to changeless nuggets of objective truth, but they do provide supportive data and supplemental insights reliable within their limits. All instruments are limited, of course, and some fail. The key question is not what narrative can't do, but what it *can* do.

Diagnosis

Diagnosis, as a technical matter of matching symptoms to diseases, may seem off limits to narrative, but who exactly sets the boundaries? And do the usual rules apply to pain? The answer might surprise a patient. Distinguished pain specialist Scott Fishman puts it this way: "When somebody comes in with 25 years of chronic pain, I might sit with them for 90 min to get the beginning of the story, to really understand what's happening. The insurers would rather pay me $1,000 to do a 20-min injection than pay me a fraction of that to spend an hour or two talking with a patient" (quoted in Wallis 2005). The decision to exclude narrative, that is, comes here not from a physician skilled in pain medicine but from an insurer—an insurer with a financial agenda who may in fact or in effect overrule the physician.

What about the insurer's legitimate concern over cost? Narrative is time-intensive when compared with an injection. If Fishman is correct about the clinical value of narrative, then there is a need to invent a cost-effective system that facilitates and advances narrative interactions: maybe a system in which paramedical aides do the more expensive preliminary narrative data-gathering. Interviews by medical sociologists or by trained doctoral candidates might reduce costs and pinpoint problems, with direct benefit (in cost and in effectiveness) to subsequent physician/patient interactions. Inventiveness in contemporary health care—so successful at discovering new technologies and new drug therapies—certainly can contrive cost-effective means to employ narrative in pain medicine if indeed narrative holds the benefits that Scott Fishman and others claim for it.

Narrative as a diagnostic instrument offers particular benefits through its privileged access to particularity and subjectivity: helping, specifically, to elucidate the irreducible differences in individual pain response. Age, gender, race, and ethnicity are well known to affect personal pain responses (Morris 2001), and narrative permits clinicians to probe behind such generic categories. The same age and race, for example, may hold different meanings for different individuals. It does not invalidate narrative as a limited instrument if, as happens rarely in medical settings, patients lie. (Then the clinical question, which narrative has crucially helped to elicit, is *why* the patient lied.) Narrative data, like all clinical data, also requires careful evaluation, but careful evaluation differs from hasty dismissals that misrepresent narrative as merely subjective, always unreliable, and medically insignificant. A patient narrative, albeit uncertain, intersubjective, and interactive, may often prove indispensable: the best evidence available.

A diagnosis in pain medicine already involves identifying what specialists call "pain beliefs." Especially important are beliefs about cause, control, duration, outcome, and blame (Williams and Thorn 1989; Jensen et al. 1991), as well as beliefs about the need to protect individual identity

(Eccleston et al. 1997). Such beliefs affect not only chronic pain but also acute pain and even postoperative pain (Williams 1996). Researchers find that patients function better who believe they have some control over their pain, who believe in the value of medical services, who believe that family members care for them, and who believe that they are not severely disabled (Jensen and Karoly 1992). In fact, specific pain beliefs can predict pain intensity (Williams and Keefe 1991) and correlate directly with treatment outcomes (Shutty et al. 1990). Quality of life in chronic pain is more associated with beliefs and perceptions, it turns out, than with pain intensity (Lame et al. 2005). An effective diagnosis simply cannot focus on tissue damage alone and ignore what patients think and feel. The brain—including its built-in cognitive, behavioral, emotional, conscious, and nonconscious capacities to alter any nociceptive stimulus—is the organ responsible for all pain (Loeser 1991).

The diagnostic value of narrative, as providing access to beliefs, coincides with its value in improved medical communication, and narrative is especially useful for identifying uncommon or idiosyncratic beliefs, hybrid beliefs, or conflicting beliefs. Narrative also proves useful for diagnotic purpose in identifying areas in which communication fails. The unsaid—as in the blocked out experience that torture victims cannot put into words—is sometimes just as important from a clinical perspective as what is said (Waitzkin and Magaña 1997). Narrative, as an instrument that registers significant absences, also points toward the social circumstances (including economic systems) under which speech occurs or fails to occur (Macherey 1978). Patients whose pain stops them from working, for example, may be unable to imagine a life without paid work. A conflict of narratives creates a mental-emotional dissonance worth noting, in a diagnostic spirit, for its possible impact on health.

Narrative can make an especially useful diagnostic contribution to pain medicine in focusing on emotion. Stories from King Lear to Little Red Riding Hood serve to express and to evoke feelings. Pain patients may tell stories in which emotions matter more than plot—stories, for example, that convey helplessness or guilt or anger. Although the manifest content (physician neglect, bureaucratic roadblocks, family strife) may be familiar, the latent emotional content of patient narratives can lead in strange, significant directions. Further, in addition to registering an absence of speech, stories may also expose telltale absences of emotion, perhaps indicating where depression imprints its blank signature on pain. Narrative in its close links to emotion thus proves sensitive to subtextual nuances of feeling that elude the broad net of "code-able" content. What is the code for the emotions—not the content or actions—reflected in a teenager's bland half-truth about how he put out cigarettes on the back of his hand or how she razor-cut her upper arms?

Treatment

Narrative competence as it affects diagnosis almost always holds implications for treatment, but implications move toward specific treatment options when narrative competence implies the skill not only to identify patient stories but also to address and even to alter them. As if a patient were addressing a doctor, physician Howard Brody (1994) subtitled an essay "My Story Is Broken; Can You Help Me Fix It?" Narrative skills, as Kearney also argues, permit us to identify stories that are harmful or confining, as a necessary step toward altering or replacing them. New replacement stories can free us from old patterns. Harmful narratives, as Kearney proposes, have imprisoned the English and the Irish in ancient antagonistic stereotypes of national identity, with untold cost in wasted lives, injuries, and death. Chronic pain, for the individual patient, is an old story, a confining pattern, often tied up with imprisoning narratives of disability and of spoiled identity. Narrative skills allow a health professional to help patients develop nontoxic and even beneficial personal stories that alter their expectations about living with pain.

Expectation as a psychological state is crucial both to pain and to the placebo effect (Pollo and Benedetti 2011). Indeed, expectation alone is enough to generate reports of pain among experimental subjects told they might receive a painful stimulus (Bayer et al. 1991), and narratives regularly embody and develop patterns of expectation. Even the *forms* of stories generate expectations. We expect comedies to reach a happy ending, and we expect tragedies to end badly. Researchers studying the neurobiology of expectation confirm that mental representations of an impending sensory event, such as pain or pain relief, can significantly shape neural processes that underlie the actual sensory experience (Koyama et al. 2005). In effect, positive expectations diminish the severity of chronic disease states. What expectations or narratives of expectation are associated with chronic pain? There is certainly need for additional research to demonstrate how new treatment narratives might alter expectations in ways that also relieve pain.

Narrative alone—almost any narrative that gives pleasure—might eventually find a respected place among treatment options. Recent research used brain scans on college students who professed to be deeply in love (Younger et al. 2010). A heated probe on the palm of the hand provided a constant stimulus producing pain. The act of looking at a picture of the beloved reduced moderate pain by about 40%, and such love-induced analgesia was associated with the brain's reward centers. (Distraction, by contrast, was associated mostly with cognitive pathways.) Pain specialist Sean Mackey, senior author of the study, says that the findings suggest, generally, that pleasurable activities can relieve pain. "Find the things to give you pleasure in life," he recommends, "whether it be through the one you love or going and listening to great music or reading a good book" (quoted in Parker-Pope 2010). On a serious note, in 2009 and 2010 a group called the Theater of War presented readings of Sophocles's pain-centered tragedies *Philoctetes* and *Ajax* to military audiences, under contract from the U. S. Defense Centers of Excellence for Psychological Health and Traumatic Brain Injury. Nearly 20,000 service members, veterans, and their families have attended and participated in Theater of War performances and discussions to date (www.philoctetesproject.org). There is no inherent reason why such innovative experiments with therapeutic narrative could not be extended to chronic pain patients and especially to veterans, whose unusually high incidence of pain constitutes a significant public health problem (Kazis et al. 1999).

Pain narratives that patients bring to the clinic are often not only short on pleasure but also at violent odds with facts and statistics. Overly optimistic narratives of surgical intervention so favored by patients, for example, can lead to damage and disillusionment. An alarming percentage of surgeries for back pain fail to provide long-term relief or to prove more effective than cognitive intervention and exercise (Brox et al. 2006). Many adults with back pain have lumbar disk disease, but many adults with lumbar disk disease are pain-free. (Jensen et al. 1994), and in America, long-term functioning of patients treated for back pain is similar whether doctors prescribe medication and bed rest—or emphasize self-care and education (Von Korff et al. 1994; see also May 2011). The erroneous patient narrative holding that pain is a reliable alarm system for injury not only encourages unnecessary surgeries but it cannot explain why the two strongest signs predicting that American workers will develop chronic back pain are job dissatisfaction and unsatisfactory social relations in the workplace (Bigos et al. 1991; Dwyer and Raftery 1991). Some lumbar surgeries actually increase pain. Fact-based narratives addressing unlikely expectations, then, offer a low-cost intervention that promises benefit and surely does no harm.

Ethics

Ethics is an important aspect of pain medicine—not least because institutional research projects require an ethical review. More important, pain raises distinctive ethical questions not identical with the questions raised by pain-free illnesses and medical procedures (see also Rich 2011; see also Fine 2011). Professional pain associations respond with specific guidelines, and guidelines are a fascinating subgenre of technical narrative designed to enunciate ruling principles and to eliminate (or tightly circumscribe) uncertainties. Narrative competence, by contrast, offers help valuable particularly in "gray areas": specific situations where official guidelines do not apply or where equally valid principles, as happens with regularity in medicine, come into conflict (Morris 2003).

Narrative ethics, then, is not about the application of general principles but about an attention to individual cases and to the ways in which the narratives we construct around individual cases influence what we choose, how we act, and whose values win-out (Nelson 1997; Charon and Montello 2002; Bennett and Gibson 2006). Although bioethics since its inception in the 1970s has focused on principles, principalism (as a principle-based bioethics is called) no longer rules supreme. A newer "narrative ethics" operates effectively in the twilight zone where regularly raise difficult and often unprecedented dilemmas clinical cases. It not only focuses on the individual case but also calls attention to narrative as a shaping force in ethical decisions. As bioethicist Tod Chambers puts it (1996), there are no artless narrations. Even the thumbnail ethical cases prized in textbooks are a specific narrative subgenre in which brevity (e.g.,) is a formal feature that crucially influences understanding. In effect, narrative ethics insists that we cannot conduct ethical inquiry outside the context of narrative. The important question, then, is how narrative competence might come to alter the discussion of ethical issues related to pain.

Narrative ethics holds a special relevance to pain when ethics is understood to concern values. Every encounter between physician and patient necessarily involves language, and our words—selected from a wider available vocabulary—always carry connotations that escape authorial control. Words also convey values. Patients regularly complain that doctors do not believe their pain is real, and differences in language and in culture doubtless compound verbal misunderstandings with a clash of values, perhaps also contributing to observed disparities in pain management and treatment (Palermo 2011; Green 2011; Hallenbeck 2011). The use of narrative to uncover values is clear in a study on patient autonomy in end-of-life decisions (Blackhall et al. 1995). Questionnaire data left troubling puzzles, so, faced with an impasse, the research team sent in anthropologists. The anthropologists discovered via narrative interviews that Korean-Americans and Mexican-Americans in Los Angeles, unlike whites and blacks, transferred end-of-life decisions to the family. Their discovery also illustrates how narrative can probe beyond statistical data to expose an ethical substrate. A bioethics of pain that focuses on values and that also stays sensitive to cultural differences as expressed in language will find principles less important or less applicable than the skills developed through narrative analysis.

Ethics is certainly at issue in the unequal treatment of pain in patients from cultural, ethnic, and racial minorities (Todd 2001; Green et al. 2003; Green 2011). In a social world where privilege and prejudice are facts of life, narrative remains a valuable tool for uncovering and for exploring such ethical dilemmas in pain medicine. Narrative sources, for example, strongly support the claim that in the United States pain holds a distinctive emotional, cognitive, historical status within the African-American community (Wailoo 2006; King 2008). An ethics of pain medicine sensitive to the cultural heritage of specific minority populations—a heritage that included an ongoing history of undertreatment for pain—cannot rely on general principles alone but also needs access to social and historical data that is fundamentally narrative in its reconstruction of the past (Green 2011). An ethics of pain may also draw upon narrative to convey the importance of emotion-rich face-to-face encounters in the choice of what, in any particular case, constitutes right action (Morris 2002). Ethics committees that meet behind closed doors to consider "documents" may in fact deprive themselves of the data obtainable only through the face-to-face encounters of a present-tense living in-person narrative.

Education

Medical education cannot dispense with narrative, even if it wanted to, but the prominence of data, graphs, statistics, and visual aids sometimes overshadows the use and power of a well-told story.

A roomful of weary medical students assembled for a lecture on medical error snapped awake when a senior physician, after first securing the doors, explained in detail how as a resident he had killed a patient. Not intentionally, and the patient had a terminal disease—but the resident's error proved as fatal as a bullet. Cardiac surgeon Larry Zaroff (2009) writes about a famous colleague whose error led to the death of a patient. The surgeon walked out of the operating suite, Zaroff reports, never to return. Medical error is an important topic in medical education, thoroughly analyzed in the professional literature, but such stories that focus on like-minded individuals in a moment of crisis tend to command attention and to change behavior in ways that statistics do not. The well-known studies and statistics concerning medical undertreatment of pain proved oddly powerless to change professional behavior. The American Pain Society Quality of Care Committee (1995) reported an absence of improvement despite "decades of effort" spent providing clinicians with information about analgesics. Threats of lost institutional accreditation—a different narrative subgenre—appear more effective in changing professional behavior than numbers.

Patient education, as distinct from the education of health professionals, is another neglected area where narrative offers to make a significant contribution. The new era of online information gives patients a license for medical self-education, and pain specialists have a special interest in correcting erroneous information and harmful beliefs circulating over the internet, which can negatively affect treatment. The positive education of patients about pain—in the manner of wellness programs in corporations or simply through the distribution of effective video materials—remains an almost unexplored resource with an opportunity to reduce the alarming number of people in the developed world who suffer from chronic pain. Figures from The National Center for Health Statistics (2009) show that nonacute pain affects more Americans than diabetes, heart disease, and cancer combined.

Narrative knowledge, because of its inherent limitations, will never attain the certainty of randomized double-blind controlled experiments. We should not expect it to. Still, within its limits, narrative is a patient-centered medical resource especially valuable for its attention to individual differences in an era of standardized best practices and medicine by guidelines. Narrative, whatever its satellite benefits, always returns to the central individual consciousness of a specific person, in a particular time and place, marked by a particular gender, race, ethnicity, and socioeconomic status. Despite its inherent uncertainties, narrative is an ordinary act performed almost nonstop in daily life—someone telling someone about something—and its medical value is implicit in its everydayness. In its everydayness, it might even suggest a new model to describe the most humdrum and widespread of all human maladies, pain.

An Integrative Model: Narrative as Analogue

The right question is not how pain resembles narrative. The differences are obvious. No sane person suffering from an inflamed appendix ever went to a narratologist. The right question is how can thinking about narrative illuminate thinking about pain? Like pain narrative is layered, nuanced, and multidimensional, and like pain it is also interactive and intersubjective. It takes four gospels to narrate what Christians call the greatest story ever told, and theologians are still arguing about it, while back pain, neck pain, and carpal tunnel syndrome all generate controversy over diagnostic criteria and optimal treatment. Narrative is a cultural product dependent upon biological properties of human brains, and human pain is the product of biological processes inflected by culture (Morris 1991, 1998; Coakley and Shelemay 2007). Most important, thinking about narrative helps point to the need for an integrative model of pain (weaving together both biological and cultural phenomena) that is centered in a storytelling and suffering human consciousness.

A new model of pain is clearly needed. The famous Melzack-Wall "gate-control" theory dating from the late 1960s now uneasily coexists alongside various cognitive/behavioral approaches (which rarely articulate a conceptual model of pain). Meanwhile the well-known 1970s biopsychosocial framework—often applied to pain—has recently come under attack in psychiatry (Ghaemi 2009), perhaps ultimately exposing its limits as a conceptual model for pain. Co-founder of the gate-control theory, Ronald Melzack, has proposed a subsequent neuromatirix model that goes far beyond biopsychosocialism (1999). Discussions of pain within the emerging discipline of integrative medicine so far focus mainly on complementary and alternative therapies (Audette and Bailey 2008; Kutner and Smith 2011). Thinking about narrative offers the advantage of a blank slate for rethinking models of pain.

Narrative has the disadvantage, however, of seeming to highlight linguistic features, so there is benefit to invoking a technology that seems at first to lie outside the realm of storytelling. No analogy or metaphor fits perfectly: the dorsal horn of the spinal column does not really contain a tiny gate, does it? In a postmodern context where narrative interpenetrates nonnarrative forms from dance and photography to TV ads, the storytelling human consciousness has no trouble colonizing the popular computer mapping application Google Earth. It is, like cinema (as a medium) or like travel literature (as a genre), almost a machine for the perpetual generation of potential narratives.

Google Earth, as a proto-narrative technology, is both integrative and interactive: it does not simply speed up traditional linear fact-retrieval but rather integrates multiple levels of data. It does not tell a single static story but rather provides the model for generating multiple changing narratives that require users or receivers to participate in their construction. Thus, in a nonlinear process of clicks and jumps, the user swoops down from a satellite-eye view to find, say, a specific address. In a photographic sequence, lets you see a single house on a single street in the context of a city, state, and region. As the technology improves, users might zoom in further via hypertext links to a virtual reality that shows deeds, blueprints, or wiring diagrams. Or—in a leap sideways—links might identify previous owners, building permits, or legal documents from local codes to state laws. The zoom feature in effect redefines any specific house less as an object-like brick-and-mortar structure than as the intersubjective product of a multilevel integrative, network, like the time-lapse film of a rosebush. The zoom technology, of course, depends crucially on human consciousness.

Consciousness and An Integrative Model of Pain

Consciousness must be the center for any new model of human pain. Pain can exist in the absence of tissue damage (Merskey and Bogduk 1994), but not without consciousness. Consciousness, including its almost nonstop internal first-person narration, is what distinguishes human pain from pain in lower animals, where tail flicks indicate nociception, say, but tell us nothing about

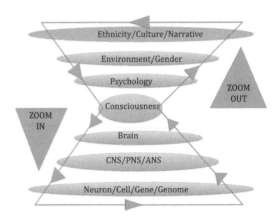

Fig. 38.1 A fully representative diagram would be three-dimensional, with interpenetrating layers, in continual motion

intersubjective, psychological, emotional states. An integrative model of human pain, then, would locate its conceptual center in human consciousness, with a circumference or periphery extending both inward and outward: inward toward the microscopic recesses of cell biology and outward toward the macroscopic cultural environments (including families, nations, religions, and other human groups). Here is what an integrative model of pain might look like (Fig. 38.1):

Consciousness is of course a complex problem that continues to resist neuroscientists and philosophers, although their renewed attention is significant. Some regard consciousness as an emergent property of human brains, like the v-formation that emerges when geese take flight, fragile and contingent rather than rock solid, but nonetheless a crucial element. The absence of final answers, however, does not change the fact that, as a logician might put it, consciousness is a "necessary condition" for human pain: that is, without consciousness there is no pain to account for.

Consciousness nonetheless is also a necessary condition for many human states—from love to guilt—so a new model of human pain will be accurate precisely to the degree that it identifies cultural and biological forces distinctive to pain. In this sense, the model belongs to a larger movement toward "biocultural" understanding (Davis and Morris 2007). An integrative model moreover must allow the various cultural and biological forces to vary in prominence, depending on a specific pain syndrome. It must even allow for what narratologists describe as varying "points of view" (POV). Clinicians, cell biologists, and geneticists will zoom in—to trace in detail and ever-finer resolution the molecular processes that from their POV correlate with a consciousness of pain. Psychologists, medical anthropologists, cultural historians, and narratologists will zoom out—to explore the personal and/or cultural relations that correlate from their POV with a consciousness of pain. An integrative model of pain, while inescapably biocultural, does not imply that biological or cultural facts always get an equal share. Proportions will differ.

Pain certainly accommodates significant biological differences, and the differences extend to culture as well. While the neurobiology of pain differs in migraine, in childbirth, in trigeminal neuralgia, and in cancer pain (among cancer's 100 varieties), for example, cultural differences prove equally significant. Childbirth and its pains usually include an emotional resonance quite different from the feelings of patients with trigeminal neuralgia. Negative emotions such as anger and sadness, at least in laboratory experiments, are known to increase pain in women (Van Middendorp et al. 2010; see also Keogh 2011). Stigma, guilt, blame, and access to medication affect the seriously undertreated pain of people with HIV/AIDS (Breitbart et al. 1996). Biofeedback alone demonstrates how directed mental activity can alter pain states. In short, complex relations between mind and body, between culture and biology, require a model of pain that connects distant layers of relevant data. An integrative model predicts that significant changes at one layer will affect changes elsewhere.

Narrative in this new integrative model is not off floating in cultural hyperspace, unconnected to the brain and cut free from human consciousness. Not only are human brains genetically fitted to produce narrative but also, as confabulation suggests, they seem unable not to produce it (Hirstein 2006). Storytelling is what human organisms cannot help doing. Some psychologists believe that human conduct is always "storied" (Sarbin 1986). If so, the storied conduct of being human is nowhere clearer (from catastrophizing to quality of life) than in people with pain.

Success Stories: A Concluding Example

A new narratized zoom model of pain ought to endorse at least one unexplored instance in which storytelling might materially assist patients. The concept of patient is more or less taken for granted inside pain medicine, but clearly patienthood is a role enfolded in narratives that change across time and cultures, and it is significant that the vast majority of medical research on chronic pain depends on study populations composed of people self-identified as patients and situated inside the culture of medicine.

Uncounted numbers of people with chronic pain, however, do not accept the narrative of patienthood and do not seek medical help, or only intermittently, like reluctant visitors, re-enter the subculture of medicine. Their experience is rarely reflected in medical research. How do many such people manage to live healthy and (by their own accounts) successful, happy lives despite chronic pain? What is their secret? What might a patient learn from their success stories? (Palermo 2011).

The medical literature on success stories—including the literature in pain medicine—is almost nonexistent (Morris 2005). Recent work in positive psychology (Lopez and Snyder 2009) and in psychotraumatology (Tedeschi and Calhoun 2004) suggests that people respond to crisis with a variety of individual strategies that point toward increased knowledge, deepened spiritual awareness, compassion for fellow sufferers, and other forms of personal growth. Chronic pain, while unwanted and even debilitating, is for some people a crisis that paradoxically generates potent individual mini-narratives of successful living.

A study of oral narratives by people with chronic pain—only intermittently defined as patients—promises to illuminate the relations between narrative and successful living.[1] Consider, for example, the person who opposes chronic pain with the metaphor of life as a poker game ("I still have a few chips left"), or the person who describes pain through the narrative metaphors of a journey, an education, background noise, or even a gift. The metaphor or mini-narrative of pain as struggle can evoke for some a life-affirming determination to resist. For others, metaphors of letting-go permit the entry into a zenlike state of acceptance. People often speak of pain as a challenge or trial, a ritualized initiation into a mystery, or an experience they must, on their own, figure out how to "handle"—as if pain were an unstable explosive device or a mechanism missing its control stick. Narratives of victimhood are sometimes countered with humor—funny stories or simply an optimism that uses joking language to generate laughter—while some people prefer to emphasize healing, growth, trade-offs, or a saving immersion in nature, in music, in the visual arts, or in the wordless bodily space time of dance.

Presence is a term applied to body-centered states, beyond meaning, that maintain a sensuous contact with the material world (Gumbrecht 2004), and dance is paradigmatic of activities or esthetic forms that evoke presence. There are success stories to be told about the importance of presence in chronic pain. Intractable pain can profoundly disorder the ordinary (brain-based) sense of time, for example, erasing past and future, transforming the present into unending torment (Morris 2010a). Time experienced as presence, for example, even while a dance performance lasts, is time redeemed from the blankness of all-encompassing pain. It offers not simply a distraction—which any abrupt change could provide—but a temporary release from pain and a healing engagement with bodily presence.

Narrative is an enduring folk remedy against loss—stories that heal (Remen 1996)—but, as Kearney observed, narrative also contains the power to harm. Susan Sontag's classic *Illness as Metaphor* (1978) describes how tuberculosis in the nineteenth century and cancer in the twentieth century accumulated damaging cultural metaphors and mini-narratives that added to the affliction of people with cancer or TB. Chronic pain in the late twentieth- and twenty-first centuries has also accumulated its own damaging set of afflictive cultural mini-narratives. Sontag's response was a call to strip medicine of all metaphor: to eliminate narrative and to replace it with pure science and sheer fact. No one legitimately turns away from facts, so Sontag's call is always part of the medical dialogue.

Narrative and metaphor, however, hold a power for good that Sontag ignored Psychologist Timothy D. W. Wilson (2011) describes the neuroscience that underlies a new clinical practice callled "story editing"--which encourages the replacement of harmful personal narratives with beneficial stories. Medical sociologist Alan Radley in *Works of Illness* (2009) provides an important counterpoint by

[1] See the research-in-progress, "Wisdom in Medicine: Mapping the Path through Adversity to Wisdom." Funded by the John Templeton Foundation. Margaret Plews-Ogan, MD, Principal Invesigator, and Justine E. Owens, PhD, Co-Principal Investigator.

showing in detail how people respond to various debilitating and life-threatening illness or bodily trauma by creating tangible social artifacts, from digging gardens to making stories (see also Palermo 2011). Such artifacts, he shows persuasively, serve as a "medium for survival." Pain medicine in the twenty-first century might well explore—under the aegis of a new integrative model—the narrative survival strategies and tacit or explicit success stories that permit some people in pain to create successful lives, inside or outside the fee-for-service, insurer-dominated, overcrowded world of pain medicine.

It is folly to see narrative as a panacea for the complex problems surrounding chronic pain. Chronic pain patients, however, as almost an initial question to a doctor or specialist want to know what their chances are of getting better (Thernstrom 2011). It seems legitimate and ethical to respond that the epidemiological odds may be discouraging, but here is a specific success story: the narrative of a patient, much like you, who beat the odds. Yes, it is merely a single instance, occupying the lowest rank in the hierarchy of evidence-based medical knowledge, but on what ethical grounds does a physician destroy hope and withhold evidence? An integrative model, which views narrative as a significant element in the complex biocultural construction of pain, provides strong incentive for research that discovers ways to enlist narrative as a positive support and as an invaluable medium for survival.

References

American Pain Society Quality of Care Committee. (1995). Quality improvement guidelines for the treatment of acute pain and cancer pain. *Journal of the American Medical Association, 274*(23), 1874–1880.

Audette, J. F., & Bailey, A. (Eds.). (2008). *Integrative pain medicine: The science and practice of complementary and alternative medicine in pain management.* New York: Humana Press.

Barnard, D., Towers, A., Boston, P., & Lambrinidou, Y. (2000). *Crossing over: Narratives of palliative care.* New York: Oxford University Press.

Bates, D. (2009). Woman with two wombs gives birth to a one-in-a-million baby girl. *Mail Online,* 16 July. Retrieved December 10, 2009, from http://www.dailymail.co.uk/health/article-1199831/Woman-wombs-gives-birth-million-baby-girl.html.

Bayer, T., Baer, P. E., & Early, C. (1991). Situational and psychophysiological factors in psychologically induced pain. *Pain, 44*(1), 45–50.

Bennett, M. D., & Gibson, J. M. (2006). *A field guide to good decisions: Values in action.* New York: Praeger.

Bigos, S. J., Battié, M. C., Spengler, D. M., Fisher, L. D., Fordyce, W. E., Hansson, T. H., Nachemson, A. L., & Wortley, M. D. (1991). A prospective study of work perceptions and psychosocial factors affecting the report of back injury. *Spine, 16*(1), 1–6.

Blackhall, L. J., Murphy, S. T., Frank, G., Michel, V., & Azen, S. (1995). Ethnicity and attitudes toward patient autonomy. *Journal of the American Medical Association, 274*(10), 820–825.

Breitbart, W., Rosenfeld, B. D., Passik, S. D., McDonald, M. V., Thaler, H., & Portenoy, R. K. (1996). The undertreatment of pain in ambulatory AIDS patients. *Pain, 65*(2–3), 243–249.

Brody, H. (1994). "My story is broken; can you help me fix it?" Medical ethics and the joint construction of narrative. *Literature and Medicine, 13*(1), 79–92.

Brox, J. I., Rejkeras, O., Nygaard, O., Sorensen, R., Indahl, A., Holm, I., et al. (2006). Lumbar instrumented fusion compared with cognitive intervention and exercises in patients with chronic back pain after previous surgery for disc herniation: A prospective randomized controlled study. *Pain, 122*(1–2), 4–5.

Bruner, J. (1990). *Acts of meaning.* Cambridge: Harvard University Press.

Carr, D. B. (2005). Memoir of a meta-analyst: On the silent "I" in "qualnitative". In D. B. Carr, J. D. Loeser, & D. B. Morris (Eds.), *Narrative, pain, and suffering* (pp. 325–354). Seattle: IASP Press.

Carr, D. B., Loeser, J. D., & Morris, D. B. (Eds.). (2005). *Narrative, pain, and suffering.* Seattle: IASP Press.

Carter, B. (2004). Pain narratives and narrative practitioners: A way of working "in-relation" with children experiencing pain. *Journal of Nursing Management, 12*(3), 210–216.

Cassel, E. J. (1982). The nature of suffering the goals of medicine. *The New England Journal of Medicine, 306*(11), 639–645.

Chambers, T. (1996). From the ethicist's point of view: The literary nature of ethical inquiry. *The Hastings Center Report, 26*(1), 25–33.

Charon, R. (2001). Narrative medicine: A model for empathy, reflection, profession, and trust. *Journal of the American Medical Association, 286*(15), 1897–1902.

Charon, R. (2005). A narrative medicine for pain. In D. B. Carr, J. D. Loeser, & D. B. Morris (Eds.), *Narrative, pain, and suffering* (pp. 29–44). Seattle: IASP Press.

Charon, R., & Montello, M. (Eds.). (2002). *Stories matter: The role of narrative in medical ethics*. New York: Routledge.

Coakley, S., & Shelemay, K. K. (Eds.). (2007). *Pain and its transformations: The interface of biology and culture*. Cambridge: Harvard University Press.

Corbett, M., Foster, N. E., & Ong, B. N. (2007). Living with low back pain: Stories of hope and despair. *Social Science & Medicine, 65*(8), 1584–1594.

DasGupta, S., & Hurst, M. (2007). *Stories of illness and healing: Women write their bodies*. Kent, OH: The Kent State University Press.

Davis, L. J., & Morris, D. B. (2007). Biocultures manifesto. *New Literary History, 38*(3), 411–418.

Diedrich, L. (2007). *Treatments: Language, politics, and the culture of illness*. Minneapolis: University of Minnesota Press.

Dwyer, T., & Raftery, A. E. (1991). Industrial accidents are produced by social relations of work: A sociological theory of industrial accidents. *Applied Ergonomics, 22*(3), 167–178.

Eakin, J. P. (1999). *How our lives become stories: Making selves*. Ithaca: Cornell University Press.

Eccleston, C., Williams, A. C., & Rogers, W. S. (1997). Patients' and professionals' understandings of the causes of chronic pain: Blame, responsibility and identity protection. *Social Science & Medicine, 45*(5), 699–709.

Fine, P. (2011). Recognition and resolution of ethical barriers to palliative care research. In R. J. Moore (Ed.), *Handbook of pain and palliative care*. New York: Springer.

Fireman, G. D., McVay, T. E., Jr., & Flanagan, O. J. (Eds.). (2003). *Narrative and consciousness: Literature, psychology, and the brain*. New York: Oxford University Press.

Fordyce, W. E. (Ed.). (1995). *Back pain in the workplace: Management of disability in nonspecific conditions*. Seattle: IASP Press.

Foucault, M. (1973). *The birth of the clinic: An archaeology of medical perception* (A. M. S. Smith, Trans.). New York: Pantheon Books. (First published in French in 1963).

Frank, A. W. (1995). *The wounded storyteller: Body, illness, and ethics*. Chicago: University of Chicago Press.

Gawande, A. (2002). *Complications: A surgeon's notes on an imperfect science*. New York: Henry Holt and Company.

Ghaemi, S. N. (2009). *The rise and fall of the biopsychosocial model: Reconciling art and science in psychiatry*. Baltimore: Johns Hopkins University Press.

Goldberg, D. S. (2010). Job and the stigmatization of chronic pain. *Perspectives in Biology and Medicine, 53*(3), 425–438.

Gottschall, J., & Wilson, D. S. (Eds.). (2005). *The literary animal: Evolution and the nature of narrative*. Evanston: Northwestern University Press.

Green, C. (2011). Disparities in pain management and palliative care. In R. J. Moore (Ed.), *Handbook of pain and palliative care*. New York: Springer.

Green, C. R., Anderson, K. O., Baker, T. A., Campbell, L. C., Decker, S., Fillingim, R. B., et al. (2003). The unequal burden of pain: Confronting racial and ethnic disparities in pain. *Pain Medicine, 4*(3), 277–294.

Greenhalgh, T., & Hurwitz, B. (1998). *Narrative based medicine: Dialogue and discourse in clinical practice*. London: BMJ Books.

Gumbrecht, H. L. (2004). *Production of presence: What meaning cannot convey*. Stanford: Stanford University Press.

Hallenbeck, J. (2011). Pain and intercultural communication. In R. J. Moore (Ed.), *Handbook of pain and palliative care*. New York: Springer.

Herman, D. (Ed.). (2007). *The Cambridge companion to narrative*. Cambridge: Cambridge University Press.

Hirstein, W. (2006). *Brain fiction: Self-deception and the riddle of confabulation*. Cambridge: The MIT Press.

Holloway, I., Sofaer-Bennett, B., & Walker, J. (2007). The stigmatisation of people with chronic back pain. *Disability and Rehabilitation, 29*(18), 1456–1464.

Holstein, J., & Gubrium, J. (2000). *The self we live by: Narrative identity in a postmodern world*. New York: Oxford UP.

Hunter, K. (1991). *Doctors' stories: The narrative structure of medical knowledge*. Princeton: Princeton University Press.

Hyvärinen, M. (2006). Towards a conceptual history of narrative. In M. Hyvärinen, A. Korhonen, & J. Mykkänen (Eds.), *The travelling concept of narrative* (pp. 20–41). Helsinki: Helsinki Collegium for Advanced Studies.

Iser, W. (1978). *The act of reading: A theory of aesthetic response*. Baltimore: Johns Hopkins University Press. (First published in German in 1976).

Jauss, H. R. (1982). *Toward an aesthetic of reception* (T. Bahti, Trans.). Minneapolis: University of Minnesota Press.

Jensen, M. C., Brant-Zawadzki, M. N., Obuchowski, N., Modic, M. T., Malkasian, D., & Ross, J. S. (1994). Magnetic resonance imaging of the lumbar spine in people without back pain. *The New England Journal of Medicine, 331*(2), 69–73.

Jensen, M. P., & Karoly, P. (1992). Pain-specific beliefs, perceived symptom severity, and adjustment to chronic pain. *The Clinical Journal of Pain, 8*(2), 123–130.

Jensen, M. P., Turner, J. A., Romano, J. M., & Karoly, P. (1991). Coping with chronic pain: A critical review of the literature. *Pain, 47*(3), 249–283.

Kazis, L. E., Ren, X. S., Lee, A., Skinner, K., Rogers, W., Clark, J., & Miller, D. R. (1999). Health status in VA patients: Results from the Veterans Health Study. *American Journal of Medical Quality, 14*(1), 28–38.

Kearney, R. (2002). *On narrative*. New York: Routledge.

Keogh, E. (2011). Sex differences in pain across the life course. In R. J. Moore (Ed.), *Handbook of pain and palliative care*. New York: Springer.

King, D. W. (2008). *African Americans and the culture of pain*. Charlottesville: University of Virginia Press.

Kleinman, A. (1988). *The illness narratives: Suffering, healing and the human condition*. New York: Basic Books.

Koyama, T., McHaffie, J. G., Laurienti, P. J., & Coghill, R. C. (2005). The subjective experience of pain: Where expectations become reality. *Proceedings of the National Academy of Sciences of the United States of America, 102*(36), 12950–12955.

Kutner, J., & Smith, M. (2011). CAM in chronic pain and palliative care. In R. J. Moore (Ed.), *Handbook of pain and palliative care*. New York: Springer.

Lame, I. E., Peters, M. L., Vlaeyen, J. W., Kleef, M., & Patijn, J. (2005). Quality of life in chronic pain is more associated with beliefs about pain, than with pain intensity. *European Journal of Pain, 9*(1), 15–24.

Loeser, J. D. (1991). What is chronic pain? *Theoretical Medicine, 12*(3), 214–215.

Lopez, S. J., & Snyder, C. R. (Eds.). (2009). *Oxford handbook of positive psychology* (2nd ed.). New York: Oxford University Press.

Macherey, P. (1978). *A theory of literary production* (G. Wall, Trans.). London: Routledge and Kegan Paul. (First published in French in 1966).

Madigan, S. (2010). Narrative therapy. Washington, DC: American Psychological Association.

Markovic, M., Manderson, L., & Warren, N. (2008). Endurance and contest: Women's narratives of endometriosis. *Health (London), 12*(3), 349–367.

Mattingly, C., & Garro, L. C. (2000). *Narrative and the cultural construction of illness and healing*. Berkeley: University of California Press.

May, S. (2011). Chronic low back pain. In R. J. Moore (Ed.), *Handbook of pain and palliative care*. New York: Springer.

McGowan, L., Luker, K., Creed, F., & Chew-Graham, C. A. (2007). "How do you explain a pain that can't be seen?" The narratives of women with chronic pelvic pain and their disengagement with the diagnostic cycle. *British Journal of Health Psychology, 12*(Pt 2), 261–274.

McKee, R. (1997). *Story: Substance, structure, style, and the principles of screenwriting*. New York: HarperCollins.

Meldrum, M. L., Tsao, J. C.-I., & Zeltner, L. K. (2009). "I can't be what I want to be": Children's narratives of chronic pain experiences and treatment outcomes. *Pain Medicine, 10*(6), 1018–1034.

Melzack, R. (1999). From the gate to the neuromatrix. *Pain, 82*(Suppl 1), S121–S126.

Mendelson, G. (1992). Compensation and chronic pain. *Pain, 48*(2), 121–123.

Merskey, H., & Bogduk, N. (Eds.). (1994). *Classification of chronic pain: Descriptions of chronic pain syndromes and definitions of pain terms* (2nd ed.). Seattle: IASP Press.

Michael, M., & Sengers, P. (2003). *Narrative intelligence*. Amsterdam: John Benjamins.

Miller, J. H. (1998). *Reading narrative*. Norman: University of Oklahoma Press.

Morone, N. E., Lynch, C. S., Greco, C. M., Tindle, H. A., & Weiner, D. K. (2008). "I felt like a new person". The effects of mindfulness meditation on older adults with chronic pain: Qualitative narrative analysis of diary entries. *The Journal of Pain, 9*(9), 841–848.

Morris, D. B. (1991). *The culture of pain*. Berkeley: University of California Press.

Morris, D. B. (1998). *Illness and culture in the postmodern age*. Berkeley: University of California Press.

Morris, D. B. (2001). Ethnicity and pain. *Pain Clinical Updates, 9*(4), 1–4.

Morris, D. B. (2002). Narrative, ethics, and pain: Thinking with stories. In R. Charon & M. Montello (Eds.), *Stories matter: The role of narrative in medical ethics* (pp. 196–218). New York: Routledge.

Morris, D. B. (2003). Ethics beyond guidelines: Culture, pain, and conflict. In J. O. Dostrovsky, D. B. Carr, & M. Koltzenburg (Eds.), *Proceedings of the 10th world congress on pain* (pp. 37–48). Seattle: IASP Press.

Morris, D. B. (2005). Success stories. In D. B. Carr, J. D. Loeser, & D. B. Morris (Eds.), *Narrative, pain, and suffering* (pp. 269–285). Seattle: IASP Press.

Morris, D. B. (2008). Narrative medicines: Challenge and resistance. *The Permanente Journal, 12*(1), 88–96.

Morris, D. B. (2009). Foreword. In L. Heshusius. *Inside chronic pain: An intimate and critical account* (pp. xii–xvii). Ithaca: Cornell University Press.

Morris, D. B. (2010a). Intractable pain and the perception of time: Every patient is an anecdote. In C. Stannard, E. Kalso, & J. Ballantyne (Eds.), *Evidence-based chronic pain management* (pp. 52–58). Oxford: Blackwell Publishing.

Morris, D. B. (2010b). Sociocultural dimensions of pain management. In J. C. Ballantyne, J. P. Rathmell, & S. M. Fishman (Eds.), *Bonica's management of pain* (4th ed., pp. 133–145). New York: Lippincott Williams and Wilkins.

National Center for Health Statistics. (2009). *Health, United States, 2009 with special feature on medical technology.* DHHS publication no. 2010–1232. Washington: Department of Health and Human Services.

Nelson, H. (Ed.). (1997). *Stories and their limits: Narrative approaches to bioethics.* New York: Routledge.

Newman, K. (2005). The case for the narrative brain. In Y. Pisan (Ed.), *Proceedings of the Second Australasian Conference on Interactive Entertainment* (pp. 145–149). Sydney, Australia: Creativity and Cognition Studios Press, University of Technology.

Nicolaidis, C. (2002). The Voices of Survivors documentary: Using patient narrative to educate physicians about domestic violence. *Journal of General Internal Medicine, 17*(2), 117–124.

Palermo, Y. (2011). The art of pain: The patient's perspective of chronic pain. In R. J. Moore (Ed.), *Handbook of pain and palliative care.* New York: Springer.

Parker-Pope, T. (2010). *Love and pain relief.* New York Times, 13 October 2010. Retrieved October 13, 2010, from http://www.plosone.org/article/info%3Adoi%2F10.1371%2Fjournal.pone.0013309.

Pollo, A., & Benedetti, F. (2011). Pain and the placebo/nocebo effect. In R. J. Moore (Ed.), *Handbook of pain and palliative care.* New York: Springer.

Radley, A. (2009). *Works of illness: Narrative, picturing and the social response to serious disease.* Ashby-de-la-Zouch, UK: InkerMen Press.

Råheim, M., & Håland, W. (2006). Lived experience of chronic pain and fibromyalgia: Women's stories from daily life. *Qualitative Health Research, 16*(6), 741–761.

Remen, R. (1996). *Kitchen table wisdom: Stories that heal.* New York: Riverhead Books.

Rich, B. A. (2011). The delineation and explication of palliative options of last resort. In R. J. Moore (Ed.), *Handbook of pain and palliative care.* New York: Springer.

Sacks, O. (1985). *The man who mistook his wife for a hat and other clinical tales.* New York: Simon and Schuster.

Sarbin, T. R. (Ed.). (1986). *Narrative psychology: The storied nature of human conduct.* New York: Praeger.

Shutty, M. S., Jr., DeGood, D. E., & Tuttle, D. H. (1990). Chronic pain patients' beliefs about their pain and treatment outcomes. *Archives of Physical Medicine and Rehabilitation, 71*(2), 128–132.

Sontag, S. (1978). *Illness as metaphor.* New York: Farrar, Straus and Giroux.

Steihaug, S., & Malterud, K. (2008). Stories about bodies: A narrative study on self-understanding and chronic pain. *Scandinavian Journal of Primary Health Care, 26*(3), 188–192.

Taylor, J. B. (2006). *My stroke of insight: A brain scientist's personal journey.* New York: Viking.

Tedeschi, R. G., & Calhoun, L. (2004). Posttraumatic growth: A new perspective on psychotraumatology. *Psychiatric Times, 21*(4). Retrieved February 23, 2009, from http://www.psychiatrictimes.com/display/article/10168/54661.

Thernstrom, M. (2011). *The pain chronicles: Cures, myths, mysteries, prayers, diaries, brain scans, healing and the science of suffering.* New York: Picador.

Todd, K. H. (2001). Influence of ethnicity on emergency department pain management. *Emergency Medicine, 13*(3), 274–278.

Tompkins, J. P. (Ed.). (1980). *Reader-response criticism: From formalism to post-structuralism.* Baltimore: Johns Hopkins University Press.

Turner, M. (1996). *The literary mind: The origins of thought and language.* New York: Oxford University Press.

Van Middendorp, H., Lumley, M. A., Jacobs, J. W. G., Bijlsma, J. W. J., & Geenen, R. (2010). The effects of anger and sadness on clinical pain reports and experimentally-induced pain thresholds in women with and without fibromyalgia. *Arthritis Care & Research (Hoboken), 62*(10), 1370–1376.

Vegni, E., Mauri, E., & Moja, E. A. (2005). Stories from doctors of patients with pain: A qualitative research on the physicians' perspective. *Supportive Care in Cancer, 13*(1), 2–4.

Von Korff, M., Barlow, W., Cherkin, D., & Deyo, R. A. (1994). Effects of practice style in managing back pain. *Annals of Internal Medicine, 121*(3), 187–195.

Wailoo, K. (2006). Stigma, race, and disease in 20th century America. *Lancet, 367*(9509), 531–533.

Waitzkin, H., & Magaña, H. (1997). The black box in somatization: Unexplained physical symptoms, culture, and narratives of trauma. *Social Science & Medicine, 45*, 811–825.

Wallis, C. (2005). The right (and wrong) way to treat pain. *Time.* Retrieved August 11, 2010, from http://www.time.com/time/magazine/article/0,9171,1029836-1,00.html.

Werner, A., Isaksen, L. W., & Malterud, K. (2004). "I am not the kind of woman who complains of everything": Illness stories on self and shame in women with chronic pain. *Social Science & Medicine, 59*(5), 1035–1045.

White, M. (2007). *Maps of narrative practice.* New York: Norton.

White, M., &Epson, D. (1990). *Narrative means to Therapeutic Ends.* New York: Norton.

Williams, D. A. (1996). Acute pain management. In R. J. Gatchel & D. C. Turk (Eds.), *Psychological approaches to pain management: A practitioner's handbook* (pp. 55–77). New York: Guilford Press.

Williams, D. A., & Keefe, F. J. (1991). Pain beliefs and the use of cognitive-behavioral coping strategies. *Pain, 46*(1), 185–190.

Williams, D. A., & Thorn, B. E. (1989). An empirical assessment of pain beliefs. *Pain, 36*(3), 351–358.

Wilson, T. D. (2011). . New York: Little, Brown.*Redirect: The surprising new science of psychological change*

Winslow, M., Seymour, J., & Clark, D. (2005). Stories of cancer pain: A historical perspective. *Journal of Pain and Symptom Management, 29*(1), 22–31.

Younger, J., Aron, A., Parke, S., Chatterjee, N., & Mackey, S. (2010). Viewing pictures of a romantic partner reduces experimental pain: Involvement of neural reward systems. *PLoS ONE, 5*(10), e13309. Retrieved October 14, 2010, from doi: 10.1371/journal.pone.0013309.

Zaroff, L. (2009). Learning compassion, learning forgiveness. *Hektoen International: A Journal of Medical Humanities, 4*, np.

Chapter 39
Representations of the Body in Pain: Anthropological Approaches

Nora L. Jones

Practitioners and chronic pain sufferers inhabit distinct symbolic worlds. Their expectations of what pain, if visualized, would look like, their understandings of how pain can be represented, and their views on the relationship between vision and knowing differ fundamentally. The ways that chronic pain sufferers and the practitioners who treat them visualize pain are influenced by why they want to see and visually represent pain and by their understanding of valid and applicable evidence. Thus, the visual representation of the body in pain cannot take a singular form, but is instead a multifaceted collection of images created from the unique positions, needs, and motivations of the viewers and creators of the image. While medicine often works as if it's convinced itself that pain is entirely a medical problem (Morris 1991:1–2), in many respects it is also very much a symbolic problem.

To understand this symbolic problem this essay will consider two distinct but intimately related endeavors: the effort by medical practitioners to create specific, technologically mediated images of the source of a patient's pain, and the parallel efforts by pain sufferers to use visual imagery to make sense of and communicate their experiences. Over a decade ago anthropologist Arthur Kleinman and colleagues wrote that we live in an age of the picture, and that experience has become "mediatized" (Kleinman et al. 1996: xiii). The first years of the twenty-first century will most likely go down as some of the most visually documented and mediated in history. Experience in these years has also become more medicalized than ever before, and these two related influences on experience are at the heart of the symbolic problem of pain. The twenty-first century finds us seeking and granting authority to underlying medical explanations for an increasingly vast range of conditions, and submitting our bodies to an array of "medical vision machines" that not only dictate our relations with practitioners, but "drive and maintain popular narratives of selves, bodies, death and life" (Kuppers 2004:123), and I would add, pain, as well.

The symbolic problem of pain stems from the fact that a pain sufferer in many ways lives in the world of medicine, but the medicalized and mediatized realm of medicine cannot encompass the embodied totality of the sufferer. In other words, while the patient and her practitioner both turn to the technologies and images of medicine to diagnose and treat pain, our patient is limited by the medical terms of the setting from truly expressing the personal embodied experience of pain. Simultaneously, but in parallel, our patient, who independent of the medical realm is also embedded in the larger mediatized climate of the twenty-first century, turns to nondiagnostic visual and artistic outlets in order to craft more personally authentic images of herself and her pain. The paradox of the

N.L. Jones, PhD (✉)
Department of Medical Ethics, University of Pennsylvania, Philadelphia, PA, USA
e-mail: noralj@upenn.edu

R.J. Moore (ed.), *Handbook of Pain and Palliative Care: Biobehavioral Approaches for the Life Course*, DOI 10.1007/978-1-4419-1651-8_39, © Springer Science+Business Media, LLC 2012

symbolic problem of pain is that while the verbal and visual languages of medicine are poorly equipped to incorporate the embodied person, the languages and worlds of medicine affect the embodiment of the sufferer, but in return the verbal and visual languages of the embodied person cannot penetrate the medical. The sufferer is caught between two symbolic systems with very little overlap.

The world of pain is in many ways an ideal subject for anthropological inquiry, with its disciplinary attention to embodiment and the range of worlds – physical, biological, social, and symbolic – that humans inhabit. While neuroscientists and a myriad of other clinician researchers strive to uncover the physical and biological secrets of chronic pain, social scientists and humanities scholars study the ways in which pain affects the sufferer's social and symbolic worlds (Kleinman 1992; Morris 1991; Scarry 1987). Pain renders a fault line in a sufferer's life (Morris 1991:31) that disrupts the totality of the sufferer by affecting her physical, biological, social, and symbolic worlds (see also, Morris 2011). Diagnostic imaging is one way practitioners seek to understand the physical and biological elements of pain, and pain art is a means through which sufferers seek to address and redress the fissure in their social and symbolic worlds.

Images of pain, both those produced in the clinical quest to treat pain and those produced by sufferers as they live with pain, should be thought of as key players in the conversations that practitioners, sufferers, and the nonpain suffering public undertake (see also Palermo 2011). The social and symbolic worlds of medicine are implicated in the manner in which the physical and biological are understood, and the clinical management of the physical and biological worlds is implicated in the social and symbolic lives and art products of the sufferers. Visual images of pain act as a nexus in how pain is communicated, experienced, and integrated into a person's life. The images thus take on interest not only because of the reason behind their creation or their subsequent interpretations and uses. It is the complex of the myriad roles they play in social relations that is revealing. Images of pain speak to the larger lived experiences of sufferers, the practitioners who treat them, and to the role and identity of pain and pain patients in society in general. Because of this, the nonpractitioner and nonsuffering public are involved in the conversation as well. This chapter surveys these various visualizations of pain and concludes with a proposal for an ethics for looking. I begin with pain visualized in medicine, as it is the dominant mode to which much of visual symbolic work of sufferers reacts.

Pain Visualized in Medicine

The evolution of the role of vision in medicine from Renaissance anatomists to computer scanning through the course of the eighteenth to the twenty-first century marks a radical shift from a text-dependent to a visually dependent system of knowledge and authority. The power and authority of the medical way of seeing has in large part derived from medical technology's increasingly sophisticated and exclusive methods of visualizing the hidden reaches of the body (Delehanty 2010:167; Spiro 2009). Our traditional understanding of technology is that it is developed and adopted because it is efficient at solving a problem: better imaging technology aids the development of increasingly sophisticated treatments. What is often neglected is the need to also look at how the technology changes how we view the world (Spiro 2009).

One such consequence of the development of diagnostic pain imaging technology is a linkage between such testing and the medical legitimization of pain (Spiro 2009). This relationship between diagnostic imaging testing and the legitimization of pain stems in large part from a set of cultural assumptions, shared by both practitioners and patients, that make seeing into the body the apex of legitimizing and confirming patient syndromes, and from the general appeal of the concreteness of diagnostic images (Rhodes et al. 1999; Spiro 2009). This hegemonic link between "seeing" and "reality" has become so engrained that the technology of medical imaging has fundamentally changed the nature of the relationship between patient and provider. The patient is no longer the subject/object of attention; the reproduction of the patient in the form of a visual image has become a stand-in for the patient, and has affected how the patient is communicated with (Spiro 2009). Given that pain, in our current state of the art of knowledge, often does not prove amenable to the diagnostic imaging tools available, when pain cannot be seen, when there are no visual documents to communicate with, the patient is often left adrift (Spiro 2009).

The literature is replete with patient stories documenting their practitioners' search for the diagnostic imaging test that will locate the source of the pain. Such a search produces a symbolical representation of the body (Zwart 1998:108). These representations do not, however, reflect an independent reality. While we as a culture may assume that medical images such as CT scans or MRIs are pictures of a person, they are in fact symbols that we have all agreed to agree represent the person. In this assumption we have placed great power, for in this role the images, these symbols, do not reflect but structure our reality (Zwart 1998:108; Spiro 2009; see also Palermo 2011). When images are used in diagnosis, they become an indelible part of a story. They create the where and how stories of pain, not just describing or representing pain, but establishing that experience and reality in both the clinic setting and in pain sufferers' extra-clinic lives (Good 1994). Sometimes, when the source of pain is located in the diagnostic image, the symbolization of the clinic matches that of lived reality. Other times, when the pain cannot be located in a symbolic form that medicine recognizes, the symbolic stories do not match, a condition with consequences for the lived reality of pain.

Diagnostic imaging leads to different stories about our insides than the narratives a patient's senses can see and make knowable, a problem of a "noncoincidence of visual evidence" (Kuppers 2004:125). In the medical realm, chronic unrelieved pain patients who lack a diagnostic image to accompany their diagnosis often must depend solely on words. But words without a form of concomitant proof that makes sense in the symbolic world of medicine fall flat. As seen in the example of one patient whose pain was eventually "found" in a diagnostic image, "what she had been saying to her doctor could not be heard, until to her joy, it could be seen" (Rhodes et al. 1999:1195).

When pain cannot be seen through diagnostic imaging modalities, practitioners sometimes will call on nondiagnostic images in their treatment plans. Similar to the way that some pain specialists use music as therapy, looking at pictures and guided imagery have been pursued as a nonpharmacological intervention in pain management (Tse et al. 2005; Moore and Spiegel 2000). Also common in the literature on pain are studies addressing the benefits of making pictures. These studies fall into two camps. The first camp considers art as a therapeutic modality, and the benefit is balanced between a tool for practitioner interpretation and the benefits of the action itself for the patient. Researchers write of the creation of art as a means for pain sufferers to make sense of the lived experience of their pain (Moore and Spiegel 2000) or to assist in self-expression of experiences that are too stressful to put in words (Reynolds and Prior 2006).

The second camp asks patients to draw self-portraits, pictures of their pain, or portraits of themselves in pain, as entry to practitioner interpretation, analogous to practitioners' use of an X-ray – as entry to a hidden realm inside the body, only in this case into the mind. It makes sense that in cases of chronic unrelieved pain, medicine would turn to both art therapy and art as therapy. Practitioners and researchers, when pain cannot be seen in ways understood by the symbolic modalities of medicine, exhibit a rising enthusiasm for the psychological interpretations of art therapy (Rhodes et al. 1999: 1196). The goal is to produce art that the practitioner can use in several ways: to understand the patient's experience (Unruh et al. 1983; Stefanatou and Bowler 1997; Kortesluoma et al. 2008), to learn about the patient's expectations of and hopes for their doctor visits (Lewis et al. 1996), and as a conduit to sufferer's subconscious fears and inner emotions (Bayrakci et al. 2009).

The terms of such art-mediated encounters are most often those of the practitioners: patients draw and practitioners interpret. One exception is a small 2003 study of 14 adult patients in pain management programs in New Zealand who were given assorted art supplies and materials and asked to make a drawing, sketch, or picture collage of their pain (Henare et al. 2003). They then shared their image and story in the group and taped a one-on-one interview with the researchers about their image and story. The authors did much more than report on their own thematic analysis, giving equal weight to the patients' own words about their paintings. Art became a means of communication, considered as equally complex as verbal language. As one participant stated, "as I started drawing myself, I started to relate very personally to myself … it's a media that's been able to clarify" (Henare et al. 2003: 516). The under-examined question, however, is clarify to whom, and clarify what? For this participant the process was clarifying to her, and this indeed is one of the keys to this study. The primary lesson of this study is that patients want a way to express their pain, in addition to relief, of course. It is unclear, although one can guess based on medicine's affinity for epidemiological, large-scale, double-blind, and multisited studies, to what extent this study's findings will resonate within the field as a whole. It is a question of being heard and seen in ways medicine is unfortunately often incapable of. With or without medical visual "proof" of pain, pain is not something that can just be suffered, it has to be made sense of (Morris 1991: 18). Akin to the allure of visuals in medical diagnostics, there is something generally appealing in the nonclinical visual depiction and communication of pain as well. So whether a pain sufferer finds herself in a situation in which medicine and diagnostic testing have failed and her words about pain have fallen on deaf ears, or in cases when testing has succeeded and practitioners "know" exactly why someone is in pain but cannot translate that knowledge into an authentic and shared understanding of the experience of pain, she may turn to self-made visual representations of her pain.

The Allure of the Visual in Communicating Pain

The allure of the visual for artists, as for practitioners, is the presumed direct relationship between images and evidence and vision and knowledge, that seeing something is key to knowing it and proving its existence. What distinguishes the approach to visuals by artists and practitioners is their understandings of what is considered valid visual evidence and the divide between what is labeled objective vs. subjective data. The embodied experience of the pain sufferer leads to a blurring of the traditional boundaries between subjective and objective that are a hallmark of the system of medical evidence and symbolizing.

There are two key reasons why pain sufferers turn to self-made visual representations of their pain. The first stems from the well-analyzed incommunicability of pain, a situation in part the result of medicine's ideological linkage of evidence with images over language, a form of data that is often deemed inadequate or insufficient subjective evidence. The literature on the social and symbolic realms of pain is replete with discussions of the language of pain. It is said that because language falls short, sufferers must resort to inadequate metaphors (Biro 2010; Das 1996; Scarry 1987). A danger of this inadequacy of words is that when words are not believed or understood, then worlds are not believed or understood as well. Going even further, pain can become such an assault on the body and self, and on language and communication, that the point is reached in which there is nothing at all that can be said (Morris 1991:73). In such cases, a communication void exists that needs to be filled, and the visual stands ready to step in. As the editor-in-chief of the journal *Pain* wrote, "You can't articulate it, and you can't see it. There is no question people often try to illustrate their pain" (Parker-Pope 2008).

Which brings us to the second, interrelated factor in the allure of the visual – the assumptions we as a culture make about visuals, an assumption nicely encapsulated by the adage "a picture is worth a thousand words." As Mark Collen, curator of the online "PAIN Exhibit" writes, "Words are limiting, but art elicits an emotional response. … People don't believe what they can't see. But they see a piece of art an individual created about their pain and everything changes" (Parker-Pope 2008).

Similarly, the initiator of a 1989 "Images of Pain" exhibit, a collection of solicited work from migraine sufferers, said that it was his concern that doctors were not hearing their patients when it came to headache pain that led him to the idea that visual art could be used as a tool to "allow patients to *speak* to us" about their pain (Wickelgren 1989: 136, emphasis mine).

Speaking of, or otherwise representing pain, is a means of moving the intimate personal experience of pain to an interpersonal arena. The extent to which this is possible is debated by pain scholars, however. Some argue that pain is such a powerful force that it cannot be shared by others as it is incapable of being communicated across the pain/painless border (Scarry 1987). This phenomeno-logical perspective seems to say that you cannot understand something unless you have personal experience with it. Others claim that pain is universal (Sandblom 1982), and that it is only our unex-amined standard dichotomies of social and individual that serve as a barrier to understanding the fact that pain is a social experience, both collective and individual (Morris 1991: 38, Moore and Spiegel 2000; Kleinman et al. 1996:xii).

Even if others do not fully understand the personal experience of pain, the act of putting yourself out there either through speech or art holds value and is liberating because the speaker or artist is in control (see also Palermo 2011). This is one of the appeals for pain patients to create their own images. In the clinic the patient is a relatively passive recipient of others' imaging; as an artist the individual herself is in control of the image's creation and display. She initiates the encounter of communicating pain. Speaking of or showing pain should not be considered an indicative statement, but the beginning of a "language game, ... making a claim for acknowledgment, which may be given or denied" (Das 1996: 70). In the New Zealand pain study, the act of sharing the story with the group was done on the premise that "declaring oneself publicly" is a key part of the process of healing from, even if not being treated for, pain (Henare et al. 2003: 512). Analogous to the signifying role of diagnostic images in the medical story of a patient's symptoms, pain sufferers are turning to their own works of art to create and share their own story on their own terms (Radley 2002; see also Palermo 2011). It is to these works that I now turn.

The Work of Art

One of the most common lines of study about the relationship between pain and art is the effect of pain on the artist and her work. Paul Klee, for example, suffered from scleroderma, and reached a point where he could hardly paint for hand and finger pain. As he became sicker, his style became simpler, less colorful, and dominated by thick black lines, changes said to reflect in two dimen-sions the lived agony he was feeling (Aronson and Ramachandran 2010). With Frieda Kahlo as a notable exception, it is less common to see pain itself represented in art. Because the production and consumption of a picture is culturally framed, and because pain in contemporary North American culture is conceptualized as a uniquely personal experience, the public expression of the body in pain can be regarded as inappropriate, and is relatively uncommon in the cannon of American art history (Annus 2008: 111; the extent to which Kahlo's status as an exception is due to her Mexican heritage is beyond the scope of this chapter). As with illnesses generally, contem-porary American culture actively tries to hide pain and teaches us to confront it with silence and denial (Morris 1991: 71). Illness and pain run counter to most symbols and metaphors of what being an American is – strong, industrious, and uncomplaining. Thus, the pain that is represented is often of a particular kind, characterized as heroic or spiritual (Annus 2008; Morris 1991). Pain can be depicted, for example, if the sufferer encounters the pain in a heroic battle, common in late eighteenth-century battle scenes, or as is seen in the second half of the nineteenth century, if the suffering is of a more spiritual nature, as in the pain of those on the margins, such as slaves and women (Annus 2008: 102, 107).

When pain is depicted more literally, in the form of crumpled bodies or mangled flesh, it often expresses defiance towards medicine, representing pain as a demon that medicine cannot alleviate or exorcise (see Morris 1991, Chap. 2). Goya's famous capricho, *De que mal morira*? (Of what ill will he die?), showing a sick man being treated by a physician in the form of a donkey, was created when a doctor's ministrations could be worse than the disease and in fact kill you. Today patients generally do not die from a treatment, but medicine's focus on curing the disease to the detriment of healing the illness (Kleinman 1981) has led to a new form of patient defiance, a defiance of the dehumanizing effects of the mechanical eyes of diagnostic technology and the overwhelming bureaucracy of the institution of medicine (Spiro 2009; see also Palermo 2011). Pain art further defies the silence that living in pain has traditionally entailed, as well as the very notion of restricted or privileged imaging of pain. Pain art is a visual statement that draws its viewers into a dialogue that defies the general lack of attention given to the lived realities of illness.

One of the most startling examples of the invisibility of the lived reality of illness and pain is found in the beautiful and powerful *Exploding into Life*, a visual and textual chronicle of Dorothea Lynch's experiences with and death from breast cancer (Lynch and Richards 1986). Lynch provided the words, while her friend, photographer Eugene Richards, took the photographs. The anecdote that stands out is Lynch's recounting of asking the American Cancer Society for images of mastectomy procedures and postoperative appearance as she herself prepared to undergo the surgery. She was told that such images were not suitable for a nonmedical audience. Whether this is a problem of the medical establishment of the early 1980s or in general is hard to discern. But the ironic situation that finds patients not considered appropriate witnesses to the symbolic realm of medicine remains today.

Jo Spence is a contemporary of Lynch and another sufferer of breast cancer who visually documented her experiences with cancer and the associated physical, social, and symbolic pain. Unlike Lynch, Spence was a photographer before her illness. Upon her diagnosis she turned her eyes and lens to her own body in attempts to navigate and make sense of her experiences. In many of her early images she stands facing the camera with her breasts exposed, adding text to her body to interrogate herself and the viewer. In one of her most famous images she has written on the side of her breast the words "Property of Jo Spence?" The question mark at the end is a key to the viewer about the symbolic rift that has occurred to Spence as she has moved through the medical system. Is her body still her own?, the image asks. Particularly in her direct gaze to the viewer, Spence's work defied the authoritative and overpowering gaze of the medical imaging machines and practitioners.

The work that Lynch and Spence did in the relative privacy of their own social networks, being spread to the public only later through publishing houses and art galleries, is being done now on a daily basis by the "everyday" sufferers of pain and illness. The Internet has been integral to democratizing imaging pain. Increasing public outlets provide more space for taking back the visual images of pain, defying not only patients' forced passivity in the medical realm but the general invisibility of pain as well. One of the most comprehensive of these public sites is the online PAIN exhibit, the mission of which is "to educate healthcare providers and the public about chronic pain through art, and to give voice to the many who suffer in abject silence" (painexhibit.com). The gallery is broken into nine sections: Portraits of Pain, Suffering, But You Look So Normal, Pain Visualized, God and Religion, Miscellaneous, Isolation and Imprisonment, Unconditional Love, and Hope and Transformation. In keeping with the theme of this chapter, I will focus here on the work related to "Pain Visualized."

The central theme of the works categorized in the "Pain Visualized" section is encapsulated in the words of contributing artist Joan Crutcher, who writes, "No one can see the agony inside of me. This is my only way to show what it is like." Many of the artists' statements in the exhibit include statements about how empowering the act of creating pain art is and the therapeutic benefits to the art. Akin to the ways in which art therapy is used in clinical settings for unrelieved pain, artist Jennifer Shifflet writes that her "internal landscape" paintings, inspired by the MRIs undertaken in the efforts to locate and treat her pain, became a "means for me to transform and find meaning in what cannot otherwise be healed through conventional medicine" (see also Palermo 2011). Resonating with this theme of the therapeutic importance of presenting pain visually is the statement from Heather Davulcu, who writes that painting is the only means for her to communicate the true depth of her pain and isolation: "It has been therapeutic, not only in creating the piece, but also in sharing it with others" (see also Palermo 2011).

While many of the themes that were found in the medical research on the therapeutic benefits of patients making art are in evidence here as well, there is a key difference between the artists and the researchers in terms of the notion of visual evidence. Whereas the medical researchers used the visual products of their subjects and patients as therapy, whether or not the images "proved" anything was not considered. The notion that art is a form of visual proof is distinct to the social and symbolic worlds of art, and perhaps the public as well. As artist Christine Feterowski wrote on her piece *See what I feel*, "See what I feel. Chronic pain uncovered," in this work the intent of pain art is made explicit – see what I feel, see me, see my world. The reception of the work of art and the obligations incurred by the viewer upon being presented with this invitation is the topic to which I now turn (see also Palermo 2011).

An Ethics of Looking

It is my contention that communicating pain visually should be approached as a conversation. What I mean by this is that what is interesting and informative about pain pictures is not *only* the creators' intent, nor *only* the viewers' interpretations, but the complex of creator, work, viewer, and sociohistorical context. Pain art, like pain itself, exists in multiple worlds. It is not unified or unitary, but polyvocal, coming from and speaking to sufferers' lives, medicine and its practitioners, the art world, and popular culture. The key unifying question here is how images made by ill people do their work (Radley 2009). In other words, visuals are more than pictures, more than documents of reality. We can look through them to better understand makers, viewers, and their contexts and interrelations (see also Palermo 2011).

In intent, pain art for sufferers is equivalent to a physician's use of an X-ray; it gives the sufferer the ability to say, "see, right here, here is my pain and this is what it looks like." Despite not carrying weight in a clinical diagnostic sense, pain art is considered by practitioners, exhibit curators, and patients as authoritative statements of experience. The public display of pain pictures is an invitation to engage in a conversation about that experience. Our obligation as viewers is to participate.

Science has also addressed the connection between viewers and images of pain in its own terms. Researchers asked nonpain experiencing people to look at painful images while in an fMRI machine, and found that when looking at images of recognized painful situations, the subjects experienced changes in their brains in regions known to play a role in pain processing (Jackson et al. 2005). Their conclusion was that perceiving the pain of others leads to a state of "intersubjective empathy" where we feel others' pain ourselves (see also Hallenbeck 2011; Moore and Hallenbeck 2010). I have no basis to doubt or question these findings, but as an anthropologist I am less interested in the behavior of brains in controlled research settings than I am with the behavior of people in real-world situations, such as choosing to visit the PAINexhibit website or viewing and engaging with any other pain art on public display.

As with all art or visual products, when we look, we are not just looking at the person, object, or image itself, but at the relationship between the person, object, or image, and *ourselves* (Berger 1972). Thus, looking at pictures of pain engages the viewer directly with the creator of the image. Similarly, people's responses to representations depicting illness tell us about the relationship of individuals to medicine and to each other (Radley 2009: 17). A viewer needs some knowledge or interpretive framework to see something *as* something, rather than just a mixture of different colored areas (Delehanty 2010: 162). In other words, viewers cannot leave images uninterpreted. We apply our own framework and attribute meaning. Depending on the subject position of the viewer, looking at images of pain may elicit sympathy, disgust, gratitude for one's own lack of pain, or any other of a myriad of responses, based on the viewer's own health and history and attitudes about pain, health, and medicine in general. This suggests that the art of pain should be looked at not only in terms of beauty and therapy, but in the context of ideology and politics of care as well.

Siebers, writing more generally about late twentieth-century body art, which he defines as art that implicates the body in direct ways (using the body or bodily products as the raw material of art, for example), a genre in which pain art can be included, says that this "new art" is "ugly and terrifying at first, but we are compelled to accept it as beautiful if we are to remain human ourselves" (Siebers 2000: 222). The question of looking at and seeing images of pain, and by extension people in pain, is a question of spirit, of recognizing, being open to listening to and engaging with the work, and to not disconfirming the worlds and lives implicated in the images. The number of blogs, websites, and academic articles on living with untreatable pain indicate that the subjective evidence for pain is overwhelming; the time has come to conceptualize new forms of evidence for it (Biro 2010: 661). If, epistemologically, seeing is believing, then new ways of seeing, such as evidenced in the pain art of today, should lead us to thinking about and believing in these new ways of seeing (Delehanty 2010: 168).

Though, while art allows sufferers to put pain into forms that "speak" to a universal audience, the societal bias towards medicine drives many to attempt to image, and thus validate, pain using diagnostic imaging devices. This makes the question of the meaning of images of pain not only an epistemological question, but also a question of power. Because medicine's technologies and treatments are able to diagnose and alleviate much pain, we do not know what to do with pain that remains. The symbolic realm of medicine does not reach far enough. The visual representation of pain speaks to how we privilege and what knowledge system we are working in. And in this way I mean that pain is a symbolic problem. Practitioners and patients are not just speaking a different language, they are seeing in different ways.

And this is where the disciplinary framework of anthropology can add a valuable voice. Anthropologists are in many ways cultural translators, attempting to reword and represent one lifeway for another audience. And this translation can work both ways, helping practitioners to understand and see the patient's life course and worldview, and likewise helping pain patients to understand the medical system in which they are embedded. The challenge is harder on the practitioner side, for what this framework is asking is for the field of medicine to look critically at itself, be reflexive about its own biases, and to then be open to validating alternative ways of seeing the world in general and pain in particular. So if anthropology, and anthropologists specifically working in and with the medical arena, can help lend credence and validity to alternative ways of seeing, showing that the two systems exist and work in tandem, and not that one system should supplant the other, then anthropology can help the field of medicine to take visuals seriously, in the way that their patients are.

References

Annus, I. E. (2008). Seeing pain: The visual representation of pain in American painting. In N. Pascual & A. B. Gonzales (Eds.), *Feeling in others: Essays on empathy and suffering in modern American culture* (pp. 101–116). Berlin: Wien Zürich Berlin Münster Lit.

Aronson, J. K., & Ramachandran, M. (2010). The diagnosis of art: Scleroderma in Paul Klee – and Rembrandt's scholar? *Journal of the Royal Society of Medicine, 103*(2), 70–71.

Bayrakci, B., Forouz, A., Sahin, A. B., Abali, M., & Aliyeva, G. Z. (2009). Disease painting or painting disease: How does illness and hospitalisation affect children's artistry? *Perception, 38*, 1721–1727.

Berger, J. (1972). *Ways of Seeing*. London: British Broadcasting Corporation and Penguin Books.

Biro, D. (2010). Is there such a thing as psychological pain? And why it matters. *Culture, Medicine and Psychiatry, 34*(4), 658–667.

Das, V. (1996). Language and body: Transactions in the construction of pain. *Daedalus, 125*(1), 67–91.

Delehanty, M. (2010). Why images? *Medicine Studies, 2*, 161–173.

Good, B. (1994). *Chapter 3: How medicine constructs its objects, in meaning, rationality, and experience: An anthropological perspective* (pp. 65–87). Cambridge: Cambridge University Press.

Henare, D., Hocking, C., & Smythe, L. (2003). Chronic pain: Gaining understanding through the use of art. *British Journal of Occupational Therapy, 66*(11), 511–518.

Jackson, P. L., Meltzoff, A. N., & Decety, J. (2005). How do we perceive the pain of others? A window into the neural processes involved in empathy. *NeuroImage, 24*(3), 771–779.

Kleinman, A. (1981). *Patients and healers in the context of culture*. Berkeley: University of California Press.

Kleinman, A. (1992). Pain and resistance: The delegitimation and relegitimation of local worlds. In B. Good et al. (Eds.), *Pain as human experience: An anthropological perspective* (pp. 169–197). Berkeley: University of California Press.

Kleinman, A., Das, D., & Lock, M. (1996). Introduction, social suffering. *Daedalus, 125*(1), XI–XX.

Kortesluoma, R., Punamaki, R., & Nikkonen, M. (2008). Hospitalized children drawing their pain: The contents and cognitive and emotional characteristics of pain drawings. *Journal of Child Health Care, 12*(4), 284–300.

Kuppers, P. (2004). Visions of anatomy: Exhibitions and dense bodies. *Differences: A Journal of Feminist Cultural Studies, 15*(3), 123–156.

Lewis, D. W., Middlebrook, M. T., Mehallick, L., Rauch, T. M., Deline, C., & Thomas, E. (1996). Pediatric headaches: What do the children want? *Headache: The Journal of Head and Face Pain, 36*(4), 224–230.

Lynch, D., & Richards, E. (1986). *Exploding into Life*. New York: Aperture.

Moore, R. J., & Spiegel, D. (2000). Uses of guided imagery for pain control by African-American and white women with metastatic breast cancer. *Integrative Medicine, 2*(2–3), 115–126.

Moore, R. J., & Hallenbeck, J. (2010). Narrative empathy and how dealing with stories helps: Creating a space for empathy in culturally diverse care settings. *Journal of Pain and Symptom Management, 40*(3), 471–476.

Morris, D. B. (1991). *The culture of pain*. Berkeley: University of California Press.

Parker-Pope, T. (2008). *Pain as an Art Form*. The New York Times, April 22. Retrieved November 1, 2010, from http://well.blogs.nytimes.com/2008/04/22/pain-as-an-art-form/.

Radley, A. (2002). Portrayals of suffering: On looking away, looking at, and the comprehension of the illness experience. *Body & Society, 8*(3), 1–23.

Radley, A. (2009). *Works of illness: Narrative, picturing, and the social response to serious disease*. London: InkerMen Press.

Reynolds, F., & Prior, S. (2006). The role of art-making in identity maintenance: Case studies of people living with cancer. *European Journal of Cancer Care, 15*, 333–341.

Rhodes, L. A., McPhillips-Tangum, C. A., Markham, C., & Klenk, R. (1999). The power of the visible: The meaning of diagnostic tests in chronic back pain. *Social Science & Medicine, 48*, 1189–1203.

Sandblom, P. (1982). *Creativity and disease: How illness affects literature, art and music*. Philadelphia: George F. Stickley Publisher.

Scarry, E. (1987). *The body in pain: The making and unmaking of the world*. Oxford: Oxford University Press.

Siebers, T. (2000). The new art. In T. Siebers (Ed.), *The body aesthetic: From fine art to body modification*. Michigan: University of Michigan Press.

Spiro, H. (2009). Narrative approaches to understanding the meaning of the pain experience. In R. J. Moore (Ed.), *Biobehavioral approaches to pain*. New York: Springer Press.

Stefanatou, A., & Bowler, D. (1997). Depiction of pain in the self-drawings of children with sickle cell disease. *Child: Care, Health and Development, 23*(2), 135–155.

Tse, M. M., Pun, S. P., & Benzie, I. F. (2005). Affective images: Relieving chronic pain and enhancing quality of life for older persons. *Cyberpsychology & Behavior, 8*(6), 571–579.

Unruh, A., McGrath, P., Cunningham, S. J., & Humphreys, P. (1983). Children's drawings of their pain. *Pain, 17*, 385–392.

Wickelgren, I. (1989). Images of pain; headache art lends a hand to science. *Science News, 136*(9), 136–137.

Zwart, H. (1998). Medicine, symbolization and the "real" body – Lacan's understanding of medical science. *Medicine, Health Care and Philosophy, 1*(2), 107–117.

Morris, D. B. (2011). Narrative and pain: Towards an integrative model. In R. J. Moore (Ed.), *Handbook of pain and palliative care*. New York: Springer.

Palermo, Y. (2011). The art of pain: The patient's perspective of chronic pain. In R. J. Moore (Ed.), *Handbook of pain and palliative care*. New York: Springer.

Hallenbeck, J. (2011). Pain and intercultural communication. In R. J. Moore (Ed.), *Handbook of pain and palliative care*. New York: Springer.

Chapter 40
The Art of Pain: The Patient's Perspective of Chronic Pain

Yvonne Palermo

The Art of Pain

As a terminal chronic pain patient, and I say terminal because it is just that. Never letting up, never going away, and yes I will die with this degeneration and torture known as pain.

I find myself learning that my accomplishments are trivial to the basic need to just get up in the morning. However, I am very thankful that my art is an outlet for advocacy to the public. Bringing awareness is a necessity, we are grossly overlooked, and patients with pain are neglected and misunderstood. This must change, and that is my goal in this chapter to teach you about the depth of what health care providers are doing whether incorrect or wonderful, and to visually see pain as I experience the torture.

I find it interesting that I was a healer in the health care field and then found myself changing roles from healing others to being the one in the hospital bed. It is a lesson, and has opened my mind, and broke my heart to see how bad our health care system truly is toward managing chronic pain. I love creating and expressing my journey through my art. I accomplish something every day, just by getting up and moving out of bed. The simple becomes the majestic. All people need to know that they are one accident away from walking in my shoes, so be aware that the simple things in life should be enjoyed just as much as the bigger ideals in life. I will continue to paint, create my life through visual means to enforce that we exist, the massive amount of pain patients, and stop the ignorance and stigmas that have swarmed those three words – "Chronic Pain Patient."

Healing truly begins by listening, taking the time to understand, believe even through doubt, and stop the ongoing bullying known as a stigma. Thank you for reading a bit of my life and viewing my art to understand the depth of chronic pain, living with it, and how we need to change everything in order to help all those that suffer.

Who I Was Before the Pain

I do not know. My memory of this person is gone. I feel a definite death of her, but to describe my original self copy would be acknowledging someone that does not and never will exist, and since I have worked through the stages of death I am not able to tell you much more. In this paper, I describe how my life and art have been transformed by the experience of chronic pain.

Y. Palermo (✉)
Seattle, WA, USA
e-mail: ydpalermo@comcast.net

R.J. Moore (ed.), *Handbook of Pain and Palliative Care: Biobehavioral Approaches for the Life Course*,
DOI 10.1007/978-1-4419-1651-8_40, © Springer Science+Business Media, LLC 2012

My background: I have worked as an Emergency Medical technician (EMT) certification, in an Emergency Room (ER) and have done ambulance work. I also worked in a Microbiology & Virology Clinical Laboratory technician dabbling in the phenomenal aspects of Histology and dissection of all bodily parts whenever I got the chance. I gained experience in Specimen collection in house hospital; Veterinary testing and dissection; served as an Alzheimer's clinic manager; a Psychology technician; and in Cadaver care. I left nursing school due to my drive to combine art and science. And, I received my B.F.A. Magna Cum Laude from ASU 1998 in Art Education with minors in painting, fiber arts, and sculpture.

Who I am Now

Yvonne 2011. Twenty years of pain on my warrior sleeve. To know me now is to learn that the original persona of me died, and I am now a daily survivor of chronic pain. I am 42 years old, intelligent, an artist, a mother, and a warrior. I am more than my pain. I am an advocate, crusader, and very wise to the reality of a failing health care system. I am one soul, but I am not alone in this battle of living with chronic pain, therefore, I am many. I light up a room with my inner being, my personality greatly exuberant, now muted at times, but I am still here. I am damaged and scarred from battles. I have a reason for my tears.

I have a family, and two new life long partners since 2003, my neck brace and my back brace. They stabilize the mess that I have become.

My day starts new, everyday, never knowing how I will feel when I awake. I am writing this with my braces on, in beautiful pain. I say beautiful pain, in reference to find beauty in everything, even pain. This does not mean I love my pain. I just think finding beauty in what it brings is better than finding disgrace. When I am at my lowest with pain, is when I create my finest in beauty on canvas.

When I can, I am consistently documenting my reality through drawing and painting. The words "easy" and "happy" do not enter my mind, nor do I feel them. Does this mean I am depressed? Well, I am sure I have been at times. I get snippets of happy, but the truth in that feeling is not there. I am in my armor fighting every day. If you walked in my shoes for a day, getting out of them couldn't happen fast enough. If you told me my pain would go away 100% if I cut off my arm, no question, I would do it. I am resourceful, persistent, and problem solving. I feel this had to happen to me because most people would not have made it this far. That may sound pompous, but it is true. Mostly the only thing on my "to do" list is: (1) survive the day.

What Happened: Encounters

In my early 20s, my first encounter with pain was with hiking. I fell and landed on a boulder, hearing the loud, gushy pop of my first lumbar disc blown. The pain was so severe; I had to be carried to the car to get to the hospital. I couldn't feel my legs. My lower half torso also felt disconnected. So, of course this led to surgery and my first prescription of vicodn.

The next encounter was with my shoulder not quite feeling right. Something was always hurting and I felt severely disabled. I ended up having a right shoulder surgery due to my bursa sac in the shoulder being blown out; I blamed it on my job which was as a foam sculptor. About two years after the bursa surgery and continuous injections I continued having severe pain, swelling, and numbness in arm and hands, and muscle spasms that I never knew could exist thereafter my bursa was removed. The doctor continued with the barbaric relentless needle injections, trigger injections, and more injections.

I've endured over at least a thousand injections to this date, which consist of trigger injections, steroid injections, Botox injections (not for cosmetic but severe muscle spasm) and anesthetic injections. Injections themselves are a completely different type of pain, but severe pain at the start nonetheless. When you get use to the process, it is like chewing gum.

In the fall of 1997 I conceived a baby. My experience finding out tells the early tales of our inadequate health care system. I missed my period for a week. I went to the college campus doctor. He told me that I needed to take some steroid meds for my breast pain and wrote a prescription, along with commenting that his good friend does breast implants. He then proceeded to give me his phone number. I walked out in shock: (a) I needed steroids for breast pain? (b) I have a missing period? And (c) now I needed implants because I am a b cup and flat as a pancake in his words? With my EMT and medical background, thankfully I knew better.

I went back to the college health clinic the next day, listening to my intuition and knowledge.

I demanded to see another doctor and showed her what I was given and what I had been told. She was stunned. I did a pee test and BLAM! I tested pregnant. I imagine what would have happened if I had taken the steroids with a baby on board! Frightening.

Medication, Motherhood, and the Medicalization of Pain

I was preparing to be a mom. The pregnancy was not easy from the get go. I had Hyper emesis gravid arum which is a severe form of morning sickness, with "unrelenting, excessive pregnancy-related nausea and/or vomiting that prevents inadequate intake of food and fluids." So, with that said, I endured while awake mind you, this giant X-ray machine above my entire body, a tube inserted into my right arm's artery, yes artery, which was fed close to my heart. I had to carry around a tank that fed me and the baby constantly with calories and vitamins. That was for the first 4 or 5 months of the pregnancy. I carried it to college every day. This marks the beginnings of me as the warrior and crusader of pain. I graduated college, B.F.A. Magna Cum Laude and I was 5 months pregnant.

I was due in late August 1998, but delivered in September. A petite 5'2", 30-year-old woman, I was two weeks over due. My normal weight was around 110 lbs. I weighed 168 lbs. It was a searing hot day in Arizona, over 115°, when I, swollen beyond belief, headed to the hospital in a bumpy old Jeep with no air conditioning.

September 3rd, 1998 I was induced with pitocin and all hell broke loose. I had an allergic reaction to the drugs they gave me at the hospital. I went straight off the charts with labor pains, enduring them for 8 hours before they gave me an epidural. The epidural pressure was horrid as it went through the first layer of scar tissue from my first lamenectomy. I remember asking for a sonogram to see if my daughter was fine and if she was ever going to pass through the small exit. They did not grant my request. Had the medical staff listened, I do not think what ended up happening to me would have occurred.

I was in for the long haul. The doctor left for the night and I was left to hopefully dilate. Morning arrived and the results were "no dilation." Nothing happened for the next 28 hours. I later learned they had stopped the intravenous infusion of the inducing medicine overnight so the doctor could sleep. My water bag was broke with a hook stick, and with the fluid gates opened, I learned that I was schedule for a c-section by 1 pm.

One pm came and went with no sonogram, no dilation, and no nothing. After 28 hours of hard labor, swollen beyond recognition, I was wheeled into the OR and assumed the crucified position on the surgical bed. I felt like Jesus at the cross. Arms strapped down, legs spread and strapped, and the wonderful blue drape positioned so I could not see the birth of my daughter. At 1:41 pm my new life proceeded to begin. I felt like complete crap, exhausted, looking at my now ex-husband who was watching anxiously as they proceeded to begin the extraction of my daughter. Two doctors were on either side of the table, there was a nurse next to the right of my head. My husband at the time was near the left side of my head, and the anesthesiologist was keeping track, and others were running around the operating room. The hospital bangs, bleeps, smells, lights, taste of saline in my mouth, drugs, and pure mayhem. Game on.

My table started to move. Oddly, my head was aimed toward the floor and my feet toward the ceiling. I knew something was not right. I yelled for the doctor to get their foot off of the table control peddles. "Stop tilting me!" The movement of the table caused my baby to shift toward my head, and I screamed "my neck, my neck, pick up my neck!" My ex-husband and the nurse grabbed my head and held it up. The nurse told the doctor that the table was at a tilt. In that moment, the shift, caused a domino effect with my vertebrae system and the inertia needed a way out which was through my neck. It felt like someone took a machete and chopped my neck from the back. The nurse was grabbing for intubation gear, my blood pressure was dropping. I was mumbling about my neck, and I felt a huge amount of pressure relief out of my lower region. Baby crying, mom disappearing, and dad stunned. Four years later, I learned that I had endured what amounted to a backward head on collision in that operating room which should have killed me.

I awoke in a room, by myself, confused, shaking tremendously, drugged, tired, and lost. No one was around. Not knowing where I was, where people were, my baby gone, and this caused me to panic. Alarms went off, and around the corner came my mom. She jumped up on the bed holding me and screaming for help. I don't quite remember all the details. I just remember that I was left alone and uncared for and my mom was screaming for help. I was in recovery, and I don't recall a nurse ever showing up. I just remember my mom looking all over for help and me worrying about where the hell my daughter was. Was I dying?

Four long hours later, a nurse for the postoperation came in the room, obviously not caring she never showed up to help. She then rolled me around the hospital on my way up to the NICU, to pass by my daughter and hug her. I recall seeing my face in a reflection of a glass window, and I was in awe, I did not recognize the person that I saw. I don't even recognize myself in those photos. I remember holding my daughter for a moment and then going to my room. I felt numb. My daughter had a blood collection at the top of her head from the pressure of being pushed down for 28 hours. She could have died as well.

Days later in the hospital, finally alert due to the trauma, is all I remember. I was holding a joyous little girl, in a daze, and frankly in shock. Not quite feeling right because I had developed flu-like symptoms and my neck still felt like it was just not connected to my body. Five days later, I was sent home.

From that moment onwards, I continued to complain of pain in my neck, both shoulders and lower back. I was told it was from the surgery and my milk coming in. As crazy as it sounds, I went from a 30 B cup to a 30 K! I had to special order the bra off the internet. I saved it for proof. Then I was told by my doctors that "it" would go away after time and healing.

Well time did pass. My surgery "healed" but still I was in great pain and suffering from flu-like symptoms. I moved to Seattle in 1999, not by choice, but following my then husband when he found a new job and new beginning for himself. I supported him, and came along with our daughter. She was 5 months old when we moved to Seattle.

I started to see some doctors to discuss my issues.

My issues consisted of flu-like symptoms, dizziness, nausea, and a lack of feeling in my arms, loss of pulse in arms, loss use of arms for 6 months, and an unrelenting pain like you cannot imagine. There are many types and categories of pain. What I know from experience with pain I have endured these are the types: nerve pain, bone pain, surgical pain, open wound pain, phantom pain, hearing pain, smelling pain, tactile pain, mental pain, trauma pain, stabbing pain, throbbing pain, stigma pain, pins ad needles pain, IV pain and/or vein pain, tolerance pain, environmental pain.

I also felt disconnected from my body.

The first doctor gave me a prescription for 250 pills of Vicodin. Me, small little ol'me: 250 mg pills of Vicodin. So, I went to another doctor, then another, and another. I was diagnosed with multiple sclerosis (MS), an extra rib in my chest which they were ready to surgically remove (second opinion doctor said I HAVE NO EXTRA RIB!, among other crazy notions such as my milk and growth of breast size that was the cause of my pain). Seems a woman complaining about anything, with or without pain, just gets a load of narcotics, instead of help solving the issue(s). Finally, I found a doctor, an anesthesiologist that injected Botox (different from cosmetic Botox) into my neck and shoulder muscles. This released the pain enough to live. However, he felt it was necessary for me to see one of the surgical docs at his hospital for my enlarged neck. He wasn't sure why it was so large. This I did, and the next thing I learned was that I had a condition called Thoracic Outlet Syndrome, or TOS. TOS is a syndrome involving compression at the superior thoracic outlet and the compression of a neurovascular bundle passing between the anterior scalene and middle scalene. It can affect the brachial plexus (nerves that pass into the arms from the neck), and/or the sub-clavian artery or vein (blood vessels that pass between the chest and upper extremity). The compression can be positional (caused by movement of the clavicle (collarbone) and shoulder girdle on arm movement) or static (caused by abnormalities or enlargement of the various muscles surrounding the arteries, veins and brachial plexus).

I ended up having a major surgery, and two incisions were made, one on each clavicle bone. The surgeon also went in and shaved every muscle in my neck down to at least half its size. I was told my neck muscles were the size of a professional football player's. The immense size of my muscles resulted in cutting off my pulse with both arms. I told them my neck still hurt and that wasn't all. I always told my doctors that my neck hurt regardless of whom I saw, or what they did. They said to heal and I will be better. This surgery was one of the top three worst ever for healing. Severe pain, lots of time in bed, and the introduction to being a patient with patience. For someone who is use to living life and having fun, it was time to sit still and do nothing.

I never heard from that surgeon again. He never even called me back. He never checked up on me and never responded to my inquiries as to why neck still hurt. This is an example of a failure in pain management and in medical care.

After this surgery, I created a plan. The next part of my plan was to research the top five neurosurgical doctors. I completed this task. One in particular was an angel in disguise.

This neurosurgeon ordered yet another MRI, but this time it was a different type of MRI where you flex and sub flex. This type of MRI causes severe pain, and so of course meds were on board. I had MRI's and CT scans before but no one could see anything due to my neck size.

I drove to the radiologist's for my MRI. As I lay down on the MRI bed again, my stomach churned. I'd truly started to hate these machines, and with my nausea, and the enclosed machine didn't help. They do not prepare you to lie still in a tomb. I remember being in the machine longer than usual, with all its bangs, clanks and rhythmic chaos. Then it ended. I was slowly let out by the bed.

Upon coming out on the automated sterile bed, I realized about ten people surrounded me. This was a first. Receiving attention from the health care team was new and I was puzzled. They proceeded to tell me my surgeon was on his way, which was in my experience highly unusual, so I knew something was wrong. Two people proceed to take hold of my head, one was talking that they were stabilizing my head and neck and they needed to call my husband. I was remarried at this point. I married 1 month before the TOS surgery. I was confused, because I had driven there and didn't quite understand what they were doing. I saw the other medical staff who did not introduce themselves looking at my scans and they ignored me. I asked to see them, and was told I could not move and my doctor was on his way to explain. The doctor arrived and he crunched down to my level in a soft voice, grabbed my hand and proceeded to tell me that I had a broken neck. That I was not suppose to be alive, and I was to have surgery first thing in the morning. They called my husband to pick me up. I was in shock. The doctor explained how the birth caused my neck to break. It was the same type of force that had caused many of the deaths from motor vehicle accidents he had seen; it was like a head on collision, but mine was backwards. I wanted to see the MRI's but they had caged me up to not move my head or neck. To my surprise, I was told that my spinal cord was completely cut off, gone.

There are no words, feelings, or emotions that I could use to explain to you that moment other than I was supposed to be dead, and for four years I had been living with a disconnected head.

I was told my neck size was so large from my body building its own neck brace. So, on top of having TOS, I had a broken neck. I had seen 21 doctors before figuring out this what was wrong with me.

I was scheduled for another surgery, with a higher risk of death and not enough time to even compute the reality of it. I ended the surgery with another scar on my neck; a donated neck bone was inserted in between the break. I am not sure whose bone is in me, and titanium screws with plating in my neck! I now only have 205 bones instead of 206. I spent the next 6 months in a neck brace for stabilization and healing. I wore it night and day and in the shower. Pain medication, and escaping death again, I truly had no idea that this was not the end but rather the beginning of a long battle with myself, pain, medication and the health care system.

Becoming a Warrior

What ensued after this was the realization that I was put back together, but with a curse called pain. No doctor, health care facility, no one, knows how to manage pain. When you have it you will do anything to cure it, control it, or lessen it. It sounds rather simple but it is rather complex.

After my neck healed, I realized my lower back was in pain. The neck pain situation was so severe it masked that I had completely blown out several discs in my lumbar back. So, more surgeries were pursued with the same neurosurgeon. I did not want a fusion; so he went in different intervals and fixed each disc.

Then I was sent out to live life. Living life doesn't happen when you are in a health care system that fails you. The new life and new self you acquire is not explained to you either. The doctor was wonderful but the physical therapy that was supposed to happen was random, and the management of pain meds is tricky due to the doctors being afraid to give them out and the doctors who don't know how to manage the medication. As a legitimate patient of chronic pain, who needs the pain medication to function, I find this mismanagement atrocious and dehumanizing. I did my best to walk and participate in light exercise. While what I could do was not much physically, it was something. I began to realize my life was not the same as it once was. It was a guessing and learning game, discovering what made my pain worse, what set it off, and what I could do without worrying about inviting more pain.

But it was not over, yet. The next years were hell itself.

The art of pain:
I always had a spiral notebook to draw. In the hospital, out of the hospital, in the waiting room, in the doctor's room, in the car, in bed, I pulled from my knowledge of the working with cadavers and my own transformed body into my drawings. Thank God for art! If I did not know creativity, I think I would be dead. You have to be a very ruthless, strong, and an engaged person to survive chronic pain and the people you have to deal with on a daily basis. The drawings, turned into paintings. The paintings turned into the Art of Pain.

The Art That Resulted from Being a "Patient"

The following art was created out of the chaos, the Hell, torture, pain, mistreatment and grieving my own death. Every brush stroke, manipulation, figure, title, everything, deals with being "patient." The art speaks for itself but I will guide you on my interactions.

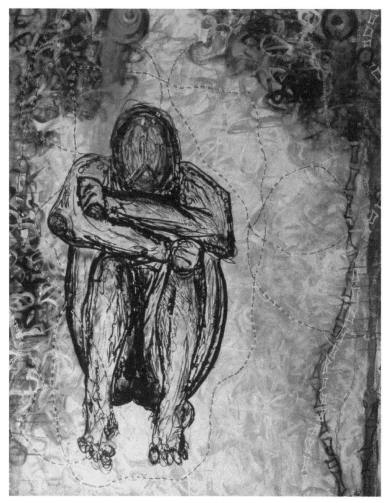

"Defeat"

This picture titled *Defeat* depicts the moment of realization that I am forever changed. The figure is in the fetal position, a ball of fear, the tender moment of losing the self through defeat. Thank God I am strong willed, Italian, and determined to pull out of this pose. The American health care system has made me like this. In the painting, I am surrounded by vertebral barbwire, intense heat, darkness, and pure death. Not showing my face, burying it into despair, but deep in my soul trying to bring forth the person, human, and soul that I know. The person I was. Most people would die. I say that, but it is true. When faced with Hell and lots of narcotic temptation is handed to you. I believe this is a moment we all faced whether it is with pain or just dealing with life. We can all relate to moments like this. To those doctors who are as cold as those caretakers I've met in our health care system, you don't understand, my goal is to make you understand this type of defeat. Never tell someone "they can't."

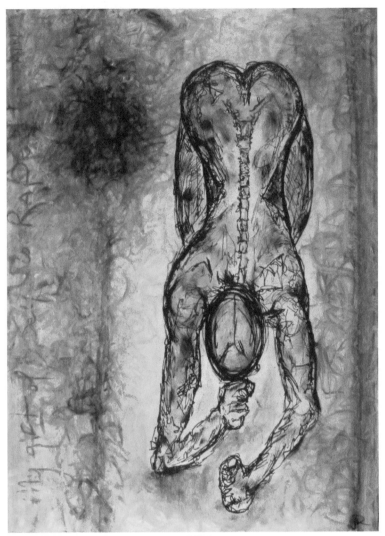

"The Gift"

The Gift is one of my most raw and emotionally charged paintings. Its creation stems from emotions of a victim in chronic pain: physical agony, frustration, and the feeling that our health care system, with its aloof doctors and careless surgeons, has raped me of my gifts of life and my spirit. Shunned by the medical world and seen as a drug addict rather than a victim of physical pain, there is no help to heal or to find solace from the loneliness of chronic pain that engulfs me. I chose to hide the figure's face from the viewer to play on the imagination of the viewer. There is no way to express the intensity and agony of chronic pain. It can only be experienced.

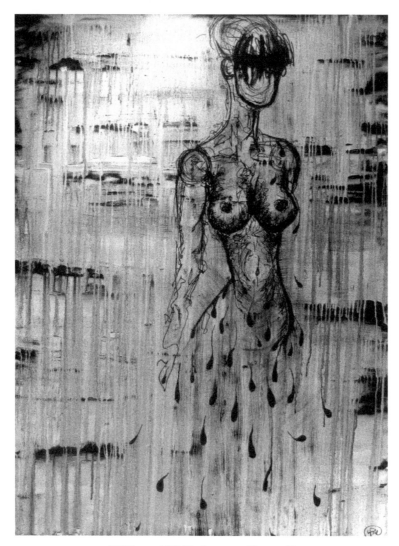

"When <u>YOU</u> do not listen"

The title says it all. This is directed toward dr. d. I will not capitalize that name nor will I capitalize any dr.'s name unless they have fulfilled their oath as a provider. The oath a person takes when they get their diploma as a health care provider. This oath is a document that reflects that that person is responsible for our health in the utmost professional manner. We need to care, to provide, to help us direct our bodies in the best possible way without judgment. A Doctor is someone who will call you in person to check on you, to listen, to provide you with your life.

When You Do Not Listen is directed to you dr. d: you did not listen. That is how I felt. You are retired now. But to me, you failed your whole life as a Doctor.

At this stage of my search to find a solution to a pain cure I was convinced of my chance to live again free of pain was to get a pain pump implant. It looks like a tuna can, implanted into your lower abdomen and a catheter runs around your body into the intrathecal cavity. It is introduced into the space under the membrane which covers the brain and spinal cord of your spinal system. The thought is that the medication in the pump runs in the spinal space instead of your organs. I am a thin person so the tuna can stuck out like a knob. The medication had to be put in every month or few months depending on the rate of the medication dispersal. They take a six inch needle, thick, lay you on a table, and try to find the port in the pain pump with the hope that they find the port to stick the needle in, through the skin in the implant and when they hit the bottom you can feel it. Like a rock sinking into a glass tank, the noise it makes is felt. Not fun at all, and its very nerve racking. The pump was a torturous nightmare. Having it on my person was like having a dark cloud that followed me every-where. I always worried about whether or not the catheter was going to slide out of my spinal cavity. With every movement I made, I would worry about the catheter.

One morning I woke up not feeling well and I felt my back, I could feel the coiled up catheter at the base of my back. Fear set in with a fierce rage. I had a major headache and I knew spinal fluid was leaking into my system causing my extremely painful spinal headache, by the time I got to the dr. d's office I knew I needed surgery. The catheter had slipped out of the intrathecal cavity! The dr. came in, and I told him I had a spinal headache, the catheter was out, and I was with-drawing. He laughed. He literally laughed at me. I said, "I know my body and you need to listen." He responded, "I will send you up stairs for an x-ray to make you feel better." Then he walked out. Alone, I went upstairs, the stairs were spinning, the halls were long, and I was vomiting. The X-ray tech took the images and sent me back downstairs with a look of terror in his eyes. The tech said to go straight back to the dr. d's, I need immediate attention. The look in the technician's eye's told me everything I already knew. As I approached the office, to my surprise my dr d. was rapidly sneaking away. And I say "sneaking" because his body was crunched in fear that I would spot him, I called his name, and he ran out. I know he heard me and I was stunned. I went in the office only to hear from receptionist say, "He is gone for the day." Well, I demanded to speak to the RN, and she was the saving grace to this practice. She would be at the office first thing in morning. They were faxed my information to her. I knew that the catheter was out and stated to the manager of the office it is an atrocity that a dr. would run away not knowing what would happen to me, his patient, suffering withdrawing, with immense neck–back pain, and a severe spinal headache.

That evening the RN called me, she said, "sorry, Yvonne you are right, the catheter is completely out and come in first thing." I couldn't go to the ER, because they do not know a thing about implanted pumps and catheters. By the morning I knew I was close to convulsions and needed a ride. My friend drove me and her face told me more than I needed to know. We arrived at the office and the RN put me in the emergency bed that they had, and told me the surgery was scheduled for 1:30 pm. They got an IV of pain medication going to try to help my massive headache, pain and with-drawl symptoms. I went in and out of consciousness, the pain was fierce, and during this time dr. d came in and started a fight. Yes, a fight, with me and the RN. dr. d yelled at her saying he was not doing the surgery due to his vacation the next day. The RN told him that this kind of situation is why we have back up doctors on call. But instead, he said, "No," and canceled my surgery. Yes, that is what he did. He bolted out of the room where I was shivering so hard, shivering as if I were naked in an Alaskan winter. I was vomiting, barely conscious, my head felt as if it was going to explode, my body ached like shards of glass were stabbing me repeatedly, and then he came back into my room and proceeded to talk to me as if I was fully functional and alert. I told him I wanted the nurse in the room with me and he said no. I said, yes, it is my right to have a witness. In response he dead bolted the doors so the nurse could not get in! The dr. said he would be back in a week to deal with me and wrote me eight prescriptions of narcotics. *Please Note: when you are beyond a point of catching up to a spinal headache, and in withdrawal, there is no way taking pills will even make a dent in your situation. So, with all my strength, I took him on. I told him he has failed his oath as a dr., and he had failed me from the start. Laughing at my proposal that the catheter was out from the beginning and running away just to go on vacation is spineless. I said the surgery was set and the on call Dr. could take over and that he was just was not doing his job. The dr. was so irate he yelled at me. He literally threw the prescriptions at me. They fell to the floor beside my bed. When he opened the door, the RN saw that I had fallen off the table, and was on the floor trying to collect what the dr.

called "care on paper." The RN tried to take the dr. on in the hallway. She said the same things I had, that it too was my right to have her as a witness in the office. The RN went to get the office manager and explain. Finally, she stepped up to the plate, went and got a wheel chair, QUIT her job, and took me about 30 yards to the ER. At this point with her it was ok to go to the ER, because she was educated about the pumps. She stayed with me, got me in immediately, and then called the on-call Dr. for the surgery. They quickly put medication in my new IV and knocked me out. I looked dead, felt dead, and I wanted this monstrous apparatus fixed. Thanks to a rare RN who took her oath seriously, my life was saved.

I now had a new Dr., a repaired catheter, and never heard from the other dr. again. He went on his vacation. I never filled the prescriptions. I stashed them away to use in an art project. From this experience, all I can say is, another surgery, another failed system, and a joke of a dr. that is world-famous for his innovation in pain pumps.

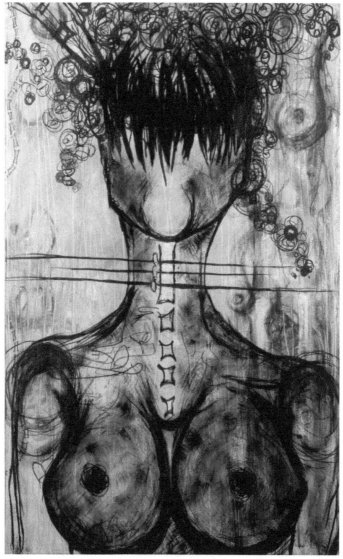

"EX-Ray"

This painting titled *Ex-Ray* makes a simple yet overwhelming point about my experience with many doctors. Many times with doctors' visits, the doctor would tend more to my physical beauty and sexuality than my overall health. This piece came from what an assisting doctor said while he thought, or perhaps "thought," I was still under anesthesia. Tolerance against anesthesia builds with surgery, and he should have known that I was alert. Alert or not, what was spoken should never even be heard. This was surgery #8, and he said, "You would think after all these surgeries she would at least get implants by now." Here I am waking up from major surgery and this idiot only thinks of me sexually. For the second time in my life, another doctor thinking my boobs just aren't big enough! I have no words but a painting for the crazy-talk that came out of his mouth.

A lot of my drawings and paintings have the cheeks darkened in, and it wasn't until a recent X-ray that I looked up in the light of the machine, and there before me was my face reflected perfectly divided with shadow lines and my cheeks darkened, like a super hero. All this time, and that subconscious creativity was working!

Why do I blacken out the eyes, and what is that black cover? A question asked frequently and only one person has figured it out. That was a great day for me in my studio/gallery; and it turns out he is in the health care system. He got it, and I thank this viewer, for understanding the depth of my art. Someday I will tell all, but for now, until I get my awareness out, I will let you try to figure it out.

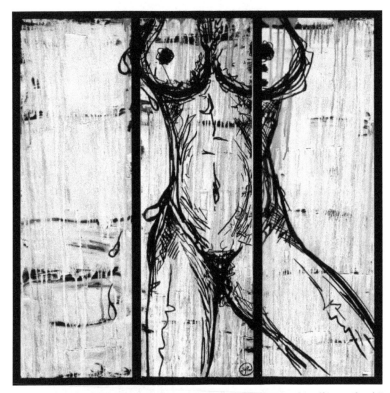

"**They See Us As Meat (trilogy of panels to express the dissection)**"

This piece titled *They See US As Meat* speaks for itself. This painting comes from the notion that after being a patient for so long, and coming to terms with the reality that most doctor's use you, dissect your body, soul, and mind, and the medical world still continues to concentrate on the idealism of physical beauty in the bodies of women. Beauty is placed above health on a surgeon's list of priorities. Each person regardless of gender should be seen as human and not separated into categories.

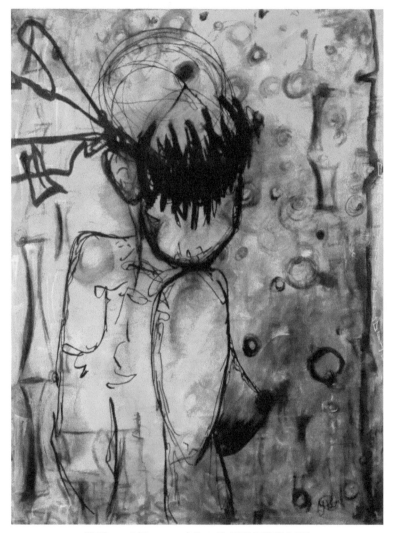

"I Heard You and So did MY CELLS"

Simply put: every part of the human body hears you, feels you, and is affected down to the smallest atomic particle, the cell. Treat me with compassion, not with disgrace. All of me is watching, listening and feeling.

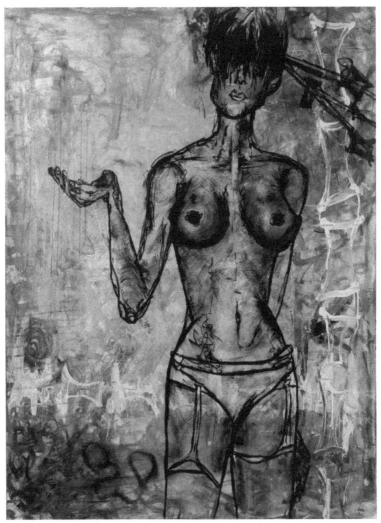

"Re-Configured"

Re-Configured examines the irony between the fiber artist I was trained to be and many of the surgeons I have known. As a fiber artist, I created clothing by carefully cutting up fabric and sewing it together in a new configuration to create a functional garment or a thing of beauty. My garments emphasized precision and care for each pattern I worked with to create the best possible garment. In comparison, surgeons supposedly cut up people and put them back together again in the hope of making our bodies more useful to us. Yet, in my experience, many of the surgeons who have operated on me have been rude, aloof and careless during and after the surgery.

This painting also illustrates our medical culture's emphasis on cosmetic beauty and money over health, supportive care, and helping each other. While I create fiber art in the name of self-expression, many of these doctors objectify bodies by seeing surgery as a moneymaker. It's absurd to think I have put more care into my garments than many surgeons have put into my body.

"Too BE on the Other Side"

This painting titled *Too BE on the Other Side* represents the pain that is always haunting me. It expresses the want, the need, to be on the other side of life. On the other side there is color and life; where I exist, it is dark and wounding. I am constantly trying to hold on to myself as a woman, and as the tears of pain trickle down my cheeks, I hope only that God will put me back into the light.

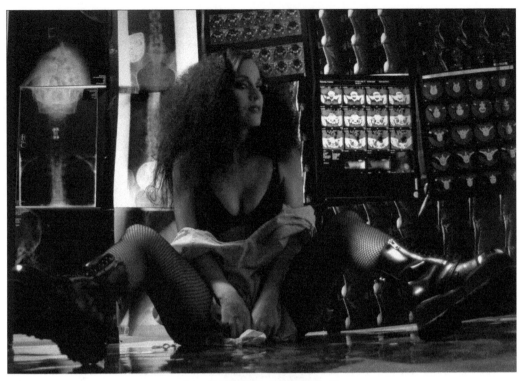

"Walking in my Shoes"

I currently have a passion for photography and ideas. I draw on and use my enormous amount of MRIs, CT scans, and other X-rays, and myself as a model to convey my experiences and communicate the irony of pain and health care, through the lens of a camera.

To create this photograph, titled *Walking in my Shoes* I created a wall of my MRIs, put on one of my hospital gowns from my DR. H (love you) and called my friend Theresa who captures the beauty in women through her lens. Theresa I thank you for your patience with my intensity and I love your willingness to understand what my mind was creating. I also appreciate you using me as your MUSE.

This photography symbolizes the beginning of many new ideas as I seed to portray the irony of beauty and pain. Many dr.'s have told me, "you are too pretty to have pain." To which I always respond, "You cannot have pain with beauty?" Well, you can. Here I am. All people should be seen as humans needing help and guidance from the health care and never judged by their reasons for needing medical aid. Beauty and pain can co-exist because *we are all beautiful*.

Advocacy

As an artist I am utilizing my studio space to exhibit artwork that is derived from pain. My goal is awareness through my art, while my art saves me. I think our nation has gone too long without addressing that over 116 million people suffer daily with chronic pain, and this is every age group. One must remember: "WE ARE ALL JUST ONE ACCIDENT AWAY FROM CHRONIC PAIN." This could be you tomorrow. There are so many of us that silently suffer. We have no colored ribbon to display that we exist and how much we suffer. If we did I would say it would be a black and grey ribbon. Pain to me can be defined within the color black, no matter how much light color you add, it will always be grey.

Where Medicine Needs to Go and What Changes Need to Take Place

If you are going to choose to work in the health care field, know this and you will go far with your career: follow through with your promise to honestly care for each and every person that you are gifted to meet. People are not numbers for a research test, not guinea pigs for money making industries, not here to make you fast cash, people coming to you are walking in with the trust that you care. Honestly care.

If You Cannot Care, Do Not Practice Medicine

I don't know how many countless times I was handed a prescription of narcotics after just 5 min with no caring interaction but just physical motions that made me feel like a rock.

When you enter the room, look directly at the patient's eyes and say hello with an introduction. No matter who is coming in the room; med tech, nurse, someone getting stocking supplies, and the doctor. Basic stuff right? But surprisingly this does not happen much and from my experience I usually would ask, "who are you?"

All health care workers need to listen and consult with new patients for at least 45 min before they start to medicate them. The goal during this time is to get to know your new patient, create a bond, and to figure out what category of patient has walked through your practice. To me, there seems to be three types of chronic pain patients: the drug addicts, the chronic pain authentic patient, or the chronic pain drug addict. So to spend time listening and getting a relationship will surely give you ample time to make a decision to base your care plan upon.

The drug addicts are there simply to get drugs. I would think within a smaller time frame and observation one can figure out what their motive for care is: To get high. This is where a chronic pain patient has received the stigma. So let's understand there is a GREAT difference. If you have a patient seeking drugs, send them to rehab, refuse medication, talk to the family and figure out how to care for this person.

The authentic chronic pain patient, will have chart notes from their GP usually, tests done or needed, and will obviously show true pain. Although with drug addicts withdrawling one does have pain, there is a difference, after their withdrawal they are not living in physical pain, but with the mental and emotional challenges of their disease. So, with the chronic pain patient, take your time to listen. Truly listen, don't jump into implantation devices, steroids and surgery. Ask the patient what they have been through, what they are taking, what have they taken, who they were before the pain and what they would like from you? The patient usually knows their body better than anyone. I know I do. Prescribe medication needed to lessen the suffering and hopefully make the patient's life functional. Make sure flare up medication is dispensed as well. Since pain is so unpredictable on what causes flare ups, it is crucial to have those meds. Also understand that tolerance will happen. When you have been a long term patient like me, VICODIN are like PEZ. This does NOT mean I am an addict. It means my body has biochemically adjusted. So work with that and make adjustments. Sometimes one must switch meds every few months just to keep the body from getting to use to the medication. Open communication is an imperative, and if you and your caregiver can discuss anything with no judgment but pure and compassionate care then the results will be much better. I know many patients out their afraid to discuss their medication tolerances due to the stigmas and this is just wrong. So as the health care provider, you bring it up! Break down that wall and create a safe place, to heal or deal with the pain. It is important that you discuss getting a lock box and a pad of paper to keep track of medication. In fact, hand it out with your prescriptions! Also jot down when you have a flare up and what you think ignited it so you can remember and you can tell your provider.

There are many dysfunctional pain management facilities out there and this has to stop! Again, from my experience if you are here to judge me or lecture me, then don't waste your time with me. I hired you and I can fire you, but I just cannot get my money or time back!

Lastly, there are people with authentic pain that are also drug addicts. This is a major dilemma. Doctors should be able to discern chronic pain patients through listening, through the exam and by looking at the patient's medical records and charts. A chronic pain patient with an addiction is another story. You have to decide if they are addicts first or if they just need management to get them care similar to other chronic pain patients. This brings us to the question of what to do with addicts with pain? Treat them; with a close eye, and close management like the rest of us, no one should suffer. It is a slippery slope, but one thing one cannot do is judge a book by its cover. We are all human, and we can have acute pain. Treat us as you wish to be treated and stop the excuse that you are "overworked." If pain management is done properly, everyone can save lots of money and time. Make follow-up calls to the patient to find out how the medication is working, and how they are feeling, if any changes in the medication should be part of the new treatment plan. And yes that means pick up the phone, not texting or emailing! Personalizing your treatment means more than you could ever understand. Don't wait for a time bomb to blow. That is not advocacy for your patients, nor is it care. We are undertreated with medication due to fear of government grips, and medication was created to help those who truly suffer, not to get high. If the government controls the supply of medication for pain patients, which is starting to happen, there will be an increase in suicides, street drug use to escape the pain and a lot more psychiatric hospital visitations. What legitimate chronic pain people have to know is that we are in this current health care environment between drug addicts and chronic pain abuse patients. You have to know where you are, who you are and get help as needed.

So, my point here for the physician is: listen, empathize, reiterate what you heard, come up with what category your patient fits in, and then start creating a treatment plan, a wellness plan, together. In this plan, all the cards should be on the table. I have been navigating this circus of health for 20 years, and just last month I learned about a medication I could have tried years ago, of which no one had bothered informed me. Doctors should let us know all of the choices that are available, no matter how long the list, so that I, the patient, can have an active say in what my management and treatment will be and what medication will be pumped through my organs. Learning how to listen is an art. Accept that the patient may know more than you. Use the patient's information as a learning tool and say "Thank you."

The Stigma of Substance Abuse

Many people predetermine that if you are living with pain then you are a drug addict. This ignorance is a very touchy subject with me so tune in closely. It seems from the time one mentions they have pain to saying you have chronic pain, in the health care field you automatically have an invisible tattoo on your forehead that says "DRUG ADDICT."

Hundreds of times I can tell you first hand of the mistreatment from people in the health care profession from receptionists to nurses to surgeons that see this imagined tattoo and treat me like dirt as a result. If you try to discuss this bullying from them they see you angry and attach that to a symptom of a drug seeker.

STOP stigmatizing everyone with chronic pain. It should not matter whether the patient is a drug addict or not; such judgments should not be tolerated in the health care environment and in life. I am sick of hearing from nurses that they are burnt out from the addicts coming to the ER for their fix. Well, this is where you should send them; to rehab, not to pass judgment. If you want to be mad at someone then be mad at the people that got them hooked or at their disease, not at legitimate chronic pain patients.

Stigmatization and a lack of empathy diminish the care authentic chronic pain patients receive. When one is perceived to be a drug addict before even getting in the door, the care one receives is not just. Care is lessened and what a patient deserves as care will not happen. It is not your oath as a health care provider to stigmatize, it is cruel, it is harsh and it hurts sometimes more than the pain because it creates an altered reality for the pain patients that affects self and mood, and the patient will battle constantly with their personal mind and soul, asking, "well am I a drug addict?"

I am not a drug addict. I have dealt with the biochemical addiction that is one consequence of having this many surgeries under one's belt, and I have gotten off of the medication. I have a Doctor that manages my pain, and I am responsible, smart, strong and refuse to submit to the stigmatization of "chronic pain patient AKA drug addict" perpetuated by many in the medical world. Propaganda from television as well infiltrates people's minds, introducing how children are getting high from their parent's medications. Well use a lock box and be smart about where you put the key! It is as if the Government is trying to scare society about people in pain, and that is discrimination. Trust me, if the President of the United States, took a fall, ended up with chronic pain, do you think he or she would just take aspirin?

The Role of Family and Significant Others

Families can help and or destroy a person living in pain. To help a loved one in pain, first hug them and let them know you are there for them with no judgment. Understand what the diagnosis(s) is, and if there is no understanding due to lack of health care then find an answer. When you live with pain, you are tired to begin with and besides being the patient through being tired you have to be the warrior and find answers. Hopefully you have a family system or friends that can attend your appointments with you and take notes. If you do not, you can do it, just be strong and do not give up. If you give up there is a chance you will not make it.

Families must understand the implication of pain upon the sufferer, and upon the family. Pain affects everyone. Empathy is needed. But do not baby the person, more than likely the person in pain wants to be their old self, the acceptance and grieving process can be long. If the person wants to try let them. Take notes on what flares up the pain.

Make sure you have a lock box for medications. Make sure you keep track of when you take your medicines, this is very important! Do not drive with meds on board.

Do not remind the person of what they use to be like. What they use to do. You are dealing with a different person now, so get to know that person and love them unconditionally.

I have seen and hear people say, "oh just rest you'll get better." "take an aspirin." "get over it." "I feel so depressed for you." THESE are not things you say to someone living in pain. These words will eat them alive. If an aspirin helped my pain don't you think I would take that instead of a stronger narcotic? Or is it the stigma that allows those words to pass your lips?

Surgery, Foreign Objects and the Medical Gaze

I was in the ER again in 2006. I had complained about stomach pain, due to my belief that a foreign object was left in my abdomen. I knew the doctors on the medical staff from all my several trips to the ER for the same complaint. Of course I got the nurse who had RN Stigma. She approached the door of the room, stood in its threshold and would not come in the room, she said, "You again, huh?" I was stunned. I am a human being and this RN would not come into the room. Is this health care? I told her to go take another look at my chart and see that I am not here to get high. I am here for help because there is a foreign object in my body (which was in for 16 months), an open wound, acute pain, and she said "Oh, that is a good one!" I was in the grips of acute pain and all she still saw the tattoo on my forehead: Drug Addict-Do Not Deserve Help.

The doctor came in, and I responded that yes it was me again, and I am telling you there is something left in my body from surgery and that the nurse is stigmatizing me as a drug addict.

So, let me take you back a bit to the foreign object story (which I had previously discussed under the painting "When you do not listen.") In the throes of trying to find solace with pain a patient will do anything if it means stopping the pain. I tried pain clinics and never will again go to one. I felt like a lab rat. The doctor that treated me was more akin to a butcher than a pain doctor as he implanted a morphine pain pump in me. The morphine pump was like a giant tuna can that stuck out of my abdomen. It lay just under the skin with a catheter running around to my back, and a port going into my intrathecal cavity to deliver medication directly to the source, instead of taking oral meds that might harm my organs. The implants are usually given to elderly people or terminally ill patients with the expectation that they will stay on them till death. I was 33 when I got mine. The catheter was complete hell, and I, done being a lab rat, had it removed. Shortly after, the gates of hell opened a bit wider as a staphylococcus infection (Staph) took over my abdomen as a result of the pain pump's shoddy removal. Once again the word "listen" did not apply to anyone around me. Two days after the implanted device and tubing was removed, I woke up at home in a bed soaked with a mix of blood and yellow curdles of what looked like rubber cement. The smell was disgusting! Off to the hospital I went. I tested positive for Staph at the ER. I was put on a borage of antibiotics, and sent home! The next day, I went back to the surgeon who removed the implant and he poked around the wound then did another surgery to clean out my abdomen in the hopes of resolving the problem.

Well, it didn't work. I ended up back at the ER again, with fever, antibiotics on board, exhausted, and just felt death's grasp on my shoulders. The doctor in the ER did not come in the room, glanced at the door, lectured me on drugs, wouldn't give me an IV, and told me the surgeon in the OR is coming down. They ordered my friend out of the room, told me to lie back, the dr. took a scalpel and cut me open 6 in. wide by 2½ in. deep. No IV, the only medication used other than an antibiotic was one small injection of lidocaine. My screams didn't compute with my ears. Everything was in slow motion. The ER doctor who wouldn't step in the room before, now knew she was in a bunch of trouble all from the lecturing and stigmatizing me as a drug addict and not listening. The OR doc who cut me open, took a poker and poked around inside my body, as if I were a cadaver, and just said, "Nope, don't see anything." That was a 1 min poke by the way. He then packed my open wound, which I would now learn I would have to heal from the inside out, and had to be packed twice a day till it finally healed. When someone packs your open wound on the inside cavity, there are no words in the human dictionary to describe the horrid event. I felt like I was dead, and I a science cadaver in class but I was awake watching the lesson. One truly disassociates from their body to survive.

They sent me home.

The next day, shock started to take effect. I was oozing blood??? Puss?? all over, my dear husband was also in shock, and I needed to go back to the hospital. This time I was going to see the head chief. As I got to the ER, the same group was there, and I could see that they were in fear, as to their error in judgment and treatment, which they should be. I was escorted to the back in a room, given an IV, and I told them I want to see the head doctor. NO one else! They knew as well as I that this was very wrong. Luckily, the head Dr. was in the ER because his wife hurt her foot, and he walked in the room. His eyes said it all to me and my husband. He went in the hall and all I could hear was anger, and raised voices, and basically what the hell did you all do? He came in the room, suited me up with medications of all types, and admitted me to the hospital for dehydration, shock, staph infection, pain, and an open wound.

I do not remember much after being admitted. I was in and out of consciousness. I do remember the head Dr. apologizing for the mess. At this point, I just wanted to live.

It took 16 months of rest and having that open wound changed twice a day by my husband for me to slowly recover. A nurse visited once a week to check up on me, and I lost over 22 lbs. To this day, I still cannot look at raw meat. My abdomen looked like a piece of filet mignon partially butter filleted. Every time the wound was changed there is no word that exists for what I felt. The whole time, my body was trying to push out the foreign object left in which caused the Staph infection to begin with. The wound care team couldn't figure out why it took me so long to heal. The whole time I insisted it is because there is something in there. No one listened.

Everyone just thought I wanted medication. Actually, all I wanted help, care, and a resolution. There were points when I did not even take the medication given to me just to prove to them I was coherent and thinking clearly that there was something in my body! Listen!

At this point, I am going to take you back to one of the ER visits with the nurse who would not come in the room. After talking to the doctor about my open wound, and what I thought was causing my pain, they did a CT scan which showed a plaque-like substance exactly where I was hurting and pointing the whole time. During the time I was sent to the CT scan the nurse that stigmatized me was really was out to get me. She had the gall to order a test without the doctors' approval, which was for THC, and when I got back from the CT scan she smiled ear to ear with this news. She stood in the doorway saying "So, you aren't a druggie, eh? Well you tested positive for THC!" I had never heard her sound so cheery. I actually think I saw butterflies and balloons around her head from the happiness.

I had in private told the dr. in the ER without her knowledge that due to the open wound and losing so much weight my GP was worried. I had tried marijuana which had caused me to eat like a football player on the NFL team. Again, as I said, I had lost 22 lbs. and my 5'2" frame was withering away. I discussed this natural medication in depth with my private Dr.'s and they agreed to try it to see if we can get past the open wound feeling, the nerve pain in order to eat. And I ate.

I made a legal complaint to the board about this nurse, who went behind the dr.'s orders to label and stigmatize me. Who the hell was she? To think: that it was her happiest moment, trying to take me down, instead of healing me. I did get a different nurse after the doctor found out from me about her disrespect. The RN I got in her place was incredible, she had on tie dye scrubs, she came to my ear and she said, no worries, 98% of all patients test positive for this THC.

To those in the health care system when you stigmatize a legitimate chronic pain patient you are bullying us and not helping to cure us. End it and heal it!

I have worked in the health care system, and now, on the other side of it, and I am appalled at the treatment. We as a society with our health care cards think we are safe when in reality it is false hope. If we do not start paying attention and making a difference in the lives of others I cannot imagine the atrocities that will occur at the expense of other human beings.

After the long 6 months of agonizing wound healing, I still continued to feel deeply sick, and hurting in my lower abdomen. It took a total of 16 months to get someone to listen and help me heal. I saw another surgeon and explained to her that I believed that I had a foreign object in me. I had gone through a tremendous amount of ridiculous tests: colonoscopy, barium X-rays, steroid injections into the cavity where my morphine pump was and all very barbaric. I told her, as crazy as you may believe I am, I want you to take out the object. She admitted that she part thought of me as crazy but wanted to help, and I told her when she finds the foreign object to wake me up in the OR.

Well I was woken up in the OR. The surgeon was getting ready to close when seeing an odd mass of tissue around something, and with some dissecting she found a mass of left over pouch from the morphine pump implant that should have been removed to begin with. This was the cause of the massive staph infection. She woke me up, and showed me, and I had to touch it. All this time, over 14 visits to the ER in pain, everyone thinking I was crazy but that plaque that showed in the CT scan, was the foreign object! Thank God this doctor took a chance. She was my last hope, and she saved me. The histology report said that the Dacron pouch was covered in white blood cells and this explains the constant sick feeling I continually had, and the severe pain and infection.

Don't Judge Me by Appearance: I Can Park in the Disability Space

I have lost count upon how many times I have had the police called on me for parking in a space that I am legally entitled to. Again, do not judge me by appearance only. You have no idea what hell wracks my body. I have had post it notes left on my windows that just spewed anger; one man grabbed the grill of my car. I revved up the engine to protect myself and I had the car in park and emergency brake on mind you and I had locked the doors. One person said "you don't look disabled!" Are you kidding me? I had no idea there was a "disabled look." I have had glass left under all the tires of my car, one person kicked my car, and the list goes on of the stupidity from judgment. The crazy part is they must have been watching me to know what to write on the post it notes, and to pass judgments. Apparently I do not look disabled enough. Not only am I dealing with pain and the health care system; but now I have to fend for myself in the public due to discrimination by appearance.

One time I had a good 2 hours to actually go out and spend time with my daughter, so we went to the mall. I parked in the disabled space, I had a cane, and this woman stood right in front of us and shook her head at me. My daughter was scared. I cracked my window and asked "You have a problem?" She said, "You cannot park here!" I was in awe. Trying to think fast to say something jolting I replied, "Shall I show you my scars, and take off my fake leg for your approval?" (Forgive me to those that have prosthetics. I am not here to make you feel bad.) I just wanted to jolt her and give her a visual to understand all of us that are disabled. She had a grave look upon her face. I told her to back off so I can take my daughter in, or I am calling the police. I got my cane and got out ready to protect my cub if needed, but I was not going to the let fear from her uneducated brain scare me from my time with my child. We got in the mall, and she followed us through the first store. When I got back to the car, the mall cops were there ready to pounce, she was there with her big attitude of judgment, the "cops" looked at my disability license, which I carry everywhere now, and they told her to leave me alone. I could have gotten her on harassment but I wanted to have a good time with my daughter and teach her not to be afraid, because she was afraid. The woman was cited.

The Reality of Pain

Having pain you quickly learn you do not know how you will feel when you wake up, do not know what will activate the pain, nor do you know what your life is anymore, you become unreliable, which can make you feel helpless.

In this unstable situation, a person in pain not only starts to lose their identity, they start to lose their family and friends. You quickly learn you truly are alone. If you do not have a loving family and an understanding partner you will have to deal with the fact that even with them, you are still alone with your pain.

You have to be a strong willed person to get through this life with chronic pain. Otherwise I do fear for those who are alone with a bottle of pills. Those bottles are a double edge sword. You learn that they are a part of your life, and you are strong enough to walk through this threshold of pain without the pills' grasp taking your soul. The darkness that surrounds you is overwhelming. When you meet the devil and cannot run because of the pain, you end up sitting still feeling every part of the pain and its intensity, while the devil watches. That is the darkness that can come with pain. Again, you have to be strong to get yourself out of the hell you are in and into some grey. It doesn't matter how much light you mix with dark it will always be grey. This is what life is with pain.

Support groups, (which I ran for a year), are hard due to the fact you are in pain and driving is not easy for me or anyone in pain. So, you may be the only one there.

I still cannot get disability. My Dr.'s are as baffled by this as am I. The judge said the state sees me as disabled, but I chose to give birth and leave the work place to do that, so that is why I cannot get disability. I chose to give birth yes, but I did not choose to break my neck!

What *Chronic Pain* Really Means Coming from The Patient Living with It!

Chronic pain falls under things you didn't sign up for and need to endure, accept, and live with. This includes the pain itself, the new you, losing friends, not being able to make plans, losing your spirit, losing loved ones, not being able to love intimately, hardening of the soul, experiencing the stages of death with yourself, not getting the care and understanding you need from health care professionals, learning you have to become a doctor; nurse; pharmacist; health insurance agent; X-ray technician, medical assistant; nurse assistant; self pain manager; naturopath; masseuse; counselor; fighter; disability agent; drug addiction counselor; physical therapist; advocate for yourself; anatomy expert; and enforcer.

You realize how alone you really are, and how over time, how lonely you become, you are a test rat for so-called new medical ingenuity, and you will always have to prove yourself with a daily test of will. You will suffer daily, experience uncertainty; learn to trust people you don't know to care for you. You must learn to be still, learn to sit, learn to be without doing, fight depression, and deal with the intolerable joke of a system: Take for example, Pain charts. The most demeaning device of them all for a patient with pain is to give them colored pens to fill in a chart to determine what level of pain you are experiencing. The cold comments, knowing your body more than any doctor ever will and getting them to understand that, learning you are paying the doctors and medical system and you have a right to fire them. You have a right to ask questions and to say NO, to learn how not to give up while dealing with excruciating pain, to not be treated like you are stupid, how protected the system is with mishaps, misdiagnosis and when things go wrong – you can lose.

You truly learn what it means to be patient as the patient and what life is all about. In a way, you grow further than most people but it always comes at a price.

What Doctor's Offices Are Missing

One of the basic things any doctor's office is missing, and I have been too many, is a welcoming environment. This comfort starts from the ease of the door opening, the smell in the air, the sounds, the comfort of chairs, the magazines provided, and most importantly how friendly is the receptionist is to the person in pain. I cannot tell you how many times I have had to deal with the rude and unhelpful counter agents when experiencing the worst pain. The last thing I need is a smartass receptionist under the age of 20 stigmatizing me, and telling me in her I–know–it–all snotty voice to "hold."

Pain management environments need nurses who will take time to triage the reception area. I myself have passed out twice, and ended up in the ER during a routine doctor exam. If there was a nurse on duty watching over those in the waiting room, things may have ended better.

When you have pain, driving can be difficult, so most times one needs a ride to the office. If the doctor is running late or called away, the receptionist should call patients and inform them they have extra time before the appointment. There is nothing harder than to sit in an uncomfortable environment while you wait for the one person that may help you only to find out they are late or not coming. If you had to sit on an ice pick that is angled straight up for an hour, how would you feel? What kind of chair would you like? Or, would you prefer a standing area? Give us some respect, because we pay you. Give us some respect, because we are human beings.

Being Defined by Pain

Many times I have heard from chronic pain people that they are not defined by their pain. I understand this idea or type of grasping on to some control over it, but I am defined by my pain. It encompasses my daily life and I am not afraid to say pain defines me, I feel I don't want to grasp on to any new definition. My name is Yvonne Palermo, and I am a daily survivor of chronic pain. Pain can control me. When I define myself, include pain. If I ignore pain as a significant part of my life, then I ignore myself and who I truly am and who I have become.

Medicinal Marijuana

I see no problem with medical marijuana. It's a natural substance that everyone should have the chance to try to see if it helps. I believe God put it here for a reason. Opium flowers are used for opioid medications, so why not THC? Opioid's affect your organs. THC when smoked affects your lungs. It is a trade off. Marijuana has in the past helped me eat when I needed to and current nauseating medications did not work. Marijuana saved my life. If you are against marijuana, the moment you step in my shoes or in the shoe of a person suffering from chronic pain, you will want more options, and THC is one of them. I do not smoke marijuana anymore. I only used it when I needed to eat. I do have chronic pain friends that do smoke it and from what I hear it is a savior.

Pain Charts

Pain charts have to be one of the most ridiculous and belittling, terrorizing, and mentally stirring jolts of them all. When I walk in to an office, with shaking hands, a neck brace and/or back brace on, a cane, pain so severe that I cannot see, and throwing up, this is the last thing I want to fill out, color in, or even see. If I see one more smiling face that still fails to describe my pain, I think I will lose my mind. Please stop showing charts to people that have noted chronic pain. You are reducing our mentality and our spirits. The biggest waste of paper to patients, when all you have to do is: look and then listen. I intend on doing an art piece about these charts. Tune in.

Learning to Become a Patient

As a patient, you have to learn to be patient. If you never mastered patience, with the hell you experience, you soon will.

You learn to sit, breathe and to do nothing quickly, yet learn to master the need for action when needed. For example, when you are having an MRI and you have to stay so steady, but when you know your body best and the injection of contrast is going to cause severe vomiting, you master the transition of becoming calm to taking control of the situation even if the technicians do not care. I have found with my severe nausea, and my neck fusion, that the idea of even vomiting cause's pain from extending the neck and hardware that is inside. When I knew I was going to project vomit, I didn't sit still as the technician's said or hold it as long as they wanted. I turned and let the vomit go otherwise. I learned that the vomit is contained in those coffins and that is not a pleasant.

So, doctors and nurses please don't act like you have walked in my shoes. Until you do, learn from your patient's, patience and listen. Hopefully you will never walk in my shoes but if you do, I pray you will try to grasp the art of patience because it has and will make a difference like I intend to in the lives of others who live in chronic pain.

The Madness of Pain

When you are in the darkest place with pain and realize how that shouldn't happen with the care we think we have, you then realize that you have walked through the door, the threshold of pain and that the health care is not prepared for you, and you in turn are not prepared for the door you just walked through.

This Madness is so deep and dark, you can smell pain, see pain, feel pain, see death, feel the hand of evil, your control can be gone, and your heart can even stop while beating. It is a place of fear, anger, disbelief, heartache, and you look so hard for that light to guide you out of this hell. This is where patience, a fantastic Doctor, and your purpose of strength come to the battle. I put my armor on, all shields up, and the war is on: daily. When having a severe flare up of pain (there are different levels of flare ups) the light you are looking for is like finding a firefly during the day. With those odds, the strength needs to kick in and one needs to know they have purpose. This is the time when I paint. It saves me and painting is my purpose besides advocacy, awareness and motherhood.

When you have the urge to stab yourself in a different area to create a distraction, you are in the belly of chronic pain. I have never acted upon this idea, but I have talked to many patients who have, and many have used these terms to talk about the belly of chronic pain. The sad part is we should have medication enough to not go to this place.

I am not crazy. I do not need to be in a psych ward. I need effective pain management with no worries of running out of medication. It is ridiculous to think that with health care, you still do not get your complete care. Doctors have to be able to prescribe flare up medication on top of the daily medication. With flare ups there are different levels of intensity so you need a supply of different meds. In a lock box mind you. Doctors are getting scared to even write narcotic prescriptions. If a Doctor cannot prescribe medication, what did they go to school for? Doctors should not be scared to care and follow through with their oath to provide care. I hear the Government (federal or state or both since both regulate these drugs) is trying to control who can prescribe medication and if this is true, we are all in grave danger.

Many doctors are also not knowledgeable about tolerance, nor are they prepared to treat long-term chronic pain patients. As I have said before, with taking medication, you build a tolerance, and this does not mean that you are an addict. You have to have a system where you can switch off meds and go on others along with not always being in control of tapering off when not needing the medication.

I had to have a colonoscopy. I stressed to everyone that they needed to know my surgical history due to my fear of waking up during the procedure due to high tolerance. This was when I still had the foreign object in me, and it was one of prescribed tests because instead of listening to me and what I knew was in me they went to look in my intestinal system. So having this colonoscopy which I did not need, I proceeded to tell them about my high tolerance, again I was stigmatized and again no one listened. And I woke up during the colonoscopy.

A similar situation also when I had a tube stuck down my throat to get an image of my heart and I awoke. The doctor was in shock to see me looking at her trying to pull out my tubing, even after describing my history.

Taking a medical history is imperative: so pay attention and listen to your patient.

With all this madness, psychological medical chaos, and still coming this far with my fierce strength, I beg anyone reading this to learn from it.

December 2010. I am currently awaiting a decision about my latest MRI. I have two lumbar collapsed discs. I am in the belly and I am fully armed. My MRI from 2008 compared to Dec 2010 is amazingly different. My body is changing again and I am in transition. My body ages, changes, and my brain follows. The good news is: I am in control.

I continue to paint in my studio, have my art shows, write and advocate. I would like to publicly speak to health care facilities about my story, and what they can do better for people like me. I would like to write a handbook for chronic pain patients to guide them. I would love to write my full story and get that published as well and this is a huge step, so thank you. Someday I hope to get my disability check, but I am not holding my breath.

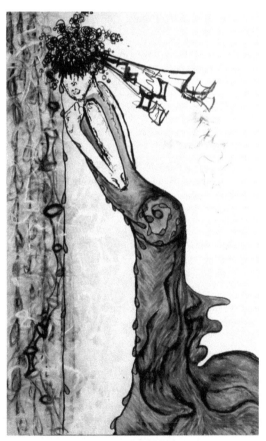

"Elegant Pain"

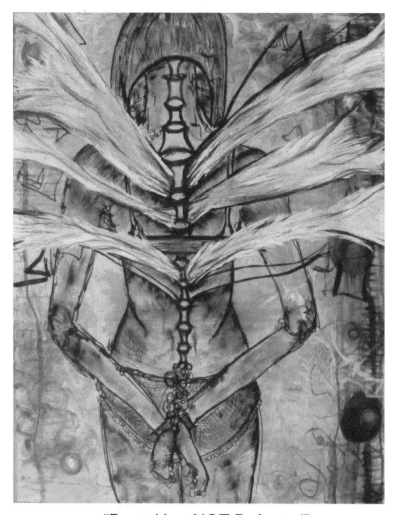

"Bound but NOT Defeated"

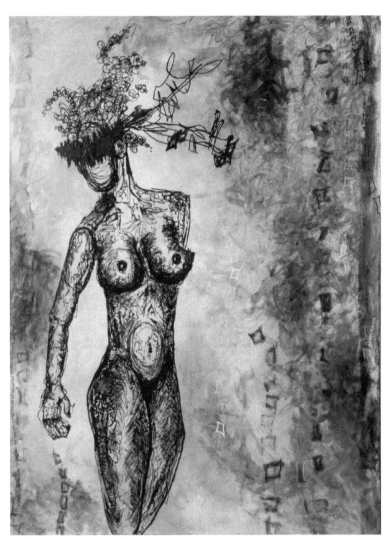

"Between darkness and light"

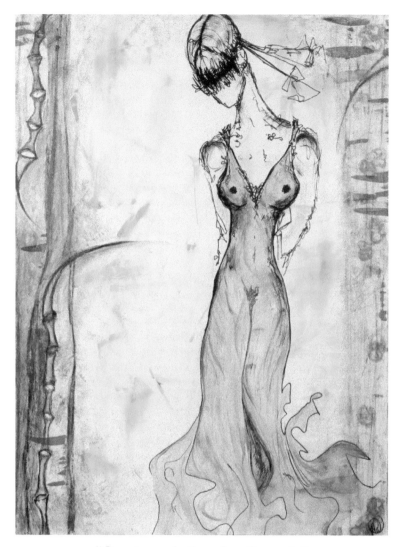

"Contemplation for Growth"

Acknowledgments This chapter was supported in part by the generous donation of *Dragon Naturally Speaking PROFFESIONAL VERSION*. Their generous support allowed me to write this chapter, with pain typing has become a pain trigger, and one thing of the abilities I am really good at now is gone. But with *Dragon Naturally Speaking ,*I can speak what I want written and it does it all for you pain free! I would also like to thank my daughter, without her I wouldn't have fought as hard, and remember NONE of this is your fault. To the child I lost due to my broken body not being able to give us both life, I think of you every day. I would like to acknowledge Dr. Hagedorn of Seattle, Washington, for being a Doctor first, and for saving my life. Jim without your believing in me I would have thought I was crazy, and thanks for staying true to your vows, that is a Man. Also I would like to thank Mark, this was quite a gift you gave me. To Judy, thank you for taking away the fog and allowing me to see the light of God. I am thanking myself, for being able to walk through the threshold of pain and keep going strong for myself and to help others. Dad, thanks for supporting me and listening when I needed help. And lastly, Dr. Moore, thanks for taking a chance on a stranger and letting her tell a scary story that should open some eyes up to many truths about chronic pain, our health care system and make some changes for the better for people living in pain.

Part VIII
Ethical Issues and Future Directions

Chapter 41
Disparities in Pain Management and Palliative Care

Carmen R. Green

Defining Health Disparities

An operational definition of disparities is the difference in health, disease burden, or clinical decisions or outcomes associated with disadvantage (Institute of Medicine 1999). Disparities in health status and health care based upon race and ethnicity prompted the United States Congress to request the Institute of Medicine (IOM) of the National Academies of Science to assess the extent of racial and ethnic differences in health care in a range of diseases and health service categories, evaluate potential sources of racial and ethnic disparities in health care, and to provide recommendations regarding interventions to eliminate health disparities (Institute of Medicine 1999). In the final report, *Unequal Treatment: Confronting Racial and Ethnic Disparities in Healthcare*, the IOM concluded that racial and ethnic disparities in health care existed and were unacceptable (Institute of Medicine 2002a). In this and other reports, they also identified that health systems, health care providers, and patients as well as bias, stereotyping, and prejudice all contributed to health care disparities (Institute of Medicine 1999, 2002a). The IOM also concluded that health care disparities occur within an historical and contemporary context that includes persistent racial and ethnic discrimination.

The Historical Context of Health and Pain Care Disparities

Discussions focusing on disparities must incorporate an historical perspective. From an historical perspective, disparities in health status and health care as well as pain care have been present for generations. Many point to the well-known Tuskegee syphilis study as the *classic example* for medical experimentation without consent on people of color (Gamble 1997). However, scholarly documents reveal medical experimentation on people of color without their consent since colonial times in the United States (Washington 2007). For instance, the health and well-being, and the quality of life of African-American slaves (and former slaves) in the United States in the peri-slavery period was significantly diminished due to the harsh legacy of slavery, poverty, and persistent discrimination. During this same time period, women (enslaved and free women alike) were also dying in childbirth or suffered many negative sequelae following childbirth such as pain or urinary incontinence

C.R. Green, MD (✉)
Departments of Anesthesiology, Obstetrics and Gynecology, and Health Management and Policy,
University of Michigan, 1H247 University Hospital, 1500 E. Medical Center Drive, Ann Arbor, MI 48109, USA

R.J. Moore (ed.), *Handbook of Pain and Palliative Care: Biobehavioral Approaches for the Life Course*,   795
DOI 10.1007/978-1-4419-1651-8_41, © Springer Science+Business Media, LLC 2012

that also impaired their quality of life (Gamble 1997). For example, women with incontinence due to vesicovaginal fistulas which developed following traumatic or prolonged labor became social outcasts. J. Marion Sims, MD developed new techniques to repair vesicovaginal fistulas by experimenting on three slave women in Alabama who had fistula problems: Anarcha, Betsy, and Lucy (Gamble 1997; Ojanuga 1993; Wall 2006; McGregor 1989; Sartin 2004; O'Leary 2004). Dr. Sims operated on Anarcha 30 times without anesthesia prior to successfully repairing her vesicovaginal fistulas. After successfully perfecting his technique on slave women, Dr. Sims began performing the procedure with anesthesia on Caucasian-American women with vesicovaginal fistulas. For his success, J. Marion Sims earned international acclaim for his operative skills. He also started a woman's hospital in New York City, successfully repaired vesicovaginal fistulas for aristocratic women in Europe, became president of the American Medical Association, and is known as the father of obstetrics and gynecology (O'Leary 2004). The debate regarding the ethics of using powerless and vulnerable women to improve the quality of care for incontinence continues and has not been adequately addressed in the literature.

Calls to improve the health status of minorities especially African-Americans began after the Civil War and continued into the turn of the twentieth century. There was clear recognition by the African-American leaders of the day and the health care community that sociopolitical and economic advances could not occur for African-Americans unless their health status also improved. These efforts led to the development of hospitals for African-Americans and increased training of African-American physicians. Persistent poverty and discrimination continues to contribute to diminished health care access and lesser quality of care for African-Americans and other racial and ethnic minorities when compared to whites.

Other discriminatory practices within the health care system, including segregating patients in hospitals based upon race and excluding African-American physicians from practicing in many hospitals also occurred (Hunter-Gault 1997; Baker et al. 2008; Davis 2008). In fact, the many examples of ingrained widespread discrimination and medical experimentation without consent, ultimately led to national apologies from both a health professional organization and a President of the United States (Hunter-Gault 1997). Thus, health and health care disparities based upon race exist in the shadows of important historical events and misplaced cultural norms.

In October 1985, during the Regan administration, U.S. Secretary of Health and Human Services, Margaret Heckler described 60,000 excess deaths annually among African-Americans, Native Americans, Hispanics, and Asia Pacific Islanders compared to whites, highlighting racial and ethnic disparities in health care (DHHS 1985). The landmark report of the Secretary's Task Force on Black and Minority Health (a.k.a. the Heckler Report) detailed deaths that occurred in minority populations that would not occur in white populations. Among the 60,000 excess deaths for blacks each year 18,181 were attributed to heart disease and stroke, 8,118 to cancer, 6,178 to infant mortality, 2,154 to cirrhosis and 1,850 to diabetes (Time 1985). Although Heckler did not propose new remedies she set aside a $3 million monitoring fund to ensure that minorities received their fair share of public health money and created the Office of Minority Health in January 1986. These efforts were the beginning of many health disparities and policy initiatives.

Nonetheless, the Department of Health and Human Services continues to report disparities in health care. Federal, state, and local authorities have uniformly endorsed the goal of reducing and eliminating disparities in health care and have incorporated these goals into their strategic plans and visions for health promotion (U.S. Department of Health and Human Services 2000, 2009). Today racial and ethnic minority Americans also face additional barriers to optimal access to quality health care and are at risk for variability in clinical decision-making that may jeopardize their health status (Travis and Lyness 2002; Travis et al. 2002; Krakauer et al. 2002).

Changing Demographics in the United States

Despite numerous references to an aging and diversifying America, there is less attention directed at the specific populations that are aging. Today, 16.1% of all Americans 65 years or older are racial and ethnic minority Americans, with the majority being African-American. Looking forward to the year 2050, an 81% increase of white elders and 217% increase in racial and ethnic minority elders is expected (http://www.aoa.gov/AoARoot/Aging_Statistics/future_growth/future_growth.aspx#hispanic). In addition, estimates project increases of 128, 301, 322, and 193% for African-Americans, Asian-Americans, Hispanic-Americans, and American-Indian and Alaska-Native elders respectively. All are populations at significant risk for health status and health care disparities(http://www.aoa.gov/AoARoot/Aging_Statistics/future_growth/future_growth.aspx#hispanic). Among those 85 years of age and older, women will continue to significantly outnumber men, the relative growth of racial and ethnic minority older adults will be less due to lower survival differences making aging (regardless of race and ethnicity) a woman's health issue (http://www.aoa.gov/AoARoot/Aging_Statistics/future_growth/future_growth.aspx). Given the predicted shifts in the U.S. population, understanding the impact of cancer pain (i.e., pain associated with the disease or due to the treatment of cancer) in racial and ethnic minority Americans is critically important (Juarez et al. 1998; Bates et al. 1993).

Currently, racial and ethnic minority Americans have higher morbidity and mortality rates for most major diseases and chronic illnesses such as cancer, hypertension, and diabetes (Satcher 2001). In addition, accelerated aging is more prevalent amongst racial and ethnic minority Americans even when they have equivalent health insurance and equal access to health care (AHRQ AfHRaQ 2001). The reasons for accelerated aging, increased morbidity, and decreased longevity for racial and ethnic minority Americans are complex but include social and economic determinants, lifestyle factors, poverty and historical inequalities.

Racial and ethnic minority Americans are more likely than Caucasian-Americans of similar socioeconomic status to rate their health as poor, more likely to use the emergency room for health care, less likely to have a primary care physician, and are less likely to receive a referral for specialty care including pain medicine specialists (Collins et al. 1999).[-12] Thus, race, ethnicity, gender, and class continue to impact health care access and quality.

Health, Pain, and Cancer Disparities

The IOM addressed these topics in a scholarly fashion through several reports. In "Unequal treatment: Confronting racial and ethnic disparities in health care," the IOM described discrimination such as biases, stereotypes, and variability in decision-making as well as health system factors such as legal and regulatory scrutiny as major causes of health disparities (Institute of Medicine 2002b). In 2010, cancer remains the second leading cause of death amongst all Americans and significant disparities exist with racial and ethnic minority Americans more likely to experience increased morbidity and mortality than Caucasian-Americans when they are diagnosed with cancer (Satcher 2001; U.S. Department of Health and Human Services 2000). In the *Unequal Burden of Cancer*, the IOM identified stark differences in the incidence, morbidity, and mortality associated with most solid tumors (e.g., breast, prostate, colorectal, and lung cancer) when racial and ethnic minority Americans were compared to Caucasian-Americans (Satcher 2001; Institute of Medicine 1999). For instance, African-American women have a lower incidence of breast cancer, but are more likely to die from breast cancer than Caucasian-American women diagnosed at the same stage (Bach et al. 1999, 2002; Eyre and Feldman 1998; Silliman and Lash 2002; Merrill and Lyon 2000; Nelson et al. 2001;

Thompson et al. 2001; Jones and Chilton 2002; Krieger 2002; Payne et al. 2003; Stromgren et al. 2004). In addition, African-American men are diagnosed with and die of prostate cancer at higher rates than Caucasian-American men (Satcher 2001; Eyre and Feldman 1998; Merrill and Lyon 2000; Thompson et al. 2001). Although the literature on quality of care consistently reveals racial and ethnic minority Americans are at risk for decreased quality of care, it also provides support that disparities in health care reflect lapses in health care quality. Despite the increasing prevalence and cost of pain, relatively little is known about differences in the experience of pain and disparities in pain care. Most of the literature on this subject in the United States emphasized disparities based upon race and ethnicity in acute and cancer pain, and not chronic pain or cancer-related chronic pain in racial and ethnic minority Americans. Nonetheless, a significant health status lag persists for racial and ethnic minority Americans.

The elimination of health and health care disparities was a goal in *Healthy People 2010* and remains a goal in *Healthy People 2020* (U.S. Department of Health and Human Services 2000, 2009). The increasing prevalence of pain has reached epidemic rates (Green et al. 2003, 2005b; Anderson et al. 2009). Pain complaints are the major reason for health care utilization and disability in the United States. In fact, the World Health Organization has called pain the third largest global health problem due to its impact on physical, social, and emotional health and well-being. Pain complaints are the most common symptom associated with cancer and most people with advanced cancer report severe and persistent pain that diminishes overall quality of life (Nelson et al. 2001; Foley 1989; Breslow 1972). There is also emerging data that pain complaint varies based upon social determinants (Poleshuck and Green 2008). Although effective pain management modalities exist, cancer pain (i.e., pain associated with the disease or due to the treatment of cancer) is often poorly assessed and treated leading to increased health care costs (Sapir et al. 1999; Turk and Okifuji 1999; Anderson et al. 2000, 2002; Mercadante et al. 2000; Vallerand and Polomano 2000; Weinstein et al. 2000; Caraceni and Weinstein 2001; Caraceni 2001; Acierno et al. 2010; Milligan et al. 2001; Weiner and Hanlon 2001; Wilkie et al. 2001; Cepeda et al. 2003; Hemstapat et al. 2003; Hwang et al. 2003; Morley-Forster et al. 2003; Di Palma et al. 2004; Slavin et al. 2004; Lynch 2005; Vallerand et al. 2005; Green et al. 2010). For instance, 14–26% of unscheduled hospital admissions at a cancer hospital were due to uncontrolled pain leading to approximately $10 million in expenditures (Fortner et al. 2002). The literature suggests that racial and ethnic minority American patients with cancer are more likely to receive lesser quality pain care in all treatment settings, thereby putting them at risk for admission, morbidity, and mortality (Green 2006). Thus, there is increasing interest regarding the impact of cancer and pain in racial and ethnic minority Americans as a cancer survivorship issue (Green 2008).

Breakthrough pain (i.e., a transitory increase in pain intensity despite a fixed analgesic regimen) is estimated to occur in 19–95% of cancer patients and is associated with poorer outcomes (Green and Hart-Johnson 2009, 2010; Montague and Green 2009). When breakthrough pain occurs it is associated with increased hospitalizations and expenditures, health care utilization, emergency department visits, physician visits, and mortality (Fortner et al. 2002). Besides causing discomfort for the patient, cancer pain is associated with decreased emotional health, patient satisfaction, diminished quality of life, and psychological symptoms, however only a few studies have looked at breakthrough pain in a diverse population (Green and Hart-Johnson 2009, 2010; Montague and Green 2009). Recent studies reveal that both consistent and breakthrough pain severity is greater for racial and ethnic minority Americans and women with cancer pain leading to further diminutions in their quality of life (Portenoy and Lesage 1999; Portenoy et al. 1999; Portenoy 2000; Bruera and Portenoy 2003). This is particularly important since racial and ethnic minorities in general are at increased risk for diminished access to quality health and pain care, suboptimal pain assessment, and under-treatment of pain (Satcher 2001; Krakauer et al. 2002; Schulman et al. 1999; Cleeland et al. 1997; Richards et al. 2000; van den Hout et al. 2001; Edwards et al. 2001). Recent studies by Green and Montague, in a diverse population reveal that racial and ethnic minority Americans and women are at significant risk for having consistent and breakthrough pain (Green and Hart-Johnson 2009, 2010; Montague and Green 2009). This puts them at further risk for diminished quality of life, increased health care utilization and expenditures, and increased psychological symptoms such as anxiety and depression.

Pain, Coping, and Quality of Life

The experience of chronic pain often has a deleterious impact on the health, well-being, and quality of life of individuals. It often limits their ability to work, maintain social relationships and role functions, and to lead a productive life. Recent work by Green revealed disparities in cancer-related chronic pain and its impact on QOL in adult black and white cancer survivors with breast, colorectal, lung, and prostate cancer and multiple myeloma in Michigan State Cancer Registry (Green et al. 2010). Twenty percent of cancer survivors had cancer-related chronic pain and 43% had experienced pain since diagnosis. Women experienced significantly more pain and greater pain severity than men while blacks experienced more pain interference and disability than whites. Experiencing pain was related to greater depressive symptoms, poorer functioning, more symptoms, and poorer quality of life when compared to those without pain. Thus, breakthrough pain and cancer-related chronic pain represent an unaddressed clinical, survivorship, research, and policy issue.

Both coping styles, social support, and attitudes influence the pain experience (Folkman et al. 1986). For instance, maladaptive coping styles such as catastrophizing, repression, and denial as well as passivity and poor information seeking are important predictors of diminished health when an individual has cancer (Powe 1994; Keefe et al. 2000) (see also Donovan et al. 2011; Ransom et al. 2011). In addition, psychological symptoms such as depression, anxiety and post-traumatic stress disorder are known to affect pain symptoms and coping (Olfson and Marcus 2002; Drossman et al. 2000; Kelsen et al. 1995). Previous studies found an increased prevalence of post-traumatic stress disorder and depression as well as increased pain severity and decreased ability to cope with pain in African-Americans with chronic noncancer pain (Green et al. 2001; Ashburn et al. 2004). The presence of social support networks and psychological support are extremely important for coping with any disease (Dilworth-Anderson et al. 2002). However, the literature also suggests that social support systems decline over time for individuals with chronic disease such as cancer and pain. In addition, reduced access to fiscal, human, and physical resources also influence health and well-being leading to increased disability and diminished quality of life. Despite the high prevalence of mood disorders such as depression, the ability to treat these conditions, racial and ethnic minority Americans may have an increased toll and be reluctant to seek mental health care. This places minority individuals with cancer and pain as well as mood disturbances at risk for substantially more impairment in their health and quality of life due to cancer pain than Caucasian-Americans (Ruiz et al. 1995). This is particularly important as more Americans survive their cancer and are living with both acute, chronic, and cancer pain. However, large epidemiologic studies designed to determine the prevalence of chronic pain following cancer is not well defined for diverse populations.

Barriers to Quality Pain Care: Patient, Physician, and System-Related Factors

Attitudinal differences among racial and ethnic minority persons regarding their health care have been demonstrated contributing to heal care disparities (Baker et al. 2005; LaVeist et al. 2000). Both patient and physician perspectives and concerns about side effects of analgesics (e.g., addiction) affect pain management decision-making (Anderson et al. 2000). An increased risk for addiction may be falsely attributed to racial and ethnic minority people (Friedman et al. 2003). These perceptions may impact physician willingness to prescribe opioid analgesics and pharmacy manager's willingness to stock opioid analgesics (Morley-Forster et al. 2003; Fullen et al. 2008; Houben et al. 2005; Turk et al. 1994; Dobscha et al. 2008; Joranson and Gilson 2001). In addition, patient concerns about becoming addicted may affect their willingness to ask for better pain control and accept opioid analgesics potentially leading to increased morbidity and further disparities in the health of racial and ethnic minority Americans with cancer. In addition, some patients may be concerned about discussing their pain complaints because they felt that it was a sign that their cancer was worsening, others may believe that the pain something they should be able to bear (Green et al.).

Differences in the physician–patient relationship and communication, pain assessment, clinician pain management decision-making strategies, and access to pain care including obtaining pain medications are noted for racial and ethnic minority Americans (Anderson et al. 2002; Green 2005). Overall, the medical care received by racial and ethnic minority Americans has been repeatedly shown to be less than that received by Caucasian Americans (Institute of Medicine 2002b; Bierman and Clancy 2001). More specifically, poor pain assessment and the under-treatment of pain have been shown to diminish quality of life, increase morbidity, and contribute to mortality (Owen et al. 2000; Ferrell 1995; Ferrell et al. 1999). Inadequate cancer pain care has also been consistently shown to increase physical and emotional symptoms while contributing to greater distress for patients and families (Portenoy and Lesage 1999). While the literature continues to document the benefits of optimizing pain control, it unfortunately remains undertreated. Optimizing cancer pain care involves evaluating many complex cultural, social, and spiritual issues. Many different therapeutic modalities are available to treat cancer pain: (1) over-the-counter drugs (e.g., acetaminophen), (2) nonpharmacologic techniques (e.g., physical therapy, counseling), (3) complementary techniques (e.g., ibuprofen), and (4) opioid analgesics (e.g., codeine). The potential for physiologic (e.g., physical dependence) and social (e.g., diversion) side-effects often limit the use of prescription opioid analgesics in patients with cancer pain. Low income and racial and ethnic minority American patients may be particularly at risk for stereotyping by clinicians thereby limiting their access to opioid analgesics to legitimately treat their pain, although there are no data to suggest that they abuse prescription opioid analgesic more so than Caucasions (Weinstein et al. 2000; Greenwald et al. 1999; Turk 1996). However, there are data suggesting that patients with pain as well as low income individuals are at risk for stigma, further jeopardizing the quality of their pain care (Othieno 2007).

Advanced techniques (e.g., nerve blocks, surgical procedures) may also provide benefits for cancer patients but are generally more costly (see also Adler et al. 2011; Zhao and Cope 2011). Given increased use of emergency service and decreased access to specialty care, it is not surprising that minorities have less access to advanced techniques and are less likely to use hospice and palliative care (Ndao-Brumblay and Green 2010; Green et al. 2004). However, there is a dearth of literature that examines access to specialty pain care or the efficacy, effectiveness, and efficiency of these modalities in a racial and ethnically diverse population with cancer. Surprisingly, the literature reveals contradictions in the use of educational interventions to reduce disparities in pain care. Anderson showed that brief educational strategies directed at the patient did not reduce disparities in cancer pain care. On the other hand, Kalauokalani showed that providing patients with individualized education and coaching increase pain management knowledge and improved their care (Anderson et al. 2004; Kalauokalani et al. 2007). Unfortunately, studies have not specifically addressed interventions directed at physicians to reduce disparities. Future studies should use large representative samples to address patient and physician educational interventions in reducing disparities.

Disparities in Pain Assessment and Treatment

The literature reveals disturbing variability in the assessment and treatment of pain based upon the patient, age, gender, race and ethnicity, and class (Green et al. 2001, 2002, 2003, 2006; Green and Wheeler 2003; Baker and Green 2005). All in all, most physicians have received little if any pain management education during medical school, residency, or via continuing medical education. Physician responses to a series of clinical vignettes revealed considerable variability in their knowledge, perceptions, and goals regarding acute, chronic and cancer pain management yet physicians report that they frequently treat pain complaints (Green et al. 2003; Green and Wheeler 2003). While physicians expressed confidence and satisfaction with the pain care they provide they also reported lesser goals for chronic pain. Unfortunately, these studies did not examine the physician's reasons or the role of their perceptions regarding pain or other co-morbidities such as addiction or substance abuse in their goals for treating patients living with pain. The good news is that most physicians report a goal of absolute and complete pain relief or adequate pain relief without distress for patients with cancer pain, although their knowledge and care may be less than optimal (Green et al. 2001, 2002, 2003; Green 2000). However, it is unclear as to how their acute, chronic and cancer pain treatment goals change based upon the patient's minority or elder status. This suggests that strategies designed to improve physician education may improve the quality of pain care as well as the need for more work examining physician and patient factors in their roles in order to reduce disparities in health status and health care.

Schulman et al. and other investigators have identified disturbing differences in the treatment of pain based upon the patient's age, race, and gender (Schulman et al. 1999; Neuhauser and Jean-Baptiste 1999; Lurie et al. 1993; Fillingim 2000). However, little is known about how patient demographic and cultural factors influence pain-seeking behavior and treatment (Ortega et al. 1999). Cleeland et al. identified that racial and ethnic minorities with cancer were at increased risk for the under-treatment of cancer pain (Anderson et al. 2000). In a study using 31 racial and ethnic minority persons (14 of whom were African-Americans), Anderson reported that some patients were concerned about discussing their pain because they thought it was something that they should be able to bear (Anderson et al. 2000). Bernabei's study of 13,625 elderly nursing home residents highlights the challenges of optimizing care with minority patients (Bernabei et al. 1998). Bernabei revealed that African-Americans were 63% more likely than Caucasian-Americans to receive no pain medications whatsoever (Bernabei et al. 1998). Up to 40% of the African-American residents reported daily pain and 25% received no analgesics whatsoever (Bernabei et al. 1998). Furthermore, Green and Wheeler demonstrated considerable gender-based variability in physician treatment of cancer pain and the pain of terminal illness (Green et al. 2001, 2003). Using clinical vignettes, significant differences in physician assessment and treatment of acute, chronic and advanced cancer pain are noted. For example, better treatment (including referral to a pain management specialist) was chosen for men more frequently than for women despite similar cancer pain problems. Morrison et al. revealed that when New York City pharmacies were adjusted for crime rates, those in minority neighborhoods were significantly less likely to stock opioid analgesics than those in non-minority neighborhoods (Morrison et al. 2000). In a statewide study, Green et al. showed that minority and low-income neighborhoods were less likely to stock sufficient opioid analgesic supplies than nonminority (Green et al. 2005a). Green further showed that regardless of income, minorities were less able to access opioid analgesics suggesting that socio-economic status did not influence access for minorities but had a significant impact for nonminorities (Green et al. 2005a). Thus, minorities are at risk for poor pain assessment while physician variability, suboptimal treatment strategies, and decreased ability to obtain pain medications may also adversely affect health and well-being for minorities with cancer pain. So clinician's perceptions may lead to variability and in decision-making and the unintentional under-treatment of pain (especially for minority persons). These studies emphasize the importance of physician variability in pain management, while supporting the need to improve the quality of pain care.

Considering the increasing prevalence of pain and cancer, the adequate assessment and treatment of cancer pain is critically important to improving the overall health, function, coping, and quality of life for an increasingly diverse and aging nation. Although the pain care and health care disparities literature has primarily focused on the experience of African-Americans, similar disparities exist for other racial and ethnic minority Americans such as Native-Americans, Asian-Americans or Hispanic-Americans. However, as interventions are designed to improve health for all Americans these populations may need to be examined separately to ensure that these interventions improve their health and well-being and are culturally sensitive and appropriate, while addressing their needs and concerns and experience as well as those of other underserved and vulnerable populations. Patient level access factors and satisfaction with care also need to be addressed. Cultural beliefs, decision-making needs, health literacy as well as chronic diseases and co-morbidities such as depression also need to be examined. Special attention is needed to address potential stereotypes and stigma. Long-term outcome data are also needed. It is conceivable that the presence of breakthrough pain is a marker for decreased quality pain care. Efforts are needed to assess and measure all types of pain. Clearly, to fully understand differences in accessing and delivering quality pain care there is a need for innovative multidisciplinary teamwork where the patient is a full partner in their health care.

Conclusion

The World Health Organization views pain relief as a human right. Yet, despite evidence supporting the critical importance of race and ethnicity, gender, and class in the health care experience, most studies of the cancer pain experience have not used diverse populations. There is limited awareness of the role of race and ethnicity on pain and symptom management in racial and ethnic minorities with advanced cancer (Bewick et al. 2001a, b). The adequate assessment and treatment of cancer pain is critically important to improving the overall health, coping, and quality of life. Further investigations into pain assessment measures that are culturally and linguistically sensitive are needed. The role of patient level factors such as coping differences, attitudes, access and satisfaction with care, cultural beliefs, and decision-making amongst racial and ethnic minority patients are also necessary. Additional research on clinician decision-making as well as variability in decision-making is necessary to understand the role of race and ethnicity in minorities with cancer pain. Long-term outcome data are extremely limited and racial and ethnic identifiers should be incorporated to understand and to monitor progress in eliminating disparities. It remains unclear whether breakthrough pain is more pronounced in minorities or whether minorities are at increased risk for chronic pain. By understanding differences in the provision of pain care in an increasingly diverse and aging society, interventions can be developed to facilitate healthier lives for all Americans thereby reducing the unequal burden of pain in racial and ethnic minorities with cancer. Clearly, innovative multidisciplinary and pain care research in combination with advocacy and public policy efforts are necessary to adequately address this significant public health problem (Brooks et al. 2002; Lorig et al. 1996).

Based upon the evidence, health care providers and patients need to be educated about health care disparities in general and pain care disparities in particular. Racial and ethnic identifiers should be used to monitor progress in addressing disparities (APS 2005). Consistent with goals to reduce and eliminate disparities, policies and procedures are needed to support quality pain care for all (especially vulnerable populations). In addition, more research is needed to determine which intervention works best to reduce racial and ethnic disparities in pain care. Toward that end, researchers should make certain that their samples are representative of the general population. Efforts should also be directed to increasing cultural sensitivity and active listening to improve understanding. Lastly, with all deliberate speed and to the extent possible, researchers and health care providers should more closely reflect and understand the diversity of the population they serve to ensure the generalizability and quality of their research findings to improve the quality of pain care (Institute of Medicine 2004).

References

Acierno, R., Hernandez, M. A., Amstadter, A. B., et al. (2010). Prevalence and correlates of emotional, physical, sexual, and financial abuse and potential neglect in the United States: The National Elder Mistreatment Study. *American Journal of Public Health, 100*(2), 292–297.

Adler, B., Yarchoan, M., & Adler, J. R. (2011). Neurosurgical interventions for the control of chronic pain conditions. In R. J. Moore (Ed.), *Handbook of pain and palliative care: Biobehavioral approaches for the life course*. New York: Springer.

AHRQ AfHRaQ. (2001). *Reducing ethnic and racial inequities in health care: AHRQ resources for research.* Rockville: Agency for Healthcare Research and Quality, 02-P009.

Anderson, K. O., Green, C. R., & Payne, R. (2009). Racial and ethnic disparities in pain: Causes and consequences of unequal care. *The Journal of Pain, 10*(12), 1187–1204.

Anderson, K. O., Mendoza, T. R., Payne, R., et al. (2004). Pain education for underserved minority cancer patients: A randomized controlled trial. *Journal of Clinical Oncology, 22*(24), 4918–4925.

Anderson, K. O., Mendoza, T. R., Valero, V., et al. (2000). Minority cancer patients and their providers: Pain management attitudes and practice. *Cancer, 88*(8), 1929–1938.

Anderson, K. O., Richman, S. P., Hurley, J., et al. (2002). Cancer pain management among underserved minority outpatients: Perceived needs and barriers to optimal control. *Cancer, 94*(8), 2295–2304.

APS. (2005). Racial and ethnic identifiers in pain management: The importance to research, clinical practice and public health policy. *APS Bulletin 15*(2).

Ashburn, M. A., Caplan, R. A., Carr, D. B., et al. (2004). Practice guidelines for acute pain management in the perioperative setting: An updated report by the American Society of Anesthesiologists Task Force on Acute Pain Management. *Anesthesiology, 100*, 1573–1581.

Bach, P. B., Cramer, L. D., Warren, J. L., & Begg, C. B. (1999). Racial differences in the treatment of early-stage lung cancer. *The New England Journal of Medicine, 341*(16), 1198–1205.

Bach, P. B., Schrag, D., Brawley, O. W., Galaznik, A., Yakren, S., & Begg, C. B. (2002). Survival of Blacks and Whites after a cancer diagnosis. *Journal of American Medical Association, 287*(16), 2106–2113.

Baker, D. W., Carmeron, K. A., Feinglass, J., et al. (2005). Patients' attitudes toward health care providers collecting information about their race and ethnicity. *Journal of General Internal Medicine, 20*, 895–900.

Baker, R. B., Washington, H. A., Olakanmi, O., et al. (2008). African American physicians and organized medicine, 1846–1968: Origins of a racial divide. *Journal of American Medical Association, 300*(3), 306–313.

Baker, T. A., & Green, C. R. (2005). Intrarace differences among black and white Americans presenting for chronic pain management: The influence of age, physical health, and psychosocial factors. *Pain Medicine, 6*(1), 29–38.

Bates, M., Edwards, W. T., & Anderson, K. O. (1993). Ethnocultural influences on variation in chronic pain perception. *Pain, 52*, 101–112.

Bernabei, R., Gambassi, G., Lapane, K., et al. (1998). Management of pain in elderly patients with cancer. SAGE Study Group. Systematic assessment of geriatric drug use via epidemiology. *Journal of American Medical Association, 279*(23), 1877–1882.

Bewick, M., Conlon, M., Gerard, S., et al. (2001a). HER-2 expression is a prognostic factor in patients with metastatic breast cancer treated with a combination of high-dose cyclophosphamide, mitoxantrone, paclitaxel and autologous blood stem cell support. *Bone Marrow Transplantation, 27*(8), 847–853.

Bewick, M., Conlon, M., Parissenti, A. M., et al. (2001b). Soluble Fas (CD95) is a prognostic factor in patients with metastatic breast cancer undergoing high-dose chemotherapy and autologous stem cell transplantation. *Journal of Hematotherapy & Stem Cell Research, 10*(6), 759–768.

Bierman, A. S., Clancy, C. M. (2001). Health disparities among older women: Identifying opportunities to improve quality of care and functional health outcomes. *Journal of American Medical Womens Association, 56*(4), 155–159, 188.

Breslow, L. (1972). A quantitative approach to the World Health Organization definition of health: Physical, mental and social well-being. *International Journal of Epidemiology, 1*(4), 347–355.

Brooks, S. E., Mullins, C. D., Guo, C., Chen, T. T., Gardner, J. F., & Baquet, C. R. (2002). Resource utilization for patients undergoing hysterectomy with or without lymph node dissection for endometrial cancer. *Gynecologic Oncology, 85*(2), 242–249.

Bruera, E., & Portenoy, R. K. (2003). *Cancer pain: Assessment and management*. New York: Cambridge University Press.

Caraceni, A. (2001). Evaluation and assessment of cancer pain and cancer pain treatment. *Acta Anaesthesiologica Scandinavica, 45*(9), 1067–1075.

Caraceni, A., Weinstein, S. M. (2001). Classification of cancer pain syndromes. *Oncology*. 2001;15(12):1627–1640, 1642; discussion 1623–1642, 1627–1646.

Cepeda, M. S., Africano, J. M., Polo, R., Alcala, R., & Carr, D. B. (2003). Agreement between percentage pain reductions calculated from numeric rating scores of pain intensity and those reported by patients with acute or cancer pain. *Pain, 106*(3), 439–442.

Cleeland, C. S., Gonin, R., Baez, L., Loehrer, P., & Pandya, K. J. (1997). Pain and treatment of pain in minority patients with cancer. The Eastern Cooperative Oncology Group minority outpatient pain study. *Annals of Internal Medicine, 127*(9), 813–816.

Collins, K., Hall, A., & Neuhaus, C. (1999). *U.S. minority health: A chartbook*. New York: The Commonwealth Fund.

Davis, R. M. (2008). Achieving racial harmony for the benefit of patients and communities: Contrition, reconciliation, and collaboration. *Journal of American Medical Association, 300*(3), 323–325.

DHHS. (1985). Black and minority health: Report of the secretary's task force (Vol. 1).

Di Palma, M., Poulain, P., & Pichard, E. (2004). What's new in the treatment of cancer pain? *Bulletin du Cancer, 91*(1), 95–98.

Dilworth-Anderson, P., Williams, I. C., & Gibson, B. E. (2002). Issues of race, ethnicity, and culture in caregiving research: A 20-year review (1980–2000). *The Gerontologist, 42*(2), 237–272.

Dobscha, S. K., Corson, K., Flores, J. A., Tansill, E. C., & Gerrity, M. S. (2008). Veterans affairs primary care clinicians' attitudes toward chronic pain and correlates of opioid prescribing rates. *Pain Medicine, 9*(5), 564–571.

Donovan, K. A., Thompson, L. M. A., & Jacobsen, P. B. (2011). Pain, depression and anxiety in cancer. In R. J. Moore (Ed.), *Handbook of pain and palliative care: Biobehavioral approaches for the life course*. New York: Springer.

Drossman, D. A., Leserman, J., Li, Z., Keefe, F., Hu, Y. J., & Toomey, T. C. (2000). Effects of coping on health outcome among women with gastrointestinal disorders. *Psychosomatic Medicine, 62*(3), 309–317.

Edwards, R. R., Doleys, D. M., Fillingim, R. B., & Lowery, D. (2001). Ethnic differences in pain tolerance: Clinical implications in a chronic pain population. *Psychosomatic Medicine, 63*(2), 316–323.

Epstein, A. M., & Ayanian, J. Z. (2001). Racial disparities in medical care. *The New England Journal of Medicine, 344*(19), 1471–1473.

Eyre, H. J., & Feldman, G. E. (1998). Status report on prostate cancer in African Americans: A national blueprint for action. *CA: A Cancer Journal for Clinicians, 48*(5), 315–319.

Ferrell, B. R. (1995). The impact of pain on quality of life. A decade of research. *The Nursing Clinics of North America, 30*(4), 609–624.

Ferrell, B. R., Juarez, G., & Borneman, T. (1999). Use of routine and breakthrough analgesia in home care. *Oncology Nursing Forum, 26*(10), 1655–1661.

Fillingim, R. B. (2000). Sex, gender, and pain: Women and men really are different. *Current Review of Pain, 4*(1), 24–30.

Fiscella, K., Franks, P., Gold, M. R., & Clancy, C. M. (2000). Inequality in quality: Addressing socioeconomic, racial, and ethnic disparities in health care. *Journal of American Medical Association, 283*(19), 2579–2584.

Foley, K. (1989). Controversies in cancer pain. Medical perspectives. *Cancer, 63*(11 Suppl), 2257–2265.

Folkman, S., Lazarus, R. S., Dunkel-Schetter, C., DeLongis, A., & Gruen, R. J. (1986). Dynamics of a stressful encounter: Cognitive appraisal, coping, and encounter outcomes. *Journal of Personality and Social Psychology, 50*(5), 992–1003.

Ford, E. S., & Cooper, R. S. (1995). Implications of race/ethnicity for health and health care use. *Health Services Research, 30*, 237–252.

Fortner, B. V., Okon, T. A., & Portenoy, R. K. (2002). A survey of pain-related hospitalizations, emergency department visits, and physician office visits reported by cancer patients with and without history of breakthrough pain. *The Journal of Pain, 3*(1), 38–44.

Friedman, R., Li, V., & Mehrotra, D. (2003). Treating pain patients at risk: Evaluation of a screening tool in opioid-treated pain patients with and without addiction [comment]. *Pain Medicine, 4*(2), 182–185.

Fullen, B. M., Baxter, G. D., O'Donovan, B. G., Doody, C., Daly, L., & Hurley, D. A. (2008). Doctors' attitudes and beliefs regarding acute low back pain management: A systematic review. *Pain, 136*(3), 388–396.

Gamble, V. N. (1997). Under the shadow of Tuskegee: African Americans and health care. *American Journal of Public Health, 87*(11), 1773–1778.

Gaskin, D. J., & Hoffman, C. (2000). Racial and ethnic differences in preventable hospitalizations across 10 states. *Medical Care Research and Review, 57*(Suppl 1), 85–107.

Green, C. (2000). An overview of acute postoperative pain management: Past, present, and future. *Pharmacology in Anesthesia Practice, 1*(1), 7–12.

Green, C., & Hart-Johnson, T. (2009). A longitudinal examination of neighborhood socioeconomic status and cancer pain. *The Journal of Pain, 10*(4), S5.

Green, C., Todd, K. H., Lebovits, A., & Francis, M. (2006). Disparities in pain: Ethical issues. *Pain Medicine, 7*(6), 530–533.

Green, C. M., Hart-Johnson, T., Ndao-Brumblay, S. Impact of an abuse history on the health outcomes among Blacks and Whites with chronic pain.

Green, C. R. (2005). Unequal burdens and unheard voices: Whose pain? Whose narratives? In D. B. Carr, J. D. Loeser, & D. B. Morris (Eds.), *Narrative, pain, and suffering, progress in pain research and management* (Vol. 34, pp. 195–214). Seattle: IASP Press.

Green, C. R. (2006). The quality of cancer pain management for racial and ethnic minority Americans: Unequal burdens and unheard voices. *Journal of Cancer Pain and Symptom Palliation, 2*(1), 19–27.

Green, C. R. (2008). The healthcare bubble through the lens of pain research, practice, and policy: Advice to the new president and congress. *The Journal of Pain, 9*(12), 1071–1073.

Green, C. R., Anderson, K. O., Baker, T. A., et al. (2003). The unequal burden of pain: Confronting racial and ethnic disparities in pain. *Pain Medicine, 4*(3), 277–294.

Green, C. R., Baker, T. A., & Ndao-Brumblay, S. K. (2004). Patient attitudes regarding healthcare utilization and referral: A descriptive comparison in African- and Caucasian Americans with chronic pain. *Journal of the National Medical Association, 96*(1), 31–42.

Green, C. R., & Hart-Johnson, T. (2010). The adequacy of chronic pain management prior to presenting at a tertiary care pain center: The role of patient socio-demographic characteristics. *The Journal of Pain, 11*(8), 746–754.

Green, C. R., Hart-Johnson, T., & Loeffler, D. R. (2010). Cancer related chronic pain. *Cancer, 10*.

Green, C. R., Ndao-Brumblay, S. K., West, B., & Washington, T. (2005a). Differences in prescription opioid analgesic availability: comparing minority and white pharmacies across Michigan. *The Journal of Pain, 6*(10), 689–699.

Green, C. R., Tait, R. C., & Gallagher, R. M. (2005b). Introduction: The unequal burden of pain: Disparities and differences. *Pain Medicine, 6*(1), 1–2.

Green, C. R., & Wheeler, J. R. (2003). Physician variability in the management of acute postoperative and cancer pain: A quantitative analysis of the Michigan experience. *Pain Medicine, 4*(1), 8–20.

Green, C. R., Wheeler, J. R., LaPorte, F., Marchant, B., & Guerrero, E. (2002). How well is chronic pain managed? Who does it well? *Pain Medicine, 3*(1), 56–65.

Green, C. R., Wheeler, J. R., Marchant, B., LaPorte, F., & Guerrero, E. (2001). Analysis of the physician variable in pain management. *Pain Medicine, 2*(4), 317–327.

Greenwald, B. D., Narcessian, E. J., & Pomeranz, B. A. (1999). Assessment of physiatrists' knowledge and perspectives on the use of opioids: Review of basic concepts for managing chronic pain. *American Journal of Physical Medicine & Rehabilitation, 78*(5), 408–415.

Hemstapat, K., Monteith, G. R., Smith, D., & Smith, M. T. (2003). Morphine-3-glucuronide's neuro-excitatory effects are mediated via indirect activation of N-methyl-D-aspartic acid receptors: Mechanistic studies in embryonic cultured hippocampal neurones [comment]. *Anesthesia and Analgesia, 97*(2), 494–505.

Houben, R. M., Gijsen, A., Peterson, J., de Jong, P. J., & Vlaeyen, J. W. (2005). Do health care providers' attitudes towards back pain predict their treatment recommendations? Differential predictive validity of implicit and explicit attitude measures. *Pain, 114*(3), 491–498.

Hunter-Gault. (1997). An apology 65 years late – The legacy of Tuskegee.

Hwang, S. S., Chang, V. T., & Kasimis, B. (2003). Cancer breakthrough pain characteristics and responses to treatment at a VA medical center. *Pain, 101*(1–2), 55–64.

Institute of Medicine. (1999). *The unequal burden of cancer: An assessment of NIH research and programs for ethnic minorities and the medically underserved.* Washington: National Academy Press.

Institute of Medicine. (2002a). *Unequal treatment: Confronting racial and ethnic disparities in health care.* Washington: The National Academies Press.

Institute of Medicine. (2002b). *Goal to eliminate health care disparities: Guidance for the national healthcare disparities report.* Washington: National Academies Press.

Institute of Medicine. (2004). *In the Nation's compelling interest – Ensuring diversity in the health care workforce.* Washington: National Academy of Sciences.

Interim State Projections of Population for Five-Year Age Groups and Selected Age Groups by Sex: July 1, 2004 to 2030 (2005). Retrieved June 10, 2010, from http://www.aoa.gov/AoARoot/Aging_Statistics/future_growth/future_growth.aspx.

Jones, L. A., & Chilton, J. A. (2002). Impact of breast cancer on African American women: Priority areas for research in the next decade. *American Journal of Public Health, 92*(4), 539–542.

Joranson, D. E., & Gilson, A. M. (2001). Pharmacists' knowledge of and attitudes toward opioid pain medications in relation to federal and state policies. *Journal of the American Pharmaceutical Association, 41*(2), 213–220.

Juarez, G., Ferrell, B., & Borneman, T. (1998). Influence of culture on cancer pain management in Hispanic patients. *Cancer Practice, 6*(5), 262–269.

Kalauokalani, D., Franks, P., Oliver, J. W., Meyers, F. J., & Kravitz, R. L. (2007). Can patient coaching reduce racial/ethnic disparities in cancer pain control? Secondary analysis of a randomized controlled trial. *Pain Medicine, 8*(1), 17–24.

Keefe, F. J., Lefebvre, J. C., Egert, J. R., Affleck, G., Sullivan, M. J., & Caldwell, D. S. (2000). The relationship of gender to pain, pain behavior, and disability in osteoarthritis patients: The role of catastrophizing. *Pain, 87*(3), 325–334.

Kelsen, D. P., Portenoy, R. K., Thaler, H. T., et al. (1995). Pain and depression in patients with newly diagnosed pancreas cancer. *Journal of Clinical Oncology, 13*(3), 748–755.

Krakauer, E. L., Crenner, C., & Fox, K. (2002). Barriers to optimum end-of-life care for minority patients. *Journal of the American Geriatrics Society, 50*, 182–190.

Krieger, N. (2002). Is breast cancer a disease of affluence, poverty, or both? The case of African American women. *American Journal of Public Health, 92*(4), 611–613.

LaVeist, T. A., Nickerson, K. J., & Bowie, J. V. (2000). Attitudes about racism, medical mistrust, and satisfaction with care among African American and White cardiac patients. *Medical Care Research and Review, 57*(Suppl 1), 146–161.

Lillie-Blanton, M., Brodie, M., Rowland, D., Altman, D., & McIntosh, M. (2000). Race, ethnicity, and the health care system: Public perceptions and experiences. *Medical Care Research and Review, 57*(1), 218–235.

Lorig, K., Stewart, A., Ritter, P., Gonzalez, V., Laurent, D., & Lynch, J. (1996). *Outcome measures for health education and other health care interventions.* Thousand Oaks: SAGE Publications.

Lurie, N., Slater, J., McGovern, P., Ekstrum, J., Quam, L., & Margolis, K. (1993). Preventive care for women. Does the sex of the physician matter? *The New England Journal of Medicine, 329*(7), 478–482.

Lynch, M. E. (2005). A review of the use of methadone for the treatment of chronic noncancer pain. *Pain Research & Management, 10*(3), 133–144.

Mayberry, R. M., Mili, F., & Ofili, E. (2000). Racial and ethnic differences in access to medical care. *Medical Care Research and Review, 57*(Suppl 1), 108–145.

McGregor, D. (1989). Sexual surgery and the origins of gynecology: J. Marion Sims, his hospital, and his patients. *The Journal of Southern History.*

Mercadante, S., Casuccio, A., Pumo, S., & Fulfaro, F. (2000). Factors influencing the opioid response in advanced cancer patients with pain followed at home: The effects of age and gender. *Supportive Care in Cancer, 8*(2), 123–130.

Merrill, R. M., & Lyon, J. L. (2000). Explaining the difference in prostate cancer mortality rates between White and Black men in the United States. *Urology, 55*(5), 730–735.

Milligan, K., Lanteri-Minet, M., Borchert, K., et al. (2001). Evaluation of long-term efficacy and safety of transdermal fentanyl in the treatment of chronic noncancer pain. *The Journal of Pain, 2*(4), 197–204.

Montague, L., & Green, C. R. (2009). Cancer and breakthrough pain's impact on a diverse population. *Pain Medicine, 10*(3), 549–561.

Morley-Forster, P. K., Clark, A. J., Speechley, M., & Moulin, D. E. (2003). Attitudes toward opioid use for chronic pain: A Canadian physician survey. *Pain Research & Management, 8*(4), 189–194.

Morrison, R. S., Wallenstein, S., Natale, D. K., Senzel, R. S., & Huang, L. L. (2000). "We don't carry that" – failure of pharmacies in predominantly nonwhite neighborhoods to stock opioid analgesics. *The New England Journal of Medicine, 342*(14), 1023–1026.

Ndao-Brumblay, S. K., & Green, C. R. (2010). Predictors of complementary and alternative medicine use in chronic pain patients. *Pain Medicine, 11*(1), 16–24.

Nelson, J. E., Meier, D. E., Oei, E. J., et al. (2001). Self-reported symptom experience of critically ill cancer patients receiving intensive care. *Critical Care Medicine, 29*(2), 277–282.

Neuhauser, D., & Jean-Baptiste, R. (1999). Differential provision or acquisition of health care is related to one's race or gender. *Ethnicity & Disease, 9*(1), 145–146.

O'Leary, J. J. (2004). Marion Sims: A defense of the father of gynecology. *Southern Medical Journal, 97*(5), 427–429.

Ojanuga, D. (1993). The medical ethics of the "father of gynaecology," Dr. J. Marion Sims. *Journal of Medical Ethics, 19*(1), 28–31.

Olfson, M., & Marcus, S. C. (2002). National trends in the outpatient treatment of depression. *Journal of American Medical Association, 287*(2), 203–209.

Ortega, R., Youdelman, B., & Havel, R. (1999). Ethnic variability in the treatment of pain. *The American Journal of Anesthesiology, 26*(9), 429–432.

Othieno, J. (2007). Understanding how contextual realities affect African born immigrants and refugees living with HIV in accessing care in the twin cities. *Journal of Health Care for the Poor and Underserved, 18*, 170–188.

Owen, J. E., Klapow, J. C., & Casebeer, L. (2000). Evaluating the relationship between pain presentation and health-related quality of life in outpatients with metastatic or recurrent neoplastic disease. *Quality of Life Research, 9*(7), 855–863.

Payne, R., Medina, E., & Hampton, J. W. (2003). Quality of life concerns in patients with breast cancer: Evidence for disparity of outcomes and experiences in pain management and palliative care among African-American women. *Cancer, 97*(1 Suppl), 311–317.

Poleshuck, E. L., & Green, C. R. (2008). Socioeconomic disadvantage and pain. *Pain, 136*(3), 235–238.

Portenoy, R. K. (2000). Current pharmacotherapy of chronic pain. *Journal of Pain and Symptom Management, 19* (1 Suppl), S16–S20.

Portenoy, R. K., & Lesage, P. (1999). Management of cancer pain. *The Lancet, 353*, 1695–1700.

Portenoy, R. K., Payne, D., & Jacobsen, P. (1999). Breakthrough pain: Characteristics and impact in patients with cancer pain. *Pain, 81*(1–2), 129–134.

Powe, B. D. (1994). Perceptions of cancer fatalism among African Americans: The influence of education, income, and cancer knowledge. *Journal of National Black Nurses Association, 7*(2), 41–48.

Projected Population by Single Year of Age, Sex, Race, and Hispanic Origin for the United States: July 1, 2000 to July 1, 2050 (NP2008_D1) (2008). Retrieved June 10, 2010, from http://www.aoa.gov/AoARoot/Aging_Statistics/future_growth/future_growth.aspx#hispanic.

Ransom, S., Pearman, T. P., Philip, E., & Anwar, D. (2011). Adult cancer-related pain. In R. J. Moore (Ed.), *Handbook of pain and palliative care: Biobehavioral approaches for the life course.* New York: Springer.

Richards, H., McConnachie, A., Morrison, C., Murray, K., & Watt, G. (2000). Social and gender variation in the prevalence, presentation and general practitioner provisional diagnosis of chest pain. *Journal of Epidemiology and Community Health, 54*(9), 714–718.

Ruiz, P., Venegas-Samuels, K., & Alarcon, R. D. (1995). The economics of pain: Mental health care costs among minorities. *Psychiatric Clinics of North America, 18*(3), 659–670.

Sapir, R., Catane, R., Strauss-Liviatan, N., & Cherny, N. I. (1999). Cancer pain: Knowledge and attitudes of physicians in Israel. *Journal of Pain & Symptom Management, 17*(4), 266–276.

Sartin, J. S. (2004). J. Marion Sims, the father of gynecology: Hero or villain? *Southern Medical Journal, 97*(5), 500–505.

Satcher, D. (2001). The unequal burden of cancer. *Cancer, 91*(S1), 205–207.

Schulman, K. A., Berlin, J. A., Harless, W., et al. (1999). The effect of race and sex on physicians' recommendations for cardiac catheterization. *The New England Journal of Medicine, 340*(8), 618–626.

Silliman, R. A., & Lash, T. L. (2002). Do variations in breast cancer care matter? *Medical Care, 40*(3), 177–180.

Slavin, K. V., Tesoro, E. P., & Mucksavage, J. J. (2004). The treatment of cancer pain. *Drugs of Today (Barcelona, Spain), 40*(3), 235–245.

Stromgren, A. S., Groenvold, M., Petersen, M. A., et al. (2004). Pain characteristics and treatment outcome for advanced cancer patients during the first week of specialized palliative care. *Journal of Pain and Symptom Management, 27*(2), 104–113.

Thompson, I., Tangen, C., Tolcher, A., Crawford, E., Eisenberger, M., & Moinpour, C. (2001). Association of African-American ethnic background with survival in men with metastatic prostate cancer. *Journal of the National Cancer Institute, 93*(3), 219–225.

Time. (1985). *Time.*

Travis, L. A., & Lyness, J. M. (2002). Minor depression. Diagnosis and management in primary care. *Geriatrics, 57*(5), 65–66.

Travis, S. S., Bernard, M., Dixon, S., McAuley, W. J., Loving, G., & McClanahan, L. (2002). Obstacles to palliation and end-of-life care in a long-term care facility. *The Gerontologist, 42*(3), 342–349.

Turk, D. C. (1996). Clinicians' attitudes about prolonged use of opioids and the issue of patient heterogeneity. *Journal of Pain and Symptom Management, 11*(4), 218–230.

Turk, D. C., Brody, M. C., & Okifuji, E. A. (1994). Physicians' attitudes and practices regarding the long-term prescribing of opioids for non-cancer pain. *Pain, 59*(2), 201–208.

Turk, D. C., & Okifuji, A. (1999). Does sex make a difference in the prescription of treatments and the adaptation to chronic pain by cancer and non-cancer patients? *Pain, 82*(2), 139–148.

U.S. Department of Health and Human Services. (2000). *Healthy people 2010: Understanding and improving health.* Washington: Department of Health and Human Services, Government Printing Office.

U.S. Department of Health and Human Services. (2009). *Healthy people 2020, objectives new to healthy people 2020, OA HP2020-8: Increase the proportion of older adults with reduced physical or cognitive function who engage in light, moderate, or vigorous leisure-time physical activities.* Washington: U.S. Department of Health and Human Services.

Vallerand, A. H., Hasenau, S., Templin, T., & Collins-Bohler, D. (2005). Disparities between Black and white patients with cancer pain: The effect of perception of control over pain. *Pain Medicine, 6*(3), 242–250.

Vallerand, A. H., & Polomano, R. C. (2000). The relationship of gender to pain. *Pain Management Nursing, 1* (3 Suppl 1), 8–15.

van den Hout, J. H., Vlaeyen, J. W., Houben, R. M., Soeters, A. P., & Peters, M. L. (2001). The effects of failure feedback and pain-related fear on pain report, pain tolerance, and pain avoidance in chronic low back pain patients. *Pain, 92*(1–2), 247–257.

Wall, L. (2006). The medical ethics of Dr. J. Marion Sims: A fresh look at the historical record. *Journal of Medical Ethics, 32*(6), 346–350.

Washington, H. (2007). Medical apartheid.

Weiner, D. K., & Hanlon, J. T. (2001). Pain in nursing home residents: Management strategies. *Drugs & Aging, 18*(1), 13–29.

Weinstein, S. M., Laux, L. F., Thornby, J. I., et al. (2000). Physicians' attitudes toward pain and the use of opioid analgesics: Results of a survey from the Texas cancer pain initiative. *Southern Medical Journal, 93*(5), 479–487.

Wilkie, D. J., Huang, H. Y., Reilly, N., & Cain, K. C. (2001). Nociceptive and neuropathic pain in patients with lung cancer: A comparison of pain quality descriptors. *Journal of Pain and Symptom Management, 22*(5), 899–910.

Zhao, Z., & Cope, D. K. (2011). Nerve blocks, trigger points, and intrathecal therapy for chronic pain. In R. J. Moore (Ed.), *Handbook of pain and palliative care: Biobehavioral approaches for the life course*. New York: Springer.

Chapter 42
The Delineation and Explication of Palliative Options of Last Resort

Ben A. Rich

Delineation and General Overview of Palliative Options of Last Resort

The Dominant Model of the Health Professional–Patient Relationship

The dominant model of the health professional–patient relationship is curative, which is often characterized in contradistinction to palliative. The primary focus of the curative model is arriving at a diagnosis and then selecting and implementing an appropriate therapeutic intervention. The primary focus of the palliative model is the relief of pain, suffering, and other forms of distress associated with the manifestation of the disease in a particular patient. The patient's experience of illness is a more important consideration than the label attached to the psychopathophysiological aspects of the disease process. The curative paradigm has shaped the modern medical school curriculum and has been identified as a major barrier to the provision of timely and effective palliative measures (Fox 1997). It is important to avoid simplistic categorizations, for example, that the curative model is only concerned about quantity of life and the avoidance of death while the palliative model is only concerned about the quality of life and the avoidance of pain and suffering at the end of life. Nevertheless, until fairly recently there has been a silo approach to the two models, with exclusively aggressive curative measures pursued until they manifestly fail to achieve their goal, and then their complete abandonment, whereupon there is an abrupt and often untimely shift to entirely palliative measures provided by a completely new cast of professional characters. At about the time of the massive study of intensive care in the United States in the mid-1990s, which revealed a plethora of problems with the palliative aspects of care in this setting (SUPPORT 1995), thought leaders began to call for a transition to what might be characterized as "simultaneous care," in which curative and palliative measures are routinely provided at the same time rather than a rigid sequence of curative only followed by palliative only (Myers and Linder 2003).

B.A. Rich, JD, PhD (✉)
Davis Medical Center, University of California, 4150 V Street, Suite 2500, Sacramento, CA 95817, USA
e-mail: barich@ucdavis.edu

R.J. Moore (ed.), *Handbook of Pain and Palliative Care: Biobehavioral Approaches for the Life Course*,
DOI 10.1007/978-1-4419-1651-8_42, © Springer Science+Business Media, LLC 2012

Palliative Care and Hospice Care

Palliative care and hospice care are related yet distinct concepts and approaches to patient care. Because hospice is provided pursuant to the qualification of the patient for hospice benefits under the Medicare program, requiring certification by a physician that the patient has 6 months or less to live, hospice care is necessarily focused on patients with a terminal condition and the needs of their families during the dying and bereavement processes. Palliative care has no such limitations and may be appropriate for any patient experiencing distress arising out of a medical condition. Nevertheless, there is much overlap in the nature of interventions provided in hospice and palliative care settings, and in extreme cases those interventions may include what is the special concern of this chapter – palliative options of last resort.

It is important to note that routine palliative and hospice measures, many of which are covered in great detail in other chapters of this volume, are effective in achieving their objects in the management of the patient in roughly 95% of cases in which it is provided (see also, Section V, this volume). Data continue to show that too many patients who should be receiving and would benefit from quality palliative care do not receive it in a timely way, and sometimes not at all. This, however, is a separate issue from the roughly 5% of patients whose pain, suffering, and distress at the end of life are refractory to the usual and customary palliative measures (IOM 1998). Making palliative options of last resort available to these patients is a clinical and ethical obligation (Pellegrino 1998). Indeed, from a clinical standard of care perspective, some have argued that "a painful death is a presumptively mismanaged death" (Annas 1995).

There is no broad and solid consensus either in the health care professions or in American society concerning what should be considered a palliative option of last resort or when such options are clinically and ethically appropriate. One often-cited article on this topic considered the following measures under this rubric: voluntarily stopping eating and drinking (VSED), terminal sedation (sedation to unconsciousness), physician-assisted suicide (PAS) (lethal dose of medication administered by patient), and voluntary active euthanasia (lethal dose of medication administered by a third person at the patient's request) (Quill et al. 1997). For reasons that will be discussed in subsequent sections of this chapter, neither the terms "terminal sedation" not "physician-assisted suicide" will be used in this chapter to refer to such practices. VSED is a right which can be asserted by any patient with decisional capacity, and can more aptly be described as a means of controlling the time and manner of one's own death rather than a form of palliation. Voluntary active euthanasia will be considered only briefly at the end of this chapter because it is not a legal option in any U.S. jurisdiction or in most other countries of the world.

The critical distinction made by most clinicians between palliative measures and euthanasia is that the former are provided with the intent to relieve pain and suffering while the latter are provided with the intent to cause the patient's death. In the section on lethal prescriptions, we will consider a counter argument that has been offered by some highly respected moral philosophers that in responding to the request for a lethal medication from a dying patient with decisional capacity a clinician may indeed have a palliative rather than homicidal intent. We must now consider how challenging it can be to discern intent solely from actions taken in the context of caring for patients with intractable end-of-life distress.

Doctrine/Principle/Rule of Double Effect

The Doctrine/Principle/Rule of Double Effect (DDE) is often invoked in the context of discussions about palliative options of last resort and therefore must be briefly reviewed at this point in the discussion. The origins of the doctrine lie in medieval Roman Catholic theology, and credit for its initial formulation is given to Thomas Aquinas in his *Summa Theologica*. In light of this, it is quite remarkable that DDE is so frequently invoked in contemporary secular discussions of end-of-life care across the domains of medicine, law, and ethics. The widespread references to DDE have tended to convey an impression that its tenets are beyond any reasonable dispute. Both the medical (Quill et al. 1997) and the philosophical (Mcintyre 2004) literatures contain robust critiques of DDE, and debates about its efficacy have been the subject of entire books (Woodward 2001).

The ostensible purpose of the doctrine is to ascertain the conditions under which it is morally acceptable to engage in an action that has both a good and a bad consequence. The doctrine consists of four essential elements:

- The action itself must be morally good or morally neutral
- The bad effect must not be intended (though it may be foreseen)
- The good effect must not be produced by means of the bad effect
- There must be proportionality between the good and bad effects (trivial good effects will not support major bad effects)

The doctrine presupposes that those who propose to use it as a heuristic device for morally assessing a particular action will have a consensus view as to such matters as whether the action under review is morally good or morally neutral in and of itself (element 1), and whether the requirement of proportionality between the good and bad effects exists (element 4). In order to appreciate how elusive such a consensus may be, particularly in the care of the dying, consider the concept of a medical fate worse than death. Palliative options of last resort may reasonably be viewed by patients as a means of delivery from such a fate, as may be the withholding or withdrawing of life-sustaining treatment. Frequently cited examples of such fates include: survival in a permanent vegetative state, protracted dying in intractable pain or distress, or being afflicted by the locked-in syndrome (Pearlman et al. 1993). However, other individuals, including some physicians, would dispute that there could be such a thing as a medical fate worse than death because death is the ultimate harm or evil (Nagel 1970).

DDE also appears to take a rather simplistic view of two very complex and nuanced concepts – intent and causation. DDE maintains that there is a distinction with a critical moral difference between that which we intend when we act and that which we merely foresee. It is actually quite remarkable that the U.S. Supreme Court opinions in the PAS cases suggested that such a distinction was consistent with traditional legal distinctions between actions taken because of a given end and actions taken in spite of unintended but foreseen consequences (Glucksberg and Quill 1997). That is because it is a common jury instruction in the criminal law that "a person is presumed to intend the natural and probable consequences of his actions." The burden of proof in such situations shifts to the defendant to rebut that presumption by competent and credible evidence. This presumption runs directly counter to the second element of DDE.

Those who invoke DDE often assert categorically that one who provides a lethal prescription at the request of a terminally ill patient necessarily intends to bring about the patient's death, whereas one who disconnects a ventilator from a patient who is dependent upon it may merely intend to respect the patient's right to refuse life-sustaining treatment, and in such instances neither the clinician nor the patient intend to bring about the patient's death and that disconnecting the ventilator is not, in fact or in law, the cause of the patient's death. Rather the underlying medical condition that necessitated ventilator support in the first instance is said to be the cause. Completely lost in the DDE calculus are the vagaries of intent, the interplay between the intent of the clinician and that of the patient, and the inescapable conclusion that but for the withdrawal of ventilator support, the ventilator-dependent patient would not die when and as she does (Miller et al. 2010).

The bottom line is that sound arguments in the philosophical and professional literature can be found supporting the proposition that DDE does not provide a litmus paper test as to whether any act or omission by a health care professional associated with end-of-life decisions is ethically and legally defensible or not. Of particular concern in arriving at such an ethical assessment are such critical considerations as whether accurate information has been conveyed to those involved and whether the patient's wishes are respected.

Aggressive Administration of Opioid Analgesics

Goals of Pain and Symptom Management at the End of Life

Most pain and symptom distress experienced by patients at the end of life can be effectively managed utilizing a combination of pharmacological and nonpharmacological measures that constitute the hallmark of quality hospice and palliative care. There are chapters of this volume addressing many types of pain and strategies for the management and treatment of pain across clinical contexts (see also, Section V, this volume). Therefore, this section will only briefly address related ethical and professional issues. On an optimistic note, at long last we may be coming to the end of the life span for the persistent and pernicious myths that appropriately aggressive pain and symptom management carries a high risk of depressing respiration to the point of actually causing or hastening death. Indeed, quite to the contrary, recent data suggest that terminally ill patients who receive hospice care in a timely way actually survive longer and with a better quality of life (Connor et al. 2007).

Prescribing medications as a part of a palliative care plan is always a risk–benefit calculation. Respect for patient autonomy and dignity require that whenever possible the patient's wishes and values be an important factor in assessing risk and benefit. Some patients wish to prioritize comfort over alertness, while others will bear significant and otherwise relievable distress in order to maintain the ability to interact with family and friends as long as possible. What is critical is that those providing care be competent to utilize available palliative measures consistent with a care plan tailored to the patient's diagnosis, prognosis, and achievable goals of care.

Such a palliative care plan can be set out in general terms in the advance directive that every adult patient should execute and periodically review and update as appropriate. Upon the diagnosis of a serious or potentially life-threatening condition, the patient's medical record should reflect more detailed provisions reflecting the patient's goals and values concerning comfort measures. Does the efficacy of care plans differ across populations? There is some evidence that there are persistent racial/ethnic disparities that persist in advanced care plans? There are definitely values disparities among racial, ethnic, and religious groups, particularly with regard to withholding or withdrawing life-sustaining treatment and utilization of palliative options of last resort. Such disparities make individualized care planning all that much more important so as to insure that the care provided is consistent with patient wishes.

Several legal cases between 1990 and 2005 reveal tragic situations in which elderly cancer patients in the advanced stages of their illness were subjected to days or weeks of unnecessary pain and distress because of the failure or refusal of clinicians to provide adequate analgesia (Estate of Henry James v. Hillhaven Corporation 1991; Bergman v. Chin 2001; Compassion in Dying v. Washington 1994; Tomlinson v. Bayberry Care Center et al. 2002). In each of these cases, clinician ignorance concerning the relative risks and benefits of opioid analgesia in the care of patients with advanced cancer may have resulted in substandard care and legal liability. What can be done to enhance prescribing for pain control in these specific environments? Patients and their family members and/

or close friends must be adequately informed about both the benefits and risks of pain and symptom management and empowered to advocate for them (Rich 2010).

Persistent and Pervasive Myths About Opioid Analgesia

For too long a significant number of clinicians have subscribed to myths and misinformation suggesting that opioids pose many dangers and offer meager benefits except, perhaps, for patients who are actively dying. Even in the care of patients at or near the end of life, some clinicians and family members view the mere possibility that an escalated dose of morphine might play any causal role in the timing of death as ethically unacceptable and potentially the basis for criminal prosecution. These exaggerated concerns reflect a failure to grasp an essential element of quality palliative care – prioritizing the relief of pain and suffering because death is imminent. When addressing the issue of PAS/aid in dying, the U.S. Supreme Court, through the words of then Justice O'Connor, noted that: "a patient who is suffering from a terminal illness and who is experiencing great pain has no legal barriers to obtaining medication, from qualified physicians, to alleviate that suffering, even to the point of causing unconsciousness and hastening death" (Washington v. Glucksberg 1997). Similarly, a seminal medical journal article by a group of 12 distinguished physicians admonishes that in the care of hopelessly ill patients: "Doses [of analgesics] should be brought promptly to levels that provide a reliable pain-free state … To allow a patient to experience unbearable pain or suffering is unethical medical practice" (Wanzer et al. 1989).

The federal Drug Enforcement Administration and the Federation of State Medical Boards have published formal statements and policies seeking to reassure physicians that they are not at risk of civil or criminal action so long as they prescribe controlled substances for legitimate medical purposes and consistent with recognized clinical practice guidelines (Fishman 2007).

Just before the turn of the twenty-first century, the American Medical Association (AMA), with the support of the Robert Wood Johnson Foundation, initiated the Education for Physicians on End-of-Life Care (2010) (EPEC) project. Its goals were to develop – through a series of national "train-the-trainer seminars" – and promulgate a set of core competencies in end-of-life care that should be learned by all physicians (not just hospice and palliative care physicians) who may at some time be involved in the care of the dying. The EPEC program materials include 12 teaching modules on a range of topics including advance care planning, whole patient assessment, pain management, goals of care, and managing the last hours of life. The pain management module materials note that the relief of pain is necessary but not sufficient for the relief of suffering (EPEC project website). Other measures may well be necessary to adequately address suffering and it is these measures that we consider in subsequent sections of the chapter.

A controversial and problematic term – "slow euthanasia" – has been introduced into the medical and legal setting to characterize the practice involving IV infusion of increasing doses of morphine (Billings and Block 1996). The suggestion here is that rather than following the standard procedure of titrating the morphine does to effect, the dosage continues to be escalated to the point of somnolence, obtundation, or even obvious respiratory depression. When the article introducing this term appeared, it was accompanied by a series of critical commentaries the analysis of which is beyond the scope of this chapter. However, one very important point to note here is that escalating doses of morphine that may impair the patient's alertness and/or respiratory drive are not the common and accepted means of providing palliative sedation for many forms of intractable distress. Similarly, the intent of the clinician in aggressively managing pain with opioids or by the administration of palliative sedation is not to cause or hasten the patient's death but rather to insure comfort. More on this point follows in the next section.

Palliative Sedation for Intractable Distress

Clarifying the Terminological Confusion

Early discussions of sedation to unconsciousness for intractable distress invoked the term "terminal sedation," which rapidly became the common characterization of this palliative strategy. Such a characterization is problematic for a number of reasons that warrant discussion at the outset. First, it is unclear to what the word terminal applies. At first glance, it would seem to be to the process of sedation itself. The most commonly used medications are barbiturates such as pentobarbital. However, properly administered and monitored, such drugs neither cause nor hasten death (Cherny and Radbruch 2009).

Upon further reflection, the word terminal does aptly describe the patient's prognosis, as sedation to unconsciousness with no expectation that the patient will subsequently be brought back to a state of consciousness is only offered to patients in the advanced stages of a terminal illness whose distress has proven refractory to standard approaches to relief. Finally, the word "terminal" may be invoked because many, but not all patients who undergo sedation to unconsciousness in the final stages of a terminal condition, do not continue to receive artificial nutrition and hydration. Consequently, some of these patients may die of dehydration before the terminal event(s) of their underlying condition occur. However, the decision whether artificial nutrition and hydration will be provided following sedation to unconsciousness is completely separate and independent from the decision to actually initiate sedation. Not only would it often be quite difficult to accurately determine in such cases whether the primary cause of death was dehydration or complications of the terminal condition, but more importantly the decision not to provide artificial nutrition and hydration can be motivated by reasons other than to hasten the patient's inevitable death.

For all of these reasons, the consensus view is that palliative sedation is the most appropriate term by which to characterize all forms of sedation for patient comfort, including sedation to unconsciousness until death. The adoption of this term is not an effort, as some have suggested, to euphemize what is really being done or why (Battin 2008). Furthermore, those clinicians who provide palliative sedation for patients consistent with national or international guidelines do not intend, to offer such patients a legalized form of slow euthanasia (Orentlicher 1997).

The Role of Artificial Nutrition and Hydration in Decisions About Palliative Sedation

The decision not to provide artificial nutrition and hydration following the initiation of palliative sedation can be reached for precisely the same reason as when it is discontinued in other clinical settings involving patients with advanced terminal illness or patients in a vegetative state. In such circumstances, patients and/or families and clinicians agree that this intervention no longer provides any medical benefit (from the patient's perspective) and is merely prolonging the dying process or mere physiological persistence (in the case of the vegetative patient). Patients who are quite near death from a terminal condition have a significantly altered capacity to benefit from nutrition and hydration, such that in some instances it may undermine rather than promote good end-of-life care. Dehydration is a natural part of the dying process. Fully sedated patients cannot experience thirst or hunger, and artificial fluids and nutrition can exacerbate such conditions as edema, ascites, pulmonary or other secretions, and dyspnea (EPEC Trainer's Guide, Withholding, Withdrawing Therapy 1999). Thus there may be sound clinical reasons to support a decision not to provide such interventions.

Intractable End-of-Life Distress as a Precondition for Palliative Sedation

Existing clinical practice guidelines on palliative sedation commonly limit the appropriateness of sedation to unconsciousness (in contradistinction to sedation sufficient only to reduce awareness of distress) to patients with intractable suffering at the very end, e.g., last days of life (AAHPM Statement on PS 2006). In cases where the patient is not imminently dying, there is a perception or belief that the proportionality provision of DDE cannot be met. That is, the prospect that the patient might survive more than a few days, perhaps for several weeks or more, renders the harm resulting from permanent unconsciousness disproportionate to the relief of intractable suffering. Examined closely, however, the contention that a longer period of unrelenting suffering from intractable distress provides less of a warrant for sedation to unconsciousness than a shorter period is difficult to comprehend and certainly to justify on secular grounds. The insistence that total sedation until death be offered only to the imminently dying appears to flow from significant clinical ambivalence about the concept of a medical fate worse than death, as well as uncertainty about how or whether intractability can be definitively determined and the extent to which a patient's protestations that their distress is unbearable must be accepted as true and clinically significant.

Recent guidelines have fallen into two distinct camps – those that make no clear distinction between types of intractable terminal suffering and those that seek to set different standards of practice depending upon whether the suffering is characterized as clinical or non-clinical, or alternatively between that which is physiological and that which is spiritual or existential. For example, in 2008 the AMA promulgated a policy statement based upon a report by its Council on Ethical and Judicial Affairs (AMA 2010) entitled "Sedation to Unconsciousness in End-of-Life Care" (AMA CEJA Report 2008). The policy declares that sedation to unconsciousness is an acceptable palliative option of last resort for terminally ill patients who are experiencing intractable "clinical" suffering. Clinical suffering is described as including pain, nausea, vomiting, and dyspnea. Interestingly, clinical suffering is also said to include severe intractable psychological distress. This is declared to be in contradistinction to severe, intractable existential suffering, which the policy characterizes as "non-clinical" in nature and for which sedation to unconsciousness is never appropriate on the grounds that it can be more appropriately addressed by other (unspecified) interventions. The critical distinction between psychological suffering that is purportedly clinical in nature and existential suffering that not appears to be whether a psychiatric label can be attached to explain the symptoms. What remains ambiguous in the AMA policy is the ethical justification for denying the possibility that so-called existential suffering might be as genuinely severe and intractable as psychological distress. In such instances, withholding palliative sedation would be to deprive the patient of a readily available means of removing the patient's capacity to experience the distress that would otherwise continue to afflict them. In the next section we will consider another critique of the AMA's distinction that goes to the very nature of human suffering.

Recently the European Association for Palliative Care (EAPC) published a "recommended framework for the use of palliative sedation" (Cherny et al. 2009). However, unlike the AMA policy, the framework does not preclude the provision of sedation to unconsciousness for intractable existential suffering. Rather, in an appendix it suggests that both refractory psychological symptoms and existential distress are different in ways that warrant special consideration. Thus both the AMA and the EAPC positions presuppose the existence of multiple types of intractable terminal distress and the need for different approaches to palliative sedation depending upon type. In contrast, the American Academy of Hospice and Palliative Medicine (2010) makes no such distinction and simply states that palliative sedation may be medically indicated and ethically appropriate when necessary to relieve otherwise intractable suffering. In the final segment of this section we consider whether or not there is a conceptual basis for such distinctions between or among types of suffering.

The Nature of Suffering and Constraints on Palliative Sedation at the End of Life

A seminal paper on the nature of suffering and the responsibilities of physicians appeared in 1982 (Cassell 1982). In it, Eric Cassell offered a conceptual analysis of human suffering as engendered by illness. Almost 10 years later, he elaborated on this analysis in a definitive book on the subject now in its second edition (Cassell 1991, 2004). Cassell's analysis is grounded on the proposition that human suffering is by its very nature a subjective experience. The nature of suffering is inextricably linked to the nature of human beings, i.e., embodied persons whose defining attributes (*qua* persons) include a sense of self (personal identity), of temporality (a remembered past, lived present, and anticipated future about which there is reasonable self-concern), familial ties and personal relationships, and societal roles, among other things. Importantly, in articulating his analysis of human persons and the nature of their suffering, Cassell discredits Cartesian mind–body dualism, insisting that "person is not mind," and that "bodies do not suffer; persons suffer." He also notes that lamentably, modern medicine continues to be afflicted by dualistic thinking that prioritizes diagnosis of disease processes and sophisticated treatment interventions while discounting the significance of the patient's subjective experience of illness.

According to Cassell, "suffering occurs when an impending destruction of the person is perceived and continues until the threat of disintegration has passed or until the integrity of the person can be restored in some other manner" (Cassell 1982). Cassell's analysis of suffering is categorically inconsistent with any subdividing of suffering into physical and mental or clinical and nonclinical. The unity of the person as an embodied mind experiences suffering in all aspects of being. It is important to acknowledge that to dispute the contention that human suffering can be divided into types or categories that track the mind–body distinction is not inconsistent with an acknowledgement that there are many potential sources or dimensions of suffering, one of which might aptly be characterized as existential in nature. Recognition of these various sources of suffering might have a bearing upon efforts to alleviate that suffering, but it would not constitute a basis for insisting, as some of the policies and guidelines noted above do, that palliative sedation should not be an option of last resort for any manifestation of suffering at the end of life that is refractory to other available measures for relief.

The medical and philosophical literatures are devoid of any serious challenge to or alternative formulation of human suffering. Yet that is what is required to support the policies that purport to distinguish among the various types of human suffering and prohibit the provision of palliative sedation for some, but not others.

Physician-Assisted Suicide/Aid-in-Dying

Brief Overview of the History of Physician-Assisted Suicide/Aid in Dying (PAS/PAD)

The so-called "Death With Dignity" movement is international in scope. The Netherlands has been considered to be at the epicenter of the movement because medicine, law, policy, and the general public have generally accepted the appropriateness of aid-in-dying that includes not only making a lethal prescription available to terminally ill patients who request it but also physician administration of a lethal dose under certain circumstances. This section will discuss the situation in the United States.

Between 1994 and 2009, a number of major developments in case and statutory law have determined the legal status of this practice in the United States. During roughly the same period, the academic and professional literatures as well as policy and position statements by professional organizations also framed the debate on the subject. In 1994, voters in the State of Oregon approved a ballot initiative (by a vote of 51–49%) that enacted into law the Oregon Death with Dignity Act (2010) (ODWDA). Before the act could take effect, opponents sought and obtained a preliminary injunction. For the next several years the challenge to the new law worked its way through the federal court system. Ultimately the act was upheld and the Supreme Court refused to consider the case. Then, the Oregon Legislature caused the issue to come before the electorate a second time in 1997, whereupon the voters supported the act by a much wider margin of 60–40%. Later in this section we will consider the data that has been accumulated in the 12 years that the ODWDA has been operational.

That same year the U.S. Supreme Court ruled in two companion cases from New York and Washington that the U.S. Constitution does not recognize either a legal right to nor a prohibition of PAS/PAD (Washington v. Glucksberg 1997; Vacco v. Quill 1997). Thus the matter is one for each individual state to determine as a matter of public policy. In 2006, yet another challenge to the ODWDA came before the Supreme Court in the form of an argument by the Attorney General of the United States that writing a lethal prescription constituted a violation of the federal Controlled Substances Act since there was no "legitimate medical purpose" to support such a practice. The Supreme Court ruled that the Attorney General would be exceeding his legal authority in prosecuting a physician on these grounds (Gonzales v. Oregon 2006), noting that what constitutes legitimate medical practice is a matter that has been traditionally left to the states to determine, primarily through their medical boards.

The key provisions of the ODWDA are the following:

- The patient must be over the age of 18 and a resident of Oregon
- The patient must have decisional capacity and the ability to communicate his/her desire for a prescription that if taken will bring about death
- The patient must make two verbal request at least 15 days apart and one written request at least 48 hours prior to the writing of the prescription
- The patient must have been determined to have a terminal condition (one that will lead to death in 6 months) that is confirmed by a second physician
- The prescribing physician may be present when the medication is taken but the patient must be capable of taking it him/herself
- If the physician believes the patient may suffer from a mental disorder or depression that would impair judgment, s/he must refer the patient to a mental health professional
- The prescribing physician must comply with the reporting requirements of the act

Semantic Issues Concerning PAS/PAD

One interesting aspect of the debate over this most controversial aspect of end-of-life care is the gradual change among some professionals concerning how we think about death and dying and how we tend to characterize the practice. Heretofore one could easily discern whether a person was a supporter or opponent of the practice depending upon whether they used the term PAS or some alternative without the word "suicide" such as physician-assisted dying. However, in the last few years a number of major national health care professional organizations have issued formal policies or position statements challenging the appropriateness of the term PAS to describe the provision of a prescription by a physician to a terminally ill patient who has decisional capacity and who has requested it for the purpose of controlling the time and manner of his/her death. Included among these organizations are: the American Academy of Hospice and Palliative Medicine, the American College of Legal Medicine, the American Medical Student Association, the American Public Health Association, and the American Medical Women's Association.

The stance taken by many of the above organizations does not necessarily reflect a shift from opposition to advocacy of lethal prescriptions at the request of terminally ill patients, but rather of "studied neutrality" (Quill and Cassel 2003). Other major national medical organizations, such as the AMA and the American College of Physicians, maintain their long-standing opposition to legalization and regulation of the practice as well as their insistence that use of terminology such as "physician-assisted dying" is misleading and constitutes an attempt to gloss over the practice's ethical implications.

The debate over the proper terminology with which to describe the practice in question continues in the courts as well. When the Ninth Circuit Court of Appeals decided the case of Glucksberg v. Quill, the majority framed the issue as whether or not terminally ill patients have a constitutional right to determine the time and manner of their own death. When the U.S. Supreme Court reversed that decision, a plurality of the justices reframed the issue as whether terminally ill patients have a constitutional right to commit suicide with the assistance of a physician. Late in 2009, the Montana Supreme Court ruled that current state law and policy does not preclude physicians from honoring the request of a decisionally capacitated terminally ill patient for a lethal prescription (Baxter v. Montana 2009). The court majority not only rejected the use of the term "physician-assisted suicide" to describe the practice, but also, as we will consider further in a subsequent section of this chapter, challenged the long-standing and widely accepted view that a physician who provides such a prescription is more directly implicated in the patients subsequent death than is a physician who discontinues a life-sustaining intervention such as mechanical ventilation or artificial nutrition and hydration. Clearly, not only the language but also professional attitudes toward the practice are in a continuing state of evolution.

Arguments in Support of PAS/PAD

There are a number of arguments frequently offered by proponents of legalizing and regulating the practice of providing a lethal prescription at the request of patients with a terminal condition. We will consider these without suggesting any priority, rank, or relative significance among them, or any effort to argue in support of or in opposition to their merits. The first argument is that providing a lethal prescription at the request of a decisionally capable patient is consistent with the well-accepted bioethical principle of respect for individual patient autonomy. Recognizing this autonomy does not entail imposing an obligation on the part of any particular physician to accede to the request if s/he believes the clinical circumstances do not warrant it or s/he conscientiously objects to the practice. Several phrases that have been used to characterize the patient's interests in influencing their dying process, such as "On Our Own Terms" and "A Death of One's Own" implicitly suggest that whenever possible how one dies should be consistent with his/her own personal values and priorities. For some this may be struggling against their terminal illness as long as possible, while for others it may be pursuing a peaceful death with the aide of palliative options of last resort including a lethal prescription.

A second argument is grounded on the recognition that a small percentage of dying patients will experience intractable distress that cannot be relieved by any means other than sedation to unconsciousness, or by a lethal prescription. Among this small subset of patients, there are those who find the option of palliative sedation to be unacceptable because, for example, it subjects their family and loved ones to an indefinite though protracted period of days to a week or more in where they must stand by as the patient dies from either dehydration or from their underlying terminal condition.

To such patients, being able to achieve a prompt and peaceful death by ingesting a lethal prescription seems much more rational and humane.

A third argument is grounded on the ethical principle of justice and often invokes the 14th amendment to the U.S. Constitution, more particularly its equal protection clause. This argument was central to the case of Vacco v. Quill, in which the Second Circuit Court of Appeals concluded that New York state's criminal statute precluding assisted suicide violated the equal protection of terminally ill patients who were not on life support but who wished to end their life. Those on life support had a recognized right to insist that it be discontinued thereby resulting in their death, whereas the criminal law precluded those not on life support from securing a lethal prescription from a willing physician. The U.S. Supreme Court reversed the Second Circuit, holding that there was no equal protection violation because all terminally ill patients in New York were treated the same, i.e., those on life support could cause it to be discontinued, while no one was allowed to secure a lethal prescription from a physician.

Arguments in Opposition to PAS/PAD

As with the previous section, the arguments in opposition will be considered without any effort to establish a priority ranking or analyze their relative strengths and weaknesses. Two arguments appear most often in opposition to PAS/PAD. The first is grounded in belief about the sanctity of human life. This argument carries an ineluctable religious dimension by virtue of our common understanding of sacred. A more secular characterization would be the inviolability of human life which is the basis for the prohibitions on killing. It is important to note that this argument is based on the presupposition that there is a legitimate moral distinction with a difference between providing patients with a lethal prescription on the one hand and withholding or withdrawing life-sustaining interventions on the other. We will address this distinction further in the next section.

A second argument maintains that actively participating in bringing about a patient's death is categorically inconsistent with the physician's professional responsibility to the patient. The provision of the Hippocratic Oath often translated: "I will not give a drug that is deadly to anyone if asked, nor will I suggest the way to such a counsel". Those who have engaged in critical historical analysis of the Oath are in disagreement about its origins as well as its interpretation. For example, it has been suggested by some that what appears to be a prohibition of PAS/PAD or euthanasia is in fact a prohibition of physicians participating in capital punishment (Miles 2004).

A third argument is based upon the slippery slope concept. In this context it maintains that while we may begin with laws such as that in Oregon and Washington, limiting lethal prescriptions to decisionally capable and terminally ill patients who request it, inexorably the practice will lead to offering it to patients who are not terminally ill or imposing it upon patients who do not wish it, particularly the frail elderly and the mentally or physically disabled.

Experience with the Oregon Death with Dignity Act (ODWDA)

What is most striking about the experience to date with the ODWDA is how starkly the data contrast with the parade of horrors predicted by the opponents to the law. Those groups, spearheaded by the Roman Catholic Church and disability rights organizations such as "Not Dead Yet," insisted that were the initiative to become law, those accessing and utilizing lethal prescriptions would be overwhelmingly the poor, the uninsured, the disabled, the marginally educated, and those without reasonable access to hospice services (Lindsay 2009). Based upon 12 years of reporting data on those who obtained and utilized a lethal prescription, a portrait of the typical patient utilizing a lethal prescription has emerged:

- Well-educated (48.3% had baccalaureate degree)
- Diagnosed with some form of cancer (77%)
- Health insurance coverage (98.7% in 2009 had some form)
- Enrolled in hospice at the time of death (91.5%)
- Died at home – the stated preference of the majority of individuals when surveyed (98.3%)

Finally, under treatment of pain and other forms of distress was not among the most commonly stated reasons for seeking and utilizing a lethal prescription. Rather, the three most commonly stated reasons were: loss of autonomy (96.6%), loss of dignity (91.5%), and decreasing ability to participate in activities that make life enjoyable (86.4) (Oregon DHS 2010).

One of the primary ongoing critiques of the ODWDA is that very few of the patients who request a lethal prescription are carefully scrutinized for clinical depression or other decisional capacity-limiting psychiatric problems. The presupposition behind this critique appears to be that only profoundly depressed or otherwise mentally compromised individuals would seek to hasten death even in the face of grave and terminal illness and profoundly diminished quality of life. One prominent palliative care specialist has advocated for the identification of a new category of mental disorder ("demoralization syndrome"), an important aspect of which is a desire for death (Kissane 2001). However, recent data suggest that most patients who avail themselves of the ODWDA do not suffer from depression (Ganzini et al. 2008). Nevertheless, many palliative care specialists strongly advocate that with the timely and adept provision of what have come to be characterized as "dignity-preserving" therapies, most terminally ill patients would not choose to hasten their death with a lethal prescription even if it were an available option (Chochinov 2006).

Euthanasia

Conceptual Analysis of Euthanasia

Within the philosophical realm, euthanasia is not a unitary concept. Rather, distinctions are made between "active" and "passive" euthanasia and among voluntary, non-voluntary, and involuntary varieties. Active euthanasia would be the administration of a lethal dose of medication for the purpose of ending the patient's life. Passive euthanasia would be discontinuing a life-sustaining intervention. Either instance is voluntary if it is in response to the patient's request, non-voluntary if the patient cannot now and has not previously expressed a preference, and involuntary if doing so is contrary to the known wishes of the patient. Nowhere in the perennial debate over euthanasia can one find any serious proponents of involuntary euthanasia.

The analysis above is in marked contradistinction to the clinical realm, in which the term euthanasia is generally applied to the act of administering a lethal medication, whereas withdrawing life-sustaining treatment is not considered to be a form of euthanasia at all. Great ethical significance is attached to the active–passive distinction, which is also characterized as that between "killing" and merely "allowing the patient to die." As we shall now consider in more depth, the distinction relies heavily on certain flawed presuppositions about causation and intent.

Voluntary active euthanasia is legal only in the Netherlands and Belgium (Lewis 2007). Interestingly, however, when the Ninth Circuit Court of Appeals issued it *en banc* ruling in the case of Compassion in Dying v. Washington, holding that a Washington statute criminalizing assisted suicide violated a terminally ill patient's 14th Amendment liberty interest in determining the time and manner of one's own death, a ruling subsequently reversed by the U.S. Supreme Court, the majority opinion included the following *dictum* (statements not essential to deciding the case before the court):

> …we view the critical line in the right-to-die cases as the one between the voluntary and involuntary termination of an individual's life. In the first case – volitional death – the physician is aiding a patient who wishes to exercise a liberty interest, and in the other – involuntary death – another person is acting in his own behalf, or, in some instances society's, is determining that an individual's life should no longer continue. We consider it less important who administers the medication than who determines whether the terminally ill person's life shall end (Compassion in Dying v. Washington 1996).

In making this point the Ninth Circuit majority embraced the argument that has been made by a small but distinguished group of moral philosophers and bioethicists that what determines the moral valence of acts or omissions that result in the death of a patient is not whether death results from active vs. passive measures, but rather whether it furthers an interest of the patient from that patient's perspective.

Issues of Causation and Intent in End-of-Life Care

Consider, for example, a hypothetical situation postulated in a recent article. Two motorcyclists (John and Sam) are rendered quadriplegic by an accident. During the next few years John remains ventilator dependent, whereas Sam has been successfully weaned from the ventilator. However, neither has come to terms with their total dependency on others and both find their quality of life unacceptable. Each one expresses a wish to die and requests the assistance of health care professionals. In the case of John, all that would be required to accede to his request is to discontinue mechanical ventilation and provide palliative measures as he dies. Sam, however, requests that he be administered a lethal dose of medication so that his death is neither painful nor prolonged. The prevailing view among health care professionals is that John is not committing suicide in seeking to discontinue mechanical ventilation, and respecting his refusal of treatment by discontinuing the ventilator is neither active euthanasia nor assisted suicide. Furthermore, the cause of John's death would be the underlying medical condition necessitating mechanical ventilation for survival (Miller et al. 2010).

In stark contrast, Sam would be viewed as asking for a health care professional to kill him by engaging in voluntary active euthanasia, and the cause of Sam's death would be the lethal dose of medication administered by a willing health care professional whose presumed intent was to kill Sam (albeit in response to his request). The authors of the article in which this hypothetical appears maintain that it is a moral fiction that there is a distinction with a moral difference between meeting John's and Sam's respective requests to die. The authors argue that the cause of both John and Sam's death is an act by a health care professional (turning off a ventilator or administering a lethal dose of medication) and the intent of both professionals was not to kill the patient but to respond to the request to help them die in a manner that respected their wishes and personal values. It is only by constructing the mythology involved in what we label as suicide and how we determine causation and intent in end-of-life practices that one can arrive at the considered judgment that helping John to die as he requested did not involve suicide on his part nor an intent to end his life on the professional's part, and the cause of his death was some "terminal" condition, whereas helping Sam to die as he requested involved suicide on his part, a specific intent to kill him on the part of the professional, and that the cause of his death by lethal prescription might be properly characterized as criminal homicide.

There is of course a risk inherent in the argument that the killing vs. allowing the patient to die distinction that lacks logical rigor and is inconsistent with an objective examination of the operative facts. That risk is that we may revert to a position in which patient requests to discontinue life support will no longer be respected because health care professionals refuse to be actively involved in bringing about a patient's death, even when that is consistent with the patient's wishes. For purposes of this chapter, it is sufficient to make the point that there exist in the academic literature solid and sustained critiques of certain basic presuppositions that go to the heart of the ethics of end-of-life care.

Concluding Observations Concerning the Relief of Pain and Suffering at the End of Life

The long-standing and overheated debate over the range of acceptable options for responding to patients whose end-of-life suffering has failed to respond to the usual and customary palliative measures has been complicated by a complex web of semantic problems and myths and misunderstandings about the nature and role of causation and intent in ascertaining the ethical legitimacy and legal acceptability of actions that are perceived to be more directly linked to the patient's imminent and inevitable death. The goal of this chapter is not necessarily to change any reader's prior views on the issues, but rather to emphasize how important unambiguous language and clear reasoning are to thoughtful and deliberate engagement with the issues. This clarity must not only characterize the discussion among leaders and policy makers, but also between clinicians, patients, and their families in the context of each individual case.

References

American Academy of Hospice and Palliative Medicine Position Statements. (2010). *Statement on palliative sedation.* Approved by the Board of Directors September 15, 2006, Glenview, IL. Retrieved June 16, 2010, from http://www.aahpm.org/positions/sedation.html.

American Medical Association Council on Ethical and Judicial Affairs. (2010). *Sedation to unconsciousness in end-of-life care.* CEJA report 5-A-08. Retrieved June 16, 2010, from http:www.ama.org/2201a.pdf.

Annas, G. J. (1995). How we lie. *The Hastings Center Report, 25,* S12–S14.

Battin, M. P. (2008). Pulling the sheet over our eyes. *The Hastings Center Report, 38,* 27–30.

Baxter v. Montana. (2009). 224 P.3d 1211, 2009, WL 5155363 (Mont).

Bergman v. Chin. (2001). No. H205732-1 (Alameda County Ct., June 13).

Billings, J. A., & Block, S. D. (1996). Slow euthanasia. *Journal of Palliative Care, 12,* 21–30.

Cassell, E. J. (1982). The nature of suffering and the goals of medicine. *The New England Journal of Medicine, 306,* 639–645.

Cassell, E. J. (2004). *The nature of suffering and the goals of medicine.* New York: Oxford University Press.

Cherney, N. I., Radbruch, L., & Board of the European Association for Palliative Care. (2009). European Association for Palliative Care (EAPC) recommended framework for the use of sedation in palliative care. *Palliative Medicine, 23,* 581–593.

Chochinov, H. M. (2006). Dying, dignity, and new horizons in palliative end-of-life care. *CA: A Cancer Journal for Clinicians, 56,* 84–103.

Compassion in Dying v. Washington. (1994). 850 F. Supp. 1454 (W.D. Wash).

Connor, S. R., Pyenson, B., Fitch, K., Spence, C., & Iwaski, K. (2007). Comparing hospice and nonhospice patient survival among patients who die within a three -year window. *Journal of Pain and Symptom Management, 33,* 238–246.

Education for Physicians on End-of-Life Care. Trainer's Guide, modol withholding, withdrawing therapy (1999). In: Emanuel LL, von Gunter CG, Ferris FD. EPEC project.

Estate of Henry James v. Hillhaven Corporation. (1991). No. 89 CVS 64 (N.C. Super. Ct. January 15).

Field, M. J., Cassel, C. K. (Eds.). (1998). Institute of Medicine. In *Approaching death: improving care at the end of life*. Washington: National Academies Press.

Fishman, S. M. (2007). *Responsible opioid prescribing: A physician's guide*. Dallas: Federation of State Medical Boards.

Fox, E. (1997). Predominance of the Curative model of medical care – A Residual Problem. *JAMA, 278*, 761–763.

Gonzales v. Oregon. (2006). 546 U.S. 243.

Institute of medicine (1998). Approaching Death: Improving Care at the End of Life. Washington, D.C.: National Academy Press.

Lewis, P. (2007). *Assisted dying and legal change*. Oxford: Oxford University Press.

Lindsay, R. A. (2009). Oregon's experience: Evaluating the record. *The American Journal of Bioethics, 9*, 19–27.

McIntyre, A. (2004). The double life of double effect. *Theoretical Medicine, 25*, 61–74.

Miles, S. H. (2004). *The hippocratic oath and the ethics of medicine*. New York: Oxford University Press.

Miller, F. G., Truog, R. D., & Brock, D. W. (2010). Moral fictions and medical ethics. *Bioethics, 24*(9), 453–460.

Myers, F. J., & Linder, J. (2003). Simultaneous care: Disease treatment and palliative care throughout illness. *Journal of Clinical Oncology, 21*, 1412–1415.

Nagel, T. (1970). Death. *Noûs, 4*, 73–80.

Oregon Death With Dignity Act. (2010). Oregon revised statutes 127.505, et. Seq. Retrieved June 16, 2010, from http://www.leg.state.or.us/ors/127.html.

Oregon Department of Health Services. (2010). 2009 Summary of Oregon death with dignity act. Retrieved June 16, 2010, from http://www.oregon.gov/DHS/ph/pas/docs/year12.pdf.

Orentlicher, D. (1997). The Supreme Court an physician-assisted suicide: Rejecting assisted suicide but embracing euthanasia. *The New England Journal of Medicine, 337*, 1236–1239.

Pearlman, R. A., Cain, K. C., Patrick, D. L., Appelbaum-Maizel, M., Starks, H. E., Jecker, N. S., et al. (1993). Insights pertaining to patient assessments of states worse than death. *The Journal of Clinical Ethics, 4*, 33–41.

Pellegrino, E. D. (1998). Emerging ethical issues in palliative care. *Journal of American Medical Association, 279*, 1521–1522.

Quill, T. E., & Cassel, C. K. (2003). Professional organizations' position statements on physician-assisted suicide: A case for studied neutrality. *Archives of Internal Medicine, 138*, 208–211.

Quill, T. E., Dresser, R., & Brock, D. W. (1997). The rule of double effect – A critique of its role in end-of-life decision making. *The New England Journal of Medicine, 337*, 1768–1771.

Quill, T. E., Lo, B., & Brock, D. W. (1997). Palliative options of last resort: A comparison of voluntarily stopping eating and drinking, terminal sedation, physician-assisted suicide, and voluntary active euthanasia. *Journal of American Medical Association, 278*, 2099–2104.

Rich, B. A. (2010). A patient's guide to pain management. In T. Kushner (Ed.), *Surviving health care* (pp. 246–263). New York: Cambridge University Press.

SUPPORT Principal Investigators. (1995). A controlled trial to improve care for seriously ill hospitalized patients. The study to understand prognoses, preferences for outcomes, and risks of treatments (SUPPORT). *Journal of American Medical Association, 274*, 1591–1598.

Tomlinson v. Bayberry Care Center, et al. (2002). No. C 02-00120, Superior Court, Contra Costa Co, CA.

Vacco v. Quill. (1997). 521 U.S. 793.

Wanzer, S. H., Federman, D. D., Adelsein, S. J., Cassel, C. K., Cassem, E. H., Cranford, R. E., et al. (1989). The physician's responsibility toward hopelessly ill patients – A second look. *New England Journal of Medicine, 320*, 844–849.

Washington v. Glucksberg. (1997). 521 U.S. 702.

Woodward, P. A. (Ed.). (2001). *The doctrine of double effect – Philosophers debate a controversial moral principle*. Notre Dame: Notre Dame University Press.

Chapter 43
Recognition and Resolution of Ethical Barriers to Palliative Care Research

Perry G. Fine

Introduction

Palliative care research can be defined as research related to understanding and improving the quality of life of patients near the end of life. Historically, there has been a paucity of research in this field for two over-arching reasons: primarily, medical interest—including research—related to relieving burden of illness, rather than primary mechanisms and treatments of disease, per se, is relatively new; and, secondarily, patients nearing the end of life have either been marginalized (i.e., viewed as not worthy of "investment" of scarce research dollars) or viewed as too vulnerable to undergo the rigorous processes of formalized research (Field and Cassell 1997). Ironically, concerns about such vulnerabilities have created an ethical paradox. In order to protect this patient population from potential harms, including coercion, exploitation, and the possibility of imposing additional suffering at the end of life, terminally ill patients have been deprived of the opportunity to participate in research afforded to other patient populations: the frank withholding of an ethical prerogative. As a result, innovation and empirical developments in the field have been seriously curtailed.

This chapter will explicate these barriers and misconceptions, and address the ways in which research can—and should—proceed, following normative ethical imperatives. Currently, two of the most intractable barriers to high-quality research in palliative care patients that bear mentioning, but are beyond the scope of this chapter, include severe limitations in research funding (especially in proportion to other high-impact clinical areas) and disparities in access to care (which includes access to research trials) among various populations (Foley et al. 2001). The self-same issues that are described by Dr. Carmen Green on health disparities in pain also pertain to the domain of pain and palliative care research as well. Conversely, ethical challenges to research in palliative care patients may pertain to other vulnerable populations, including the very young, the very old, pregnant women, prisoners, and psychiatrically and cognitively impaired persons, among others. Patients with far-advanced medical illness provide a good paradigm to explore ethical concerns about vulnerable populations insofar as they embody some of the greatest challenges to unencumbered decision-making: a high symptom burden (including fatigue, pain, mood disturbance, nausea, dyspnea), cognitive impairment and imminent mortality (Brechtl et al. 2006). As such, the tenets brought forth in this chapter may pertain to barriers to, and the provision of, ethical research in other vulnerable populations.

P.G. Fine, MD (✉)
Department of Anesthesiology, University of Utah, Salt Lake City, UT, USA
e-mail: perry.fine@hsc.utah.edu

R.J. Moore (ed.), *Handbook of Pain and Palliative Care: Biobehavioral Approaches for the Life Course*, DOI 10.1007/978-1-4419-1651-8_43, © Springer Science+Business Media, LLC 2012

Ethical Challenges and Tensions in Recruiting and Performing Research in Patients with Far-Advanced Illness

It has been authoritatively stated that "being ill brings with it a multitude of pressures, and a patient suffering from a life-threatening disease may feel as though she has little choice regarding treatment." Physicians should be aware of how vulnerable patients may be to the coercive influence of unrealistic hope especially those suffering from chronic, life-threatening disorders (Berg et al. 2001). Importantly, there is no distinction made in this appeal between actions around routine clinical care and those that involve research, nor should there be. But within the context of the ethical principle of autonomy, under which the doctrine of informed consent logically falls, the meaning of terms such as "vulnerability" and "coercion" must be thoroughly considered and well understood. The implication of these terms, and concern for palliative care patient well-being and self-determination that is inherent to their use in a research context, is that exploitation may occur when there is so much at stake as life itself, since life for these patients is short.

It is also noteworthy that the traditional arguments for patient protection against exploitation rely upon loss of life as the greatest perceived risk of either intervention or nonintervention, whereas quality of remaining life may be of greater importance for palliative care patients. A patient's priorities need to be unambiguously determined at the outset of any discussion regarding potential benefits vs. harms of being involved in a research protocol. For example, if a protocol involving a potent analgesic for breakthrough pain is being discussed, and the patient's greatest concern is adequate pain control without excessive sedation, and in their view an imminent comfortable death is preferable to a prolonged, agonizing one, this is an important starting point for discussion of potential risks. If the Institutional Review Board fails to attend to or understand this type of nuance, and requires an informed consent "script" that focuses excessively on potential risks of respiratory depression, subjects may be unwittingly exploited into agreeing to participate since "the worst outcome" is, for them, a preferred outcome, under exigent circumstances of poorly controlled pain.

What Exactly Makes a "Vulnerable Person" Vulnerable as a Human Subject in Clinical Research?

The Federal Regulations on the Protection of Human Subjects require that IRBs take into account the "special problems of research involving vulnerable populations" (US Department of Health and Human Services 2003). Vulnerability in the context of human subjects research implies that individuals are less able to make informed decisions on their own behalf, or protect themselves from external influences. Sensory, cognitive, language and other barriers make people vulnerable, since they may not understand what is going on or the implications of enrollment in a trial. So, in considering palliative care patients as a group, there are concerns about vulnerability, due to the myriad influences of advanced disease on comprehension, communication, thought processes, and emotions. But individuals within this group may have no vulnerabilities in this regard. So, in evaluating vulnerability within this population, each individual needs to be assessed on the basis of what they are vulnerable to, rather than a generalization that will likely have limited applicability to individuals, and deter, rather than facilitate, voluntary participation in clinical research trials.

Voluntariness, Vulnerability, Coercion, Exploitation, and Informed Consent

Voluntariness is a necessary but far from sufficient safeguard to the ethical conduct of research. Whereas it is a prerequisite to self-determined decision-making and informed consent, it does

Table 43.1 Distinguishing voluntariness from vulnerability, coercion, and exploitation (US Department of Health and Human Services 2003) reprinted with permission, Elsevier, New York

Concept	Definition	Relationship to voluntariness	Safeguard	Responsible part for safeguard
Vulnerability	Increased potential that one's interests cannot be protected	Not necessarily related to voluntariness; potentially related to issues of informed consent depending on the circumstance	Varies depending on what the participant is vulnerable to	Investigator or IRB—varies depending on the circumstances
Coercion	A credible and irresistible force exerted by one person that negatively limits the options of another person	Direct violation of voluntariness	Keep participant free from the threat	Investigator– participant (team effort by investigators, nurses, social work)
Exploitation	The unfair distribution of the benefits and burdens from a transaction	Not related to voluntariness; related to issues of risk and benefit	Ensure favorable risk–benefit ratio for all involved participants	IRB

not ensure against exploitation of vulnerable persons (see Table 43.1) (Agrawal 2003). In the orchestration of research activities involving vulnerable persons, genuine threats to voluntariness need to be clearly identified, and articulated, as do other distinctly unethical activities, whether deliberate or unintended.

Voluntariness

"Voluntariness" has been defined as a choice or action that is free from coercion and undue influence from other people (Nelson and Merz 2002). Contemporary tenets of ethical research conduct, as canonized in the Nuremberg Code and the Helsinki Declaration require the voluntary consent of human subjects (The Nuremberg Code 1996). In vulnerable populations, such as palliative care patients, it is clear that the requirement for voluntariness can be met, but other requirements for the ethical conduct of research, including social or scientific value, scientific validity, fair subject selection, favorable risk–benefit ratio, independent review, informed consent, and respect for subjects (privacy protection, opportunity to withdraw, etc.) (Emmanuel et al. 2000). However, it is voluntariness that most commonly becomes the foremost pragmatic barrier to enrolling subjects into palliative care research, including clinical trials (Lehan-Mackin et al. 2009; Kirchhoff and Kehl 2008) (see also Currow, this volume). As will be discussed in more detail shortly, coercion undermines voluntariness, but it is more feasible to identify and actively prevent coercive influences in vulnerable populations than it is to gain access to and ensure their voluntary enrollment into clinical trials. Several types of impasses or barriers that impact directly or indirectly upon voluntariness have been identified by Lehan-Mackin et al. (2009), including societal attitudes toward death, research procedures, health care organizations, agency staff, patients' families and caregivers, and patient characteristics. These, singly and collectively, pose high hurdles for palliative care patients to overcome. Proposed solutions to these formidable barriers are not simple, and require a multipronged approach. Chiefly, though, systems of care and the professionals who work within them where such patients reside, including hospitals, nursing homes, assisted living facilities and hospice programs must view palliative care research as a legitimate and important *potential* opportunity for patients. This will likely only occur through wholesale cultural change that includes a demand for improvements in evidence-based care, both by healthcare professionals and patients and their families alike. Simply put, voluntariness depends upon having a comprehensible choice, and that choice can only be made if the conversation about options, including research opportunities, is available to be had without extreme prejudice.

Coercion

Coercion is something that one person does to another that limits the choice a research participant makes in a particular way, and one that is usually negative for the research subject. One of the major constraints on research in palliative care has been the view that life-limiting disease in and of itself is a coercive influence, disallowing freedom of choice. This highly paternalistic point of view has had a back-firing effect on this vulnerable population, preventing them from voluntarily participating in research activities. Difficult choices, absent direct contrivance by another person to create a "no-win" circumstance for the patient/subject, do not create a coercive situation in and of themselves. Palliative care patients commonly face difficult choices, brought on by their medical conditions, and although these strongly influence and weigh heavily on decisions that they must make, they do not preclude against voluntary choices, if given the opportunity to choose. Extending the earlier example, a decision to enroll in an analgesic trial, weighing the risks vs. benefits, opportunity costs, and so on may be very difficult for a patient with pain that is difficult to control using conventional means. However, this is not the same as if it were implied that unless the patient enrolls in the clinical trial, access to pain medications will be strictly limited. This latter case is clearly coercive and is a direct violation of voluntarism.

Exploitation

In the context of clinical subjects research, exploitation, namely taking unfair advantage of someone's bad situation, must be differentiated from voluntariness because it can only be dealt with at the IRB level, in contrast to the informed consent process. A person may freely choose an unfair proposition, believing that it is in her best interest to do so, but it is the unfairness of the proposition that creates the ethical problem of exploitation. It is easy to see why there is serious concern about exploitation of palliative care patients as research subjects. Going back to the example where pain is poorly controlled, and especially where specialized pain care (or high-cost analgesics or interventions) is limited, the prospect of access to "new and improved" analgesics or therapies, albeit unproven, may seem to be better than the alternative. A similar concern over exploitation and potential patient burden would exist if the contingency of enrollment required several trips to a medical center for blood draws, where the whole trip might take several hours. Although unencumbered and voluntary consent can be given, is this "fair" to an individual with limited life expectancy, who is burdened by fatigue, pain, and nausea? The determination of exploitation must be made on the balance of risks (harms, burdens) vs. benefits. Researchers and clinicians who are knowledgeable about the proposed study population and the research methodology need to make a determination about the contingencies in advance of finalizing the protocol, in order to assure an overall favorable risk–benefit ratio, in order to obviate concerns about exploitation. As important as this is, this is one of the least well understood and poorly studied areas of human subjects research (US Department of Health and Human Services 2003).

Cognitively Impaired Individuals

Cognitive impairment can also impede the ability to provide informed consent are common in the palliative care patients (Schaeffer et al. 1996; Cassarett 2003).

As vulnerable as this population might be to unethical research practices, these people are also vulnerable to unjust discrimination against participation in research that might provide direct benefit to them. Means to identify and enroll potential subjects and to provide safeguards for ethical conduct of research in these patients must be sought prior to the initiation of any study and at other intervals in order to improve the evidence base for therapeutics for these self-same patients (Karlawish 2003a).

Assessing Decision-Making Capacity

Due to the high prevalence of cognitive impairment and other barriers to the provision of informed consent in the palliative care population, an informal assessment of decision-making capacity should be built into subject recruitment screening processes for all studies that involve anything more than minimal risk (for which waiver of consent would normally be granted in healthy patients). Based upon the results of screening, a more formal assessment of decision-making capacity should be made using a series of evidence based and standard, validated questions, such as those in the MacArthur Competency Assessment Tool of Clinical Research (Cassarett 2003; Grisso and Appelbaum 1995). The results should be used to make a determination about a potential subject's ability to provide independent informed consent, assent, or dissent (Grisso and Appelbaum 1995).

Added Patient Protections

Added measures at the time of enrollment are required to ensure that cognitively impaired patients' rights and well-being are protected. The ground rules for enrolling cognitively impaired patients into a research study are based upon an assessment of risk associated with participation. Minimal risk is defined as "the probability and magnitude of physical or psychological harm or discomfort anticipated in the research are not greater in and of themselves than those ordinarily encountered in daily life, or during the performance of routine physical or psychological examinations or tests (Berg et al. 2001)." Additional protections include the provision of assent, not dissent, or they need to have provided an informed consent while able, in anticipation of losing capacity. In addition to these provisions, the consent of a proxy is required.

Great controversy exists over what is considered to be "minimal risk" in potential subjects such as palliative care patients or others who are critically ill who already have a very high "baseline" of risk, compared with healthy individuals. It is generally agreed that any research involving more than minimal risk at least require advance consent. But again, what is the basis of comparison for minimal risk? Recent interpretations of minimal risk tend to use the patient's clinical circumstances as the basis for comparison, rather than measures for healthy individuals. As such, for many palliative care patients, and especially those with cognitive impairment, their risk status is so high, that the baseline for "minimal risk" might be construed as equally high. Take the example of a cognitively impaired patient with metastatic bone disease who appears to be in severe pain when turned in bed for bathing, but otherwise appears comfortable. A clinical trial of a low-dose of a potent, noninvasively delivered, rapidly absorbed transmucosal analgesic is proposed with this population in mind: i.e., opioid naïve patients without intravenous access who appear to be experiencing rapidly developing and severe episodic pain. The risks of this intervention involve opioid toxicity, which would be appreciable in opioid naïve healthy patients. However, the risks of other approved modalities and of inadequate pain management are as high or higher in this patient population, making the risk of opioid toxicity relatively "minimal" in comparison, especially in a monitored setting.

The argument against this "relativism" in risk assignment is that the need for added protections is thereby undermined. This is a quandary that continues to generate controversy, both among ethicists and in regulatory policy. In order to proceed against a stalemate, the IRB needs to determine the value of the knowledge that can be reasonably expected to result and the likelihood that the subjects will benefit from the knowledge. Risks that are greater than minimal should only be pursued if the research will produce knowledge that will benefit the subjects of the research (Casarett 2005; Wendler and Miller 2007). The case above would appear to satisfy this criterion, based upon knowledge gleaned from studies in cognitively capable subjects. Nonetheless, obtaining proxy consent provides an additional safeguard, regardless of the level of risk. Additionally, since mental status changes commonly occur in palliative care patients due to disease or treatment-related reasons, assignment by the cognitively capable patient of a proxy at the time or consent may prevent ethical dilemmas as the study progresses (Dresser 1984).

Proxy Consent

Advance directives for clinical decision-making exist in all states, but advance directives for research purposes may not have a clear legal status or may not be allowed in some states. Paragraph 46.117 of US Department of Health and Human Services Protections of human subjects (US Department of Health and Human Services 2003) specifies that "informed consent shall be documented by the use of a written consent form approved by the IRB and signed by the subject *or the subject's legally authorized representative*" (italics by author). This seems rather straightforward, except that proxy consent for research in the absence of formal guardian designation or advance directives may also not have clear status under some states' laws. Since a subject's legally authorized representative is defined variously by each of the 50 state's statutory codes researchers must assure that their respective state's requirements are met in order to comply with ethical standards.

The Role of Proxies/Surrogates in Human Subjects Research

Once statutory requirements for ensuring that a proxy is authorized to act on behalf of the prospective subject, the role that the proxy plays goes beyond signing the consent document. It is recommended that consent forms include a section that both describes why they are acting as a proxy and the substituted judgment and best interests standards of proxy decision-making (Karlawish 2003b). The proxy should have ample understanding of the patient and her/his condition, such as a record of assisting the patient in activities of daily living, acting as decision-maker and serving as a knowledgeable informant to health care professionals. Therefore, some subjects may be best served by two proxies, if feasible: one who is "official," as recognized under the law, and one who is more functional, for the purposes of the activities of the research study.

In view of the absence of clarity within Federal Regulations and State Codes in matters pertaining to research involving cognitively impaired subjects, The American Geriatrics Society has recently put forward a position statement (Sachs 2007). In this document, they conclude that surrogates should be allowed to refuse to enroll potential subjects or to withdraw a subject from an ongoing trial on the basis that the surrogate believes that the research protocol is not in the best interests of the subject or is not what the subject intended, even if that decision would conflict with the subject's advance directive.

This position is taken on the basis that instructions in advance directives for research are likely to be imperfect at best as they will be based on knowledge at one point in time, but will be applied perhaps several years in the future. The individual's condition, available treatments, and other factors may change in the intervening years, making it safer to allow surrogates to decline enrollment or withdraw the subject from a trial if the surrogate determines that enrollment would either not be in the subject's best interests or would not be consistent with what the subject intended.

Therapeutic Trials

Palliative care research lends itself to the full spectrum of investigational designs with therapeutic objectives, which include cohort, cross-sectional, case control, and randomized controlled trials (RCTs) (Tables 43.2–43.4) (Fine 2003) (see also Currow, this volume). However, a significant obstacle to adjudicating the relative benefits vs. risks of therapeutic research in patients with far-advanced disease is the contextual knowledge and perceptions of contemporary palliative care by members of IRBs.

Table 43.2 A "cost of care" study

Study design	Key feature	Example	Ethical implications/risks
Observational designs			
Cohort study	A group followed over time	Comparison of Medicare costs accrued by a cohort of patients with stage IV heart disease from time of diagnosis until death	None
Cross-sectional study	A group examined at one point in time	Comparison of Medicare costs for the last 48 h of care prior to death for patients with stage IV heart disease in different settings (hospice, nursing home, hospital)	None
Case–control study	Two groups, based on the outcome	Comparison of Medicare costs accrued by patients with stage IV heart disease who elect hospice (the "cases") with a group who do not (the "controls")	None
Experimental design			
Randomized blinded trial	Two groups created by a random process, with or without a blinded intervention	Medicare beneficiaries with cardiac disease are randomly allocated to receive hospice care or "traditional" care when they develop stage IV disease; costs accrued to Medicare are compared	Informed consent required, to include full disclosure of differences between hospice care and "traditional" Medicare Part A coverage. Freedom of patients to change care path without prejudice. "Hospice Care" must be predefined; e.g., will home intravenous dobutamine therapy be provided?

There are innumerable variations on these research paradigms, and endless examples of different types of epidemiological investigations, therapeutic outcomes studies, and open-ended mechanistic or basic clinical science research studies. These tables serve only as a means of providing some guidance in formulating different approaches to answering very different, but all important, types of questions pursuant to end of life care

Table 43.3 A "psycho-social outcomes" study

Study design	Key feature	Example	Ethical implications/risks
Observational designs			
Cohort study	A group followed over time	Incidence of depression among surviving spouses of deceased cardiac patients who died in either hospice or nonhospice settings	Consent to undergo screening evaluations on a regular basis; results may be biased by differences among those who agree and those who do not
Cross-sectional study	A group examined at one point in time	Prevalence of depressive symptoms 1 month post-death in spouses of deceased cardiac patients who died in either hospice or nonhospice settings	Consent to undergo screening evaluation; results may be biased by differences among those who agree and those who do not
Case–control study	Two groups, based on the outcome	Examines a group of widowed Medicare beneficiaries being treated for depression (the "cases") and compares them with a group of widowed Medicare beneficiaries in a general medical setting (the "controls"), asking about setting of their deceased spouses' end-of-life care	Consent to undergo interview; assurance of privacy; possibility of exacerbating symptoms or undermining therapy
Experimental design			
Randomized trial	Two groups created by a random process, with or without a blinded intervention	Spouses of patients with stage IV heart disease are randomly allocated to a standardized bereavement care program; incidence of post-death depression between groups is measured by an investigator blinded to the intervention	Informed consent required Would referral for counseling and/or psychotherapy for those with depressive findings be a moral imperative?

With reference to methodological concerns, IRBs must be able to critically analyze how societal biases and taboos serve as a barrier to making improvements through research. IRB members may, in fact, be contributory to ongoing cultural misconceptions and their practices may reinforce existing taboos. An example of this is the commonly held injunction against the use of opioids in patients with respiratory disease who are experiencing severe dyspnea, for fear of overtly hastening death. Only through keen and candid introspection, open-mindedness toward the spectrum of exigent literature, along with highly informed leadership and the courage to challenge precepts, will break through this barrier to progress.

Palliative Care Research and Comiogenesis

One of the more interesting, and even compelling aspects of the importance of doing research in the palliative care population centers around the distinction between disease and illness. Disease refers to objectively measureable consequences of pathology, whereas illness refers to the patient's experience of pathophyiological conditions and their consequences (Fine 2003). It is the focus on illness

Table 43.4 A "symptom burden" study

Study design	Key feature	Example	Ethical implications/risks
Observational designs			
Cohort study	A group followed over time	Incidence, progressive nature, and management approaches to dyspnea—at a level defined as "shortness of breath or air hunger beyond my level of comfort"—among patients at various stages of amyotrophic lateral sclerosis (ALS)	Consent and willingness to keep and provide a "dyspnea diary." More or less symptom burden associated with study participation, due to individual responses to focusing attention on symptoms
Cross-sectional study	A group examined at one point in time	Comparison of prevalence of symptomatic dyspnea (see above) in advanced ALS patients treated in either hospice or nonhospice care settings	Consent and willingness to keep and provide a "dyspnea diary." More or less symptom burden associated with study participation, due to individual responses to focusing attention on symptoms
Case–control study	Two groups, based on the outcome	Measurement of frequency, duration, severity of dyspnea in hospice patients with ALS (the "cases") with similarly advanced ALS patients in other settings (the "controls")	Consent to undergo repeated assessments. More or less symptom burden associated with study participation, due to individual responses to focusing attention on symptoms
Experimental design			
Randomized trial	Two groups created by a random process, with or without a blinded intervention	Similarly staged ALS patients are randomly assigned to receive inhalational (nebulized) fentanyl, an opioid, vs. placebo for treatment of dyspnea	Risk of exacerbation of respiratory distress is possible in either group—a "rescue" protocol would need to be in place, that would consist of "conventional" therapy. Need to "break the double-blind" code under defined circumstances (patient's best interest) would need to be codified

in this population that invites a discussion of comiogenesis. Comiogenic illness refers to the negative effects that a disease process brings to bear on a patient's life, including treatment effects. This can be broadly applied to patients' families as well, since family members will inevitably experience additional life stress both during the patient's terminal illness and through grief. Involvement in research can either add to or mitigate comiogenic harms. Since the essential purpose of palliative care is to reduce suffering, great care must be taken to assure that involvement in research comports with this overarching goal.

In this light, it is important to recognize and to intentionally optimize the opportunity for anticomiogenic effects that involvement in palliative care research can provide for patients and their families. Instead of additive burdens and sacrifice, in the negative sense, there can be perceived benefit, as a result of a sense of being helpful, useful, purposeful, and through increased contact with others. This may also be a portal through which hope can be redefined or reshaped at the end of life. Participation in research can serve as a way to derive meaning from difficult existential circumstances, as long as great care is taken not to use this as a coercive device (Appelbaum et al. 2009; Fine and Peterson 2002; Todd et al. 2009).

Placebo-Controlled Trials in Palliative Care Patients

The randomized, placebo-controlled clinical trial paradigm came into favor at a time when there were few, if any, empirically proven efficacious pharmacological therapies. After nearly half a century of scientific investigations employing this methodology as a "gold standard," and shunning other methodologies as being inadequate, there has been some rethinking of the ethics and interpretability of RCTs using placebos (Temple and Ellenberg 2000) (see also Pollo and Benedetti 2011). The latest revision of the Declaration of Helsinki strongly supports the use of active controls in lieu of placebos in controlled clinical trials, except in cases where there are not any proven prophylactic, diagnostic, or therapeutic methods (Enserink 2000).

The polemic of "placebo orthodoxy" (i.e., placebos are the gold standard in RCTs) vs. "active control orthodoxy" (i.e., placebos are not ethical and should be eschewed in favor of comparator treatments in clinical trials) has been thoroughly and effectively reviewed (Emanuel and Miller 2001). From an analysis of the ethical and pragmatic implications for both individual patients and the population at risk, it can be concluded that the decision to employ a placebo control is best viewed as a contextual one, rather than an absolute requirement or prohibition.

On the surface, it would seem that in palliative care it would be easier to cope with the current Helsinki rules, since there are so few proven therapies, thereby justifying the use of placebos. However, the complication is that anecdotal therapies, whose efficacies have not been *disproved*, have become normalized in modern palliative care (Vase et al. 2002). In effect, this has created a standard of care, and the sympathy involved in witnessing the suffering of patients is so great, that it "feels" unethical to use a placebo while "withholding" a normally used comparator treatment when a patient is symptomatic. The seemingly perilous dilemma of "damned if you do, damned if you don't" set up by this argument represents a false impasse for patients with decision-making capacity. It is inconsistent (and arguably unethical) to advocate for patient self-determination through all manner of processes (advance directives, informed consent, etc.) while discounting patient autonomy by creating prohibitions against participation in well-constructed RCTs. There is no justifiable basis for withholding participation in such trials from capable and appropriately informed patients; they should retain the opportunity to decide for themselves what is in their best interests. Notwithstanding other ethical considerations, in these cases decisions about methodology should be based upon scientific merits.

The crucial difference between patients with decision-making capacity and those without, for whom proxy consent would need to be obtained in order to participate in a clinical study, hinges on the willingness of self-reporting patients to submit to anything more than predictably trivial burdens associated with a study protocol. Since this is rarely the case in palliative medicine there are few instances where placebo trials could be sanctioned in nonself-reporting patients. This is because a surrogate decision-maker is not able to determine when the threshold has been crossed at which time the patient (subject), if she or he were able, would request a protocol-approved alternative therapy (i.e., "rescue dose") or drop out of the study.

Insights into current understanding of placebo effects make arguments in favor of placebos in controlled clinical trials even more compelling. It must be appreciated that the effects of placebos and active drugs alike are strongly influenced by certain types of cognitive and oftentimes subliminally induced neurophysiological changes. These are established by preconditioning of a cause–effect response or by "empowerment" of the placebo/drug through suggestion and attribution of effects. These effects can be powerful and enduring but are highly variable and require the investigator to adopt specific behaviors that help promote effectiveness of the placebo (Fine et al. 1994). Ideally, under blinded conditions, communication with the research subject is devoid of bias through unawareness of whether the subject will be receiving (or has received) investigational or placebo treatment. What is said and the manner in which the message is communicated become exquisitely important. This is because although placebos are pharmacologically nonspecific, the context and way in which they are administered make them highly malleable forces whose potential capabilities need to be understood and used thoughtfully. In research, they can only be used ethically if the way their use may affect outcomes is appreciated and managed accordingly. As proven in pain and analgesic studies, subjects' knowledge and understanding of the therapeutic intervention are fundamental to the placebo analgesic effect. Perceptions and expectations greatly influence the outcomes in placebo-controlled trials, including the failure to recognize and manage this can, and most certainly will, influence conclusions reached about investigational agents (see also Pollo and Benedetti 2011).

Although these concepts about placebo effects are not new, the evidence to support them has only recent empirical support (Petrovic et al. 2002). The current scientific understanding of placebo mechanisms and influences have developed to the point where investigators, IRB members, grant reviewers, and peer reviewers must be even more keenly aware of methodology—especially the means by which subjects are apprised of protocol information, processes, and procedures. Even when communications are scripted and processes are choreographed to try and minimize variance, different patients may respond variously to different cues and nuances of the "milieu," adding yet another degree of complexity to an already challenging process. What this suggests is that even when a placebo, per se, is not employed, such as in a comparator or equivalence study, powerful placebo-like effects can still be created, either wittingly or unwittingly, influencing or confounding results.

In a clinical setting, when a treating physician intentionally employs a placebo (an ethically dubious enterprise) s/he can only optimize the desired therapeutic effect by engaging in a purposeful charade, which increases the deception. In contrast, in a research setting, the intent behind "empowering" the placebo and the investigational drug, is not so much to determine how effective a placebo might be, but to equalize these effects. This determines how suggestible each subject is, creating a means to ascertain pharmacologically specific differences between this degree of suggestibility and the true efficacy of the investigational agent.

The decision to do a study with an "active comparator" (equivalence study) vs. a placebo must be based on several considerations that involve both ethical and methodological concerns. Questions to be considered include:

- With a placebo control, what are the likely frequencies, intensities, and durations of harms that can occur while awaiting "rescue" therapy?
- How many more patients would need to be enrolled in an equivalence trial than a placebo-controlled trial in order to demonstrate a certain level of response of the investigational agent compared with "standard therapy?"

Ethical dilemmas may be found in those studies where there are treatments that are known to be at least somewhat effective and there is a relatively high likelihood that absence of these specific therapies (i.e., use of a placebo control) will more likely than not cause preventable harm or distress. In these circumstances, in order to justify placebo use, methodology that allows for immediately available "rescue" therapy, and an analysis of potential harms that might come from the potentially larger number of subjects required to demonstrate a difference between standard therapy and an investigational treatment, must be carried out. A "least worst" choice of methodology should then be made in consultation with a capable review committee.

This is a particularly important duty of review committees, which requires both a willingness and capability (knowledge, experience, time) to become involved in difficult and complex methodological determinations. The informed consent process must apprise subjects of foreseeable risks and what will be done to minimize them. The manner in which information is given and the degree to which it is understood during the consent process will determine the ethical integrity of the recruitment process. All of this presumes a protocol that assures sufficient monitoring in a setting that precludes avoidable suffering or harms unacceptable to the patient (or family). These provisos are not unique to palliative care research or research involving patients who are near to death, but they require highlighting. With increasing recognition that improvements are needed in end of life care, due attention and constant vigilance to ethical conduct, as applied to all other areas of clinical research, must be fostered and maintained.

Conclusions and Recommendations

Research in palliative care patients is constrained more by pragmatic, social, cultural, and financial constraints than ethical issues that preclude the application of typical research methodologies. When normally accepted and ethically sound protections for subjects (especially for those who lack independent decision-making) are in place, exclusion of patients with far-advanced disease from research is in and of itself unethical. Involvement in research may have a therapeutic, anticomiogenic effect on dying patients and their families. Institutional review boards must be educated to evaluate research protocols involving this group of vulnerable patients with an eye toward assuring that ethical safeguards are in place, conflicts of interest are transparent and resolved, and that the proposed methodology has duly considered all practical exigencies so that resources and peoples' time and emotional investments are not squandered. Investigators and research review committees must be knowledgeable about placebo effects and under what types of circumstances their use is justifiable, preferred or requisite to fulfill both ethical and scientific imperatives. A brief list of actionable items, based on rational hypothesis and best evidence, that would lead to significant improvement in the care of patients with far-advanced illness includes:

- Tax-based research funds need to be apportioned to reflect the magnitude of the national public health problem of inadequate provision of palliative care and the insufficient evidence base that results from historically meager research funding.
- Clinical research needs to expressly involve patients with far-advanced and life-limiting illness, incorporating methodologies that prospectively evaluate palliative care outcomes.
- Clinical care venues, including hospitals, long-term care facilities, and hospice programs need to be specifically targeted, encouraged, and incentivized to become involved (e.g., allied with academic centers) in legitimate, ethically performed palliative care research. Conversely, grant appropriations to academic centers should include provisions for community-based alliances.
- Palliative care researchers need to be educated to design protocols that appropriately anticipate and manage rapidly changing clinical conditions (including mental capacity), cohort mortality, and the unique variable of limited life expectancy.
- Institutional Review Boards must be educated to manage the nuances of research in patients near the end of life. Alternatively, they need to include expertise that is both sensitive to and knowledgeable about end-of-life care ethics and the unique methodological issues pursuant to research in this vulnerable population (e.g., informed consent processes, potential comiogenic and anticomiogenic effects, appropriateness of placebo vs. active comparator methodology in the context of particular clinical trials).
- Institutional Review Boards should be audited to determine that specific and well-defined justification has been provided whenever there is a decision to exclude patients near the end of life from research.

I submit that any combination of these actionable items would not only begin to eliminate an unacknowledged but ongoing form of discrimination within the province of publically funded research, but such changes would likely lead to wholesale improvements in the care of patients with far-advanced disease.

References

Agrawal, M. (2003). Voluntariness in clinical research at the end of life. *Journal of Pain and Symptom Management, 25*(4), S25–S32.

Appelbaum, P. S., Lidz, C. W., & Klitzman, R. (2009). Voluntariness of consent to research: A preliminary empirical investigation. *IRB: Ethics & Human Research, 31*(6), 10–14.

Berg, J. W., Appelbaum, P. S., Lidz, C. W., & Parker, L. S. (2001). *Informed consent: Legal theory and clinical practice*. New York: Oxford University Press.

Brechtl, J., Murshed, S., Homel, P., & Bookbinder, M. (2006). Monitoring symptoms in patients with advanced illness in long-term care: A pilot study. *Journal of Pain and Symptom Management, 32*(2), 168–174.

Casarett, D. (2005). Ethical considerations in end-of-life care and research. *Journal of Palliative Medicine, 8*(Suppl 1), S148–S160.

Cassarett, D. (2003). Assessing decision-making capacity in the setting of palliative care research. *Journal of Pain and Symptom Management, 25*(4), S6–S13.

Dresser, R. (1984). Bound to treatment: The Ulysses contract. *The Hastings Center Report, 12*, 3–38.

Emanuel, E. J., & Miller, F. G. (2001). The ethics of placebo-controlled trials—a middle ground. *The New England Journal of Medicine, 345*(12), 915–919.

Emmanuel, E. J., Wendler, D., & Grady, C. (2000). What makes clinical research ethical? *Journal of the American Medical Association, 283*, 2701–2711.

Enserink, M. (2000). Helsinki's new clinical rules: Fewer placebos, more disclosure. *Science, 290*, 418–419.

Field, M. J., & Cassell, C. K. (1997). *Approaching death: Improving care at the end of life* (pp. 235–258). Washington: National Academies Press.

Fine, P. G. (2003). Maximizing benefits and minimizing risks in palliative care research that involves patients near the end of life. *Journal of Pain and Symptom Management, 25*(4), S53–S62.

Fine, P. G., & Peterson, D. (2002). Caring about what dying patients care about caring. *Journal of Pain and Symptom Management, 23*, 267–268.

Fine, P. G., Roberts, W. J., Gillette, R. G., & Child, T. R. (1994). Slowly developing placebo responses obscure results of the intravenous phentolamine test in subjects with idiopathic chronic low back pain. *Pain, 56*, 235–242.

Foley, K. M., Gelband, H., For the National Cancer Policy Board, Institute of Medicine and Commission on Life Sciences, & National Research Council. (2001). *Improving palliative care for cancer: Summary and recommendations*. Washington: National Academy Press.

Grisso, T., & Appelbaum, P. S. (1995). The MacArthur treatment-competence study III. *Law and Human Behavior, 19*, 149–174.

Karlawish, J. H. T. (2003a). Conducting research that involves subjects at the end of life who are unable to give consent. *Journal of Pain and Symptom Management, 25*(4), S14–S24.

Karlawish, J. H. T. (2003b). Conducting research that involves subjects at the end of life who are unable to give consent. *Journal of Pain and Symptom Management, 25*(4), S14–S24.

Kirchhoff, K. T., & Kehl, K. A. (2008). Recruiting participants in end-of-life research. *The American Journal of Hospice & Palliative Care, 24*, 515–521.

Lehan-Mackin, M., Herr, K., Fine, P. G., Sanders, S., Bergen-Jackson, K., & Forcucci, C. (2009). Research participation by older adults at the end-of-life: Barriers and solutions. *Research in Gerontological Nursing, 2*(3), 162–171.

Nelson, R. M., & Merz, J. F. (2002). Voluntariness of consent for research: An empirical and conceptual review. *Medical Care, 40*, V69–V80.

Petrovic, P., Kalso, E., Petersson, K. M., & Ingvar, M. (2002). Placebo and opioid analgesia—imaging a shared neuronal network. *Science, 295*(5560), 1737–1740.

Pollo, A., & Benedetti, F. (2011). Pain and the placebo/nocebo effect. In R. J. Moore (Ed.), *Handbook of pain and palliative care*. New York: Springer.

Sachs, G. A. (2007). *AGS Ethics Committee Position Statement Informed Consent for Research on Human Subjects with Dementia*. Retrieved, American Geriatrics Society, archive records, 2007.

Schaeffer, M. H., Krantz, D. S., Wichman, A., et al. (1996). The impact of disease severity on the informed consent process in clinical research. *The American Journal of Medicine, 100*(3), 261–268.

Temple, R., & Ellenberg, S. S. (2000). Placebo-controlled trials and active-control trials in the evaluation of new treatments. *Annals of Internal Medicine, 133*(6), 455–470.

The Nuremberg Code. (1996). *The Journal of the American Medical Association, 276*, 1691. Retrieved, from http://ohsr.od.nih.gov/guidelines/nuremberg.html. Accessed October 14, 2011.

Todd, A., Laird, B., Boyle, D., Colvin, L., & Fallon, M. (2009). A systematic review examining the literature on attitudes of patients with advanced cancer toward research. *Journal of Pain and Symptom Management, 37*(6), 1078–1085.

US Department of Health and Human Services. (2003). *Protections of human subjects*. Accessed October 14, 2011
Vase, L., Riley, J. L., & Price, D. D. (2002). A comparison of placebo effects in analgesic trials versus studies of placebo analgesia. *Pain, 99*(3), 443–452.
Wendler, D., & Miller, F. G. (2007). Assessing research risks systematically: The net risks test. *Journal of Medical Ethics, 33*, 481–486.

Chapter 44
How Health Care Reform Can Improve Access to Quality Pain and Palliative Care Services

Amber B. Jones and Diane E. Meier

Health Care Reform

The Patient Protection and Affordable Care Act (ACA) provides a framework and a set of expectations for testing new delivery models and payment options. The ACA goals are to enhance health care quality while at the same time limiting spending. Efforts to address quality include investment in comparative effectiveness research and rewarding quality of care through the mechanism of value-based purchasing – known also as Pay for Performance.

What Do Patients and Their Families Want?

If Health Care Reform is to achieve its goals, it must begin and end with the patient and family – what do they want, what do they need? Does the provider community effectively convey diagnostic and treatment options to enable and elicit informed decisions? How do we assure that the patient, her/his family, and the providers who care for them realize a coordinated journey that results in the right care at the right time for the right patient?

Singer et al. (Scott and Hughes 2006) identified the preferences of patients with serious illnesses: pain and symptom control, avoidance of the prolongation of the dying process, achievement of a sense of control, relief of burdens on the family, and strengthening of relationships with loved ones.

In a study of 475 family members who cared for their loved ones and were surveyed 1–2 years post bereavement, Tolle et al. (Thorpe and Howard 2006) found consensus about their wishes: honor the loved one's preferences and include the loved one in the decision-making process; provide support and assistance in the home; make available assistance with practical needs (transportation, medicines, equipment); offer help with personal care needs (bathing, feeding, toileting); convey honest information about the patient's condition and circumstances; assure access to health care

A.B. Jones, M.ED (✉)
Palliative and Hospice Care Consultant, Center to Advance Palliative Care, New York, NY, USA

D.E. Meier, MD, FACP
Center to Advance Palliative Care, Hertzberg Palliative Care Institute, New York, NY, USA

Departments of Geriatrics and Palliative Medicine and Internal Medicine, Mount Sinai School of Medicine, New York, NY, USA

R.J. Moore (ed.), *Handbook of Pain and Palliative Care: Biobehavioral Approaches for the Life Course*,
DOI 10.1007/978-1-4419-1651-8_44, © Springer Science+Business Media, LLC 2012

advice all day every day; listen to family member/care-giver input; honor patient and family caregiver privacy; and remember and contacted family caregivers after the patient's death.

What Are Palliative Care and Hospice?

Given these statements from patients and family caregivers, how can providers best shape their practices to achieve those goals? Optimizing palliative care is one strategy that will contribute to this outcome. The Center for Medicare and Medicaid Services defines palliative care as follows: *Palliative care means patient and family-centered care that optimizes quality of life* by anticipating, preventing, and treating suffering. Palliative care *throughout the continuum of illness* involves addressing physical, intellectual, emotional, social, and spiritual needs and facilitates patient autonomy, access to information, and choice (73 Federal Register 32204 2008).

Hospice, a specialized form of palliative care has been effectively caring for patients with limited life expectancies and their families for many years. The success of hospice is characterized by its remarkable utilization statistics. According to the National Hospice and Palliative Care Organization as of 2009, there were 3,400 programs of which 93% were Medicare-certified. These programs served 1.56 million Americans, primarily in their homes (56% of days), nursing homes (29% of days), or assisted living facilities (10.9% of days). In 2009, over 40% of Medicare decedents utilized hospice in their care, an increase from 23% in 2000 (National Hospice and Palliative Care Organization 2010; MedPAC 2010). It is noteworthy that more than 80% of hospice beneficiaries are over age 65 and more than a-third are over 85 years of age. Ten years ago, the majority (53%) of hospice patients died from cancer. By 2008, that percentage had dropped to 31% reflecting a pattern of utilization increasingly correlated with the current leading causes of death (cancer accounts for less that 25% of U.S. deaths) (MedPAC 2010; National Hospice and Palliative Care Organization 2008). This shift demonstrates that hospices are responding to the circumstances and needs of Medicare beneficiaries.

Unlike the hospice community, palliative care as a recognized specialty service is a relative newcomer to the health care arena. Palliative care embraces the interdisciplinary focus of hospice and extends expert pain and symptom management and supportive care to patients with complex chronic illnesses who are not yet eligible for, or who have not elected hospice.

What is it about palliative care and hospice care services that makes them a good fit for the needs of patients and families and with the challenges of health care reform? According to the National Consensus Project Clinical Practice Guidelines for Quality Palliative Care, "the goal of palliative care is to prevent and relieve suffering and to support the best possible quality of life for patients and their families, regardless of the stage of the disease or the need for other therapies. Palliative care is both a philosophy of care and an organized, highly structured system of delivering care. Palliative care expands traditional disease-model medical treatments to include the goals of enhancing quality of life for patient and family, optimizing function, helping with decision-making, and providing opportunities for personal growth. As such, it can be delivered concurrently with life-prolonging care or as the main focus of care" (National Quality Forum 2006).

The Guidelines continue: "Palliative care is operationalized through effective management of pain and other distressing symptoms, while incorporating psychosocial and spiritual care with consideration of patient/family needs, preferences, values, beliefs, and culture. Evaluation and treatment should be comprehensive and patient-centered with a focus on the central role of the family unit in decision-making. Comprehensive palliative care services often require the expertise of various providers to adequately assess and treat the complex needs of seriously ill patients an their families. Leadership, collaboration, coordination and communication are key elements for effective integration of these disciplines and services" (National Quality Forum 2006).

Growth in Palliative Care

The growth of hospital palliative care programs has been dramatic. As of 2008, 58.5% of U.S. Hospitals (with at least 50 beds) and 81% of hospitals with more than 300 beds reported the presence of a palliative care program – an increase of 125% from 2000 (American Hospital Association 2009; Goldsmith et al. 2008; Center to Advance Palliative Care 2010). As the demand for services grew, so did recognition of the need for an appropriately trained workforce of providers. In 2008, the American Board of Medical Specialties formally recognized the specialty of palliative medicine, sponsored by ten parent specialty Boards. The first hospice and palliative medicine subspecialty board examination, sponsored by the American Boards of Internal and Family Medicine, was given in 2008. Graduate medical education in palliative medicine is now accredited by the Accreditation Council for Graduate Medical Education (ACGME). The profession of nursing has also adopted specialty training as have other members of the palliative care interdisciplinary team including social work, pharmacists, and the clergy. The Joint Commission is currently considering recommendations to offer a certification to hospitals with a palliative care program.

Palliative Care and the Quality Movement

In 2006, the National Quality Forum (NQF) identified the "increasingly important role of palliative care and hospice services by identifying them as priority areas for healthcare quality improvement" (National Quality Forum 2006). In its 2008 report, *National Priorities and Goals – Aligning our Efforts to Transform America's Healthcare* (National Priorities Partnership 2008), the National Priorities Partnership (NPP) identified six national priorities that if addressed, would significantly improve the quality of health care delivered to Americans. In recognition of evidence of poor health care quality despite high expenditure among patients with multiple chronic conditions, functional impairment and serious life-threatening illness, the NPP cited the impact of both palliative care and hospice services on improving key patient-centered, population health, and utilization outcomes.

The Case for Palliative Care

Why do we need palliative care? Despite enormous expenditures, studies demonstrate that patients with serious illness and their families receive poor-quality medical care, characterized by untreated symptoms, unmet psychosocial and personal care needs, high caregiver burden, and low patient and family satisfaction (Field and Cassel 1997; Thorpe and Howard 2006; Foundation 2005; Foundation 2009; Teno et al. 2004). The patients served by palliative care providers are those with chronic complex illnesses. This population of represents more than 95% of all health care spending. About 64% of all Medicare spending is for the 10% of beneficiaries with 5 or more chronic conditions. However, despite the heavy allocation of health care dollars spent on this population of patients, the data in these studies offer abundant evidence that the care they receive is poor.

Impact of Palliative Care and Hospice

How do we know that palliative care and hospice help to conserve health care dollars? Based on recent findings, the per patient net costs saved by hospital palliative consultations are $2,659

(Morrison et al. 2008). This figure is clearly an underestimate of the potential savings as many hospitalized patients with advanced and chronic illnesses do not have access to a palliative care consultation referral.

Hospices have also been shown to contribute significant cost-savings among the majority (70%) of Medicare beneficiaries (Taylor et al. 2007; Taylor 2009). Using propensity score analysis to control for selection bias, an estimated $2,300 is saved per beneficiary on average. Extrapolating this average savings across the number of hospice patients served each year yields overall savings of more than $3.5 billion a year. The savings attributed to hospice patients persisted through 233 days of hospice care for cancer patients and 154 days of care for noncancer patients (ASPE et al. 2010). In addition, recent analysis have found that the costs of care for patients who disenrolled from hospice were nearly 5 times higher than for patients who remained with hospice. Patients who disenroll from hospice are far more likely to use emergency department care and to be hospitalized (Carlson et al. 2010).

Health Care Reform Opportunities

The confluence of the emergence of palliative care and the passage of health care reform legislation has significant synergistic potential. The need for new approaches to high-quality patient-centered cost-effective care has been the stimulus for both. As a result, palliative care and hospice are uniquely well-qualified to address several of legislative initiatives including the following ACA HR 3590 provisions: Hospital Value-Based Purchasing (3001), Hospital mortality reporting (MIMA 501b), Hospital readmission reporting (3025), National Health Care Workforce Council (5101–3), Medicare Hospice Concurrent Care Demonstration (3140), Concurrent Care for Children (2302), the Center for Medicare and Medicaid Innovation (3021) and Tests of new delivery and payment models such as: Accountable Care Organizations (3022), Medical Homes, Health Homes (2703), Community health teams to support medical homes (3502), Bundling (3023), Care coordination for the dually eligible (2601–2), and Independence at Home (3024).

There are also opportunities for more effective utilization of palliative care and hospice expertise to be realized in ACA implementation strategies. Inclusion of the perspectives and skills of this field will add otherwise unrealized perspectives to the on-going planning processes. Examples include but are not limited to:

1. Welcome to Medicare, Annual Wellness Visits to include regular review/update ACP/POLST (Physicians Orders for Life-Sustaining Treatment).
2. Meaningful Use – inclusion of meaningful, easy, timely availability of the content of ACP/POLST.
3. New shared decision-making program at the Agency for Healthcare Research and Quality (AHRQ).
4. The development of the Secretary's National Quality Strategy.
5. Inclusion of meaningful palliative care metrics in the National Health Quality Report (AHRQ).
6. PQRI (physician quality reporting – measures requiring timely referral to palliative care and hospice).
7. Assurance that access to palliative care and hospice services are included in the conditions of participation for Exchange Criteria.
8. Careful review of the definition and assessment of the impact Quality reporting measures for hospice, mandated for implementation as of 2014.
9. Assurance of provisions for workforce development – especially training for palliative care nursing/medicine where short supply is already a problem.
10. Integration of elements yielding a continuum of palliative care such as those evidenced in the Hospice Concurrent Care and Transitional Care Demonstration developing models (Meier 2010a).

Barriers to Delivery of Palliative Care and Hospice

If palliative and hospice care effectively meet the needs of patients and families while at the same time addressing cost considerations, why is distribution of the services a struggle? The primary barriers to the delivery of quality palliative care and hospice are variability in access by geographic and other characteristics, inadequate workforce and workforce pipeline to meet the needs of patients and their families, an inadequate evidence base to guide and continue the evolution of the field, and the lack of public knowledge of and demand for the benefits of these services.

Variability in Access

In both palliative care and hospice delivery models, location can facilitate or preclude service availability. For-profit, southern U.S., and small safety net hospitals (under 100 beds) are less likely to offer palliative care services as compared to for-for-profit hospitals, hospitals outside the South, and larger hospitals (Center to Advance Palliative Care 2010). Even in settings where palliative care is available, there is a great deal of variability in the services to which patients have access, ranging from (for example) a 0.5 FTE RN to a full interdisciplinary team . Hospice penetration is also highly variable, from a low of 6.7% of all deaths in Alaska, to a high of 44.7% in Arizona, based on 2006 data (Atlas 2006).

Workforce Shortfall

The demand for palliative care workforce exceeds the supply. An inadequate medical and nursing workforce with expertise in palliative care is among the most important barriers. A report commissioned by HRSA in 2002 predicated a significant shortfall in palliative medicine specialists and called for policy focused on increasing training in palliative medicine across all clinical specialties serving patients with chronic and eventually fatal illness; expanded funding and reimbursement to attract young physicians into the field; and examination of the appropriate roles of nonphysicians (such as nurse practitioners, clinical social workers, and physicians' assistants) in strengthening access to palliative care across health care settings (Salsberg ECfHWSS 2002). Another physician workforce study commissioned by the American Academy of Hospice and Palliative Medicine in 2010 conservatively estimated a shortfall of at least 2,787 FTE (or approximately 6,000 palliative medicine physicians given the frequency of part-time participation in the field) (Lupu 2010).

This workforce shortfall has had a dramatic impact on the hospice community. Growth in the number of programs and patients served has rapidly outstripped the growth in the number of trained professionals. More recently, the CMS requirement for face-to-face visits by physicians or nurse practitioners for recertification of hospice services (MedPAC 2008, 2009, 2010) has heightened the mismatch between workforce capacity and clinical needs.

Several Institute of Medicine reports have called for policy changes aimed at strengthening the palliative care workforce (Field and Cassel 1997). It was in part as a response to these concerns that Hospice and Palliative Medicine was approved as a sub-specialty by the American Board of Medical Sub-specialties (American Board of Hospice and Palliative Medicine 2006). Subsequently, the Accreditation Council of Graduate Medical Education (ACGME) has certified (American Academy of Hospice and Palliative Medicine 2008) the first 63 postgraduate training fellowship programs to develop the workforce necessary to meet the nation's needs (Casarett 2000; Scharfenberger et al. 2008; Scott and Hughes 2006; von Gunten 2006; Portenoy et al. 2006).

A significant impediment to physician specialty training in palliative medicine is the cap on Graduate Medical education (GME) slots in teaching hospitals (Association of American Medicl Colleges CfwS 2009). Despite a 30% growth in population and a doubling of the number of Americans over 65 since 1997, the total number of funded graduate medical education training slots has been capped at 110,000 since the passage of the Balanced Budget Act of 1997 (AmMedNews 2009). At present, distribution of GME training slots is entirely within the purview of each teaching hospital; there is no federal mandate based on priority or need. A new subspecialty such as palliative medicine has little power to secure GME-funded slots from long-standing and preexisting training programs. As a result, specialty training in palliative medicine is largely dependent on private sector philanthropy. In recognition of the need for data to inform federal training programs, the August 2010 U.S. Senate Appropriates Committee report for the Departments of Labor, Health and Human Services, and Education for FY 2011 included language in its section on Health Professions Workforce and Analysis calling for HRSA-sponsored research on the adequacy of the palliative care workforce.

> The (U.S. Senate Appropriations) Committee is aware that hospice and palliative medicine (HPM) improves quality, controls cost, and enhances patient and family satisfaction for the rapidly expanding population of patients with serious of life-threatening illness. Therefore, the Committee encourages HRSA to study workforce trends, training capacity, and need for HPM physicians, physician assistants, and nurse practitioners in our National's academic medical centers, hospice organizations and palliative care programs (U.S Senate Appropriations Committee 2010).

Inadequate Research Funding

Much improved research funding for palliative care and hospice is necessary to assure that care is based on reliable evidence and to test promising delivery models in a range of patient populations and settings. Despite the fact that the U.S. population is aging and that persons with chronic illnesses and multiple impairment drive well over 2/3 of health care spending (ASPE et al. 2010), a recent study (Gelfman and Morrison 2008) found that less than 1% of total NIH extramural funding between 2003 and 2005 went to palliative care-related research. Reflecting awareness of this problem, the August 2010 U.S. Senate Appropriations Committee Report for the Departments of Labor, Health and Human Services and Education for 2011 included report language (U.S Senate Appropriations Committee 2010) in its section on the National Institutes of Health calling for a trans-Institute strategy aimed at increasing funding for palliative care research.

> Palliative Care – The (Senate Appropriations) Committee strongly urges the NIH to develop a trans-Institute strategy for increasing funded research in palliative care for persons living with chronic and advanced illness. Research is needed on: treatment of pain and common nonpain symptoms across all chronic disease categories, which should include cancer, heart, renal and liver failure, lung disease, Alzheimer's disease and related dementias, methods to improve communications about goals of care and treatment options between providers, patients, and caregivers; care models that maximize the likelihood that treatment delivered is consistent with patient wishes; and care models that improve coordination, transitions, caregiver support, and strengthen the likelihood of remaining at home.

The Social Marketing Challenge

Although providers are becoming increasingly well informed about the benefits of palliative care and hospice offer, the general public has much to learn. Fear of the unknown (what exactly is palliative care?) and of misperceptions (I don't want to die, therefore I don't want hospice or palliative care) impede the referral process. This barrier is well-characterized by the data on hospice utilization. The Medicare Hospice Benefit provides care for patients with a life prognosis of 6 months or less if the disease follows its expected course (and also provides for extension beyond 6 months if the clinical condition continues to support the required prognostic timeframe). Utilization findings tell us that in 2009, 34.4% of patients received this specialized interdisciplinary care for 7 days or less (National Hospice and Palliative Care Organization 2008).

As further evidence of the barriers confronted by the field, as the ACA was drafted, a provision were promulgated that would require physicians to discuss patients' advance care planning preferences during annual physical examinations. This focused effort to support healthy and sick patients and families as they consider, select, and articulate their personal preferences for care was inaccurately dubbed as a "death panel." Misinformation carried the day and the provision was dropped from the proposed legislation – not because it was accurate but because the rhetoric surrounding the allegation was deemed as constituting a significant liability to ACA passage.

The ACA does afford opportunities for integration and participation of palliative care and hospice programs as a component of new payment and delivery models including Accountable Care Organizations (ACO's), Patient-Centered Medical Homes (PCMH's) – also known as Health Homes and bundling of payments for a single episode of care. Each of these models aims to improve quality and control cost for high-need patient populations by focusing on patient-centered, goal-driven services, and intensive care coordination. Also included is the identification of treatment problems before crises prompt Emergency Department visits or hospitalizations and shifting of payment incentives from fee-for-service drivers for quantity to payment based on quality.

The Economics of Change

A major challenge to the success and scaling of new delivery and payment models is the fact that the skills necessary to care for high-risk, high-need patients with serious and advanced illness, multi-morbidity and functional dependency are not widely available among health care providers in the U.S. This is due both to lack of training in the care for seriously and chronically ill, as well as long experience with the current fee-for-service incentives for acute and specialist level care.

However, the needed skills are available in the staff of the nation's 1,500 palliative care and 3,400 hospice programs. The rapid growth of these provider types in the last decade is a response to unmet needs of seriously and chronically ill patients. Linkage of hospice and palliative care teams to implementation of new delivery models may increase the likelihood that these interventions will achieve their quality and health care value objectives (Rodgers 2010).

Solutions and Drivers of Change

To assure access to palliative and hospice care for all patients who might benefit requires that an evidence base exists to assure quality, that the providers who deliver the services are well-trained, that health care organizations have the capacity to deliver it and that the public understand what palliative care and hospice are and demands access to these specialized services.

Policies aimed at achieving these goals fall into four categories:

1. Research to build the evidence base necessary for assuring quality care
2. Workforce education and training
3. Financial and Regulatory incentive devised to encourage and support access to needed services
4. Public education campaigns designed to improve awareness and sustain service access

Conclusion

The ACA and related government directives and planning initiatives are positioned to support the directions outlined here. However, governmental and private sector efforts must be aligned to enable the allocation of needed intellectual, health care personnel, and financial resources to the achieve the stated goals. These efforts should build on the enormous investment of private philanthropy that has been instrumental in fostering the growth and development of hospice and palliative care as providers for our most vulnerable citizens. We have before us an unprecedented congruence of need, policy options, and provider commitment. The future of our field will be predicated on our ability to welcome and leverage the opportunities presented.

References

73 Federal Register 32204. (2008). *Medicare Hospice Conditions of Participation, Final Rule.*

American Academy of Hospice and Palliative Medicine. (2008). *Fellowship Program Directory.* Chicago.

American Board of Hospice and Palliative Medicine. (2006). *ABMS votes to make Hospice and Palliative Medicine an ABMS subspecialty.* Retrieved October 9, 2006, from http://www.abhpm.org/gfxc_119.aspx.

American Hospital Association. (2009). *AHA hospital statistics.* Chicago: American Hospital Association.

AmMedNews. (2009). *Bill would raise cap on Medicare-funded residency slots.* Retrieved October 19, 2010, from http://www.ama-assn.org/amednews/2009/05/25/prse0528.html.

ASPE, Evaluation OotASfPa, Services USDoHaH, Group TL. (2010). *Individuals living in the community with chronic conditions and functional limitations: A closer look.* Washington.

Association of American Medicl Colleges CfwS. (2009). *Recent studies and reports on physician shortages in the U.S.* Retrieved September 19, 2001, from http://www.aamc.org/workforce/.

Atlas, T. D. (2006). *Hospice days per decedent during last 6 months of life, 2001–2005.* Retrieved September 19, 2010, from http://www.dartmouthatlas.org/data/map.aspx?ind=4.

CAPC. (2008). *State-by-State Report Card on Access to Palliative Care.* Retrieved September 19, 2010, from http://www.capc.org/reportcard/.

Carlson, M., Herrin, J., Du, Q., et al. (2010). Impact of hospice disenrollment on health care use and medicare expenditures for patients with cancer. *Journal of Clinical Oncology, 28,* 4371–4375.

Casarett, D. J. (2000). The future of the palliative medicine fellowship. *Journal of Palliative Medicine, 3,* 151–155.

Center to Advance Palliative Care. (2010). *Analysis of U.S. hospital palliative care programs, 2010 snapshot.* Retrieved September 19, 2010.

Field, M. J., & Cassel, C. K. (Eds.). (1997). *Approaching death: Improving care at the end of life.* Washington: National Academy Press.

Foundation THJKF. (2005). *Kaiser Family Foundation analysis of the CMS Medicare Current Beneficiary Survey Cost & Use file.* Retrieved August 1, 2009, fron http://facts.kff.org/chart.aspx?ch=382.

Foundation THJKF. (2009). *Kaiser Commission on Medicaid and the Uninsured.* http://facts.kff.org/chart.aspx?ch=463.

Gelfman, L. P., & Morrison, R. S. (2008). Research funding for palliative medicine. *Journal of Palliative Medicine, 11,* 36–43.

Goldsmith, B., Dietrich, J., Du, Q., & Morrison, R. S. (2008). Variability in access to hospital palliative care in the United States. *Journal of Palliative Medicine, 11,* 1094–1102.

Lupu, D. (2010). Estimates of current hospice and palliative medicine physician workforce shortage. *Journal of Pain and Symptom Management, 40*(6), 899–911.

MedPAC. (2008). *Evaluating medicare's hospice benefit, in reforming the delivery system, a report to the congress* (pp. 203–232). Washington: MedPAC.

MedPAC. (2009). *Reforming the medicare hospice benefit, in medicare payment policy: Report to the congress* (pp. 347–373). Washington: MedPAC.

MedPAC. (2010). *Report to the congress: Medicare payment policies* (p. 148). Washington: MedPAC.

Meier, D. (2010a). *Center to advance palliative care presentation: Palliative care and health care reform: Connecting the dots.*

Meier, D. (2010b). *Improving Health Care Quality through Increased Access to Palliative Care and Hospice, Invited Paper, National Quality Forum.*

Morrison, R. S., Penrod, J. D., Cassel, J. B., et al. (2008). Cost savings associated with US hospital palliative care consultation programs. *Archives of Internal Medicine, 168*, 1783–1790.

National Hospice and Palliative Care Organization. (2008). *Hospice Facts and Figures 2008 Edition.* Retrieved September 19, 2010, from http://www.nhpco.org.

National Hospice and Palliative Care Organization. (2010). *NHPCO Facts and Figures: Hospice Care in America 2010 Edition.* Accessed October 17, 2010, from http://www.nhpco.org.

National Priorities Partnership. (2008). *National priorities and goals – aligning our efforts to transform America's healthcare.* Washington: National Quality Forum.

National Quality Forum. (2006). *A national framework and preferred practices for palliative and hospice care quality.* Washington: National Quality Forum.

Portenoy, R. K., Lupu, D. E., Arnold, R. M., Cordes, A., & Storey, P. (2006). Formal ABMS and ACGME recognition of hospice and palliative medicine expected in 2006. *Journal of Palliative Medicine, 9*, 21–23.

Rodgers, P. (2010). Palliative care in the patient-centered medical home. *Journal of Pain and Symptom Management, 39*, 426 (abstract).

Salsberg ECfHWSS. (2002). *The supply, demand and use of palliative care physicians in the U.S.: A report prepared for the Bureau of HIV/AIDS, HRSA.* Albany: Center for Health Workforce Studies.

Scharfenberger, J., Furman, C. D., Rotella, J., & Pfeifer, M. (2008). Meeting American Council of Graduate Medical Education guidelines for a palliative medicine fellowship through diverse community partnerships. *Journal of Palliative Medicine, 11*, 428–430.

Scott, J. O., & Hughes, L. (2006). A needs assessment: Fellowship Directors Forum of the American Academy of Hospice and Palliative Medicine. *Journal of Palliative Medicine, 9*, 273–278.

Singer, P. A., Martin, D. K., & Keiner, M. (1999). Quality end-of-life care: Patients' perspectives. *Journal of the American Medical Association, 281*, 163–168.

Taylor, D. (2009). Effect of hospice on Medicare and informal care costs: The United States experience. *Journal of Pain and Symptom Management, 38*, 110–114.

Taylor, D. H., Jr., Ostermann, J., Van Houtven, C. H., Tulsky, J. A., & Steinhauser, K. (2007). What length of hospice use maximizes reduction in medical expenditures near death in the US Medicare program? *Social Science & Medicine, 65*, 1466–1478.

Teno, J. M., Clarridge, B. R., Casey, V., et al. (2004). Family perspectives on end-of-life care at the last place of care. *Journal of the American Medical Association, 291*, 88–93.

Thorpe, K. E., & Howard, D. H. (2006). The rise in spending among medicare beneficiaries: The role of chronic disease prevalence and changes in treatment intensity. *Health Affairs, 25*, 378–388.

Tolle, et al. (1999). *Oregon Report Card.* http://www.ohsu.edu/ethics.

U.S Senate Appropriations Committee. (2010). *Report for the Departments of Labor, Health and Human Services, and Education for FY 2011.*

von Gunten, C. F. (2006). Fellowship training in palliative medicine. *Journal of Palliative Medicine, 9*, 234–235.

Index

A

Abbreviated Injury Severity Scale (AISS), 180, 182
Acupuncture, 260–261
Acute and chronic pain syndromes, 477
Adult cancer-related pain
  barriers, pain treatment, 261–262
  BTP (*see* Breakthrough pain)
  co-analgesics
    biphosphonates, 256
    defined, 255
  combination drugs, 253–254
  complementary treatments
    acupuncture, 260
    massage, 261
  ethnic differences, 262
  fentanyl, 254
  initiation, treatment and titration, 254
  methadone, 256
  opioid drugs
    "equianalgesic ratio", 252
    mixed agonist–antagonists, 252
    substances/equivalences, 252
    tolerance, 253
  opioid side effects, 256–257
  palliative and supportive medicine, 262–263
  pharmacological treatment, 251–252
  psychological and behavioral treatments
    CBT, 260
    cognitive restructuring, 260
    oncology support services, 259–260
  psychological influences
    catastrophizing, 258
    coping, 258–259
    emotional distress, 259
  radiation therapy, 257
  situations
    chemotherapy-related pain, 255
    impaired renal function, 255
    neuropathic pain, 255
  temporal variations
    axillary lymph node dissection and radiotherapy,
      251
    breast cancer, 251
    physician-assisted suicide, 250
  types
    neuropathic, 249–250
    somatic, 248–249
    visceral, 249
Advanced dementia
  assessment
    anxiety, 134
    back pain, 134
    behavioral observation tools, 133
    behaviors, 132
    bilateral knee pain, 133–134
    comorbid problems, 133
    self-report, 132
  cognitive impairment, 131
  STI (*see* Serial trial intervention)unresolved
    physical pain, 131
American college of chest physicians (ACCP)
  acupuncture, 659
  dietary supplements, 687–688
  mind-body modalities, 652
  MT, 671
American college of physicians (ACP), 652, 659, 671
Analgesia, stress, 374–375
Analgesic medications, pediatric chronic pain
  antiepileptic drugs, 158–159
  off-label medication use, 156
  tramadol, 156–157
  transdermal fentanyl, 157–158
  tricyclic antidepressants, 158
Anterior cingulate cortex (ACC)
  endogenous opioid binding, 440
  increased activity, 441
  labeling, 447
Anthropological approach
  allure, communication, 754–755
  diagnostic imaging, 752
  ethics, looking, 757–758
  medicalized and mediatized realm, 751
  "medical vision machines", 751
  visualization, medicine

Anthropological approach (*cont.*)
 art therapy, 753–754
 diagnostic imaging, 753
 "seeing" and "reality", hegemonic link, 752
 visual representation, body, 751
 work of art, 755–757
Antiepileptic drugs, pediatric chronic pain, 158–159
Anxiety, cancer patients
 assessment
  beck anxiety inventory (BAI), 626
  single symptom approach, 625
 etiology, 625
 management
  clinical practice guidelines, management, 628
  pharmacologic approaches, 628–629
  psychosocial approaches, 629–631
 and pain relationship, 627
 prevalence, 626
Appraisal of Guidelines for Research and Evaluation
  (AGREE), 114
Army Substance Abuse Program (ASAP), 200
Art, chronic pain
 advocacy
  drug addicts, 778
  health care workers, 777
  medication tolerances, 777–778
  medicines and changes, 777
  silently suffering, 776
 charts, 784
 defined, pain, 784
 doctor's offices, 783–784
 EMT certification, 762
 encounters, 762–763
 failing health care system, 762
 family, role, 779
 learning, become patient, 784–785
 madness
  Bound but Not Defeated, 787
  Contemplation for Growth, 789
  Between darkness and light, 788
  Elegant pain, 786
  flare ups, 785
  health care facilities, 786
  tolerance, 785
 medical ingenuity, 783
 medication, motherhood and medicalization
  broken neck, 766
  flu-like symptoms, 764
  Hyper emesis gravid arum, 763
  TOS surgery and MRI scan, 765
 medicinal marijuana, 784
 parking, disability space, 782
 patient
  Defeat, 767
  Ex-Ray, 771, 772
  The Gift, 768
  I Heard you and So did My Cells, 773
  implanted pumps and catheters, 769, 770
  Re-Configured, 774

  They See US As Meat, 772, 773 *Too BE on the
   Other Side*, 775
  Walking in my Shoes, 776
  When You Do Not Listen, 769–770
 reality, 782–783
 stigma, substance abuse, 778–779
 surgery, foreign objects and medical gaze
  CT scan, 781
  Dacron pouch, 782
  morphine pump, 780
  nurse, RN stigma, 779–780
  open wound, 780–781
  staph infection, 781–782
 warrior, 766
Assessment tools, cancer
 BPI, 79, 82
 BTP, 84
 classification systems
  formal systems, 74
  formal, validated, 73
  IASP, 74
  OEI, 73
  regional multicentre study, 74
 definitions, 76
 ECS-CP, 75
 ESAS and MSAS, 82
 international research groups, 75
 management, factors, 72
 methods, 76–77
 multidimensional tools, 79–81
 NP, 84–88
 NRS, VRS and visual rating scale, 82, 83
 pain intensity, 83
 prevalence rates, 71
 psychometric requirements and tool development
  EPCRC data collection study, 78, 79
  ideal symptom criteria, self-report, 77
  oncology and palliative care, 77–78
  properties, 77
  steady flow, 78
 research and clinical practice, 73
 symptom assessment, 90

B
Battlefield injured pain
 LBP (*see* Low back pain) NBI (*see* Nonbattle
  injuries)polytrauma
  acute pain, 198–199
  alternatives, opioid analgesia, 200–201
  blast injuries, 196
  defined, 196
  management, acute pain, 196–198
  opioids, 199–200
Biological markers, stress, 370
Biopsychosocial (BPS) approach
 acute pain to chronic pain, 6–7
 chronic pain
  assessment, 7–8

and disability, 10–13
management, 8–10
comorbidity, chronic pain and mental health
disorders
anxiety disorders, 5
major depressive disorder
(MDD), 4–5
screening, 6
substance use disorders, 5–6
disease and illness, 4
neuromatrix model, pain, 2–3
physical disorders, 3
theories
gate control theory (*see* Gate control
theory)"pattern response", 1
specificity theory, 1
Bio-psycho-social-spiritual model
culture and religion-specific factors, 703
gate control/neuromatrix theory, 702
images and symbols religious, 703–705
opioids and clarity, mind, 703
Botulinum toxin (BTX), 488
BPS approach. *See* Biopsychosocial approach
Breakthrough pain (BTP)
adult cancer-related pain, 251
assessment, cancer, 84, 85
CPACS classification system, 89
defined, 84
treatment, 84
Brief pain inventory (BPI), 79, 81, 89

C
CAM, chronic pain and palliative care
acupuncture
ACCP, 659
evidence, 659–661
uses, 659
biologically based therapies, 687–688
categories, NCCAM, 649
chiropractic
description, 671
RCTs, spinal manipulation, 672–674
SMT, 672
treatment, 672, 675
energy fields manipulation
HT, 685–686
magnetic therapy, 679, 684
Qi therapy, 686–687
Reiki, 686
research, biofield therapies, 679–683
spiritual healing, 687
TT, 684–685
health care providers, 650–651
massage and lymphatic drainage
cancer, 663
methods classification, 662
palliative effects, 662
research, MT, 663–670

meditation
defined, 652
evidence, 652–656
NCCAM-specified categories, 651
NHIS, 650, 659, 662
practices, 649–650
reflexology
defined, 675
evidence, 675–678
use, cancer patients, 650
yoga
defined, 652
evidence, 652, 657–658
Cancer pain assessment and classification system
(CPACS)
BTP, 89
ECS-CP, 75
pain mechanism, 89
Cancer patients, pain
adverse effects, 615
etiology, 615
prevalence, 616
psychological factors, 615
Carpal tunnel syndrome, 671–672
Catastrophizing, defined, 257
Catechol-*O*-methyltransferase (COMT), 432–433
CBT. *See* Cognitive behavioral therapy
Central factors, phantom limb pain
brainstem, thalamus, and cortex
"bottom-up" model, sensory processing, 420
cortical reorganization, 420–421
neurotransmitters mechanism, 421
vs. sensations, 420
somatosensory (SI) cortex, 420
spinal cord
central sensitization, 419
degeneration, projection axons, 419
GABA and BDNF, 419
NMDA receptors, 419
Central neuropathic pain (CNP)
PET, 440
treatment, 442
Cerebral spinal fluid (CSF)
choroid plexus, 548
local anesthetic, 529
Cervical spine pain, 205–206
Chemotherapy-induced peripheral neuropathy (CIPN),
255
Child Depression Inventory (CDI), 153
Child Health Questionnaire (CHQ PF50), 154
Cholecystokinin, 338–339
CHQ PF50. *See* Child Health Questionnaire
Chronic headache syndrome, 672
Chronic low back pain (CLBP)
aerobic capacity, 586
biopsychosocial concept
barriers, recovery, 235
central sensitisation, 235
cognitive behavioural approach, 238

Chronic low back pain (CLBP) (*cont.*)
    interruption, normal activities, 235–236
    programme features, 239
    psychological factors, 235
    social issues, 235
  causes
    centralisation, 234
    classification systems, 234
    directional preference subgroup patients, 235
    "nonspecific low back pain", 234
  characteristics, 240–241
  description, 231
  dynamic trunk muscle endurance, 595
  epidemiological cohorts, 232
  healthcare, 233
  osteoporosis, 585
  randomised controlled trials, 240
  recurrence rate, 232
  self-management
    depression, 240
    exercises and postural modifications, 239
    self-efficacy, 240
    "talking therapies", 239
  structural diagnosis, 231
  treatment
    manual therapy, 238
    MRI, 236
    NICE Guidelines, 237
    self-care options, 237
Chronic non-cancer pain (CNCP), 497
Chronic opioid therapy
  addiction, 514
  CNCP, 503
  discontinuation, 515
  opioid rotation, 515
  respiratory depression, 504
  Chronic pain. *See also* Chronic pain and
      opioids; Evidence-based pharmacotherapy,
      chronic painassessment
    imaging techniques, 7
    neuroendocrine system, 7
    step-wise approach, 8
  and disability
    activity adjustment, 11
    catastrophizing, 12
    cognitive distortion model, 12
    depression, 11
    passive and active coping, 11
    psychological therapies, 12–13
    psychosocial stressors, 10
    stress and anger, 10
  management
    cogntive-behavioral therapy, 10
    functional restoration programs, 9
    primary and secondary care, 8
    tertiary care, 8–9
    tolerance, 9
Chronic pain and opioids
  adverse effects
    drug interactions, 504–505

    respiratory depression, 504
    side effects, 504
  analgesic properties, 498
  approach, CNCP
    addressing problems, chronic therapy,
      514–515
    biopsychosocial assessment, 512–513
    principles, analgesics, 513–514
  benefits, CNCP, 502–503
  history, 498
  imaging studies, 502
  long-term consequences
    effects, endocrine systems, 506–507
    opioid-induced hyperalgesia, 505–506
  ORL-1 receptor, 516
  pharmacology
    buprenorphine, 501
    codeine, 499
    cytochrome P450 (CYP) system, 498
    fentanyl, 500
    hydrocodone, 499
    methadone, 500
    morphine, 499
    oxycodone, 500
    terminology, 499
    tramadol, 501
  side effects, 503
  therapy, 497
  tolerance and physical dependence
    aberrant drug-related behaviors (ADRB), 511
    addiction, 508
    DSM-IV, 509
    epidemiology, 510–511
    patients identification, 511–512
    problematic opioid use, 510
Chronic pain syndromes, 663, 671, 672, 675, 685
Chronic post-surgical pain (CPSP)
  definition, 296
  epidemiology
    incidence rate, 298
    phantom limb pain, 297
    surgeries, 297
  nonpharmacologic treatments
    behavioral medicine, 320–321
    interventional procedures, 320
    physical medicine and rehabilitation, 319–320
  pathophysiology
    activation-dependent plasticity, 298
    activation threshold, 299
    behavioral factors, 309
    central sensitization, 305–307
    descending tracts, 307–308
    electrophysiological concepts, neuroplasticity,
      301–303
    modulation and modification, 298
    NS and WDR neurons, 299–300
    parabrachial nucleus, 301
    peripheral nerve injury, 305
    peripheral sensitization, 303–305
    sensitization, 298

spinothalamic tract, 300–301
transduction, 299
pharmacological management
    alpha-2 receptor agonists, 317
    anticonvulsants, 314–315
    antidepressants, 313–314
    local anesthetics, 315
    N-methyl-D-aspartate receptor antagonists,
        316–317
    NSAIDs, 317–318
    opioids, 316
    topical agents, 319
preventative therapies, 312–313
risk factors
    biopsychosocial, 311–312
    procedural, 309–310
syndromes
    postamputation pain, 322
    postmastectomy pain, 322
    postthoracotomy pain, 322–323
Cingulotomy
    emotional factors, 571
    limbic system, 570
CIPN. *See* Chemotherapy-induced peripheral
    neuropathy
CLBP. *See* Chronic low back pain
Clinical infometrics
    cultural disparities, 127–128
    definition, 125
    design
        computerized adaptive testing platform, 127
        item bank development, 126
    diverse patients, 127
    integrated methods
        accurate pain assessment, 122
        culturally sensitive pain assessment, 122
        health, economic and societal impacts, 122
        tools, limitations, 122–123
    measurement issues, 127
    multidimensional pain, 124
    psychometrics and informatics, 123–124
    STATE care process model
        cycle, 124, 125
        steps, 124
    system architecture, 126
    team science approach, 128
CNCP. *See* Chronic non-cancer pain
Co-analgesics, 255–256
Cognitive behavioral therapy (CBT)
    chronic pain, 12–13
    components, 260
    description, 457–458
    mechanism, 459
    treatments, 460
Cognitive distortion model, 11
Communication and palliative care
    and delivery, health
        active lines, 45
        cancer patients, 45
        description, 44

effective consumer–provider, 45
symptom management model,
    45, 46
E-Health, 46–49
nature, pain, 43–44
Compassionate solidarity, 727–728
Complementary and alternative medicine (CAM)
    description, 389
    patients belief, 389
    pediatric chronic pain, 160
    practitioner-patient relationship, 390
    quality of life, source, 389–390
Complex regional pain syndrome (CRPS)
    preoperative anxiety, 311
    subdivisions, 552
    type I, 152, 188
COMT. *See* Catechol-*O*-methyltransferase
Consciousness and integration
    cultural and biological forces, 745
    human pain, 744
    negative emotions, 745
Consolidated Standards of Reporting Trials
    (CONSORT), 114
Cordotomy
    complication rate, 567
    spinothalamic tract, 565
    treatment of chronic pain, 566
Cortical pain processing, 281–282
Cortical plasticity treatment, phantom limb pain
    central stimulation, 426
    imagery, 425
    mirrors and virtual reality, 425
    prosthesis use, 424
    sensory discrimination, 424–425
CRPS. *See* Complex regional pain syndrome
CSF. *See* Cerebral spinal fluid
Current opioid misuse measure
    (COMM), 479–480
Cytochrome P450, CYP2D6, 433

D
DC. *See* Dorsal column
"Death With Dignity" movement, 814
Deep brain stimulation
    paralysis, 576
    relief, chronic pain symptoms, 575
    thalamic stimulation, 576
Defense and Veterans Brain Injury Center
    (DVBIC), 185
Dehydroepiandrosterone (DHEA), 370
Delineation and explication
    DDE, 808–810
    euthanasia (*see* Euthanasia) health
        professional–patient relationship, 807
    intractable distress, palliative sedation
        artificial nutrition and hydration, 812
        end-of-life distress, precondition, 813
        nature, suffering and constraints, 814
        terminological confusion, 812

Delineation and explication (*cont.*)
  opioid analgesics
    pain and symptom, end of life, 810
    persistent and pervasive myths, 811
  palliative and hospice care, 807–808
  PAS/PAD
    arguments, 816–817
    "Death With Dignity" movement, 814
    ODWDA, 815, 817–818
    opposition arguments, 817
    semantic issues, 815–816
  relief, pain and suffering, 820
Depression, cancer patients
  assessment, 617–618
  clinical practice guidelines, management, 620
  etiology, 616–617
  and pain relationship
    psychiatric disorders, 618
    psychological factors, 619
  pharmacologic approaches
    antidepressants, 620–621
    psychostimulants, 621–622
  prevalence, 618
  psychosocial approaches
    effectiveness, intervention, 625
    efficacy, cognitive therapy, 623
    meta-analyses, 622
    metastatic cancer, 624
DHEA. *See* Dehydroepiandrosterone
Diagnostic and statistical manual (DSM-IV), 200, 509
Diathesis stress model, 3
Diffusion tensor imaging (DTI), 444
Disparities, pain management and palliative care
  assessment and treatment
    chronic diseases and co-morbidities, 800
    patient demographic and cultural factor, 799
    physician variability, 799–800
    series, clinical vignette, 799
  cancer and health
    epidemic rates, 796
    IOM description, 795
    racial and ethnic minorities, 796–797
  coping and quality of life, 797
  definition, 793
  demographics, United States, 795
  health
    civil war, 794
    people, color, 793
    vesicovaginal fistulas, 794
  patient, physician and system-related factors
    educational interventions, 798
    racial and ethnic minority, 798
    side effects, analgesics, 797–798
Dorsal column (DC)
  commissural myelotomy, 278
  PSDC, 278, 279
  splanchnic afferents, 279
  visceral nociceptive fibers, 278
Dorsal root ganglion (DRG), 418–419
DRG. *See* Dorsal root ganglion

Drug Enforcement Administration (DEA), 141, 811
Drug response, genetics
  analysis methods
    environmental *vs.* genetic
        contribution, 434–435
    sex and ethnic variations, 434
  cytochrome P450, CYP2D6, 433
  gene polymorphism, 433
  interpersonal genetic variations, 433
  OPRM1 118G, 433
Dynamic pain assessment. *See* Clinical infometrics

E
Ectopy, 305, 315
Edmonton classification system for cancer
        pain (ECS-CP)
  ESS, 74
  international validation study, 74
  uses, 75
EGAPP. *See* Evaluation of Genomic Applications
        in Practice and Prevention
E-Health communication
  advantages, 46–47
  defined, 46
  electronic channels, 47
  interventions and pain management
    computer-based intervention programs,
        48–49
    consumers, 47
    creative technology developers, 49
    electronic pain questionnaires, 48
    nanotechnology, 49
    online support groups, 48
    self-report systems, 47
    telehealth information systems, 48
    web sites, 47
Electroencephalography (EEG)
  and MEG
    description, 445
    evoked potentials, 445–446
    spectral analyses, 445
  placebo analgesia, 336
EMs. *See* Extensive metabolizers
End-stage renal disease (ESRD), 659
Epidural steroid injection
  caudal, 545, 547
  interlaminar approach, 542–543
  subpedicular/retroneural approach, 543, 545
  superior articular process, 542, 543
  transforaminal approach, 543–544
Episodic pain syndromes, 663, 679
"Equianalgesic ratio", 252
Euthanasia
  "active" and "passive", 818
  causation issues and end-of-life care, 819–820
  Ninth Circuit majority, 819
  voluntary active, 818–819
Evaluation of Genomic Applications in Practice and
        Prevention (EGAPP), 436

Evidence-based pharmacotherapy, chronic pain
  antidepressants
    norepinephrine and serotonin reuptake
      inhibition, 483–484
    TCAs, 481–483
  BTX, 488
  description, 471
  fibromyalgia, treatment considerations, 489–490
  gabapentin and pregabalin
    acute and chronic pain, 485
    drug interactions, 484
    pain relief, 485
    plasma concentrations, 484–485
  NNT, 471–472
  nonopioid analgesics
    acetaminophen, 472–473
    agents, 472
    COX-2 inhibitors, 474
    traditional NSAIDs, 473
    tramadol, 474
  nonpharmacologic approaches, 490
  older persons treatment considerations, 490
  opioids (*see* Opioids)skeletal muscle
    relaxants, 485–486
  sources, information, 471
  spinal analgesics, 488
  topical analgesics
    capsaicin, 486
    high concentration capsaicin patch, 487–488
    lidocaine 5% patch, 486
    NSAIDs, 486–487
  treatment considerations, NP, 489
Extensive metabolizers (EMs), 433

F
Family stress model, 149–150
Fbromyalgia syndromes, 669
FDA. *See* Food and Drug Administration
Fear-Avoidance model, 11
fMRI. *See* Functional magnetic resonance imaging
Food and Drug Administration (FDA), 140, 158, 260,
    435, 472, 483–485, 488, 490
Functional Disability Inventory (FDI), 152
Functional magnetic resonance imaging (fMRI)
  advantages, PET, 442
  analysis, 456
  maladaptive cortical reorganization, 376
  phMRI, 444
  resting state, 457
  studies, 443
  WAD, 215
Functional restoration programs (FRP), 601

G
γ-Aminobutyric acid (GABA), 419
Gasserian ganglion and trigeminal nerve block
  CSF, 528
  radiofrequency rhizotomy, 529

Gate control theory, 2, 662, 702
Generalizability and applicability, hospice and
    palliative care. *See* Palliative and hospice
    care
Glasgow Coma Scale (GCS) score, 180–181
GME. *See* Graduate medical education
Goal-Directed Therapy Agreements (GDTA), 478
Graduate medical education (GME)
  long-standing and preexisting training
    programs, 842
  teaching hospitals, 842
Grounded theory, 654
Guillain-Barre syndrome, 485

H
Healing
  compassionate solidarity, 727
  defined, 717
  natural human resource, 728
  touch (HT)
    vs. MT, 686
    vs. RCTs, 685
    TT, 685
Health care reform
  access variability, 841
  barriers, 841
  economics, change, 843
  growth, 839
  and hospice
    continuum, illness, 838
    philosophy, care and structured
      system, 838
  and hospice impact, 839–840
  opportunities
    ACA implementation, 840
    synergistic potential, 840
  patients and families
    diagnostic and treatment, 837
    post bereavement consensus, 837–838
  and quality movement
    health care dollars, 839
    hospices, cost-saving, 840
    patients, serious illness, 839
    potential savings, 839–840
  research funding, 842
  social marketing, 842–843
  solutions and drivers, change, 843
  workforce shortfall
    chronic and fatal illness, 841
    CMS requirement, 841
    GME, 842
Health-related quality of life (HRQoL), 151–152
Heterotopic ossification, 188
High and low context communication
  acute and chronic pain, 23
  affect, 25–26
  cross-cultural misunderstandings, 20
  description, 20
  discrete encounters, 24

High and low context communication (*cont.*)
    empathy and mutual understanding, 26–27
    IASP, 21
    illness, 21
    legitimacy, 27
    metaphors, 27
    obligation, 25
    patients care, 26
    power, 27–28
    relational goals, 20
    respect, 25
    specialness, 26
    subtext, 28–29
    tissue damage, 21
    trust, 24
Hope
    clinician and patient
      characteristics, 724
      clinical empathy, 726
      compassionate solidarity, 727–728
      detached concern, 725–726
      empathy to compassion, 726–727
      goal, 725
      hope-enhancing and hindering features, 724
    deep, the song without words
      defined, 724
      Dickinson's observations, 723
      transcendence/religious dogma, 723
    false
      impression, 723
      palliative care physicians, 722
      physician–patient–family relationship, 722
      therapeutic privilege, 723
    medical beliefs
      diagnosis, 721
      empirical and moral assumption, 721
      palliative medicine, 722
    and patient outcomes
      and survival length, 387–388
      and survival quality, 388
Hope, pain and palliative care
    biobehavioral intervention
      adrenergic and steriodal effects, 387
      lymphocyte proliferative response, 386
      significance and relationship, 386
      T-cell proliferation, 386–387
    biology, 386
    CAM (*see* Complementary and alternative medicine
      (CAM)) and cancer
      illness and diagnosis, vulnerable, 383
      patient and survivor's ability, 384
    CBT, 385
    defined, 383
    "good health and life", 391
    heterogeneity, 385–386
    and honesty, ethics, 390
    hopelessness hurts, 388–389
    impact, behavior, 385–386
    and patient outcomes, 387–388

    psychology
      adequate pain relief and symptom control, 385
      age and illness stage, 384
      collusion, patient and clinician, 384
      gender/ethnicity literature, 385
      researches, 384
    social networks, cancer, 388
    and spirituality
      definitions, occupational therapy literature, 391
      description, 391
      dimensions, concept, 391–392
      distress, symptoms, 392
      "strength", 392
HPA. *See* Hypothalamic-pituitary-adrenal
HRQoL. *See* Health-related quality of life
Hyperalgesia, 375
Hyperpathia, 303
Hypothalamic-pituitary-adrenal (HPA),
    370, 372, 375

I
IASP. *See* International Association for the Study
    of Pain
Ideal body weight (IBW), 594
IMs. *See* Intermediate metabolizers
Intercultural communication
    acute and chronic, evolutionary
      caregivers, 23
      concordance, 23
      description, 21–22
      temporal longevity, 22
    assessment instrument
      experience, 29
      importance, dimensions, 29
      relational issues, 29
      standard analogue scales, 30
      visual analogue pain score, 30
    biologic veracity, 20
    cross-cultural work, 19
    description, 19
    high and low context, 20–21, 23–29
    management, skills
      awareness, 30–31
      expansion, truncation, and switch, 31–32
      highlight relational issues, 31
      task-oriented and relational events, 31
      texts and subtexts raise *vs.* subtext address,
        32–33
      therapeutic relationship, 30
    survey instrument, 20
Intermediate metabolizers (IMs), 433
International Association for the Study of Pain (IASP)
    classification, chronic pain, 74
    development, 73
    pain
      definition, 21
      women, 347
Intrathecal therapy, chronic pain

complications
    postprocedural epidural hematoma, 554
    vasovagal reaction, 555
efficacy, diseases
    abdominal pain, pancreatic cancer, 553–554
    CRPS, 552
    interventional pain procedures, 548
    intrathecal therapy, 552–553
    myofascial pain syndrome, 549
    pain, spinal origin, 549–551
    sacroiliac joint pain, 551–552
epidural steroids, 526
intrathecally administered drugs, 527–528
nerve blocks, 526–527
neuraxial and sympathetic blocks
    celiac plexus, splanchnic nerve block and
        neurolysis, 539–540
    epidural steroid injection, 541–545
    ganglion impar block, 541
    gasserian ganglion and trigeminal nerve,
        528–529
    genitofemoral nerve, 532
    ilioinguinal/iliohypogastrick nerve, 531–532
    intercostal, 530–531
    intrathecal therapy, 548
    lateral femoral cutaneous, 531
    lumbar, 540
    occipital nerve, 528
    radiofrequency treatment, 533–538
    sacroiliac joint block, 532–533
    sphenopalatine ganglion, 529–530
    stellate ganglion, 538–539
    superior hypogastric plexus, 540–541
    trigger point injection, 545–547
pain relief, 556
physiological basis, 525
radiofrequency treatments, 527
trigger point release, 526
IRT. See Item response theory
Item response theory (IRT)
    based models, 126
    clinical outcome assessment, 123

K
KCNK18, 432
Kinesiophobia, 219

L
LBP. See Low back pain
Leeds assessment of neuropathic symptoms
        and signs (LANSS), 171
Locus of control model, 11
Low back pain (LBP)
    cervical spine pain, 205–206
    CT scans, 204
    ESI, 203–204
    facetogenic, 204

myofascial, 205
nonradicular leg pain, 206
sacroiliac (SI) joint pain, 204–205
spinal stenosis and degenerative disc
        disease, 205

M
Magnetic resonance imaging (MRI)
    CLBP, 236
    DTI, 444
    fibromyalgia patients, 378
    fMRI, 442–443
    MRS, 444
    phMRI, 444
    structural, 443
    WAD, 215
Magnetoencephalography (MEG). See
        Electroencephalography
Maslow's model
    love and connection, 699
    physiologic, 699
    safety, 699
McGill Pain Questionnaire (MPQ), 171
Mechanically insensitive afferents (MIAs), 304
Medial branch nerve block and radiofrequency
        treatment
    fluoroscopic images, 536, 537
    pulsed radiofrequency, medial branch, 538
    spinal nerves, 535
    superior articular process, 533
    third occipital nerve (TON), 534
Melanocortin-1 receptor (MC1R) gene, 434
Meta-Analysis of Observational Studies in
        Epidemiology (MOOSE), 114
Methadone, 256
Military table of organization and equipment
        (MTOE), 199
Mindfulness-based stress reduction (MBSR)
        program, 652
Modulation, pain
    cognition
        correlations, PCS scores and brain
            activity, 455
        fMRI, 455–456
        pain catastrophizing, brain regions, 454–455
    effect, attention and distraction
        brain activity, 450–451
        and concurrent cognitive demand, SI activity,
            449, 450
        immersive VR, 449–450
    emotions effect
        anxiety and depression, 453
        combined fMRI, 454
        fibromyalgia, 454
    expectation
        brain activity, amygdala, 451–452
        influence, midazolam, 452
    hypnosis, 452–453

Modulatory mechanisms, FMD and TMS
central, 406–407
characteristics, muscle fiber type, 404
CNS mechanism, 403–404
peripheral, 404–406
Morphine, battlefield pain control, 197
Motor cortex stimulation, 577
Motor vehicle crash (MVC)
cadaveric studies, 214
physiological stress response systems, 218
PTSD, 219–220
stressful, 219
trauma, 215
MRI. *See* Magnetic resonance imaging
MVC. *See* Motor vehicle crash
Myelotomy
anatomical discovery, 569
respiratory dysfunction, 568
Myofascial pain syndrome, 187–188

N
Narrative and pain, integrative model
cognition, 733
consciousness and integration, 744–745
definition, 734
interactive and intersubjective
communicative action, 736
epistemological foundation, 735
human interactive structure, 735
medicine
epistemological foundation, 735
Western biomedical procedures, 734–735
narrative, analogue
Google Earth, 744
pain model, 743
predictable uncertainties
communicative, 738–739
communicative action, 736
content analysis, 737
diagnosis, 739–740
education, 742–743
ethics, 741–742
treatment, 740–741
success stories
evidence-based medical knowledge, 747
presence, 746
psychotraumatology, 745–746
National Center for Biotechnology Information
(NCBI), 436
National Center for Complementary and Alternative
Medicine (NCCAM)
CAM, categories, 649
defined, 662
energy medicine, 679
National consensus project (NCP)
domains, 96
and NQF, 97
National Health Interview Survey (NHIS),
650, 651

National Hospice and Palliative Care Organization
(NHPCO), 99, 101
National Institutes of Health (NIH), 435
National quality forum (NQF)
criteria, 98
NCP, 96, 97
NBI. *See* Nonbattle injuries
NCBI. *See* National Center for Biotechnology Information
Nerve growth factor (NGF), 304
Neuroanatomy, pain pathways
central
dorsal (posterior) quadrant, 277–279
lamina I, 275
ventral (anterior) quadrant, 276–277
descending modulatory, 282
gender differences, pain processing, 284
molecular
ion channels, nociceptors, 283
presynaptic voltage-gated calcium channels, 284
sensitization, 283
nociceptive sensation, brain
cortical pain processing, 281–282
thalamic representation, 280–281
peripheral
nociceptors, 273–274
sensitization and primary hypersensitivity, 274
sensory nerves, 273
somatic and visceral afferents, 274–275
translational research, 285
Neuromatrix model, pain
chronic pain and stress, 3
self neuromatrix, 3
Neuromatrix theory, pain, 372–373
Neuropathic pain (NP)
assessment tools, 86–88
characteristics and treatment, 85
chronic, 485
defined, 84
intensity reduction, 476
intravenous opioids, 475–476
objective, 86
TCAs, 483
treatment considerations, 489
Neuropathic Pain Scale (NPS), 171
Neuroplasticity
behavioral factors, 309
defined, 298
electrophysiological concepts
hyperesthesia and sensitization, 301–302
hyperpathia, 303
noxious stimulus, 302
zone, primary and secondary hyperalgesia, 302
Neurosurgical interventions, chronic pain conditions
destructive/ablative surgeries
cingulotomy, 570–571
cordotomy, 565–567
dorsal root entry zone (DREZ) lesioning,
569–570
hypophysectomy, 571–572
myelotomy, 568–569

intraspinal analgesic pumps
    opiates, 572
    respiratory depression and hypotension, 573
    treatment, pain
        motor cortex stimulation, 575–577
        SCS, 573–575
Neurotrophins, definition, 304
NIH. *See* National Institutes of Health
N-methyl-D-aspartate (NMDA) receptors, 419, 423
Nonbattle injuries (NBI)
    female soldiers, 202
    Gulf War veterans, 202
    return-to-duty rate, 202–203
    treatments, 201
Nonradicular leg pain, 206
"Nonspecific low back pain", 234
Nonsteroidal anti-inflammatory drugs (NSAIDs)
    topical diclofenac, 487
    topical salicylate, 487
    traditional, 473

O
Older person
    assessment
        depression, 171
        nociceptive pain, 171
        tools, measurement, 171
    management, end of life, 174
    medical attention, 173
    minimalistic approach, 174
    neurophysiology, aging, 170
    osteoarthritis, 170
    self-management
        elevation, serum lipids, 172
        Kaiser health plan, 172–173
        overweight, 172
    transitions
        level, 173–174
        psychosocial environment, 173
OMIM. *See* Online mendelian inheritance in man
Oncologist assisted spiritual intervention study
        (OASIS), 709–710
Online mendelian inheritance in man (OMIM), 436
Opioid analgesia, 200–201
Opioid risk tool (ORT), 511
Opioids
    adverse effects
        chronic, trial agreements, 479
        COMM, 479–480
        GDTA, 478
        informed consent, 479
        maintenance, chronic opioid-therapy
            documentation, 479
        POPP, 478
        UDT, 480–481
    antinociceptive system, 335–336
    battlefield injury, 199–200
    endogenous, 335
    inclusion criteria and classification, 476

NNH, 476
rotation, 475
tapentadol hydrochloride
    analgesia, dual mechanism, 476
    doses, 476–477
uses and side effects, 475
OPRM1 118G, 433
Orbitofrontal cortex (OFC)
    and insular cortex, 440
    ipsilateral medial, 440
Oregon Death with Dignity Act (ODWDA)
    lethal prescription, 818
    mental disorder, 818
    "Not Dead Yet", 817
    provisions, 815
ORT. *See* Opioid risk tool
OTC. *See* Over-the-counter
Over-the-counter (OTC), 377–378

P
Pain imaging
    matrix (*see* Pain matrix, imaging)methods
        brain structure and function, 439
        EEG and MEG, 445–446
        limitations, 446–447
        MRI, 442–444
        PET, 440–442
    modulation (*see* Modulation, pain)patients
        CBT effect, 457–459
        effects, placebo, 459
        resting state fMRI, 457
        structural analysis, 456–457
    research, neuroimaging, 439
    "suffering", 439
Pain matrix, imaging
    affective-motivational aspects, 449
    brain imaging research, 447
    lateral and medial system, 448
    role, 448
    sensory and affective components, 447
    sensory-discriminative aspects, 448–449
Pain memory, phantom limb pain
    afferent nociceptive input, 423
    description, 422
    long-term noxious input, 422
    psychological and genetic susceptibility, 423
Pain processing
    candidate gene
        COMT, 432–433
        IL-1, 432
        KCNK18, 432
        SC9NA, 432
        TRPV, 431–432
    cortical pain processing, 281–282
    DNA polymorphism, 431
    gender differences, 284
Palliative and hospice care
    discipline-specific checklists
        internal validity evaluation, 114

Palliative and hospice care (*cont.*)
  methodology-based checklists, 114
  services, 115
  evidence
    appraisal skills, 112
    base, 111
  evidence-based practice, 109–110
  generalizability
    clinicians and service planners, 116, 117
    domains, 115–116
    pharmacokinetic study, medication, 116
  genesis
    health systems, 111
    phase III studies, 111
    requirements, 110
  process application, 116–117
  progression, 115
  referral-based speciality, 113–114
  research
    definitions, 112
    generalizability and applicability, 112–113
    randomized controlled trials, 113
  tools, methodological checklists, 114
Palliative care research and comiogenesis
  coercive device, 831
  measureable consequences, pathology, 830
  "symptom burden" study, 831
Parent proxy-reported health-related quality of life
    scores (PedsQL Total Score), 153
Patient controlled analgesia (PCA), 351
Patient dignity inventory (PDI), 701, 710, 711
Patient-reported outcomes (PROs)
  data collection, 105
  measures, 104
Patients and caregivers education, pain management
  arthritis, 55
  health information, guide education efforts
    persistent pain, 59
    traditional information sources, 59
  knowledge is power
    decision making process, 54–55
    primary care physicians (PCPs), 55
  leveraging, health professional, 64–65
  pain-specific brochures, 56
  patient education frameworks, 53
  role, 55
  skills building, 56
  tools, healthcare providers
    community-based strategies, 60–61
    enhancement, pain communication, 62–64
  translating education, practice
    effective pain management, 57, 58
    pain myths, 57, 58
PCA. *See* Patient controlled analgesia
Pediatric chronic pain
  biopsychosocial characteristics, 152–153
  consensus, factors, 150–151
  family stress model, 149–150
  HRQoL (*see* Health-related quality of life)
    management

biomedical modalities, 156–159
  pragmatic goal, 155
  psychosocial modalities, 159
multidimensional biobehavioral model
  anxiety and psychosocial stress, 149
  description, 147–148
  JIA, 148
qualitative nature
  adaptive and passive children, 155
  CHQ PF50, 154
  narratives, 155
  themes, experience, 155
race and ethnicity, 153–154
Perceived stress scale (PSS), 369
Peripheral factors, phantom limb pain
  DRG, 418–419
  ectopic signals, 418
  electrical properties, cell membranes, 418
Peripheral nerve injury, 305
Peripheral pathways, pain
  nociceptors, 274
  peripheral sensitization and primary
    hypersensitivity, 274
  somatic and visceral afferents, 274–275
Phantom limb pain
  accidental/clinical amputation, 417
  central factors, 419–421
  congenital limb deficiency, 417–418
  cortical plasticity, 424–426
  intensity and quality, 417
  pain memory, 422–423
  perceptual illusions
    incongruence, sensory modalities, 422
    neuropsychological amputations, 421
    RHI and fMRI, 421
    telescoping, 422
  peripheral factors, 418–419
  pharmacological treatments, 423
  pre- and perioperative treatment, 418
  therapy, 423
Pharmacogenetics, personalized medicine
  chronic pain conditions, 436
  drug response, 433–435
  health databases, 436
  implications, clinical practice
    genotype variants, 435
    opioid response, 435
    toxicity and adverse reactions, patient, 435
  pain processing, 431–433
  public-private partnerships, 436
  treatment *vs.* risk, 436
Pharmacological MRI (phMRI), 442, 444
Physician-assisted suicide/aid in dying (PAS/PAD)
  arguments, 816–817
  "Death With Dignity" movement, 814
  ODWDA (*see* Oregon Death with Dignity
    Act)opposition arguments, 817
  semantic issues, 815–816
Placebo-controlled trials
  vs. active comparator, 833

vs. active control orthodoxy, 832
empirical support, 833
gold standard, 832
palliative care research, 833–834
potential capabilities, 832–833
protocol-approved alternative therapy, 832
Placebo/nocebo effect
clinical practice
deception, 340
non-verbal clues, 341
social observational learning, 341
clinical trials, 341–342
definition, 332
existsence, continuum, 340
mechanisms
conditioning, 333, 334
expectations, 333
immune functions, 335
reflex control, immunity, 335
reward system, 334
neurobiology, placebo analgesia
CCK system, 335
dopamine, 336
images, 336–338
opioid antinociceptive system, 335–336
nocebo hyperalgesia
images, 339
molecules, cholecystokinin, 338–339
PMs. *See* Poor metabolizers
Poor metabolizers (PMs), 433
Positron emission tomography (PET)
description, 440
neural metabolism indirect measurement, ^{18}FDG,
442
radiolabeled receptor ligands
analysis, opioids and opioid receptors, 440–441
analysis, serotonin and serotonin receptors, 441
dopamine and dopamine receptors analysis, 441
regional cerebral blood flow measurement, 441–442
Postconcussion syndrome, 186–187
Postpolio syndromes, 683, 684
Postsynaptic dorsal column pathway (PSDC), 279
Postthoracotomy pain, 322–323
Posttraumatic headache. *See* Postconcussion syndrome
Post-traumatic stress disorder (PTSD), 199, 370
Posttraumatic stress disorder Diagnostic Scale (PDS),
220
Proxy consent, cognitively impaired individuals, 828–829
PSA. *See* Public service announcements
PSDC. *See* Postsynaptic dorsal column pathway
PSS. *See* Perceived stress scale
Psychosocial stress
acute and chronic, 370
comorbidity, stress and pain
acute, 370–371
chronic, 371
traumatic and PTSD, 370
description, 367–368
and emotional aspects, pain
anxiety disorders, 373–374

depression, 373
description, 373
economic disparity, 374
fear and anger, 373
in humans, 369
management, patient-based
description, 377
OTC, 377–378
pain catastrophizing, defined, 378
management, provider-based, 378
treatment approach, 377
PTSD. *See* Posttraumatic stress disorder
Public service announcements (PSA), 644

Q
Qi therapy, 686–687
Quality indicators
classification, 95
defined, 95
development and implementation
assessment, 103
categorization, 104
pain indicators, 104
frameworks, palliative care
care process and outcomes steps, 97–98
developing and assessing, cancer, 96, 97
end-of-life cancer care and hospice projects, 96
evaluation criteria, 98
identification, 97
population and broad quality domains, 97
seminal US initiatives, 96
specific target areas, 97
limitations, 105
palliative care and pain
cancer quality-ASSIST project, 99, 102
cancer-specific, 99, 100
development and characteristics, 98
noncancer-specific, 99, 101
patient-centered measures, pain management, 105
PROs, 105, 106
selected palliative care research
follow-up/outcome, 103
screening, 102–103
treatment, 103
Quality of Reporting of Meta-Analyses (QUORUM),
114

R
Radiation therapy, 257
Randomized controlled trial (RCT)
capsaicin patch, 487
impact, yoga, 652
MT, 662
placebo-controlled, 472, 483
quasi-experimental designs, 663
Recognition and resolution, ethical barriers
cognitive impairment and imminent mortality, 823
cognitively impairment

Recognition and resolution, ethical barriers (*cont.*)
    decision-making capacity, 827
    patient protections, 827–828
    proxy consent, 828–829
  ethical paradox, 823
  far-advanced illness research
    coercion, 826
    exploitation, 826
    voluntariness, 825–826
    vulnerable person, 824
  rational hypothesis, 834
  therapeutic trials
    "cost of care" study, 829
    IRB members, 830
    palliative care research and comiogenesis, 830–831
    placebo-controlled trials, 832–834
    psycho-social outcomes, 829, 830
Recruiting and performing research, patients
  coercive influence, unrealistic hope, 824
  distinguishing, voluntariness, 824–825
Reflex sympathetic dystrophy. *See* Complex regional pain syndrome
Rehabilitation exercises
  cardiovascular fitness, 599–600
  CLBP, 602–603
  flexibility, 595–596
  FRP, 601
  functional, 599
  IBW, 594
  muscle conditioning, 596–598
  proprioceptive training, 598–599
  work hardening, 600–601
Rehabilitation treatments, chronic musculoskeletal pain
  adverse physical consequences
    altered biomechanics, 585–586
    bone health, 585
    cardiovascular fitness, 586
    muscle disuse and deconditioning, 584–585
  cost-effectiveness
    CLBP and osteoarthritis, 604
    manual therapy and exercises, 603
  exercises, 594–603
  hydrotherapy, 603
  modalities
    bracing, 593
    contrast baths, 587
    electrotherapeutic, 592–593
    heat wraps, 587
    physical, 587, 588
    randomized clinical trials, 587, 589–591
    traction, 593
    ultrasound, 592
  musculoskeletal disorders, 586
  statistical databases, 605
Reward system, brain, 334
RHI. *See* Rubber hand illusion
Rubber hand illusion (RHI), 421

S
Sacroiliac (SI) joint pain, 204–205
SASC. *See* Social Anxiety Scale for Children
SC9NA, 432
SCS. *See* Spinal cord stimulation
Self-hypnosis, 260
Serial trial intervention (STI)
  analgesic administration, 138–140
  challenges and barriers
    experience and reporting, 141
    vital signs, 140
  competence, staff, 141
  description, 135
  environmental stress, 137–138
  nonpharmacological comfort treatments, 138
  passive behaviors, 136
  physical assessment, 137
  positive response, 137
  steps, 135, 136
  training program components, 136
Serotonin syndrome, 474, 477
SES. *See* Socioeconomic status
Sex differences
  cognition, role
    catastrophizing, pain-related, 355
    gender role expectations, 355
    self-efficacy reports, 355–356
  emotions and pain
    anxiety, 354
    depression, 353–354
    female adolescents, 354
  epidemiology
    age-related differences, 348
    hormones, 349
    postoperative pain, 348–349
    women, susceptibility, 348
  intervention responses
    adolescents, 352
    analgesic effects, 350–351
    nonpharmacological treatment, 352
    pharmacological studies, 351
  laboratory-based studies
    gender roles, 350
    older adults, 350
    sensitivity, female, 349
  pain behavior
    healthcare utilization, 352
    pharmacological behaviors, 353
    social and emotional support, 353
  social context and communication, 356–357
Single-nucleotide polymorphisms (SNPs), 431
SNPs. *See* Single-nucleotide polymorphisms
Social Anxiety Scale for Children (SASC), 154
Socioeconomic status (SES), 373, 374
"Somatic focus", 333
Somatosensory (SI) cortex, 420
Spasticity, 188
Spinal cord stimulation (SCS)
  anterior–posterior x-ray, 575, 576
  intraspinal electrodes, 575

metanalysis, 574
pulse generator, 573
sensation, pain, 574
Spinal manipulation therapy (SMT)
    chiropractic therapies, 675
    meta-analysis, RCTs, 672
Spinal origin
    radicular
        MRI, 549
        pulsed radiofrequency treatment, 550
        zygapophyseal joint pain, 550–551
Spinocervical pathway, 277
Spinothalamic tract (STT)
    axons, 276
    description, 276
    primate cells, 277
Spiritual dimensions, pain and suffering
    adaptive and maladaptive religious-spiritual
        coping, 707–708
    bio-psycho-social-spiritual model, 702–705
    hierarchy needs, palliative care
        love and connection, 699
        Maslow's heirarchy, 699
        physiologic, 699
        safety, 699
        self-actualization, 700
        significant stressors, 698
        "situational pain", 699–700
        truncated life, 700
    logotherapy, 701, 702
    management, 711
    and personhood, 700–701
    qualitative assessments
        FICA, 709
        HOPE survey, 708–709
        OASIS, 709–710
    and quantitative assessments, 710–711
    severity vs. tolerance, 708
    spiritual well-being assessment tools, 708
    stages, grief, 706
    total pain, 697–698
Standards for Reporting of Diagnostic Accuracy
        (STARD), 114
StarT Back, 236
STATE care process model
    cycle, 124, 125
    steps, 124
STI. See Serial trial intervention
Strengthening the Reporting of Observational Studies
        in Epidemiology (STROBE), 114
Stress and pain
    acute to chronic pain, transition
        maladaptive cortical reorganization, 376
        pervasive and long-term nature, 376
        psychosocial mechanisms, 375
        secondary consequence, 376
    analgesia, 374–375
    biological relationships
        absence, condition, 372
        disorders, 372

neuromatrix theory, 372–373
neuropeptides, 372
comorbidity, psychosocial explanations,
        370–371
defined, psychosocial, 367–368
hyperalgesia, 375
predictors
    resilience factor, 379
    treatment interventions, 378
psychosocial and emotional, 373–374
and stressors
    behavioral and report measure, 370
    biological markers, 370
    event-driven measure, 369
    patient-reported measure, 369
treatment, 377–378
STT. See Spinothalamic tract
Stump pain, 322
Suffering
    defined, 717–718
    and dignity
        dying, 720–721
        physical and mental deterioration, 720
        physiological and psychological challenges,
            721
    phenomenology
        Daudet's reflections, 718
        expression, Requiem, 718–719
        initial response, calamity, 720
        Lawrence's central metaphors, 719
        mute and expressive, 719–720
        old and new self, 720
Support groups, chronic pain
    establishment, logistics, 643–644
    formation, peer lead, 642–643
    funding, 642
    governance, 641–642
    identifcation, goals, 643
    maintainance, long term, 646
    meaningful meetings
        integrity, organization, 644
        validation, 645
    meetings, types, 647
    peer lead groups, needed, 639–640
    problem, pain, 639
    publicizing group meetings, 644
    resources, starting and maintain, 647–648
    traps
        subgroups, 646
        support group, 645
    types, 641
    value, peer, 640
    window, hope, 640
Symbolic nature, pain management, 43–44

T
"Talking therapies", 239
TBI. See Traumatic brain injury
tDCS. See Transcranial direct current stimulation

Temporomandibular disorders (TMD)
  clinical characteristics, 402
  definitions and prevalence, 400–401
  description, 400
  environmental and genetic factors, 403
  modulatory mechanisms, 403–407
  treatment implications, 408–409
  vice versa, subjects, 401
Thalamic representation, pain
  microstimulation, 281
  visceral inputs, 281
  VPL nucleus, 280
Therapeutic touch (TT)
  defined, 684
  HT, 685
  practice, 684
  uses, 686
TMS. *See* Transcranial magnetic stimulation
Tools, healthcare providers
  in-practice and community-based strategies
    health literacy, 60–61
    teachable moments, 60
    written educational materials, 60
  pain communication enhancment
    advocate, educate, 63–64
    diaries and intensity scales, 62–63
    information sharing, 63
    questions handy, 62
Tramadol, 156–157
Transcranial direct current stimulation (tDCS), 426
Transcranial magnetic stimulation (TMS), 426
Transdermal fentanyl, 157–158
Transforaminal epidural steroid injections
    (TFESI), 204
Transient receptor potential vanilloid (TRPV), 431–432
Traumatic brain injury (TBI)
  biomarkers
    disparities research, 190
    microRNAs, 190
  biopsychosocial factors/comorbidities
    coping, 188
    depression, 189
    mood disorders, 189
  causes
    alcohol use, 180
    CDC data, 179
    pediatric populations, 179–180
    risk factors, 180
  chronic pain, after
    cognitive impairment, 186
    treatment strategies, 190
  classification methods, 180–181
  defined, 177–178
  diagnosis, 182
  diagnostic features, 178
  direct and indirect costs, 179
  epidemiology, 177–178
  incidence and prevalence, 178
  injury mechanism and pathologic features

    acceleration–deceleration injury, 181
    contusion and mild edema, 182
    diffuse axonal injury, 181–182
  mild, 181
  moderate and severe, 181
  mortality, 178–179
  nonfatal, 178
  pain syndromes
    CRPS, 188
    heterotopic ossification, 188
    myofascial pain syndrome, 187–188
    spasticity, 188
  populations
    disability and litigation, 185–186
    geriatric, 184–185
    military, 185
    pediatric, 184
  posttraumatic headache, 186–187
  predictors, mortality and prognosis, 184
  prevention, 180
  signs and symptoms, 182
  treatment
    cognitive and behavioral changes, 182
    complications and comorbidities, 183
    neuropsychological assessment, 183
    persistent symptoms, 183
Tricyclic antidepressants (TCAs)
  medications classification, 481
  multiple placebo-controlled RCTs, 483
  pediatric chronic pain, 158
  tertiary and secondary amine, 482–483
Trochanteric bursitis (TB), 206
TRPV. *See* Transient receptor potential vanilloid
Truth and palliative care
  caregivers, 37
  clinician's own discomfort, 37
  cognitive
    impairment, 40
    roadmaps, 39
  compassionate and empathetic clinicians, 38–39
  description, 35
  diagnostic and prognostic information, 38
  doctor–patient relationship, 36
  ethnographic study, patients, 37
  integrity and dignity, 40
  minimizing/omitting, 37
  parameters, optimal dosing, 36
  patient advocacy organizations, 36
  philosophers and clinicians, 36
  repercussions, protective buffering, 38
  treatment, patients, 35–36

U
Ultra-rapid metabolizers (UMs), 433
UMs. *See* Ultra-rapid metabolizers
Urine drug testing (UDT)
  algorithmic approach, 481, 482
  caveats, use, 480

V

Verbal Descriptor Scales (VDS), 171
Visual Analog Scale (VAS), 171

W

WAD. *See* Whiplash-associated disorders
Whiplash-associated disorders (WAD)
    Cochrane review, 222
    description, 213
    education and advice, management, 223
    motor and muscles changes
        dysfunction, sensorimotor control, 216
        neuromuscular control changes, 215–216
        upper cervical flexion, 215
    multifactorial nature, 222
    nociceptive processing
        augmented central, 217
        cold hyperalgesia, 217–218
        hypersensitivity, 218
        sensory disturbances, 216, 217
        spread, pain, 217

peripheral pathology
    damaged structures, 214
    MRI and fMRI, 215
    nerve tissue, 215
    zygapophyseal arthropathy, 214–215
pharmacotherapy, 222–223
psychological features
    depressive symptoms, 219
    fear of movement/kinesiophobia, 219
    PTSD, 219–220
relationship, biological and psychological
    factors
    adrenaline, 221
    central hyperexcitability, 221
    sensory hypersensitivity and psychological
        distress, 220
    trajectory modelling analyses, 221
stress system responses
    autonomic nervous system dysfunction, 218
    COMT, 219
symptoms
WHO Cancer Pain Ladder, 251

Lightning Source UK Ltd.
Milton Keynes UK
UKHW052216291222
414563UK00003B/39